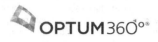

OPTUM360°®

DESK REFERENCE

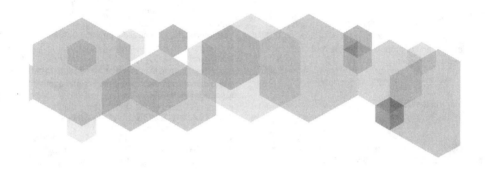

2018

Coders' Desk Reference for ICD-10-CM Diagnoses

Clinical descriptions with answers to your toughest ICD-10-CM coding questions

Notice

Coders' Desk Reference for Diagnoses is designed to be an authoritative source of information about coding and reimbursement issues. Every effort has been made to verify accuracy and all information is believed reliable at the time of publication. Absolute accuracy cannot be guaranteed, however. This publication is made available with the understanding that the publisher is not engaged in rendering legal or other services that require a professional license. If you identify a correction or wish to share information, please email the Optum360 customer service department at customerservice@optum360.com or fax us at 801.982.4033.

Copyright

Our Commitment to Accuracy

Optum360 is committed to producing accurate and reliable materials. To report corrections, please visit www.optum360coding.com/accuracy or email accuracy@optum.com. You can also reach customer service by calling 1.800.464.3649, option 1.

Acknowledgments

The following staff contributed to the development and/or production of this book:

Lauri Gray, RHIT, CPC, AHIMA-approved
    ICD-10-CM/PCS Trainer, *Product Manager*
Karen Schmidt, BSN, *Technical Director*
Stacy Perry, Manager, *Desktop Publishing*
Lisa Singley, *Project Manager*
Peggy Willard, CCS, AHIMA-approved ICD-10-CM/PCS
    Trainer, *Clinical Technical Editor*
Karen Krawzik, RHIT, CCS, AHIMA-approved
    ICD-10-CM/PCS Trainer, *Clinical Technical Editor*
Kristin Bentley, BS, CPC, *Clinical Technical Editor*
Tracy Betzler, *Senior Desktop Publishing Specialist*
Hope M. Dunn, *Senior Desktop Publishing Specialist*
Katie Russell, *Desktop Publishing Specialist*
Kimberli Turner, *Editor*

Clinical/Technical Editors

Peggy Willard, CCS, AHIMA-approved ICD-10-CM/PCS Trainer

Ms. Willard's expertise is in ICD-10-CM and PCS including in-depth analysis of medical record documentation, ICD-10-CM/PCS code and DRG assignment as well as clinical documentation improvement (CDI). In recent years she has been responsible for the creation and development of several print products and e-books for Optum Coding Solutions that are designed to assist with appropriate application of ICD-10-CM and PCS coding system. Willard has several years of prior experience in Level I Adult and Pediatric Trauma hospital and inpatient rehab (IRF) coding, specializing in ICD-9-CM, Diagnosis and Procedural coding, with emphasis in conducting coding audits, conducting coding training for coding staff and clinical documentation specialists. Ms. Willard is an AHIMA approved ICD-10 CM/PCS Trainer and is an active member of the American Health Information Management Association (AHIMA) and the Minnesota Health Information Management Association (MHIMA).

Kristin Bentley, BS, CPC

Ms. Bentley has more than 15 years of experience in the health care profession. She has an extensive background in professional component coding, with expertise in radiation therapy, chemotherapy, radiology, and ambulatory surgery procedure coding. She has conducted chart-to-claim audits and physician education. Ms. Bentley has most recently functioned as an auditing compliance consultant, as well as a product assessment coordinator, billing specialist, and she has extensive denial management experience. She is an active member of the American Academy of Professional Coders (AAPC).

Karen Krawzik, RHIT, CCS, AHIMA-approved ICD-10-CM/PCS Trainer

Ms. Krawzik has expertise in ICD-10-CM, ICD-9-CM, and CPT/HCPCS coding. Her coding experience includes inpatient, observation, ambulatory surgery, and ancillary and emergency room records. She has served as a DRG analyst and auditor of commercial and government payer claims, and as a contract administrator. Most recently, she was responsible for the conversion of the ICD-9-CM code set to ICD-10 and for analyzing audit results, identifying issues and trends, and developing remediation plans. Ms. Krawzik is credentialed by the American Health Information Management Association (AHIMA) as a Registered Health Information Technician (RHIT) and a Certified Coding Specialist (CCS) and is an AHIMA-approved ICD-10-CM/PCS trainer. She is an active member of AHIMA and the Missouri Health Information Management Association.

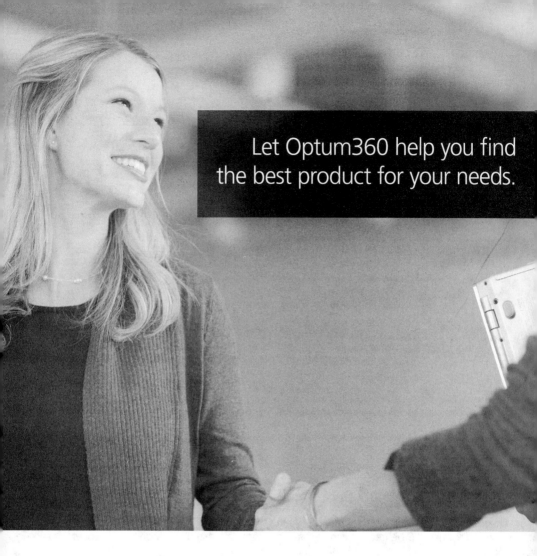

Let Optum360 help you find the best product for your needs.

Together with you, Optum360® can help drive financial results across your organization with industry-leading resources that cut through the complexity of medical coding challenges.

Let us help you find the best coding solution, at the best price.

Contact your Medallion representative directly or call Customer Service at 1-800-464-3649, option 1.

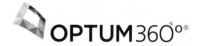

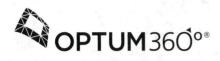

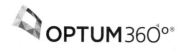

OPTUM360°®

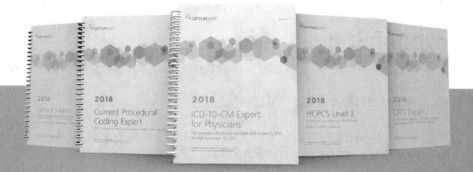

2018
General Surgery/
Gastroenterology

2018
Current Procedural
Coding Expert

2018
ICD-10-CM Expert
for Physicians
The complete official code set Codes valid October 1, 2017
through November 30, 2018

2018
HCPCS Level II

2018
DRG Expert

Keep your go-to coding resources up to date.

Stay current and compliant with our 2018 edition code books.
With more than 30 years in the coding industry, Optum360® is proud to
be your trusted resource for coding, billing and reimbursement resources.
Our 2018 editions include tools for ICD-10-CM/PCS, CPT®, HCPCS, DRG,
specialty-specific coding and much more.

SAVE UP TO 25% ON ADDITIONAL CODING RESOURCES

Visit us at optum360coding.com
and enter promo code **FOBA18ED**
to save 25%.

Call 1-800-464-3649, option 1,
and be sure to mention promo
code **FOBA18ED** to save 20%.

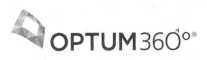

OPTUM360°®

Optum360 Learning

Earn your CEUs with US

You've worked hard for your coding credentials, and now you need an easy way to maintain your certification.

Optum360® offers the most complete training in the marketplace, designed to address exactly what you and your organization need. We offer eLearning courses you can take online at your desk; you can invite a specialist to your office for on-the-job preparation; or ask our consulting professionals to create a tailor-made program specific for your organization.

Our strategy is simple — education must be concise, relevant and accurate. Choose the delivery method that works best for you:

- **eLearning:** Web-based courses offered at the most convenient times for your learners. eLearning courses are interactive, task-focused and developed around practical scenarios. These self-paced courses include "try-it" functionality, knowledge checks and downloadable resources.

- **Instructor-led training (ILT):** On-site or remote courses, built specifically for your organization.

- **Webinars:** Online courses, geared toward a broad market of learners, delivered in a live or recorded setting.

- **Podcasts and videos:** Physician-focused online courses available when and where convenient.

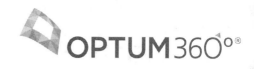

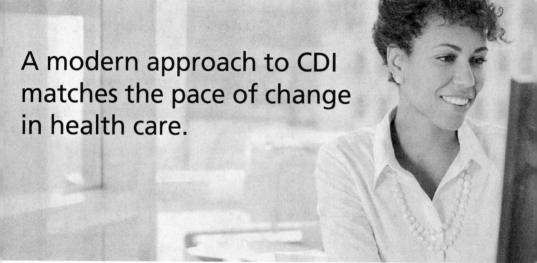

A modern approach to CDI matches the pace of change in health care.

The move to value-based care increases the need for accuracy in clinical documentation—across every patient and payer. A modern CDI approach makes the work of CDI specialists more efficient by automatically reviewing every patient record and prioritizing those that require intervention.

Using case-finding logic and state-of-the-art natural language processing, Optum CDI 3D connects clinical indicators to identify records with gaps or deficiencies and enables timely documentation improvement, cleaner claims, faster reimbursement and accurate reporting.

Optum CDI 3D, together with Optum's market-leading Enterprise CAC, provides unmatched capabilities in a single, fully integrated CDI and coding solution.

Modernizing your CDI program starts here. Visit optum360.com/CDI3D to learn more.

OPTUM CDI 3D

* Automates 100-percent record review and identifies clinical documentation improvement opportunities

* Identifies co-morbidities, HACs and patient safety indicators

* Streamlines the query loop between CDIS and physicians

* Enhances code assignment efficiency, compliance and quality reporting

Visit: optum360.com/CDI3D
Email: optum360@optum.com

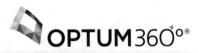

OPTUM360°®

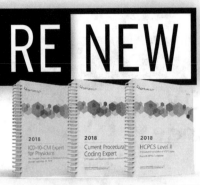

Contents

Introduction

Coders' Desk Reference for Diagnoses is an ICD-10-CM coding reference that provides comprehensive lay descriptions of diseases, injuries, poisonings, and other conditions. It has been developed for coders, billers, and other health care professionals in all health care settings, including medical offices, hospitals, post-acute care settings, and health insurance companies. It is also a valuable reference for educators and students who seek to expand their understanding of diagnostic coding. The goal is to enrich the user's clinical understanding of ICD-10-CM so that code selection becomes more accurate.

It should be noted that this diagnostic coding reference is intended to be used with an official ICD-10-CM code book. The *Coders' Desk Reference for Diagnoses* does not include the comprehensive index or guidelines found in the official ICD-10-CM, nor does it include coding instructions from the tabular section. Information related to includes and excludes notes have also been omitted as providing this information would be redundant to what is readily available in an official ICD-10-CM code book. For these reasons, *Coders' Desk Reference for Diagnoses* does not replace an official code book; however, used in conjunction with a code book, this reference provides an unparalleled clinical roadmap to code selection.

Format

The *Coders' Desk Reference for Diagnoses* follows the organization of the tabular section of ICD-10-CM with the same 21 chapters beginning with Chapter 1: Certain Infectious and Parasitic Diseases and ending with Chapter 21: Factors Influencing Health Status and Contact with Health Services.

Each chapter is organized using a format similar to the tabular section of ICD-10-CM with chapters subdivided into blocks, alphanumeric categories, subcategories, and codes. Chapters begin with a general overview of diseases and other conditions classified to the chapter. Following the chapter overview, each chapter is divided into the various blocks where information is provided related to categories included in the block. This is followed by the lay descriptions. Lay descriptions may be provided at the category, subcategory, or code level.

Not all categories, subcategories, or codes have been represented in the *Coders' Desk Reference for Diagnoses*. The 2018 edition of *Coders' Desk Reference for Diagnoses* focuses on:

- A subset of the new fiscal year 2018 diagnosis codes released by the National Center for Health Statistics (NCHS) and the Centers for Medicare and Medicaid Services (CMS).

- Codes regularly encountered in various health care settings

- Codes that require in-depth clinical information in order to differentiate the represented condition from similar conditions that would be captured with other, more specific codes

Additional codes and lay descriptions will gradually be incorporated into future editions. Due to the structure of ICD-10-CM, many categories, subcategories, and codes have been updated with more robust official descriptions. In some cases, official code descriptions supply enough information about the disease process and any associated manifestations that provide additional narrative would be redundant. Also, codes in many categories and subcategories provide information related to site and/or laterality. Although site and laterality are important for valid code selection, they do not need additional explanations beyond the related disease process provided at the category or subcategory level.

ICD-10-CM Codes and Lay Descriptions

The codes in *Coders' Desk Reference for Diagnoses* are based on the official version of the *International Classification of Diseases, 10th Revision, Clinical Modification* effective October 1, 2018.

Coders' Desk Reference for Diagnoses is organized in a hierarchical context, similar to how the ICD-10-CM code book is organized with lay descriptions provided at the three, four, five, and/or six character level. Lay descriptions at the category level provide a broad overview of diseases or other conditions classified to the category. Category-level lay descriptions may be followed by subcategory and/or code level lay descriptions. Lay descriptions at the subcategory and code levels build on the information provided at the category level. The category level will be the most general and provides information relevant to all subcategories and codes in the category. The subcategory is more specific with the code level lay description providing the most detailed information about the disease, injury, or other condition.

Because some lay descriptions are not carried to the code level, the book uses a dash (-) to differentiate invalid codes from valid codes.

Valid Code

A valid code in the *Coders' Desk Reference for Diagnoses* is any code for which a dash (-) is **not** appended to the end of an alphanumeric code. Valid codes may be three characters to seven characters long.

Example: Lay description for valid three-character code

B20   Human immunodeficiency virus [HIV] disease

HIV is a blood-borne virus in that it is transmitted through body fluids containing blood or plasma. Transmission of HIV can occur sexually or nonsexually through the exchange of body fluids infected with a high concentration of the virus, mainly blood, semen, or vaginal/cervical secretions. Initially, HIV may be present in the body, but may be asymptomatic. During this period, the patient is HIV positive but does not have HIV disease. In symptomatic HIV, also called ARC (AIDS related complex), symptoms of a weakened immune system are present, including general lymphadenopathy, anorexia, fever, malaise, diarrhea, anemia, oral hairy leukoplakia, and oral candidiasis, but the patient does not have full blown AIDS. A diagnosis of AIDS requires an AIDS-defining condition (e.g., an opportunistic infection or certain types of cancer) or a CD4 count of less than 200 cells/mm^3. HIV is divided into two categories: HIV-1 and HIV-2. HIV-1 is seen worldwide; HIV-2 is limited to Africa and other countries and is seldom seen in the United States. HIV-1 has far-ranging health effects and manifestations. This code is reserved for patients with symptomatic HIV-1 infections, ARC, or AIDS.

Example: Lay description for valid five-character code

O86.81   Puerperal septic thrombophlebitis

Septic thrombophlebitis is inflammation of a vein (phlebitis) due to an infected blood clot (thrombus). Puerperal septic thrombophlebitis is when the infected thrombus develops during the postpartum period. In most cases, these occur as a complication from a puerperal infection (e.g., endometritis). Septic embolism is a potential complication.

Invalid Code

An invalid code, one that needs additional characters, has a dash (-) appended to the alphanumeric code. The dash informs the user that the code is not a complete code, and the ICD-10-CM code book should be referenced to determine the appropriate valid code selection. Any lay description information supplied at this level applies to all subcategories and/or codes that would be found indented under this code in the tabular section of an official ICD-10-CM code book.

Example: Category level lay description requiring additional characters

D57.-   Sickle-cell disorders

Sickle-cell disorders are severe, chronic diseases caused by a genetic variation in the hemoglobin protein in the red blood cell. These are the most common types of inherited blood disorders in the United States and are found most predominantly in African Americans. A red blood cell is normally disc shaped, which allows it to move through the blood vessels easily. In sickle-cell disorders, the gene mutation causes the red blood cell to become hard, sticky, and crescent or sickle shaped. These changes make it harder for red blood cells to travel through the bloodstream disrupting blood flow and decreasing oxygen transport to tissues. Sickle-cell disorders are classified based on the specific type of sickle cell disease and whether the individual is experiencing a crisis. Crisis in sickle-cell disorders refers to recurring acute episodes of pain most often due to a vasoocclusive process that can involve any body system, but manifestations usually involve the chest, bones, or abdomen. The pain comes on without warning and can last hours or days. Specific forms of crises include:

- Acute chest syndrome: In young children this is characterized by chest pain, fever, cough, tachypnea, leukocytosis, and pulmonary infiltrates in the upper lobes. Adults are less symptomatic but may have dyspnea, severe chest pain, and multilobar or lower lobe disease.

- Splenic sequestration: This is characterized by rapid enlargement of the spleen and occurs most often during the first five years of life but can occur at any age.

- Unspecified or not otherwise specified crisis.

Example: Subcategory level lay description requiring additional characters

D57.0-   Hb-SS disease with crisis

This is the most common type of the sickle-cell disorder and occurs when both parents pass on a hemoglobin S gene. A code from this subcategory is assigned when the patient is currently experiencing a crisis.

Coders' Desk Reference for Diagnoses provides a clinical description of the Hb-SS sickle-cell disease with a dash after the code to indicate that there are more codes indented under the four-character code D57.0-, and to which the lay description will also apply. Upon referencing an official ICD-10-CM code book, the user will see that there are three valid code options for Hb-SS disease with crisis as follows:

D57.00   Hb-SS disease with crisis, unspecified

D57.01   Hb-SS disease with acute chest syndrome

D57.02   Hb-SS disease with splenic sequestration

As is demonstrated in the examples above, the lay description found at each character level (category and subcategory) provides unique information, with more general information at the category level and additional, more specific information at subsequent levels (subcategory and code). In this case the category level lay description provides important information related to sickle-cell disorders of which Hb-SS disease is one type. The category level lay description also describes the various types of crisis associated with sickle cell disorders because crisis and crisis manifestations are components of all types of sickle cell disorders described as "with crisis."

It is important that the user not only review the information at the specific code level but also refer to the subcategory and category levels within which a code is classified for a full understanding of the disease process.

Code Ranges

Lay descriptions may be written for a single category, subcategory, or code or for a range of codes. Code ranges are used when two or more categories, subcategories, and/or codes share a similar disease process and the lay description applies to all the codes in the range.

When a range applies, two or more categories, subcategories, and/or codes are listed along with their official ICD-10-CM descriptions. The lay description follows the last code in the range. In addition, the same formatting is used to differentiate valid codes in the range from codes that require additional characters. Valid codes do not have a dash appended while invalid codes are displayed with a dash (-). In the example below, code H90.0, all codes under the subcategory H90.1-, and code H90.2 represent the disease process of conductive hearing loss and have been grouped together in a range with a single lay description.

Example: Code range with both valid and invalid codes

H90.0   Conductive hearing loss, bilateral

H90.1-   Conductive hearing loss, unilateral with unrestricted hearing on the contralateral side

H90.2   Conductive hearing loss, unspecified

Conductive hearing loss is the inability of sound waves to move from the outer (external ear) to the inner ear. This may be due to things like a blocked external auditory canal, fluid or abnormal bone growth in the middle ear, or a rupture of the eardrum. Each of these conditions in some way limits the movement of the structures in the middle ear, inhibiting transmission of the sound wave from the middle ear to the inner ear. Although the sound is typically not distorted, the sounds are much quieter. The most common cause of conductive hearing loss in children and adults is otitis media infection and otosclerosis respectively.

Focus Point

Some lay descriptions are followed by *Focus Point* information. The *Focus Point* sections provide additional information that differentiate between clinically similar disease processes and/or provide coding guidance that cannot be easily garnered from the index or tabular section of the official ICD-10-CM code book.

Example: Focus point differentiating between similar disease processes

A74.81   Chlamydial peritonitis

Chlamydial peritonitis is a complication of female pelvic inflammatory disease caused by *Chlamydia trachomatis* infection. It is characterized by inflammation of the peritoneum, which is the membrane that lines the intraabdominal wall. In some cases, the membrane covering the liver also becomes inflamed (perihepatitis) causing a condition called Fitzhugh-Curtis disease, which is also classified here. Symptoms include severe upper right quadrant abdominal pain, fever, chills, and headache.

> **Focus Point**
>
> *Fitzhugh-Curtis Syndrome can be classified to two different codes depending on the causal infection. Infection caused by* Chlamydia trachomatis *is classified to A74.81 Chlamydial peritonitis in contrast to infection caused by* Neisseria gonorrhoeae *which is classified to code A54.85 Gonococcal peritonitis.*

Example: Focus point providing coding guidance

A02.0   Salmonella enteritis

Salmonella enteritis, also known as salmonella gastroenteritis, is an infection of the gastrointestinal tract that is caused by the ingestion of contaminated foods, eggs, and poultry being the most common sources. Symptoms typically occur within hours to two days and typically last no more than seven days even without the use of antibiotics.

> **Focus Point**
>
> *Dehydration (E86.0) is a complication of* Salmonella enteritis *and should be reported additionally when documented.*

When a category is referenced in a *Focus Point*, no dash is used as it is understood that the codes within that category must be consulted for the appropriate code.

Example: Focus point referring to category level rather than specific code

I15.- Secondary hypertension

Secondary hypertension is caused by renovascular or other diseases, such as renal parenchymal diseases, oral contraceptives, primary aldosteronism, Cushing's syndrome, pheochromocytoma, hyperparathyroidism, hyperthyroidism, and acromegaly.

Focus Point

Codes in category I15 do not include any reference to chronic kidney disease or renal failure. If chronic kidney disease is documented, an additional code from category N18 should be assigned.

Illustrations

Several new illustrations are provided at the category or code level. Illustrations promote a better understanding of the anatomical nuances associated with specific codes. The illustrations usually include a labeled anatomical view and may include narrative that discusses specific conditions or anatomic sites. The illustrations are almost always simplified schematic representations. In many instances, some detail is eliminated to make a clear point about the anatomic site that is the focus of the depiction.

Supplementary Sections

In addition to the 21 chapters containing the lay descriptions, there are three additional sections that follow the introduction.

Prefixes and Suffixes

The uniquely efficient language of medicine is based on prefixes and suffixes attached to root words to modify their meaning. Medical prefixes and suffixes evolved from the Greek and Latin used by pioneering physicians. Common prefixes and suffixes are included in this section along with their meanings.

Abbreviations, Acronyms, and Symbols

The medical profession has its own shorthand for documentation, including abbreviations, acronyms, and symbols. The second reference provided in the front of this book identifies and defines abbreviations, acronyms, and symbols commonly seen in the medical record.

Anatomy Charts

Understanding human anatomy greatly improves coding accuracy. A compilation of anatomy charts is the third supplementary reference provided. These anatomy charts illustrate the body systems as well as organs and organ structures within each body system.

Prefixes and Suffixes

The uniquely efficient language of medicine is possible thanks to the prefixes and suffixes attached to roots. Changing prefixes and suffixes allows subtle and overt changes in meaning of the terms. The following prefixes and suffixes are paired with their meanings.

Prefixes

Prefixes are one half of the medical language equation and are attached to the beginning of words. For example, the prefix "eu-," meaning good or well, combined with the Greek word for death, "thanatos," produces euthanasia — a good death.

a-, an-	without, away from, not
ab-	from, away from, absent
acanth/o-	thorny, spine
acro-	extremity, top, highest point
ad-	indicates toward, adherence to, or increase
adeno-	relating to a gland
adip-	relating to fat (also adipo-)
aero-	relating to gas or air
agglutin-	stick together, clump
alb-	white in color
alge-	awareness to pain (also algesi-)
all/o-	indicates difference or divergence from the norm
ambi-	both sides; about or around (also amphi-)
ambly-	dull, dimmed
an-	without
andro-	male
angi-	relating to a vessel
aniso-	dissimilar, unequal, or asymmetrical
ankylo-	bent, crooked, or two parts growing together
ante-	in front of, before
antero-	before, front, anterior
anti-	in opposition to, against
antro-	relating to a chamber or cavity
aphth/o-	ulcer
arch-	beginning, first, principal (also arche-, archi-)
archo-	relating to the rectum or anus
arterio-	relating to an artery
arthro-	relating to a joint
astro-	star-like or shaped
atelo-	incomplete or imperfect
auto-	relating to the self
axio-	relating to an axis (also axo-)
balano-	relating to the glans penis or glans clitoridis
baro-	relating to weight or heaviness
basi-	relating to the base or foundation (also basio-)
bi-	double, twice, two
blasto-	relating to germs
blenn-	relating to mucus (also blenno-)
blepharo-	relating to the eyelid
brachi-	relating to the arm (also brachio-)
brachy-	short
brady-	meaning slow or prolonged
broncho-	relating to the trachea
bucc/o-	relating to the cheek
cac-	meaning diseased or bad (also caci-, caco-)
cardio-	relating to the heart
cari/o-	rot, decay
carpo-	relating to the wrist
cathar/o-	purging, cleansing
cata-	down from, down, according to
caud/o-	lower part of body
celo-	indicating a tumor or hernia; cavity
cervico-	relating to the neck or neck of an organ
chilo-	relating to the lip (also cheilo-)
chole-	relating to the gallbladder
choledocho-	relating to the common bile duct
chondr/o-	relating to cartilage
chromo-	color
cirrho-	yellow in color
cleid/o-	relating to the clavicle
coel-	cavity, ventricle
coen/o-	common, shared
cole/o-	sheath

colp/o-	relating to the vagina
cryo-	frozen, cold
crypto-	hidden
cyst-	relating to the urinary bladder or a cyst (also cysto-)
cyto-	in relation to cell
dacry-	pertaining to the lacrimal glands
dactyl-	relating to the fingers or toes
demi-	half the amount
desmo-	relating to ligaments
desicco-	drying
deuter-	secondary or second
dextro-	meaning on or to the right
dorsi-	relating to the back (also dorso-)
dys-	painful, bad, disordered, difficult
echo-	reverberating sound
ecto-	external, outside
ectro-	congenital absence of something
endo-	within, internal
entero-	relating to the intestines
eosino-	red in color
epi-	on, upon, in addition to
eu-	well, healthy, good, normal
erythr/o-	red in color
esthesio-	sensation (also esthesia-)
exo-	outside of, without
ferr-	iron
fibro-	relating to fibers or fibrous tissue
galacto-	relating to milk
gastro-	relating to the stomach and abdominal region
genito-	relating to reproduction
glauco-	gray in color
gloss/o-	relating to the tongue
gnath/o-	relating to the jaw
gono-	relating to the genitals, offspring, origination
gyn-	relating to the female gender
hema-	relating to blood (also hemato-)
hemi-	half
hepato-	relating to the liver
hetero-	different
hidr/o-	sweat

histo-	relating to tissue
homeo-	indicates resemblance or likeness (also homo-)
hydro-	relating to fluid, water, or hydrogen
hyper-	excessive, above, exaggerated
hypo-	below, less than, under
hypophyso-	relating to the pituitary gland
hyster-	relating to either the womb or hysteria (also hystero-)
idio-	distinct or individual characteristics
ileo-	relating to the ileum (part of the small intestine)
ilio-	relating to the pelvis
infra-	meaning inferior to, beneath, under
irid-	relating to the iris
ischio-	relating to the hip
iso-	equal
jejuno-	relating to the jejunum (part of the small intestine)
juxta-	next to, near
karyo-	relating to the nucleus of a cell
kerato-	relating to the cornea or horny tissue
laparo-	flank, loins; operations through the abdominal wall
laryngo-	relating to the larynx
leio-	smooth
leuk/o-	white in color
levo-	left
lien-	relating to the spleen
lip-	relating to fat (also lipo-)
lith-	relating to a hard or calcified substance (also litho-)
lumbo-	relating to the loin region
macro-	meaning oversized, large
mal-	bad, poor, ill
medull/o-	middle, inner section
melano-	dark or black in color
meningo-	relating to membranes covering the brain and spine
mer/o-	relating to the thigh; part or portion
mesio-	toward the middle; secondary (also meso-)
meta-	indicates a change
metopo-	relating to the forehead

mis-	bad, improper
muta-	change
my-	relating to muscle (also myo-)
myc-	relating to fungus (also myco-)
myelo-	relating to bone marrow or the spinal cord
myring-	relating to the eardrum/tympanic membrane
narco-	indicates insensate condition or numbness
necro-	indicates death or dead tissue
nephr-	relating to the kidney
noci-	relating to injury or pain
nulli-	none
nycto-	relating to darkness or night
odont-	relating to the teeth
oligo-	indicates few or small
omo-	relating to the shoulder
omphalo-	relating to the navel
onco-	relating to a mass, tumor, or swelling
onycho-	relating to the finger- or toenails
oophor-	relating to the ovaries
opistho-	indicates behind or backwards
orchi-	relating to the testicles (also orchido-)
oscheo-	relating to the scrotum
osphresi/o-	sense of smell
osteo-	having to do with bone
oto-	relating to the ear
oxysmo-	sudden
pachy-	indicates heavy, large, or thick
pali-	repetition, back again, recurring (also palin-)
palp-	touch gently, feel (also palpat-)
panto-	indicates the whole or all
para-	indicates near, similar, beside, or past
patho-	indicates sensitivity, feeling, or suffering
pector-	relating to the chest
ped-	relating to the foot (also pedi-)
peri-	about, around, or in the vicinity
pero-	indicates being maimed or deformed
phaco-	relating to the lens of the eye
phago-	relating to eating and ingestion

pharyngo-	relating to the pharynx
phlebo-	relating to the vein
phreno-	relating to the diaphragm; head or mind
pimel-	relating to fat
platy-	indicates wide or broad
pleio-	more, additional
pleur-	relating to the side or ribs
pneum-	relating to respiration, air, the lungs
pod-	relating to the feet (also podo-)
polio-	gray in color
poly-	indicates much or many
primi-	first
procto-	relating to the rectum and/or anus
proso-	indicates toward the front, anterior, forward
pseudo-	indicates false or imagined
psor-	itch
ptyal/o-	saliva
pulmo-	relating to the lungs and respiration
purpur-	purple in color
pyelo-	relating to the pelvis
pygo-	relating to the buttocks or rump
pyle-	relating to an opening/orifice of the portal vein
pyloro-	relating to the pylorus, the stomach opening into the duodenum
pyo-	relating to pus
pyreto-	indicates a fever, heat
rachi-	relating to the spine (also rachio-)
radiculo-	relating to the nerve root
recto-	meaning straight or relating to the rectum
retro-	indicates behind, backward, in a reverse direction
rhabd/o-	rod, stick
rheo-	indicates a flow or stream of fluid
rhino-	relating to the nose
sacro-	relating to the sacrum, the base of the vertebral column
salpingo-	relating to the fallopian or eustachian tubes
sangu-	relating to blood
sarco-	relating to flesh

scapho-	indicates deformed condition, shaped like a boat
scapulo-	relating to the shoulder
schisto-	indicates cleft or split; a fissure
scoto-	relating to darkness; visual field gap
sial-	relating to saliva
sinistro-	meaning on or to the left
somato-	relating to the body
spheno-	relating to the sphenoid bone at the base of the skull
sphygm/o-	relating to the pulse
splanch-	relating to the intestines; viscera
spondyl/o-	relating to the vertebra
squam-	scaly
staphyl/o-	clusters
steato-	relating to fat
stetho-	relating to the chest
stomato-	relating to the mouth
strept/o-	twisted chains
sym-	indicates together with, along with, beside
syn-	indicates being joined together
tachy-	indicates swift or fast
tarso-	relating to the foot; margin of the eyelid
teleo-	indicates complete or perfectly formed
teno-	relating to tendons
terato-	indicates being seriously deformed, esp. a fetus
tetra-	four
thalamo-	relating to the thalamus, origin of nerves in the brain
thanato-	relating to death
thoraco-	relating to the chest
thrombo-	relating to blood clots
thymo-	relating to the thymus
toco-	relating to birth
trachelo-	relating to the neck
trichi-	relating to hair; hair-like shape (also tricho-)
tympano-	relating to the eardrum
typhlo-	relating to the cecum; relating to blindness

vaso-	relating to blood vessels
ventro-	relating to the abdomen; anterior surface of the body
verruc-	wart
vesico-	relating to the bladder
viscero-	relating to the abdominal organs
xantho-	yellow in color
xeno-	relating to a foreign substance
xero-	indicates a dry condition

Suffixes

Suffixes are the other half of the equation. These are attached to the ends of words.

-agra	indicating severe pain
-algia	pain
-artresia	closure, occlusion
-ase	denoting an enzyme
-blast	incomplete cellular development
-capnia	carbon dioxide
-cele	hernia
-centesis	puncture
-cephal	having to do with the head
-chalasia	relaxation (also -chalasis)
-clasis	to break (also -clast)
-cle	meaning small or little (also -cule)
-clysis	washing, irrigating
-cusis	hearing
-cyesis	pregnancy
-cyte	having to do with cells
-dactyl	having to do with fingers or toes
-desis	binding or fusion
-ectasia	dilation, widening (also –ectasis)
-ectomy	excision, removal
-eurysm	widening
-ferous	produces, causes, or brings about
-fuge	drive out or expel
-genic	indicates production, causation, generation
-gram	drawn, written, and recorded
-graphic	written or drawn
-hexia	habit
-ia	state of being, condition (abnormal)

-iasis	condition
-itis	inflammation
-lipsis	omit or fail
-listhesis	with stones
-lysis	release, free, reduction of
-malacia	softening
-metry	scientific measurement
-para	live births, bear (also -parous)
-phthisis	wasting away
-phylaxis	protection
-ptosis	protrude, prolapse
-ptysis	spitting
-odynia	indicates pain or discomfort
-oid	indicates likeness or resemblance
-ology	study of
-oma	tumor
-orraphy	suturing
-oscopy	to examine
-osis	condition, process
-ostomy	indicates a surgically created artificial opening
-otomy	indicates a cutting
-pagus	indicates fixed or joined together
-pathic	indicates a feeling, diseased condition, or therapy
-penia	indicates a deficiency; less than normal
-pexy	fixation

-philia	inordinate love of or craving for something
-phobia	abnormal fear of or aversion to something
-plasty	indicates surgically formed or molded
-plegia	indicates a stroke or paralysis
-poietic	indicates producing or making
-praxis	indicates activity, action, condition, or use
-rhage	indicates bleeding or other fluid discharge (also -rhagia)
-rhaphy	indicates a suture or seam joining two structures
-rrhagia	indicates an abnormal or excessive fluid discharge
-rrhexis	splitting or breaking
-spadia	to cut or tear
-spasm	contraction
-stalsis	contraction
-taxy	arrangement, grouping (also -taxis)
-tomy	indicates a cutting
-tresia	opening
-trophy	relating to food or nutrition
-tropic	indicates an affinity for or turning toward
-tropism	responding to an external stimulus
-tumesc/o	swelling (also -tumescence)
-ule	small

Abbreviations, Acronyms, and Symbols

The acronyms, abbreviations, and symbols used by health care providers speed communications. The following list includes the most often seen acronyms, abbreviations, and symbols. In some cases, abbreviations have more than one meaning. Multiple interpretations are separated by a slash (/). Abbreviations of Latin phrases are punctuated.

<	less than
>	greater than
@	at
6-PGD	deficiency of 6 phosphogluconate dehydrogenase
A	assessment/blood type
a (ante)	before
a fib	atrial fibrillation
a flutter	atrial flutter
A2	aortic second sound
AA	aggregative adherence
AAA	abdominal aortic aneurysms
AAL	anterior axillary line
AAMI	age-associated memory impairment
AAROM	active assistive range of motion
ATT	alpha-1 antitrypsin
ab	abortion
AB	blood type
abd	abdomen
ABE	acute bacterial endocarditis
ABG	arterial blood gas
abn.	abnormal
ABO	referring to ABO incompatibility
ACD	absolute cardiac dullness
ACDMPV	alveolar capillary dysplasia with misalignment of pulmonary veins
ACE	angiotensin converting enzyme/ adrenal cortical extract
ACL	anterior cruciate ligament
ACLS	advanced cardiac life support
ACP	acid phosphatase
acq.	acquired
ACS	acute coronary syndrome
ACTH	adrenocorticotropic hormone
ACVD	acute cardiovascular disease

a.d.	right ear/to, up to
ADA	adenosine deaminase
ADD	attention deficit disorder acute disseminated encephalomyelitis
ADH	antidiuretic hormone
ADHD	attention deficit hyperactivity disorder
ADL	activities of daily living
adm	admission, admit
ADM	alcohol, drug or mental disorder
ADO	autosomal dominant osteopetrosis
ADP	adenosine diphosphate
AE	above the elbow
AED	antiepileptic drugs
AF	atrial fibrillation
AFB	acid fast bacilli
AFF	atypical femoral fracture
AFH	angiofollicular lymph node hyperplasia
AFP	alpha-fetoprotein
A/G	albumin-globulin ratio
AGA	appropriate (average) for gestational age
AGC	atypical glandular cells
AGN	acute glomerulonephritis
AgNO3	silver nitrate
AGUS	atypical glandular cells of undetermined significance
AHA	American Hospital Association
AHC	acute hemorrhagic conjunctivitis
AHIMA	American Health Information Management Association
AHTR	acute hemolytic transfusion reaction
AI	aortic insufficiency/aromatase inhibitor
AICD	automatic implant cardioverter defibrilator
AID	artificial insemination donor/acute infectious disease
AIDS	acquired immunodeficiency syndrome
AIH	artificial insemination by husband

Abbreviations, Acronyms, and Symbols

AIM	abnormal involuntary movement
AIN	anal intraepithelial neoplasia
AIP	acute interstitial pneumonitis
AIPHI	acute idiopathic pulmonary hemorrhage in infants
AIS	androgen insensitivity syndrome
AK	above the knee
AKA	above knee amputation
a.k.a.	also known as
AKI	acute kidney injury
AL	amyloid light chain
ALA	aminolevulinic acid
ALCL	anaplastic large cell lymphoma
alk. phos.	alkaline phosphatase
ALL	acute lymphocytic leukemia/anterior longitudinal ligament
ALP	alkaline phosphatase
ALPS	autoimmune lymphoproliferative syndrome
ALS	advanced life support/amyotrophic lateral sclerosis
ALT	alanine aminotransferase
ALTE	apparent life threatening event
a.m.	morning
ama	against medical advice
AMA	American Medical Association
amb	ambulate
AMH	anti-Müllerian hormone
AMI	acute myocardial infarction
AML	acute myelogenous leukemia
AMML	acute myelomonocytic leukemia
AMP	adenosine monophosphate/ampule
ANA	American Nursing Association/antinuclear antibodies
ANC	absolute neutrophil count
ANS	autonomic nervous system
ant	anterior
AOD	arterial occlusive disease
AODM	adult onset diabetes mellitus
A&P	auscultation and percussion
A-P	anterior posterior
Ap	apical
AP	antepartum/anterior-posterior
APD	auditory processing disorder
APF	arterio-portal fistula

APM	arterial pressure monitoring
approx	approximately
appy.	appendectomy
APS	antiphospholipid syndrome
ARC	AIDS-related complex
ARD	acute respiratory disease
ARDS	adult respiratory distress syndrome
ARF	acute respiratory/renal failure
ARFID	avoidant/restrictive food intake disorder
ARO	autosomal recessive osteopetrosis
AROM	active range of motion/artificial rupture of membranes
ARPKD	autosomal recessive polycystic kidney disease
art.	artery, arterial
AS	aortic stenosis/arteriosclerosis/Asperger's syndrome
a.s.	left ear
ASAP	as soon as possible/atypical small acinar proliferation
ASC	ambulatory surgery center
ASC-H	atypical squamous cell cannot exclude high grade squamous intraepithelial lesion
ASC-US	atypical squamous cell of undetermined significance
ASCVD	arteriosclerotic cardiovascular disease
ASD	atrial septal defect
ASE	aortic saddle embolus
ASHD	arteriosclerotic heart disease
ASM	aggressive systemic mastocytosis
ASO	antistreptolysin-O
ASR	age/sex rate
Asst	assistance (min= minimal; mod= moderate)
AST	aspartate aminotransferase
ATIN	acute tubulointerstitial nephritis
ATP	adenosine triphosphate
ATS	arterial tortuosity syndrome
a.u.	each ear/both ears
AUB	anovulatory bleeding
A-V	arterioveneous
AV	atrioventricular
AVF	arteriovenous fistula
AVM	arteriovenous malformation

AVSD	atrioventricular septal defect		C	centigrade/complements/cervical vertebrae
ax	auxiliary		C-collar	cervical collar
AZT	azidothymidine		CA	cancer
Ba	barium		CA 125	cancer antigen 125
B&B	bowel and bladder		Ca	calcium/cancer
BAV	bicuspid aortic valve		CAA	cerebral amyloid angiopathy
BBB	bundle branch block		CABG	coronary artery bypass graft
BCC	basal cell carcinoma		CAD	coronary artery disease
BCP	birth control pill		CAL	clinical attachment loss
BE	barium enema/below the elbow		CALME	childhood asymmetric labium majus enlargement
BGL	blood glucose level		CA-MRSA	community acquired methicillin-resistant Staphylococcus aureus
BI	biopsy			
bib.	drink		CAPD	continuous ambulatory peritoneal dialysis
BK	below the knee			
BKA	below knee amputation		CAPS	cryopyrin-associated periodic syndrome
BLS	basic life support			
BM	bowel movement		CAT	computerized axial tomography
BMI	body mass index		cath	catheterize
BMR	basal metabolic rate		CBC	complete blood count
BMT	bone marrow transplant		CBD	corticobasal degeneration
BO	body order		CBF	cerebral blood flow study
BOO	bladder outlet obstruction		CBR	complete bed rest
BOW	bag of water		cc	chief complaint
BP	biophosphonate/blood pressure		CCE	congenital cystic eyeball
BPD	bronchopulmonary dysplasia		CCPD	continuous cycling peritoneal dialysis
BPH	benign prostatic hypertrophy		CCU	coronary care unit
Br	breastfeeding		CD	Castleman disease
BRAO	branch retinal artery occlusion		CDA	congenital dyserythropoietic anemia
BRBPR	bright red blood per rectum		CDC	Centers for Disease Control
BrC	breast care		CDG	congenital disorder of glycosylation
BRUE	brief resolved unexplained event		CDGS	carbohydrate-deficient glycoprotein syndrome
BRVO	branch retinal vein occlusion			
BS	bachelor of science/breath sounds/ bowel sounds		CDH	congenital dislocation of hip
BSA	body surface area		CE	cardiac enlargement
BSC	bedside commode		CEA	carcinoembryonic antigen
BSD	bedside drainage		CF	cystic fibrosis
BTD	biotinidase		CFS	chronic fatigue syndrome
BUN	blood urea nitrogen		CFTR	cystic fibrosis transmembrane conductance regulator
BUR	back-up rate (ventilator)			
BUS	Bartholin urethra skenes		CFC	cardiofasciocutaneous syndrome
bx	biopsy		CGF	congenital generalized fibromatosis
BXO	balanitis xerotica obliterans		CH,Chol	cholesterol
C&S	culture and sensitivity			

CHD	congenital heart disease/congestive heart disease
CHF	congestive heart failure
CI	confidence interval/chloride
CIC	chronic idiopathic constipation
CIDP	chronic inflammatory demyelinating polyneuropathy
CIN	cervical intraepithelial neoplasia
CIS	carcinoma in situ/cold injury syndrome
CJD	Creutzfeldt-Jakob disease
CK	creatine phosphokinase
CKD	chronic kidney disease
CLABSI	central line-associated bloodstream infection
CLD	chronic lung disease/chronic liver disease
CLL	chronic lymphatic leukemia
CLPC	contact lens–induced papillary conjunctivitis
cm	centimeter
cm2	square centimeters
CMC	carpometacarpal
CME	cystoid macular degeneration
CMG	cystometrogram
CMHC	community mental health center
CML	chronic myelogenous leukemia
CMML	chronic myelomonocytic leukemia
CMRI	cardiac magnetic resonance imaging
CMS	circulation motion sensation
CMS	Centers for Medicare and Medicaid Services
CMTC	cutis marmorata telangiectatica congenita
CMV	cytomegalovirus
cn	cranial nerves
CNP	continuous negative airway pressure
CNS	central nervous system
co	cardiac output
CO2	carbon dioxide
COLD	chronic obstructive lung disease
conc.	concentration
cont.	continue
COP	cryptogenic organizing pneumonia
COPD	chronic obstructive pulmonary disease
COSR	combat operational stress reaction
CP	cerebral palsy
CPAP	continuous positive airway pressure
CPB	cardiopulmonary bypass
CPD	cephalopelvic disproportion
CPK	creatine phosphokinase
CPM	continuous passive motion
CPPD	calcium pyrophosphate dihydrate crystal deposition
CPR	cardiopulmonary resuscitation/ computer-based patient record
CPRCA	constitutional (pure) red blood cell aplasia
CPT	chest physical therapy/Physicians' Current Procedural Terminology
CPT 1, CPT 2	carnitine palmityltransferase
CQI	Continuous Quality Improvement
CR	creatine
CRBSI	catheter related blood stream infection
CRC	community rating by class
CRF	chronic renal failure
CRH	corticotropic releasing hormone
crit.	hematocrit
CRMO	chronic recurrent multifocal osteomyelitis
CROS	contralateral routing of signals
CRP	C-reactive protein
CRPC	castrate-resistant prostate cancer
CRPS	complex regional pain syndrome
CRVO	central retinal vein occlusion
C/S	cesarean section
CSD	cat-scratch disease
CSF	cerebrospinal fluid
CT	computerized tomography/corneal thickness/ carpal tunnel syndrome
CTEPH	chronic thromboembolic pulmonary hypertension
CTIN	chronic tubulointerstitial nephritis
CTLSO	cervical-thoracic-lumbar-sacral-orthosis
CTZ	chemoreceptor trigger zone
CV	cardiovascular
CVA	cerebral vascular accident/ cerebrovascular accident/ costovertebral angle

CVD	cardiovascular disease, cerebrovascular disease
CVI	chronic venous insufficiency
CVID	common variable immunodeficiency
CVL	central venous line
CVP	central venous pressure
CVU	cerebrovascular unit
CXR	chest x-ray
cysto	cystoscopy
D&C	dilation and curettage
DA	diffuse adherence
DAEC	diffusely adherent Escherichia coli
D/C	discharge/discontinue
DC'd	discharged/discontinued
DCIS	ductal carcinoma in-situ
DCR	dacrocytstorhinostomy
DDD	degenerative disc disease/dense deposit disease
decub.	decubitus ulcer/lying down
DES	diethylstilbestrol
DEXA	dual energy x-ray absorptiometry
dexter	Latin for right
dextra	on the right
DHEA	dehydroepiandrosterone
DHT	dihydrotestosterone
DHTR	delayed hemolytic transfusion reaction
DI	diabetes insipidus
DIC	disseminated intravascular coagulopathy
DIF	direct immunofluorescence
DIP	distal interphalangeal (joint)/ desquamative interstitial pneumonia
DIRA	deficiency of interleukin 1 receptor antagonist
DISH	diffuse idiopathic skeletal hyperostosis
DJD	degenerative joint disease
DKA	diabetic ketoacidosis
DLE	discoid lupus erythematosus
DM	diabetes mellitus
DMAC	disseminated mycobacterium avium-intracellulare complex
DMD	Duchenne muscular dystrophy
DMDD	disruptive mood dysregulation disorder

DME	durable medical equipment
DNA	deoxyribonucleic acid
DNR	do not resuscitate
DOA	dead on arrival
DOB	date of birth
DOE	dyspnea on exertion
DPD	dihydropyrimidine dehydrogenase deficiency/dihydropyrimidine dehydrogenase disease
DPT	diphtheria - pertussis - tetanus
Dr	doctor
DS	Down syndrome
DSAP	disseminated superficial actinic porokeratosis
Dsg	dressing
DSM-5	Diagnostic and Statistical Manual of Mental Disorders, Fifth Edition
DSS	dioctyl sulfosoccinate
DTs	delirium tremens
DTRs	deep tendon reflexes
DU	depleted uranium
DUB	dysfunctional uterine bleeding
DUE	drug use evaluation
duo	two
DVT	deep vein thrombosis
D/W	dextrose in water
dx	diagnosis
DX	diagnosis code
dz	disease
EAEC	enteroaggregative Escherichia coli
EAggEC	enteroaggregative Escherichia coli
EBL	estimated blood loss
EBV	Epstein-Barr virus
ECCE	extracapsular cataract extraction
ECF	extended care facility/extracellular fluid
ECD	Erdheim-Chester Disease
ECG	electrocardiogram
ECHO	enterocytopathogenic human orphan virus/echocardiogram
ECMO	extracorporeal membrane oxygenation
ECP	extracorporeal photopheresis
ECT	electro-convulsive therapy/emission computerized tomography
ectopic	ectopic pregnancy (OB)

ED	emergency department/effective dose/erectile dysfunction
EDI	electronic data interchange
EEE	eastern equine encephalitis
EEG	electroencephalogram
EENT	eye, ear, nose, and throat
EFA	essential fatty acid
EGA	estimated gestational age
EGD	esophagus, stomach and duodenum
EGID	eosinophilic gastrointestinal disorders
EHEC	enterohemorrhagic Escherichia coli
EIEC	enteroinvasive Escherichia coli
EIN	endometrial intraepithelial neoplasia
EKC	epidemic keratoconjunctivitis
EKG	electrocardiogram
E/M	evaluation and management
EM	erythema multiforme
EMG	electromyogram
EMS	eosinophilic myalgia syndrome
en bloc	in total
ENG	electronystagmogram
ENT	ear, nose, and throat
EO	elbow orthosis
EOG	electrooculography
EOM	extraocular motion
EOMI	extraocular motion intact
EOP	external occipital protuberance
EPEC	enteropathogenic Escherichia coli
EPI	exocrine pancreatic insufficiency
Epis.	episiotomy
EPO	epoetin alfa/erythropoietin
EPS	electrophysiologic stimulation/electrophysiological study
ER	emergency room
ER-	estrogen receptor negative status
ER+	estrogen receptor positive status
ERC	endoscopic retrograde cholangiography
ERCP	endoscopic retrograde cholangiopancreatography
ERD	estrogen-receptor down regulators
ERG	electroretinogram
ESR	erythrocyte sedimentation rate
ESRD	end stage renal disease
EST	electroshock therapy

ESWL	extracorporeal shockwave lithotripsy
ET	endotracheal/eustachian tube
ETEC	Enterotoxigenic Escherichia coli
ETN	erythema toxicum neonatorum
ETOH	alcohol
Ex	examination
ext.	extremity
F	Fahrenheit/female
FA	Fanconi's anemia
FAS	fetal alcohol syndrome
FAZ	foveal avascular zone
FB (fb)	fingerbreadth
FB	foreign body
FBR	foreign body removal
FBS	fasting blood sugar
FDP	fibrin degradation products
Fe	female/iron
FEV	forced expiratory volume
FFI	fatal familial insomnia
FFP	fresh frozen plasma
FGR	fetal growth retardation
FH	familial hypercholesterolemia/family history
FHL	familial hemophagocytic lymphohistiocytosis
FHM	familial hemiplegic migraine
FHR	fetal heart rate
FHT	fetal heart tone
FI	firm one finger down from umbilicus
fl	fluid
fluro	fluoroscopy
FM	face mask
FMF	familial Mediterranean fever
FMRP	fragile X mental retardation protein
FNHTR	febrile nonhemolytic transfusion reaction
FP	family planning/family practitioner
FPH	female pseudohermaphroditism
FPIES	food protein-induced enterocolitis syndrome
FR	family relationship
FSE	fetal scalp electrode
FSGS	focal and segmental glomerulosclerosis
FSH	follicle stimulating hormone

FTND	full term normal delivery	HAA	hepatitis antigen B
FTSG	full thickness skin graft	HAAb	hepatitis antibody A
FTT	failure to thrive	HaAg	hepatitis antigen A
F/U	follow-up	HAI	hemaglutination test
FUI	functional urinary incontinence	HAV	hepatitis A virus
FUO	fever of unknown origin	HB	headbox/hepatitis B
fx	fracture	HBsAb	hepatitis surface antibody B
G	gram	HBcAg	hepatitis antigen B
G6PD	glucose-6-phosphate dehydrogenase	HBD	hydroxybutyril dehydrogenase
GA	gastric analysis	HbF	fetal hemoglobin
GABA	gamma-aminobutyric acid	Hbg	hemoglobin
GAD	generalized anxiety disorder	HBO	hyperbaric oxygen
GALD	gestational alloimmune liver disease	HbO2	oxyhemoglobin
gav.	gavage	HBP	high blood pressure
GAVE	gastric antral vascular ectasia	HBS	hungry bone syndrome
GB	gallbladder	HBsAg	hepatitis antigen B
GDM	gestational diabetes mellitus	HBV	hepatitis B vaccine/hepatitis B virus
GERD	gastroesophageal reflux disease	HCG	human chorionic gonadotropin
GFR	glomerular filtration rate	HCl	hydrochloric acid
GGO	ground-glass opacities	HCM	hypertrophic cardiomyopathy
GH	growth hormone	HCPCS	Healthcare Common Procedural Coding System
GI	gastrointestinal	Hct	hematocrit
GIFT	gamete intrafallopian transfer	Hctz	hydrochlorothiazide
GISA	glycopeptide intermediate Staphylococcus aureus	HCV	hepatitis C virus
GIST	gastrointestinal stromal tumor	HCVD	hypertensive cardiovascular disease
GLC	gas liquid chromatography	HD	hip disarticulation
GMP	guanosine monophosphate	HDL	high-density lipoproteins
GN	glomerulonephritis	HDV	hepatitis D virus
GnRH	gonadotropin-releasing hormone	HEENT	head, eyes, ears, nose, and throat
grav	number of pregnancies	HEV	hepatitis E virus
GSRA	glycopeptide resistant Staphylococcus aureus	HGH	human growth hormone
		Hg/Hgb	hemoglobin
GSS	Gerstmann-Straussler-Scheinker syndrome	HGSIL	high grade squamous intraepithelial lesion
gsw	gunshot wound	HH	hard of hearing
GU	genitourinary	HHNS	hyperosmolar hyperglycemic nonketotic syndrome
Gu	guiac	HHS	hyperosmolar hyperglycemic state
GVHD	graft-versus-host disease	HHV-6	human herpesvirus 6
H&P	history and physical	HHV-7	human herpesvirus 7
H2O	water	HIAA	hydroxyindolacetic acid
H2O2	hydrogen peroxide	Hib	Hemophilus influenzae vaccine/ Haemophilus influenzae type b
H5N1	avian influenza		
HA	headache/hearing aid/hemagglutinin	HIE	hypoxic-ischemic encephalopathy

HIT	heparin-induced thrombocytopenia
HIV	human immunodeficiency virus
HLA	human leukocyte antigen
HLHS	hypoplastic left heart syndrome
HLV	herpes-like virus
HMD	hyaline membrane disease
hMPV	human metapneumovirus
HMS	hepatosplenomegaly
HNPCC	hereditary nonpolyposis colorectal cancer syndromes
HORF	high output renal failure
HPA	human platelet antigen
HPF	high power field
HPFH	hereditary persistence of fetal hemoglobin
HPG	human pituitary gonadotropin
HPI	history of present illness
HPIV	human parainfluenza virus
HPS	Hantavirus pulmonary syndrome/ hepatopulmonary syndrome
HPV	human papillomavirus
HR	Harrington rod/heart rate/hour
HRCT	high resolution computerized tomography
HRIG	human rabies immune globulin
HRPC	hormone-refractory prostate cancer
HRT	hormone replacement therapy
HS	heelstick/hour of sleep
HSG	hysterosalpingogram
HSIL	high-grade squamous intraepithelial lesion
HSV	herpes simplex virus
HTLV	human T-cell lymphotropic virus
HTN	hypertension
HTR	hemolytic transfusion reaction
HUS	hemolytic-uremic syndrome
HVA	homovanillic acid
Hx	history
hypo	hypodermic injection
IA	intra-arterial
IAA	interruption of aortic arch
IAB	intra-aortic balloon
IABC	intra-aortic balloon counterpulsation
IABP	intra-aortic balloon pump
IAO	intermediate autosomal osteopetrosis

IAPP	idiopathic atrophoderma of Pasini and Pierini
IBM	inclusion body myositis
IBS	irritable bowel syndrome
IBW	ideal body weight
ICCE	intracapsular cataract extraction
ICD-9-CM	International Classification of Diseases, 9th Revision, Clinical Modification
ICD-10	International Classification of Diseases, 10th Revision, WHO
ICD-10-CM	International Classification of Diseases, 10th Revision, Clinical Modification, U.S.
ICD-10-PCS	International Classification of Diseases, 10th Revision, Procedure Coding System
ICH	intracranial/cerebral hemorrhage
ICP	intracranial pressure
ICS	intercostal space
ICSH	interstitial cell stimulating hormone
ICU	intensive care unit
I&D	incision and drainage
Id31	radioactive iodine
IDDM	insulin dependent diabetis mellitus
IDH	isocitric dehydrogenase
IDM	infant of diabetic mother
IEED	involuntary emotional expression disorder
IFIS	intraoperative floppy iris syndrome
Ig	immunoglobulin, gamma
IgE	immunoglobulin E
IgG	immunoglobulin G
IgM	immunoglobulin M
IGRA	interferon gamma release assay
IH	infectious hepatitis
IHSS	idiopathic hypertrophic subaortic stenosis
ILD	interstitial lung disease
IM	internal medicine/intramuscular/ infectious mononucleosis
IMV	intermittent mandatory ventilation
inc.	incision
indep	independent
INF	inferior, infusion
INH	inhalation solution
INJ	injection

INPH	idiopathic normal pressure hydrocephalus
instill	instillation
IOL	intraocular lens
IOP	intraocular pressure
IP	intraperitoneal/interphalangeal
IPD	intermittent peritoneal dialysis
IPF	idiopathic pulmonary fibrosis
IPP	induration penis plastica
IPPB	intermittent positive pressure breathing
IQ	intelligence quotient
ISC	infant servo-control
ISD	intrinsic sphincter deficiency
ISG	immune serum globulin
IT	intrathecal administration
ITP	idiopathic thrombocytopenia purpura
IU	international units
IUD	intrauterine device
IUGR	intrauterine growth restriction/retardation
IV	intravenous
IVC	inferior vena cava/intravenous cholangiogram
IVF	in vitro fertilization
IVH	intraventricular hemorrhage
IVP	intravenous pyelogram
JC	John Cunningham (polyomavirus)
JODM	juvenile onset diabetes mellitus
JRA	juvenile rheumatoid arthritis
JVP	jugular venous pressure
K	potassium
Kcal	kilocalorie
KCL	potassium chloride
kg	kilogram
KO	keep open/knee orthosis
KUB	kidneys, ureters, bladder
KVO	keep vein open
L	left/lumbar vertebrae
LA	left atrium
LAC	lupus anticoagulant
LAD	left anterior descending
LAM	lymphangioleiomyomatosis
LAP	leucine aminopeptidase
LAT	lateral

LAV	lymphadenopathy associated virus
LAVH	laparoscopic assisted vaginal hysterectomy
LBB	left bundle branch
LBBB	left bundle branch block
LBP	lower back pain
LCAD	long chain acyl CoA dehydrogenase deficiency
LCAV	La Cross encephalitis virus
LCBI	laboratory-confirmed bloodstream infections
LCDD	light chain deposition disease
LCHAD	long chain 3-hydroxyacyl CoA dehydrogenase deficiency
LCP	licensed clinical psychologist
LD	lethal dose
LDH	lactate dehydrogenase
LDL	low-density lipoproteins
LE	lower extremity/lupus erythematosis
LEEP	loop electrocautery excision procedure
LEMS	Lambert-Eaton myasthenic syndrome
LES	Lambert-Eaton syndrome
LFT	liver function test
LIP	lymphoid interstitial pneumonia
LGA	large for gestational age
LGSIL	low grade squamous intraepithelial lesion
LH	luteinizing hormone
LHF	left heart failure
LHR	leukocyte histamine release
Li	lithium
lido	lidocaine
LKS	liver, kidneys, spleen
LLL	left lower lobe
LLQ	left lower quadrant
LML	left medio lateral position
LMP	last menstrual period
LMS	left mentum anterior position (chin)
LMT	left mentum transverse position
LOC	level of consciousness/loss of consciousness
LOM	limitation of motion
LOP	left occiput posterior position
LOPS	loss of protective sensation
LOT	left occiput transverse position

LP	lumbar puncture
LPM	liters per minute
LR	lactated Ringer's/log roll
LS fusion	lumbar sacral fusion
LSA	left sacrum anterior position
LSB	left sternal border
LSIL	low-grade squamous intraepithelial lesion
LSO	lumbar sacral orthosis
LSVC	left superior vena cava
LT	left
lul	left upper lobe
luq	left upper quadrant
LUTS	lower urinary tract symptoms
LV	left ventricle
lymphs	lymphocytes
lytes	electrolytes
M	manifest refraction/male
M1	mitral first sound
M2	mitral second sound
MA1	volume respirator
MAC	maximum allowable cost
MAD	monoamine oxidase (inhibitor)
MALT	mucosa associated lymphoid tissue
MAP	mean arterial pressure
MAS	macrophage activation syndrome
MASER	microwave amplification by stimulated emission of radiation
MBC	minimum bactericidal concentration/ maximum breathing capacity
MBD	minimal brain dysfunction
mcg	microgram
MCAD	medium chain acyl CoA dehydrogenase deficiency
MCAS	mast cell activation syndrome
MCC	Merkel cell carcinoma
MCH	mean corpuscular hemoglobin
MCI	mild cognitive impairment
MCKD	medullary cystic kidney disease
MCL	midclavicular line
MCP	metacarpophalangeal
MCR	modified community rating
MCT	mediastinal chest tube
MCV	mean corpuscular volume
MD	medical doctor
MD	muscular dystrophy/myocardial disease/manic depression
MDD	manic-depressive disorder
MDMA	methylenedioxymethamphetamine (Ecstasy)
MDS	myelodysplastic syndrome
Mec	meconium
MED	minimal effective dose
med/surg	medical, surgical
meds	medications
MELAS	mitochondrial encephalopathy, lactic acidosis and stroke-like episodes
MEN	multiple endocrine neoplasia
MERRF	myoclonus with epilepsy and with ragged red fibers
MFD	minimum fatal dose
MFT	muscle function test
mg	milligram
Mg	magnesium
MG	myasthenia gravis
MGUS	monoclonal gammopathy of undetermined significance
MH/CD	mental health/chemical dependency
MH/SA	mental health/substance abuse
MHC	major histocompatibility complex
MI	myocardial infarction
MID	multi-infarct dementia
min	minimum/minimal/minute
misce.	miscellaneous
ML	midline
ml	milliliter
MLC	midline catheter
mm	millimeter
MMAS	monoclonal mast cell activation syndrome
MMD	myotonic muscular dystrophy
mmHg	millimeters of mercury
MMN	multifocal motor neuropathy
MMRV	measles, mumps, rubella vaccine
MOD	multiple organ dysfunction
MOH	medication overuse headache
MOM	milk of magnesia
mono	monocyte/mononucleosis
MOTT	mycobacteria other than tuberculosis
MPD	maximum permissible dose

MPH	male pseudohermaphroditism
MR	mitral regurgitation
MRA	magnetic resonance angiography
MRI	magnetic resonance imaging
MS	morphine sulfate/multiple sclerosis
MSLT	multiple sleep latency testing
MSRA	methicillin-resistant Staphylococcus aureus
MSSA	methicillin susceptible Staphylococcus aureus
MTC	medullary carcinoma of the thyroid
MTD	right eardrum
mtDNA	mitochondrial deoxyribonucleic acid
MTHFR	methylenetetrahydrofolate reductase
MTP	metatarsophalangeal
MTS	left eardrum
multip.	multipara - pregnant woman who has more than one child
MVA	motor vehicle accident
MVD	microvillous inclusion disease
MVP	mitral valve prolapse
MWS	Mickety-Wilson syndrome
MZL	marginal zone lymphoma
N	nitrogen
N2O	nitrous oxide
Na	sodium
NA	neuraminidase
NaCl	sodium chloride (salt)
NASH	nonalcoholic steatohepatitis
NAT	nonaccidental trauma
NB	newborn
NBICU	newborn intensive care unit
NBT	nitroblue tetrazolium
NC	neurogenic claudication
NCA	neurocirculatory asthenia
NCPR	no cardiopulmonary resuscitation
NCR	no cardiac resuscitation
NCV	nerve conduction velocity
NDC	national drug code
NDM	neonatal diabetes mellitus
NDPH	new daily persistent headache
NE	neonatal encephalopathy
NEC	necrotizing enterocolitis/not elsewhere classified
NEHI	neuroendocrine cell hyperplasia of infancy
NF	National Formulary/ neurofibromatosis
NFD	nephrogenic fibrosing dermopathy
NG	nasogastric
NGU	nongonococcal urethritis
NH	neonatal hemochromatosis
NHL	non-Hodgkin lymphoma
NICU	neonatal intensive care unit
NID	neuronal intestinal dysplasia
NIDDM	non-insulin dependent diabetes mellitus
NIHSS	National Institutes of Health Stroke Scale
NJ	nasojejunal
NK	natural killer (cells)
NKA	no known allergies
NKHHC	nonketotic hyperglycemic-hyperosmolar coma
NKMA	no known medical allergies
NMDA	N-Methyl-D-aspartate
NMS	neuroleptic malignant syndrome
NOMID	neonatal onset multisystem inflammatory disease
NOS	not otherwise specified
novem.	nine
NP-CPAP	nasopharyngeal continuous positive airway pressure
NPN	non-par not approved/nonprotein nitrogen
n.p.o.	nothing by mouth
NS	normal saline/not significant
NSAID	nonsteroidal anti-inflammatory drug
NSIP	nonspecific interstitial pneumonitis
NSR	normal sinus rhythm
NST	nonstress test
NSTEMI	non-ST elevation myocardial infarction
NSVB	normal spontaneous vaginal bleeding
NSVD	normal spontaneous vaginal delivery
NT	nasotracheal/nontender
NTE	neutral thermal environment
NTM	nontuberculous mycobacteria
NTP	normal temperature and pressure
N&V	nausea and vomiting

Abbreviations, Acronyms, and Symbols

O	blood type/oxygen		PAC	premature atrial contraction
O2	oxygen		PACU	post anesthesia care unit
OA	occiput-anterior/open access/osteoarthritis		PAD	pulmonary artery diastolic
OAG	open angle glaucoma		PAH	pulmonary arterial hypertension/phenylalanine hydroxylase
OB	obstetrics		PAM	pulmonary alveolar microlithiasis
OB-GYN	obstetrics and gynecology		PAP	Papanicolaou test or smear/pulmonary artery pressure
OC	open crib/oral contraceptive/office call		PAPA	pyogenic arthritis, pyoderma gangrenosum, and acne syndrome
OCD	obsessive-compulsive disorder		PAPVC	partial anomalous pulmonary venous connection
OCT	ornithine carbamyl transterase/oxytocin challenge test		PAPVR	partial anomalous pulmonary venous return
octo.	eight		PAR	post anesthesia recovery/parenteral
o.d.	right eye		para	alongside of/number of pregnancies, e.g., para 1, 2, 3, etc.
ODD	oppositional defiant disorder			
OFC	occipitofrontal circumference		PARR	post anesthesia recovery room
OHS	obesity hypoventilation syndrome		PAT	paroxysmal atrial tachycardia
oint	ointment		path	pathology
o.m.	every morning/otitis media		PAVM	pulmonary arteriovenous malformation
ONH	optic nerve head/optic nerve hypoplasia		PBA	pseudobulbar affect
ONJ	osteonecrosis of the jaw		PBI	protein-bound iodine
O&P	ova and parasites		PC	packed cells
OPG	oculoplethysmography		PCA	patient controlled analgesia
ophth	ophthalmology		PCB	postcoital bleeding
OPV	oral polio vaccine		PCD	polycystic disease
OR	operating room		PCG	phonocardiogram
ORIF	open reduction internal fixation		PCN	penicillin
ortho.	orthopedics		PCOS	polycystic ovarian syndrome
o.s.	left eye		PCS	primary ciliary dyskinesia
os, oris	mouth		PCTA	percutaneous transluminal angioplasty
OSA	obstructive sleep apnea			
OST	oxytocin stress test		PCV	packed cell volume
OT	occupational therapy		PCW	pulmonary capillary wedge
OTC	over-the-counter		PD	postural drainage/Parkinson's disease
OTD	organ tolerance dose		PDA	patent ductus arteriosus
OTH	other routes of administration		PDD	pervasive developmental disorder
o.u.	each eye/both eyes		PDS	polyglandular deficiency syndrome
ov.	ovum/office visit		PE	physical examination/pulmonary embolism/pulmonary edema
oz.	ounce			
P	plan/after/pulse/phosphorus		PEA	pulseless electrical activity
P2	pulmonic 2nd sound		PEC	pre-existing condition
PA	physician assistant/posteroanterior/pulmonary artery		Peds	pediatrics
			PEG	pneumoencephalogram
PAB	premature atrial beats			

PEN	parenteral and enteral nutrition	POAG	primary open angle glaucoma
PENS	percutaneous electrical nerve stimulation	polys	polymorphonuclear neutrophil leukocytes
PERRLA	pupils equal, regular, reactive to light and accommodation	POS	place of service/point of service/point of sale
PET	positron emission tomography	pos.	positive
PFAPA	periodic fever, aphthous stomatitis, pharyngitis, and adenopathy syndrome	post or PM	postmortem exam or autopsy
		PP	postprandial
PFC	persistent fetal circulation	PPD	percussion and postural drainage/ purified protein derivative
PFT	pulmonary function test	PPE	palmar plantar erythrodysesthesia
PG	prostaglandin	PPH	postpartum hemorrhage/primary pulmonary hypertension
PH	past history/pulmonary hypertension		
pH	potential of hydrogen	PPHN	persistent pulmonary hypertension of the newborn
PI	present illness		
PICC	peripherally inserted central catheter	PPP	palmoplantar pustulosis/pentose phosphate pathway/protamine paracoagulation
PID	pelvic inflammatory disease		
PIG	pulmonary interstitial glycogenosis	PR	pityriasis rosea
PIN	prostatic intraepithelial neoplasia	PRBC	packed red blood cells
PIP	proximal interphalangeal (joint)	PRCA	pure red cell aplasia
PKU	phenylketonuria	PRES	posterior reversible encephalopathy syndrome
PLCH	pulmonary Langerhans cell histiocytosis		
		PREs	progressive resistive exercises
PLEVA	pityriasis lichenoides et varioliformis acuta	PRF	postprocedural respiratory failure
		preg	pregnant
PLL	posterior longitudinal ligament	previa	placenta previa
PLMD	periodic limb movement disorder	primip	primipara - a woman having her first child
PLS	primary lateral sclerosis		
PMDD	premenstrual dysphoric disorder	PRIND	prolonged reversible ischemic neurologic deficit
PMHx	past medical history		
PML	progressive multifocal leukoencephalopathy	p.r.n.	as needed for
		PRNP	prion protein
PMN	polvmorphonuclear neutrophil leukocytes	PROM	premature rupture of membranes
		PROMM	proximal myotonic myotonia
PMP	pseudomyxoma peritonei	PSA	prostate specific antigen
PMS	premenstrual syndrome	PSMA	progressive spinal muscle atrophy
PMT	premenstrual tension syndrome	PSP	phenolsulfonphthalein/primary spontaneous pneumothorax
PNC	premature nodal contraction		
PND	paroxysmal nocturnal dyspnea/ post nasal drip	PSVT	paroxysmal supraventricular tachycardia
PNDM	permanent neonatal diabetes mellitus	PT	physical therapy/prothrombin time
PNH	paroxysmal nocturnal hemoglobinuria	Pt	patient/prothrombin time
		PTA	prior to admission/percutaneous transluminal angioplasty
PNP	purine nucleoside phosphorylase		
PNS	peripheral nervous system	PTB	patellar tendon bearing (cast)
p/o	by mouth	PTCA	percutaneous transluminal coronary angioplasty
PO	(per os) by mouth/postoperative		

PTCL	peripheral T-cell lymphoma
PTE	pulmonary thromboendarterectomy/posttraumatic epilepsy
PTH	parathyroid hormone
PTLD	posttransplant lymphoproliferative disorder
PTP	posttransfusion purpura
PTS	posttraumatic seizures
PTSD	post-traumatic stress disorder
PTT	partial thromboplastin time
PUD	peptic ulcer disease
PUPPP	pruritic urticarial papules and plaques of pregnancy
PVA	poikiloderma vasculare atrophicans
PVC	premature ventricular contraction
PVD	peripheral vascular disease/posterior vitreous detachment/premature ventricular depolarization
PVF	pulmonary vascular resistance
PVL	paraventricular leukomalasia
PVT	paroxysmal ventricular tachycardia
Px	prognosis
QFT	QuantiFERON tuberculosis test
R	respiration/right atrium
R/O	rule out
RA	rheumatoid arthritis/refractory anemia
RAEB-1	refractory anemia w/excess blasts-1
RAEB-2	refractory anemia w/excess blasts-2
RARS	refractory anemia w/ringed sideroblasts
RBB	right bundle branch
RBBB	right bundle branch block
RBC	red blood cell
RB-ILD	respiratory bronchiolitis interstitial lung disease
RBOW	ruptured bag of water
RCD	relative cardiac dullness
RCMD	refractory cytopenia w/multilineage dysplasia
RCMD-RS	refractory cytopenia w/multilineage dysplasia and ringed sideroblasts
RDS	respiratory distress syndrome
REM	rapid eye movement
RESA	radial cryosurgical ablation
resp	respiration, respiratory
Rh neg	Rhesus factor negative

Rh	Rhesus
RHD	rheumatic heart disease
RHF	right heart failure
RIA	radioimmunoassay
RIND	reversible ischemic neurological deficit
RL	Ringer's lactate
RLE	right lower extremity
RLF	rentrolental fibroplasia
RLL	right lower lobe
rlq	right lower quadrant
RLS	restless legs syndrome
RML	right middle lobe
RMLS	right middle lobe syndrome
RN	registered nurse
RNA	ribonucleic acid
RND	reflex neurovascular dystrophy
ROA	right occiput anterior position
ROM	range of motion
ROP	retinopathy of prematurity/right occiput posterior position
ROS	review of systems
RPE	retinal pigment epithelium
RPG	retrograde pyelogram
RR	recovery room
RRR	regular rate and rhythm
RSD	reflex sympathetic dystrophy
RSI	repetitive strain injury
RSV	respiratory syncytial virus
RT	recreational therapist/respiratory therapist/resting tracing/right
RUL	right upper lobe
ruq	right upper quadrant
RV	right ventricle
Rx	take (prescription; treatment)
RxN	reaction
s.c.	subcutaneous
s.l.	under the tongue, sublingual
S/P	status post
SAH	subarachnoid hemorrhage
SALT	serum alanine aminotransferase
SARS	severe acute respiratory syndrome
SAST	serum aspartate aminotransferase
SB	sinus bradycardia

SBFT	small bowel follow through		SSNRI	selective serotonin and norepinephrine reuptake inhibitors
S-C disease	sickle cell hemoglobin-c disease		SSP	secondary spontaneous pneumothorax
SCAD	short chain acyl CoA dehydrogenase deficiency		SSPE	subacute sclerosing panencephalitis
SCD	sudden cardiac death		SSRI	selective serotonin reuptake inhibitors
SCI	spinal cord injury		ST	sinus tachycardia
SCID	severe combined immunodeficiency		staph	staphylococcus
SED	selective eating disorder		stat	immediately
sed rate	sedimentation rate of erythrocytes		STC	slow transit constipation
SEI	subepithelial infiltrates		STD	sexually transmitted disease
SEM	systolic ejection murmur		STEC	shiga toxin-producing Escherichia coli
SERM	selective estrogen receptor modulator		STEMI	ST elevation myocardial infarction
sex	six		STH	somatotrophic hormone
SG	Swan-Ganz		strep	streptococcus
SGA	small for gestational age		STS	serology test for syphilis
SGOT	serum glutamic oxaloacetic acid		STSG	split thickness skin graft
SH	social history		subcu	subcutaneous
SHBG	sex hormone binding globulin		SUNCT	short lasting unilateral neuralgiform headache with conjunctival injection and tearing
SHM	sporadic hemiplegic migraine			
SHOX	short stature homeobox (gene)		SVAS	supravalvular aortic stenosis
SIADH	syndrome of inappropriate antidiuretic hormone		SVC	superior vena cava
SIDS	sudden infant death syndrome		SVCS	superior vena cava syndrome
SIRS	systemic inflammatory response syndrome		SVT	supraventricular tachycardia
			Sx	sign/symptom
SISI	short increment sensitivity index		T	temperature/tender/thoracic vertebrae
SJS	Stevens-Johnson syndrome			
SLE	systemic lupus erythematosus		T&A	tonsils and adenoids
SLEV	St. Louis encephalitis virus		T3	triiodothyronine
SMA	spinal muscular atrophy		T4	thyroxine
SMCAS	secondary mast cell activation syndrome		TAA	thoracic aortic aneurysm/ tumor-associated antigen
SMCD	systemic mast cell disease		TAC	trigeminal autonomic cephalgia
SMZL	splenic marginal zone lymphoma		TACO	transfusion associated circulatory overload
SNF	skilled nursing facility			
SNS	sympathetic nervous system		TAH	total abdominal hysterectomy
SOB	shortness of breath		TAPVC	total anomalous pulmonary venous connection
SPD	semantic pragmatic disorder/ summary plan description		TAR	thrombocytopenia with absent radii syndrome
SPN	solitary pulmonary nodule			
SQ	status quo/subcutaneous		TAT	tetanus antitoxin/turnaround time
SROM	spontaneous rupture of membranes		Tb	tubercule bacillus
SRSV	small round structured viruses		TB	tuberculosis
SRV	small round viruses		TBG	thyroxine/thyroid binding globulin
SSA	senile systemic amyloidosis		TBI	total body irradiation/ traumatic brain injury

TBSA	total body surface area		TUR	transurethral resection
TC&DB	turn, cough, and deep breathe		TURP	transurethral resection of prostate
Td	tetanus		Tx	treatment
temp	temperature		U/A	urinalysis
TEN	toxic epidermal necrolysis		UAC	umbilical artery catheter/catheterization
TENS	transcutaneous electrical nerve stimulation		UE	upper extremity
TFT	transfer factor test		UFR	uroflowmetry
THA	total hip arthroplasty		UGI	upper gastrointestinal
Thal	thalassemia		UMN	upper motor neuron
THC	tetrahydrocannabinol		UPJ	ureteropelvic junction
TI	tricuspid insufficiency		UPP	urethra pressure profile
TIA	transient ischemic attack		URI	upper respiratory infection
TKA	total knee arthroplasty		URTI	upper respiratory tract infection
TLS	tumor lysis syndrome		US	unstable spine/ultrasound
TM	tympanic membrane		UTI	urinary tract infection
TMI	transient myocardial ischemia		UV	ultraviolet light
TMJ	temporomandibular joint		UVC	umbilical vein catheter
TNDM	transient neonatal diabetes mellitus		V Fib	ventricular fibrillation
TNS	transcutaneous nerve stimulator/stimulation		V tach	ventricular tachycardia
TOA	tubo-ovarian abscess		VAHS	virus-associated hemophagocytic syndrome
TORCH	toxoplasmosis, other (includes syphilis), rubella, cytomegalovirus, and herpes virus		VAIN	vaginal intraepithelial neoplasia
			VBAC	vaginal birth after cesarean
TP	total protein		VC	vena cava
tPA	tissue plasminogen activator		VCFS	velo-cardio-facial syndrome
TPN	total parenteral nutrition		VCG	vectorcardiogram
TPR	temperature, pulse, respiration		vCJD	variant Creutzfeldt-Jakob disease
TRALI	transfusion-related acute lung injury		VD	venereal disease/voiding dysfunction
TRAM	transverse rectus abdominos musculocutaneous		VDH	valvular disease of the heart
			VDRL	venereal disease report
trans	transverse		VEP	visual evoked potential
TRF	thyrotropin releasing factor		VF	visual field/ventricular fibrillation
TRH	thyrotropin releasing hormone		VHL	Von Hippel-Lindau
TSA	tumor specific antigen		VIN	vulvar intraepithelial neoplasia
TSD	Tay-Sachs disease		VIP	vasoactive intestinal peptide
TSE	testicular self-exam/transmissible spongiform encephalopathy		VLBW	very low birth weight
			VLCAD	very long chain acyl CoA dehydrogenase deficiency
TSH	thyroid stimulating hormone			
TSS	toxic shock syndrome		VLDL	very low-density lipoproteins
TTN	transient tachypnea of newborn		VMA	vitreomacular adhesion
TTR	transthyretin		VO2	maximum oxygen consumption
TTTS	twin-to-twin transfusion syndrome		VP	vasopressin/voiding pressure
TULIP	transurethral ultrasound guided laser induced prostate		VPC	ventricular premature contraction

VPI	velopharyngeal incompetence
VPRC	volume of packed red cells
VS	vital signs/vesicular sound
VSD	ventricular septal defect
VUR	vesicoureteral-reflux
vv	veins
vWF	von Willebrand factor
VZV	varicella zoster virus
w/HSBH	warmed heelstick blood gas
WAS	Wiskott-Aldrich syndrome
WASP	Wiskott-Aldrich syndrome protein
WB	whole blood
WBC	white blood count

WC	wheelchair
WEE	western equine encephalitis
WHO	World Health Organization
WLS	wet lung syndrome
WNL	within normal limits
WPW	Wolff-Parkinson-White syndrome
Wt	weight
WTTA	wild-type transthyretin amyloidosis
YLDV	yaba-like disease virus
YMTV	yaba monkey tumor virus
ZIFT	zygote intrafallopian transfer

Anatomy Charts

Skeletal System

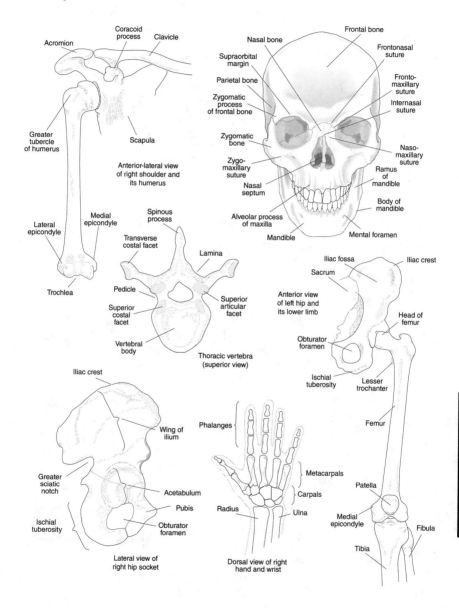

Acromion
Coracoid process
Clavicle
Greater tubercle of humerus
Scapula

Anterior-lateral view of right shoulder and its humerus

Lateral epicondyle
Medial epicondyle
Trochlea

Frontal bone
Nasal bone
Frontonasal suture
Supraorbital margin
Parietal bone
Fronto-maxillary suture
Zygomatic process of frontal bone
Internasal suture
Zygomatic bone
Zygo-maxillary suture
Naso-maxillary suture
Nasal septum
Ramus of mandible
Body of mandible
Alveolar process of maxilla
Mental foramen
Mandible

Spinous process
Transverse costal facet
Lamina
Superior articular facet
Pedicle
Superior costal facet
Vertebral body

Thoracic vertebra (superior view)

Iliac fossa
Iliac crest
Sacrum
Anterior view of left hip and its lower limb
Head of femur
Obturator foramen
Ischial tuberosity
Lesser trochanter
Femur

Iliac crest
Wing of ilium
Phalanges
Greater sciatic notch
Acetabulum
Pubis
Metacarpals
Carpals
Patella
Radius
Ulna
Medial epicondyle
Fibula
Ischial tuberosity
Obturator foramen
Tibia

Lateral view of right hip socket

Dorsal view of right hand and wrist

Anatomy Charts

Lymphatic System

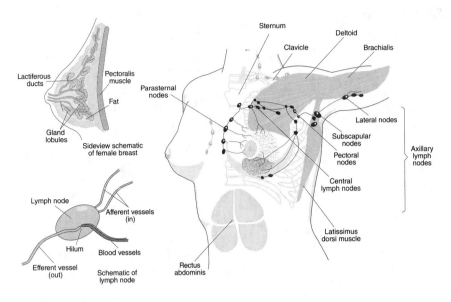

Sternum
Deltoid
Clavicle
Brachialis

Lactiferous ducts
Pectoralis muscle
Parasternal nodes
Fat

Gland lobules
Sideview schematic of female breast

Lateral nodes

Subscapular nodes

Pectoral nodes

Axillary lymph nodes

Central lymph nodes

Lymph node
Afferent vessels (in)

Hilum
Blood vessels

Efferent vessel (out)
Schematic of lymph node

Rectus abdominis

Latissimus dorsi muscle

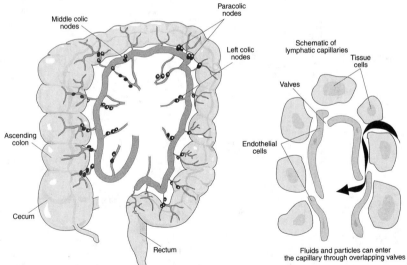

Paracolic nodes
Middle colic nodes

Left colic nodes

Schematic of lymphatic capillaries
Tissue cells

Valves

Ascending colon

Endothelial cells

Cecum

Rectum

Fluids and particles can enter the capillary through overlapping valves

Lymphatic drainage of the colon follows blood supply

Endocrine System

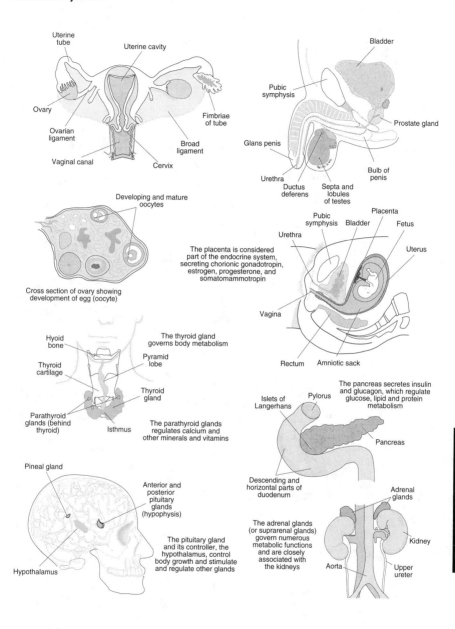

Uterine tube

Uterine cavity

Ovary

Ovarian ligament

Vaginal canal

Fimbriae of tube

Broad ligament

Cervix

Bladder

Pubic symphysis

Prostate gland

Glans penis

Urethra

Ductus deferens

Septa and lobules of testes

Bulb of penis

Developing and mature oocytes

Cross section of ovary showing development of egg (oocyte)

Pubic symphysis

Bladder

Placenta

Fetus

Urethra

Uterus

The placenta is considered part of the endocrine system, secreting chorionic gonadotropin, estrogen, progesterone, and somatomammotropin

Vagina

Rectum

Amniotic sack

Hyoid bone

The thyroid gland governs body metabolism

Thyroid cartilage

Pyramid lobe

Thyroid gland

Parathyroid glands (behind thyroid)

Isthmus

The parathyroid glands regulates calcium and other minerals and vitamins

The pancreas secretes insulin and glucagon, which regulate glucose, lipid and protein metabolism

Islets of Langerhans

Pylorus

Pancreas

Pineal gland

Anterior and posterior pituitary glands (hypophysis)

Descending and horizontal parts of duodenum

Adrenal glands

The pituitary gland and its controller, the hypothalamus, control body growth and stimulate and regulate other glands

The adrenal glands (or suprarenal glands) govern numerous metabolic functions and are closely associated with the kidneys

Kidney

Hypothalamus

Aorta

Upper ureter

Digestive System

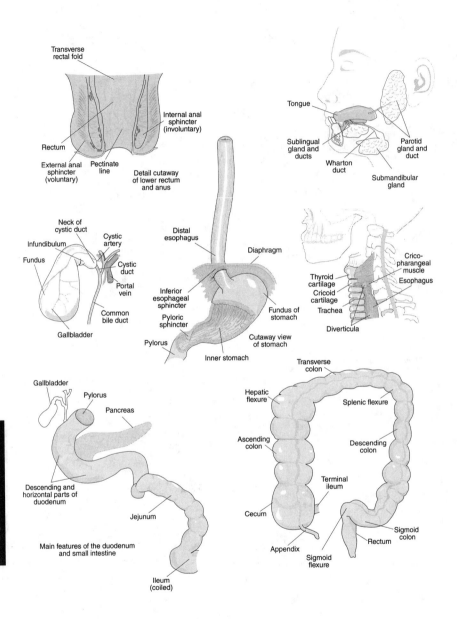

Transverse rectal fold

Internal anal sphincter (involuntary)

Rectum

External anal sphincter (voluntary)

Pectinate line

Detail cutaway of lower rectum and anus

Tongue

Sublingual gland and ducts

Wharton duct

Parotid gland and duct

Submandibular gland

Neck of cystic duct

Infundibulum

Fundus

Cystic artery

Cystic duct

Portal vein

Common bile duct

Gallbladder

Distal esophagus

Inferior esophageal sphincter

Pyloric sphincter

Pylorus

Inner stomach

Diaphragm

Fundus of stomach

Cutaway view of stomach

Thyroid cartilage

Cricoid cartilage

Trachea

Diverticula

Crico-pharangeal muscle

Esophagus

Gallbladder

Pylorus

Pancreas

Descending and horizontal parts of duodenum

Jejunum

Main features of the duodenum and small intestine

Ileum (coiled)

Transverse colon

Hepatic flexure

Ascending colon

Cecum

Appendix

Splenic flexure

Descending colon

Terminal ileum

Sigmoid flexure

Sigmoid colon

Rectum

Anatomy Charts

Nervous System

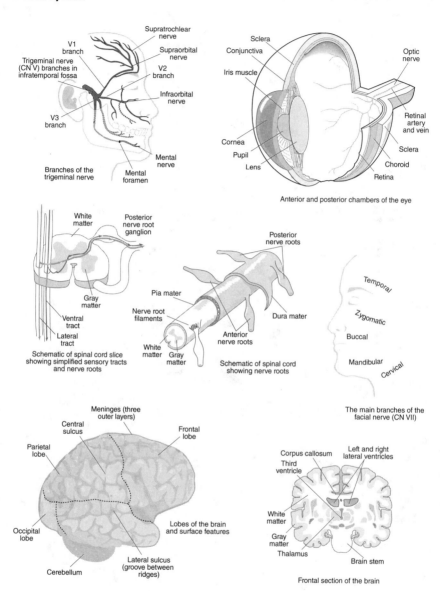

Branches of the trigeminal nerve

Anterior and posterior chambers of the eye

Schematic of spinal cord slice showing simplified sensory tracts and nerve roots

Schematic of spinal cord showing nerve roots

The main branches of the facial nerve (CN VII)

Lobes of the brain and surface features

Frontal section of the brain

Circulatory System: Arterial

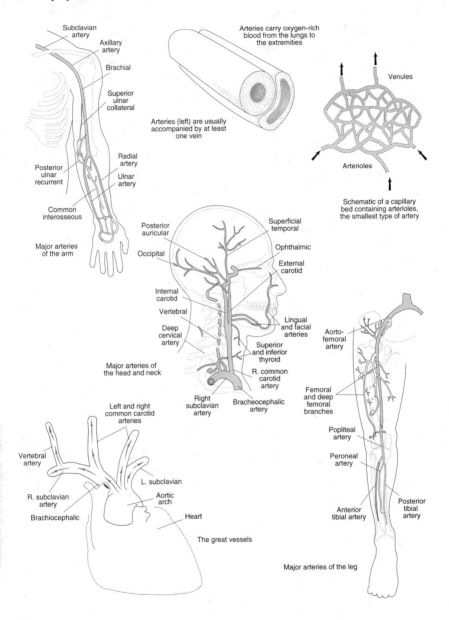

Subclavian artery

Axillary artery

Brachial

Superior ulnar collateral

Posterior ulnar recurrent

Radial artery

Ulnar artery

Common interosseous

Major arteries of the arm

Arteries carry oxygen-rich blood from the lungs to the extremities

Arteries (left) are usually accompanied by at least one vein

Venules

Arterioles

Schematic of a capillary bed containing arterioles, the smallest type of artery

Posterior auricular

Occipital

Internal carotid

Vertebral

Deep cervical artery

Major arteries of the head and neck

Superficial temporal

Ophthalmic

External carotid

Lingual and facial arteries

Superior and inferior thyroid

R. common carotid artery

Right subclavian artery

Bracheocephalic artery

Left and right common carotid arteries

Vertebral artery

R. subclavian artery

Brachiocephalic

L. subclavian

Aortic arch

Heart

The great vessels

Aorto-femoral artery

Femoral and deep femoral branches

Popliteal artery

Peroneal artery

Anterior tibial artery

Posterior tibial artery

Major arteries of the leg

Circulatory System: Venous

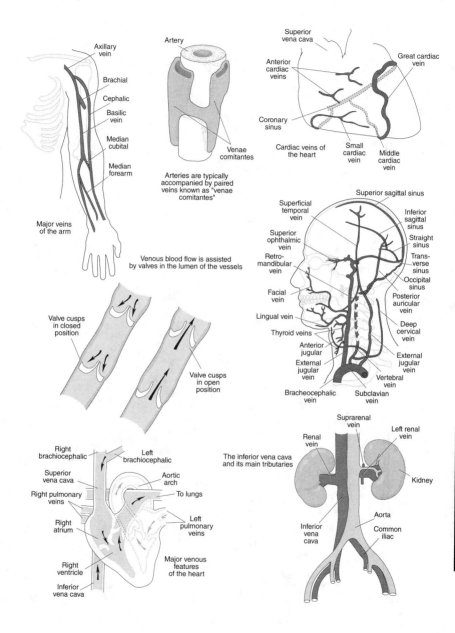

Axillary vein

Brachial

Cephalic

Basilic vein

Median cubital

Median forearm

Major veins of the arm

Artery

Venae comitantes

Arteries are typically accompanied by paired veins known as "venae comitantes"

Venous blood flow is assisted by valves in the lumen of the vessels

Valve cusps in closed position

Valve cusps in open position

Superior vena cava

Anterior cardiac veins

Great cardiac vein

Coronary sinus

Cardiac veins of the heart

Small cardiac vein

Middle cardiac vein

Superior sagittal sinus

Superficial temporal vein

Inferior sagittal sinus

Superior ophthalmic vein

Straight sinus

Retro-mandibular vein

Trans-verse sinus

Occipital sinus

Facial vein

Posterior auricular vein

Lingual vein

Deep cervical vein

Thyroid veins

Anterior jugular

External jugular vein

External jugular vein

Vertebral vein

Bracheocephalic vein

Subclavian vein

Right brachiocephalic

Left brachiocephalic

Superior vena cava

Aortic arch

Right pulmonary veins

To lungs

Right atrium

Left pulmonary veins

Right ventricle

Major venous features of the heart

Inferior vena cava

Suprarenal vein

Left renal vein

Renal vein

The inferior vena cava and its main tributaries

Kidney

Aorta

Inferior vena cava

Common iliac

Anatomy Charts

Urogenital Tracts

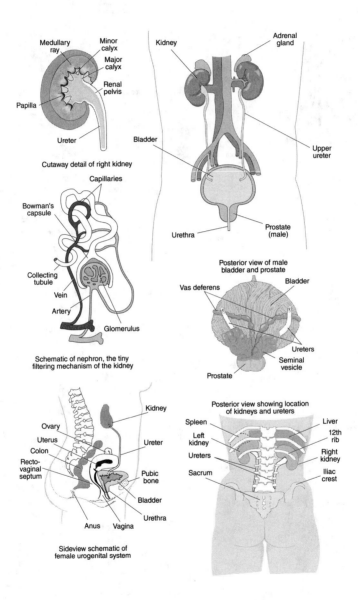

Medullary ray

Minor calyx

Major calyx

Renal pelvis

Papilla

Ureter

Cutaway detail of right kidney

Kidney

Adrenal gland

Bladder

Upper ureter

Urethra

Prostate (male)

Capillaries

Bowman's capsule

Collecting tubule

Vein

Artery

Glomerulus

Schematic of nephron, the tiny filtering mechanism of the kidney

Posterior view of male bladder and prostate

Vas deferens

Bladder

Ureters

Seminal vesicle

Prostate

Ovary

Uterus

Colon

Recto-vaginal septum

Kidney

Ureter

Pubic bone

Bladder

Urethra

Anus   Vagina

Sideview schematic of female urogenital system

Posterior view showing location of kidneys and ureters

Spleen

Left kidney

Ureters

Sacrum

Liver

12th rib

Right kidney

Iliac crest

Respiratory System

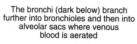

The bronchi (dark below) branch
further into bronchioles and then into
alveolar sacs where venous
blood is aerated

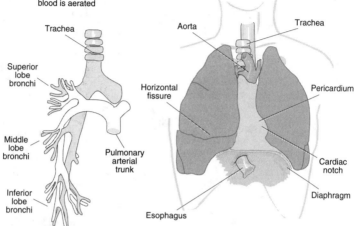

Trachea

Superior
lobe
bronchi

Middle
lobe
bronchi

Inferior
lobe
bronchi

Pulmonary
arterial
trunk

Aorta

Trachea

Horizontal
fissure

Pericardium

Cardiac
notch

Diaphragm

Esophagus

The pulmonary arteries (white above)
deliver venous blood to the lungs where
it is oxygenated and converted into
arterial blood

The right lung is larger and heavier than
its counterpart due to space lost to the
bulge of the heart at the cardiac notch

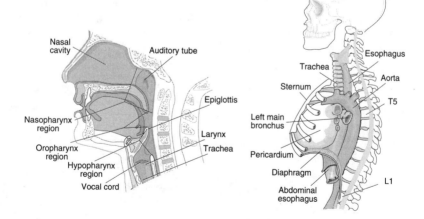

Nasal
cavity

Auditory tube

Nasopharynx
region

Epiglottis

Oropharynx
region

Hypopharynx
region

Vocal cord

Larynx

Trachea

Esophagus

Trachea

Sternum

Aorta

Left main
bronchus

T5

Pericardium

Diaphragm

Abdominal
esophagus

L1

Chapter 1: Certain Infectious and Parasitic Diseases (A00-B99)

This chapter covers diseases caused by infectious and parasitic organisms, which include diseases generally recognized as communicable or transmissible. Only a small percentage of organisms in the environment cause disease. Most bacteria, viruses, fungi, and other microorganisms found in the external environment (e.g., air, water, and soil) or the internal environment (e.g., on or within our bodies) are harmless or even beneficial. Disease is caused almost exclusively by microorganisms that are human pathogens, also referred to as pathogenic microorganisms, except in persons or hosts whose immune systems are weakened, which allows normally harmless microorganisms to cause opportunistic infections.

This chapter is organized primarily by the type of infectious organism or parasite, such as infections caused by bacteria, viruses, and mycoses and parasitic diseases caused by protozoa and helminthes. There are also some code blocks organized by site of infection, such as intestinal infectious diseases, and other code blocks organized by mode of transmission, such as infections with a predominantly sexual mode of transmission, arthropod-borne viral fevers, and viral hemorrhagic fevers.

The chapter is broken down into the following code blocks:

A00-A09	Intestinal infectious diseases
A15-A19	Tuberculosis
A20-A28	Certain zoonotic bacterial diseases
A30-A49	Other bacterial diseases
A50-A64	Infections with a predominantly sexual mode of transmission
A65-A69	Other spirochetal diseases
A70-A74	Other diseases caused by chlamydiae
A75-A79	Rickettsioses
A80-A89	Viral infections of the central nervous system
A90-A99	Arthropod-borne viral fevers and viral hemorrhagic fevers
B00-B09	Viral infections characterized by skin and mucous membrane lesions
B10	Other human herpesviruses
B15-B19	Viral hepatitis
B20	Human immunodeficiency virus [HIV] disease
B25-B34	Other viral diseases
B35-B49	Mycoses
B50-B64	Protozoal diseases
B65-B83	Helminthiases
B85-B89	Pediculosis, acariasis and other infestations
B90-B94	Sequelae of infectious and parasitic diseases
B95-B97	Bacterial and viral infectious agents
B99	Other infectious diseases

There are a few infectious conditions that are excluded from this chapter, including certain localized infections that are classified in specific body-system chapters. For example:

- Suppurative otitis media is classified in Chapter 8 Diseases of the Ear and Mastoid Process

- Influenza and other acute respiratory infections are classified in Chapter 10 Diseases of the Respiratory System

- Pyogenic arthritis is classified in Chapter 13 Diseases of the Musculoskeletal System and Connective Tissue

Intestinal Infectious Diseases (A00-A09)

Intestinal infectious diseases are caused primarily by ingestion of contaminated food or water. Less common means of infection include handling contaminated food products or other contaminated items or coming in direct contact with infected animals.

The first symptoms of intestinal infectious diseases usually involve the gastrointestinal tract and may include abdominal pain or cramping, nausea, vomiting, and/or diarrhea, although some microorganisms may produce other initial symptoms. For example, *Clostridium botulinum* causes foodborne botulism poisoning and often produces neurological symptoms initially.

Intestinal infections usually remain localized to the intestinal tract and often resolve without medical treatment. In most cases, infections requiring treatment only need supportive care such as replacement of lost fluids and maintenance of electrolyte balance. In some cases, particularly the very young, the elderly, or individuals with immune system disorders or chronic health conditions, a localized intestinal infection becomes disseminated causing infection of other sites. Some manifestations of a disseminated infection include meningitis, pneumonia, endocarditis or myocarditis, arthritis, osteomyelitis, and pyelonephritis.

The categories in this code block are as follows:

A00	Cholera
A01	Typhoid and paratyphoid fevers
A02	Other salmonella infections
A03	Shigellosis
A04	Other bacterial intestinal infections
A05	Other bacterial foodborne intoxications, not elsewhere classified
A06	Amebiasis
A07	Other protozoal intestinal diseases
A08	Viral and other specified intestinal infections
A09	Infectious gastroenteritis and colitis, unspecified

A00.-   Cholera

Cholera is an infection of the entire bowel due to *Vibrio cholerae*. Risk of mortality is related to severe dehydration, acidosis, and hypovolemic shock secondary to profuse diarrhea. *V. cholerae* contains pathogenic and nonpathogenic strains. Pathogenic strains of cholera are endemic to parts of Asia, Africa, the Middle East, and also portions of the Gulf Coast of the United States. In endemic areas, outbreaks are usually limited to warm seasons. If the infection is imported to other locales, an outbreak can occur in any season.

A00.0   Cholera due to Vibrio cholerae 01, biovar cholerae

A00.1   Cholera due to Vibrio cholerae 01, biovar eltor

Biovar cholerae and eltor are two specific biotypes of the *Vibrio cholerae* bacteria and are commonly associated with epidemic outbreaks.

A01.-   Typhoid and paratyphoid fevers

Typhoid fever is a systemic bacterial disease caused by the unique human strain of salmonella, *Salmonella typhi*. Paratyphoid is similar in presentation to typhoid, though usually milder, and is caused by any of several organisms: *S. paratyphi* (paratyphoid A), *S. schottmülleri* (paratyphoid B), or *S. hirschfeldii* (paratyphoid C). The means of infection, clinical course, pathology, and treatment are similar for typhoid and paratyphoid.

A01.0-   Typhoid fever

Salmonella typhi is the responsible bacterial agent of typhoid fever and is generally transmitted by the ingestion of food or water that is contaminated with feces from an infected person. The microorganism moves through the gastrointestinal tract and enters the bloodstream through the lymphatic system.

A02.-   Other salmonella infections

This category classifies infections related to all salmonellas—more than 1,500 serotypes—except congenital, typhoid, and paratyphoid salmonella. *Salmonella* serotypes most often seen in humans include *S. enteritidis*, *S. Newport*, and *S. typhimurium*. Salmonella infection is a significant health problem and is the most common food-borne infectious disease diagnosed in the United States. Meat, poultry, raw milk, eggs, fruits, and vegetables are the most common sources of infection. Other reported sources include infected pet turtles or lizards, infected dyes, or contaminated marijuana. The bacteria pass through the stomach and colonize the intestines. The bacteria invade enterocytes, epithelial cells, and dendritic cells in the intestine resulting in an inflammatory response. Bacteria may cross the epithelial layer of the intestine and replicate in Peyer patches (bundles of lymphatic tissue in the small intestine), mesenteric lymph nodes, and the spleen. Salmonella infections can become disseminated causing sepsis or infections of the central nervous system, lungs, joints, bone, kidneys, and other sites. About 85 percent of salmonella infections present as gastroenteritis, with the other 15 percent as septicemia or with other manifestations. About one-third of all untreated infections result in complications.

A02.0   Salmonella enteritis

Salmonella enteritis, also known as salmonella gastroenteritis, is an infection of the gastrointestinal tract that is caused by the ingestion of contaminated foods, eggs and poultry being the most common sources. Symptoms typically occur within hours to two days and typically last no more than seven days even without the use of antibiotics.

> **Focus Point**
>
> *Dehydration (E86.0) is a complication of Salmonella enteritis and should be reported additionally.*

A02.1   Salmonella sepsis

Sepsis is a complication of a localized infection caused by a systemic or bodywide response to the infectious agent. Symptoms of sepsis include a body temperature above 101 degrees or below 96.8 degrees Fahrenheit, rapid heart rate (above 90 beats per minute), and rapid respiratory rate (above 20 breaths per minute). Some *Salmonella* serovars (strains) are more apt to cause a systemic response than others.

A02.2- Localized salmonella infections

Localized infection occurs as a result of salmonella bacteria crossing the epithelium of the small intestine and entering the bloodstream, which allows colonization to other sites. The most common sites of localized infection include meninges of the spinal cord and brain, lungs, joints, bone and bone marrow, and kidneys. Other sites of localized infection include the heart, arteries, lymphatic cells (macrophages and monocytes), lymphatic tissue, and the genital region.

A02.21 Salmonella meningitis

Salmonella meningitis, an infection of the membranes covering the brain and spinal cord, is a rare complication of salmonella infection and a rare type of bacterial meningitis. It occurs predominantly in newborns, although immunocompromised individuals are also at risk. Symptoms indicative of meningitis include stiff neck, photophobia (intolerance to bright light), confusion or delirium, sleepiness or difficulty waking, and seizures.

A02.22 Salmonella pneumonia

Salmonella pneumonia is a rare complication of a salmonella infection occurring most often in infants, the elderly, immunocompromised individuals, and individuals with previous lung pathology such as lung cancer. Symptoms indicative of pneumonia include fever, shortness of breath (dyspnea), elevated heart rate (tachypnea), noncardiac chest pain, and productive cough.

A02.23 Salmonella arthritis

Salmonella arthritis occurs when salmonella bacteria cross the epithelium of the small intestine, enter the bloodstream, and colonize in one or more joints causing acute suppurative arthritis.

Focus Point

Reactive arthritis, also known as Reiter's disease or syndrome, is a chronic condition that can occur weeks or months after salmonella gastroenteritis. Reactive arthritis is classified to Chapter 13 Diseases of the Musculoskeletal System and Connective Tissue, with codes in category M02.

A02.24 Salmonella osteomyelitis

Infection of bone and bone marrow due to *Salmonella* is a rare complication that occurs primarily in children. Osteomyelitis symptoms include localized pain and inflammation at the site of the bone or bone marrow infection, as well as systemic symptoms such as fever, irritability, and malaise. *Salmonella* osteomyelitis may be diagnosed by puncture aspiration at the site of the infection or by positive blood cultures. X-rays may also be obtained and typically show bone changes characteristic of osteomyelitis.

A02.25 Salmonella pyelonephritis

Pyelonephritis due to *Salmonella* is an infection of the renal pelvis and renal parenchyma. The renal pelvis and renal parenchyma are composed of cells called nephrons that make up the functional tissue of the kidneys. Acute pyelonephritis can result in abscess formation, scarring, and can permanently damage the kidney with resultant kidney failure.

A02.29 Salmonella with other localized infection

Localized endocarditis due to Salmonella is classified here.

A03.- Shigellosis

Shigellosis is a bacterium that causes an acute infection of the bowel with fever, irritability, drowsiness, anorexia, nausea, vomiting, diarrhea, abdominal pain, and distension. Blood, pus, and mucus are found in the stool. Ingestion of food contaminated by feces of infected individuals is the most common source of infection. Incubation period is one to four days. There are four species in the *Shigella* genus and they differ according to their biochemical reactions.

A04.- Other bacterial intestinal infections

Bacterial intestinal infections are caused by the ingestion of pathogenic bacteria that then colonize the gastrointestinal tract. Other bacterial causes of enteritis, also called gastroenteritis, are classified here, including *Escherichia coli, Campylobacter, Yersinia enterocolitica*, and *Clostridium difficile*. Unspecified bacterial enteritis is also included in this category.

A04.0 Enteropathogenic Escherichia coli infection

A04.1 Enterotoxigenic Escherichia coli infection

A04.2 Enteroinvasive Escherichia coli infection

Escherichia coli (E. coli) are a copious and diverse group of bacteria that range from relatively harmless to those that cause serious, life-threatening gastrointestinal illness. Enteropathogenic, enterotoxigenic, and enteroinvasive are three types of pathogenic *E. coli* that are non-Shiga toxin producing strains that can cause acute gastroenteritis. All three of these strains are transmitted by consumption of food or water contaminated with animal or human feces containing the infectious bacteria. Enteropathogenic *E. coli* infection (EPEC) primarily affects infants and young children in developing countries. The virulence of EPEC strains is its ability to efface microvilli of the epithelial cells lining the intestines. Once the microvilli are effaced, two genes in EPEC act together to allow intimate attachment of the bacteria to the epithelial cells. Enterotoxigenic *E. coli* infection (ETEC) is the most common cause of travelers' diarrhea. It is also an important cause of diarrhea in infants in underdeveloped countries. This strain produces heat labile and heat stable toxins increasing its virulence. Enteroinvasive *E. coli* infection (EIEC) causes acute gastroenteritis and bacillary dysentery. As their name implies, these bacteria have the ability to invade epithelial cells of the colon, which increases its virulence.

Focus Point

There is a fourth common non-Shiga toxin producing E. coli strain called enteroaggregative E. coli (EAEC); however, this strain was not given its own individual code in category A04 but instead is coded to A04.4 Other intestinal Escherichia coli infections.

A04.3 Enterohemorrhagic Escherichia coli infection

Enterohemorrhagic *E. coli* (EHEC) infection, which causes acute bloody diarrhea and severe abdominal cramps, is caused by Shiga toxin-producing *Escherichia coli* (STEC), most often the serotype *E. coli* O157:H7. The O157:H7 *E. coli* strain is a devastating infection, particularly in the pediatric and elderly population. This strain is particularly virulent and likely to lead to permanent renal damage, including hemolytic uremic syndrome (HUS). STEC transmission can occur by the consumption of contaminated food (e.g., ground beef, unpasteurized juice, raw milk, and raw produce) or by direct contact with contaminated animals or surfaces. Known routes of direct contamination include contact with an asymptomatic animal carrier, contact with contaminated surfaces in an animal care environment, or from hand-to-hand transmission of fecal contaminants. Prompt, accurate diagnosis of STEC infection is imperative to expedite appropriate treatment early in the course of infection, and prevent potentially fatal illnesses (e.g., gastrointestinal, urinary tract, respiratory) and complications. Furthermore, early, accurate detection assists in epidemiology efforts to ensure effective management response in the event of infectious outbreaks.

A04.4 Other intestinal Escherichia coli infections

Two types of *Escherichia coli* (E. coli) infections that do not have more specific codes include enteroaggregative [*E. coli* (EAEC, EAggEC) and diffusely adherent *E. coli* (DAEC). Enteroaggregative *E. coli* infection, is most common among immunocompromised individuals and may cause chronic diarrhea. EAEC is characterized by the ability to adhere to the surface of epithelial cells in an aggregative adherence (AA) or stacked pattern. Diffusely adherent *E. coli* causes diarrhea primarily in children in developing countries. DAEC is characterized by a diffuse adherence (DA) pattern meaning that the bacteria cover the entire epithelial cell surface in a uniform pattern.

A04.5 Campylobacter enteritis

Campylobacter is a gram negative bacterium that causes diarrhea and abdominal pain sometimes accompanied by nausea and vomiting. Diarrhea is often bloody. The species *C. jejuni* is responsible for most infections, although there are a number of other species that also cause enteritis in humans. The infection is spread by eating or drinking contaminated food or beverages including chicken, raw milk, and water; handling infected farm or domestic animals; or from person-to-person by the fecal to oral route.

Focus Point

Guillain-Barre syndrome can occur as a sequela of Campylobacter enteritis. This is reported with code G61.0 Guillain-Barre syndrome, as the first listed diagnosis followed by B94.8 Sequelae of other specified infectious and parasitic diseases.

A04.6 Enteritis due to Yersinia enterocolitica

Enteritis, also referred to as yersiniosis, is caused by the bacterium *Yersinia enterocolitica*. Symptoms differ depending on the age of the patient, with young children experiencing fever, abdominal pain, and bloody diarrhea, and older children and adults presenting with symptoms similar to appendicitis, including fever and right-sided abdominal pain. Infection typically results from eating contaminated raw or undercooked pork or drinking contaminated raw milk or untreated water.

A04.7- Enterocolitis due to Clostridium difficile

Clostridium difficile, also called *C. diff*, is part of the normal flora found in the intestines of healthy individuals. Inflammation of the small bowel and colon due to *C. diff* results from overgrowth of the bacteria with subsequent release of toxins. This is a common complication of prolonged antibiotic use and can be a one-time occurrence or a recurrent condition.

A04.8 Other specified bacterial intestinal infections

Bacterial infections of the intestines that are not classified to a more specific code include *Aerobacter aerogenes*, *Enterobacter aerogenes*, *Helicobacter pylori*, and *Pseudotuberculosis enterocolitis*.

Focus Point

Bacterial foodborne intestinal tract infections and bacterial foodborne intoxications (food poisoning) are not synonymous. Bacterial foodborne intoxication is not a true infection, as the related symptoms are due to preformed toxins produced by the bacteria and not due to the bacteria. Staphylococcus aureus and Clostridium perfringens (Clostridium welchii) are two toxin-producing bacteria; the appropriate category to consult is A05.

A05.- Other bacterial foodborne intoxications, not elsewhere classified

Bacterial foodborne intoxication is caused by ingestion of food contaminated with pathogenic bacteria that produce toxins in or on food. It is the toxin produced by the bacteria, not the bacteria itself, that causes the symptoms.

A05.0 Foodborne staphylococcal intoxication

Staphylococcal enterotoxin is a common cause of food poisoning that can occur when an infected food handler introduces the *S. aureus* bacteria into food or when contaminated milk or dairy products are ingested. An acute bout of diarrhea and vomiting usually occurs within a few hours of ingestion and resolves within several hours. Dehydration (hypovolemia) poses the greatest risk to the elderly, the young, and the immunosuppressed, but this form of food poisoning rarely is fatal.

Focus Point

Staphylococcal infection of the intestinal tract that is not due to S. aureus toxins and transmitted by ingestion of contaminated food is reported with code A04.8 Other specified bacterial intestinal infections.

Focus Point

Staphylococcal intoxication caused by ingestion of toxins produced by S. aureus bacteria in contaminated food is reported with code A05.0 Bacterial staphylococcal intoxication. Clostridium perfringens, also called C. welchii or C. perfringens Type A, caused by toxins transmitted by ingestion of contaminated food, is reported with code A05.2 Foodborne Clostridium perfringens [Clostridium welchii] intoxication.

A05.1 Botulism food poisoning

Clostridium botulinum is a bacterium found in the soil that produces a neurotoxin that when ingested can result in food poisoning. The most common sources of botulism food poisoning are improperly home or commercially canned foods with low acid content, home canned or fermented fish, herb infused oils, bottled garlic, aluminum foil wrapped baked potatoes, and foods held at room temperature for long periods of time. Botulism food poisoning is a public health emergency because the contaminated food may still be available to persons other than the patient. Following ingestion of the toxin, symptoms may occur within as little as a few hours or as long as two weeks, although symptoms typically begin between 12 and 36 hours. Symptoms include double vision, blurred vision, drooping eyelids, slurred speech, difficulty swallowing, dry mouth, and muscle weakness. Muscle weakness always descends through the body: shoulders are affected, then upper arms, lower arms, thighs, calves, etc. Paralysis of breathing muscles may

be fatal unless assistance with breathing (mechanical ventilation) is provided. Gastrointestinal symptoms including vomiting and diarrhea may precede neurological symptoms.

A05.2 Foodborne Clostridium perfringens [Clostridium welchii] intoxication

C. perfringens is a gram positive bacterium commonly found in soil, air, and water and is one of the most common causes of food poisoning. The bacterium forms spores, and some strains produce a toxin in the gastrointestinal tract when ingested. Meat and poultry are the most common sources of pathogenic strains. Symptoms, which include severe abdominal cramping and diarrhea, typically occur within six to 24 hours of eating food contaminated with large amounts of the bacteria and resolve within 24 hours, but milder symptoms of gastroenteritis may persist for one to two weeks.

Focus Point

Clostridium perfringens may cause bacterial infection or intoxication depending on the specific type of C. perfringens. For Type C and Type F C. perfringens bacterial intestinal infection, where the infection is caused by the bacteria itself and is not due to toxins produced by the bacteria, report code A04.8 Other specified bacterial intestinal infections.

A05.3 Foodborne Vibrio parahaemolyticus intoxication

Vibrio parahaemolyticus is a bacterium that is found in salt water and is naturally present along the coasts of the United States and Canada. During the warmer months, the concentration of *V. parahaemolyticus* bacteria in the water increases. The bacteria contaminate shellfish, particularly oysters, and people become infected by eating raw or undercooked contaminated shellfish. Symptoms, which include watery diarrhea, abdominal pain and cramping, nausea, vomiting, fever, and chills, usually occur within 24 hours of eating contaminated shellfish and may last up to three days.

A05.4 Foodborne Bacillus cereus intoxication

When ingested, *Bacillus cereus* causes gastrointestinal symptoms: nausea and vomiting typically occur within 30 minutes to six hours of ingestion and/or diarrhea occurs between six and 15 hours. *B. cereus* is commonly found in soil, milk, and dried food such as cereals, herbs, and spices. Meat pies, fried rice, and puddings are also frequently implicated in outbreaks.

A05.5 Foodborne Vibrio vulnificus intoxication

Vibrio vulnificus is a bacterium found in sea water. Eating raw seafood can result in severe gastroenteritis that may be fatal to persons with liver disease or depressed immune systems.

A06.- Amebiasis

Amebiasis is caused by the protozoa *Entamoeba histolytica* and most commonly occurs in tropical areas where crowded living conditions and poor sanitation exist. In the United States, most cases of amebiasis are seen in individuals arriving from other parts of the world where the disease is prevalent, such as Africa, Latin America, Southeast Asia, and India. In addition to recent travel to a region where the disease is prevalent, other individuals at risk include immunosuppressed populations, people living in institutions, people with disabilities, and male homosexuals. In amebiasis, protozoa can live in the large intestine without causing symptoms or they can invade the colon wall causing colitis, acute dysentery, or chronic diarrhea. The infection may spread through the blood to the liver and, rarely, to the lungs, brain, or other organs. Transmission occurs through ingestion of feces in contaminated food or water, use of human feces as fertilizer, or person-to-person contact. Malnutrition and alcoholism predispose a person to more severe disease, as does immunosuppression.

A07.- Other protozoal intestinal diseases

Protozoa are unicellular microorganisms that live in moist environments of water and soil. Most protozoa are nonpathogenic; however, there are a few that cause disease in humans, including *Balantidium (B. coli)*, *Cryptosporidium*, *Giardia*, and *Toxoplasma*. The types of protozoa that cause disease in humans are able to survive by encapsulating themselves in protective coatings called cysts. The cyst protects the protozoa from extreme temperatures and chemicals, which enables them to survive in adverse environments for long periods of time.

A07.0 Balantidiasis

Balantidiasis is caused by the protozoa *Balantidium coli*. These microorganisms are found in feces and are transmitted by the fecal-oral route, usually in contaminated food or water. *B. coli* infection is typically asymptomatic in healthy individuals. However, people with compromised immune systems or systemic diseases can experience persistent diarrhea, abdominal pain, and in rare instances perforation of the colon.

A07.1 Giardiasis [lambliasis]

Giardia lamblia is the most common intestinal parasite in the United States. Giardiasis is an infection of the lumen of the small intestine, spread by contaminated food and water or by direct contact. Contaminated water from lakes or streams is commonly a source of the disease. Most cases are asymptomatic, but those with symptoms experience diarrhea, nausea, lassitude, anorexia, and weight loss

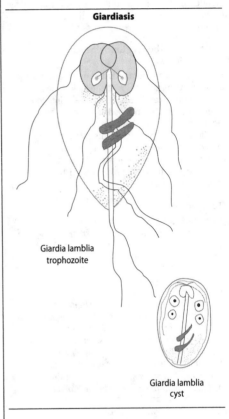

Giardiasis

Giardia lamblia trophozoite

Giardia lamblia cyst

A07.2 Cryptosporidiosis

Cryptosporidium is a microscopic parasite found in water and is one of the most common causes of waterborne gastrointestinal infectious disease in the United States. The infection, called cryptosporidiosis or crypto for short, is usually transmitted via drinking water or recreational water. Symptoms are mild and self-limited in a healthy population. However, cryptosporidiosis is frequently seen as an opportunistic infection in acquired immune deficiency syndrome (AIDS), causing profound dehydration and electrolyte imbalances. There is no specific antibiotic therapy for cryptosporidiosis.

A07.3 Isosporiasis

Isosporiasis is caused by two species of *Isospora*, *I. belli* and *I. hominis*, with the majority of infections caused by *I. belli*. Although found worldwide, most infections occur in tropical and subtropical regions. It is spread by the ingestion of contaminated food or water.

Isosporiasis is characterized by profuse watery diarrhea, flatulence, abdominal pain, and cramping that may last up to three weeks. Immunocompromised individuals may experience long-term symptoms unless treated.

A07.4   Cyclosporiasis

Cyclosporiasis is an intestinal illness caused by the parasite *Cyclospora cayetanensis*. *C. cayetanensis* is endemic to tropical and subtropical regions, although outbreaks linked to importation of contaminated produce have occurred in the United States. The parasite is passed by fecal-oral route by ingestion of contaminated food or water. Cyclosporiasis is characterized by profuse watery diarrhea, flatulence, abdominal pain, and cramping that may last from a few days to several weeks. Other symptoms include low grade fever, malaise, nausea, vomiting, loss of appetite, headache, and body aches.

A07.8   Other specified protozoal intestinal diseases

The following protozoal species are classified here: *Chilomastix* (chilomastigiasis), *Dientamoeba*, *Embadomonas* (embadomoniasis), and trichomonal types of dysentery, including *Microsporidial* enteritis (microsporidiosis), *Retortamonis intestinalis* (retortamoniasis), and *Sarcocystis* (sarcosporidiosis).

A08.-   Viral and other specified intestinal infections

Intestinal infections described as viral colitis, viral enteritis, or viral gastroenteritis are characterized by inflammation of the lining of the small and/or large intestines and sometimes the stomach and are due to a viral pathogen. Gastroenteropathy is a more generalized term referring to any disorder of the gastrointestinal tract, such as nausea and vomiting, but is categorized here when specifically due to Norwalk agents or other small round viruses.

A08.0   Rotaviral enteritis

Rotavirus infection of the small intestine is a common cause of severe diarrhea in infants and children worldwide. Rotavirus infects the cells of the villi, the minute fingerlike projections that cover the entire lining of the small intestine. Rotaviral infection causes inflammation of the villi, which impairs digestion of carbohydrates and absorption of fluids and electrolytes causing severe watery diarrhea. A vaccine was introduced in the United States in 1998, which has significantly reduced the number of rotaviral infections in infants and children.

A08.1-   Acute gastroenteropathy due to Norwalk agent and other small round viruses

Norwalk agent and other small round viruses (SRV), also called small round structured viruses (SRSV), are classified in the family of viruses called Caliciviridae or caliciviruses. Viruses in this family are subclassified by morphology as "typical," which means the calicivirus has the typical 32 cup-shaped depressions on its surface, or as small round viruses. Only small round viruses in the Caliciviridae family are classified here, including Norwalk agent, Norwalk-like agent, Norovirus.

> **Focus Point**
>
> *Norwalk agent and other small round viruses (SRV), also called small round structured viruses (SRSV), are classified in the family of viruses called Caliciviridae or caliciviruses. Viruses in this family are subclassified by morphology as "typical," which means the calicivirus has the typical 32 cup-shaped depressions on its surface, or as small round viruses. Only small round viruses in the Caliciviridae family are classified here, including Norwalk agent, Norwalk-like agent, Norovirus.*

A08.11   Acute gastroenteropathy due to Norwalk agent

Norwalk agent, also called Norwalk-like agent or Norovirus, causes gastrointestinal illness with symptoms that include nausea, vomiting, diarrhea, and abdominal cramps, along with fever, chills, headache, and body aches. It is transmitted primarily via fecal-oral route, although it may also be airborne.

A08.19   Acute gastroenteropathy due to other small round viruses

Gastrointestinal illness due to small round viruses (SRV) not specifically identified as Norwalk agent, Norwalk-like agent, or Norovirus is classified here. Symptoms are similar to that of Norovirus primarily involving nausea, vomiting, and diarrhea. Gastroenteropathy due to an SRV may also be referred to as Bradley's, Goodall's, or Spencer's disease.

A08.2   Adenoviral enteritis

There are many adenoviruses that cause infection of a variety of sites in humans; however, types 40 and 41 are the two that are most often associated with infections of the gastrointestinal tract. Although adenoviral enteritis can occur in any age group, most adenoviral intestinal infections occur in infants and children younger than age 2. The virus is passed by fecal-oral route. Common symptoms include nausea, vomiting, and watery diarrhea. Other symptoms include fever, headache, and body aches.

A08.3-   Other viral enteritis

Mode of transmission for most viruses in this subcategory involves a fecal-oral route. Symptomology is also, for the most part, the same with nausea, vomiting, diarrhea, fever, and abdominal pain being the most common.

A08.31   Calicivirus enteritis

This code captures what is referred to morphologically as "typical" caliciviruses. The only caliciviruses that are not included in this code are the Norwalk-like viruses and small round viruses, which are a genus within the Caliciviridae family. Typical calicivirus infection of the gastrointestinal tract occurs most often in infants and children.

Focus Point

For acute gastroenteritis due to caliciviruses described as Norwalk agent, Norwalk-like agent, Norovirus, or small round virus (SRV), see codes in subcategory A08.1- Acute gastroenteropathy due to Norwalk agent or other small round viruses.

A08.32   Astrovirus enteritis

Astrovirus was identified in the 1970s as a cause of gastroenteritis in infants and young children. At the time it was believed to be a rare cause, but recent advances in identification of causative agents in infectious diseases now identify astrovirus as a common cause of gastroenteritis in children. Most cases are mild and resolve without complications.

A08.8   Other specified intestinal infections

Intestinal infections that are due to a specified organism that is not classified as a bacterium, protozoa, parasite, or virus are classified here.

A09   Infectious gastroenteritis and colitis, unspecified

Often symptoms consistent with infectious colitis, enteritis, or gastroenteritis do not require identification of the specific causative agent because treatment for many types of infectious intestinal illnesses focuses on relieving the symptoms and replacing fluids and electrolytes.

Tuberculosis (A15-A19)

Tuberculosis (TB) is a bacterial infection that usually attacks the lungs, but may also affect other organs. The disease is caused by *Mycobacterium tuberculosis* or *Mycobacterium bovis*, with *M. tuberculosis* being the most common type causing 98 percent of all infections in humans.

The mode of transmission is the principal difference between these two types of TB. *M. tuberculosis* is transmitted primarily by inhaling air droplets exhaled by an infected person, although it may also be absorbed through the skin or enter through an open wound. *M. bovis* is found in cattle and other animals including bison, elk, and deer. It is transmitted to humans by ingestion of contaminated dairy products or in the case of bison, elk, and deer through the skin or an open wound during the slaughtering process.

The categories in this code block are as follows:

A15	Respiratory tuberculosis
A17	Tuberculosis of nervous system
A18	Tuberculosis of other organs
A19	Miliary tuberculosis

Focus Point

Some TB infections are resistant to one or more antimycobacterial drugs, also called tuberculostatics. Drug resistant status is reported separately. For TB resistance to one tuberculostatic, report Z16.341; for resistance to multiple tuberculostatics, report Z16.342.

A15.-   Respiratory tuberculosis

The most common site of tuberculosis (TB) infection is the respiratory system.

A15.0   Tuberculosis of lung

Tuberculosis (TB) is a bacterial infection that usually attacks the lungs but may also affect other organs. The disease is caused by *Mycobacterium tuberculosis*. Lung tuberculosis, referred to as pulmonary TB, is transmitted by inhaling air droplets exhaled by an infected person. If the bacteria multiply, active tuberculosis develops along with typical symptoms of TB: coughing, night sweats, weight loss, and fever. Most often at high risk for pulmonary TB are the elderly, young, or the immunocompromised population. Active pulmonary TB does not go away on its own but requires treatment with multiple drugs. A chest x-ray typically shows shadows or fluid collection between the lung and its lining.

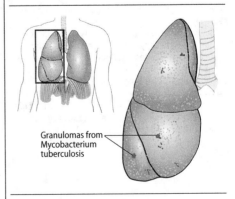

Granulomas from Mycobacterium tuberculosis

A15.7   Primary respiratory tuberculosis

Primary tuberculosis, usually appearing in children, refers to the initial TB infection when TB bacteria first enter the lungs and there are no noticeable symptoms. Upon presentation of TB bacteria, the body responds by containing the bacteria in tubercles (granulomas) and/or macrophages, the latter of which travel to the hilar lymph nodes. This collection of granulomas, together with granulomatous hilar lymph nodes, form the Ghon complex. Following containment, the body may be able to eliminate the bacteria completely or the bacteria may stay encapsulated but dormant. At this primary stage of TB, the disease does not progress, but bacteria may remain dormant in the body for many years. Most patients recover without further evidence of disease, but others develop a reactivation of the disease with symptoms.

Focus Point

Code A15.7 Primary respiratory tuberculosis, is not appropriate for reactivation or reoccurrence of a respiratory tuberculosis infection. Report a code from category A15–A19 that more specifically describes the type of tuberculosis.

Focus Point

In many cases, patients test positive for or have a nonspecific reaction to a tuberculosis diagnostic test but without any evidence of active tuberculosis; this is known as latent TB. In latent TB, the immune system is able to contain the infection and the individual is not contagious. For documented latent TB, code R76.11 Nonspecific reaction to tuberculin skin test without active tuberculosis, should be used.

A17.-   Tuberculosis of nervous system

Tuberculosis (TB) infection of the nervous system is a rare manifestation associated with a high rate of mortality. Those who survive often suffer from severe neurological sequela. Central nervous system TB may manifest with inflammation or with round, tumor-like masses called tuberculomas, both of which can occur in the brain and spinal cord, the membranes around the brain and spinal cord, or both. Most peripheral nervous system manifestations include only inflammation of one or more peripheral nerves (neuritis).

A18.-   Tuberculosis of other organs

Tuberculosis (TB) of other organs is clinically differentiated as primary or secondary. Primary TB originates in the affected site, while secondary TB has spread from the primary infection site, usually the lungs, to another site via the bloodstream. TB can affect virtually all body systems, including sites in the musculoskeletal system, genitourinary system, lymph system, gastrointestinal system, integumentary system, endocrine glands, and the eyes and ears.

A19.-   Miliary tuberculosis

Miliary tuberculosis (TB) is a disseminated form of active TB that may involve just a single site, such as the lungs, or may be more widespread and affect multiple sites. Miliary TB spreads through the bloodstream to sites that are remote from the primary infection site. In contrast to the typical granulomatous formations, miliary TB is characterized by multiple millet-sized lesions throughout the affected organs or sites. Like other forms of TB, it can occur as a primary infection when the body's immune system fails to effectively contain and eradicate the mycobacterium or it can occur when a previously dormant infection becomes active.

Certain Zoonotic Bacterial Diseases (A20-A28)

Zoonotic diseases are those that are passed from animals to humans. Zoonotic bacterial diseases are spread in three ways: direct contact with an infected animal, particularly the saliva, blood, urine, or feces of the animal; by vectors such as mosquitos or ticks; or by ingesting food or water contaminated with bacteria from an infected animal.

The categories in this code block are as follows:

A20	Plague
A21	Tularemia
A22	Anthrax
A23	Brucellosis
A24	Glanders and melioidosis
A25	Rat-bite fevers
A26	Erysipeloid
A27	Leptospirosis
A28	Other zoonotic bacterial diseases, not elsewhere classified

A20.-   Plague

Plague is an acute bacterial infection caused by the bacillus *Yersinia pestis*. It is transmitted to humans by fleas that first bite an infected rodent and then bite humans or by the direct handling of infected rodents. Plague has been called "black death" because in untreated cases, respiratory failure precedes death by several hours, and during this time, the hypoxic victim's skin may turn deep purple. In the United States, sporadic infections are seen primarily in the Southwest.

A20.0 Bubonic plague

Bubonic plague is the most common manifestation of plague. It is transmitted by the bite of insects, typically the rat flea *Xenopsylla cheopis*, that are normally rodent parasites. Bubonic plague is characterized by buboes, which are enlarged, inflamed lymph nodes in the groin, armpit, or neck.

A20.1 Cellulocutaneous plague

Cellulocutaneous plague is an inflammation and infection of the skin caused by *Y. pestis* usually at the site of the flea bite.

A20.2 Pneumonic plague

Pneumonic plague occurs when *Y. pestis* infects the lungs. It is the least common but also the most deadly form and is particularly dangerous because it can be transmitted from person-to-person. Primary pneumonic plague is typically transmitted by inhaling bacteria-carrying air droplets exhaled by an infected person. Secondary pneumonic plague begins as another form of plague before infecting the lungs. The first signs of illness in pneumonic plague are fever, headache, weakness, and cough productive of bloody or watery sputum. The pneumonia progresses over two to five days and may cause septic shock and, without early treatment, death.

A20.3 Plague meningitis

Plague meningitis is a rare complication of *Y. pestis* infection with inflammation of cerebral and spinal meninges, which are the membranes that cover the brain and spinal cord.

A20.7 Septicemic plague

Septicemic plague arises when *Y. pestis* multiply in the bloodstream. Like other forms of plague, the first symptoms are typically fever and chills. The patient may also experience gastrointestinal symptoms such as abdominal pain, diarrhea, and vomiting. This may be followed by bleeding from the mouth, nose, or rectum or bleeding under the skin as well as gangrene of the extremities. Septic shock may also occur. The fatality rate of untreated septicemic plague is nearly 100 percent.

A21.- Tularemia

Tularemia is a bacterial infection caused by *Francisella tularensis*. It is a fairly uncommon disease seen in the United States mostly in Oklahoma, Missouri, and Alaska. The infectious organism may be spread by tick and deer fly bites or by direct contact with the skin. The bacillus can penetrate unbroken skin, and can therefore be transmitted by handling tainted meat or cleaning wild game, usually rodents such as squirrels or rabbits. Less common routes of infection include ingestion of contaminated water and inhalation of contaminated dusts or aerosols. Once infected, the patient develops immunity.

A21.0 Ulceroglandular tularemia

Ulceroglandular tularemia is the most common type of *Francisella tularensis* infection and is characterized by a skin ulcer at the site of infection and inflammation of surrounding tissues and regional lymph nodes.

A21.1 Oculoglandular tularemia

Oculoglandular tularemia is an infection of the conjunctiva due to *Francisella tularensis* that may spread to the cornea and lacrimal systems, as well as to the lymph nodes in front of the ear. Symptoms include inflammation, nodules, and ulcers of the involved structures of the eye and enlarged lymph nodes in the region in front of the ears. Oculoglandular tularemia is typically spread by handling of tainted meat or wild game and then touching the eye area.

A21.2 Pulmonary tularemia

Pulmonary tularemia is a less common but more serious form of *Francisella tularensis* infection that affects the bronchi and lungs. It is characterized by cough, chest pain, and shortness of breath. This form is most often caused by inhalation of dust or aerosols that contain the bacteria, although it can also develop as a complication of untreated tularemia of other sites.

A21.3 Gastrointestinal tularemia

Gastrointestinal tularemia results from eating meat or other foodstuffs or drinking water tainted with *F. tularensis*. Gastrointestinal symptoms range from mild to severe diarrhea to extensive ulceration of the bowel, the latter of which may be fatal.

A21.7 Generalized tularemia

Generalized tularemia is a more severe form of infection with *Francisella tularensis* and is characterized by fever, chills, muscle aches (myalgia), malaise, and weight loss. Patients also often present with pneumonia but are less apt to manifest ulcers or lymph node enlargement. Generalized tularemia is also referred to as typhoidal or septicemic tularemia.

A21.8 Other forms of tularemia

Classified here is oropharyngeal tularemia, which is characterized by sore throat, tonsillitis, and ulceration of the oropharyngeal mucosa. The oropharyngeal mucosa may also develop a yellow-white pseudomembrane.

A22.- Anthrax

Anthrax is caused by the gram-positive, rod-shaped bacterium *Bacillus anthracis*, which once inside the body emerges from the dormant spore phase, begins to reproduce, and in the process of reproduction, produces toxins that can lead to organ failure. Anthrax is found in the soil and can infect domestic and wild animals. Infection of humans is rare. Anthrax can also be manufactured in a laboratory and has been used in bioterrorism attacks in the United States. DNA analysis can determine the strain of anthrax in an outbreak and whether the strain has been genetically manipulated in a laboratory. A vaccine is available but is reserved for individuals at high risk for exposure to anthrax.

A22.0   Cutaneous anthrax

In cutaneous anthrax, the anthrax bacterium enters a cut or abrasion on the skin. Skin infection begins as a raised itchy bump that resembles an insect bite. The bump develops into a vesicle and, from there, a painless ulcer, usually 1 to 3 centimeters in diameter, within 48 hours. Lymph glands in the adjacent area may swell. Not long afterward, the lesions turn black, a hallmark of skin anthrax, as tissue begins to die.

A22.1   Pulmonary anthrax

Pulmonary anthrax, also called inhalation anthrax, is caused by inhalation of the anthrax bacterium. It generally takes two to five days for symptoms to appear, though in some cases spores lodged in the lungs may take up to 60 days to germinate. Initially, symptoms mimic those of the flu with fever, nausea, muscle aches, and cough. After several days, as the immune system fails to rid the body of the bacteria, more severe signs appear, including difficulty breathing, high fever, and shock. Fatality is 90 percent if left untreated.

A22.2   Gastrointestinal anthrax

The intestinal form of anthrax is rare, and may follow the consumption of contaminated meat or water. Intestinal anthrax is characterized by an acute gastroenteritis progressing to septicemia. A variant of GI anthrax included here is oropharyngeal anthrax. Throat pain and swallowing difficulties may be experienced, as well as ulcers at the entry site.

A22.7   Anthrax sepsis

Anthrax sepsis is a complication of anthrax infection originating at another site, usually the lungs or gastrointestinal tract, and causes a systemic response that can lead to septic shock and organ failure.

A22.8   Other forms of anthrax

Anthrax meningitis is a complication most often associated with pulmonary anthrax but can be secondary to any initial anthrax insult. Typical meningitis symptoms occur including stiff neck, headache, and intolerance to bright light. Mortality rates are high even with prompt diagnosis and aggressive treatment. Also included here is cerebral anthrax, although in most cases any cerebral manifestations are a direct consequence of anthrax meningitis.

A23.-   Brucellosis

Brucellosis, also known as "undulant fever" or "Bangs disease," is a systemic bacterial infection caused by exposure to any of several Brucella species. Humans contract brucellosis from infected animals or contaminated animal products, with the bacteria entering the body through a break in the skin. Onset of symptoms can be within three days to 30 days. Symptoms of brucellosis infection include fever, night sweats, fatigue, anorexia, weight loss, headache, and arthralgia.

A23.1   Brucellosis due to Brucella abortus

Brucella abortus is a brucellosis causing bacteria that primarily affects cows, although bison, buffalo, and elk can also be infected. Humans who come in contact with infected animals or ingest contaminated meat or unpasteurized dairy products can contract *B. abortus*. The most common presentation is flu-like symptoms including intermittent fever, headache, malaise, back pain, and generalized body aches although some may have no symptoms. Complications include arthritis, spondylitis, chronic fatigue, anemia, internal abscesses, uveitis, optic neuritis, nephritis, endocarditis, dermatitis, and in males inflammation of the epididymis and testes. Some individuals develop neurologic complications including meningitis.

A24.-   Glanders and melioidosis

Glanders is an equine (horse) disease communicable to man and caused by *Burkholderia mallei* (formerly *Pseudomonas mallei*). Melioidosis, also known as Whitmore's disease or pseudoglanders, is a rare infection caused by *Pseudomonas pseudomallei*. Melioidosis is classified as acute and fulminating, subacute and chronic, other, and unspecified. Patients with melioidosis may suffer relapses years after the initial infection has resolved.

A24.0   Glanders

Glanders is an equine (horse) disease communicable to man and caused by *Burkholderia mallei* (formerly *Pseudomonas malle*). Nearly all cases of glanders in the United States occur among people who are professionally or recreationally exposed to horses, although glanders can be transmitted from human to human and in the laboratory. Glanders cases have been extremely rare in the United States since the 1940s. Outbreaks do occur in South America, Asia, Africa, and the Middle East. Symptoms of glanders include headache, chills, fever, and vomiting.

A24.1   Acute and fulminating melioidosis

Also known as Whitmore's disease or pseudoglanders, melioidosis is a rare infection caused by *Burkholderia pseudomallei* (formerly *Pseudomonas pseudomallei*). Most cases are limited to Southeast Asia and northern Australia. The disease is acquired through exposure to contaminated soil or water and the infectious organism enters the body through a break in the skin. Acute infections may present as a localized infection, such as a skin lesion, ulcer, or abscess; a respiratory infection, such as pneumonia; or a disseminated infection such as sepsis.

A24.2   Subacute and chronic melioidosis

Duration of symptoms most often defines chronic melioidosis, which can present in a variety of ways most often as skin or pulmonary issues.

A25.-   Rat-bite fevers

Rat-bite fever begins with a bite or scratch from an infected rodent, handling an infected rodent, or ingestion of food or water contaminated with the bacterium that causes rat-bite fever. Rodents that can spread rat-bite fever include rats, mice, and gerbils. When the bacteria are introduced by a bite or scratch, the initial wound may heal without signs or symptoms of infection; however, it usually becomes swollen and painful again within a few weeks of the bite. At that time, regional lymph nodes may swell and there may be chills, fever, and a skin rash. Periods of relapse may subside and recur. When the bacteria are introduced by handling an infected rodent or via ingestion of contaminated food or water, symptoms may include fever, headache, vomiting, muscle and joint pain, and skin rash.

A25.Ø   Spirillosis

The bacterium *Spirillum minus* is responsible for rat-bite fever that occurs primarily in Asia. Onset of illness is typically seven to 21 days following infection. The most common symptoms of *S. minus*, also called spirillary rat-bite fever and Sodoku, are intermittent fever, ulceration at the site of the bite or scratch, swelling at and around the site of the wound, inflammation of regional lymph nodes, and skin rash. When infection is caused by contaminated food or water, initial symptoms are typically sore throat and vomiting.

A25.1   Streptobacillosis

The bacterium *Streptobacillus moniliformis* is responsible for rat-bite fever that occurs primarily in North America. Onset of illness is typically three to 1Ø days following exposure, but in some cases symptoms may not present for up to three weeks. The most common symptoms of *S. moniliformis* are fever, vomiting, headache, muscle and joint pain, and skin rash. When infection is caused by contaminated food or water, the condition may be referred to as Haverhill fever and initial symptoms are typically sore throat and vomiting.

A27.-   Leptospirosis

Leptospirosis is an infection due to any serotype of *Leptospira*. Dogs and rats are the most common carriers of leptospirosis and, in the United States, the most common source of infection is swimming in contaminated water. The infection usually enters the host through mucous membranes or injured skin. Less than 1ØØ cases are reported in the United States annually.

A28.-   Other zoonotic bacterial diseases, not elsewhere classified

Other zoonotic diseases passed from animals to humans included here with specific codes are pasteurellosis, cat-scratch disease, and extraintestinal yersiniosis.

A28.1   Cat-scratch disease

Cat-scratch disease (CSD) is a bacterial infection caused by *Bartonella henselae*. As the name implies, mode of transmission largely occurs when an infected animal, usually a cat, scratches or bites. However, rare incidents of dog bites have been known to cause cat-scratch disease. CSD causes self-limited local enlargement of the lymph nodes (lymphadenopathy) and is the most common adenopathy in children. Typically, within a couple of weeks an area close to the scratch or bite becomes red with swelling and tenderness. The lymph nodes surrounding the area also become enlarged. At some point, the lymph nodes may fill with pus and drain.

Other Bacterial Diseases (A3Ø-A49)

A wide variety of bacterial diseases are classified here. Some like leprosy are rare in the United States. Others, like diphtheria and whooping cough, can be prevented by vaccines. Two categories classify sepsis due to bacterial infections. Many of the codes for bacterial infections in this code block are combination codes that identify the bacterial agent and the site, manifestation, and/or complication.

The categories in this code block are as follows:

A3Ø	Leprosy [Hansen's disease]
A31	Infection due to other mycobacteria
A32	Listeriosis
A33	Tetanus neonatorium
A34	Obstetrical tetanus
A35	Other tetanus
A36	Diphtheria
A37	Whooping cough
A38	Scarlet fever
A39	Meningococcal infection
A4Ø	Streptococcal sepsis
A41	Other sepsis
A42	Actinomycosis
A43	Nocardiosis
A44	Bartonellosis
A46	Erysipelas

A48	Other bacterial diseases, not elsewhere classified
A49	Bacterial infection of unspecified site

A30.- Leprosy [Hansen's disease]

Leprosy, also known as Hansen's disease, is a chronic infectious disease caused by *Mycobacterium leprae* that affects the peripheral nerves, skin, upper respiratory tract, eyes, and nasal mucosa. The bacterium is parasitic in nature requiring a host cell to survive and reproduce. Leprosy is not easily transmitted, and the mode of transmission is not well understood, but one possible mode is person-to-person transmission through nasal droplets released from an infected person. Less than 5 percent of people who are infected with *M. leprae* actually develop leprosy. For most, the immune system fights off infection. There is a wide spectrum of clinical manifestations that are tied to the individual immune response at the cellular level. Patients with good T-cell immunity to *M. leprae* develop milder forms while those with poor T-cell immunity develop more severe forms. All patients with leprosy experience some peripheral nerve damage characterized by loss of sensation and muscle weakness, particularly in the extremities. The loss of sensation is a risk factor for injury, particularly of the hands and feet. Treating leprosy using multidrug therapy can halt the progression of the disease, though there are side effects. Untreated leprosy results in progression of the disease with permanent damage to the skin, peripheral nerves, and eyes.

A30.1 Tuberculoid leprosy

Tuberculoid leprosy, also called TT leprosy or paucibacillary leprosy, is seen in patients with good T-cell immunity to *M. leprae*. These patients develop a mild form of leprosy characterized by discoloration at the site of the skin lesion. The skin lesions are few in number, small in size, and with few bacteria present.

A30.5 Lepromatous leprosy

Lepromatous leprosy, also called LL leprosy, is a more severe disease seen in patients with poor T-cell immunity to *M. leprae*. This form is characterized by widespread skin lesions and significant bacteria present. The skin lesions are symmetric with nodules, plaques, and thickening of the dermis. Often the nasal mucosa is involved with resultant congestion and nosebleeds.

A31.- Infection due to other mycobacteria

Mycobacteria are widespread in the environment. Most do not cause illness and those that do affect primarily immunocompromised individuals. Mycobacterial infections classified here include all types other than *M. leprae* and *M. tuberculosis* and may be referred to as nontuberculous mycobacteria (NTM),

mycobacteria other than tuberculosis (MOTT), or atypical mycobacteria. Mycobacterial infections in category A31 are classified by site of infection rather than by the specific infectious organism.

A31.0 Pulmonary mycobacterial infection

Atypical mycobacteria that cause pulmonary infections include *Mycobacterium avium, Mycobacterium intracellulare*, and *Mycobacterium kansasii*. When *M. avium* and *M. intracellulare* occur together in a localized infection of the lungs, the infection is referred to as *M.* avium-*intracellulare* complex. *M.* avium-*intracellulare* complex affects up to 40 percent of human immunodeficiency virus (HIV)-infected people in the United States. *M. intracellulare* is also called Battey bacillus. Both *M. avium* and *M. intracellulare* are characterized by similar symptoms and are often difficult to differentiate from each other. Symptoms include productive cough, fever, night sweats, weight loss, and lethargy. *M. kansasii* causes pulmonary symptoms that are almost indistinguishable from tuberculosis including fever, chills, night sweats, productive or nonproductive cough, hemoptysis, shortness of breath, weight loss, fatigue, and chest pain. In the United States, *M. kansasii* occurs most commonly in Kansas, Texas, and Illinois. Both antibiotics and antituberculosis drugs are effective against mycobacterial infections.

A31.1 Cutaneous mycobacterial infection

Cutaneous mycobacterial infection is rare in the United States. Buruli ulcer disease caused by *M. ulcerans* and fish tank granuloma caused by *M. marinum*, formerly called *M. balnei*, are two types of cutaneous mycobacterial infection classified here.

A31.2 Disseminated mycobacterium avium-intracellulare complex (DMAC)

The disseminated form of the *Mycobacterium* avium-*intracellulare* complex (DMAC) primarily affects patients with symptomatic human immunodeficiency virus (HIV) infection and other people with severely impaired immune systems. Severe anemia, fever, night sweats, anorexia, and diarrhea characterize DMAC. It is a significant cause of morbidity in patients with symptomatic HIV infection.

A31.8 Other mycobacterial infections

Mycobacteria are widespread in the environment. Most do not cause illness and those that do affect primarily immunocompromised individuals. Conditions that are classified here include operative wound infections and lymph node infections due to *M. chelonae (chelonei), M. fortuitum, M. kakaferifu, M. haemophilum, M. kasongo, M. scrofulaceum, M. simiae, M. szulgai, M. terrae, M. triviale*, and *M. xenopi*.

A32.-   Listeriosis

Listeriosis is an infection caused by ingesting food contaminated with the bacterium *Listeria monocytogenes*. Even though listeriosis is a form of food poisoning, most people who seek medical care present with manifestations of invasive listeriosis. Invasive infections primarily affect the elderly, pregnant women, infants, and individuals with compromised immune systems. The elderly and immunocompromised individuals most often present with sepsis, meningitis, or meningoencephalitis. Pregnant women typically first experience nonspecific symptoms such as fever, fatigue, and body aches, but are at risk for miscarriage, stillbirth, and premature delivery, and newborns infected in utero may experience a life-threating infection. Healthy individuals who consume contaminated food may have typical symptoms of gastroenteritis or may be asymptomatic.

A32.0   Cutaneous listeriosis

Cutaneous listeriosis is a rare manifestation of *Listeria monocytogenes* infection that is seen most often in veterinarians and farmers who are infected by handling the products of conception of infected animals. Symptoms include a localized eruption of pus containing lesions at the site of the infection. A second form is seen in immunocompromised individuals with invasive listeriosis that is spread through the blood to the skin.

A32.1-   Listerial meningitis and meningoencephalitis

Listerial meningitis and meningoencephalitis are invasive forms of *Listeria monocytogenes* in which the infection spreads from the gastrointestinal tract to the membranes that cover the brain (meningitis) or to the membranes covering the brain and to the brain tissue (meningoencephalitis). Meningitis and meningoencephalitis share the same symptoms and are often difficult to differentiate based on symptoms alone. Listerial meningitis and meningoencephalitis are seen most often in infants, the elderly, and in immunocompromised individuals. Common symptoms in adults include fever, headache, stiff neck, nausea, vomiting, confusion or other symptoms of altered mental status, and sensitivity to bright light. Infants often have nonspecific symptoms such as lack of alertness, sleepiness, difficulty in waking up even with stimulation, irritability, high pitched or moaning cry, vomiting, refusal to feed, and loss of muscle tone or muscle stiffness.

A32.7   Listerial sepsis

Listerial sepsis is a manifestation of invasive listeriosis caused by a systemic or body-wide response to *L. monocytogenes*. The elderly, immunocompromised individuals, and infants are more likely to present with complications such as listerial sepsis. Symptoms of listerial sepsis include elevated body temperature (above 101 degrees Fahrenheit) or subnormal body temperature (below 96.8 degrees Fahrenheit), elevated heart rate (above 90 beats per minute), elevated respiratory rate (above 20 breaths per minute), along with known *L. monocytogenes* infection.

A32.8   Other forms of listeriosis

Less common manifestations of *Listeria monocytogenes* infection are classified here and include infection of the eye with local inflammation of lymph nodes (oculoglandular listeriosis), infection and inflammation of the inner lining of the heart chambers and heart valves (endocarditis), inflammation of the arteries (arteritis), and miliary granulomatosis.

A32.81   Oculoglandular listeriosis

Oculoglandular listeriosis is an infection of the conjunctiva that may spread to the cornea and lacrimal systems as well as to the lymph nodes in front of the ear. Symptoms include inflammation, nodules, and ulcers of the involved structures of the eye and enlarged lymph nodes in the region in front of the ears. Oculoglandular listeriosis is typically spread by handling contaminated food products and then touching the eye area. It may also be spread through the bloodstream.

A32.82   Listerial endocarditis

An uncommon manifestation of invasive listeriosis is infection and inflammation of the inner lining of the heart chambers and the heart valves. Symptoms of listerial endocarditis are often nonspecific and include fatigue, shortness of breath, and cardiac murmur. Some individuals develop acute congestive heart failure as a complication of the endocarditis.

A32.89   Other forms of listeriosis

Other less common manifestations of invasive *Listeria monocytogenes* infection are classified here and include arteritis commonly found in the cerebral arteries and miliary granulomatosis with the characteristic millet-sized nodular lesions most often found in the liver.

A33   Tetanus neonatorum

Tetanus neonatorum is defined as tetanus infection with onset during the first month (28 days) of life. Tetanus is a bacterial infection that affects the nervous system. It is caused by *Clostridium tetani*, and is commonly called "lockjaw" because of the tonic spasms that occur in voluntary muscles. *C. tetani* is found in soil and animal feces. Infection during the neonatal period is caused by contamination of the umbilical stump with early symptoms seen in irritability and difficulty feeding most commonly seen within three to 14 days after birth. Treatment involves administering human tetanus immune globulin to neutralize the unbound toxin and antibiotics. Supportive measures are also used to control rigidity and muscle spasms, to maintain respiratory function, and to minimize other effects on the autonomic nervous system.

A34   Obstetrical tetanus

Obstetrical tetanus is defined as tetanus infection occurring during pregnancy or within six weeks after delivery or termination of a pregnancy. Tetanus is a bacterial infection that affects the nervous system. It is caused by *Clostridium tetani*, and is commonly called "lockjaw" because of the tonic spasms that occur in voluntary muscles. *C. tetani* is found in soil and animal feces, and infection during pregnancy may result from insignificant abrasions or deep wounds or as a result of a nonsterile delivery or abortion. The infected patient may have difficulty swallowing, speaking, or breathing as a result of the tonic spasms caused by the infection. Treatment involves administering human tetanus immune globulin to neutralize the unbound toxin, antibiotics, and wound care with debridement of infected and necrotic tissue. Supportive measures are also used to control rigidity and muscle spasms, to maintain respiratory function, and to minimize other effects on the autonomic nervous system.

A35   Other tetanus

Tetanus is a bacterial infection that affects the nervous system. It is caused by *Clostridium tetani*, and is commonly called "lockjaw" because of the tonic spasms that occur in voluntary muscles. *C. tetani* is found in soil and animal feces, and infection may result from insignificant or deep wounds. The infected patient may have difficulty swallowing, speaking, or breathing as a result of the tonic spasms caused by the infection. A vaccine given in childhood with booster shots given throughout life protects against the infection and cases in the United States are rare. The highest number of tetanus cases in the United States is seen among intravenous drug abusers and in burn victims or as a complication of abortion or pregnancy. Treatment involves administering human tetanus immune globulin to neutralize the unbound toxin, antibiotics, and wound care with debridement of infected and necrotic tissue. Supportive measures are also used to control rigidity and muscle spasms, to maintain respiratory function, and to minimize other effects on the autonomic nervous system.

A36.-   Diphtheria

An acute, contagious disease, diphtheria is one of the childhood diseases that common immunizations protect against. The infective agent is *Corynebacterium diphtheriae*. Diphtheria usually presents with sore throat, with its hallmark fibrous membrane most commonly seen on the tonsil or nasopharynx. This membrane can combine with pharyngeal edema to obstruct breathing. However, diphtheria can attack other organs rather than presenting as a sore throat, and the codes are assigned based on the site of infection.

A36.81   Diphtheritic cardiomyopathy

Diphtheritic cardiomyopathy occurs when the muscle of the heart becomes inflamed due to the contagious infection *Corynebacterium diphtheriae*. This infection spreads through respiratory and nasal discharge. Overcrowded living conditions, poor health, and lack of immunization against the disease contribute to its spread.

A37.-   Whooping cough

An acute, contagious disease, whooping cough is one of the childhood diseases that common immunizations protect against. The course of whooping cough is approximately six weeks and has three stages: catarrhal (nocturnal cough, sneezing, and lacrimation); paroxysmal (thick mucus, choking spells); and convalescence, when the severity of the symptoms diminishes. Mortality for the most severe form of whooping cough, *B. pertussis*, is about 2 percent in children younger than age 1.

A37.0-   Whooping cough due to Bordetella pertussis

Several species of *Bordetella* cause whooping cough, but *Bordetella pertussis* is the infective agent most commonly associated with the infection and causes the most severe symptoms. Whooping cough complicated by pneumonia is seen most often in younger children, particularly those younger than age 1, and is the primary complication associated with death in this age group.

A37.1-   Whooping cough due to Bordetella parapertussis

B. parapertussis generally causes a milder form if whooping cough with symptoms of shorter duration. The most common symptoms are cough, including paroxysmal cough with thick mucus and choking spells, high-pitched whooping breath sounds on inhalation during and after a coughing spell, and posttussive (post-cough) vomiting. Less common symptoms include apnea and cyanosis during paroxysmal coughing spells. The paroxysmal stage typically lasts two weeks or less. Whooping cough due to *B. parapertussis* complicated by pneumonia is seen most often in younger children, particularly those younger than age 1.

A37.8- Whooping cough due to other Bordetella species

One Bordetella species classified here is *B. bronchiseptica*. It is more often found in wild and domestic animals and is the cause of kennel cough. However, it is known to cause whooping cough in humans who are severely immunocompromised and infection typically occurs as a result of exposure to infected farm or domestic animals.

A38.- Scarlet fever

Scarlet fever is a bacterial infection caused by Group A *Streptococcus*, the same bacterium that causes strep throat. Individuals with strep throat or less commonly a strep infection of the skin can develop scarlet fever particularly if the infection is not treated with antibiotics. Scarlet fever is caused by a toxin released by the *Streptococcus* bacterium and is characterized by a red blush to the skin of the chest and abdomen that blanches under pressure, as well as a red tongue. Scarlet fever typically affects children and adolescents between the ages of 5 and 15. Antibiotics are effective in treating scarlet fever. Several of the scarlet fever codes recognize a complication that may manifest with the infection.

Focus Point

Scarlet fever and acute rheumatic fever are two conditions caused by Group A Streptococcus bacteria that can have associated heart complications. In scarlet fever, associated myocarditis is a result of the bacteria moving to and infecting the heart; however, heart involvement in acute rheumatic fever is an inflammatory response unrelated to direct bacterial involvement. See category I01 for acute rheumatic fever.

A39.- Meningococcal infection

Neisseria meningitidis is a common cause of meningitis. Also called meningococcus, the bacteria may invade the spinal cord, brain, heart, joints, optic nerve, or bloodstream. A pink or petechial rash may accompany the disease. Although the bacterium is found in the nasopharynx of 5 percent of the population, only a fraction of carriers ever develop the disease. It is seen most commonly in infants or in epidemics among persons who live in close quarters (barracks, schools).

A40.- Streptococcal sepsis

Sepsis is a systemic or body-wide response to an infection with the majority of sepsis cases being due to a bacterial infection. The systemic response is characterized by certain changes in body temperature, heart rate, respiratory rate or arterial blood gases, and white blood cell count. More specifically, these include elevated body temperature (usually above 101 degrees Fahrenheit) or subnormal body temperature (usually below 96.8 degrees Fahrenheit), elevated heart rate (usually above 90 beats per minute), elevated

respiratory rate (usually above 20 breaths per minute) or arterial blood gases reflecting a reduced partial pressure of carbon dioxide PACO2, and an abnormal white blood cell count either above 12,000 cells/microliter or below 4,000 cells/microliter or greater than 10 percent bands (immature white blood cells). Two or more of these indications and a suspected or known infection are indicative of sepsis. Code selection for this category is based on the streptococcal organism, including specific codes for group A, group B, and *S. pneumoniae*.

Focus Point

Do not report sepsis due to group D Streptococcus with code A40.8 Other streptococcal sepsis. Group D streptococci have been reclassified into the new genus Enterococcus and sepsis due to the 19 species of bacteria classified in this genus are reported with code A41.81 Sepsis due to Enterococcus.

A41.- Other sepsis

Sepsis is a systemic or body-wide response to an infection with the majority of sepsis cases being due to a bacterial infection. The systemic response is characterized by certain changes in body temperature, heart rate, respiratory rate or arterial blood gases, and white blood cell count. More specifically, these include elevated body temperature (usually above 101 degrees Fahrenheit) or subnormal body temperature (usually below 96.8 degrees Fahrenheit), elevated heart rate (usually above 90 beats per minute), elevated respiratory rate (usually above 20 breaths per minute) or arterial blood gases reflecting a reduced partial pressure of carbon dioxide PACO2, and an abnormal white blood cell count either above 12,000 cells/microliter or below 4,000 cells/microliter or greater than 10 percent bands (immature white blood cells). Two or more of these indications and a suspected or known infection are indicative of sepsis.

A41.0- Sepsis due to Staphylococcus aureus

Staphylococcus aureus is a bacterium that causes a wide spectrum of infectious diseases. In recent years, some *S. aureus* strains have become resistant to a number of antibiotics. Sepsis due to *S. aureus* is classified based on susceptibility or resistance to beta lactam antibiotics.

A41.01 Sepsis due to Methicillin susceptible Staphylococcus aureus

The term methicillin-susceptible *Staphylococcus aureus* (MSSA) identifies strains of *S. aureus* that are susceptible or treatable with the traditional beta lactam class of antibiotics, such as penicillin, methicillin, and cephalosporins.

A41.02   Sepsis due to Methicillin resistant Staphylococcus aureus

Methicillin-resistant *Staphylococcus aureus* (MRSA) is a variant form of the bacterium that is resistant to the traditional beta lactam class of antibiotics, such as penicillin, methicillin, and cephalosporins. Sometimes referred to as a "superbug," MRSA is a major cause of hospital-acquired infections, as well as community-acquired infections. Community acquired MRSA infections (CA-MRSA) are generally not life-threatening. Skin and soft tissue infections are spread through direct contact. Due to clinical challenges, MRSA is more difficult and costly to combat than MSSA and generally poses a greater public health threat due to its multidrug resistance.

A41.1   Sepsis due to other specified staphylococcus

This classification includes coagulase negative staphylococcus species, including *S. hominis* and *S. epidermidis*, that inhabit the skin and *S. saprophyticus* found in the vaginal tract. When confined to these sites, these species are typically not pathogenic. However, they can cause sepsis if they are introduced into the bloodstream secondary to infection.

A41.3   Sepsis due to Hemophilus influenzae

Haemophilus influenzae is a bacterium most often associated with respiratory illnesses in infants and young children. There are six classifiable types identified with the letters a through f as well as a number of unclassifiable types that cause disease in humans. Only one type, *H. influenza* type b (Hib), is preventable with the Hib vaccine.

A41.4   Sepsis due to anaerobes

Anaerobic bacteria are part of the normal flora of the skin and mucous membranes. Most anaerobic infections originate from the patient's own flora and begin in areas of poor blood supply or tissue necrosis. An anaerobic infection may be indicative of an undiagnosed underlying disease process. Sepsis due to *Clostridium* difficile, Clostridium perfringens (C. welchii), and gram-negative anaerobes are classified here.

A41.5-   Sepsis due to other Gram-negative organisms

One method of identifying characteristics of bacteria is the use of a laboratory test called Gram staining. Bacteria are classified as Gram-positive or Gram-negative based on color retention during Gram staining. Gram-positive bacteria retain purple stain, while Gram-negative bacteria do not and instead display a red or pinkish color. A number of Gram-negative bacteria cause sepsis including *Escherichia coli*, *Pseudomonas*, and *Serratia*.

A41.51   Sepsis due to Escherichia coli [E. coli]

Escherichia coli (E. coli) are a large and diverse group of bacteria that range from the relatively harmless to those that cause serious, life-threatening illnesses.

A41.52   Sepsis due to Pseudomonas

Pseudomonas is a genus of bacteria that is widely dispersed in the environment including in soil and water. There are several species of Pseudomonas that are pathogenic to humans, but the most common is *Pseudomonas aeruginosa*. Healthy individuals sometimes develop mild *Pseudomonas* infections, such as otitis media or skin infection after exposure to inadequately treated water in public pools. Severe infections such as sepsis are typically limited to individuals with compromised immune systems.

A41.53   Sepsis due to Serratia

Serratia is a genus of bacteria that is widespread in the environment. Most species are harmless, but a few cause opportunistic infections in immunocompromised individuals. The most common opportunistic pathogenic species is *S. marcescens*, which causes a wide variety of illnesses including sepsis.

A41.81   Sepsis due to Enterococcus

Enterococcus is a relatively new genus of bacteria with more than a dozen species, including group D streptococci recently reclassified to this genus. Enterococci make up part of the normal flora of the intestinal tract in humans, but are responsible for infections of the urinary tract, heart, surgical or other open wounds, catheter sites, and intraabdominal and pelvic sites. Specific species known to be responsible for infection in humans include *E.* avium, E. casseliflavus, E. durans, E. faecalis, E. faecium, E. gallinarum, E. *mundtii*, and E. *raffinosus*.

> **Focus Point**
>
> *Some species of Enterococcus are antibiotic resistant including E. faecium, which is responsible for most vancomycin resistant Enterococcus infections. See category Z16 to capture documented resistance to antimicrobial drugs.*

A41.89   Other specified sepsis

Sepsis is defined as an infection within the bloodstream, leading to organ malfunction and potentially death. While sepsis can be caused by bacteria, fungi, or parasites, it can also be caused by a virus. Viral sepsis is reported with this code and an additional code for the specific type of viral infection. The medical community continues to explore improved assessments to evaluate for sepsis versus other less complicated infections. Providers are urged to watch for these warning signs: altered mental status, decreased systolic BP less than 100mm Hg, and/or respiration higher than 22 breaths per minute. Risk factors for acquiring sepsis include age, a weak immune system, trauma, and burns.

Focus Point

Since there currently is no specific code in ICD-10-CM to identify viral sepsis, in addition to A41.89, report a code for the specific virus if known. If the virus is unknown, code B97.89 Other viral agents, as the cause of diseases classified elsewhere, is appropriate.

A42.- Actinomycosis

Actinomycosis is a chronic type of infection caused by anaerobic bacteria that are normally found on the teeth and on mucous membranes, including the gums, tonsils, intestinal tract, and vagina. These bacteria are harmless unless they enter a break in the mucosa, which allows the bacteria to penetrate into deeper tissues. Most infections are caused by *Actinomyces israelii*, although there are other species that also cause infection in humans, including *A.* naeslundii, A. odontolyticus, A. *viscosus*, and A. *gerencseriae*. Actinomycosis is characterized by formation of deep abscesses and fistulas. The disease is most commonly seen in adult males, although it is sometimes seen as a local complication of intrauterine device (IUD) placement in women.

A42.0 Pulmonary actinomycosis

Pulmonary actinomycosis, also called thoracic actinomycosis, is caused by *Actinomyces* infection and is characterized by abscess formation beginning in the lungs and spreading to the pleura. The infection causes inflammation of the pleura and infected fluid accumulation in the pleural cavity, which is called empyema. Symptoms include chest pain, fever, and a cough that may produce sputum. Untreated infection can spread via fistula formation to the ribs, spine, chest wall, and skin.

A42.1 Abdominal actinomycosis

Abdominal actinomycosis, also called gastrointestinal actinomycosis, is caused by *Actinomyces* bacteria entering deeper tissues and the peritoneum via a break in the intestinal mucosa. The bacteria then cause abscess formation in the peritoneum and peritoneal cavity. Symptoms include abdominal pain, fever, vomiting, diarrhea, constipation, and weight loss. Fistula formation to other sites and organs in the peritoneum and to the skin of the abdomen can occur if the infection is not sufficiently treated.

A42.2 Cervicofacial actinomycosis

Cervicofacial actinomycosis is caused by a break in the mucosa of the oral cavity, which allows *Actinomyces* to infect deeper tissues in the face and neck. Abscess formation in the mouth, face, jawline, and neck is common, starting out as small hard lumps that eventually soften and open, discharging pus. If left untreated, the infection can spread to the throat, salivary glands, skull, cervical spine, meninges, and brain.

A42.7 Actinomycotic sepsis

Actinomycotic sepsis is a rare condition that occurs when an anaerobic actinomycosis bacteria infects the blood. Diagnosis is based on the presence of two or more of the following characteristics, in addition to a suspected or known *actinomyces* infection: elevated or subnormal body temperature, elevated heart rate, elevated respiratory rate, abnormal arterial blood gases, and an abnormal white blood cell count.

A42.81 Actinomycotic meningitis

Actinomycotic meningitis is an infection of the membranes covering the spinal cord and brain (meninges), which is typically caused by spread of the bacteria via fistula formation from the soft tissues of the head, neck, thorax, or abdomen or through the bloodstream.

A42.82 Actinomycotic encephalitis

Actinomycotic bacteria can enter the brain in two ways: via the bloodstream or via fistulous tracts that form between the soft tissue in the head and the brain. Once present, the bacteria can cause inflammation of the brain tissues or what is known as encephalitis.

A42.89 Other forms of actinomycosis

Other sites that may incur *Actinomyces* infection include the bones and skin, which are classified here.

A43.- Nocardiosis

This bacterial infection, found in soil, decaying plants, and standing water, most often affects those who are immunocompromised or with chronic diseases such as diabetes, HIV, cancer, or alcoholism. Men are three times more likely to contract nocardiosis than women. It generally affects the lungs (pulmonary), and can spread to the brain and/or spinal cord. Exposure of an open wound to soil can instigate a *Nocardia* skin (cutaneous) infection exhibiting nodules and skin ulcers. Pulmonary infections can present with fever, cough, weight loss, and pneumonia with confusion and seizures occurring if the nervous system is involved. Once the infection has progressed to the nervous system, the mortality rate is up to 44 percent for all people and 85 percent in the immunocompromised population. A prolonged regimen of multiple antibiotics may eventually eradicate the infection although some species are resistant to certain antibiotics.

A44.- Bartonellosis

Bartonellosis is in infection of *Bartonella* bacilliformis, transmitted by sandflies in the Andes Mountains of South America. Cases in the United States are rare.

A46   Erysipelas

Erysipelas is a skin infection affecting the upper dermis and superficial dermal lymphatics. The bright red lesion edges are well-demarcated with distinct raised borders that cause the patient to present with fevers, chills, and headache. The distinct characteristics of the lesions are generally enough to determine a diagnosis.

It is caused by group A *Streptococci* with antibiotics as the typical treatment course.

A48.-   Other bacterial diseases, not elsewhere classified

Most bacterial diseases are classified by genus or species and may be subclassified by site. A few bacterial diseases do not fit easily into those categories and are classified here.

A48.0   Gas gangrene

Gas gangrene is a severe muscle tissue infection resulting in red, extremely painful swelling of the infected site with quick progression to surrounding areas. *Clostridia* species, most often *Clostridium perfringens*, are the usual suspects with infection typically occurring at a surgical wound or injury sites. Tissue damage and the signature gas buildup is a consequence of toxins produced by these bacteria. Mortality rate is high as related tissue death and systemic effects, such as shock, renal failure, and coma, can progress rapidly.

A48.1   Legionnaires' disease

Legionnaires' disease is a type of pneumonia caused by the bacteria *Legionella*, and grows best in warm water found in hot tubs, hot water tanks, large plumbing systems, cooling towers, and decorative fountains. The disease is contracted by inhaling vapor or droplets of water contaminated with large amounts of *Legionella*. Most infections occur in the elderly, current and former smokers, individuals with chronic lung conditions such as chronic obstructive pulmonary disease or emphysema, and individuals with compromised immune systems. Following exposure to *Legionella* bacteria, there is a two to 14 day incubation period before symptoms become apparent.

A48.2   Nonpneumonic Legionnaires' disease [Pontiac fever]

Nonpneumonic Legionnaires' disease is a milder form of Legionnaires' disease with a respiratory infection that does not progress to pneumonia. Although the incubation period is the same, Pontiac fever typically only lasts two to five days and often resolves without treatment.

A48.3   Toxic shock syndrome

Toxic shock syndrome (TSS) is a rare, life-threatening complication of toxin-producing bacteria, such as *Staphylococcus aureus* or Group A *Streptococcus*. Toxic shock syndrome due to *S. aureus* toxin may be designated as STSS or TSS-toxin 1 (TSS-T1), while Group A *Streptococcus* toxin may be designated as GAS TSS. Definitive symptoms of toxic shock syndrome are fever, rash, low blood pressure, multisystem organ failure, and peeling of skin (desquamation) on the palms of the hands and soles of the feet. These symptoms typically manifest one to two weeks following onset of the acute bacterial infection. Risk factors for toxic shock syndrome are an open wound or burn, a recent surgical procedure, a recent viral infection such as influenza or varicella (chickenpox), and in women the use of super absorbent tampons or a contraceptive sponge or diaphragm.

A48.4   Brazilian purpuric fever

Brazilian purpuric fever is a rare, often fatal, systemic infection caused by *Hemophilus aegyptius*. It was originally identified in the town of Promissao in the state of Sao Paulo, Brazil in 1984. Seen primarily in children younger than age 8, it is characterized by fever, abdominal pain, vomiting, and the development of petechiae (minute hemorrhagic skin spots) and/or purpura (skin hemorrhages of variable size), all of which is preceded by purulent conjunctivitis. Only a small percentage of children with *H. aegyptius* conjunctivitis develop a systemic infection; local antibiotics used to treat the conjunctivitis do not prevent systemic involvement. Successful treatment requires diagnosis of the systemic infection prior to development of petechiae and/or purpura and the use of intravenous antibiotics.

A48.5-   Other specified botulism

Botulism, an uncommon but serious neuromuscular poisoning caused by toxins produced by the bacteria *Clostridium botulinum*, occurs in three forms: food-borne botulism, wound botulism, and infant botulism, all of which are coded to this subcategory except the foodborne form.

A48.51   Infant botulism

Infant botulism is a result of consuming the spores of the *C. botulinum* bacteria, and occurs most often in infants less than 6 months of age. The spores colonize in the large intestine, frequently resulting in constipation and progressing to neuromuscular paralysis. Infant botulism, like other forms of botulism, can be fatal, with life-threatening impairment of respiratory function being one of the greatest complications.

A48.52   Wound botulism

Wound botulism, caused by a toxin produced from a wound infected with *C. botulinum*, is frequently the result of a traumatic injury or a deep puncture wound. Often caused by abscess formation due to self-injected illegal drugs, its manifestations include neurologic symptoms with onset typically two weeks following the initial wound or trauma. Life-threatening impairment of respiratory function is one of the greatest complications.

A48.8   Other specified bacterial diseases

Some specific bacterial diseases coded here are dermatophilosis, trichomycosis axillaris, and rhinoscleroma. Dermatophilosis, also called cutaneous streptotrichosis, is a rare skin disease caused by the bacterium *Dermatophilus congolensis*. It infects wild and domestic animals and humans can contract the infection by handling infected animals. In humans, the infection is characterized by formation of pustules and sores usually on the hands that eventually drain and heal leaving scars. Trichomycosis axillaris, also called trichosis axillaris or lepothrix, is a relatively common condition in which bacteria colonize the hair shafts of the armpit forming yellow, red, or black concretions. The easiest method of treatment is hair removal by shaving or waxing. Rhinoscleroma, also called scleroma nasi, is a rare chronic granulomatous infection of the nose and upper respiratory tract caused by the bacterium *Klebsiella rhinoscleromatis*. It is endemic to certain regions in Africa, Southeast Asia, Mexico, Central and South America, and Central and Eastern Europe, but is rarely seen in the United States.

A49.-   Bacterial infection of unspecified site

Bacteria are single-celled living organisms. Most bacteria are harmless and many perform essential functions within the human body and in the external environment. Only infectious or pathogenic organisms cause disease. Most infections are localized to a specific site and produce symptoms related to the site of infection. In rare instances, the site may be unknown or unspecified; codes in category A49 are used to classify bacterial infections of an unspecified nature or site.

A49.0-   Staphylococcal infection, unspecified site

Staphylococcus is a genus of bacteria that contains several pathogenic species. Staphylococcus bacteria are gram-positive, nonspore-forming, nonmotile, facultative anaerobes that are spherical in shape and have a tendency to cluster together. Most infections are caused by the species *S. aureus*. Other species that cause infection include *S. hominis* and *S. epidermidis*, which inhabit the skin, and *S. saprophyticus* found in the vaginal tract. However these species are relatively harmless when confined to these sites, only causing infection when they are introduced into other sites such as deeper soft tissues. Infections of unspecified site specific codes are available only for *S. aureus* infections, which are further differentiated as methicillin susceptible and methicillin resistant.

A49.01   Methicillin susceptible Staphylococcus aureus infection, unspecified site

The term methicillin-susceptible *Staphylococcus aureus* (MSSA) identifies strains of *S. aureus* that are susceptible or treatable with the traditional beta lactam class of antibiotics, such as penicillin, methicillin, and cephalosporins.

Focus Point

S. aureus infection that is not specified as to whether it is susceptible to or resistant to methicillin is coded as methicillin susceptible.

A49.02   Methicillin resistant Staphylococcus aureus infection, unspecified site

Methicillin-resistant *Staphylococcus aureus* (MRSA) is a variant form of the bacterium that is resistant to the traditional beta lactam class of antibiotics, such as penicillin, methicillin, and cephalosporins. Sometimes referred to as a "superbug," MRSA is a major cause of hospital-acquired infections, as well as community-acquired infections. Due to clinical challenges, MRSA is more difficult and costly to combat than methicillin susceptible Staphylococcus aureus) MSSA, and generally poses a greater public health threat due to its multidrug resistance.

A49.1   Streptococcal infection, unspecified site

Streptococcus is one of the more common causes of infectious disease. It is a spherical, gram positive, nonmotile bacterium that clusters together to form chains. The three most common pathogenic species are *S. pyogenes*, also called group A *Streptococcus*; *S. agalactiae*, also called group B *Streptococcus*; and *S. pneumoniae*.

A49.2   Hemophilus influenzae infection, unspecified site

Hemophilus influenza is a bacterium most often associated with respiratory illnesses in infants and young children. There are six classifiable types identified with the letters a through f, as well as a number of unclassifiable types that cause disease in humans. Only one type, *H. influenza* type b (Hib), is preventable with the Hib vaccine.

A49.3   Mycoplasma infection, unspecified site

Mycoplasma bacteria are the smallest free-living (nonparasitic) organisms. This genus of bacteria is also unique in that it lacks a cell wall, a characteristic that makes it resistant to many antimicrobial medications. *Mycoplasma* typically infects mucosal surfaces such as the bronchi, lungs, and urogenital tract.

Infections with a Predominantly Sexual Mode of Transmission (A50-A64)

Infections with a sexual mode of transmission include bacterial infections, such as syphilis, gonorrhea, and chlamydia; viruses, such as herpes; and protozoal infection, such as trichomoniasis.

The categories in this code block are as follows:

A50	Congenital syphilis
A51	Early syphilis
A52	Late syphilis
A53	Other and unspecified syphilis
A54	Gonococcal infection
A55	Chlamydial lymphogranuloma (venereum)
A56	Other sexually transmitted chlamydial diseases
A57	Chancroid
A58	Granuloma inguinale
A59	Trichomoniasis
A60	Anogenital herpesviral [herpes simplex] infections
A63	Other predominantly sexually transmitted diseases, not elsewhere classified
A64	Unspecified sexually transmitted disease

A50.-   Congenital syphilis

Congenital syphilis is atypical in mode of transmission compared to acquired syphilis and the other sexually transmitted diseases in this code block. Although the causative organism is the same, *Treponema pallidum*, this bacteria is passed from an infected mother to her fetus, during the birth process or during development in the womb. Symptoms may not develop in some neonates, so diagnosis in the hospital nursery is usually the result of tests performed on the infant because of the mother's medical history. Congenital syphilis codes are classified as early or late and then as symptomatic (with manifestations) or latent (without clinical manifestations).

A50.0-   Early congenital syphilis, symptomatic

Early congenital syphilis usually manifests before 3 months of age, but if the condition is documented as early syphilis or occurs within two years of birth, it is classified here. Initial symptoms include a rash on the patient's palms and soles, swollen lymph glands, an enlarged spleen, and/or characteristic syphilitic chancres near mucous membranes. Syphilis is confirmed with serologic tests and responds to antibiotic treatment.

A50.01   Early congenital syphilitic oculopathy

Oculopathy refers to any manifestation of congenital syphilis that affects the eyes. The most common manifestation is iritis, inflammation of the iris. Other ocular manifestations occurring in early congenital syphilis include chorioretinitis, retinitis, dacryocystitis, iritis, and uveitis.

> **Focus Point**
>
> When the ocular manifestation is specified as chorioretinitis or retinitis, use code H32 Chorioretinal disorders in diseases classified elsewhere, to identify the manifestation.

A50.02   Early congenital syphilitic osteochondropathy

Osteochondropathy, as it relates to congenital syphilis, is any manifestation that affects the bones, cartilage, or joints, with most occurring in the bones. Typical manifestations include bone caries, epiphysitis, osteochondritis, osteochondrosis, osteomyelitis, oxycephaly, periostitis, and synovitis. Osteochondritis, defined as inflammation of the bone and the articular cartilage, largely affects the humerus and femur. Wegner's and Parrot's disease are two common osteochondrotic conditions. Bone caries refers to any destructive disease of the bone characterized by loss of bone tissue resulting in holes or lesions in the bone. Epiphysitis is an inflammation of the growth plates found at the ends of the long bones. Osteochondrosis refers to degenerative changes in the ossification centers of the bone that sometimes results in necrosis (death) of the bone tissue. Osteomyelitis is an inflammation of the bone marrow and surrounding bone tissue. Oxycephaly is a condition affecting the skull that is caused by early closure of the lambdoid and coronal sutures resulting in a narrow, pointed shape at the top of the skull. Periostitis is an inflammation of the periosteum, which is the outer layer of the bone. Synovitis is an inflammation of the synovial tissue that lines the joints.

A50.03   Early congenital syphilitic pharyngitis

Pharyngitis, laryngitis, and laryngotracheitis are categorized here and characterized by inflammation of the mucous membranes in the throat and/or larynx.

A50.05   Early congenital syphilitic rhinitis

Rhinitis is one of the more common manifestations of early congenital syphilis and is characterized by inflammation of the mucous membranes of the nose with secretion of mucus that is often bloody.

A50.06   Early cutaneous congenital syphilis

One of the more common early symptoms of congenital syphilis is a rash that is most severe on the palms of the hands and soles of the feet. The rash typically begins as small dark red or copper spots that fade to a dusky red or a pale copper color. There may also be a more extensive measles-like rash or nickel- and dime-sized skin lesions. Syphilitic pemphigus, blistering (bullae) of the skin of distal extremities, is also captured here.

A50.07   Early mucocutaneous congenital syphilis

Mucocutaneous lesions can take several forms, including white patches in the mucous membranes, buboes or blistering, and chancres.

A50.08   Early visceral congenital syphilis

Visceral manifestations typically involve the peritoneum (peritonitis), spleen (splenomegaly), and/ or liver (hepatitis or hepatomegaly).

A50.09   Other early congenital syphilis, symptomatic

This code captures other manifestations such as blood disorders, bulging fontanelle, seizures, and cranial nerve deficits.

A50.1   Early congenital syphilis, latent

Latent early congenital syphilis has no clinical manifestations and spinal fluid tests are negative for the bacterium. It is diagnosed solely by a positive serologic reaction on laboratory testing.

A50.3-   Late congenital syphilitic oculopathy

Congenital syphilis diagnosed at 2 years of age or later is classified as late congenital syphilis. Oculopathy refers to any manifestation of congenital syphilis that affects the eyes.

A50.31   Late congenital syphilitic interstitial keratitis

Interstitial keratitis is one of the more common late manifestations of congenital syphilis. It is characterized by inflammation of the stroma (connective tissue) of the cornea thought to be due to an immune response to antigens found in the bacterium *Treponema pallidum*, which causes syphilis.

A50.32   Late congenital syphilitic chorioretinitis

Chorioretinitis is an inflammation of the retina that extends into the choroid. The retina is the light sensitive layer of the posterior segment of the eye that converts images to electric signals that are then processed by the brain. The choroid is the vascular layer of the posterior segment of the eye.

A50.39   Other late congenital syphilitic oculopathy

Other specified ocular manifestations are reported here such as inflammation of the cornea and iris (keratoiritis) and displacement (luxation) of the lens.

A50.4-   Late congenital neurosyphilis [juvenile neurosyphilis]

Neurosyphilis is a central nervous system infection. A diagnosis of neurosyphilis requires only a positive spinal fluid test for the bacterium *Treponema pallidum*, although nervous system manifestations may also be present.

A50.41   Late congenital syphilitic meningitis

Syphilitic meningitis is an inflammation of the membranes covering the spinal cord and brain. A positive spinal fluid test for *T. pallidum*, even in the absence of other symptoms indicative of meningitis, is classified as syphilitic meningitis. Common symptoms of meningitis include headache, fever, neck stiffness, vomiting, photophobia, and cranial nerve abnormalities.

A50.42   Late congenital syphilitic encephalitis

Encephalitis is an inflammation of brain tissue and is characterized by fever, seizures, mental status changes, progressive intellectual deterioration, and other neurological signs and symptoms.

A50.43   Late congenital syphilitic polyneuropathy

Polyneuropathy may affect the cranial and/or peripheral nerves. Common sympathetic nervous system symptoms are altered sensation, pain, and weakness. Common autonomic nervous system symptoms are bowel and bladder control changes, orthostatic hypotension, and increased or decreased sweating.

A50.44   Late congenital syphilitic optic nerve atrophy

Optic nerve atrophy in congenital neurosyphilis is rare. Symptoms include a loss of visual acuity, loss of central and/or peripheral vision, and loss of color vision with eventual blindness if the congenital syphilis is not treated. Once damage to the optic nerve occurs it is irreversible. Treatment is aimed at preventing additional damage to the nerve.

A50.5-   Other late congenital syphilis, symptomatic

Other manifestations of late congenital syphilis include Clutton's joints and other bone and joint disorders, saddle nose, Hutchinson's teeth, Hutchinson's triad, and cardiovascular manifestations.

A50.51 Clutton's joints

Clutton's joints are characterized by bilateral and symmetrical joint effusion with synovial thickening but without bone involvement. The knees are most often affected, but the condition may also affect the elbows and/or ankles.

Focus Point

In late congenital syphilis, joint effusion, also called hydrarthrosis, without a specific diagnosis of Clutton's joints, is reported with code A50.55 Late congenital syphilitic arthropathy.

A50.52 Hutchinson's teeth

One of the more common manifestations of late congenital syphilis are deformities of the teeth, specifically the upper incisors, in which the teeth are wider at the top (near the gum line) and narrower at the bottom with a crescent-shaped notch.

A50.53 Hutchinson's triad

Hutchinson's triad, a typical manifestation of late congenital syphilis, is comprised of interstitial keratitis, Hutchinson's teeth, and eighth cranial nerve deafness. Interstitial keratitis is characterized by inflammation of the stroma (connective tissue) of the cornea thought to be due to an immune response to antigens found in the bacterium *Treponema pallidum*, which causes syphilis. Hutchinson's teeth are characterized by deformities of the upper incisors, in which the teeth are wider at the top (near the gum line) and narrower at the bottom with a crescent-shaped notch. Eighth cranial nerve deafness in congenital syphilis is a sudden onset sensorineural type that usually occurs between the ages of 8 and 10 years.

A50.54 Late congenital cardiovascular syphilis

Manifestations of late congenital cardiovascular syphilis include aortitis, aortic aneurysm, endarteritis, narrowing of the coronary arteries, as well as other forms of cardiovascular disease.

A50.55 Late congenital syphilitic arthropathy

Manifestations of late congenital syphilitic arthropathy include arthritis and hydrarthrosis when the hydrarthrosis is not more specifically documented as Clutton's joints.

A50.56 Late congenital syphilitic osteochondropathy

Manifestations of late congenital syphilitic osteochondropathy include saber tibia, craniotabes, kyphosis, as well as other conditions affecting the bones and cartilage.

A50.57 Syphilitic saddle nose

Syphilitic saddle nose deformity is caused by collapse of the bridge of the nose due to damage to the septal cartilage.

A50.59 Other late congenital syphilis, symptomatic

Conditions due to late congenital syphilis that do not have a more specific code are classified here, including Dubois' disease or abscess, glomerulonephritis, nephritis, gumma, hepatitis, laryngitis, laryngotracheitis, stenosis or stricture of the larynx, leontiasis, sarcocele, esophageal stenosis or stricture, stigmata congenital syphilis, nasal (nares) stricture, and syphiloma.

A50.6 Late congenital syphilis, latent

Latent late congenital syphilis has no clinical manifestations and spinal fluid tests are negative for the bacterium *Treponema pallidum*. The presence of latent late congenital syphilis is diagnosed solely by a positive serologic reaction on laboratory testing.

Focus Point

If a test of spinal fluid is positive for syphilis, the disease is not considered latent, even if the patient does not show symptoms. Instead, the condition is reported as late congenital syphilitic meningitis (A50.41).

A51.- Early syphilis

Early syphilis, unlike congenital syphilis, is transmitted person to person via direct contact with a syphilitic sore or chancre. Caused by the spirochete *Treponema pallidum,* early syphilis is divided into three stages: primary, secondary and latent. Spread of the disease can occur during the primary and secondary stages, but individuals are not contagious when in the latent stage.

A51.0 Primary genital syphilis

A51.1 Primary anal syphilis

A51.2 Primary syphilis of other sites

In primary syphilis, one or more painless chancres appear. The location of the chancre often represents the entry point of the bacteria, with typical locations being the genital or anal areas. Less often these sores may form on the lips, hand, or even the eyes.

A51.3- Secondary syphilis of skin and mucous membranes

A skin rash typically marks the start of secondary syphilis, largely appearing on the soles of the feet or palms of the hands. In addition to skin changes, fever, swollen lymph glands, patchy hair loss, headaches, and fatigue may also be present.

A51.5   Early syphilis, latent

Latent early syphilis has no clinical manifestations and negative spinal fluid tests for syphilis. To be classified as early latent syphilis, the positive serologic test is obtained within the first year of infection.

Focus Point

If at any point within the first two years of infection a test of spinal fluid is positive for syphilis, the disease is not considered early latent syphilis, even if the patient does not show symptoms. Instead, the condition is reported as secondary syphilitic meningitis (A51.41).

A52.-   Late syphilis

The late or tertiary stage of syphilis is characterized by significant and irreversible organ damage but is no longer contagious. Progression to this stage only occurs when the syphilis is left untreated throughout the early stages of the disease.

A52.0-   Cardiovascular and cerebrovascular syphilis

Codes in this subcategory are reported for acquired late syphilitic infection with cardiovascular or cerebrovascular manifestations. Manifestations are classified by site (e.g., aorta, heart, cerebral arteries) and specific manifestation (e.g., arteritis, aneurysm, endocarditis, other heart conditions). Clinical diagnosis of cardiovascular manifestations due to late syphilis is based on echocardiography (ECG) and a positive serologic test for syphilis.

A52.8   Late syphilis, latent

When symptoms related to syphilis are no longer present and spinal fluid tests are or remain negative, the disease is considered to be in a latent phase. To be classified as late latent syphilis, the positive serologic test is obtained two or more years after infection. Latent syphilis may remain asymptomatic for years.

Focus Point

If a test of spinal fluid is positive for syphilis two or more years after the initial infection, the disease is not considered late latent syphilis, even if the patient does not show symptoms. Instead, the condition is reported as late syphilitic meningitis (A52.13).

A54.-   Gonococcal infection

Gonorrhea is a bacterial infection caused by *Neisseria gonorrhoeae*. Women are often asymptomatic, while men tend to develop urinary symptoms rather quickly. Diagnosis is based on bacteriologic examination of vaginal or penile discharge or urine. Gonorrhea responds to antibiotic treatment, though several courses may be required to eradicate the disease. Gonococcal infection is classified by site. The genitourinary tract is the most common site and codes for the genitourinary tract are assigned based on site-specific manifestations. Specific codes are also available for gonococcal infections of other sites, including the eye, musculoskeletal system, throat, anus and rectum, brain and meninges, heart, lungs, and peritoneum, and infections of these sites are also assigned based on manifestation. Gonococcal infection can also cause sepsis, which is included in this category.

A54.0-   Gonococcal infection of lower genitourinary tract without periurethral or accessory gland abscess

Codes for gonococcal infection without periurethral or accessory gland abscess are specific to sites in the lower urinary tract. Symptoms in men and women include pain or burning on urination and urinary frequency or urgency. Men may also have purulent drainage from the urethra, while women may have purulent vaginal discharge.

A54.01   Gonococcal cystitis and urethritis, unspecified

This code reports *N.* gonorrhoeae infection limited to the bladder (cystitis) and urethra (urethritis).

A54.02   Gonococcal vulvovaginitis, unspecified

This code reports *N. gonorrhoeae* infection limited to the vulva and vagina.

A54.03   Gonococcal cervicitis, unspecified

This code reports *N. gonorrhoeae* infection limited to the uterine cervix (cervicitis), which is the most common site of initial infection in women.

A54.09   Other gonococcal infection of lower genitourinary tract

This code includes *N. gonorrhoeae* infection of the penis, including specific sites such as the glans penis or the foreskin and glans penis in uncircumcised males. Manifestations including balanitis (inflammation of the glans penis), balanoposthitis (inflammation of the foreskin and glans), or chordee (curvature of the penis) due to the infection are also coded here.

A54.1   Gonococcal infection of lower genitourinary tract with periurethral and accessory gland abscess

The lower genitourinary tract includes the bladder and urethra in men and women and the cervix, vagina, and vulva in the women. Infections of the lower genitourinary tract can be complicated by an abscess, which is a collection of pus around the urethra or affecting the Bartholin's gland in women or the Cowper's gland in men. The site of the abscess is painful with redness and inflammation of the surrounding soft tissue.

A54.2- Gonococcal pelviperitonitis and other gonococcal genitourinary infection

Infections of the upper urinary tract, which includes the kidney and ureter, as well as the prostate and female pelvis, are included in this subcategory.

A54.21 Gonococcal infection of kidney and ureter

Infection of the kidney and ureters typically occurs when the initial infection is not treated and the infection spreads from the lower urinary tract to the upper urinary tract. Symptoms include fever; pain in the back, flank, groin, or abdomen; pain or burning on urination and urinary frequency or urgency; pus or blood in the urine; and dark-colored or cloudy urine with a foul odor.

A54.22 Gonococcal prostatitis

Prostatitis is inflammation of the prostate, in this case related to gonococcal infection. It typically occurs when an initial infection in the lower genitourinary tract is left untreated and spreads. Symptoms of gonococcal abscess of the prostate include fever, painful defecation, and difficulty urinating.

A54.23 Gonococcal infection of other male genital organs

Infection of male genital organs, excluding the prostate, penis, and foreskin, is reported here. Infection of the epididymis and testes usually result from an untreated or unsuccessfully treated prostate infection of more than a month's duration. *N. gonorrhoeae* bacteria travel from the prostate to these sites causing pain and inflammation of the epididymis, testes, and scrotum. Infection of the epididymis can result in scarring and obstruction of the flow of sperm.

A54.24 Gonococcal female pelvic inflammatory disease

In gonococcal female PID, the infection spreads from the lower genitourinary tract to the uterus, fallopian tubes, ovaries, and peritoneum causing inflammation of the endometrium of the uterus (endometritis), inflammation of the fallopian tubes (salpingitis), tubo-ovarian abscesses, and/or inflammation of the peritoneum (peritonitis). Symptoms include fever, pelvic pain, and mucopurulent cervical or vaginal discharge.

A54.3- Gonococcal infection of eye

Gonococcal infection of the eye typically occurs during sexual contact but may also be transmitted during nonintimate contact with an infected individual. In newborns, the infection is transmitted from the mother during the birth process as the newborn passes through the infected birth canal. *N. gonorrhoeae* infections of the eye are classified based on manifestation.

A54.31 Gonococcal conjunctivitis

Following exposure and infection with *N. gonorrhoeae*, there is a two to seven day incubation period after which conjunctival inflammation, characterized by redness and a foreign body feeling in the eye, develops. There may be purulent drainage from the eye along with subconjunctival hemorrhage. Conjunctivitis is the most common manifestation of gonococcal infection in newborns.

A54.32 Gonococcal iridocyclitis

Iridocyclitis is an infection or inflammation of the iris and ciliary body, also referred to as anterior uveitis. It is exhibited by a red painful eye, sensitivity to light (photophobia), and tearing or drainage from the eye.

A54.33 Gonococcal keratitis

Keratitis is inflammation of the cornea. Keratitis due to *Neisseria gonorrhoeae* may involve the epithelial layer only or may affect the deeper tissues in which case it is called stromal or interstitial keratitis. Symptoms include inflammation and ulcerations of the cornea.

A54.39 Other gonococcal eye infection

Two manifestations classified here are blepharopyorrhea and endophthalmitis. Blepharopyorrhea is an infection and inflammation of the eyelids with purulent drainage. Endophthalmitis is a generalized inflammation of intraocular tissues.

A54.4- Gonococcal infection of musculoskeletal system

Untreated gonorrhea may become disseminated, spreading to other areas within the body, and the musculoskeletal system is a common secondary site. The musculoskeletal system is made up of bones, tendons, cartilage, ligaments, connective tissue, muscles, and joints.

A54.41 Gonococcal spondylopathy

Spondylopathy is a general term that refers to a nonspecific disease or condition affecting the vertebrae and associated tendons and ligaments. Symptoms of spondylopathy include pain and stiffness.

A54.42 Gonococcal arthritis

Two of the more common musculoskeletal system manifestations related to gonococcal infection include migratory polyarthritis and localized septic arthritis. Migratory polyarthritis usually presents with pain and inflammation in one or more joints that moves from joint to joint. The wrists, elbows, and ankles are most often affected but usually not symmetric. Septic arthritis presents with redness over the affected joint with pain and swelling. Often only one joint is affected with the knees being the most common site.

A54.43 Gonococcal osteomyelitis

This condition is defined as inflammation of the bone marrow and surrounding bone tissue secondary to gonococcal infection.

A54.49 Gonococcal infection of other musculoskeletal tissue

Bursitis is inflammation of a fluid-filled synovial sac that protects joint structures. Myositis is inflammation of muscle tissue. Synovitis is inflammation of the synovial tissue that lines the joints. Tenosynovitis is inflammation of the tendon and tendon sheath that typically presents with pain, swelling, and stiffness. Tenosynovitis symptoms may affect one or more joints but affected joints are typically asymmetric. Joints of the wrist and hand are most often affected.

A54.5 Gonococcal pharyngitis

Neisseria gonorrhoeae infection of the throat typically occurs due to oral contact with the genitourinary tract of an infected person. A sore throat (pharyngitis) may be present or the patient may be asymptomatic. Gonococcal pharyngitis may resolve on its own without antibiotic treatment.

A54.6 Gonococcal infection of anus and rectum

Any anal contact with a person infected with gonorrhea, including intercourse with or without penetration, may result in the spread of the infection. Vaginal discharge or menstrual blood containing *N. gonorrhoeae* coming in contact with the anal region can also spread infection. Symptoms are often not present but may include itching, bleeding, and abnormal rectal discharge.

A54.8- Other gonococcal infections

Typically transmitted via sexual contact, gonorrhea is largely a bacterial infection of the genitourinary tract. If left untreated, gonococcal infection may become disseminated resulting in sepsis or an infection of a remote site including the brain, cerebral and spinal meninges, heart, lungs, or peritoneum.

A54.81 Gonococcal meningitis

In rare instances, an untreated gonococcal infection may spread via the bloodstream to the cerebral and spinal meninges causing meningitis. Symptoms of gonococcal meningitis include fever, headache, stiff neck, nausea, vomiting, confusion or other symptoms of altered mental status, and sensitivity to bright light. Diagnosis is by spinal puncture to obtain cerebrospinal fluid sample for bacteriologic evaluation.

A54.82 Gonococcal brain abscess

A brain abscess is a rare complication of untreated gonococcal infection. Symptoms may include fever, headache, cranial and peripheral nerve symptoms, nausea, vomiting, confusion or other symptoms of altered mental status, seizures, and vision changes.

Diagnosis of a brain abscess requires CT or MRI scan of the brain and identification of the causative organism requires aspiration of the abscess, which is usually performed using radiologic guidance techniques along with laboratory analysis of the aspirate.

A54.83 Gonococcal heart infection

In very rare instances, an untreated gonococcal infection may spread via the bloodstream to the heart. The infection may affect the inner lining of the heart wall and heart valves (endocarditis), the heart muscle (myocarditis) or the membrane that covers the heart (pericarditis). Symptoms of heart involvement may be nonspecific and include fever, chills, night sweats, and malaise. Atypical chest pain along with respiratory symptoms such as cough and shortness of breath may also be present. Development of a new onset heart murmur along with these symptoms may suggest endocarditis. Untreated endocarditis can cause severe, life-threatening valvular damage.

A54.84 Gonococcal pneumonia

Gonococcal pneumonia, although rare, is a consequence of an untreated gonococcal infection that has spread via the bloodstream to the lungs.

A54.85 Gonococcal peritonitis

In women, untreated gonorrhea of the fallopian tubes may spread beyond the pelvic organs and pelvic peritoneum to the upper abdomen resulting in inflammation of the peritoneum covering the abdominal cavity and the visceral peritoneum covering the abdominal organs. Gonococcal peritonitis is typically diagnosed based on the presence of a current acute gonococcal infection or a history of gonococcal female pelvic inflammatory disease, along with symptoms of upper abdominal pain, fever, chills, night sweats, nausea, and vomiting. A common presentation of gonococcal peritonitis is Fitzhugh-Curtis (Fitz-Hugh-Curtis) syndrome. This syndrome is characterized by inflammation of the liver capsule with adhesions between the liver and anterior abdominal wall. The primary symptom of Fitzhugh-Curtis syndrome is right upper quadrant pain described as sharp or pleuritic in nature.

> **Focus Point**
>
> *Fitzhugh-Curtis syndrome is classified to two different codes depending on the causal infection. Infection caused by Neisseria gonorrhoeae is classified to code A54.85 Gonococcal peritonitis. Infection caused by Chlamydia trachomatis is classified to A74.81 Chlamydial peritonitis.*

A54.86 Gonococcal sepsis

In rare instances, *N. gonorrhoeae* bacteria from an untreated infection may enter the bloodstream resulting in sepsis. Sepsis is a systemic response caused by an infection resulting in certain changes in body temperature, heart rate, respiratory rate or arterial blood gases, and white blood cell counts. More specifically, these include elevated body temperature (usually above 101 degrees Fahrenheit) or subnormal body temperature (usually below 96.8 degrees Fahrenheit), elevated heart rate (usually above 90 beats per minute), elevated respiratory rate (usually above 20 breaths per minute) or arterial blood gases reflecting a reduced partial pressure of carbon dioxide PACO2, and an abnormal white blood cell count above 12,000 cells/microliter or below 4,000 cells/microliter or greater than 10 percent bands (immature white blood cells). Two or more of these indications and a suspected or known gonococcal infection are indicative of sepsis.

A54.89   Other gonococcal infections

Gonococcal keratoderma presents with skin lesions most often found on the extremities. The lesions begin as small raised lesions that become filled with pus. Infection of the lymph system typically presents as inflammation of the lymph nodes or what is referred to as Gonococcal lymphadenitis.

A55   Chlamydial lymphogranuloma (venereum)

Chlamydial lymphogranuloma is a manifestation of *Chlamydia trachomatis* characterized by ulcers at the site of infection and inguinal and femoral lymphadenopathy. The infection is endemic to Africa, Southeast Asia, India, the Caribbean, and South America. It has been diagnosed in the United States and Canada, Europe, and the United Kingdom, although it is quite rare in these regions. The first stage of infection is characterized by a small, painless papule presenting at the site of inoculation from three to 30 days after initial infection. If untreated during the initial stage, secondary infection occurs two to six weeks later with the primary symptom being painful, enlarged inguinal and/or femoral lymph nodes. There may be systemic spread of the infection to the joints, eyes, heart, lungs, meninges, or liver. Men are typically diagnosed at the second stage of the infection. Women may not have any recognizable symptoms at the first or second stage and so progress to the third stage. In the third stage, called the genitoanorectal stage, painful buboes develop in the genital, anal, and/or rectal region, and often rupture with resulting bloody purulent drainage.

A56.-   Other sexually transmitted chlamydial diseases

The most common sexually transmitted disease in the United States is chlamydial infection caused by *Chlamydia trachomatis*. Sexually transmitted *C. trachomatis* infects the columnar epithelium of the mucous membranes of the genitourinary tract, anus and rectum, and throat. The most common manifestation is urethritis, although most infections are asymptomatic. Men and women with untreated chlamydial infections can experience serious complications including infertility. Women are at higher risk of infection than men and in women infections are most common in sexually active adolescents ages 15 to 19 and in the 20 to 24 year age range. For this reason, routine screening of sexually active women under the age of 25 is recommended as is screening of all pregnant women and women at higher risk for infection.

A56.0-   Chlamydial infection of lower genitourinary tract

C. trachomatis infections of the urethra, bladder, vulva, vagina, and uterine cervix are classified here. The urethra is the most common site of infection in men while in women it most often occurs in the vagina.

A56.01   Chlamydial cystitis and urethritis

The bladder and urethra are common sites of chlamydial infection. In fact, at least 50 percent of nongonococcal urethritis cases in the United States are due to *C. trachomatis*. Chlamydial infection of the bladder or urethra may be asymptomatic or may present with common signs and symptoms of lower urinary tract infection, including urinary frequency and pain and burning on urination.

A56.02   Chlamydial vulvovaginitis

Vulvovaginitis is the most common manifestation of chlamydial infection in women. Most of the time, the infection is asymptomatic. However, when symptoms are present they include vaginal discharge, vaginal bleeding particularly following intercourse, and painful urination.

A56.09   Other chlamydial infection of lower genitourinary tract

Chlamydial cervicitis is classified here. Like other manifestations it is often asymptomatic, but poses significant risk of complications when untreated, including the development of pelvic inflammatory disease and in pregnant women the risk for premature rupture of membranes and other risks to the fetus.

A56.1-   Chlamydial infection of pelviperitoneum and other genitourinary organs

The pelviperitoneum includes the uterus, tubes, ovaries, and the lower peritoneum in women. Other genitourinary sites include the testes and epididymis in men.

A56.11   Chlamydial female pelvic inflammatory disease

In chlamydial female pelvic inflammatory disease (PID), the infection spreads from the lower genitourinary tract to the uterus, fallopian tubes, ovaries, and peritoneum causing inflammation of the endometrium of the uterus (endometritis), inflammation of the Fallopian tubes (salpingitis), and/or inflammation of the peritoneum (peritonitis).

Symptoms include fever, lower abdominal and pelvic pain or tenderness, pain on urination, painful intercourse, irregular menses, and cervical or vaginal discharge or bleeding. Chlamydial PID can cause infertility due to scarring and obstruction of the Fallopian tubes.

> **Focus Point**
>
> *For chlamydial peritonitis, also called Fitz-Hugh (Fitzhugh)-Curtis syndrome, see code A74.81.*

A56.19   Other chlamydial genitourinary infection

C. trachomatis infection in males may result in epididymitis or orchitis. Acute epididymitis develops from an untreated urethral infection that spreads to the epididymis and usually occurs unilaterally. When only the epididymis is involved, there is testicular pain, redness (erythema) of the scrotum, and tenderness and swelling of the epididymis. When infection of the epididymis is untreated, the infection may spread and become generalized in the testis (chlamydial orchitis) and is characterized by increased scrotal pain, swelling, and erythema. Untreated infection can lead to infertility due to disruption of spermatogenesis from the inflammatory process and also due to scarring and blockage of the epididymis.

A56.3   Chlamydial infection of anus and rectum

C. trachomatis infection of the anus or rectum typically occurs due to anal intercourse with an infected person. It may also occur due to anal contact without penetration and in women a secondary infection may occur from vaginal discharge or menstrual blood containing *C. trachomatis* bacteria coming in contact with the anal region.

A56.4   Chlamydial infection of pharynx

Chlamydial infection of the throat may be asymptomatic or may manifest as a sore throat (pharyngitis).

A57   Chancroid

Chancroid is a localized infection by *Haemophilus ducreyi*, causing genital ulcers and infecting the inguinal lymph nodes. Care must be taken to distinguish chancroid infection from herpes simplex infection. This diagnosis is made via cultures or microscopic examination.

A59.-   Trichomoniasis

Trichomonas vaginalis is parasitic flagellated protozoa infestation that is generally sexually transmitted, although transmission by other routes, such as moist, soiled washcloths, has been documented. Infection commonly originates at a urogenital site, such as the vagina, prostate, urethra, or cervix. Most people infected with trichomoniasis are asymptomatic. Those who do present with symptoms often experience white discharge from the genital tract and itching.

A60.-   Anogenital herpesviral [herpes simplex] infections

Herpes simplex is an infection caused by the herpes simplex virus (HSV) and includes two subtypes: HSV-1 and HSV-2. The infection causes multiple clusters of fluid-filled, inflamed blisters on the skin or mucous membranes typically transmitted by direct contact. Although both types can occur anywhere, HSV-1 is commonly seen about the mouth, lips, and conjunctiva. HSV-2 usually affects genitals and is often transmitted through sexual contact. The virus can remain dormant and be reactivated by emotional stress, fever, or photosensitivity. Typically, the virus is localized, and code selection is based on the anogenital anatomy affected.

A63.-   Other predominantly sexually transmitted diseases, not elsewhere classified

Only two codes are available in this category for reporting other STDs: one code is specific to anogenital warts and the other code reports all other STDs that are not classified elsewhere.

A63.0   Anogenital (venereal) warts

Anogenital warts, also called condylomata acuminata, are caused by the human papilloma virus (HPV). Condylomata acuminata are sexually transmitted genital warts and are distinct from other viral warts of other sites. There are more than 100 types of HPV, but most HPV infections that manifest as warts are caused by two types: HPV-6 and HPV-11. Some types of HPV are associated with an increased risk of developing malignant neoplasms of the cervix, vagina, vulva, or penis, but the types that cause anogenital warts pose a low risk for future development of dysplasia and malignancy.

Other Spirochetal Diseases (A65-A69)

Spirochetal diseases are caused by types of bacteria called spirochetes that get their name from their long, thin, coiled, or spiral shape. Another characteristic of spirochetes are axial filaments outside the cell protoplasm but contained within an outer sheath that facilitate movement by allowing the spirochetal bacterium to rotate in place. Not all spirochetes are pathogenic. Those that do cause disease include *Borrelia burgdorferi*, which causes Lyme disease.

The categories in this code block are as follows:

A65	Nonvenereal syphilis
A66	Yaws
A67	Pinta [carate]
A68	Relapsing fevers
A69	Other spirochetal infections

A65   Nonvenereal syphilis

Nonvenereal endemic syphilis is an infection of *Treponema* pallidum *endemicum* found in the Eastern Mediterranean region and Africa. It initially causes skin lesions that may progress to soft tissue and bone lesions.

A66.-   Yaws

Yaws is an infection by *Treponema* pallidum *pertenue* causing lesions of the skin, bone, and soft tissue. Upon infection, a lesion develops at the site where the yaws spirochete entered the body. This lesion is called the "mother yaw." Yaws is endemic to equatorial countries with high humidity, so cases in the United States are limited to travelers.

A67.-   Pinta [carate]

Pinta is an infection by *Treponema* pallidum *carateum* confined to the skin and causing progressive lesions. Pinta is confined to the natives of Mexico and Central and South America, so cases in the United States are limited to travelers.

A68.-   Relapsing fevers

Relapsing fever is an infection caused by *Borrelia*. Symptoms are episodic and may include fever and arthralgia. Code selection is based on the insect vector.

A69.-   Other spirochetal infections

Spirochetes are a type of gram-negative bacteria named for their tightly coiled, spiral shape. Another characteristic of spirochetes is their ability for spontaneous movement (motility), which is accomplished using axial filaments located outside the protoplasm of the cell but enclosed within a sheath that runs the entire length of the cell. These axial filaments rotate in place, which allows the bacterium to move. There are only six genera of spirochetes and, of these, the following cause disease in humans: *Borrelia, Leptospira, Spirochaeta,* and *Treponema*.

A69.0   Necrotizing ulcerative stomatitis

This is a chronic, progressive infection of the mouth caused by spirochetes from the genera *Borrelia* or *Treponema*, along with *Fusobacterium* nucleatum. It is characterized by painful ulcers of the mouth with bleeding, edema of mucosal tissue, increased salivation, and fetid breath.

A69.1   Other Vincent's infections

This code includes ulcerative gingivitis infections with or without pharyngeal involvement. When pharyngeal infection is present, it is referred to as Vincent's angina or *Fusiformis* pharyngitis. Acute ulcerative gingivitis alone is often referred to as Vincent's infection, Vincent's stomatitis, or trench mouth. This painful ulceration caused by fusiform bacteria and spirochetes is poorly understood but causes bleeding, swelling, and sloughing of dead tissue in the mucous membranes of the oral cavity. It is most common in teens and young adults residing in underdeveloped nations and those people with poor dental hygiene.

A69.2-   Lyme disease

Lyme disease is caused by the bite of a tick infected with the bacterium *Borrelia burgdorferi*. It is endemic to most parts of the United States, as well as in Russia, Australia, and the Far East. In the United States, the *Ixodes scapularis* tick, also called the blacklegged or deer tick, carries the disease; the *Ixodes pacificus* tick carries it in the west. There are three recognized stages of infection: an early localized stage, an early disseminated stage, and a late disseminated stage. The initial localized stage lasts from three to 30 days. If the infection is not treated during the localized phase, it becomes disseminated. During the disseminated stages, occurring days to weeks (early disseminated) or months to years (late disseminated) after the initial infection, neurological, musculoskeletal, and/or cardiac complications may occur.

A69.20   Lyme disease, unspecified

The early localized stage is classified here, along with Lyme disease without any documented manifestations. The initial localized stage lasts from three to 30 days following the bite of an infected tick and is characterized by a localized red expanding rash, called erythema migrans, at the site of the tick bite and flu-like symptoms.

A69.21   Meningitis due to Lyme disease

Meningitis due to Lyme disease is often seen in the early disseminated phase and is characterized by headache, stiff neck, sensitivity to bright light, and pain on eye motion. There may also be symptoms of fever, fatigue, nausea, and vomiting.

A69.22   Other neurologic disorders in Lyme disease

There are a number of Lyme disease-related neurological disorders that can occur during the early (days to weeks) and late (month to years) disseminated stages. Neurologic disorders such as encephalitis or meningoencephalitis, cranial neuritis, radiculopathy or radiculitis, and polyneuropathy are typically seen in the early disseminated phase, while late manifestations include encephalopathy and encephalomyelitis with cognitive deficits and psychiatric changes.

A69.23   Arthritis due to Lyme disease

Arthritis may appear during the early disseminated or late disseminated stage. In the early disseminated stage, pain and inflammation occurs in the large joints. This may resolve without treatment but can recur weeks to months later during the late disseminated stage with similar although more severe symptoms of joint pain and swelling in the large joints.

A69.29   Other conditions associated with Lyme disease

Conditions affecting the heart such as inflammation of the heart muscle (myocarditis) and/or the membrane covering the heart (pericarditis) are classified here and usually occur during the early disseminated phase.

A69.8   Other specified spirochetal infections

Castellani's bronchitis and spirochetal pneumonia are included here.

Other Diseases Caused by Chlamydiae (A70-A74)

Chlamydiae are a type of bacteria that requires a host cell in order to reproduce. Bacteria that cannot reproduce without a host are referred to as intracellular obligate bacteria. There are three species, *C. trachomatis*, *C. psittaci*, and *C. pneumoniae*, that cause disease in humans and all three infect mucous epithelial cells. These species often cause deep epithelial tissue damage.

The categories in this code block are as follows:

A70	Chlamydia psittaci infections
A71	Trachoma
A74	Other diseases caused by chlamydiae

A70   Chlamydia psittaci infections

Also called ornithosis or psittacosis, the disease is caused by *Chlamydia psittaci*, transmitted most commonly by parrots, parakeets, or lovebirds. Occasionally domestic birds such as pigeons, turkeys, or canaries, and even some seabirds can also be carriers. Infection usually occurs when dust or

droppings are inhaled by man or, rarely, by a bird bite. Ornithosis can also be transmitted from man to man, but this is very rare. Symptoms include fever, malaise, and cough, in the case of lung infection. Ornithosis has a 30 percent mortality rate without treatment, but responds well to antibiotics.

A71.-   Trachoma

Chlamydia trachomatis is the culprit organism in this chronic eye infection. Occurring worldwide it is primarily seen in rural areas of developing countries where crowding and poor hygiene is common. The condition is rare in the United States. The infection is spread by direct contact with secretions from the eyes, nose, or throat or with objects that are contaminated with these secretions. It can also be spread by some species of flies. The infection begins slowly as a mild conjunctivitis that if untreated develops into a more severe infection that involves the conjunctiva and cornea (keratoconjunctivitis) with symptoms of tearing, itching, mucopurulent drainage, edema, and pain. The infection resolves, but repeated infections occur from early childhood through adulthood, which is the definitive characteristic of trachoma. Eventually progressive scarring of the conjunctiva, deformities of the eyelid, and erosion, scarring, and vascularization of the cornea lead to vision loss and blindness, usually by age 40 to 50.

> **Focus Point**
>
> Trachoma is an eye condition caused by chronic infection of the eye with *Chlamydia trachomatis*. Do not confuse it with *Chlamydial conjunctivitis*, also called paratrachoma, which is a current, acute infection of the eye and is reported with A74.0.

A71.0   Initial stage of trachoma

During the earliest stage of trachoma, called trachoma dubium or suspect trachoma, there are early signs and symptoms to suggest trachoma, such as abrupt onset of conjunctivitis and pain, but there is no evidence of the characteristic follicles beneath the conjunctiva nor is there evidence of corneal involvement. Follicles result from the accumulation of lymphocytes, polymorphonuclear leukocytes, neutrophils, and macrophages that pool together under the conjunctiva. This is followed by a perifollicular stage of trachoma, in which the infection can be definitively diagnosed, but there are still no follicles present nor is there any related corneal damage. The initial stage lasts several weeks.

A71.1   Active stage of trachoma

The active stage of trachoma is represented by conjunctiva and cornea inflammation (keratoconjunctivitis) with symptoms of tearing, itching, mucopurulent drainage, edema, and pain. Follicles are clearly visible as white, yellow, or grey elevations in the conjunctiva. Minute spaces called vacuoles develop in the cornea followed by corneal pannus, which is characterized by the proliferation of fibrovascular connective tissue that causes scarring, vascularization, and opacification of the cornea.

A74.- Other diseases caused by chlamydiae

Chlamydiae are a small group of ovoid-shaped bacteria that require a host cell to provide them with the chemicals necessary for metabolism and reproduction. They can cause infections of the eyes, genital tract, and respiratory tract.

A74.0 Chlamydial conjunctivitis

This is a current acute infection of the conjunctiva due to *Chlamydial trachomatis* characterized by some or all of the following symptoms: persistent redness and inflammation of the conjunctiva, tearing, mucous or mucopurulent discharge, crusting on eyelashes, eyelids sticking together, itching or foreign body sensation, sensitivity to light, and impaired vision. There may also be follicular reaction of the bulbar conjunctiva and semilunar folds. The cornea may show evidence of epithelial infiltrates. The infection is treated with topical or systemic antibiotics.

Focus Point

Chlamydial conjunctivitis, also called paratrachoma, is a current, acute infection of the eye and is reported with A74.0. Do not confuse it with trachoma, which is an eye condition caused by chronic infection with Chlamydia trachomatis, and is reported with codes in category A71.

A74.8- Other chlamydial diseases

Chlamydiae are a small group of ovoid-shaped bacteria that require a host cell to provide them with the chemicals necessary for metabolism and reproduction. Chlamydiae cause infections of the eyes, genital tract, and respiratory tract. Chlamydial peritonitis or Fitzhugh-Curtis (Fitz-Hugh-Curtis) disease that may occur as a complication of pelvic inflammatory disease due to *Chlamydia trachomatis* and other chlamydial diseases that are not specifically excluded from this category are classified here.

A74.81 Chlamydial peritonitis

Chlamydial peritonitis is a complication of female pelvic inflammatory disease caused by *Chlamydia trachomatis* infection. It is characterized by inflammation of the peritoneum, which is the membrane that lines the intraabdominal wall. In some cases, the membrane covering the liver also becomes

inflamed (perihepatitis) causing a condition called Fitzhugh-Curtis disease, which is also classified here. Symptoms include severe upper right quadrant abdominal pain, fever, chills, and headache.

Focus Point

Fitzhugh-Curtis syndrome is classified to two different codes depending on the causal infection. Infection caused by Chlamydia trachomatis is classified to A74.81 Chlamydial peritonitis. Infection caused by Neisseria gonorrhoeae is classified to A54.85 Gonococcal peritonitis.

Rickettsioses (A75-A79)

Rickettsioses are infections caused by bacteria in the Rickettsiaceae family. There are four genuses in this family including *Rickettsia*, Ehrlichia, *Coxiella*, and *Bartonella* and of these four genuses all but *Coxiella* contain two or more pathogenic species. *Coxiella* consists of a single species, *C. burnetii*, that causes Q fever. All bacteria in this family are intracellular obligate parasites, meaning that they require a host cell in order to reproduce. Infections caused by this group of bacteria are spread by arthropod vectors, which include lice, fleas, ticks, and mites.

The categories in this code block are as follows:

A75	Typhus fever
A77	Spotted fever [tick-borne rickettsioses]
A78	Q fever
A79	Other rickettsioses

A75.- Typhus fever

Typhus fever is actually caused by several species of Rickettsia. Each species is spread by specific arthropod vectors and each species causes slightly different symptoms. Epidemic louse-borne fever caused by *R. prowazekii* and flea borne murine fever caused by *R. typhi* occur globally, while other types are limited to specific regions. Infection results from being bit by an infected vector and then scratching the bite, which releases the bacteria into the bloodstream. The predominant feature of typhus fever is a high fever, which is typically accompanied by a rash and headache.

A75.0 Epidemic louse-borne typhus fever due to Rickettsia prowazekii

Rickettsia prowazekii is transmitted by feces from the human body louse (*Pediculus humanus*), through a break in the skin, often from scratching or by entry of the louse droppings into mucous membranes. This infectious disease, also called classical typhus or epidemic typhus, causes headache, rash, and high fever, and is most dangerous to people older than age 50.

A75.1   Recrudescent typhus [Brill's disease]

Brill's disease, also known as Brill-Zinsser disease, is a reoccurrence of epidemic louse-borne typhus fever caused by *Rickettsia prowazekii*. The reoccurrence can occur years to decades after the initial infection and while the exact mechanism of reoccurrence is not known, it may be due to waning immunity, stress, or other factors. Symptoms of recrudescent typhus include fever, headache, muscle aches, and fatigue.

A75.2   Typhus fever due to Rickettsia typhi

This kind of typhus, also called murine typhus, is found worldwide in the tropics and subtropics. It is spread by fleas carried on rodents and domestic animals. All age groups are at risk in these areas but due to a longer incubation period, travelers may not experience symptoms until back home. Outbreaks have been reported in Hawaii, Texas, and California in the United States. Presenting symptoms include severe fever accompanied by rash.

A75.3   Typhus fever due to Rickettsia tsutsugamushi

This infection is generally found outside of the United States in the Asia-Pacific regions, Russia, China, Indonesia, and Australia and is contracted through travel to those areas. Also called scrub typhus or tsutsugamushi fever, it is caused by the chigger carried by rodents or encountered in high grass or brush. Symptoms include fever, headache, and muscle aches and can be accompanied by swelling of lymph nodes and encephalitis.

A77.-   Spotted fever [tick-borne rickettsioses]

These diseases typically begin with a tick bite in which a lesion develops at the site of the bite. This may be called an eschar, or, in boutonneuse fever, a tache noire. Lymphadenopathy, low fever, and a rash usually follow.

A77.0   Spotted fever due to Rickettsia rickettsii

Spotted fever, also called Rocky Mountain spotted fever or Sao Paulo fever, is endemic to the United States.

> **Focus Point**
>
> *Do not confuse spotted fever with Colorado tick fever reported with code A93.2, which is caused by an arbovirus and is also referred to as mountain tick fever or America Mountain fever.*

A77.1   Spotted fever due to Rickettsia conorii

Boutonneuse fever occurs in Africa, India, Europe, the Mideast, and near the Caspian, Black, and Mediterranean seas. Normally, Boutonneuse fever is seen in the United States only among travelers who return with an infection.

A77.2   Spotted fever due to Rickettsia siberica

North Asian tick fever is seen in the United States only among travelers who return with an infection.

A77.3   Spotted fever due to Rickettsia australis

Queensland tick typhus is seen in the United States only among travelers who return with an infection.

A77.4-   Ehrlichiosis

Ehrlichiosis is likely caused by various *Ehrlichia* species and code selection is based on the species. Infection resembles Rocky Mountain spotted fever, without a rash, and illness may extend for weeks or months. The infection responds to antibiotics.

A78   Q fever

Q fever is a rare bacterial infection caused by *Coxiella burnetii*. It normally infects farm animals but can be contracted by people breathing dust contaminated by waste or birth products of the infected animal. Symptoms are flu-like with fevers, chills, muscle aches, and fatigue. Although not all people exposed develop the infection, the risk is higher for pregnant woman where it can cause miscarriage, preterm, or stillborn delivery. A severe form called chronic Q fever develops in a small percentage of people and can lead to endocarditis or death if not treated correctly with prolonged antibiotics. Most at risk for chronic Q fever are the immunosuppressed or those with heart valve disease.

A79.-   Other rickettsioses

These codes include types of rickettsioses spread by arthropod vectors, which are not otherwise classified, such as trench fever, urban fever, and others.

A79.0   Trench fever

Trench fever was named for its discovery in soldiers fighting in trenches during World War I. It is an infection caused by *Bartonella Quintana*, a type of rickettsial organism, and is also called Quintan fever. In modern times, it is most commonly found in homeless or poor populations and referred to as urban fever. Body lice feces are transmitted into the human body via open breaks in the skin, the mucous membrane, contaminated blood or organs received by transfusion and transplantation, or contaminated IV paraphernalia used by drug abusers. Symptoms may include fever, headache, conjunctivitis, rash, and abdominal and bone pain, which may be accompanied by lymphadenopathy, endocarditis, or skin lesions. Patients with weakened immune systems are more likely to develop severe manifestations of the infection that may lead to death.

A79.1   Rickettsialpox due to Rickettsia akari

This is a mild febrile illness caused by *Rickettsia akari*, transmitted through the bites of mites found on mice and other rodents. After the initial eschar at the mite bite, symptoms occur that include fevers, chills, head and muscle aches, and a papulovesicular rash. The symptoms are self-limiting, lasting approximately two to three weeks. It is generally found in heavily populated urban areas, including those in the United States.

Viral and Prion Infections of the Central Nervous System (A80-A89)

Viral infections of the central nervous system (CNS) manifest as flaccid paralysis as seen in poliomyelitis, encephalitis, and meningitis. Some types of CNS viral infections are spread by infected animals or insects, such as rabies. Other types of viral CNS infections are complications of viral infections originating in other sites that then spread to the CNS.

Prion diseases are a family of rare progressive neurodegenerative disorders that affect humans and animals. A prion is an abnormal, transmissible agent that is able to induce abnormal folding of normal cellular prion proteins in the brain, leading to brain damage and the characteristic signs and symptoms of the disease. Prion diseases are usually rapidly progressive and always fatal.

The categories in this code block are as follows:

A80	Acute poliomyelitis
A81	Atypical virus infections of central nervous system
A82	Rabies
A83	Mosquito-borne viral encephalitis
A84	Tick-borne viral encephalitis
A85	Other viral encephalitis, not elsewhere classified
A86	Unspecified viral encephalitis
A87	Viral meningitis
A88	Other viral infections of central nervous system, not elsewhere classified
A89	Unspecified viral infection of central nervous system

A80.-   Acute poliomyelitis

Poliomyelitis is an infectious viral disease of the central nervous system that sometimes results in paralysis. The World Health Organization (WHO) declared the Western Hemisphere polio-free in 1994. Today, polio is most prevalent in areas of Africa, the Middle East, and South Asia. Three types of poliovirus have been identified: the Brunhilde (Type I), Lansing (Type II), and Leon (Type III) strains. Immunity to one strain does not provide protection against the other two. Type I causes 85 percent of paralytic infection, Type II causes 5 percent, and Type III causes 10 percent. Polio enters the body through the digestive tract and spreads along nerve cells to affect various parts of the central nervous system. The incubation period ranges from four days to 35 days. Symptoms include fatigue, headache, fever, vomiting, constipation, and stiffness of the neck. Although polio infection can cause permanent paralysis, nonparalytic cases far outnumber paralytic cases. No drug has proven effective against polio infection, so treatment is symptomatic.

A81.-   Atypical virus infections of central nervous system

Atypical virus infections of the central nervous system include prion diseases, also known as transmissible spongiform encephalopathies (TSE). Prion diseases are a family of rare progressive neurodegenerative disorders that affect humans and animals. A prion is an abnormal, transmissible agent that is able to induce abnormal folding of normal cellular prion proteins in the brain. They are distinguished by long incubation periods, characteristic spongiform changes associated with neuronal loss, and a failure to induce inflammatory response. Some prion diseases affect cervides (hoofed antlered mammals, such as deer), while other forms are specific to humans. Prion diseases are generally characterized by loss of motor control, dementia, paralysis wasting, and eventually death, typically following pneumonia. Upon autopsy, noninflammatory lesions, vacuoles, amyloid protein deposits, and astrogliosis may be present in CNS and/or lymphoid tissue.

> **Focus Point**
>
> *Conditions in category A81 Atypical virus infections of the central nervous system, often include or progress to dementia. An additional code from chapter 5, "Mental, Behavioral and Neurodevelopmental Disorders," subcategory F02.8-, must be reported for the dementia to specify whether it is with or without behavioral disturbance.*

A81.0-   Creutzfeldt-Jakob disease

Creutzfeldt-Jakob disease (CJD) is a rapidly progressive and always fatal form of transmissible spongiform encephalopathy (TSE). While rare, it is the most common type of TSE seen in humans. CJD is typically diagnosed later in life, usually age 60 or older. Infection usually leads to death within one year of onset of illness. Early symptoms include memory loss, psychiatric and behavioral changes, lack of coordination, and visual disturbances. As the disease progresses dementia becomes pronounced and is accompanied by other symptoms, including involuntary movements, extreme lack of coordination, muscle weakness, and blindness. During the late stage of the disease individuals lose the ability to move and speak and eventually become comatose.

A81.01 Variant Creutzfeldt-Jakob disease

Variant Creutzfeldt-Jakob disease (vCJD) was first identified in 1996 in the United Kingdom (UK). It is distinguished from classic CJD by certain clinical and pathologic characteristics. Median age life expectancy is roughly 28 years for vCJD, while classic CJD is around 65. Unlike classic CJD where neurological signs present early, initial symptoms of vCJD are psychiatric and behavioral. The one neurological symptom that is a prominent sign of vCJD is painful dysesthesia, which is a distortion of the sense of touch in which normal stimuli cause abnormal sensations that can range from tingling to mild or excruciating pain. As the disease progresses, additional neurological symptoms appear.

A81.09 Other Creutzfeldt-Jakob disease

Classic Creutzfeldt-Jakob disease (CJD) occurs in many forms, including sporadic (random, isolated occurrences), familial (inherited), or iatrogenic (without known cause). The most common form, sporadic, accounts for 85 percent of all cases. The familial form results from inherited mutations of the prion gene and accounts for 5 to 15 percent of all cases. Classic CJD is typically diagnosed later in life, usually age 60 or older. Infection usually leads to death within one year of onset of illness with median life expectancy after diagnosis of three to four months. Early symptoms include memory loss, behavioral changes, lack of coordination, and visual disturbances. As the disease progresses pronounced dementia is accompanied by other symptoms, including involuntary movements, extreme lack of coordination, muscle weakness, and blindness. During the late stage of the disease, individuals lose the ability to move and speak and eventually become comatose.

A81.1 Subacute sclerosing panencephalitis

Subacute sclerosing panencephalitis (SSPE) is a rare, progressive, and grave disorder, occurring months or years following measles or measles vaccination, usually before age 20. Mental faculties are diminished, seizures occur, and the patient deteriorates until death, usually within three years.

A81.2 Progressive multifocal leukoencephalopathy

Progressive multifocal leukoencephalopathy (PML) is a cerebral cortex infection typically found only in the immunosuppressed population. It is caused by the John Cunningham (JC) polyomavirus, which can be acquired in childhood and is dormant unless an immune system disease such as HIV, systemic lupus erythematosus (SLE), malignancy, or a drug that suppresses the immune system reactivates it. Symptoms include decline of mental capacity,

difficulty speaking, blindness, and gait difficulty. PML carries a mortality rate of 30 percent to 50 percent within three months of diagnosis without treatment. Even with intervention, significant neurological damage may be permanent.

A81.8- Other atypical virus infections of central nervous system

This subcategory includes other types of prion diseases not caused by bacteria, which affect the nervous system. Prion diseases or transmissible spongiform encephalopathies (TSE) are a family of rare progressive neurodegenerative disorders that affect both humans and animals. They are distinguished by long incubation periods, characteristic spongiform changes associated with neuronal loss, and a failure to induce inflammatory response. The causative agent of TSE is believed to be a prion. A prion is an abnormal, transmissible agent that can induce abnormal folding of normal cellular prion proteins in the brain, leading to brain damage and the characteristic signs and symptoms of the disease. Prion diseases are usually rapidly progressive and always fatal. Certain forms included in this subcategory have distinguishing clinical signs and symptoms.

A81.81 Kuru

Although not likely to be seen, it is an interesting prion disease that was prevalent in the 50s and 60s among a tribe in the New Guinea Highlands. It is a fatal neurological disease contracted by eating brains of their kinsmen during funeral rituals or by contact with open wounds of an infected person. The discovery assisted in the scientific research of other, more prevalent modern-day neurodegenerative diseases such as Creutzfeldt-Jakob and Gerstmann-Sträussler-Scheinker disease. Because of its prolonged incubation period, there are still reported rare appearances. As the disease affects the cerebellum, the center of coordination and balance, the symptoms mimic a stroke or Parkinson's disease. Dementia, malnutrition, and death follow.

A81.82 Gerstmann-Straussler-Scheinker syndrome

Gerstmann-Sträussler-Scheinker syndrome (GSS) is caused by mutations in the gene that encodes prion protein (PRNP). These mutations allow abnormal proteins to build up, forming amyloid plaque clumps that damage nerve cells in the brain. GSS occurs typically in patients 40 to 50 years of age and is characterized by cerebellar ataxia with concomitant motor problems. Dementia is less common, and the disease course lasts several years to death. Originally thought to be a familial condition, GSS is now known to occur sporadically, as well.

A81.83 Fatal familial insomnia

Fatal familial insomnia (FFI) is characterized by severe selective atrophy of the thalamus. Inherited genetic mutations can cause susceptibility to disease without apparent infection. FFI presents with characteristic untreatable insomnia and dysautonomia, yet the pathogenesis of the disease is largely unknown. There is no treatment, and death generally follows within 12 to 18 months from the onset of symptoms.

A82.- Rabies

Rabies, or hydrophobia, is an acute infectious disease caused by a neurotropic virus found in the saliva of rabid mammals. Canine vaccination has nearly eliminated canine rabies in the United States and cases of wild animal bites causing rabies are rare. Rabies causes restlessness, fever, excessive salivation, and painful laryngeal spasms. Exposure to rabies is usually treated successfully with immediate local wound cleansing and administration of rabies immune globulin. If the patient develops rabies, the diagnosis is no longer an imminent death sentence. Supportive treatment of respiratory system, circulatory system, and central nervous system complications can result in a positive outcome for the symptomatic rabies patient. Rabies is often described as urban or sylvan, depending on the source of infection.

A82.0 Sylvatic rabies

In sylvatic rabies, the host or infected animal is a wild, as opposed to domesticated, animal. Wild animal hosts in the United States include bats, foxes, raccoons, and skunks.

A82.1 Urban rabies

In urban rabies, the host or infected animal is a domesticated, as opposed to wild, animal. In the past, dogs were the primary domesticated animal host in the United States; however, vaccination has nearly eliminated urban rabies in the United States.

A83.- Mosquito-borne viral encephalitis

Mosquitos are a significant vector of viral illnesses, particularly viruses that can cause inflammation of the brain, what is known as encephalitis. Some mosquito species can harbor several different viruses, but it is largely the geographic location of the mosquito that dictates which virus is transmitted, as many viruses are endemic to only one specific region or area. In fact, the name of the virus often reflects the location to which it is typically found. Codes in this category are largely classified based on this viral nomenclature.

A83.0 Japanese encephalitis

Japanese encephalitis is seen in the Far East. The virus is transmitted from vertebrate hosts, most often pigs or birds to mosquitoes and then to humans. The majority of people infected do not show symptoms or develop only mild symptoms. However, small percentages develop brain inflammation characterized by headache, high fever, disorientation, and confusion, which may rapidly progress to tremors, convulsions, and coma. Approximately 25 percent of symptomatic cases are fatal. Japanese encephalitis is preventable by vaccination, which is recommended prior to travel to regions where the virus is prevalent.

A83.1 Western equine encephalitis

Western equine encephalitis (WEE) is seen in areas west of the Mississippi and is spread primarily by mosquitos from the subspecies *Culex tarsalis*, but may also be spread by the *Aedes* species of mosquitos or less often by small wild animals. Vector mosquitos are found in warm, moist regions and outbreaks generally occur in the summer months. WEE is transmitted from infected wild birds to mosquitos to humans. Initial symptoms include fever, headache, chills, nausea, and vomiting, which may last one to four days, although not all individuals develop these generalized symptoms. Especially for young children and older adults, onset of central nervous system symptoms can cause significant complications, including behavioral problems, seizure disorders, and sensory or motor nerve deficits.

A83.2 Eastern equine encephalitis

Eastern equine encephalitis (EEE) is a viral disease that originates in birds and is transmitted to humans by infected mosquito vectors. It is a rare disease, usually affecting less than 10 people per year. The species of mosquito primarily responsible for spreading this virus, *Culiseta melanura*, is found in the Atlantic and Gulf Coast states, upper New York, and western Michigan where most cases of EEE occur. Neurologic symptoms develop suddenly, and the most common initial symptoms include severe headache, high fever, chills, and vomiting. More severe symptoms often follow, including disorientation and confusion, seizures, and coma. EEE has a mortality rate higher than any other mosquito vector disease in the United States with those who do survive suffering some degree of brain damage.

A83.3 St Louis encephalitis

Birds are hosts for the St. Louis encephalitis virus (SLEV), which is transmitted to humans by several species of the *Culex* genus of mosquito. SLEV usually does not produce clinical symptoms in infected individuals. Severity of symptomatic infections is largely age dependent with older adults, 60 years or older, more likely to present with complications such as encephalitis. While cases of SLEV do occur throughout the United States, it is most common in the central and eastern United States and the Caribbean. Onset of viral symptoms is usually sudden and includes typical flu-like symptoms of fever, headache, dizziness, nausea, and malaise. Some symptomatic individuals go on to develop neurological symptoms, including stiff neck, disorientation and confusion, dizziness, tremors, and coma.

A83.5   California encephalitis

California encephalitis is caused by the La Cross encephalitis virus (LCAV), which is transmitted by the *Aedes triseriatus* mosquito from invertebrate hosts to other invertebrates including humans. Despite being named California encephalitis, the vast majority of cases occur in central and eastern United States, not in California or the west. Following a bite by an infected mosquito, the virus begins replicating at the site of the bite. The virus then enters the bloodstream and seeds reticuloendothelial cells in the liver, spleen, and lymph nodes and begins replicating. The virus enters the bloodstream a second time and seeds sites in the central nervous system. CNS symptoms are generally limited to children, who first develop flu-like symptoms that last for a few days. The early flu-like symptoms are followed by CNS symptoms, which include increased sleepiness (somnolence), seizures, focal neurologic symptoms such as asymmetric reflexes, and coma. Adults are typically asymptomatic or develop mild febrile illness. In most cases, the infection resolves within 10 to 14 days; however, approximately 20 percent of children with CNS symptoms develop epilepsy.

A84.-   Tick-borne viral encephalitis

Diseases transmitted by ticks that cause inflammation of the brain (encephalitis) are classified here. Most tick-borne encephalitis is limited to Russia, Central Europe, and Great Britain. Only Powassan encephalitis is commonly found in North America, both in New York and in Canada. Any other variety diagnosed in the United States is likely to be found among individuals who have traveled to countries where these viruses are prevalent.

A87.-   Viral meningitis

Meningitis is the inflammation of the membranes surrounding the brain or spinal cord, in this case, due to viral infection. Meningitis due to viruses are typically less severe than those caused by bacteria, although in children, the elderly, and individuals with compromised immune systems viral meningitis can cause severe symptoms and may be fatal. Typically, a viral infection of the central nervous system is suspected by default, when a culture fails to grow bacteria. A virus may be isolated in spinal fluid or other tissues, but viruses causing aseptic meningitis is identified in less than half of all cases. Symptomology is generally the same regardless of the inciting virus and include fever, headache, stiff neck (nuchal rigidity), mental status changes such as sleepiness and difficulty being awakened, nausea and vomiting, and sensitivity to light (photophobia) and typically lasts seven to 10 days. Only Powassan encephalitis is commonly found in North America, both in New York and in Canada. Any other variety diagnosed in the United States is likely to be found among individuals who have traveled to countries where these viruses are prevalent.

A87.0   Enteroviral meningitis

Most viral meningitis cases seen in the United States are caused by enteroviruses and are spread by person-to-person contact by fecal contamination or respiratory secretions. Most people who contract an enterovirus do not develop complications such as meningitis and recover without treatment. In severe cases, hospitalization may be required. Two of the more common causative agents of enteroviral meningitis are coxsackie viruses and echoviruses. Coxsackie viruses cause symptoms resembling polio, but without paralysis, and is most commonly seen in children during warm months. Echovirus is an acronym for enteric cytopathic human orphan virus and is also most prevalent during warm months.

A87.1   Adenoviral meningitis

Adenoviral meningitis is seen primarily in immunocompromised patients, especially those with human immunodeficiency virus (HIV) disease.

Arthropod-Borne Viral Fevers and Viral Hemorrhagic Fevers (A90-A99)

Arthropod-borne viral fevers are most often transmitted by mosquitoes, although there are a few types transmitted by other arthropod vectors, such as the tick.

Viral hemorrhagic fevers may also be transmitted by arthropods, most often mosquitos, but some are transmitted by direct person-to-person contact, contact with blood, body fluids, or feces from an infected person, or from contact with an infected animal or the animal's urine or feces. Symptoms vary depending on the infectious agent and the individual. As the title of this code block implies, the common symptom of diseases classified here is a fever.

The categories in this code block are as follows:

A90	Dengue fever [classical dengue]
A91	Dengue hemorrhagic fever
A92	Other mosquito-borne viral fevers
A93	Other arthropod-borne viral fevers, not elsewhere classified
A94	Unspecified arthropod-borne viral fever
A95	Yellow fever
A96	Arenaviral hemorrhagic fever
A98	Other viral hemorrhagic fevers, not elsewhere classified
A99	Unspecified viral hemorrhagic fever

A90 Dengue fever [classical dengue]

Dengue is transmitted to man by the bite of the Aedes mosquito, predominantly the *Aedes aegypti*. A secondary vector, the *Aedes albopictus* mosquito, is mainly found in Asian countries but has spread to the United States and Europe via used tires and other trade goods. The disease is endemic throughout tropical and subtropical regions, and is usually seen in the United States only when people come to this country already infected with the virus. There are four serotypes of Dengue fever: DEN-1, DEN-2, DEN-3, and DEN-4. Infection with one serotype provides lifelong immunity only to that serotype. Infection with one serotype confers only temporary partial immunity to the other serotypes. Classical dengue is characterized by a flu-like illness with fever, chills, headache, backache, and prostration. Joint and leg aches and onset of high fever are rapid. There is no specific treatment and uncomplicated Dengue fever typically resolves on its own.

A91 Dengue hemorrhagic fever

Dengue hemorrhagic fever is caused by the same virus as classical dengue, *Aedes aegypti*, but it is a more severe form of the disease. Dengue is found in most Asian and Latin American countries and in Asian countries may be referred to by the name of the city, country, or region where it is found, such as Bangkok, Philippine, Singapore, Thailand, or Southeast Asia hemorrhagic fever. There are four serotypes of Dengue fever: DEN-1, DEN-2, DEN-3, and DEN-4. Infection with one serotype provides lifelong immunity only to that serotype. Infection with one serotype confers temporary partial immunity to the other serotypes; however, once the partial immunity has worn off, a new infection with another serotype increases the risk of developing the more severe hemorrhagic form of the disease. Dengue hemorrhage fever is characterized by plasma leaking into tissues, fluid accumulation, respiratory distress, severe bleeding, and organ failure. The symptoms of disease progression from classical dengue to dengue hemorrhagic fever include decrease in temperature to below 100°F, severe abdominal pain, persistent vomiting with hematemesis, rapid respiratory rate, bleeding gums, and extreme fatigue. Dengue hemorrhagic fever requires prompt recognition and hospitalization so that the necessary acute care can be provided. The mortality rate can be as high as 10 percent but with proper care this can be reduced to 1 percent.

A92.- Other mosquito-borne viral fevers

Arthropod-borne viral fevers are most often transmitted by mosquitoes. Other viral mosquito-borne fevers are reported here, including West Nile virus.

A92.0 Chikungunya virus disease

Chikungunya is a viral disease spread from human to human by the bite of an infected mosquito. The virus originated in Africa, Asia, and India, but has since spread to Europe and the Americas. Primary symptoms are fever and joint pain, which may be accompanied by headache, muscle pain, swollen joints, rash, nausea, and fatigue.

A92.3- West Nile virus infection

West Nile virus infection is caused by an arbovirus, transmitted to humans by an arthropod; in this case, an infected mosquito. West Nile virus was first isolated 65 years ago in Uganda but was not reported in the continental United States until 1999. It affects humans, birds, and some mammals, including horses, cats, bats, skunks, chipmunks, squirrels, and rabbits. Initial symptoms following infection usually occur after an incubation period of five to 15 days. Symptoms of uncomplicated West Nile virus infection include nausea, vomiting, loss of appetite, malaise, body aches, headache, backache, eye pain, rash, and fever.

A92.31 West Nile virus infection with encephalitis

Half of all individuals infected with West Nile virus experience a neuroinvasive form of the infection with the elderly more likely to experience complications such as encephalitis (inflammation of the brain) or encephalomyelitis (inflammation of the brain and spinal cord).

A92.32 West Nile virus infection with other neurologic manifestation

West Nile virus infection can cause a number of neurological symptoms, including cranial nerve disorders, optic neuritis, radiculitis (polyradiculitis), tremors, convulsions, coma, and paralysis. Typically half of infected individuals experience some form of neurological manifestation.

A92.5 Zika virus disease

Zika virus was first identified in the late 1940s but was not recognized as a public health concern until 2016, when outbreaks began to occur throughout the world. Primary transmission is via an infected *Aedes* species of mosquito. However, the virus can also be spread from an infected mother to her fetus and from an infected individual to his or her sexual partner(s). In adults, symptoms are typical of many other viral infections with the most common symptoms being fever, rash, joint pain, conjunctivitis, muscle pain, and headache. The symptoms are also sometimes mild enough that the individual may not be aware of the infection. The primary cause of concern related to Zika virus infection is the potential for complications, especially those that affect the nervous system. Some individuals who contract the virus develop Guillain-Barré syndrome, although the link between Zika and Guillain-Barré has not yet been definitively confirmed. In female patients who are pregnant, the Zika virus has been linked to severe birth defects, including microcephaly.

Focus Point

Coding based on documentation of possible or suspected Zika virus is limited to only the symptoms present and code Z20.828 Contact with and (suspected) exposure to other viral communicable diseases. Code A92.5 is applicable only when the physician confirms Zika virus.

A93.- Other arthropod-borne viral fevers, not elsewhere classified

Classic vectors for arthropod-borne viral fevers include mosquitos and ticks.

A93.2 Colorado tick fever

Colorado tick fever, also referred to as mountain tick fever or America mountain fever, is caused by the arbovirus Colorado tick fever virus. The most common vector of the virus is the adult wood tick. The virus is found primarily in the Rocky Mountain region of the United States and in western Canada in the provinces of British Columbia and Alberta. Symptoms include fever, headache, myalgia, and malaise. Gastrointestinal symptoms of nausea, vomiting, and stomach pain may also be present along with light sensitivity, pharyngitis, and petechial rash. The symptoms, particularly the fever, may occur for several days, resolve, and then recur with greater severity a few days later.

Focus Point

Colorado tick fever should not be confused with Rocky Mountain spotted fever, which is a Rickettsia infection that causes a petechial rash in addition to fever, malaise, headache, and myalgia. Rocky Mountain spotted fever is reported with A77.0.

A95.- Yellow fever

Yellow fever is viral hemorrhagic disease transmitted from mosquito to man and is classified based on the transmission cycle (e.g., animal to mosquito to human, human to mosquito to human). In the United States, cases of yellow fever are usually limited to people who have been abroad. Yellow fever is most commonly seen in Central Africa and South and Central America. Initial presentation includes high fever, headache, loss of appetite, and muscle pain; although for most individuals clinical manifestations do not appear at all. A small percentage of patients who do manifest clinical symptoms may progress to what is known as the toxic stage of the disease. Typically this is when the classic symptoms of jaundice and hemorrhage appear. Mortality rates are also increased during this stage due to related shock and organ failure.

A95.0 Sylvatic yellow fever

Sylvatic yellow fever is transmitted from nonhuman primates to mosquitos and is found in the jungle or woods. It can then be transmitted from mosquitos to man when humans visit or work in the jungles or woods. Sylvatic yellow fever is spread by *Haemagogus* and other forest canopy mosquitoes.

A95.1 Urban yellow fever

Urban yellow fever, spread by the mosquito species *Aedes aegypti*, is usually transmitted from human to mosquito to human in cities or towns.

Viral Infections Characterized by Skin and Mucous Membrane Lesions (B00-B09)

Manifestations of viral infections that cause skin and mucous membrane lesions include rashes, blisters, and warts. Some of these viral infections remain localized to the skin or mucous membranes while others become disseminated causing manifestations and complications that may affect the central nervous system, cardiovascular system, eyes, lungs, as well as other sites.

The categories in this code block are as follows:

B00	Herpesviral [herpes simplex] infections
B01	Varicella [chickenpox]
B02	Zoster [herpes zoster]
B03	Smallpox
B04	Monkeypox
B05	Measles
B06	Rubella [German measles]
B07	Viral warts
B08	Other viral infections characterized by skin and mucous membrane lesions, not elsewhere classified
B09	Unspecified viral infection characterized by skin and mucous membrane lesions

B00.- Herpesviral [herpes simplex] infections

Herpes simplex is an infection caused by the herpes simplex virus (HSV) and includes two subtypes: HSV-1 and HSV-2. The infection causes multiple clusters of fluid-filled, inflamed blisters on the skin or mucous membranes and is usually transmitted by direct contact. HSV-1 is commonly seen about the mouth, lips, and conjunctiva. HSV-2 usually affects genitals and is often transmitted through sexual contact. The virus can remain dormant and be reactivated by emotional stress, fever, or photosensitivity. Typically, the virus is localized, and code selection is based on the site affected. Only herpesviral infections of sites other than the anogenital region are classified here.

B00.0   Eczema herpeticum

Eczema herpeticum is a form of herpes simplex virus infection that affects individuals with atopic dermatitis. It usually occurs only during the initial infection. It is characterized by itchy and/or painful blisters on the skin in areas where atopic dermatitis is or has been present. The most common sites of infection are the face and neck. After the initial outbreak, new patches may continue to appear for seven to 10 days and, in rare instances, the patches may be widely disseminated over the skin surface. The infection is typically accompanied by fever, body aches, headache, and local lymph node inflammation. While most symptoms resolve within several days to a week, the blisters resolve more slowly over a two- to six-week period.

B00.1   Herpesviral vesicular dermatitis

Herpesviral blisters of the skin, also called cold sores, are the most common manifestation related to the herpes simplex virus, with the lips and face being the most common sites of infection. Most people contract the infection during infancy or childhood from an adult who carries the virus. Carriers most often spread the virus when they are not suffering from a current outbreak. The initial infection is commonly accompanied by flu-like symptoms including fever, headache, body aches, and malaise. After the symptoms of the initial infection resolve, the virus remains dormant in the nervous system and subsequent outbreaks, triggered by stressors, can occur. Common stressors that trigger outbreaks include physical stressors such as sun exposure, extreme cold, illness or surgery, or fever; emotional stressors involving family, relationships, work, or school; and in women, hormone changes related to the menstrual cycle.

B00.2   Herpesviral gingivostomatitis and pharyngotonsillitis

Infection of the mouth and gums (gingivostomatitis) or the throat and tonsils (pharyngotonsillitis) is another manifestation of herpes simplex virus infection. Gingivostomatitis is a common manifestation in children presenting as painful blisters or sores of the mouth or gums, in addition to fever, irritability, and refusal of food and/or liquids. The main symptom of pharyngotonsillitis is sore throat due to the blisters or sores. The symptoms usually resolve over one to two weeks.

B00.3   Herpesviral meningitis

Meningitis is inflammation of the membranes that cover the brain and spinal cord. Symptoms of meningitis include fever, light sensitivity, headache, and a stiff neck.

B00.4   Herpesviral encephalitis

Approximately 10 percent of all encephalitis cases are caused by herpes simplex virus 1 or 2. Encephalitis is an infection or inflammation of the brain. Symptoms include those seen in meningitis—fever, light sensitivity, headache, and a stiff neck—along with other neurological symptoms suggesting brain involvement, such as seizures, confusion, personality and behavior changes, sleepiness, and coma.

B00.5-   Herpesviral ocular disease

Both strains of herpes simplex virus, HSV-1 and HSV-2, can cause infections involving the eye and ocular adnexa, but the majority is caused by HSV-1. The infection is spread by direct contact or from the mouth to the eye via the trigeminal nerve. Most symptomatic infections involving the eye are believed to be secondary infections caused by reactivation of the virus in the trigeminal ganglion. The most common manifestations of HSV ocular disease is conjunctivitis.

B00.51   Herpesviral iridocyclitis

Iridocyclitis is an infection or inflammation of the iris and ciliary body, also referred to as anterior uveitis. Iridocyclitis presents with a red painful eye, sensitivity to light (photophobia), and tearing or drainage from the eye.

B00.52   Herpesviral keratitis

Keratitis is an inflammation of the cornea. In herpes simplex virus infections, the inflammation is characterized by dendritic lesions that begin as small raised vesicles in the corneal epithelium and may progress to corneal ulcers. These may eventually penetrate the basement membrane of the corneal epithelium. Further damage, including corneal erosion, persistent corneal epithelial defects, stromal erosion, and necrosis, may occur and may eventually cause corneal blindness. Symptoms of HSV keratitis include pain, sensitivity to bright light, vision changes, redness, and tearing. Aggressive treatment is required to prevent progression of the disease that may result in blindness.

B00.53   Herpesviral conjunctivitis

The most common ocular manifestation of herpesviral infection is conjunctivitis and the most common type of conjunctivitis seen in herpes simplex virus infection (HSV) is follicular. Follicular conjunctivitis is characterized by the development of follicles, which are clumps of lymphocytes that function like miniature lymph nodes in response to the infection. The follicles appear as small yellowish or grayish elevations on the conjunctiva. A less common form is dendritic conjunctivitis, which affects the epithelial cells of the conjunctiva. Both strains of herpes simplex virus, HSV-1 and HSV-2, can cause conjunctivitis, but the majority is caused by HSV-1. The infection is spread by direct contact or from the mouth to the eye via the trigeminal nerve. Most symptomatic infections involving the eye are believed to be secondary infections caused by reactivation of the virus in the trigeminal ganglion.

B00.59   Other herpesviral disease of eye

Herpesviral manifestations affecting the eyelid including dermatitis and blepharitis are included here.

B00.7   Disseminated herpesviral disease

Disseminated herpesviral disease caused by Herpes simplex 1 or 2 (HSV-1 or HSV-2) is a rare occurrence. When disseminated or systemic manifestations do occur, they are typically found in infants or the immunosuppressed. Herpesviral sepsis is one form of disseminated disease. Sepsis is a systemic or body-wide response to an infection, in this case a viral infection. The systemic response is characterized by certain changes in body temperature, heart rate, respiratory rate or arterial blood gases, and white blood cell count. More specifically, these include elevated body temperature (usually above 101 degrees Fahrenheit) or subnormal body temperature (usually below 96.8 degrees Fahrenheit), elevated heart rate (usually above 90 beats per minute), elevated respiratory rate (usually above 20 breaths per minute) or arterial blood gases reflecting a reduced partial pressure of carbon dioxide PACO2, and an abnormal white blood cell count above 12,000 cells/microliter or below 4,000 cells/microliter or greater than 10 percent bands (immature white blood cells). Two or more of these indications and a suspected or known herpesviral infection are indicative of sepsis.

Focus Point

Documentation of viremia due to herpes simplex 1 or 2 is not sufficient to assign a code for disseminated herpesviral infection.

B00.8-   Other forms of herpesviral infections

This subcategory reports other forms of herpesviral infections, including herpesviral hepatitis, herpes simplex myelitis, and herpetic whitlow.

B00.81   Herpesviral hepatitis

Herpesviral hepatitis, infection/inflammation of the liver, is a rare and often fatal complication of herpesviral infection. Those at risk include infants and pregnant women, immunocompromised patients including individuals with HIV/AIDS, cancer patients, patients with myelodysplastic disease, and individuals on steroids. In herpesviral hepatitis, there is typically a rapid onset of symptoms, which include fever, abdominal pain and loss of appetite, nausea, and

vomiting. Diagnosis of herpesviral hepatitis may require a liver biopsy or may be diagnosed based on symptoms and the presence of the virus in the bloodstream.

B00.82   Herpes simplex myelitis

Herpesviral myelitis, an inflammation of the spinal cord, is a rare complication of HSV-1 and HSV-2 infection. Initial symptoms include sensorimotor deficits in the lower body affecting bladder function and sensation and movement in the lower extremities. If the myelitis is an acute ascending type, the spinal cord involvement may ascend to the cervicothoracic region causing additional sensorimotor deficits. If the myelitis is a transverse nonascending type, sensorimotor deficits remain limited to the lower half of the body.

Focus Point

Many patients experience long-term sequelae from herpes simplex myelitis. Coding a sequela of herpes simplex myelitis requires two codes. The condition resulting from the herpes simplex myelitis is reported first, such as G82.22 Paraplegia, incomplete, followed by code B94.8 Sequelae of other specified infectious and parasitic diseases, to identify the incomplete paraplegia as a sequela or late effect of the infection.

B00.89   Other herpesviral infection

Other herpesviral infections reported here include herpetic whitlow and other visceral manifestations. A whitlow is an infection of the skin of the finger, usually occurring over the distal phalanx. Herpetic whitlow is characterized by pain and swelling of the distal aspect of the finger along with fluid-filled lesions. Often systemic symptoms are also present, including fever and malaise. There may also be inflammation of the lymph vessels (lymphangitis) and lymph nodes (lymphangiopathy).

Herpesviral infection of the viscera excluding the liver are also included here. The viscera include internal organs of the digestive system, respiratory system, urogenital system, endocrine system, heart and great vessels, and spleen.

B01.-   Varicella [chickenpox]

Varicella zoster virus (VZV) causes chickenpox and herpes zoster. The initial primary phase of the disease, Chickenpox, is coded here. Chickenpox is highly contagious and usually mild, but it may be severe in infants, adults, or the immunosuppressed. Before introduction of the chickenpox vaccine in 1995, more than four million people were infected with chickenpox each year in the United States alone. Chickenpox has a characteristic itchy rash, which then forms blisters that dry into scabs. An infected person may have anywhere from a few lesions to more than 500 lesions. An adult bout of chickenpox is more likely to have complications than a childhood infection.

Complications occur when the varicella zoster virus inflames the brain, spinal cord, lungs, or other organs; when infection is accompanied by manifestations of high fever; or when the patient is immunosuppressed. Secondary infections are also considered complications.

B01.0   Varicella meningitis

Meningitis is the inflammation of the membranes surrounding the brain or spinal cord, in this case, due to the varicella virus as a complication of chickenpox. Meningitis due to varicella is not a common complication and occurs primarily in individuals with compromised immune systems. Symptoms of meningitis are often severe and may be fatal, including fever, headache, stiff neck (nuchal rigidity), mental status changes such as sleepiness and difficulty being awakened, nausea and vomiting, and sensitivity to light (photophobia).

B01.1-   Varicella encephalitis, myelitis and encephalomyelitis

Encephalitis is an inflammation of brain tissue, myelitis is an inflammation of the spinal cord, and when the inflammation affects both the spinal cord and the brain the term encephalomyelitis is used.

B01.11   Varicella encephalitis and encephalomyelitis

Central nervous system (CNS) complications due to chickenpox are rare, but when they do occur symptoms may be preceded by rash, enlarged parotid gland and lymph nodes (lymphadenopathy), and enlarged liver and spleen (hepatosplenomegaly). Common CNS symptoms of encephalitis include altered mental status, such as altered levels of consciousness, personality and/or behavioral changes, unilateral sensorimotor dysfunction such as hemiparesis, seizures, and autonomic nervous system dysfunction. Pain and stiffness of the neck, sensitivity to bright light (photophobia), and loss of muscle coordination (ataxia) may also be present.

B01.12   Varicella myelitis

Myelitis may present as acute flaccid paralysis involving only one side of the spinal cord with unilateral motor and sensory symptoms, or as acute transverse myelitis where both sides of the spinal cord are involved with bilateral motor and sensory symptoms including urinary bladder symptoms.

B01.2   Varicella pneumonia

Varicella pneumonia is a rare but serious complication of chickenpox that occurs primarily in teenagers and adults. The first symptoms of pneumonia can occur as early as two days to as many as 10 days after the initial chickenpox symptoms of fever and vesicular rash appear. Cough is the most common presenting symptom. Lung infection with the varicella virus is diagnosed based on respiratory symptoms and radiological evidence of pneumonia. Risk of associated acute respiratory failure requiring mechanical ventilation is also a concern. Those at greatest risk for developing varicella pneumonia include individuals with immune system disorders, chronic lung disease, and current or past smokers. The severity of the initial rash and pregnancy may also increase the risk of developing lung infection.

B01.8-   Varicella with other complications

Varicella (chickenpox) begins with an itchy rash, which forms blisters that dry into scabs. It is a highly contagious airborne virus that spreads from person-to-person in respiratory droplets spread by coughing or sneezing. It can also spread from direct contact with the skin lesion or from virus particles from the lesions spreading through the air.

B01.81   Varicella keratitis

Keratitis, an inflammation of the cornea, is a rare complication of chickenpox.

B01.89   Other varicella complications

Two rare complications of chickenpox that are reported here include varicella arthritis and varicella osteomyelitis. Varicella arthritis typically presents as pain and inflammation of a single joint shortly after an acute chickenpox infection. Varicella osteomyelitis presents as bone pain or limb pain following the acute infection.

B02.-   Zoster [herpes zoster]

Varicella zoster virus (VZV) causes chickenpox and herpes zoster. Chickenpox is the initial, acute phase of the disease, and herpes zoster is a reactivation of the virus in a latent stage. Herpes zoster is often referred to as shingles or zona. After resolution of the primary VZV infection, the virus particles lie dormant in nerve ganglia until immune responses decline; this may be due to age, an underlying disease process, an acute illness or other stressor. The latent VZV may then reactivate causing a variety of neurologic manifestations. The disease is classified according to manifestation, the most common of which is a unilateral localized cutaneous eruption along a nerve path.

B02.21   Postherpetic geniculate ganglionitis

Following reactivation of latent VZV along the facial nerve, inflammation of the geniculate ganglion may persist and is referred to as postherpetic geniculate ganglionitis. Ganglions are formed by a collection of nerve cell bodies. The geniculate ganglion is located in the facial nerve at the point after the motor and sensory nerve roots fuse, where the facial nerve bends before exiting the facial canal of the temporal bone. Symptoms of geniculate ganglionitis include deep seated ear pain and pain along the facial nerve, which may progress to include facial paralysis, partial loss of taste, tinnitus, hearing loss, disturbances of balance, vertigo, nystagmus, nausea and vomiting, as well as skin lesions in the ear canal. The condition may also be called aural shingles, Hunt's disease, Hunt's neuralgia, Ramsay-Hunt syndrome or disease, zoster auricularis, or zoster oticus. Gasserian ganglionitis, which is inflammation of the ganglion associated with the trigeminal nerve, is also reported with this code.

B02.22   Postherpetic trigeminal neuralgia

Postherpetic trigeminal neuralgia occurs following reactivation of VZV along the trigeminal nerve. The trigeminal nerve has three branches: the ophthalmic branch, maxillary branch, and mandibular branch. Any one of these branches may be affected, but the most common location is the first or ophthalmic branch. Postherpetic trigeminal neuralgia of the ophthalmic branch is preceded by cutaneous herpes zoster on one side of the forehead or affecting one eye. Following resolution of the cutaneous manifestations, bouts of severe pain along the affected branch of the trigeminal nerve occur. Other sensory disturbances characteristic of postherpetic trigeminal neuralgia include electrical shock sensations, deep facial pain, and burning or aching in the affected region of the face.

B02.24   Postherpetic myelitis

Herpes zoster myelitis, which is inflammation of the spinal cord, is a rare complication of an acute attack of chickenpox. Following this initial infection, the herpes zoster virus becomes dormant in cranial and spinal ganglia in a noninfectious state. The virus later reactivates in a ganglion and causes a localized, unilateral eruption of shingles, or zona, resulting in the neurologic sequela of myelitis, which typically develops days to weeks after the appearance of the rash. Common symptoms of myelitis include loss of spinal cord function, low back pain, weakness of the muscles, or altered sensations in the feet and toes. These symptoms can progress in severity and may include paralysis, urinary retention, and loss of bowel or bladder control.

B02.9   Zoster without complications

Included here is the most common manifestation of a zoster infection, which is a localized cutaneous rash consisting of blisters that scab over as the rash resolves. The rash is unilateral occurring along a nerve path. The rash may be preceded by pain (neuralgia), burning, or itching along the nerve path for several days and these symptoms may persist even after the blisters resolve.

B03   Smallpox

In 1980, the 33rd World Health Assembly declared that smallpox had been eradicated as a result of a worldwide vaccination program. The last case of naturally occurring smallpox in the United States occurred in 1949, and the last case in the world occurred in Somalia in 1977. Vaccination has been discontinued because it is no longer necessary to prevent outbreaks. This classification is maintained for surveillance purposes. The CDC maintains an emergency preparedness plan for smallpox as there is the potential for an outbreak due to bioterrorism. Smallpox is a highly contagious human disease caused by the virus variolae, of which there are two strains: variolae major, which has severe symptoms and a mortality rate of 20 percent to 40 percent; and variolae minor, which has less severe symptoms and a 1 percent mortality rate. Variola major has four recognized types: ordinary, modified, flat, and hemorrhagic. Smallpox is spread by direct person-to-person contact or direct contact with objects contaminated with body fluids from an infected person. It usually begins in the respiratory tract and local lymph nodes and then the virus enters the blood (primary viremia) and internal organs are infected. The virus reenters the blood (secondary viremia) and spreads to the skin. Symptoms appear about 12 days after exposure and mimic a gastrointestinal illness with nausea, vomiting, headache, and backache followed by severe abdominal pain and disorientation. About two to three days after the onset of illness, the true smallpox rash appears. It begins as macules, which enlarge and become raised papules. By the third day, the papules progress into blisters, 6.0 mm in diameter and deep in the skin. In two more days, the fluid inside becomes turbid; the papules shrink and dry up in the skin. Toxemia may cause death before the rash is fully developed, but more commonly death, if it occurs, is between the 11th and 15th day of the rash. In severe cases, the rash may cover the entire body.

B04   Monkeypox

Monkeypox virus is not endemic within the United States but has the potential for importation via infected travelers or imported animals.

B05.-   Measles

Measles is an acute infection caused by paramyxovirus; typical symptoms include high fever, Koplik's spots, generalized rash, and cough. Koplik's spots are white, grainy spots that can occur in the buccal mucosa and are an early symptom of measles. Pharyngitis is also a common symptom. Measles is usually transmitted from person-to-person via airborne respiratory droplets. In the United States, measles outbreaks have been greatly reduced by government immunization programs. Measles has a low mortality rate in healthy individuals; however, measles can make some patients more susceptible to secondary streptococcal infection, worsening of tuberculosis, or reactivation of an inactive mycobacterial infection. Measles are classified according to complication. In most cases, the complication occurs after the symptoms of acute measles infection have diminished.

> **Focus Point**
>
> *German measles (rubella) is a different infection, reported with codes from category B06.*

B05.0 Measles complicated by encephalitis

Postmeasles encephalitis occurs in 1 percent to 2 percent of measles cases with adolescents and adults more apt to develop this complication. Symptoms include abrupt onset of new fever, seizures, mental status changes, and other neurological signs and symptoms. Postmeasles encephalitis is believed to be an abnormal immune response to the measles infection. Postmeasles encephalitis is fatal in up to 25 percent of patients and up to 33 percent of survivors suffer from lifelong neurological sequelae, including blindness and hemiparesis.

B05.1 Measles complicated by meningitis

Meningitis is the inflammation of the membranes surrounding the brain or spinal cord.

B05.2 Measles complicated by pneumonia

During the acute phase of measles, the respiratory tract of most individuals is the primary site of infection. In about 5 percent of measles cases, the respiratory tract infection is complicated by pneumonia. Pneumonia may be due to the measles virus, a secondary viral infection such as herpes simplex virus (HSV) or adenovirus, or a secondary bacterial infection. Postmeasles pneumonia occurs most often in infants, young children, and individuals with compromised immune systems, and is also the most common complication to result in death.

B05.3 Measles complicated by otitis media

Otitis media is the most common complication of measles in young children, affecting approximately 14 percent of children younger than age 5. It is believed that otitis media is caused by inflammation of the eustachian tube resulting from the measles infection, which in turn causes obstruction and secondary bacterial infection of the middle ear. The incidence of otitis media complicating measles decreases with age.

B05.4 Measles with intestinal complications

During the acute phase of measles, the virus infects the intestinal tract of most individuals, but only 8 percent exhibit intestinal complications such as diarrhea. Measles associated diarrhea typically manifests before onset of measles rash and most measles associated diarrhea is believed to be due to the measles virus. Secondary viral or bacterial intestinal infection may cause more severe and more prolonged diarrhea in association with measles infection.

B05.8- Measles with other complications

Other measles related complications classified here include those affecting the eye, respiratory and neurological systems, and other systemic complications.

B05.81 Measles keratitis and keratoconjunctivitis

The measles virus causes conjunctivitis in most measles cases with keratitis being one of the more common ophthalmological complications. Keratitis is an inflammation of the cornea. In most individuals, the corneal inflammation heals without causing long-term damage to the cornea; however, secondary infections and Vitamin A deficiencies can cause severe inflammation resulting in impaired vision due to corneal scarring or blindness.

B05.89 Other measles complications

Other complications such as laryngotracheobronchitis, sometimes referred to as "measles croup," pneumomediastinum, and mediastinal emphysema, are classified here.

B06.- Rubella [German measles]

Rubella, also called German measles or three-day measles, is a highly contagious virus, but the symptoms are mild and short-lived in most people. Rubella during pregnancy, however, can result in abortion, stillbirth, or in congenital defects. Because of its highly contagious nature and effect upon the fetus, rubella is considered a serious health threat. In the United States, rubella outbreaks have been greatly reduced by government immunization programs.

B07.- Viral warts

More than 50 types of human papillomaviruses (HPV) cause viral warts in humans. These infections may be asymptomatic or produce warts or mucosal lesions. Viral warts may also be documented as condyloma, verruca simplex, or verruca vulgaris.

B07.0 Plantar wart

Plantar warts are caused by the human papillomavirus (HPV), which enters the body through tiny cuts and breaks in the skin. They typically occur on the sole, heel, or ball of the foot and occur most often in children and young adults between the ages of 12 and 16. Incidence is higher in people who share common bathing areas (e.g., dormitory students, gym members). According to some literature, plantar warts are responsible for one third of warts. Most plantar warts aren't a serious health concern, but they may be bothersome or painful and can be resistant to treatment. Plantar warts are often mistaken for corns or calluses. They can be identified by the presence of small, fleshy, grainy bumps on the soles of the feet, with hard, flat growths with a rough surface and well-defined boundaries. Gray or brown lumps with one or more black pinpoints of clotted blood vessels may be present. These lesions interrupt the normal lines and ridges in the skin of the feet. Plantar warts can shed the virus into the skin of the foot before they're treated, prompting new warts to grow as fast as the old ones disappear. If untreated, warts can swell and become painful, making it difficult to walk or run.

B07.8   Other viral warts

Common warts are generally found on fingers, hands, knees, and elbows. They are small, hard, dome-shaped bumps that are usually grayish-brown in color. The surface is rough and may resemble cauliflower, with black dots inside. Occasionally warts cause mild pain when on weight bearing surfaces, but usually they are asymptomatic. Flat warts, also called verruca plana and plane warts, are smoother than other types of warts and may grow in clusters with flat tops. Some may appear as skin colored papules, others can be pink, light brown, or yellow. They are usually found on the face, but they can also grow on arms, knees, or hands. They are typically asymptomatic, but can be difficult to treat.

Also reported here is a rare inherited disorder called epidermodysplasia verruciformis characterized by chronic HPV infection with multiple lesions of varying shapes and sizes that have a tendency to become malignant.

B08.-   Other viral infections characterized by skin and mucous membrane lesions, not elsewhere classified

This category classifies a number of poxviruses as well as exanthems of childhood.

B08.0-   Other orthopoxvirus infections

Orthopoxviruses cause systemic infections in humans, necessitating specific diagnosis, treatment, and infection control precautions. Not all orthopoxviruses are found in the United States; however, global travel and imported animals have increased the concern for spread of these viruses to regions where they are not endemic.

B08.010 Cowpox

Cowpox is also called vaccinia because it is closely related to variola, the causative virus of smallpox, and infection by cowpox renders the patient immune to smallpox. Cowpox infection is due to Poxvirus bovis infection from milking cattle, and is much milder than smallpox, with hard lesions and low fever. Cowpox is a rare disease and is not endemic within the United States, occurring only in Europe and Great Britain, but it does have the potential for importation via infected travelers or imported animals.

B08.02   Orf virus disease

Orf virus is primarily a disease of sheep and goats that causes sores that appear as blisters on the lips, muzzle, and mouth of these animals. Orf virus can spread to humans who have direct contact with infected sheep and goats. In humans, sores caused by Orf virus occur at the site of contact, which is typically the hands. In general, these infections are self-limited but may cause severe infections in immunocompromised hosts.

B08.1   Molluscum contagiosum

Molluscum contagiosum is a poxvirus that causes small, flesh colored bumps on the skin or conjunctiva. It is a common disease in children.

B08.2-   Exanthema subitum [sixth disease]

The sixth of the customary exanthems of childhood, roseola infantum, is typically an acute benign disease manifested by a short-lived high fever followed by the appearance of a light pink maculopapular or erythematous rash. In some children febrile seizures may occur but these are related to the fever and not the virus itself. Although typically seen only in young children, sixth disease can also occur in immunocompromised adults, such as transplant recipients or those with AIDS.

B08.20   Exanthema subitum [sixth disease], unspecified

B08.21   Exanthema subitum [sixth disease] due to human herpesvirus 6

B08.22   Exanthema subitum [sixth disease] due to human herpesvirus 7

Two etiologic agents of sixth disease have been identified: human herpesvirus 6 (HHV-6) and human herpesvirus 7 (HHV-7). There are two recognized variants of HHV-6: HHV-6A and HHV-6B. HHV-6-related sixth disease is often contracted before the age of 2. HHV-7 is closely related to HHV-6 but is rarely diagnosed and the least pathogenic of the two viruses. Sixth disease due to HHV-7 is most often acquired prior to age 5. As with other herpesvirus infections, HHV-6 and HHV-7 can become latent in the host following the primary infection, predisposing individuals to later reactivation. Complications can arise from HHV-6 and HHV-7 viruses; however, the codes in this subcategory capture only uncomplicated sixth disease.

B08.3   Erythema infectiosum [fifth disease]

The causative agent of erythema infectiosum, also called fifth disease, is human parvovirus B19. The illness occurs most frequently in childhood causing a mild rash illness occurring most commonly during childhood. Manifested by a "slapped-cheek" facial rash and a lacy red rash on the limbs and trunk, fifth disease may present with a low-grade fever, malaise, or cold symptoms prior to the presence of the rash. In adults, parvovirus B19 can result in the typical rash, or may manifest as joint pain and/or swelling. The joints most frequently affected are those in the hands, wrists, and knees, and the occurrence is typically bilateral. Although typically a mild disease that resolves on its own among healthy individuals, serious complications such as acute, severe anemia may occur in those with sickle-cell disease or comparable types of chronic anemia. Parvovirus B19 infection also poses an increased risk for serious illness in individuals with leukemia or cancer, HIV, those born with immune deficiencies, or organ transplant recipients.

B08.4 Enteroviral vesicular stomatitis with exanthem

More commonly called hand, foot, and mouth disease, this is a common viral infection that affects primarily children younger than age 5, although it can affect older children and adults. The virus is spread from person-to-person by close personal contact, respiratory secretions and fluids from mucosal sores, contact with feces, and contact with objects or surfaces contaminated with the virus. The infection is characterized by fever, sores in the mouth called herpangina that resemble blisters, and a skin rash particularly on the hands and feet. Two causative agents include coxsackievirus A16 and enterovirus 71.

B08.5 Enteroviral vesicular pharyngitis

Enteroviral vesicular pharyngitis, also called herpangina, is an acute infection of Coxsackievirus causing throat lesions, fever, and vomiting, generally seen in children during the summer months. Herpangina has a rapid onset of fever, with fevers usually higher in younger patients. Red rimmed blisters and ulcers on the soft palate, tonsils, and uvula appear with the fever or shortly afterwards, giving each lesion a ringed appearance. This virus typically lasts three to six days.

B08.6- Parapoxvirus infections

Parapox virus, a DNA virus hosted by hooved animals, can affect both humans and animals through direct or indirect contact with the infected animal. Parapoxvirus infections present as single or multiple skin lesions and can also affect the lymphatic system. These lesions are self-limiting and heal slowly on their own.

B08.61 Bovine stomatitis

Bovine stomatitis is a viral illness enzootic to cattle throughout the world and is an occupational hazard for cattle handlers. The disease presents as lesions in the animal's oral or facial mucosa or other moist, hairless areas of the body.

B08.62 Sealpox

Sealpox is from harbor seals in the North Sea or from sea lions in California and is technically both a parapoxvirus (found in hooved animals) and an orthopoxvirus (found in vertebrates). Sealpox lesions have been found on hands of marine animal handlers after contact with infected skin shed from or bites of these animals.

B08.69 Other parapoxvirus infections

Other types of parapoxviruses are from red squirrels in the United Kingdom and red deer in New Zealand and Finland. A new type attributed to white-tailed deer has emerged in the United States. These infections have generally been found on deer hunters.

B08.7- Yatapoxvirus infections

Yatapoxviruses are a small group of chordopoxviruses that include yaba-like disease virus (YLDV), tanapox virus, and yaba monkey tumor virus, which are endemic to sub-Saharan Africa. Yatapoxviruses typically only infect monkeys, but accidental infections of humans have been reported. These viruses are a concern for travelers or handlers in animal research facilities.

B08.70 Yatapoxvirus infection, unspecified

Diagnostic tests to more specifically identify some Yatapoxvirus infections are not readily available, and clinicians may not be able to make a diagnosis beyond "Yatapoxvirus."

B08.71 Tanapox virus disease

Tanapox virus is endemic to monkeys, but can spread to humans causing a relatively benign disease. In humans, the disease is characterized by one or two pock-like lesions on the upper body, fever, headache, and malaise.

B08.72 Yaba pox virus disease

Yaba pox virus causes subcutaneous pseudotumors in monkeys and thus it is more commonly called yaba monkey tumor virus (YMTV). YMTV is spread to humans by direct contact with infected monkeys and is also believed to be spread by mosquitos. In humans, the virus is characterized by slow growing nodules that may reach to 2 cm in diameter typically located on the hands and feet and regional lymphadenopathy. The infection resolves without intervention and the nodules disappear usually within a few weeks.

B08.8 Other specified viral infections characterized by skin and mucous membrane lesions

Acute lymphonodular pharyngitis, aphthous fever, Cotia virus, epidemic stomatitis, epizootic aphthous, epizootic stomatitis, foot and mouth disease, fourth disease, and other specified types of poxvirus that are not classified elsewhere are included here.

Viral Hepatitis (B15-B19)

Hepatitis is an inflammation of the liver. Viral hepatitis is caused by a group of hepatitis viruses designated as hepatitis A, B, C, D, and E. Hepatitis may be acute or chronic with the chronic form generally defined as an inflammation of the liver lasting longer than six months.

The categories in this code block are as follows:

B15	Acute hepatitis A
B16	Acute hepatitis B
B17	Other acute viral hepatitis
B18	Chronic viral hepatitis
B19	Unspecified hepatitis

B15.-   Acute hepatitis A

Hepatitis A virus (HAV) or "infectious hepatitis" is a picornavirus that is spread through fecal contamination or by eating contaminated raw shellfish and is considered to be a milder form of hepatitis. It has an incubation period ranging from 15 to 50 days with the average incubation time being 28 days. The virus replicates in the liver and is shed in large amounts in the feces from two weeks prior to the onset of symptoms to one week after symptoms occur. Common symptoms of hepatitis A include fatigue, nausea, vomiting, abdominal discomfort or pain, loss of appetite, low grade fever, muscle pain, dark urine, and jaundice. Symptoms typically last four to eight weeks, but may last as long as six months. The acute infection does not progress to a chronic condition, although relapse can occur during the six months following the initial infection. Acute HAV rarely leads to liver failure and hepatic coma, which is characterized by loss of consciousness.

B16.-   Acute hepatitis B

Hepatitis B virus (HBV) or "serum hepatitis" is a hepadnavirus that is transmitted parenterally through contaminated blood or blood products, by infected intravenous drug users sharing needles, and through sexual contact with an infected person. A high number of cases progress into chronic liver disease.

B16.0   Acute hepatitis B with delta-agent with hepatic coma

B16.1   Acute hepatitis B with delta-agent without hepatic coma

B16.2   Acute hepatitis B without delta-agent with hepatic coma

B16.9   Acute hepatitis B without delta-agent and without hepatic coma

Hepatitis delta-agent is an incomplete virus that requires the presence of hepatitis B surface antigen (HBsAg) to replicate. The severity of the liver damage increases when there is simultaneous infection of hepatitis B and hepatitis delta-agent.

B17.-   Other acute viral hepatitis

Viral hepatitis infections classified here include acute delta infection of hepatitis B carrier, acute hepatitis C infection, acute hepatitis E infection, and other acute non-A and non-B hepatitis infections.

B17.1-   Acute hepatitis C

Hepatitis C virus (HCV) is a flavivirus with six major subtypes. It has been identified as the virus responsible for most cases of parenteral non-A, non-B hepatitis. Although typically associated with blood transfusions, it has been proven to result from other types of exposure (e.g., occupational-health care related, sexual contact). It has been noted that up to 40 percent of cases with this form have no recognized cause for the infection. Patients with HCV are more likely to develop chronic liver disease and chronic manifestations such as chronic active hepatitis and/or cirrhosis.

B17.2   Acute hepatitis E

Hepatitis E virus (HEV) or enteric "fecal-oral hepatitis" is serologically different from the other known hepatitis viruses. It is caused by an RNA virus that produces symptoms similar to Hepatitis A. This type has been identified during investigations of large epidemics in developing countries. The disease is also a clinically distinct entity as one of the foremost causes of acute viral hepatitis in young to middle-aged adults in developing countries and carries a high risk of fatality among pregnant women.

B18.-   Chronic viral hepatitis

Chronic hepatitis is generally defined as an inflammation of the liver lasting longer than six months. Chronic viral hepatitis patients continue to test positive for the hepatitis virus beyond the six-month period after initial diagnosis. Individuals with chronic hepatitis are unable to clear the virus from their bodies and continue to be infectious. Chronic viral hepatitis is associated with a number of health risks, including the development of cirrhosis of the liver, liver failure, and liver cancer. Chronic forms of viral hepatitis occur in hepatitis B and hepatitis C. Chronic hepatitis B may be complicated by concurrent infection with hepatitis delta agent, also called hepatitis D.

B18.0   Chronic viral hepatitis B with delta-agent

B18.1   Chronic viral hepatitis B without delta-agent

Hepatitis B virus (HBV) or "serum hepatitis" is a hepadnavirus that is transmitted parenterally through contaminated blood or blood products, by infected intravenous drug users sharing needles, and through sexual contact with an infected person. HBV may progress to chronic liver disease and the risk of developing chronic HBV is greatest in those that contract the virus before age 6. Approximately 90 to 95 percent of newborns and infants with acute HBV develop chronic HBV. Chronic HBV infection may be complicated by concurrent infection with hepatitis delta-agent also called hepatitis D (HDV). Hepatitis delta-agent can only replicate in patients with a concurrent hepatitis B infection. Chronic HBV with concurrent delta-agent infection increases the risk of developing severe forms of chronic hepatitis with accelerated progression to cirrhosis and a high mortality rate.

B18.2   Chronic viral hepatitis C

Hepatitis C virus (HCV) is a flavivirus with six major subtypes. It has been identified as the virus responsible for most cases of parenteral non-A, non-B hepatitis. Although typically associated with blood transfusions, it has been proven to result from other types of exposure (e.g., occupational-health care related, sexual contact). Chronic HCV is defined as an inflammation of the liver lasting longer than six months with a positive blood test for HCV beyond the six-month period following the acute infection. Patients with chronic HCV are unable to clear the virus from their bodies putting them at risk for developing cirrhosis, liver failure, and liver cancer. However, many individuals with chronic HCV have no symptoms during the acute infection nor do they develop symptoms of the chronic infection until there is significant liver damage.

B18.8   Other chronic viral hepatitis

Viral hepatitis is an inflammation of the liver caused by a group of hepatitis viruses designated as hepatitis A, B, C, D, and E. Chronic viral hepatitis can lead to liver damage, including cirrhosis, liver failure, and liver cancer. Most chronic hepatitis cases are captured in other codes as typically they are related to hepatitis B and hepatitis C viral agents; however, immunosuppressed patients can develop chronic hepatitis E, which is coded here.

B19.-   Unspecified viral hepatitis

Hepatitis is an inflammation of the liver. Viral hepatitis is caused by a group of hepatitis viruses designated as hepatitis A, B, C, D, and E. Hepatitis is subclassified as acute or chronic based on the length of time that the liver has been inflamed. A viral hepatitis infection is considered acute when the liver inflammation lasts six months or less from the time of the initial infection. The chronic form is generally defined as an inflammation of the liver lasting longer than six months. This category reports only viral hepatitis for which the date of the initial infection or inflammation is not known and/or the physician has not documented whether the liver inflammation is acute or chronic.

> **Focus Point**
>
> *Hepatitis A is always classified as acute because it does not have the potential to become chronic. For unspecified hepatitis A infection use category B15.*

Human Immunodeficiency Virus [HIV] Disease (B20)

There is a single category and code in this code block for human immunodeficiency virus [HIV] disease. Conditions classified here include symptomatic human immunodeficiency virus (HIV), acquired immune deficiency syndrome (AIDS), and AIDS related complex (ARC).

B20   Human immunodeficiency virus [HIV] disease

HIV is a blood-borne virus in that it is transmitted through body fluids containing blood or plasma. Transmission of HIV can occur sexually or nonsexually through the exchange of body fluids infected with a high concentration of the virus, mainly blood, semen, or vaginal/cervical secretions. Initially, HIV may be present in the body, but may be asymptomatic. During this period, the patient is HIV positive but does not have HIV disease. In symptomatic HIV, also called ARC (AIDS related complex), symptoms of a weakened immune system are present, including general lymphadenopathy, anorexia, fever, malaise, diarrhea, anemia, oral hairy leukoplakia, and oral candidiasis, but the patient does not have full blown AIDS. A diagnosis of AIDS requires an AIDS-defining condition (e.g., an opportunistic infection or certain types of cancer) or a CD4 count of less than 200 cells/mm^3. HIV is divided into two categories: HIV-1 and HIV-2. HIV-1 is seen worldwide; HIV-2 is limited to Africa and other countries and is seldom seen in the United States. HIV-1 has far-ranging health effects and manifestations. This code is reserved for patients with symptomatic HIV-1 infections, ARC, or AIDS.

Focus Point

For HIV-2, refer to code B97.35.

Other Viral Diseases (B25-B34)

Other viral diseases that do not fit well into a more specific code block are included here.

The categories in this code block are as follows:

B25	Cytomegaloviral disease
B26	Mumps
B27	Infectious mononucleosis
B30	Viral conjunctivitis
B33	Other viral diseases, not elsewhere classified
B34	Viral infection of unspecified site

B25.- Cytomegaloviral disease

Cytomegaloviral disease (CMV), also called cytomegalic inclusion disease, is a human salivary gland virus and member of the herpes virus group, more specifically human herpesvirus type 5. It affects only humans, and the initial infection can range from benign and asymptomatic to severe with the potential to cause significant impairment or death in infants and the immunosuppressed. Like all herpes viruses, CMV remains in the body and can be reactivated, particularly in individuals with compromised immune systems due to organ or tissue transplant, chemotherapy, acquired immune deficiency syndrome (AIDS), or other conditions. In symptomatic initial cases, fatigue, lymphadenopathy, fever, loss of appetite, muscle aches, rash, and sore throat may be present. Reactivation of the virus causes similar symptoms. Complications are rare and more often associated with the reactivation of the virus than with initial infection, including pneumonitis, hepatitis, pancreatitis, pericarditis or myocarditis, colitis, and encephalitis.

B25.0 Cytomegaloviral pneumonitis

Cytomegaloviral (CMV) pneumonitis or pneumonia is a complication of CMV infection characterized by infection and inflammation of the lungs. This is a rare complication that in healthy individuals is often self-limiting. For patients with compromised immune systems or lung transplant recipients, the pneumonitis may be more severe, even life-threatening. Symptoms of CMV pneumonitis include cough and shortness of breath, along with generalized symptoms of fatigue, lymphadenopathy, fever, loss of appetite, and muscle, joint, or body aches. Diagnosis of CMV pneumonia may require bronchioalveolar lavage to obtain a fluid specimen or lung biopsy to obtain a tissue sample.

B25.1 Cytomegaloviral hepatitis

Hepatitis as a complication of CMV infection is characterized by infection and inflammation of the liver. Symptoms of CMV hepatitis include elevated bilirubin and liver enzymes on liver function tests, along with the typical generalized symptoms of CMV. Diagnosis of CMV hepatitis may require a liver biopsy to identify the virus in liver tissue.

B25.2 Cytomegaloviral pancreatitis

Cytomegaloviral (CMV) pancreatitis is a complication of CMV infection characterized by infection and inflammation of the pancreas. Symptoms of CMV pancreatitis include upper abdominal pain, nausea and vomiting, and generalized symptoms of fatigue, lymphadenopathy, fever, loss of appetite, and muscle, joint, or body aches. Diagnosis of CMV pancreatitis may require a pancreas biopsy for detection of the virus in pancreatic tissue or histologic changes in the tissue sample indicative of CMV infection.

B25.8 Other cytomegaloviral diseases

This code is assigned for other complications of CMV, which include CMV infection of the brain (encephalitis), gastrointestinal tract (enteritis/colitis), urinary tract including the kidney (nephritis) or bladder (cystitis), retina of the eye (retinitis), and heart (myocarditis/pericarditis).

B26.- Mumps

Mumps present as an acute infection of the salivary glands, usually the parotids, caused by paramyxovirus. Inhaling respiratory droplets from an infected person can spread the disease. Most cases occur in children 2 years of age or older. Mumps causes painful swelling of the salivary glands, pain upon chewing, and high fever. Complications may occur, especially in adults.

B27.- Infectious mononucleosis

Infectious mononucleosis is an active infection most commonly associated with the Epstein-Barr virus (EBV), also called gammaherpesviral mononucleosis. The virus causes fever, sore throat, enlarged lymph glands and spleen, and fatigue. It is most commonly seen in teens and young adults, and runs a mild course in most cases.

Focus Point

Cytomegaloviral mononucleosis is now classified to B27.1-, in the same category as infectious mononucleosis.

B30.- Viral conjunctivitis

Viral conjunctivitis is an inflammation of the conjunctiva, a thin transparent layer covering the surface of the inner eyelid and the front of the eye, caused by a viral infection. It is frequently referred to as "pink eye" and is a common acute eye disorder.

B30.0 Keratoconjunctivitis due to adenovirus

Keratoconjunctivitis, also called epidemic keratoconjunctivitis (EKC), is the most common cause of "pink eye." Approximately 19 documented adenoviral serotypes are known to cause EKC. The most common include adenovirus 8, 19, and 37. The viruses are easily spread by finger to eye contact. EKC is a form of adenoviral conjunctivitis and is typically self-limiting, resolving spontaneously within two to three weeks. It can be associated with significant manifestations, including subepithelial infiltrates (SEI or superficial corneal inflammatory deposits), lacrimal drainage scarring, and symblepharon.

B30.2 Viral pharyngoconjunctivitis

Viral pharyngoconjunctivitis, also called pharyngoconjunctival fever or Béal conjunctivitis or syndrome, is an infectious disease usually caused by adenovirus type 3, which is related to severe respiratory illness in children. The infection may be acute, epidemic, or sporadic and is more common among school age children. It occurs when adenovirus affects the lining of the eye and the respiratory tract. Infection can be transmitted through swimming pools.

B30.3 Acute epidemic hemorrhagic conjunctivitis (enteroviral)

Epidemic hemorrhagic conjunctivitis serological studies have shown the presence of neutralizing antibodies to Coxsackie group A24 (CA24) and enterovirus E70 (EV70) strains as the causative agent. Acute hemorrhagic conjunctivitis (AHC) is characterized by conjunctival congestion, vascular dilatation, and an onset of edema. An outbreak of AHC was first reported from Ghana in 1969 and was referred to as Apollo conjunctivitis. It is also caused by Coxsackievirus A24 variant (CA24v). Epidemics by this organism have appeared in numerous other countries, including Africa, China, India, Egypt, Cuba, Singapore, Brazil, and Japan. The disease is self-limiting and the viruses may be characterized by photophobia, watering, foreign body sensation, eyelid edema, conjunctival hemorrhages, and superficial punctate keratitis. The virus is transmitted by close person-to-person contact and fomites such as linens, water, and contaminated optical instruments.

B30.8 Other viral conjunctivitis

Included here is Newcastle conjunctivitis, a rare disorder characterized by conjunctival burning, itching, tearing, redness, and pain that is caused by Newcastle disease virus. Newcastle conjunctivitis occurs primarily in poultry workers handling birds that have been infected and veterinarians or laboratory assistants working with live vaccines or viruses.

B33.- Other viral diseases, not elsewhere classified

Only a few viral diseases that do not fit well into other categories are included here.

B33.0 Epidemic myalgia

Also referred to as Dabney's or devil's grip, epidemic pleurodynia, or epidemic diaphragm spasm, epidemic myalgia is an acute illness occurring most frequently during the summer months among adolescents and adults. It is characterized by fever, muscle spasms of the abdomen and chest, and occasionally involves other areas. The spasmodic pain varies in intensity and may last minutes or hours. During a spasm, breathing may become irregular (e.g., rapid, grunting, or shallow). The pain may disappear for a few days after the initial episode and reappear at a later time. Children have a milder illness than adults, who are often restricted to bed. The typical illness lasts four to six days.

B33.2- Viral carditis

There are a number of viral infections that can cause infection and inflammation of the heart. Code selection is based on whether the infection occurs in the outer lining of the heart (viral pericarditis), the heart cavities (viral endocarditis), or the heart muscle (viral myocarditis). In most cases, viral carditis resolves spontaneously without treatment, but some individuals experience mild to moderate heart damage and in about 20 percent of viral carditis cases, there is recurring symptoms and/or progressive heart disease.

B33.4 Hantavirus (cardio)-pulmonary syndrome [HPS] [HCPS]

Hantavirus is carried by rodents and is transmitted to humans when they come in direct contact with or inhale dust of urine or feces of infected rodents. Different rodents in different regions of the United States carry different strains of Hantavirus, all of which cause Hantavirus pulmonary syndrome (HPS). The "Sin Nombre" strain is carried by the deer mouse, which is found in all regions of the United States. The cotton rat found in the southeastern United States and Central and South America carries the Black Creek Canal Hantavirus strain. The rice rat found in the southeastern United States and Central America carries the Bayou Hantavirus strain. The white-footed mouse carries the New York Hantavirus strain and is found in most eastern and southern states, throughout the Midwest, and in Mexico. All patients with Hantavirus pulmonary syndrome (HPS) have initial symptoms of fever, fatigue, and muscle aches with some patients also experiencing headache, dizziness, chills, nausea, vomiting, diarrhea, and/or abdominal pain. Respiratory symptoms begin between four and 10 days after the initial generalized symptoms appear and include cough and shortness of breath. This can progress to severe respiratory distress due to pulmonary edema with hypoxia requiring mechanical ventilation. Most patients also develop cardiovascular symptoms including hypotension and myocardial dysfunction with cardiac rhythm disorders. The mortality rate for HPS is about 50 percent, with treatment.

Mycoses (B35-B49)

Mycoses are fungal infections. Because fungi are present in the natural environment most people come into contact with fungi on a regular basis, but very few people develop infections. Many fungi infections are classified as opportunistic meaning that they affect individuals with weakened immune systems, including people with cancer, transplant patients, and people with HIV/AIDS.

The categories in this code block are as follows:

B35	Dermatophytosis
B36	Other superficial mycoses
B37	Candidiasis
B38	Coccidioidomycosis
B39	Histoplasmosis
B40	Blastomycosis
B41	Paracoccidioidomycosis
B42	Sporotrichosis
B43	Chromomycosis and pheomycotic abscess
B44	Aspergillosis
B45	Cryptococcosis
B46	Zygomycosis
B47	Mycetoma
B48	Other mycoses, not elsewhere classified
B49	Unspecified mycosis

B35.-   Dermatophytosis

Dermatophytoses are superficial fungal infections of the skin. Ringworm, though no worm is present, and athlete's foot are common names for the disease. Dermatophytosis is classified according to the site of the lesion. This category includes infections by species of *Epidermophyton*, *Microsporum*, and *Trichophyton tinea*.

B36.-   Other superficial mycoses

These superficial infections of the skin are fungal infections other than ringworm, not elsewhere classified, or have an unknown fungal infectious agent.

B36.0   Pityriasis versicolor

Also called tinea versicolor, this is a common fungal infection native to the tropics that develops from an overgrowth of the normal yeast that grows on the skin. It typically presents in warm, humid weather as the appearance of many spots of various lighter shades of pinks, reds, or browns over the skin. These spots develop slowly, can be itchy and dry, and can disappear when the weather becomes cooler and dryer.

B36.1   Tinea nigra

Tinea (fungal) nigra (black) is a benign fungal skin infection generally affecting the soles of the feet and/or palms of the hands causing darker discoloration of the affected area. Most often caused by the *Phaeoannellomyces werneckii* fungi, also referred to as *Hortaea werneckii*, *Exophiala* werneckii, or *Cladosporium werneckii*, tinea nigra is a brown mold found on wood or in soil or compost in tropical regions. Typically no inflammation or itching is present. Treatment consists of the use of antifungals for three to four weeks.

B36.2   White piedra

White piedra, also called tinea blanca is a superficial *Trichosporon* (fungal) infection of the shaft of the hair and can be mistaken for dandruff or lice. It appears as white, cream, or brown soft nodules along the hair shaft on the face (beard, moustache), axilla, and genitals and less commonly, the scalp regions. The infection is most often felt before it is seen, feeling like gritty, detachable particles. It more frequently affects the immunocompromised populations and can be found in more temperate climates, including the United States. Treatment may include removal of affected hair along with topical antifungal medication; however, this infection may have intermittent recurrences.

B36.3   Black piedra

Black piedra is a superficial *Trichosporon* (fungal) hair infection that presents as dark-colored hard nodules that typically affect only the scalp hair and can grow into the actual shaft of the hair, causing damage and breakage at the shaft level. Black piedra is most common to the tropical and subtropical regions. Treatment may include removal of affected hair in addition to either topical or oral antifungal medications to completely treat the condition with no recurrence; however, without proper diagnosis and treatment, the condition may be present for many years.

B37.-   Candidiasis

Candidiasis is a yeast infection caused by the *Candida* species, usually *C. albicans* but also *C. tropicalis* and *C. parapsilosis*. *C. albicans* is found on mucosal tissues in the mouth and genital regions in about half the population and typically does not cause infection. Infection is present only when overgrowth occurs in the mouth or genital region or when the yeast is found in sites other than the mouth and genital areas. In healthy individuals this may be a result of medications, such as antibiotics, changing the natural environment of these areas. Most *Candida* infections are simple cases of diaper rash or vulvovaginal infection. However, *Candida* is also an opportunistic illness and significant systemic infection is seen among the immunosuppressed, including individuals receiving chemotherapy and those with acquired immune deficiency syndrome (AIDS). Candidiasis codes are classified by site and/or manifestation.

B37.0   Candidal stomatitis

Candidal stomatitis, also called oral thrush, is a yeast infection caused by *Candida*. Candidal stomatitis is diagnosed only when overgrowth occurs in the mouth and is characterized by white patches on the tongue and mucosal surfaces. The patches can resemble milk curds and when wiped off typically reveal red inflamed mucosal tissue that may bleed. Oral thrush is considered clinically significant in adults as it may be an indicator of acquired immune deficiency syndrome (AIDS) or other immune impairment.

B37.1   Pulmonary candidiasis

Pulmonary candidiasis is an opportunistic infection of the lung that occurs in individuals with impaired immune systems and may present as bronchitis or pneumonia. Symptoms of candidal pneumonia include cough, sputum production that may be tinged with blood, and pleuritic chest pain.

B37.2   Candidiasis of skin and nail

The skin and nails are common sites of candidal infection. Treatment involves keeping affected regions as dry as possible and using a topical or oral antifungal medication. The primary symptom of candidal skin infections is an itchy red rash that can occur anywhere on the skin but are most common in warm moist areas, such as under the arms, under the breasts, and in the groin region. In obese individuals it can occur in body folds, sometimes referred to as intertrigo candidiasis. When it occurs between the fingers it may be called erosio interdigitalis blastomycetica. It is also a common cause of diaper rash in infants. In rare instances *Candida* may affect deeper layers of the skin resulting in granuloma-like lesions. Nail infections may occur in the nail itself and is called *Candida* onychia or around the nail where it is called paronychia.

B37.3   Candidiasis of vulva and vagina

The vulva and vagina are common sites of candidal infection, which is also called a yeast infection when it occurs at these sites. The infection is due to an overgrowth of *Candida* that may be caused by changes in the pH of the vagina and hormonal changes. Use of systemic antibiotics or corticosteroids can also be a predisposing factor. Symptoms include a cottage cheese like discharge from the vagina and vulvar redness, burning, and itching. Local antifungal medications, in the form of vaginal suppositories or creams, are used to treat the infection.

B37.4-   Candidiasis of other urogenital sites

There are specific codes for candidiasis of the bladder (cystitis), urethra (urethritis), and glans penis (balanitis) and also a code for other specified urogenital sites, which is reported for *Candida* infections of the kidney, ureter, or prostate, as well as specified urogenital sites that do not have a more specific code.

B37.41   Candidal cystitis and urethritis

Candidal infection of the bladder (cystitis) and/or urethra (urethritis) is seen most often in patients on antibiotics who require urinary catheterization. Symptoms include urinary frequency, urgency, pain on urination, and/or suprapubic pain. Candidal infection of the bladder can be complicated by formation of fungal balls or bezoars (fungal concretions), and in rare cases the development of a severe emphysematous infection of the bladder tissue characterized by necrosis and gas formation.

B37.42   Candidal balanitis

Balanitis is an inflammation of the head of the penis, also called the glans penis. *Candida* is the most common cause of inflammation of the glans penis with associated redness, burning, and itching. Treatment involves keeping the affected area as clean and dry as possible along with topical antifungal medication.

B37.49   Other urogenital candidiasis

Candidal pyelonephritis, which is an infection of the kidney that affects the renal (kidney) parenchyma, calyces, and pelvis, is included here. Renal candidiasis may occur as a result of candidal spread through the bloodstream to the kidney or it may be a complication of a procedure, a nephrostomy tube, or renal stent. A complication of fungal infection of the kidney is the development of emphysematous pyelonephritis, which is a severe infection characterized by necrosis of the renal parenchyma and accumulation of gas in the renal tissue. Another complication of infection of the kidney and ureter includes the development of fungal balls that may cause obstruction to the flow of urine. A second manifestation included here is candidal prostatitis. Infections of the kidney and prostate sites are rare, usually occurring only in diabetics or immunocompromised individuals who have undergone a surgical procedure often involving an indwelling internal device.

B37.5 Candidal meningitis

Meningitis is a rare candidal manifestation. It may occur as a complication of neurosurgery, a systemic *Candida* infection, or in patients with compromised immune systems. Symptoms indicative of *Candida* meningitis are often nonspecific but may include fever, headache, alternated consciousness including confusion or delirium, and focal neurological signs and symptoms. Diagnosis is made by cerebrospinal fluid culture. Treatment is with intravenous administration of antifungal medications.

B37.6 Candidal endocarditis

Endocarditis is a rare manifestation of candidal infection. The infection typically involves the heart valves and may occur in a native heart valve or a prosthetic valve. Candidal infection is also associated with the presence of other cardiac devices. Risk factors for candidal endocarditis include intravenous drug abuse; indwelling cardiovascular devices such as catheters, pacemakers, and prosthetic valves; prosthetic joints; immune system suppression due to stem cell, bone marrow, or solid organ transplants or chemotherapy; HIV/AIDS, diabetes and other chronic conditions affecting the immune system; and long-term use of antibiotics. Symptoms are nonspecific but may include fever, shortness of breath, chest pain, or pressure. Fungal endocarditis increases the risk of emboli and embolism of the brain, other organs, or extremities. Diagnosis is made by blood culture and echocardiography. Treatment is a combination of intravenous antifungal medication and surgery to replace infected native valves and remove cardiovascular or other devices if they are the source of the infection.

B37.7 Candidal sepsis

While sepsis due to *Candida* is rare, it is the most common cause of fungal sepsis. Sepsis is a systemic or body-wide response to an infection. The systemic response is characterized by certain changes in body temperature, heart rate, respiratory rate and/or arterial blood gases, and white blood cell count. More specifically, these include elevated body temperature (usually above 101 degrees Fahrenheit) or subnormal body temperature (usually below 96.8 degrees Fahrenheit), elevated heart rate (usually above 90 beats per minute), elevated respiratory rate (usually above 20 breaths per minute) or arterial blood gases reflecting a reduced partial pressure of carbon dioxide PACO2, and an abnormal white blood cell count above 12,000 cells/microliter or below 4,000 cells/microliter

or greater than 10 percent bands (immature white blood cells). Two or more of these indications and a suspected or known infection due to *Candida* are indicative of candidal sepsis.

B37.8- Candidiasis of other sites

Candidiasis is a yeast infection caused by the *Candida* species, usually *C. albicans* but also *C. tropicalis* and *C. parapsilosis*.

B37.81 Candidal esophagitis

Candida is the most common cause of infectious esophagitis. *Candidal* esophagitis, which may also be called esophageal thrush, is an opportunistic infection that affects people with compromised immune systems, such as people with HIV/AIDS, cancer, people undergoing chemotherapy, and the elderly. Symptoms include white lesions in the esophagus that may be accompanied by pain or difficulty swallowing, nausea, vomiting, and loss of appetite. It is treated with antifungal medication administered orally or intravenously.

B37.82 Candidal enteritis

Candida is normally present in the digestive tract of about half of all individuals in the United States. It causes symptoms and is considered pathogenic only when overgrowth occurs and is manifested by inflammation of the intestines. Candidal enteritis typically affects only the very young, the elderly, and individuals with compromised immune systems. Common symptoms include abdominal pain, nausea, vomiting, diarrhea, bloating, loss of appetite, and weight loss. Stool specimen cultures may be used to diagnose candidal enteritis, but this is not a definitive test since *Candida* is normally present in the intestinal tract of many individuals. Antifungal medications are used to treat candidal enteritis.

B37.83 Candidal cheilitis

Candidal infection of the lips causes inflammation, usually at the sides of the mouth where the upper and lower lips meet, which may be referred to as angular cheilitis. The infection causes redness, cracking of the skin, soreness and burning at the site of the infection. Topical antifungal medication is used to treat the infection.

B37.84 Candidal otitis externa

The external ear canal is an uncommon site of candidal infection characterized by cheesy white lesions in the external ear. Symptoms include itching and a feeling of fullness due to lesions in the ear canal. Treatment involves cleaning the ear, debriding any lesions, and applying topical antifungal medication.

B37.89 Other sites of candidiasis

Candidal infections of the bone and bone marrow (osteomyelitis) are reported here.

B39.- Histoplasmosis

Histoplasmosis is a fungal disease caused by one of two *Histoplasma* species depending on the geographic location: *H. capsulatum* in the United States and *H. duboisii* in Africa, also referred to as small form histoplasmosis or large form histoplasmosis respectively. Specific codes for the American form of *H. capsulatum* capture the chronicity of the pulmonary infection (acute, chronic, or unspecified) or if it has disseminated (moved to other organs). Additional codes represent African or unspecified types of the disease.

Histoplasmosis

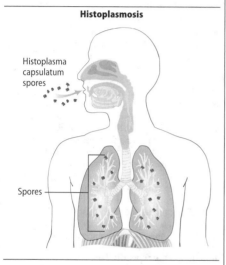

Histoplasma capsulatum spores

Spores

B44.- Aspergillosis

The fungus *Aspergillus* is commonly found in decaying leaves, stored grain, or bird droppings. There are several species including *Aspergillus flavus*, *Aspergillus terreus*, *Aspergillus nidulans*, and *Aspergillus niger*, with the most common infection causing agent being *Aspergillus fumigatus*. Although the most common site of the infection is the lungs, it may also infect the tonsils, sinuses, or skin.

B44.0 Invasive pulmonary aspergillosis

Invasive pulmonary aspergillosis is an opportunistic infection seen primarily in individuals with neutropenia (low white blood cell counts); recipients of stem cell, bone marrow, and organ transplants; patients with graft versus host disease; patients with HIV/AIDS; or patients with chronic obstructive pulmonary disease with long-term steroid use. This is an aggressive form of pulmonary aspergillosis that if not treated can lead to life-threatening respiratory failure or the disseminated form of aspergillosis.

B44.1 Other pulmonary aspergillosis

Bronchopulmonary aspergillosis, not related to an allergic reaction, as well as aspergilloma are two aspergillosis conditions included here. An aspergilloma is a fungal ball, also called a mycetoma, which fills a pulmonary cavity and is usually associated with a history of cavitating lung disease, such as tuberculosis.

> **Focus Point**
>
> *Allergic bronchopulmonary aspergillosis is reported with code B44.81.*

B44.2 Tonsillar aspergillosis

Aspergillosis of the tonsils typically presents as chronic inflammation. It is diagnosed by throat swab and culture. Antifungal medication is used to treat the infection.

B44.7 Disseminated aspergillosis

Disseminated aspergillosis is a rare but severe manifestation of aspergillosis that is typically seen only in immunosuppressed patients. Disseminated aspergillosis typically begins with a lung infection that then spreads via the bloodstream to multiple other sites.

B44.8- Other forms of aspergillosis

Other manifestations of aspergillosis classified here include an allergic bronchopulmonary response to the fungus and localized infection of sites other than sites in the respiratory tract.

B44.81 Allergic bronchopulmonary aspergillosis

Allergic bronchopulmonary aspergillosis occurs when an individual becomes sensitized to the *Aspergillus* fungus, which is widespread in the environment being present in decaying leaves, stored grain, or bird droppings. There are several species, with the most common causative agent of allergic manifestations being *Aspergillus fumigatus*. The allergic form of aspergillosis does not invade tissues of the bronchi or lung. Instead the fungus accumulates and multiplies in mucus found in the airways causing inflammation of the mucus, which if untreated can result in scarring of the lungs and widening of the bronchi. Symptoms include productive cough with blood-flecked sputum, wheezing, shortness of breath, and fever. Predisposing factors to the development of allergic bronchopulmonary aspergillosis are asthma and cystic fibrosis.

B44.89 Other forms of aspergillosis

Other localized manifestations or infections due to *Aspergillus* are classified here, including otitis externa (otomycosis).

B44.9 Aspergillosis, unspecified

Pneumonia due to aspergillosis is coded here.

B45.- Cryptococcosis

Cryptococcosis is an infection by *Cryptococcus neoformans*. The primary infection is often pulmonary in origin and can be followed by infections in organs, bones, or the nervous system. Cryptococcosis is sometimes called European blastomycosis or torulosis, after its former name, Torula histolytica.

B48.- Other mycoses, not elsewhere classified

A fungal infection in a human is called mycosis. Because fungi are present in the natural environment most people come into contact with fungi on a regular basis, but very few people develop infections. Spore inhalation or skin colonization often initiates an infection.

B48.0 Lobomycosis

Lobomycosis is a chronic fungal infection of the skin that is endemic to Central and South America. The infectious organism does not currently have a universally accepted species name. Some species names that are currently used to describe the infection include *Blastomycosis loboi* (keloidal blastomycosis), *Glenosporella loboi* (glenosporosis), and *Lacazia loboi*, *Loboa loboi* (lobomycosis). The disease is rarely diagnosed in the United States and only in individuals with a history of travel to regions where it is endemic. Lobomycosis is a slow growing fungal infection and symptoms may not present for months to years after infection. The first symptom is typically a small papule or pustule that may itch or burn. The initial lesion grows slowly over many months or years and satellite lesions may eventually develop. Systemic symptoms other than mild lymphadenopathy are rare. The lesions may regress and form scar tissue but the fungus does not disappear from the site. Oral fungicides offer only limited benefits and the treatment of choice is excision of the lesion.

B48.1 Rhinosporidiosis

Rhinosporidiosis is caused by *Rhinosporidium seeberi*. It was classified for more than 50 years as a water mold, but is now thought to be a water parasite, although there is some dispute about its exact classification because other scientists believe it may be a bacterium. Rhinosporidiosis is endemic to India, Sri Lanka, South America, and Africa. It infects the mucous membranes of the nose, sinuses, and conjunctiva forming vascular polypoid type lesions on the skin causing wart-like lesions. The lesions are treated by surgical excision.

B48.2 Allescheriasis

Allescheriasis is a rare opportunistic infection caused by a fungus that has been renamed multiple times. The organism that causes allescheriasis may be referred to as *Allescheria boydii* (allescheriasis), *Monosporium apiospermum*, *Petriellidium boydii* (petriellidiosis), or *Pseudoallescheria boydii*. It can infect the lungs, central nervous system, eye, prostate, and skin usually on the foot or external ear canal.

B48.3 Geotrichosis

Geotrichosis, which is caused by *Geotrichum candidum*, is a rare opportunistic infection that causes localized and systemic infections in immunocompromised individuals. One of the more common sites of infection is the mucous membranes of the mouth, which manifests as inflammation and ulceration.

B48.4 Penicillosis

Penicillium marneffei is a dimorphic fungus, which means that it presents in two forms: a mold that converts to yeast at body temperature. Penicillosis is an opportunistic infection that affects immunocompromised individuals, particularly those with HIV/AIDS. It is endemic to Southeast Asia and parts of China, rarely occurring outside these regions, and then usually only in individuals who have a history of travel to areas where it is endemic. Because it is an opportunistic infection, the most common manifestation of penicillosis is disseminated disease that presents with systemic symptoms of fever, skin lesions, anemia, enlarged lymph nodes (lymphadenopathy), and enlarged liver (hepatomegaly). Localized infections, such as pneumonia, are less common. Treatment is with multiple antifungal agents and once systemic symptoms resolve, patients must remain on maintenance therapy to prevent recurrence.

B48.8 Other specified mycoses

Use this code to report infection of skin, subcutaneous tissues, mucous membranes, or organs by a wide variety of fungi generally considered to be pathogenic to immunocompromised hosts only. Among the opportunistic mycoses is the species *Alternaria*, *Dreschlera*, and *Fusarium*. These infections are most likely to occur in patients after radiation therapy or during therapy with corticosteroids or immunosuppressants. People with AIDS, Hodgkin's lymphoma, or diabetes are more susceptible to opportunistic mycoses.

Protozoal Diseases (B50-B64)

Protozoa are unicellular microorganisms that live in moist environments. They are found in water and soil. Most protozoa are nonpathogenic; however, there are a few that cause disease in humans, such as several species of *Plasmodium*, which cause malaria; *Toxoplasma gondii*, which causes toxoplasmosis; and *Pneumocystis jiroveci* (previously called *Pneumocystis carinii*), which causes pneumonia.

The categories in this code block are as follows:

B50	Plasmodium falciparum malaria
B51	Plasmodium vivax malaria
B52	Plasmodium malariae malaria
B53	Other specified malaria
B54	Unspecified malaria
B55	Leishmaniasis
B56	African trypanosomiasis
B57	Chagas' disease
B58	Toxoplasmosis
B59	Pneumocystosis
B60	Other protozoal diseases, not elsewhere classified
B64	Unspecified protozoal disease

B50.-   Plasmodium falciparum malaria

Malaria is a mosquito-borne protozoan infection endemic to the tropics. It is transmitted man to mosquito to man and has largely been eradicated in the United States through insecticide programs and drugs. Most cases of malaria in the United States are seen in people who have traveled abroad. *Plasmodium falciparum*, considered the most dangerous malaria, is found in tropical and subtropical regions worldwide with concentration in Africa. This type is considered severe and carries a higher morbidity rate because it multiplies so rapidly in the bloodstream, adhering to blood vessels and causing obstructions. It initially causes malaise and headache with intermittent fever and chills, and quickly leads to severe blood loss anemia and clotting. A specific code in this category is reported for cerebral complications that occur when the parasites clog blood vessels to the brain.

B51.-   Plasmodium vivax malaria

This malaria is a mosquito-borne protozoan infection that can be found in temperate climates, including the United States, although it has largely been eradicated in the United States through insecticide programs and drugs. *Plasmodium vivax* malaria is most prevalent in Asia, with concentrations also present in Latin America and parts of Africa. Most cases of malaria in the United States are seen in people who have traveled abroad. It can lie dormant in the liver for months or years after the initial bite. Less deadly than *Plasmodium falciparum*, *Plasmodium vivax* is still a severe disease with death caused by splenomegaly. This type of malaria continues to multiply in the bloodstream well before symptoms first appear, leading to the potential for more infections in other people. Furthermore, one bite can cause six or more recurrences per year, leading to increased risk for other infections.

B52.-   Plasmodium malariae malaria

Malaria is a mosquito-borne protozoan infection endemic to the tropics and is transmitted man to mosquito to man. Although *Plasmodium malariae* malaria is present worldwide, it has largely been eradicated in the United States through insecticide programs and drugs. Most cases of malaria in the United States are seen in people who have traveled abroad. Although more benign than vivax and falciparum, if left untreated, this infection can cause lifelong infection and nephropathy.

B55.-   Leishmaniasis

Leishmaniasis is an infection by *Leishmania*, a genus of parasitic protozoa. This infection is usually seen in developing nations and is rare in the United States, although it has been seen in parts of South America. The focus of infection and the infective agent are variables that create a broad spectrum of disease associated with leishmaniasis.

B56.-   African trypanosomiasis

Several species of *Trypanosoma* protozoa are responsible for African trypanosomiasis. This chronic disease typically presents with symptoms of fever, lymphadenopathy, headache, and edema. Complications can affect the central nervous system and major organs and can be fatal. African trypanosomiasis is endemic to Africa and is found only in international travelers who return to the United States with the infection.

B57.-   Chagas' disease

Chagas' disease, also called American trypanosomiasis, is caused by the protozoa *Trypanosoma cruzi*, which is endemic only to South America. The primary mode of transmission is by insect vectors called triatomine bugs, a blood-sucking insect that becomes infected by biting an infected animal or person. The infected triatomine bug then transmits the disease in its feces to other animals and humans. Chagas' disease is classified as acute or chronic. The acute phase often goes unnoticed because the symptoms are often mild and include fever, fatigue, body aches, headache, rash, loss of appetite, diarrhea, and vomiting. Swollen glands, mild enlargement of the liver or spleen, and local swelling where the parasite entered the body are also common. A small percentage of individuals develop myocarditis due to an acute infection of the heart. The acute phase lasts for several weeks to several months. If untreated, the symptoms resolve but the infection persists and becomes chronic. Complications from chronic Chagas' disease can affect the central nervous system, heart, and digestive system and can be fatal. Chagas' disease is rarely seen in the United States being limited to international travelers who have recently returned to the United States from South America.

B58.- Toxoplasmosis

Toxoplasmosis is caused by a single-celled parasite, *Toxoplasma gondii*, that can be found throughout the world. Millions of people in the United States are infected with a *Toxoplasma* parasite, but very few have symptoms because the immune system usually keeps the parasite from causing illness. Toxoplasmosis is an opportunistic disease and a danger to the unborn and immunocompromised.

B58.81 Toxoplasma myocarditis

Inflammation of the muscular midlayer of the heart wall (myocarditis), as well as cyst formation in this muscular layer, is a rare complication of an acute toxoplasma infection. Symptoms include arrhythmia, chest pain, shortness of breath, edema, and fatigue.

B59 Pneumocystosis

Pneumocystosis is an infection by *Pneumocystis jiroveci*, previously called *Pneumocystis carinii*, which although classified as a fungus does not respond to antifungal medications. *P. jiroveci* causes pneumonia in immunocompromised patients and is the leading cause of death among AIDS patients. Patients with intact immune systems are not affected by pneumocystosis. Symptoms are nonspecific and include shortness of breath on exertion, fever, nonproductive cough, chest discomfort, weight loss, and chills. Infection outside the respiratory system is rare and typically only seen in immunocompromised patients who are receiving Pentamidine aerosol as a prophylactic treatment for pneumocystosis or those with advanced AIDS.

B60.- Other protozoal diseases, not elsewhere classified

Protozoa are unicellular microorganisms that live in moist environments. They are found in water and soil and although most are nonpathogenic, there are a few that cause disease in humans.

B60.0 Babesiosis

Babesiosis identifies a group of tick-borne diseases infected with the *Babesia* protozoa. In the United States, babesiosis occurs primarily in the Northeast and upper Midwest with most infections occurring during the summer. Most cases in the United States are caused by *B. microti*, which is spread by *Ixodes scapularis* ticks, also referred to as deer ticks. The protozoa infect the red blood cells and symptomatic infections cause fever, chills, anemia, splenomegaly, and muscle pain. The severity of the infection ranges from asymptomatic to life-threatening. People with a history of splenectomy have a high mortality rate from babesiosis. In others, it resolves within weeks.

B60.1- Acanthamebiasis

Diseases caused by the free-living ameboid protozoan *Acanthamebiasis* is classified by manifestation. The most common *Acanthamoeba* manifestations include amoebic conjunctivitis, keratoconjunctivitis, and meningoencephalitis.

B60.13 Keratoconjunctivitis due to Acanthamoeba

Acanthamoeba keratitis or keratoconjunctivitis is a rare but potentially blinding infection of the cornea. It primarily affects otherwise healthy persons who improperly store, handle, or disinfect their contact lenses (e.g., by using tap water or homemade solutions for cleaning). Symptoms are similar to other eye infections but targeted treatment is necessary to be effective. Complications include corneal scarring and loss of vision. Long-term therapy and management are often required.

B60.2 Naegleriasis

Free-living amoeba, *Naegleria*, can cause a grave form of meningoencephalitis. The infection is acquired by swimming in infested lakes.

Helminthiases (B65-B83)

Helminths are parasitic worms and helminthiases are infections caused by parasitic worms.

The categories in this code block are as follows:

B65	Schistosomiasis [bilharziasis]
B66	Other fluke infestations
B67	Echinococcosis
B68	Taeniasis
B69	Cysticercosis
B70	Diphyllobothriasis and sparganosis
B71	Other cestode infections
B72	Dracunculiasis
B73	Onchocerciasis
B74	Filiariasis
B75	Trichinellosis
B76	Hookworm diseases
B77	Ascariasis
B78	Strongyloidiasis
B79	Trichuriasis
B80	Enterobiasis
B81	Other intestinal helminthiases, not elsewhere classified
B82	Unspecified intestinal parasitism
B83	Other helminthiases

B65.- Schistosomiasis [bilharziasis]

Schistosomiasis, also known as bilharzia or blood fluke, is a water-borne parasitic disease. It is the major health risk in the rural areas of Central China and Egypt and continues to rank high in other developing countries. The main forms of schistosomiasis are caused by five species, and classification of infection is based on the species. Each schistosomiasis species survives through a complex life cycle involving two hosts: the water snail and a human/animal. The eggs of the schistosomes in the excreta of an infected host (human, animal) open on contact with water and release a parasite, the miracidium, which seeks a fresh water snail. Once the parasite has found its snail host, the miracidium produces thousands of parasite larvae (cercariae), which are excreted into the surrounding water. These larvae penetrate the skin of a human or animal where they continue the biological cycle as worms, making their way to the victim's blood vessels. Once in the blood vessels, the worms live and procreate via egg production. About half of the eggs are excreted in the feces (intestinal schistosomiasis) or in the urine

(urinary schistosomiasis), which if excreted into a water source can start the cycle all over again. The rest remain in the host, damaging vital organs. It is the eggs and not the worms that cause damage.

B67.- Echinococcosis

Echinococcosis is an infection by the tapeworm *Echinococcus*. Diseases are classified according to serotype—*E. granulosus* or *E. multilocularis*—and by site of infection. *E. granulosis* is also called cystic echinococcus due to the formation of cysts that contain the tapeworm larvae. The cysts are slow growing and the infection may remain asymptomatic for years until the cysts become large enough to produce symptoms. The most common symptoms are pain, nausea, and vomiting. Most *E. granulosis* cysts are found in the liver and lungs, but they can also occur in the spleen, kidneys, heart, bone, and central nervous system. *E. granulosis* is typically spread to humans from dogs that have eaten infected livestock, most often sheep. *E. granulosus* is endemic to Africa, Europe, Asia, the Middle East, and Central and South America, but is rare in the United States. *E. multilocularis* is also called alveolar echinococcus. This infection is characterized by vesicle formation rather than cysts with the most common sites of infection being the liver, lungs, and brain. The vesicles containing the tapeworm larva invade and destroy surrounding tissues. The most common symptoms are pain, weight loss, and malaise. *E. multilocularis* is found worldwide. In the United States, the eggs of these tapeworms are passed from wildlife, most often coyotes and foxes. Hunters, trappers, and veterinarians that care for wildlife may become infected by direct contact with infected animals. Dogs and cats that eat infected rodents are also a possible source of the infection.

B69.- Cysticercosis

Humans develop cysticercosis when larvae or eggs of the tapeworm *Taenia solium* are ingested, most commonly in fecally contaminated water or undercooked pork. In areas of poor sanitation, humans or swine may ingest the eggs and contaminate the water supply. Once ingested, the eggs may hatch and invade the bloodstream and tissues of the body, forming cysts in affected tissue (cysticerci). These cysts do not grow into adult tapeworms, unless they reach the intestine, but remain encapsulated in the tissues of the body. The infection may be subacute or chronic and the severity of symptoms depends on the severity of the host immune response, the location, and number of lesions.

B69.0 Cysticercosis of central nervous system

Neurocysticercosis is listed as a "rare disease" by the Office of Rare Diseases (ORD) of the National Institutes of Health (NIH), affecting less than 200,000 in the United States. Brain involvement of the larval parasite *T. solium* can result in epilepsy, increased intracranial pressure, and other neurologic conditions. Treatment for neurocysticercosis includes antiparasitic and antiinflammatory therapies or surgical intervention. The decision to treat neurocysticercosis is based upon the number of lesions found in the brain and the severity and presentation of symptoms. When only one lesion is found, treatment is not necessary. For more than one lesion, specific antiparasitic treatment is recommended. If the brain lesion is considered calcified (a hard shell has formed around the tapeworm larvae), the cysticerci is considered dead and antiparasitic treatment is not useful. When the cysticerci die, the lesion shrinks and the swelling and symptoms abate.

B69.1   Cysticercosis of eye

In orbital and subconjunctival cysticercosis, the cyst is usually attached to the muscle sheath and induces an inflammatory reaction. Because of its constant motility, it erodes through and leaves an opening in the conjunctiva, which ultimately heals within a short period of time. Cysticerci can lodge in any part of ocular and extraocular tissue, even though ocular localization is not frequent. Ocular dissemination of cysticercus cellulosae is a common manifestation, particularly in the vitreous and subretinal space followed by subconjunctival tissue and extraocular muscles.

B72   Dracunculiasis

In dracunculiasis, a threadlike worm up to 120 centimeters long inhabits the subcutaneous and muscle tissues of man. It is limited to Africa, India, and Arabia.

B74.-   Filariasis

Filarial infections are uncommon in the United States. Many of the filarial infections cause congestion in the lymphatic system that can lead to other manifestations, including elephantiasis or chyluria (lymphatic fluid in the urine).

B75   Trichinellosis

In the United States, the roundworm *Trichinella spiralis*, the smallest of the parasitic nematodes, is most often responsible for the infectious disease trichinellosis. *Trichinella* is found in the muscle of wild game and pig and, generally, infection occurs when undercooked meat is eaten. Infection is rare but not unknown in the United States. Patients may be asymptomatic or may have gastrointestinal symptoms, muscle pains, fever, and periorbital edema. It is more often referred to as trichinosis.

B76.-   Hookworm diseases

Hookworm is a parasite that is present in the soil. It is found primarily in areas where there is not an adequate means for human sewage disposal and where human feces are used as fertilizer. Eggs from an infected person are passed in feces, hatch, and then mature in the soil as larva. During the larval stage they develop into a form that is able to penetrate the skin. Humans are typically infected by walking barefoot in contaminated soil. Once the larva have penetrated the skin, they are carried through the blood vessels to the heart and lungs where they penetrate the alveoli of the lungs, ascend into the bronchi to the pharynx, where they are then swallowed. They pass into the intestines where they mature into adults and remain until they are eliminated in the stool, which may take several years. Several infective agents, the most common being *Ancylostoma duodenale* and *Necator americanus*, can cause hookworm. Symptoms include gastrointestinal pain and anemia, though many patients are asymptomatic.

B76.0   Ancylostomiasis

Found primarily in the Far East and the Mediterranean, the species *Ancylostoma duodenale* is one of the most common species of hookworm.

B76.1   Necatoriasis

This hookworm infection is caused by *Necator americanus*, which was widespread in the southeastern United States until the early 1900s before adequate sewage disposal was available in most areas.

B77.-   Ascariasis

Ascariasis is a roundworm (nematode) infection of which *Ascaris lumbricoides* is the largest species. Transmission occurs in several ways, including direct contact with soil or fertilizer contaminated with fertilized *A. lumbricoides* eggs (most common), person to person, and in rare cases human contact with infected pigs. Once present in the human host, the eggs hatch into larva, most often in the small intestine. The final destination for most larvae is the jejunum by way of the liver and lungs where they must be coughed up and swallowed. Symptomatic ascariasis is more common in children then in adults.

B77.0   Ascariasis with intestinal complications

Heavy infestation of the intestinal tract with *A. lumbricoides* can cause intestinal blockage resulting in severe abdominal cramping and vomiting. Blockage of the intestinal tract may also result in perforation of the intestinal wall, with resulting hemorrhage and peritonitis. In heavy infestation, the worms may also block pancreatic, hepatic, and bile ducts causing damage to the pancreas, liver, or gallbladder.

B78.-   Strongyloidiasis

Strongyloidiasis is a roundworm infection caused by *Strongyloides stercoralis* and is endemic to the tropics, although it is also found in subtropical and temperate regions. *S. stercoralis* passes through four stages: egg, rhabditiform larva, filariform larva, and adult. Only filariform larvae are infectious. Filariform larvae of *S. stercoralis* are found in the soil and are able to penetrate the skin. Walking barefoot in contaminated soil is a common cause of infection. Once the larvae have penetrated the skin, they enter the circulatory system where they are carried to the lungs and deposited in the alveoli. The larvae then penetrate the alveoli of the lungs and move into the trachea and pharynx where they are swallowed. The larvae pass through the esophagus and stomach and into the small intestine where they mature into adults. The adults lay eggs in the intestinal mucosa. The eggs hatch and the rhabditiform larvae may be excreted or they may remain in the colon where they become filariform larvae. Filariform larvae then reinfect the host by penetrating the intestinal mucosa and traveling via the circulatory system to the lungs. Excreted rhabditiform larvae mature into infectious filariform larvae in the soil.

B78.0   Intestinal strongyloidiasis

The presence of an adult *S. stercoralis* roundworm in the small intestine causes gastric pain, vomiting, and diarrhea. Treatment is with anthelmintic medications that kill the adult roundworm. Repeat dosing is often necessary given the ability of *S. stercoralis* rhabditiform larvae, which are not affected by anthelmintic medications, to remain in the colon and reinfect the host.

B78.1   Cutaneous strongyloidiasis

At initial infection, individuals may develop an itchy, red rash at the site where the larvae have penetrated the skin. Following initial infection, the patient may develop chronic strongyloidiasis with repeated autoinfection resulting in urticarial rashes of the buttock, perineal, and thigh regions and also around the waist.

B78.7   Disseminated strongyloidiasis

In disseminated strongyloidiasis, infection is not limited to the lungs and gastrointestinal tract. Large numbers of larvae invade other organs, including those of the central nervous system, and cause a wide variety of symptoms. With large numbers of larvae penetrating the intestinal wall, bacteria from the intestines also escapes and this may cause septicemia, meningitis, and endocarditis.

B80   Enterobiasis

Pinworm infection or enterobiasis is caused by the nematode *Enterobius vermicularis* and is very common in the United States. As humans are the only natural host, infection is spread from person-to-person. Eggs are ingested after handling contaminated items. The larvae hatch in the small intestine where they remain until they reach the adult stage and move to the colon. Female pinworms travel from the colon to the anal region at night to lay eggs. Reinfection can occur when an individual touches or scratches the perianal region while sleeping and then touches the face or mouth. Symptoms include anal itching, restless sleep, decreased appetite, and lack of weight gain.

Pediculosis, Acariasis and Other Infestations (B85-B89)

Pediculosis is a lice infection. Different species of lice infect different regions of the body. Acariasis refers to mite infection, such as scabies. Myasis refers to maggot infestation, which is also classified to this code block.

The categories in this code block are as follows:

B85	Pediculosis and phthiriasis
B86	Scabies
B87	Myiasis
B88	Other infestations
B89	Unspecified parasitic disease

B85.-   Pediculosis and phthiriasis

Lice infestations are classified here. Lice suck the blood of the host and cause severe itching and loss of sleep. Louse saliva or feces irritate some sensitive hosts, increasing the chance of secondary infection from excessive scratching.

B85.0   Pediculosis due to Pediculus humanus capitis

Head lice are *Pediculus* humanus *capitis*, and they live predominantly on the scalp and neck hairs of their human host. Head lice are mainly acquired by direct head-to-head contact with an infested person's hair, but may be transferred with shared combs, hats, and other hair accessories. Infestation is seen most often in children and in Caucasians more frequently than other ethnic groups. Most commonly, epidemics are seen among school children. Head lice do not transmit infectious agents from person to person.

B85.1   Pediculosis due to Pediculus humanus corporis

Body lice are *Pediculus* humanus *corporus* and are closely related to head lice, but less frequently encountered in the United States. Body lice feed on the body, though they may be discovered on the scalp and facial hair. They usually remain on clothing near the skin and generally deposit their eggs on or near the seams of garments. Body lice are acquired mainly through direct contact with an infested person or clothing and bedding, and are most commonly found on individuals who infrequently change or wash their clothes. Body lice serve as carriers of certain human pathogens, including louse-borne typhus, louse-borne relapsing fever, and trench fever.

B85.3   Phthiriasis

Pubic or crab lice are *Phthirus pubis* and have a short crab-like body easily distinguished from that of head and body lice. Pubic lice are most frequently found among the pubic hairs of the infested person, but may also be found elsewhere on the body. The infestation by pubic lice is termed phthiriasis. Pubic lice are acquired mainly through sexual contact or by sharing a bed with an infested person. Pubic lice do not transmit infectious agents from person to person.

B86   Scabies

Scabies is a mite infestation that is caused by *Sarcoptes scabiei*. Scabies causes intense itching and sometimes secondary infection.

B87.-   Myiasis

Myiasis is an infestation by fly larvae (maggots) and is most commonly seen in wound or ulcer sites. Myiasis is usually cutaneous, but is also found in nasal mucosa or in the intestines.

Sequelae of Infectious and Parasitic Diseases (B90-B94)

A sequela, also called a late effect, is a residual effect that occurs as a direct result of another condition that has since resolved. The residual effect may occur within a few days of the initial condition or years later. Sequelae of infectious and parasitic diseases do not include chronic infections, which are coded to the appropriate infectious disease.

The categories in this code block are as follows:

B90	Sequelae of tuberculosis
B91	Sequelae of poliomyelitis
B92	Sequelae of leprosy
B94	Sequelae of other and unspecified infectious and parasitic diseases

Bacterial and Viral Infectious Agents (B95-B97)

This code block provides supplementary codes to identify the infectious agents in diseases classified elsewhere.

The categories in this code block are as follows:

B95	Streptococcus, Staphylococcus, and Enterococcus as the cause of diseases classified elsewhere
B96	Other bacterial agents as the cause of diseases classified elsewhere
B97	Viral agents as the cause of diseases classified elsewhere

B95.-   Streptococcus, Staphylococcus, and Enterococcus as the cause of diseases classified elsewhere

Streptococcus, *Staphylococcus*, and *Enterococcus* are three genuses of bacteria that are common causes of infectious disease. *Streptococcus* is a spherical, gram positive, nonmotile bacterium that clusters together to form chains. *Enterococcus* is a relatively new genus of bacteria with more than a dozen species. Bacteria now classified as enterococci were previously classified as group D streptococci. Enterococci make up part of the normal flora of the intestinal tract in humans, but are responsible for infections of other sites. *Staphylococcus* is a gram-positive bacterium that clusters together to form clumps. Species of *Staphylococcus* have traditionally been grouped into coagulase positive and coagulase negative species, which identifies the ability or inability of the species to clot blood. Codes in this category are used as supplementary or additional codes to identify the infectious agent in diseases that are classified in other chapters.

B95.0   Streptococcus, group A, as the cause of diseases classified elsewhere

Streptococcus is one of the more common causes of infectious disease. It is a spherical, gram positive, nonmotile bacterium that clusters together to form chains. One common pathogenic species is *S. pyogenes*, also called group A *Streptococcus* or GAS.

B95.1   Streptococcus, group B, as the cause of diseases classified elsewhere

Streptococcus is one of the more common causes of infectious disease. It is a spherical, gram-positive, nonmotile bacterium that clusters together to form chains. One common pathogenic species is *S. agalactiae*, also called group B *Streptococcus*.

B95.2   Enterococcus as the cause of diseases classified elsewhere

Enterococcus is a relatively new genus of bacteria with more than a dozen species. Bacteria now classified as enterococci were previously classified as group D streptococci. Enterococci make up part of the normal flora of the intestinal tract in humans, but are responsible for infections of the urinary tract, heart, surgical or other open wounds, catheter sites, and intraabdominal and pelvic sites. Specific species known to be responsible for infection in humans include *E. avium*, *E. casseliflavus*, *E. durans*, *E. faecalis*, *E. faecium*, *E. gallinarum*, *E. mundtii*, and *E. raffinosus*.

B95.3   Streptococcus pneumoniae as the cause of diseases classified elsewhere

Streptococcus is one of the more common causes of infectious disease. It is a spherical, gram-positive, nonmotile bacterium that clusters together to form chains. One common pathogenic species is *S. pneumoniae*, also called pneumococcus.

B95.6- Staphylococcus aureus as the cause of diseases classified elsewhere

Staphylococcus aureus is a coagulase-positive species that causes a wide spectrum of infectious diseases. In recent years, some *S. aureus* strains have become resistant to a number of antibiotics and infections due to *S. aureus* are also classified based on susceptibility or resistance to beta lactam antibiotics. Infections due to coagulase negative staphylococci and species other than *S. aureus* are reported with the code for other *Staphylococcus*.

B95.61 Methicillin susceptible Staphylococcus aureus infection as the cause of diseases classified elsewhere

The term methicillin-susceptible *Staphylococcus aureus* (MSSA) identifies strains of *S. aureus* that are susceptible or treatable with the traditional beta lactam class of antibiotics, such as penicillin, methicillin, and cephalosporins.

B95.62 Methicillin resistant Staphylococcus aureus infection as the cause of diseases classified elsewhere

Methicillin-resistant *Staphylococcus aureus* (MRSA) is a variant form of the bacterium that is resistant to the traditional beta lactam class of antibiotics, such as penicillin, methicillin, and cephalosporins. Sometimes referred to as a "superbug," MRSA is a major cause of hospital-acquired infections and community-acquired infections. Community acquired MRSA infections (CA-MRSA) are generally not life-threatening. Due to clinical challenges, MRSA is more difficult and costly to combat than MSSA, and generally poses a greater public health threat due to its multidrug resistance.

B95.7 Other staphylococcus as the cause of diseases classified elsewhere

This code includes coagulase negative *Staphylococcus* species, as well as all other specifically identified types of *Staphylococcus* other than *S. aureus*. Coagulase negative *Staphylococcus* species include *S. hominis* and *S. epidermidis*, which inhabit the skin and *S. saprophyticus* found in the vaginal tract. When confined to these sites, these species are typically not pathogenic. However, when they invade other sites they can result in an infectious process.

B97.- Viral agents as the cause of diseases classified elsewhere

Codes listed here are for use as supplementary or additional codes to identify the specific viral agent as the cause of a disease classified elsewhere.

B97.2- Coronavirus as the cause of diseases classified elsewhere

Of the plethora of coronavirus species, only six are known to cause infection in humans. All six infectious coronaviruses manifest as upper respiratory tract infections with severity dependent upon the specific species. Almost all humans are infected with at least one of the coronavirus species in their lifetime except SARS-CoV (severe acute respiratory syndrome coronavirus) and MERS-CoV (Middle East Respiratory Syndrome coronavirus), which are very rare.

B97.21 SARS-associated coronavirus as the cause of diseases classified elsewhere

SARS-associated coronavirus (SARS-CoV) is a novel coronavirus that typically causes a severe lower respiratory infection. The virus was first identified in Southeast Asia in 2003. The vast majority of infected patients develop pneumonia or severe acute respiratory syndrome (SARS), which is where the virus gets its name. SARS-CoV infection that is not documented as causing pneumonia or as causing severe acute respiratory syndrome is classified here.

> **Focus Point**
>
> For pneumonia due to SARS virus, SARS, or severe acute respiratory syndrome, report code J12.81 Pneumonia due to SARS-associated coronavirus. This code description includes the causative agent and therefore code B97.21 does not need to be coded in addition.

B97.4 Respiratory syncytial virus as the cause of diseases classified elsewhere

Respiratory syncytial virus (RSV) is a common cause of respiratory disease during the winter months in the United States. Infants are most vulnerable to the disease. Each year, RSV causes 4,500 U.S. deaths and 90,000 hospitalizations. This code is reported only when the disease caused by RSV is in an organ or site beyond the respiratory tract.

> **Focus Point**
>
> There are specific codes for pneumonia due to RSV (J12.1), bronchitis due to RSV (J29.5), and bronchiolitis due to RSV (J21.0); code B97.4 should not be reported additionally.

Other Infectious Diseases (B99)

There is a single category in the code block B99 Other and unspecified infectious diseases, and only two codes B99.8 and B99.9. These codes should rarely be used as documentation typically provides information that allows assignment of a more specific code, such as the site of the infection.

Chapter 2: Neoplasms (C00-D49)

Neoplasms are classified primarily by site, with broad groupings for behavior such as malignant, benign, in situ, uncertain behavior, and unspecified. The Table of Neoplasms should be used to identify the correct site (topography) code. In some cases, such as malignant melanoma and certain neuroendocrine tumors, the morphology is included in the category and codes. The tabular section should be consulted for the specific code.

Malignant neoplasms have the potential to invade surrounding tissue or shed cells that seed malignancies in other body sites. Malignant neoplasms are, therefore, classified as primary, meaning the site of origin of the malignant neoplasm; secondary, meaning a remote or metastatic site; and carcinoma in situ, meaning that the malignancy is localized and has not invaded deeper or surrounding tissues at the site of origin. When a primary malignancy overlaps two or more contiguous sites, it should be coded to the subcategory/code 8 (overlapping lesion) unless the combination is specifically indexed elsewhere. If there are multiple neoplasms of adjacent sites that are not contiguous, codes for each site should be assigned. For example, tumors of different breast quadrants in the same breast should be assigned separate codes for each site.

In addition to these classifications for solid tissue malignant neoplasms, there are additional classifications for blood cancers of lymphoid, hematopoietic, and other related tissues; some specific histological types of cancer such as malignant and benign neuroendocrine tumors; and some specific types of skin cancers, such as melanoma, basal cell carcinoma, and squamous cell carcinoma.

A benign neoplasm may grow, but does not invade surrounding tissues or remote sites. Benign neoplasms remain confined to the site of origin.

Neoplasms of uncertain behavior are those that currently exhibit benign characteristics but have the potential to transform and become malignant.

Only when the nature of the neoplasm is not specified is the neoplasm classified as unspecified behavior.

All neoplasms are classified to this chapter, whether or not they are functionally active. A functionally active neoplasm is a growth that performs functions ascribed to surrounding tissue, as in a thyroid tumor that secretes thyroxine and causes hyperthyroidism in the patient. An additional code from Chapter 4 may be used to identify functional activity associated with any neoplasm.

Focus Point

In most cases, encounters for treatment of complications of a neoplasm (e.g., dehydration, pain) are reported with the neoplasm complication sequenced first, followed by the appropriate neoplasm code. However, when the neoplasm complication is anemia, an exception is made. In these cases, the malignancy code is sequenced as the first-listed diagnosis followed by code D63.0 Anemia in neoplastic disease.

The chapter is broken down into the following code blocks:

C00-C14	Malignant neoplasms of lip, oral cavity and pharynx
C15-C26	Malignant neoplasms of digestive organs
C30-C39	Malignant neoplasms of respiratory and intrathoracic organs
C40-C41	Malignant neoplasms of bone and articular cartilage
C43-C44	Melanoma and other malignant neoplasms of skin
C45-C49	Malignant neoplasms of mesothelial and soft tissue
C50	Malignant neoplasms of breast
C51-C58	Malignant neoplasms of female genital organs
C60-C63	Malignant neoplasms of male genital organs
C64-C68	Malignant neoplasms of urinary tract
C69-C72	Malignant neoplasms of eye, brain and other parts of central nervous system
C73-C75	Malignant neoplasms of thyroid and other endocrine glands
C7A	Malignant neuroendocrine tumors
C7B	Secondary neuroendocrine tumors
C76-C80	Malignant neoplasms of ill-defined, other secondary and unspecified sites
C81-C96	Malignant neoplasms of lymphoid, hematopoietic and related tissue
D00-D09	In situ neoplasms
D10-D36	Benign neoplasms, except benign neuroendocrine tumors

D3A	Benign neuroendocrine tumors
D37-D48	Neoplasms of uncertain behavior, polycythemia vera and myelodysplastic syndromes
D49	Neoplasms of unspecified behavior

Malignant Neoplasms of Lip, Oral Cavity and Pharynx (C00-C14)

Primary malignant neoplasms of the lip, oral cavity, and pharynx are classified here. A primary malignant neoplasm is defined as cells or tissue described on the pathology report as malignant or by a specific histological type that is classified as malignant, such as carcinoma. Primary malignant neoplasms represent the site of origin of the malignancy.

The categories in this code block are as follows:

C00	Malignant neoplasm of lip
C01	Malignant neoplasm of base of tongue
C02	Malignant neoplasm of other and unspecified parts of tongue
C03	Malignant neoplasm of gum
C04	Malignant neoplasm of floor of mouth
C05	Malignant neoplasm of palate
C06	Malignant neoplasm of other and unspecified parts of mouth
C07	Malignant neoplasm of parotid gland
C08	Malignant neoplasm of other and unspecified major salivary glands
C09	Malignant neoplasm of tonsil
C10	Malignant neoplasm of oropharynx
C11	Malignant neoplasm of nasopharynx
C12	Malignant neoplasm of pyriform sinus
C13	Malignant neoplasm of hypopharynx
C14	Malignant neoplasm of other and ill-defined sites in the lip, oral cavity and pharynx

C00.- Malignant neoplasm of lip

Carcinoma is a histological type of primary malignant neoplasm that occurs on the lips. Anatomically, the lips are divided into two distinct segments. The vermilion border is the pigmented, fleshy, outer lip, and may be described in the medical record as the lipstick area or external lip. The interior aspect is the second segment. Lined in buccal mucosa, the interior aspect may be described as the mucosa, buccal aspect, or frenulum. The commissure of the lip is the juncture of the upper and lower lips, whether at the vermilion border or

interior aspect. Cancer of the lip is most often caused by sun exposure with men more likely to be affected due to occupational sun exposure along with more tobacco and alcohol use. Most are detected at an early and treatable stage with low rate of metastasis. Malignant neoplasms of the lip are classified by site.

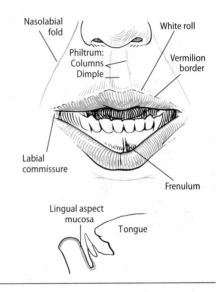

C01 Malignant neoplasm of base of tongue

C02.- Malignant neoplasm of other and unspecified parts of tongue

The tongue is a strong muscle that is attached to the floor of the mouth within the curve of the jawbone. It is anchored to muscles at the rear of the mouth, which attach to the base of the skull and to the hyoid bone. The underside of the tongue is attached to the floor of the mouth by membranes. These form a distinct vertical fold in the centerline, called the frenulum linguae. The surface of the tongue is covered with the lingual membrane, a specialized tissue with a variety of papillae protruding from it. These papillae nodules produce the characteristic rough surface of the tongue. Between the papillae are the taste buds, the sensory nerve organs that provide the sensations of flavor. The muscle fibers of the tongue are also heavily supplied with nerves to provide for manipulation and safe placement of food in the mouth and between the teeth for chewing. The tongue also aids in swallowing and in the formation of sounds of speech. Most tongue cancers develop in the thin, flat cells on the surface of the tongue called squamous cells. Cancers of the front of the tongue are often diagnosed in early stages and easily removed. Base of tongue cancers are generally diagnosed in later, more advanced stages. Base of tongue cancers are increasingly being linked with human papillomavirus (HPV). Subcategories identify the specific site of the tongue that is involved.

C03.-   Malignant neoplasm of gum

More than 95 percent of cancers of the oral cavity are squamous cell carcinomas, found most commonly in males, ages 50 to 70, with a history of tobacco and alcohol use. Smokeless tobacco or snuff and betel nut (common in India) contribute greatly to gum cancer risk. Codes for malignant neoplasms of the gum are specific to the upper and lower gum with an additional code for unspecified site.

C04.-   Malignant neoplasm of floor of mouth

The floor of the mouth is described as the horseshoe-shaped area under the tongue. A neoplasm on the mouth floor often presents as a painless ulcer that is mistaken for a canker sore. It is found most commonly in males, ages 50-70, with a history of tobacco and alcohol use with a higher risk associated with smokeless tobacco or snuff and betel nut. Exposure to human papilloma virus (HPV) has surfaced as another potential cause. Cancers of the floor of the mouth have a higher incidence of lymph node involvement than do other cancers of the inside of the mouth. Codes are specific to site.

C05.-   Malignant neoplasm of palate

The palate or roof of the mouth is divided into the hard palate in the front and the soft palate in the back of the mouth. Most palate cancers are squamous cell and present with a painless ulcer. Although a relationship to risk and use of tobacco and alcohol is clear in cancer of the soft palate, it has not been as clear for hard palate. A practice called reverse smoking, where the lit end of the cigarette is put into the mouth, has been shown to be a risk factor for hard palate cancer. Cancer of the uvula, which is a hanging conical tissue that projects from the soft palate, is also represented in this category.

C06.-   Malignant neoplasm of other and unspecified parts of mouth

This category includes cancers of the cheek mucosa and vestibule of the mouth, as well as the retromolar (space behind the molars) and other overlapping and unspecified areas of the mouth.

C06.1   Malignant neoplasm of vestibule of mouth

The vestibule of the mouth is the part of the oral cavity inside the cheeks and lips and outside the dentoalveolar structures (the teeth and gums). It includes the mucosal and submucosal tissue of the lips and cheeks and the labial and buccal frenulum, or frenum, the connecting folds of membrane that support and restrain the lips and cheeks. A neoplasm in this area often presents as a painless ulcer that is

mistaken for a canker sore. It is found most commonly in males, aged 50 to 70, with a history of tobacco and alcohol use with a higher risk associated with the use of smokeless tobacco or snuff and betel nut. Exposure to human papilloma virus (HPV) has surfaced as another potential cause.

C07   Malignant neoplasm of parotid gland

C08.-   Malignant neoplasm of other and unspecified major salivary glands

These codes report malignant neoplasms of major salivary glands, but not of surrounding tissues. Salivary glands secrete saliva to aid in mastication and to keep the mouth moist. The major salivary glands are the parotid, sublingual, and submandibular glands. The parotid is the most common site of salivary gland tumor and mucoepidermoid carcinoma is the most common type of parotid cancer.

Symptoms of parotid tumor include pain, enlargement of nodule, and sometimes facial nerve paralysis or lymphadenopathy. Other types of salivary gland tumors classified as malignant include the following carcinomas: adenoid cystic, epithelial-myoepithelial, primary squamous cell, biphasic malignancy, ex-pleomorphic adenoma, malignant oncocytoma, clear cell, or acinic cell.

> **Focus Point**
>
> *The appropriate code for malignant neoplasm of minor salivary gland unspecified is C06.9 Malignant neoplasm of mouth, unspecified.*

C09.-   Malignant neoplasm of tonsil

Tonsil cancers are typically squamous cell carcinomas, although some are lymphomas. They most often occur in the palatine tonsils, which are located on either side of the throat. Risk factors include smoking and alcohol, with the highest risk being the use of both substances in combination. Tonsil cancer has also been linked to a certain type of human papilloma virus called HPV16.

> **Focus Point**
>
> *The code for the palatine tonsil is included in the unspecified code (C09.9) and codes for the palatoglossal or palatopharyngeal arch are both included in the tonsillar pillar code (C09.1). Two other common sites of tonsillar neoplasms are the lingual tonsils reported with code C02.4 Malignant neoplasm lingual tonsil, and the pharyngeal tonsil reported with C11.1 Malignant neoplasm of posterior wall of nasopharynx.*

C10.-   Malignant neoplasm of oropharynx

The part of the pharynx that lies posterior to the oral cavity is called the oropharynx. It extends from its upper part at the soft palate down to its lower part that ends at the level of the hyoid bone. Most oropharyngeal tumors are squamous carcinomas, many with deep infiltrations. Risk factors include smoking and alcohol, with the highest risk being the use of both substances in combination. Oropharynx cancer has also been linked to the human papilloma virus (HPV).

C11.-   Malignant neoplasm of nasopharynx

Most malignant neoplasms of the nasopharynx originate in squamous cells but may spread to deeper tissues or distant sites if left untreated. The part of the pharynx that lies behind (posterior) the nasal cavity is called the nasopharynx. The nasopharynx extends from behind the nasal cavity to the soft palate. There are two openings from the nasopharynx to the nose (internal nares) and two openings to the ears (Eustachian tubes). The adenoids (pharyngeal tonsil) are located on the posterior wall of the nasopharynx. The most common tumor of the nasopharynx is squamous cell carcinoma. Malignant neoplasms of the nasopharynx are classified by site. Cancer of the nasopharynx is rare in North America with higher incidence in China, other parts of Asia, and North Africa. It most often occurs in males under 55 years of age. Some risk factors include smoking, heavy alcohol, diet rich in salt-cured fish and meat, and formaldehyde exposure. There has been some association with Epstein-Barr virus (EBV) and some genetic and family history linkage.

C12   Malignant neoplasm of pyriform sinus

C13.-   Malignant neoplasm of hypopharynx

The lowest part of the pharynx is called the laryngopharynx or hypopharynx. It extends from the hyoid bone and ends at a point where it divides into two structures: the esophagus and larynx. The pyriform sinus is a depressed area (fossa) in the hypopharynx that is located on either side of the larynx. More than 95 percent of hypopharyngeal cancers are squamous carcinoma, and the most common site is the pyriform sinus. Malignant neoplasms of the pyriform sinus account for 60 percent of hypopharyngeal cancers. Hypopharyngeal cancers usually don't present with symptoms until larger lesions are present. Because cancers of this site are not often detected until advanced stages, lymphatic involvement is seen in about 70 percent of hypopharyngeal malignancy. It is most typical in men aged 55 to 70 years old with a history of smoking and heavy alcohol use. Malignant neoplasms of the hypopharynx are classified by specific site.

C14.-   Malignant neoplasm of other and ill-defined sites in the lip, oral cavity and pharynx

This category includes primary malignancies of the pharynx that are not specified as to site, Waldeyer's ring, and overlapping sites of the lip, oral cavity, and pharynx.

C14.2   Malignant neoplasm of Waldeyer's ring

Waldeyer's ring is a ring of lymphoid tissue located in the region of the nasopharynx and oropharynx that is made up of the two palatine tonsils, the pharyngeal tonsil (adenoid), and the lingual tonsil. This lymphoid tissue grows until about 11 years of age and then decreases in size. Waldeyer's ring functions as the defense against infection and assists with the development of the immune system.

Malignant Neoplasms of Digestive Organs (C15-C26)

The digestive system is a group of organs that breaks down and changes food chemically for absorption as simple, soluble substances by blood, lymph systems, and body tissues. The digestive system begins in the mouth and continues in the pharynx and esophagus, the stomach, the small and large intestines, the rectum, and the anus.

Structures that support the digestive process from outside this continuous tube are also included in this system, including the gallbladder, pancreas, and liver. These organs provide secretions that are critical to food absorption and use by the body.

The categories in this code block are as follows:

C15	Malignant neoplasm of esophagus
C16	Malignant neoplasm of stomach
C17	Malignant neoplasm of small intestine
C18	Malignant neoplasm of colon
C19	Malignant neoplasm of rectosigmoid junction
C20	Malignant neoplasm of rectum
C21	Malignant neoplasm of anus and anal canal
C22	Malignant neoplasm of liver and intrahepatic bile ducts
C23	Malignant neoplasm of gallbladder
C24	Malignant neoplasm of other and unspecified parts of biliary tract
C25	Malignant neoplasm of pancreas
C26	Malignant neoplasm of other and ill-defined digestive organs

C15.-   Malignant neoplasm of esophagus

The esophagus is the alimentary canal connecting the pharynx to the stomach. Symptoms of carcinoma of the esophagus include difficulty swallowing, weight loss, coughing, and pain. Hoarseness is often seen. A majority of these cancers are squamous cell or adenocarcinoma. Anatomically, 20 percent occur in the upper third of the esophagus, 30 percent in the midesophagus, and 50 percent in the lower esophagus. Adenocarcinoma is most typically found in the lower esophagus, affecting primarily white males, and is the most common esophageal cancer in the United States. Squamous cell carcinoma is common in the mid to the upper esophagus and is more prevalent world-wide. It is believed that chronic irritation of the esophagus due to acid/bile reflux (GERD) can contribute to the risk of developing esophageal cancer. Other risk factors include obesity, alcohol, smoking, previous radiation, and a diet low in fruits and vegetables. Esophageal neoplasms are categorized by upper, middle, lower, overlapping, or unspecified sites.

C16.- Malignant neoplasm of stomach

The stomach has four functions: to act as a reservoir for food, to mix food, to begin the digestive process, and to allow the absorption of some substances. The stomach begins at the portal between the esophagus and the stomach—the cardia. It ends at the portal to the duodenum—the pylorus. In between is the corpus, or the body of the stomach. The corpus is divided into the upper portion, the fundus, which is served by the oxyntic gland; the lower portion or the antrum, served by the pyloric gland; and the large midportion, the body. There are no clear demarcations between the segments of the corpus. The lesser and greater curvatures of the stomach refer to the short and long walls of the organ. Also referred to as gastric cancer, stomach cancer is rarely found before age 40 and is twice as common in men as in women. It is typically slow growing with known causes linked to infection of *H. pylori*, gastritis, chronic anemia, and polyps. Risk factors include history of Epstein-Barr virus (EBV), smoking, obesity, type A blood type, exposure to asbestos, and a diet rich in salty, pickled, or smoked foods. Occupational hazards include working in coal, metal, timber, or rubber industries. The most common types of stomach cancers are ulcerating carcinomas, polypoid carcinomas, superficial spreading carcinomas, linitis plastica, and advanced carcinoma. Stomach neoplasms are classified by site.

C17.- Malignant neoplasm of small intestine

The small intestine, often called the small bowel, is the portion of the alimentary canal from the pylorus to the cecum. The duodenum lies between the pyloric valve at the exit of the stomach and the jejunum. The jejunum then leads to the ileum. There is no demarcation between the two portions of small bowel, but, generally, the jejunum resides to the left side of the peritoneum and the ileum resides to the right and into the pelvis. The main function of the small intestine is to digest and absorb nutrients. Typical tumors of the small intestine include lymphoma, sarcoma, and carcinoid, although the most common form of small intestine malignancy is adenocarcinoma in the proximal jejunum. The occurrence of small bowel cancer is less than that of the rest of the

gastrointestinal tract. The presence of Crohn's disease, celiac disease, or a family history of polyp syndromes is associated with adenocarcinoma. Celiac is also associated with lymphoma of the small intestine as is human immunodeficiency virus (HIV). Small intestine neoplasms are classified by site.

C17.3 Meckel's diverticulum, malignant

A Meckel's diverticulum is a congenital malformation of the intestine. Only a small number of people have a Meckel's diverticulum, which is a small pouch on the wall of the lower part of the small intestine that is a remainder of the formation of the digestive tract before birth. Very few people with this congenital malformation have any symptoms or problems associated with its presence and malignancies are also rare, although they may be somewhat higher in the diverticulum than in other regions of the small intestine.

> **Focus Point**
>
> *The small intestine is a common site for melanoma metastases, and these should be classified as secondary malignant neoplasms.*

C18.- Malignant neoplasm of colon

The large intestine, or colon, extends from the end of the ileum to the rectum. The rectum and rectosigmoid junction, however, are excluded from this category. The right colon consists of the cecum, ascending colon, hepatic flexure, and proximal transverse colon. The left colon consists of the distal transverse colon, the splenic flexure, the descending colon, sigmoid colon, and rectosigmoid colon.

Adenocarcinoma, which develops from adenomatous polyps from abnormal cells arising from the glands lining the colon, is the most common form of colon cancer. Adenomatous polyps often run in families as does hereditary nonpolyposis colorectal cancer syndromes (HNPCC). Other risk factors linked to colon cancer are Crohn's disease, a family history of colon cancer, and breast, uterine, or ovarian cancer. Obesity, smoking, and diet can also be factors affecting colon cancer development. Malignant neoplasms of the colon are categorized by site.

Malignant Neoplasm of Colon

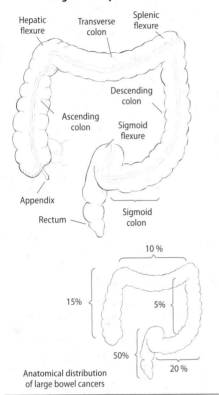

Anatomical distribution
of large bowel cancers

C19 Malignant neoplasm of rectosigmoid junction

C20 Malignant neoplasm of rectum

The rectum begins at the rectosigmoid junction and ends at the anus. The rectum and rectosigmoid junctions are the most common sites for cancer in the colon, accounting for more than 30 percent of cases. Adenocarcinoma, a cancer stemming from polyps in the mucosa, comprises the largest percentage (98 percent) of these cancers with the remainder being lymphoma, carcinoid, and sarcoma. Risk factors for developing rectal cancer include Crohn's disease, older age, smoking, high-fat diet, and a family history. Colon and rectal cancers are the third most common cancer in males and females with occurrence only slightly higher in men. The most common symptoms are rectal bleeding with bowel movement and pain upon defecation (tenesmus).

C21.- Malignant neoplasm of anus and anal canal

The anus is the opening at the end of the rectum and has a lower rate of malignancy than other parts of the gastrointestinal tract. Approximately 50 percent of cancers of the anus and anal canal are diagnosed before they have spread beyond the primary site. When diagnosed at early stages, it is highly treatable with a five-year survival rate of 82 percent. It is more common in men than women prior to age 35, but changes to women with a slightly higher incidence over the age of 50. Some associated risk factors include receptive anal intercourse, human papillomavirus (HPV) with genital warts, and immunocompromised patients such as those with HIV.

C22.- Malignant neoplasm of liver and intrahepatic bile ducts

Primary liver cancer is uncommon in the United States. About 80 percent of primary liver cancers are hepatocellular carcinoma. Others included here are hepatoblastoma, which primarily affects children, and intrahepatic bile duct cancer, most of which are cholangiocarcinomas. Chronic infection with hepatitis B (HBV) or hepatitis C (HCV) is associated with liver cancer. About 50 percent of people with hepatocellular carcinoma have cirrhosis from alcohol abuse. Other risk factors for primary liver cancer include nonalcoholic fatty liver disease, diabetes, obesity, smoking, and inherited liver diseases. Angiosarcoma, rarer than hepatocellular, is associated with hemochromatosis and exposure to other toxins such as herbicides, vinyl chloride, and arsenic.

Focus Point

The liver is a common site for metastases and secondary malignant neoplasms of the liver and intrahepatic bile ducts are reported with code C78.7.

C23 Malignant neoplasm of gallbladder

The gallbladder is a small, pear-shaped organ that sits just beneath the liver on the right side of the abdomen. Its function is to store bile. Gallbladder cancer is uncommon and usually seen only in the elderly. Most of these cancers are adenocarcinomas. Because there are generally no symptoms, most gallbladder cancers are not detected until later stages with poor prognosis. The cause of this cancer is mostly unknown, but a history of gallstones and obesity are considered slight risk factors. Gallbladder cancer occurs more often in women with frequency rising with age.

C24.0 Malignant neoplasm of extrahepatic bile duct

Extrahepatic bile duct cancer can manifest outside the liver in the hilum or distal region, the areas of the right and left bile ducts exiting the liver and entering the common hepatic duct or within the area of the common bile duct passing through the pancreas and ending in the small intestine. It is often referred to as perihilar or extrahepatic cholangiocarcinoma. This is a rare form of cancer in which colitis and some forms of liver disease may increase the risk, with symptoms of jaundice or abdominal pain. Prognosis and treatment rely on symptoms and whether the cancer has spread to other areas. Typically bile duct cancer goes undiscovered until it has spread, which eliminates the possibility of complete removal with surgery. Treatment then is focused on symptom relief and improvement of quality of life.

Focus Point

Intrahepatic bile duct carcinoma, which can also be referred to a cholangiocarcinoma, is specified with code C22.1, which differentiates between intrahepatic location and an extrahepatic site. Code C24.8 Malignant neoplasm of overlapping sites of biliary tract, is reported when the neoplasm involves both the intrahepatic and extrahepatic bile ducts.

C24.1 Malignant neoplasm of ampulla of Vater

A neoplasm of the ampulla of Vater is located in the area of the dilation at the juncture of the common bile and pancreatic ducts near the opening into the lumen of the duodenum. This form of cancer is often detected early due to symptoms leading to discovery of biliary obstruction. Surgical resection is the treatment of choice to promote long-term recovery; however the five-year survival rate remains at 40 percent to 67 percent. Other forms of treatment, such as biliary decompression, removal of gastric obstruction, and pain control, can improve quality of life but do not increase the overall survival rate. Ampullary cancer is uncommon but has increased in incidence over the last 40+ years, making up about 0.5 percent of all gastrointestinal neoplasms. It tends to affect Caucasian males, appearing most often between the ages of 50 and 70 years of age.

C25.- Malignant neoplasm of pancreas

The pancreas is a slender organ lying behind the stomach in the abdomen. The head of the pancreas is curved near the duodenum, the body is the main portion, and the tail is the portion that abuts the spleen. There are no clear demarcations between the parts of the pancreas. The pancreas (exocrine cells) produces pancreatic juice, which are enzymes that assist in digestion. The endocrine cells of the pancreas make and secrete insulin, which regulates blood glucose levels. Most pancreatic cancers start in the exocrine cells. Pancreatic cancer is aggressive and one of the most prevalent cancers in the United States, after lung cancer and colon cancer. It is most common in people aged 50 to 70. Because there are generally no symptoms, most pancreatic cancers are not detected until later stages with poor prognosis. Symptoms may include weight loss, jaundice, and

abdominal or back pain. Pancreatic cancer is most common in the head of the gland, with 66 percent of malignancies occurring there. Ductal adenocarcinoma is the most common type of malignancy in pancreatic cancer. Some risk factors include smoking, chronic pancreatitis, chronic diabetes, and inherited or familial conditions. Malignant neoplasms of the pancreas are classified by site.

C25.4 Malignant neoplasm of endocrine pancreas

Malignant neoplasms of the endocrine pancreas are sometimes referred to as malignant islet cell tumors. The islet cells are responsible for making and secreting insulin and glucagon, hormones necessary to maintain normal blood sugar levels. If the cancer is in the islets of Langerhans, production of these hormones can be affected causing elevated or decreased blood sugar levels and symptoms associated with hyper- or hypoglycemia.

Focus Point

When a neoplasm affects hormone production it is called a functional tumor and an additional code is reported from the endocrine chapter to identify the functional activity.

C26.- Malignant neoplasm of other and ill-defined digestive organs

This category includes malignant neoplasm of the spleen, which is under the ribs on the left side of the abdomen. It is part of the lymphatic system and filters blood and fights infections.

Focus Point

Most spleen malignancies are not primary but are blood cancers, such as lymphoma or leukemias, and are not coded in this category.

Malignant Neoplasms of Respiratory and Intrathoracic Organs (C30-C39)

This code block includes the larynx and the lower respiratory tract contained within the thorax, which consists of the trachea, bronchial tree, lungs, and pleura. Also classified to this subsection are malignant neoplasms of the middle ears, nasal cavity, sinuses, heart, thymus, and mediastinum.

The categories in this code block are as follows:

C30	Malignant neoplasm of nasal cavity and middle ear
C31	Malignant neoplasm of accessory sinuses
C32	Malignant neoplasm of larynx
C33	Malignant neoplasm of trachea
C34	Malignant neoplasm of bronchus and lung
C37	Malignant neoplasm of thymus
C38	Malignant neoplasm of heart, mediastinum and pleura
C39	Malignant neoplasm of other and ill-defined sites in the respiratory system and intrathoracic organs

C30.- Malignant neoplasm of nasal cavity and middle ear

This category represents malignant neoplasms of the nasal cavity including areas such as the nose cartilage, nasal concha, and internal, septum, and vestibule of the nose. Also included are uncommon malignant neoplasms of the middle ear such as antrum tympanicum, auditory and eustachian tube, tympanic cavity, inner ear, and mastoid air cells.

C30.0 Malignant neoplasm of nasal cavity

The nasal cavity opens into the vestibule, which is just inside of the nostrils and continues to the respiratory area where bone in three shelves (formed by the nasal cavity) called the superior, middle, and inferior nasal turbinates (nasal conchae) are located. The turbinates come close to the nasal septum and subdivide the nasal cavity into passageways. The largest majority of neoplasms of the nasal cavity are squamous cell carcinoma followed by adenocarcinoma. Malignant neoplasm of the nasal cavity is rare. Smoking, including second-hand smoke, and heavy alcohol use are known to increase chances of developing this cancer with recent studies showing some link to marijuana use. Other risk factors include infection with the human papillomavirus (HPV) and exposure to air pollution. Also considered risks are various inhalants from occupational environments such as dust from

wood, textile or leather industries, asbestos, rubbing alcohol, glue, formaldehyde, or solvent fumes, among others. It affects men more than women and usually doesn't present until after age 45.

> **Focus Point**
>
> *Malignant neoplasms in this category exclude melanoma (skin) and other skin cancers, as well as malignant neoplasm of many other parts of the nose.*

C31.- Malignant neoplasm of accessory sinuses

The accessory sinuses or paranasal sinuses are air spaces that surround the nasal cavity. The maxillary sinuses are located behind each cheekbone. The frontal and ethmoidal sinuses are above and between the eyes and the sphenoidal sinuses are behind the eyes on either side of the upper nose. The most common area for paranasal sinus cancer is the maxillary sinus. The largest majority of neoplasms of the paranasal sinuses are squamous cell carcinoma followed by adenocarcinoma. Malignant neoplasm of the paranasal sinuses is rare. Smoking, including second-hand smoke, and heavy alcohol use are known to increase chances of developing this cancer with recent studies showing some link to marijuana use. Other risk factors include infection with the human papillomavirus (HPV) and exposure to air pollution. Also considered risks are various inhalants from occupational environments such as dust from wood, textile or leather industries, asbestos, rubbing alcohol, glue, formaldehyde, or solvent fumes, among others. It affects men more than women and usually doesn't present until after age 45. Malignant neoplasms of the paranasal sinuses are classified by site.

C32.- Malignant neoplasm of larynx

The larynx is divided into the glottis, where the true vocal cord lie, the supraglottis, and the subglottis. The larynx has two primary functions: speech and respiration. It is commonly called the "voice box." Most laryngeal malignancies originate in the glottis and are squamous cell carcinomas, with a much higher occurrence in men than women. Hoarseness and throat pain are common symptoms. Smoking is the largest risk factor for cancer in the larynx with heavy use of alcohol also a contributing factor. Malignant neoplasms of the larynx are classified by site.

C33 Malignant neoplasm of trachea

The trachea, also referred to as the windpipe, is the tube that lies in front of the esophagus and runs from the mouth to the lungs dividing into the left and right bronchus. Tracheal cancer is uncommon, and affects men and women equally most often between the ages of 40 and 60. The most typical types are squamous cell carcinoma and adenoid cystic carcinoma. Although the exact cause is unknown for both types, smoking is linked to squamous cell carcinoma.

C34.- Malignant neoplasm of bronchus and lung

Lung cancer is the leading cause of cancer deaths in the United States for both men and women, with more than 200,000 cases diagnosed and more than 150,000 dying from the disease annually. There are three main types of lung cancer: non-small cell, which is the most common and includes squamous cell, adenocarcinoma, and large cell carcinoma; small cell, also referred to as oat cell cancer; and the least common, which is not included in this category, is lung carcinoid tumor, also referred to as neuroendocrine tumors. While the largest risk factor is smoking, other risk factors include asbestos, radon gas, radiation exposure, genetic disposition, lung disease such as COPD, and air pollution exposure. Lung cancer is considered one of the most lethal forms of cancer, with only 20 percent of patients surviving one year after diagnosis. Lung cancer is classified according to the lobe of the lung. The subcategories identify the bronchus or specific lobe of the lung affected, as well as laterality.

Focus Point

Primary neoplasms of the lung or bronchus specified as "carcinoid" or "neuroendocrine" are classified to category C7A.

C37 Malignant neoplasm of thymus

The thymus is a lymph-rich organ that produces T lymphocytes that circulate throughout the body to provide an immune function. This pyramid-shaped, double-lobed organ is located in the chest cavity, anterior to the heart, in the upper mediastinum. A malignant thymoma is a rare tumor located on the anterior mediastinum that originates from epithelial tissue in the thymus, accounting for most cases of thymus malignancies. Thymomas are most common between the ages of 40 and 60 with slightly higher occurrence in men. There are few known risk factors and many of these malignancies are asymptomatic.

Focus Point

Some lymphomas arise in thymus tissue. Lymphoma of the thymus is classified to categories C81-C85.

C38.- Malignant neoplasm of heart, mediastinum and pleura

The mediastinum is the compartment between the sternum and lungs/heart (anterior) and the spine and lungs/heart (posterior). This category also identifies malignant neoplasms of the heart and pericardium, which is the fibrous tissue membrane that surrounds the heart, and the pleura, which is the thin tissue membrane around the lungs.

Focus Point

Because of the general nature of the mediastinum in anatomical descriptions, care should be taken that a more specific site is not overlooked when coding malignant neoplasm of the mediastinum. For example, the thymus and parathyroid reside in the mediastinum and malignancies of these sites are reported with more specific codes.

C38.0 Malignant neoplasm of heart

Malignant neoplasms of the heart are rarely seen as primary neoplasms. Primary cancer of the heart occurs most commonly in children. Histological types of heart tumors classified as malignant include angiosarcoma, rhabdomyosarcoma, fibrosarcoma, and sarcoma. Complications from cardiac cancer can be grave and include heart failure, hemorrhagic pericardial effusion with tamponade, and arrhythmia. A primary cancer of the heart is also prone to metastasize to the spine and other major organs.

Focus Point

Mesothelioma of the heart is reported with code C45.7 Mesothelioma of other sites. Lymphoma of the heart is reported with a code for the appropriate type of lymphoma in categories C81-C85 with the site identified as an extranodal/solid organ site.

Malignant Neoplasms of Bone and Articular Cartilage (C40-C41)

Primary malignancies of the bone are uncommon compared to the incidence of metastases to the bone.

The categories in this code block are as follows:

C40   Malignant neoplasm of bone and articular cartilage of limbs

C41   Malignant neoplasm of bone and articular cartilage of other and unspecified sites

Focus Point

Multiple myeloma is the most common bone malignancy but this is a malignancy of the bone marrow and is reported with codes in category C90.

C40.-   Malignant neoplasm of bone and articular cartilage of limbs

C41.-   Malignant neoplasm of bone and articular cartilage of other and unspecified sites

Histological types of bone and cartilage tumors classified as primary malignancies include osteosarcoma, fibrosarcoma, malignant fibrous histiocytoma, chondrosarcoma, Ewing's sarcoma, and malignant giant cell tumor. Osteosarcoma is a malignant neoplasm most commonly seen in children and young adults. It most often develops in long bones such as the distal femur or proximal tibia with the proximal humerus being the next most common site, although it can affect any bone. Pain, swelling, limited range of motion, and pathological fractures are common symptoms. Fibrosarcomas are similar to osteosarcoma but develop fibrous rather than bone tumors. Chondrosarcomas are malignancies of cartilage and tend to occur in older adults. Ewing's sarcoma is malignancy affecting mostly children and adolescents. It is a round cell cancer that typically develops inside but can grow on the outside of the bones. Although it can affect any bone, it typically develops in the extremities and can involve the entire bone shaft. It is not hereditary, but it is linked to a specific protein-encoding gene called the EWS gene that can be switched on after birth predisposing those individuals to a variety of benign and malignant neoplasms.

Melanoma and Other Malignant Neoplasms of Skin (C43-C44)

The integumentary system is a diverse and complex organ forming the boundary and barrier between the internal environment of the body and the outside world. Although quite thin, the skin (or cutaneous membrane) is the largest human organ, usually 12 to 20 square feet in area and composing 12 percent of the total body weight. The depth of the skin varies from 0.5 mm in thin areas such as the eyelids to 5 mm or more at its thickest over the back. Malignant neoplasms in this code block are melanoma, basal cell, squamous cell, and Merkel cell and are classified by type of neoplasm and site.

The categories in this code block are as follows:

C43   Malignant melanoma of skin

C4A   Merkel cell carcinoma

C44   Other and unspecified malignant neoplasm of skin

C43.-   Malignant melanoma of skin

Melanomas are skin cancers that are usually pigmented but otherwise vary in size and presentation. They are among the most invasive of the cancers. Change is the hallmark of melanoma; adjacent tissue is usually transformed. The most common type of melanoma is superficial spreading melanoma, accounting for 65 percent of all melanomas. They are most common on women's legs or men's trunks. Other types of melanoma include nodular, with dark papules or plaques, and solar lentigo, arising as a flat tan macule on areas of skin that have had long-term sun exposure, especially on the hands and forehead. Melanoma is classified by site.

Focus Point

Melanoma begins as a skin cancer, but aggressively metastasizes to other systems or organs. These secondary sites are not classified as melanomas, but as secondary malignant neoplasms.

C4A.-   Merkel cell carcinoma

Merkel cell carcinoma (MCC) is an aggressive neuroendocrine skin cancer that arises from the uncontrolled growth of Merkel cells in the epidermal layer of the skin. MCC is a neuroendocrine tumor because the affected Merkel cells have sensory and hormonal functions. Once thought to be relatively rare, the incidence of this cancer has been steadily increasing, with approximately 1,500 new cases per year. Incidence rates have more than tripled in the past two decades. MCC is fatal in 33 percent, or one-third, of patients. Immune-suppressed (e.g., transplants, HIV, chronic immunosuppressive disease) or fair-skinned individuals 50 to 65 years of age with a history of extensive sun exposure are considered to be at the highest risk. As a result, MCC has become the most common cause of nonmelanoma skin cancer fatalities in the United States. Characteristic signs include firm, flesh, or red-violet colored bumps that develop suddenly on sun-exposed skin and tend to grow rapidly over a period of weeks or months. It occurs most frequently on sun-exposed areas of the body (e.g., head, face, neck, and limbs) but may arise from commonly sun-protected sites (e.g., back, chest, buttock). Due to the aggressive nature of MCC, immediate identification is necessary to ensure optimal treatment. MCC is classified by site.

C44.- Other and unspecified malignant neoplasm of skin

Basal cell carcinoma, squamous cell carcinoma, and other or unspecified malignant skin neoplasms are classified here. Basal cell carcinoma is the most common and least likely to metastasize form of non-melanoma skin cancer. Squamous cell carcinoma is the second most common form. Causation for both basal and squamous cell includes a combination of genetic, environmental, and other risk factors (e.g., immunosuppression status, age, sex, medical history). However, lesions most commonly develop on sun-exposed areas of the skin, due to long-term exposure to ultraviolet (UV) radiation from sunlight. The UV radiation is thought to damage the DNA within the skin. As a result, the normal cellular regeneration process is disrupted, causing cells to grow abnormally, thereby forming a cancerous tumor.

Basal cells are the regenerative cells located at the bottom layer of the epidermis. The appearance of basal skin lesions varies in color and characteristics, from colorless or white, waxy bumps or crusty, scar-like lesions to flesh colored or darkened brown or black patches. Some lesions contain visible blood vessels at the site of a nonhealing wound-like lesion, which may bleed or ooze. These lesions may be easily confused with an ordinary nonhealing sore or scar and can grow rapidly in diameter.

Squamous cells are flat, brick-like cells situated just above the basal cell layer. Squamous cell skin lesions vary in appearance from white to reddened lesions that may present as firm nodules or scaly, flat crusted lesions or ulcerations.

Although both types of cancers are easily treated, basal cell lesions have a high recurrence rate. Both lesions can invade adjacent tissues and can cause extensive damage if not removed.

Malignant Neoplasms of Mesothelial and Soft Tissue (C45-C49)

The categories in this code block are as follows:

C45	Mesothelioma
C46	Kaposi's sarcoma
C47	Malignant neoplasm of peripheral nerves and autonomic nervous system
C48	Malignant neoplasm of retroperitoneum and peritoneum
C49	Malignant neoplasm of other connective and soft tissue

C45.- Mesothelioma

Malignant mesothelioma is most often caused by asbestos exposure. It is a rare cancer that affects the lining that protects the internal organs, most commonly the pleura, but can also develop in the pericardium and peritoneum. Most mesotheliomas involve the epithelial cells and are most common in men older than age 60.

C46.- Kaposi's sarcoma

Kaposi's sarcoma is a malignancy characterized by numerous vascular skin tumors. Kaposi's sarcoma was once found only rarely, in aging men, usually of Italian or Jewish decent. Today, incidence is common in the United States, as a manifestation of Acquired Immune Deficiency Syndrome (AIDS). A diagnosis of Kaposi's sarcoma of the skin is significant because it is often the first clinical manifestation of AIDS in a Human Immunodeficiency Virus (HIV) positive patient, though Kaposi's sarcoma itself is rarely a cause of death. Disseminated Kaposi's sarcoma can involve lymph nodes, viscera, and the gastrointestinal tract.

C47.- Malignant neoplasm of peripheral nerves and autonomic nervous system

Malignant nerve sheath tumor, also referred to as neurofibrosarcoma, is a type of malignant neoplasm classified here. It is characterized by the development of tumors in the cells that surround the peripheral nerves. People with neurofibromatosis type 1, a genetic condition that causes benign fibrous tumors of the nerves, are at increased risk of developing neurofibrosarcoma. Neurofibrosarcomas are aggressive tumors that require aggressive treatment.

C48.- Malignant neoplasm of retroperitoneum and peritoneum

The retroperitoneum is the space behind the peritoneum and in front of the spine. The peritoneum is the membrane that holds the abdominal organs. Retroperitoneal tumors are usually of mesodermal tissue.

Focus Point

A majority of peritoneal malignancies are secondary, with the exception of peritoneal mesothelioma, a rare cancer arising in the mesodermal lining of the peritoneum and reported with code C45.1

C49.- Malignant neoplasm of other connective and soft tissue

Malignant neoplasms of the connective tissue and other soft tissue are classified according to site rather than specific type of tissue. These codes can be used to classify malignant neoplasms of blood vessels, bursa, cartilage (except articular, laryngeal, and nasal), fascia, fat, ligament (except uterine), muscle, synovia, or tendons. Cartilage is a type of dense connective tissue. Soft tissue generally includes the deep fascia, muscles, tendons, and ligaments. Deep fascia lies beneath the second layer of subcutaneous tissue (hypodermis) of the integumentary system. Deep fascia in the musculoskeletal system lines extremities and holds together groups of muscles.

C49.A- Gastrointestinal stromal tumor

Malignant gastrointestinal stromal tumor (GIST) is an uncommon tumor found in the GI tract that originates from interstitial cells of the autonomic nervous system. These interstitial cells regulate the muscle contractions that move the food through the digestive process. Although GIST can start anywhere in the GI tract, it most often begins in the stomach. It can occur at any age but is seen mostly in people older than age 50 and affects slightly more men than women.

Focus Point

If documentation specifies stromal tumor of digestive system but of uncertain behavior, the appropriate code would be D48.1. If the documentation specifies stromal tumor of digestive system that is benign, the appropriate code would be D21.4.

Malignant Neoplasms of Breast (C50)

This code block represents malignant neoplasms of the breast and surrounding connective tissue of females and males.

The categories in this code block are as follows:

C50   Malignant neoplasm of breast

C50.- Malignant neoplasm of breast

Breast cancer develops primarily in the milk ducts (ductal carcinoma) or glands (lobular carcinoma). Invasive breast cancer has spread from the ducts or lobules to surrounding breast tissue. Even though it is known that certain risk factors exist, many at high risk never develop it while others with none of the risks do develop it. Some of the known risk factors include older age, family history, history of benign lumps, and previous breast, endometrial, ovarian, or colon cancer. Research has found that a factor responsible for some familial breast cancer is presence of the BRCA1 or BRCA2 gene, which has been shown to predispose women to breast cancer along with other cancers. The BRCA2 also increases that risk in males, although men still only make up 1 percent of all breast cancers. Researchers also think that estrogen hormone exposure increases a woman's susceptibility to develop breast cancer. A large majority of men that develop breast cancer have estrogen receptors in the cell membranes. Klinefelter syndrome, a condition where infant boys are born with higher than normal estrogen, is a major risk factor. Studies also show that family history of a first-degree male relative with breast cancer also increases risk.

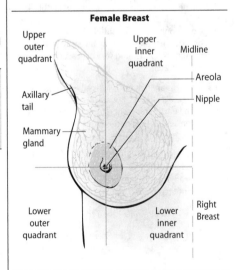

Female Breast

Upper outer quadrant

Upper inner quadrant

Midline

Areola

Axillary tail

Nipple

Mammary gland

Lower outer quadrant

Lower inner quadrant

Right Breast

Malignant Neoplasms of Female Genital Organs (C51-C58)

This code block includes primary malignancies of the female genital organs including the placenta.

The categories in this code block are as follows:

C51	Malignant neoplasm of vulva
C52	Malignant neoplasm of vagina
C53	Malignant neoplasm of cervix uteri
C54	Malignant neoplasm of corpus uteri
C55	Malignant neoplasm of uterus, part unspecified
C56	Malignant neoplasm of ovary
C57	Malignant neoplasm of other and unspecified female genital organs
C58	Malignant neoplasm of placenta

C52   Malignant neoplasm of vagina

Primary vaginal cancers are described as arising solely from the vagina, with no involvement of the cervix or vulva. It is considered rare, although the incidence is increasing as women live longer. The most common type is squamous cell carcinoma, occurring in the upper third of the vagina and accounting for about 85 percent of cases. It is suggested that the HPV virus has shown some association with development of vaginal cancer. Other risk factors include history of cervical intraepithelial neoplasia (CIN), in utero exposure to diethylstilbestrol (DES), a drug used prior to 1971 to prevent miscarriages, and prior hysterectomy.

C53.-   Malignant neoplasm of cervix uteri

Cancer of the cervix uteri may be asymptomatic or may cause vaginal discharge, pain, or postcoital bleeding. Most cervical cancers are squamous cell cancers. Cervical cancer is classified as endocervix (opens into the uterus), exocervix (protrudes into the vagina), or involving overlapping sites.

C54.-   Malignant neoplasm of corpus uteri

C55   Malignant neoplasm of uterus, part unspecified

The uterus is the muscular female organ where the fetus develops until delivery. Normally only three inches long and the shape of a pear, the uterus expands greatly during pregnancy. Malignant neoplasms of the body of the uterus are classified according to site: the body of the uterus, including the fundus and endometrium; and the isthmus of the uterus, the narrow, distal portion of the uterus between the main body, endometrium, or myometrium. Endometrial carcinoma is a common malignancy that affects primarily postmenopausal women. Symptoms include postmenopausal bleeding, though symptoms may not be present until metastases become symptomatic. If the site is not specified, the code for part unspecified is assigned.

C56.-   Malignant neoplasm of ovary

The ovary is the female gonad and produces the ova. The organs are situated on either side of the uterus and lie near bilateral fallopian tubes, which carry the ova from the ovary to the uterus. Ligaments secure the female reproductive organs in the abdominal cavity. Ovarian malignancies often present as an abdominal mass. Common types of ovarian malignancies include mucinous cystadenocarcinoma and endometrioid carcinoma. Other ovarian cancers are hormone producing and include Sertoli-Leydig cell tumors, adrenal cell rest tumors, and granulosa-theca cell tumors. Use an additional code to report any functional activity associated with the ovarian malignancy.

C58   Malignant neoplasm of placenta

The placenta is an organ of pregnancy, operating as an exchange point for waste from the fetus and nourishment from the mother. In rare cases, an anomalous placenta may develop when no viable fetus exists, as in the case of hydatidiform mole. Use this code to report choriocarcinoma, also called chorioepithelioma. Hydatidiform mole or pregnancy precedes choriocarcinoma. It is an epithelial malignancy that metastasizes rapidly.

Malignant Neoplasms of Male Genital Organs (C60-C63)

Primary malignant neoplasms of the male genital organs, including malignancies of the skin of these sites, are classified here.

The categories in this code block are as follows:

C60	Malignant neoplasm of penis
C61	Malignant neoplasm of prostate
C62	Malignant neoplasm of testis
C63	Malignant neoplasm of other and unspecified male genital organs

C60.- Malignant neoplasm of penis

The penis has two functions in males: sexual and excretory. The urethra may convey semen or urine. The tip of the penis is called the glans penis and is covered in mucous membrane. The prepuce, or foreskin, is a fold of skin at the juncture where the body of the penis meets the glans penis; this extra skin is removed in circumcision. The corpora cavernosa are twin cylinders that extend the length of the organ called the body of the penis. Cancer of the penis usually occurs in uncircumcised males and human papillomavirus infection has been linked to penile cancer rates.

C61 Malignant neoplasm of prostate

The prostate is a singular, walnut-sized gland in the male. It surrounds the neck of the bladder and its ducts empty into the prostatic portion of the urethra. The prostate contributes fluid that helps to liquefy semen. Adenocarcinoma of the prostate is the most common form of cancer in males older than age 50 in the United States. Symptoms are uncommon until late in the disease course, when urethral obstruction and hematuria may occur.

C62.- Malignant neoplasm of testis

The testes are a pair of male gonads found in the scrotum and produce spermatozoa for fertilization. Leydig cells in the testes produce testosterone. Most testicular masses are malignant and testicular cancer is more common among males with a history of undescended testes, even if the condition has been corrected surgically.

Malignant Neoplasms of Urinary Tract (C64-C68)

The kidneys are paired organs between the parietal peritoneum and the posterior abdominal wall (retroperitoneal). They are located in the area of the last thoracic vertebrae to the third lumbar vertebrae and function as the body's blood filter. Items no longer needed are removed from the blood by the filter (kidneys) and eliminated in the form of urine, and elements needed are put back into the blood to be used by the cells and tissues of the body. Some of the blood the heart outputs with each cardiac cycle is sent to the kidneys to be filtered via two renal arteries (one to each kidney). In the kidneys, the renal arteries drain into other small arteries, then even smaller arterioles and capillary networks called glomeruli where filtration takes place. Once the blood has been filtered and cleaned in the kidneys, it goes through venous capillaries that change into small veins called venules. Venules drain into larger veins that finally drain into the renal veins. The renal veins return the blood that has been filtered to the heart via the inferior vena cava.

Cup-like projections in each of the kidneys, called the renal calyces, drain the urine. Urine that has collected in the renal pelvis is transported via a process called peristalsis to storage in the bladder. The ureters enter the bladder (one at each side) at its base and deposit the urine they carry into the bladder. Each ureter includes a valve that prevents urine that has been placed into the bladder from backing up into the ureters and the renal pelvis. This section identifies malignant neoplasms of specific sites in the kidney, renal pelvis, ureter, and bladder. Also included are malignant neoplasms of urethra and paraurethral glands.

The categories in this code block are as follows:

C64	Malignant neoplasm of kidney, except renal pelvis
C65	Malignant neoplasm of renal pelvis
C66	Malignant neoplasm of ureter
C67	Malignant neoplasm of bladder
C68	Malignant neoplasm of other and unspecified urinary organs

C64.- Malignant neoplasm of kidney, except renal pelvis

Renal cell carcinoma is the most common kidney malignancy. It develops in the lining of the small tubes of the filtering system that lead to the bladder. Sarcoma is the more rare type; it can grow large but it doesn't spread to other parts of the body as often as the other types. Wilms' tumor or nephroblastoma is a childhood malignancy of the kidney. The tumor begins in utero and may be asymptomatic for years, though it is usually diagnosed before age 5. Risk factors for kidney cancer include smoking, obesity, hypertension, long-term dialysis, and Von Hippel-Lindau (VHL) syndrome, an inherited condition caused by an abnormal gene. Men are more likely to develop renal malignancies and higher risk is associated with certain occupations with exposure to asbestos or cadmium or coke oven workers in steel and iron industries.

C65.- Malignant neoplasm of renal pelvis

C66.- Malignant neoplasm of ureter

Primary malignant neoplasms of the renal pelvis, in the lower part of each kidney, and the ureter start in the lining of the renal pelvis or the ureter. The renal calyces, also included in the renal pelvis code, are the urine collection chambers in the lower kidney. The calyces meet at the renal pelvis where the urine is funneled into the ureter. Transitional cell carcinoma, also referred to as urothelial carcinoma, is a type of malignancy that develops in tissues of the renal pelvis and ureter. However, malignancies of the renal pelvis and ureters are uncommon and rarely occur before age

65. It affects more men than women and generally only affects one side of the renal pelvis or ureter. Some suggested risk factors are smoking and kidney damage from long term use of pain killers.

C67.- Malignant neoplasm of bladder

The bladder lies in front (anterior) of the rectum in men and in front (anterior) of the vagina in women. As the bladder fills with urine, impulses from voluntary and involuntary nerves signal that the bladder is full. When full, the bladder releases the urine it has stored through urination (voiding) via a tube called the urethra that connects the bladder floor to the outside of the body. Internal and external urinary muscle sphincters control the urine flow and stop the urine. Malignant neoplasms of the bladder are classified by site. The dome of the bladder is the ceiling and the trigone is the triangular lower portion of the bladder bounded by the ureteral and urethral openings. Symptoms of malignant neoplasm of the bladder include hematuria, urinary urgency or frequency, or secondary infection at the tumor site. Pain or urinary retention may be present. Males are twice as likely to develop bladder cancers as are females, and more than 90 percent of these cancers are transitional cell carcinomas. The most common site for cancer in the bladder is in the trigone.

Malignant Neoplasms of Eye, Brain and Other Parts of Central Nervous System (C69-C72)

This section includes malignant neoplasms of the eye and adnexa, brain and spinal meninges, brain, spinal cord, and the nerves of the central nervous system such as optic, acoustic, and olfactory.

The categories in this code block are as follows:

C69	Malignant neoplasm of eye and adnexa
C70	Malignant neoplasm of meninges
C71	Malignant neoplasm of brain
C72	Malignant neoplasm of spinal cord, cranial nerves and other parts of central nervous system

C69.- Malignant neoplasm of eye and adnexa

The eye is made up of three main parts: the eyeball or globe, the orbit, and the adnexal structures. There are several types of malignant neoplasms that affect the eye. These types vary by the part of the eye or adnexal structures where the malignancy arises.

C69.0- Malignant neoplasm of conjunctiva

C69.1- Malignant neoplasm of cornea

C69.2- Malignant neoplasm of retina

C69.3- Malignant neoplasm of choroid

C69.4- Malignant neoplasm of ciliary body

The main part of the eye or globe includes a thin, vascular mucous membrane that covers the inner eyelids and the white outer shell of the eye (sclera). This membrane is called the conjunctiva. The cornea is the bulging "window" through which we see, and the retina is the light-sensitive "viewing screen" at the back of the eye. The choroid is a vascular pigmented layer of the inside of the eyeball that supplies blood to the retina and front of the eye. The ciliary body contains the muscles inside the eye that enable the eye to focus on near or far objects by controlling and changing the shape of the lens. The ciliary body also contains the cells that make the aqueous humor. Since they develop within the eyeball, these cancers are called "intraocular cancers." Although rare, melanoma is one of the main types of primary malignant intraocular neoplasms in adults. Most melanomas develop in the choroid or ciliary body and usually present as a dark spot on the iris that begins to grow. They are typically slow growing and rarely spread.

> **Focus Point**
>
> *A congenital cancer that is usually detected before age 2, retinoblastoma is reported here with a code from subcategory C69.2-. Retinoblastoma is a malignancy of the retina and occurs bilaterally in 25 percent of patients with the disease.*

C69.5- Malignant neoplasm of lacrimal gland and duct

The lacrimal system provides tears and is also an agent in their disposal. Tears are produced in the lacrimal glands, located bilaterally behind the eyebrow, and the lacrimal ducts carry the tears to the eye or away from the eye to the nose. This area is considered an adnexal structure and malignant neoplasms here are called adnexal cancers.

C69.6- Malignant neoplasm of orbit

The eyeball rests in fatty tissue in the bony orbit of the skull where it is protected from jarring actions. A malignant neoplasm of the orbit lies in these fatty and other tissues between the eyeball and the skull and is called an orbital cancer.

C70.- Malignant neoplasm of meninges

Meningioma is a primary cancer tumor that develops in the cerebral or spinal meninges, which are the membranes that cover the brain or spinal cord. Most meningiomas are benign and slow growing but approximately 10 percent are malignant and grow much more quickly. They tend to occur more often in women and often spread to the brain and lungs. Much is unknown about the cause of meningioma, although two risk factors that have been identified are exposure to radiation and neurofibromatosis Type 2. With a higher incidence noted in middle aged women, a link to the use of the progesterone hormone is suspect.

Focus Point

The majority of meningeal cancer is secondary and is not coded here.

C71.- Malignant neoplasm of brain

Primary brain cancers are generally named for the part of the brain cell that they arise from or the part of the brain where they develop. There are more than 120 different types of brain tumors as classified by the National Brain Tumor Society. The most common is a group called gliomas that arise from the glial cells. This group has many subgroups including astrocytomas, which can develop anywhere in the brain or spinal cord but in adults it often occurs in the cerebrum. A grade IV astrocytoma is also called a glioblastoma or glioblastoma multiforme. These account for more than half of astrocytomas occurring typically in adults between ages 50 and 70. This type is aggressive and rapidly spreading. Brainstem gliomas are also high-grade astrocytomas and are difficult to treat. An ependymoma is a glioma that occurs in the lining of the ventricles of the brain. There are many more types of gliomas as well as other types of brain cancers that do not arise from glial tissue such as medulloblastomas, which are usually found in children and young adults and develop from the neurons in the cerebellum. Much is unknown about the cause of primary brain cancer but some suggested risk factors include smoking, radiation to the head, HIV infection, genetics, and environmental toxins.

Malignant Neoplasms of Thyroid and Other Endocrine Glands (C73-C75)

This section includes malignancies of the thyroid, parathyroid, adrenal, pituitary, and pineal glands. Also included are neoplasms of craniopharyngeal duct, carotid body, and aortic body.

Focus Point

Malignancies of the endocrine glands can create functional activities in those glands. For example, adrenal tumors can cause virilizing or feminizing symptoms. Pituitary cancers can cause gigantism, Cushing's disease, amenorrhea or galactorrhea, or acromegaly. Report these functional activities in addition to the cancer.

Neuroendocrine tumors are excluded from this code block.

The categories in this code block are as follows:

C73	Malignant neoplasm of thyroid gland
C74	Malignant neoplasm of adrenal gland
C75	Malignant neoplasm of other endocrine glands and related structures

C73 Malignant neoplasm of thyroid gland

The thyroid gland is located just below the cricoid cartilage near the larynx and its purpose is to secrete thyroxine and triiodothyronine. Thyroxine and triiodothyronine increase the rate of cell metabolism.

Papillary adenocarcinoma accounts for 85 percent of thyroid cancers and usually appears in young adults. Though the only symptom of thyroid cancer may be a palpable node, some patients with thyroid cancer present with symptoms of hypothyroidism or hyperthyroidism.

Focus Point

Sipple's syndrome, characterized by medullary carcinoma of the thyroid, pheochromocytoma, and parathyroid disease, requires assignment of multiple codes. The syndrome itself is classified as multiple endocrine neoplasia (MEN) type II A and is reported with code E31.22. The medullary carcinoma of the thyroid is captured by code C73. Pheochromocytoma is a medullary tumor of the adrenal gland that is most often benign, but there are also malignant forms. The benign form is the type most often seen in Sipple's syndrome and is reported with a code from subcategory D35.0-. Malignant pheochromocytoma is reported with a code from subcategory C74.1-.

C74.- Malignant neoplasm of adrenal gland

The adrenal glands are situated above each kidney and are made up of two parts: the outer part is the cortex and the inner part is the medulla. Malignant neoplasms of the adrenal gland are classified by site and laterality. Adrenal gland neoplasms may be functional, meaning they produce excessive amounts of hormones, or nonfunctional.

Focus Point

Most adrenal gland tumors are functional. If the adrenal gland tumor is described as functional, additional codes are required to report the functional activity.

C74.0- Malignant neoplasm of cortex of adrenal gland

The function of the adrenal cortex is making steroid hormones, which include cortisol, aldosterone, and dehydroepiandrosterone (DHEA). These hormones affect metabolism and body characteristics, such as hair growth and body shape. Although adrenal gland malignancies are extremely rare, the most common type is adrenal cortical carcinoma and it occurs in the cortex. There are few known risk factors for adrenal cancer with average age of occurrence in the mid-40s, although it can affect people at any age including children.

C74.1- Malignant neoplasm of medulla of adrenal gland

The adrenal medulla secretes adrenaline. One type of malignant neoplasm found in the medulla is pheochromocytoma. Neoplasms of the adrenal gland can be life-threatening because they can cause severe hypertensive symptoms.

Focus Point

Most pheochromocytomas of the adrenal medulla are benign. The benign form is reported with a code from subcategory D35.0-.

Malignant Neuroendocrine Tumors (C7A)

This section represents primary malignant neuroendocrine tumors (carcinoid) of the digestive system, lung and bronchus, kidney, and thymus gland. Neuroendocrine tumors arise from neuroendocrine cells, which have traits of nerve cells and endocrine cells.

The categories in this code block are as follows:

C7A   Malignant neuroendocrine tumors

C7A.- Malignant neuroendocrine tumors

Neuroendocrine cells produce and secrete regulatory hormones. Tumors comprised of these cells are consequently capable of producing hormonal syndromes (e.g., carcinoid syndrome), in which the normal hormonal balance required to support body system functions is adversely affected. Symptoms caused by neuroendocrine tumors are caused by the abnormal secretion of hormones due to the presence of neoplastic growth and its affected tissues. As a result, many of these tumors are associated with a diverse range of characteristic hormonal syndromes. Although many neuroendocrine tumors are slow-growing by comparison to other pathologies, some manifestations present aggressively and may be recalcitrant to conventional treatment. Carcinoid tumors have different expected outcomes than more common neoplasms and require different treatments. The most common metastatic sites for neuroendocrine tumor are the peritoneum, liver, the lymph nodes, and the bones. Liver metastasis is of particularly high incidence in certain primary neuroendocrine tumors

(e.g., intestines, pancreas). The treatment of liver metastases may dominate the cancer treatment due to the prominent blood supply, risk for hepatic failure, and surgical risk included in debulking of the tumor.

Focus Point

Neuroendocrine tumor of the pancreas is called islet cell tumor (islets of Langerhans) and is properly represented with code C25.4 Malignant neoplasm of endocrine pancreas.

C7A.0- Malignant carcinoid tumors

Carcinoid tumors are a specific type of slow-growing malignant neoplasm originating in the cells of the neuroendocrine system. Although the terms "carcinoid" and "neuroendocrine" may be used interchangeably in the clinical environment to describe specific types of neoplasm, carcinoid tumor is one type of neuroendocrine neoplasm. In adults, carcinoid tumors are the most commonly occurring neuroendocrine tumors. Carcinoid tumors occur most commonly in the respiratory and gastrointestinal tracts and usually originate in hormone-producing cells in the linings of these organs. They can also occur in the pancreas, testes, ovaries, or lungs. Gastrointestinal carcinoid tumors are classified according to the presumed embryonic site of origin. If the specific site of origin is known, the code for the site is reported.

Focus Point

Instructional notes indicate to code additionally E34.0 for carcinoid syndrome, if applicable. Carcinoid syndrome is the most common systemic syndrome associated with carcinoid tumors. Carcinoid syndrome causes patients to have flushing, diarrhea, and heart disease. It is caused by an abnormally high concentration of serotonin secretion.

Secondary Neuroendocrine Tumors (C7B)

This section represents secondary neuroendocrine tumors that have originated from another body site and have now spread to a secondary site. Codes in this section identify the metastatic or secondary site of the neuroendocrine tumor.

The categories in this code block are as follows:

C7B   Secondary neuroendocrine tumors

C7B.- Secondary neuroendocrine tumors

Neuroendocrine cells produce and secrete regulatory hormones. Secondary sites of functional neuroendocrine tumors produce the same hormones as the primary neuroendocrine tumor. Symptoms caused by neuroendocrine tumors are caused by the abnormal secretion of hormones due to the presence of neoplastic growth and its affected tissues. As a result, many of these tumors are associated with a diverse range of characteristic hormonal syndromes.

Focus Point

Functional secondary tumors comprised of neuroendocrine cells are capable of producing hormonal syndromes (e.g., carcinoid syndrome), in which the normal hormonal balance required to support body system functions is adversely affected. Any associated endocrine syndrome caused by secondary tumors is reported additionally.

Malignant Neoplasms of Ill-Defined, Other Secondary and Unspecified Sites (C76-C80)

All malignant neoplasms have the potential to shed cells into the patient's circulation. When these cells adhere to the vascular endothelium and begin to multiply into new tumors at new sites, the malignant neoplasm is said to have metastasized. The new cancers are considered secondary malignancies, the primary malignancy being the "mother" site.

Focus Point

When a cancer recurs at the site of the original malignancy, it is still considered a primary malignancy and should not be reported with secondary malignancy codes. If the cancer recurs at a different site, secondary neoplasm codes are appropriate.

The categories in this code block are as follows:

C76	Malignant neoplasm of other and ill-defined sites
C77	Secondary and unspecified malignant neoplasm of lymph nodes
C78	Secondary malignant neoplasm of respiratory and digestive organs
C79	Secondary malignant neoplasm of other and unspecified sites
C80	Malignant neoplasm without specification of site

C77.- Secondary and unspecified malignant neoplasm of lymph nodes

Metastases of malignant neoplasms to lymphatic sites are fairly common since lymphatic fluid circulates throughout the body and is filtered in the lymph nodes. The primary cancer may be near the affected lymph tissue or distant from it.

C78.- Secondary malignant neoplasm of respiratory and digestive organs

This category includes neoplasms that originate at a site other than digestive or respiratory sites and metastasize to the lung, pleura, mediastinum, liver, peritoneum, retroperitoneum, intestine, or other gastrointestinal organs.

C78.6 Secondary malignant neoplasm of retroperitoneum and peritoneum

Malignant neoplasms may spread to the retroperitoneum and peritoneum by direct invasion from a primary malignancy of an organ or structure in the abdomen or pelvis or from a remote site most often via the bloodstream (hematogenous spread) but also via the lymphatic system. This subcategory includes pseudomyxoma peritonei (PMP), a rare but increasingly seen condition characterized by the appearance of mucin-producing tumors in the abdominal cavity. Much about this condition is unknown but the primary malignancy is usually located in the appendix and less often in other parts of the intestine, the ovaries, or the urinary bladder. Malignant mucinous cells are believed to leak into the peritoneum attaching to the peritoneal membrane and other abdominal organs. The end result of this metastatic process is abdominal-wide mucinous ascites (jelly belly) with bloating and potential damage to organs. PMP is often initially misdiagnosed in women as ovarian cancer and in men as a hernia.

C80.- Malignant neoplasm without specification of site

Three codes are available in this category that designate the following: a disseminated or generalized malignant neoplasm with an unknown or unspecified primary site, a primary malignant neoplasm of an unspecified site, and a malignant neoplasm associated with an organ transplant.

C80.0 Disseminated malignant neoplasm, unspecified

Up to 7 percent of cancer patients are diagnosed with a secondary malignancy for which the primary site cannot be found, which may be designated as UPO for unknown primary origin.

C80.2 Malignant neoplasm associated with transplanted organ

Organ recipients are routinely placed on immunosuppressive drugs to prevent rejection of the transplanted organ, but this immunosuppression also renders them vulnerable to infection and disease, including malignancy. Additionally, a transplanted organ may contain malignant cells that were undetected prior to transplant.

Malignant Neoplasms of Lymphoid, Hematopoietic and Related Tissue (C81-C96)

Malignant neoplasms of the lymphatic and hematopoietic tissues are considered primary neoplasms. The malignant cells circulate to other areas through the lymphatic or blood systems. In fact, one primary difference between lymphoid, hematopoietic, and other related malignancies is that the tumor cells typically circulate in large numbers in the bloodstream.

Lymphoma is the most common blood cancer and occurs when the lymphocytes in the white blood cells that regulate the immune system multiply uncontrollably. Lymphomas are divided into two broad types: Hodgkin and non-Hodgkin lymphomas. Both are named after Dr. Thomas Hodgkin who originally identified some of the specific characteristics of these types of tumors. Hodgkin and non-Hodgkin lymphomas have a number of subtypes.

Hematopoietic refers to the stem cells that are located in the red blood marrow and are responsible for the formation of the blood and blood cells. Hematopoietic neoplasms include multiple myeloma, various types of leukemia, as well as other malignant neoplasms of these cells and tissue types.

Focus Point

Because malignant cells that originate in the blood and lymphatic systems circulate throughout the body, multiple lymph node sites are often involved. When lymphoma involves multiple sites, all sites are classified as primary and reported with codes in this code block, not with codes for secondary neoplasms. Codes from this code block are also used when there is bone marrow, extranodal, and solid organ involvement.

The categories in this code block are as follows:

C81	Hodgkin lymphoma
C82	Follicular lymphoma
C83	Non-follicular lymphoma
C84	Mature T/NK-cell lymphomas
C85	Other specified and unspecified types of non-Hodgkin lymphoma
C86	Other specified types of T/NK-cell lymphoma
C88	Malignant immunoproliferative diseases and certain other B-cell lymphomas
C90	Multiple myeloma and malignant plasma cell neoplasms
C91	Lymphoid leukemia
C92	Myeloid leukemia
C93	Monocytic leukemia
C94	Other leukemias of specified cell type
C95	Leukemia of unspecified cell type
C96	Other and unspecified malignant neoplasms of lymphoid, hematopoietic and related tissue

C81.- Hodgkin lymphoma

The two main forms of lymphoma are Hodgkin and non-Hodgkin lymphoma, which are differentiated by the type of cells that are involved. A diagnosis of Hodgkin's disease or lymphoma can be confirmed by the presence of Reed-Sternberg cells. Non-Hodgkin lymphoma includes more than 50 subgroups and is much more common than Hodgkin's, which accounts for only about 1 percent of all cancers in the United States. Although both types can occur at any age, Hodgkin's lymphoma generally affects people in two different age groups: younger adults ages 20 to 30 and then again later in life, 55 years of age or older. Non-Hodgkin's is most often diagnosed in people older than age 60. Both lymphomas involve swelling of the lymph nodes that can occur anywhere in the body; however, Hodgkin's is more likely to originate in the upper body such as the neck, axiliary, and chest. Although largely unknown, a few risk factors are suspected. A link between a history of infectious mononucleosis from the Epstein-Barr virus (EBV) genome has been identified in a large number of Hodgkin cases. Familial association, including having a same-sex sibling, identical twin, or parent diagnosed with Hodgkin lymphoma, also increases the risk. Also thought to be an increased risk is the lack of exposure at an early age to bacterial or viral infections, such as noted in children with smaller families or fewer playmates.

C81.0- Nodular lymphocyte predominant Hodgkin lymphoma

This rare subtype of Hodgkin, referred to as NLPHD, comprises only about 5 percent of Hodgkin disease and is identified by a variant of the Reed-Sternberg cell called popcorn cells because of their large size and shape. It is more common in men; generally appears in the lymph nodes of the neck and axila, and carries the most favorable prognosis.

C81.1- Nodular sclerosis Hodgkin lymphoma

This subtype is the most common type of Hodgkin lymphoma in developed countries and can occur at any age, but occurs most often in teenagers and younger adults. It is characterized by large tumor nodules of classic Reed-Sternberg cells, reactive lymphocytes, eosinophils, plasma cells, and collagen fibrosis (sclerosis) that usually start in the lymph nodes of the neck or chest.

C81.2- Mixed cellularity Hodgkin lymphoma

This subtype is the second most common and most often occurs in older adults. It is characterized by the presence of many classic Reed-Sternberg cells mixed with reactive lymphocytes, eosinophils, and plasma cells without the collagen fibrosis (sclerosis). This usually develops in the lymph nodes in the upper body although it can start in any lymph node. This type is most often linked to a history of Epstein-Barr virus (EBV) infection.

C81.3- Lymphocyte depleted Hodgkin lymphoma

The rarest subtype of Hodgkin lymphoma, lymphocyte-depleted classical Hodgkin lymphoma typically affects older people. It often originates in the lymph nodes in the abdomen, liver, and bone marrow where it is likely to be in advanced stages by the time of discovery.

C81.4- Lymphocyte-rich Hodgkin lymphoma

This subtype is uncommon, accounting for about 5 percent of Hodgkin cases. It is seldom found in more than a few lymph nodes and usually occurs in the upper body.

C82.- Follicular lymphoma

Follicular lymphoma is the most common subgroup of non-Hodgkin lymphomas (NHL) accounting for 20 to 30 percent of all NHLs. NHL is classified based on the type of lymphocyte cell that is malignant: B-cell or T-cell. Follicular NHL is a B-cell lymphoma that is characterized as indolent, which means slow growing. Follicular lymphoma is further characterized by the circular pattern of malignant cell growth with the cells clustered into identifiable nodules or follicles.

C82.0- Follicular lymphoma grade I

C82.1- Follicular lymphoma grade II

C82.2- Follicular lymphoma grade III, unspecified

C82.3- Follicular lymphoma grade IIIa

C82.4- Follicular lymphoma grade IIIb

Even though follicular lymphoma is an indolent, slow-growing type of lymphoma, the aggressiveness of this type of lymphoma varies somewhat based on the characteristics of the malignant cells, which are divided into several grades. The grades relate to the number of the large, more aggressive cells that appear under a microscope. Grade I and II have fewer large cells and are considered less aggressive and more treatable with Grade III being more aggressive. Grade III is generally thought to be related to a worse survival rate; however, since controversy exists in studies of Grade III, it is broken into IIIa and IIIb. Grade IIIa compares similarly with the outcomes of Grade I and II, while Grade IIIB has a poorer prognosis.

> **Focus Point**
>
> *Lymphoma grade is not the same as lymphoma stage. Grade identifies the relative aggressiveness of the particular type of lymphoma. Three grades are defined, including low-grade (indolent), medium-grade, and high-grade (aggressive). All follicular lymphomas are low-grade (indolent) types but follicular lymphoma is subdivided into grades I, II, and III (IIIa, IIIb). Staging relates to the spread of the disease throughout the body. Stage is based on the number of lymph node regions involved; the distribution of lymph node involvement, whether situated above or below the diaphragm or both; and whether there is any involvement outside the lymph nodes in extranodal or solid organ sites. Stage also uses a number system with four stages designated as Stage I, II, III, and IV.*

C83.- Non-follicular lymphoma

This category includes other types of non-Hodgkin lymphoma subgroups that are not of the follicular family, such as small cell B-cell, mantle cell, diffuse large B-cell, lymphoblastic, and Burkitt lymphoma, as well as codes for other or unspecified non-follicular lymphomas.

C83.0- Small cell B-cell lymphoma

Nodal marginal zone B-cell lymphomas and splenic marginal zone lymphoma are reported here. Nodal marginal-zone B-cell lymphomas (MZL) are rare, slow growing, and mostly found in older women. The majority of nodal MZL cases lack splenic or extranodal involvement, staying only in the lymph nodes. This type is often curable if diagnosed early. Splenic marginal zone lymphoma (SMZL) is a slow-growing B-cell lymphoma affecting primarily older men. It is characterized by spleen involvement with bone marrow infiltration and occasionally liver or mesenteric lymph node involvement. Symptoms include discomfort from splenomegaly. Risk factors have been linked to the hepatitis C virus.

C83.1- Mantle cell lymphoma

Mantle cell lymphoma is a rare type of non-Hodgkin's lymphoma of the small to medium B-lymphocytes. It occurs more commonly in those older than age 50, and is three times more likely to affect men than women. Even though it is considered slow growing, it is often in advanced stages by the time of diagnosis with spread to other lymph nodes, bone marrow, or spleen. Initial symptoms include lymph node enlargement in the neck, axilla, or groin. Other symptoms, known as B symptoms, include night sweats, fever, and weight loss.

C83.3- Diffuse large B-cell lymphoma

Large B-cell lymphoma is one of the more common types of lymphoma. The cells are fast growing and appear larger under a microscope. It can affect any age but is most typically found in older people with an average age of 60. It typically presents as a fast-growing mass in the lymph node. One third of cases remain localized.

C83.5- Lymphoblastic (diffuse) lymphoma

This subcategory includes lymphoblastic T-cell lymphoma, which is a type of non-Hodgkin lymphoma that can be considered lymphoma or leukemia—the determination is made based on the amount of bone marrow involvement. The cells are small to medium immature T-cells that often originate in the thymus where many of the T-cells are made. It can develop into a large tumor in the chest that interferes with breathing by impinging on the trachea or pressing on the superior vena cava (SVC) and can cause swelling of the face or arms. It is fast growing and most often affects younger men.

C83.7- Burkitt lymphoma

Burkitt's tumor or lymphoma is a fast growing form of non-Hodgkin lymphoma characterized by an undifferentiated B-cell tumor. There are two variants: endemic (African) and sporadic. The endemic variant is associated with Epstein-Barr virus infection and has a variable diagnosis. Jaw and orbital involvement is typical in endemic Burkitt's lymphoma and a large abdominal mass predominates in sporadic Burkitt's lymphoma. It is most common in children and young adults, especially males, and is rare in the United States, predominantly occurring in central Africa. AIDS has also been noted as an associated risk for Burkitt lymphoma.

C83.8- Other non-follicular lymphoma

Intravascular lymphoma is a rare subtype that is classified here. The distinctive feature of intravascular lymphoma is the presence of clonal lymphocytes in the small blood vessels rather than the bone marrow or lymph nodes.

C84.- Mature T/NK-cell lymphomas

T-cell lymphomas comprise about 15 percent of non-Hodgkin lymphomas in the United States. Natural killer (NK) cells are lymphocytes that are similar to T-cells. When NK cells become cancerous, they are grouped with T-cell lymphoma.

C84.0- Mycosis fungoides

Mycosis fungoides, although rare, is the most common of the skin lymphomas. It is a persistent, slow growing, chronic T-cell lymphoma affecting the skin and sometimes internal organs, usually in men 50 years or older. It begins as scaly, red, itchy patches and can turn into plaques and invade lymph nodes and organs.

Focus Point

When mycosis fungoides affect the blood, it is classified as Sézary disease and reported with codes in subcategory C84.1-.

C84.1- Sezary disease

Sézary disease is an extension of mycosis fungoides that affects the blood. It also affects all of the skin, appearing as sunburn, rather than patches. It spreads to the lymph nodes and is often linked to a weakened immune system. It grows faster than mycosis fungoides and is also harder to treat.

C84.4- Peripheral T-cell lymphoma, not classified

Peripheral T-cell lymphoma, not classified (PTCL-NOS) is a group of diseases that don't fit into the other subtypes; it is the most common of all the T-cell lymphomas. It is most often localized to the lymph nodes, although it can be found in other sites such as the liver, bone marrow, gastrointestinal tract, and skin. This is an aggressive form of lymphoma.

C84.6- Anaplastic large cell lymphoma, ALK-positive

C84.7- Anaplastic large cell lymphoma, ALK-negative

Anaplastic large cell lymphoma (ALCL) is a high-grade (fast-growing) lymphoma. It typically originates in the lymph nodes and spreads to the skin. ALCL is typically made up of T-lymphocytes, although some cases are null-cell type, meaning the type of cell (B or T) that makes up the lymphoma is unclear. It is a rare lymphoma that is differentiated based on the presence or absence of an abnormal surface protein called anaplastic lymphoma kinase. When this abnormal protein is present the term ALK-positive is applied and when it is absent the term ALK-negative is applied. ALK-positive most often occurs in children and young adults and has a better prognosis.

C85.- Other specified and unspecified types of non-Hodgkin lymphoma

This category identifies other and unspecified types of non-Hodgkin lymphoma subtypes, including mediastinal large B-cell.

C85.2- Mediastinal (thymic) large B-cell lymphoma

Mediastinal (thymic) large B-cell lymphoma is a subtype of diffuse large B-cell lymphoma with fibrosis in the background of the large cells. It is usually localized to the mediastinum and can cause breathing problems if it presses on the trachea or face and arm swelling if it obstructs the superior vena cava. Most affected are young women generally in their 30s. It is fast growing but responds well to treatment.

C86.- Other specified types of T/NK-cell lymphoma

This category includes several types of T/NK-cell lymphomas that do not fit into other categories. Because of the similarities of the features of T-cell and natural killer (NK) cells, they are both categorized into the same lymphoma groups.

C86.0 Extranodal NK/T-cell lymphoma, nasal type

This rare type of lymphoma can originate in the T-cells or the natural killer (NK) cells. Although it generally occurs in the nose or sinuses, it can occur in the skin. It is fast growing and has been linked to the Epstein-Barr virus (EBV). It is mainly found in Asia and Central and South America.

C86.3 Subcutaneous panniculitis-like T-cell lymphoma

This slow growing type of lymphoma is rare but affects both men and women of all age groups. It is characterized by the formation of lumps in the deep layers of the skin most often on the legs. It has a good prognosis.

C86.6 Primary cutaneous CD30-positive T-cell proliferations

This category includes primary cutaneous anaplastic large cell lymphoma (ALCL), which presents as single or multiple tumors on the skin of various sizes that can turn into ulcers. It occurs mainly in middle aged men but can affect children. It does not spread and has a good prognosis. Lymphomatoid papulosis is also classified here, which starts as a chronic skin disease with histological features consistent with malignant lymphoma. It is characterized by pruritic papules on the trunk and limbs that heal over time but leave scarring. What is interesting about this condition is that it is histologically malignant, exhibiting the clinical features of a lymphoma. However, its benign clinical course and fairly spontaneous resolution make clinicians reluctant to classify this as a malignancy. Treatment usually includes oral and/or topical medications.

C88.- Malignant immunoproliferative diseases and certain other B-cell lymphomas

This category includes various types of rare lymphomas such as Waldenström's, which is characterized by the formation of large amounts of a protein called macroglobulin; heavy chain disease, which is a proliferation of plasma cells; and immunoproliferative small intestinal disease, which is a small intestinal form of heavy chain disease affecting predominately young adults in underdeveloped countries.

C88.4 Extranodal marginal zone B-cell lymphoma of mucosa-associated lymphoid tissue [MALT-lymphoma]

MALT is a mucosa-associated lymphoma that originates in lymphoid tissue found in the lining of the gastrointestinal tract, thyroid, lung, salivary glands, eye, skin, breast, or soft tissues. Most patients are diagnosed with early-stage 1 or 2, localized extranodal disease. MALT is often associated with inflammatory disease caused by infection, such as *Helicobacter pylori* infection of the gastrointestinal tract, or autoimmune disorders, such as Sjögren's syndrome or Hashimoto's thyroiditis. The average age of occurrence is about 60 years old. It is slow growing and highly curable if caught in early stages.

C90.- Multiple myeloma and malignant plasma cell neoplasms

These neoplasms affect the plasma cells and include multiple myeloma, extramedullary plasmacytoma, plasma cell leukemia, and solitary plasmacytoma.

C90.0- Multiple myeloma

Multiple myeloma is an uncontrolled proliferation of plasma cells and results in a number of organ dysfunctions and symptoms of bone pain or fracture, renal failure, infection, anemia, hypercalcemia, as well as clotting and neurologic or vascular abnormalities. Relapse or recurrence of multiple myeloma occurs when the disease returns during therapy or after being successfully treated (remission). Relapse during or soon after the completion of treatment is generally considered less favorable than relapse after remission has been achieved. Interventions and treatments of relapses may vary from induction (primary) therapy and may be more aggressive in nature.

Focus Point

Multiple myeloma is sometimes described as metastatic to the bone, but because this is part of the disease, the bone metastases should not be reported separately as a secondary malignant neoplasm.

C91.-   Lymphoid leukemia

Lymphoid leukemia is a malignant proliferation of immature lymphocytes called lymphoblasts. The acute condition is common in children and fatal if untreated. The chronic condition is a generalized, progressive form of lymphocytic leukemia predominantly affecting men older than age 50. It is the least malignant form of leukemia. Relapse or recurrence of leukemia occurs when the disease returns during therapy or after being successfully treated (remission). Relapse during or soon after the completion of treatment is generally considered less favorable than relapse after remission has been achieved. Interventions and treatments of relapses may vary from induction (primary) therapy and may be more aggressive in nature. Relapse of a primary leukemia especially is associated with a greater risk of additional morbidity and mortality because aggressive chemotherapy, radiation, or bone marrow transplantation may be required.

C91.4-   Hairy cell leukemia

This rare type is often also considered a type of lymphoma. The small B-cell lymphocytes appear with "hairy" projections under a microscope and are found mostly in the bone marrow, spleen, and blood. It occurs more often in men with an average age of 50. It is slow growing and often does not need treatment, but if it does, prognosis is good.

C92.-   Myeloid leukemia

Myeloid leukemia is a rapid and malignant proliferation of immature myelocytes called myeloblasts. These are the cells that become white blood cells (except lymphocytes), red blood cells, or platelet making cells. The acute condition is common in children and fatal if untreated. The chronic condition is a fatal disease characterized by abnormal proliferation of premature granulocytes called myeloblasts, promyelocytes, metamyelocytes, and myelocytes in bone marrow, peripheral blood, and body tissues. Relapse, or recurrence of leukemia, occurs when the disease returns during therapy or after being successfully treated (remission). Relapse during or soon after the completion of treatment is generally considered less favorable than relapse after remission has been achieved. Interventions and treatments for relapse may vary from induction (primary) therapy, and may be more aggressive in nature. Relapse of a primary leukemia especially is associated with a greater risk of additional morbidity and mortality because aggressive chemotherapy, radiation, or bone marrow transplantation may be required.

Focus Point

Blast crisis is characterized by an abrupt, severe change in the course of chronic myelocytic leukemia that resembles acute myelocytic leukemia, with an increase in the proportion of myeloblasts. In some cases, the cells may be lymphoblasts. There is no code to separately identify the blast crisis as it identifies progression of chronic myelogenous leukemia and is captured by codes in subcategory C92.1- Chronic myeloid leukemia, BCR/ABL positive.

C93.-   Monocytic leukemia

Monocytic leukemia starts in the blood forming cells in the bone marrow. When monocytes, a type of white blood cell, leave the bone marrow and enter the bloodstream, they become macrophages, a cell that destroys and eats bacteria. In chronic myelomonocytic leukemia (CMML), the monocyte count in the bone marrow becomes abnormally high and dysplastic. CMML is a rare condition with the majority of cases in males 60 years and older.

C95.-   Leukemia of unspecified cell type

Use these leukemia codes when documentation does not provide sufficient information or when the patient's specific diagnosis has not yet been established although leukemia is certain. Relapse, or recurrence of leukemia, occurs when the disease returns during therapy or after being successfully treated (remission). Relapse during or soon after the completion of treatment is generally considered less favorable than relapse after remission has been achieved. Interventions and treatments for relapse may vary from induction (primary) therapy and may be more aggressive in nature. Relapse of a primary leukemia especially is associated with a greater risk of additional morbidity and mortality because aggressive chemotherapy, radiation, or bone marrow transplantation may be required.

C96.-   Other and unspecified malignant neoplasms of lymphoid, hematopoietic and related tissue

Malignant neoplasms of the lymphatic and hematopoietic tissues are considered primary neoplasms. The malignant cells circulate to other areas through the lymphatic or blood systems. In fact, one primary difference between lymphoid, hematopoietic and other related malignancies is that the tumor cells typically circulate in large numbers in the bloodstream. Hematopoietic refers to the stem cells that are located in the red blood marrow and are responsible for the formation of the blood and blood cells.

C96.2-   Malignant mast cell neoplasm

Mast cells, also known as mastocytes, are a type of white blood cell of the immune system present in connective tissues that release the chemicals histamine and heparin in response to disease or irritants. They are instrumental in initiating parts of the immune defense system as well as promoting healing of wounds. Mast cells originate in the bone marrow and contain small sacs called granules that contain mediators that are dispersed into connective tissues such as skin and the linings of organs. Studies have never found anyone with too few mast cells, leading research to believe that a certain number must be maintained for survival; however, an overabundance of mast cells can be problematic.

Focus Point

Mastocytosis is the overabundance of mast cells and is broadly categorized in three different groups: systemic, cutaneous, and mast cell sarcoma. Two types of mastocytosis—aggressive systemic and mast cell sarcoma—are discussed in this subcategory. Others such as cutaneous and systemic are explained in subcategory D47.0-. Another condition called mast cell activation syndrome (MCAS) occurs when there is a normal amount of mast cells but they are overly sensitive to triggers such stings, stress, heat, cold, foods, etc. They prematurely release their contents causing many unwanted symptoms such as rashes, flushing, vomiting, pains, and even anaphylaxis. This condition is coded in subcategory D89.4-.

C96.21   Aggressive systemic mastocytosis

Aggressive systemic mastocytosis (ASM) is defined as systemic mastocytosis, which is the abnormal growth of mast cells in one or multiple systems, with the addition of skin involvement and one or more of the following conditions: cytopenia, liver impairment (hepatomegaly, ascites, portal HTN), skeletal lesions or pathological fractures, malabsorption, and weight loss. Treatment with chemotherapy is often required for this condition.

C96.22   Mast cell sarcoma

Mast cell sarcoma is an extremely rare, aggressive, highly malignant tumor with poor prognosis. The tumor is a solitary mass comprised of mast cells that can infiltrate surrounding tissues and can metastasize to other body systems. It has presented in adults and children and because of its rare nature, little is known about its origin or treatment options.

C96.A   Histiocytic sarcoma

Histiocytic sarcoma, also called malignant histiocytosis, presents with progressive, abnormal histiocytes in the blood.

In Situ Neoplasms (D00-D09)

The word "in situ" means "in the original place," thus an in situ neoplasm is defined as a malignant neoplasm that has not invaded neighboring tissue. Once microscopic extension of malignant cells is found in tissue adjacent to an in situ lesion, it is no longer "in situ," and malignant neoplasm codes should be used.

The categories in this code block are as follows:

D00	Carcinoma in situ of oral cavity, esophagus and stomach
D01	Carcinoma in situ of other and unspecified digestive organs
D02	Carcinoma in situ of middle ear and respiratory system
D03	Melanoma in situ
D04	Carcinoma in situ of skin
D05	Carcinoma in situ of breast
D06	Carcinoma in situ of cervix uteri
D07	Carcinoma in situ of other and unspecified genital organs
D09	Carcinoma in situ of other and unspecified sites

D05.-   Carcinoma in situ of breast

Carcinoma in situ of the breast is a noninvasive type of breast cancer that can originate in the milk glands (lobular), milk ducts (intraductal), or in both sites (lobular with intraductal). This category includes ductal carcinoma in situ (DCIS), the most common type of noninvasive breast cancer. In DCIS, the abnormal cells begin in the milk ducts and do not invade the surrounding tissues. Because it is a risk factor for developing invasive breast cancer, it is generally treated with excision and some types are also treated with additional hormonal therapy.

Focus Point

While most types of DCIS are classified to D05.1- Intraductal carcinoma in situ of breast, noninfiltrating comedocarcinoma, a slightly more aggressive type of intraductal CIS is classified to D05.8- Other specified type of carcinoma in situ of breast.

D06.-   Carcinoma in situ of cervix uteri

Dysplasias of the cervix are cellular deviations from the normal structure and function of the cells of the cervix of the uterus. Dysplasias are considered a precursor to carcinoma. Cervical dysplasia is classified to one of three levels of cervical intraepithelial neoplasia (CIN). Only CIN III, the most severe of the three levels, is classified here.

D07.- Carcinoma in situ of other and unspecified genital organs

This category includes carcinoma in situ of the endometrium, vulva, and vagina in the female genitourinary system and the penis and prostate in the male genitourinary system.

D07.1 Carcinoma in situ of vulva

D07.2 Carcinoma in situ of vagina

In situ carcinoma of the vulva and vagina is linked to human papilloma virus and occurs more frequently in premenopausal women.

Benign Neoplasms, Except Benign Neuroendocrine Tumors (D10-D36)

Benign neoplasms are tumors characterized by dividing cells that adhere to each other so that the mass remains a circumscribed lesion. Benign neoplasms are classified according to site.

The categories in this code block are as follows:

D10	Benign neoplasm of mouth and pharynx
D11	Benign neoplasm of major salivary glands
D12	Benign neoplasm of colon, rectum, anus and anal canal
D13	Benign neoplasm of other and ill-defined parts of digestive system
D14	Benign neoplasm of middle ear and respiratory system
D15	Benign neoplasm of other and unspecified intrathoracic organs
D16	Benign neoplasm of bone and articular cartilage
D17	Benign lipomatous neoplasm
D18	Hemangioma and lymphangioma, any site
D19	Benign neoplasm of mesothelial tissue
D20	Benign neoplasm of soft tissue of retroperitoneum and peritoneum
D21	Other benign neoplasms of connective and other soft tissue
D22	Melanocytic nevi
D23	Other benign neoplasms of skin
D24	Benign neoplasm of breast
D25	Leiomyoma of uterus
D26	Other benign neoplasms of uterus
D27	Benign neoplasm of ovary
D28	Benign neoplasm of other and unspecified female genital organs
D29	Benign neoplasm of male genital organs
D30	Benign neoplasm of urinary organs
D31	Benign neoplasm of eye and adnexa
D32	Benign neoplasm of meninges
D33	Benign neoplasm of brain and other parts of central nervous system
D34	Benign neoplasm of thyroid gland
D35	Benign neoplasm of other and unspecified endocrine glands
D36	Benign neoplasm of other and unspecified sites

D17.- Benign lipomatous neoplasm

A lipoma is a soft nodule of fat that can occur subcutaneously or in any organ system. Treatment is not usually required, unless the lipoma is causing discomfort or compression. Lipomas are also known as angiolipoma, fibrolipoma, hibernoma, myelolipoma, and myxolipoma. Lipomas are classified by site.

D18.- Hemangioma and lymphangioma, any site

Hemangiomas are neoplasms arising from vascular tissue or malformations of vascular structures. Many are congenital. They can occur topically (on the skin) or within any organ system. Common topical hemangiomas include strawberry nevus, nevus vasculosus, capillary hemangioma, port wine stain, and nevus flammeus. Hemangiomas are classified according to site. A lymphangioma is a benign, congenital malformation in the lymphatic system.

D25.- Leiomyoma of uterus

A leiomyoma, also referred to as a myoma, fibromyoma, or fibroid, is a benign tumor of the smooth muscle tissue and is the most common type of benign tumor of the uterus. Most leiomyomas are detected during the course of routine pelvic exam; there are often no symptoms. If there are symptoms, they might include abdominal discomfort, urinary frequency, and constipation. Uterine leiomyomas usually occur in multiples. They are classified according to where they establish within the wall of the uterus.

D27.- Benign neoplasm of ovary

The ovary is the female gonad and produces the ova. Benign neoplasms of the ovary include endometrioid, mucinoid and serous adenofibroma and cystadenofibroma, Sertoli cell adenoma, benign androblastoma, benign arrhenoblastoma, and teratoma, as well as others. Some benign ovarian neoplasms are hormone-producing.

Focus Point

Use an additional code to report any functional activity associated with the ovarian neoplasm.

D31.- Benign neoplasm of eye and adnexa

The eye is basically a fluid-filled ball. Even though benign neoplasms do not spread, when they occur in the eye they can impair vision or cause blindness by disrupting the visual field or by compressing tissue and impairing the flow of blood or aqueous. In addition, a benign neoplasm can result in significant irritation or pain.

D33.- Benign neoplasm of brain and other parts of central nervous system

While benign neoplasms of the brain do not metastasize, even slow-growing benign neoplasms can cause systemic and often life-threatening complications, such as compression of intracranial structures and obstruction to blood flow and intracerebral fluid. Symptoms of a neoplasm of the brain include headache, seizures, personality changes, impaired mental or physical functions, or in children, an enlarged head.

D34 Benign neoplasm of thyroid gland

The thyroid gland is located just below the cricoid cartilage near the larynx. Its purpose is to secrete thyroxine and triiodothyronine, which increase the rate of cell metabolism. Benign thyroid tumors are adenomas, cysts, or involutionary nodules, and the majority are follicular. In many cases, the patient with a benign thyroid growth undergoes surgery because of suspicion of cancer, to improve cosmetic appearance, or to alleviate functional activity.

D35.- Benign neoplasm of other and unspecified endocrine glands

Benign neoplasms of the endocrine glands can create functional activities in those glands. For example, adrenal tumors can cause virilizing or feminizing symptoms. Pituitary cancers can cause gigantism, Cushing's disease, amenorrhea or galactorrhea, or acromegaly.

Focus Point

Use an additional code to report any functional activity associated with the neoplasm.

D35.0- Benign neoplasm of adrenal gland

The adrenal glands are situated above each kidney and the pituitary gland is located in the sella turcica of the sphenoid bone.

D35.1 Benign neoplasm of parathyroid gland

The parathyroid glands come in pairs—the superior and inferior pair—and they are embedded in the posterior thyroid.

D35.4 Benign neoplasm of pineal gland

The pineal gland, located at the base of the corpus callosum, secretes melatonin.

Benign Neuroendocrine Tumors (D3A)

Benign neuroendocrine tumors are a rare type of tumor composed of cells that produce and secrete regulatory hormones. Tumors comprised of these cells are consequently capable of producing hormonal syndromes (e.g., carcinoid syndrome), in which the normal hormonal balance required to support body system functions is adversely affected. Symptoms caused by neuroendocrine tumors are caused by the abnormal secretion of hormones due to the presence of neoplastic growth and its affected tissues. As a result, many of these tumors are associated with a diverse range of hormonal syndromes. However, not all neuroendocrine tumors secrete hormones. Those that do secrete hormones are referred to as functional tumors, while those that do not are called nonfunctional tumors. Benign neuroendocrine tumors are generally slow-growing and take many years before becoming symptomatic.

The categories in this code block are as follows:

D3A   Benign neuroendocrine tumors

Neoplasms of Uncertain Behavior, Polycythemia Vera and Myelodysplastic Syndromes (D37-D48)

Uncertain behavior is a histomorphological determination indicating that while the current behavior of the neoplasm is benign, the neoplasm possesses certain characteristics giving it the potential to transform into a malignant neoplasm. Neoplasms of uncertain behavior are classified by site or organ system. Polycythemia vera, myelodysplastic syndromes, and neoplasms of lymphoid, hematopoietic, and related tissues of uncertain behavior, such as mast cell tumors, are also classified in this block.

The categories in this code block are as follows:

D37	Neoplasm of uncertain behavior of oral cavity and digestive organs
D38	Neoplasm of uncertain behavior of middle ear and respiratory and intrathoracic organs
D39	Neoplasm of uncertain behavior of female genital organs
D40	Neoplasm of uncertain behavior of male genital organs
D41	Neoplasm of uncertain behavior of urinary organs
D42	Neoplasm of uncertain behavior of meninges
D43	Neoplasm of uncertain behavior of brain and central nervous system
D44	Neoplasm of uncertain behavior of endocrine glands
D45	Polycythemia vera
D46	Myelodysplastic syndromes
D47	Other neoplasms of uncertain behavior of lymphoid, hematopoietic and related tissue
D48	Neoplasm of uncertain behavior of other and unspecified sites

D45   Polycythemia vera

Polycythemia vera is the most common of the myeloproliferative disorders and is characterized by the increase in all blood cells—red, white, and platelets. Because of the increase in the number of blood cells, the risk of thrombosis increases, which can result in complications such as stroke, myocardial infarction (MI), or other ischemic attacks. Abnormal behavior in platelets can also cause increased bleeding. It affects men slightly more than women and is rare in children, generally appearing around age 60. This slow growing disorder carries an increased risk of developing more aggressive blood cancers such as acute leukemia or myelofibrosis.

D46.-   Myelodysplastic syndromes

Myelodysplastic syndromes are diseases in which the bone marrow functions abnormally. The immature stem cells formed in the bone marrow do not mature into normal red and white blood cells and platelets. These immature cells, called blasts, die in the bone marrow or shortly after entering the bloodstream, leaving less room for the development of healthy cells. This may result in infection, anemia, or bleeding. Symptoms include shortness of breath, weakness, pallor, easy bruising, petechiae, fever, or frequent infections. Diagnosis of the various forms of myelodysplastic syndrome is based on specific changes in the blood cells and bone marrow. Cutaneous lesions in myelodysplastic syndromes may indicate transition to acute myeloid leukemia and are associated with poorer prognoses. The most common lesions include petechiae and purpura, cutaneous infections, vasculitis, and neutrophilic dermatoses. A dermal infiltrate of malignant hematopoietic cells, which is the specific cutaneous manifestation of myelodysplastic syndromes, is rare.

D47.-   Other neoplasms of uncertain behavior of lymphoid, hematopoietic and related tissue

Neoplasms of the lymphatic and hematopoietic tissues whose behavior is considered uncertain are classified here. Lymphoid tissue refers to the tissue of the lymphatic system, such as white blood cells, and hematopoietic refers to the stem cells that are located in the red blood marrow and are responsible for the formation of the blood and blood cells.

D47.0-   Mast cell neoplasms of uncertain behavior

Mast cells, also known as mastocytes are a type of white blood cell of the immune system present in connective tissue that release the chemicals histamine and heparin in response to disease or irritants. They are instrumental in initiating parts of the immune defense system as well as promoting healing of wounds. Mast cells originate in the bone marrow and contain small sacs called granules that contain mediators that are dispersed into connective tissues such as skin and the linings of organs. Studies have never found anyone with too few mast cells, leading research to believe that a certain number must be maintained for survival;

however, an overabundance of mast cells can be problematic. The neoplastic conditions in this subcategory are considered to be of uncertain behavior instead of a malignancy.

Focus Point

Mastocytosis is the overabundance of mast cells and is broadly categorized in three different groups: systemic, cutaneous, and mast cell sarcoma. Two types of mastocytosis—cutaneous and systemic—are explained in this subcategory. Others such as aggressive systemic and mast cell sarcoma are discussed in subcategory C96.2-. Another condition called mast cell activation syndrome (MCAS) occurs when there is a normal amount of mast cells but they are overly sensitive to triggers such stings, stress, heat, cold, foods, etc. They prematurely release their contents causing many unwanted symptoms such as rashes, flushing, vomiting, pains, and even anaphylaxis. This condition is coded in subcategory D89.4-.

D47.01   Cutaneous mastocytosis

Urticaria pigmentosa is the most common form of cutaneous mastocytosis and includes maculopapular, which presents with dark, itchy patches on the skin and is most common in children and dissipates in teenage years. If developed later in life, it usually progresses to systemic mastocytosis. A localized form also predominantly found in children is solitary cutaneous, which also resolves in the teen years and appears as thickened itchy, brown patches that may blister when scratched. Telangiectasia macularis eruptiva perstans, also included here, is rare and most often affects adults with formation of telangiectasia in addition to dark patches. The most severe type of cutaneous mastocytosis is called diffuse as it affects most of the skin, appearing thick, leathery, and blistered. Gastrointestinal problems and even hypotensive shock may be present.

Focus Point

Urticaria pigmentosa that is documented as congenital is not reported here but with code Q82.2 Congenital urticaria pigmentosa in Chapter 17.

D47.02   Systemic mastocytosis

Systemic mastocytosis is a proliferation of mast cells in the internal tissues and organs including bone marrow and is generally found in adults. A subtype is indolent systemic mastocytosis, which is a slow, benign form that mainly involves the bone marrow and includes relatively minor symptoms such as itching, headache, vomiting, and diarrhea, with no aggressive or malignant features. Another slowly progressing type is smoldering mastocytosis which can also include hepatomegaly or splenomegaly. Smoldering is considered intermediate between the more mild indolent and the more aggressive forms. Both indolent and smoldering subtypes are captured with this code.

D47.2   Monoclonal gammopathy

Monoclonal gammopathy of undetermined significance (MGUS) is a condition that although not always harmful, can lead to other forms of blood cancer. It presents as abnormal monoclonal protein cells (M protein) in the blood that are produced by the plasma cells in the bone marrow. It should be monitored to ensure that it is not increasing and pushing out normal healthy cells and to provide earlier treatment if it turns into a blood cancer.

D47.4   Osteomyelofibrosis

This condition is also known as myelofibrosis with myeloid metaplasia, chronic idiopathic myelofibrosis, agnogenic myeloid metaplasia, primary myelofibrosis, and myelosclerosis with myeloid metaplasia. Osteomyelofibrosis is characterized by the replacement of bone marrow with fibrous tissue. This progressive, chronic disease is manifested by splenomegaly and worsening anemia. Since the bone marrow has been replaced by fibrous tissue, blood is made in organs such as the liver and spleen. Symptoms include pain or a full sensation on the left side beneath the ribs, early satiety, fatigue, shortness of breath, easy bruising, petechiae, fever, night sweats, or weight loss.

D47.Z1   Post-transplant lymphoproliferative disorder (PTLD)

Post-transplant lymphoproliferative disorder (PTLD) is a disease of uncontrolled proliferation or production of B cell lymphocytes, often following infection with the Epstein-Barr virus. Clinical presentation of PTLD varies and may present asymptomatically or with localized or systemic symptoms. Localized presentation may include one or more nodal or extranodal tumors. Systemic presentations may range from an unexplained infectious syndrome or mononucleosis-like illness with or without lymphadenopathy to a disseminated sepsis-like syndrome. However, some patients may be relatively asymptomatic, whereby diagnosis is made on the basis of an incidental, clinical, or radiographic finding. Most patients with PTLD present with at least one tumor. About two thirds of these tumors are extranodal and about one third are nodal. Symptoms of PTLD are related to the site of tumor growth. Gastrointestinal tumors can cause abdominal pain with hemorrhage and may perforate. Central nervous system tumors cause symptoms secondary to local necrosis and tumor mass effect. However, PTLD can occur at any site. Patients with PTLD present with distinct histologic findings, a more aggressive clinical course as compared to other malignant lymphomas, and are less likely to respond to conventional lymphoma treatments. PTLD may regress spontaneously after reduction or cessation of immunosuppressant medication, and can also be treated with antiviral therapy. If untreated, PTLD may form tumor masses with resultant bowel obstruction or progress to a non-Hodgkin's lymphoma.

D47.Z2   Castleman disease

Castleman disease (CD), also known as giant lymph node hyperplasia and angiofollicular lymph node hyperplasia (AFH), is a rare disease of lymph nodes and lymphoid tissues. CD is a lymphoproliferative disorder that closely mimics lymphoma and is often treated with chemotherapy and radiation therapy although it is not itself a cancer. There are many types and subtypes of CD, but classification is primarily based on the extent of the disease. Localized CD typically affects a single lymph node group while multicentric CD affects several groups of lymph nodes and/or lymphoid tissue containing organs.

Focus Point

Patients with multicentric Castleman disease often go on to develop lymphoma.

D48.-   Neoplasm of uncertain behavior of other and unspecified sites

This category includes sites such as bone and articular cartilage, connective and soft tissue, nerves, skin, retroperitoneum and peritoneum.

D48.1   Neoplasm of uncertain behavior of connective and other soft tissue

Included in this code is stromal tumor of uncertain behavior of the digestive system, which is an uncommon tumor found in the gastrointestinal tract that originates from interstitial cells of the autonomic nervous system. These interstitial cells regulate the muscle contractions that move the food through the digestive process. Although stromal tumors can start anywhere in the gastrointestinal tract, they most often begin in the stomach. It can occur at any age but occurs most often in people older than age 50 and it affects slightly more men than women.

Focus Point

For documentation stating malignant gastrointestinal stromal tumor (GIST), the appropriate code is found in subcategory C49.A- Gastrointestinal stromal tumor.

Chapter 3: Diseases of the Blood and Blood-forming Organs and Certain Disorders Involving the Immune Mechanism (D5Ø-D89)

This chapter classifies diseases of the blood, including anemia and those disorders that affect the cellular constituents in the blood. There are three major groups of cellular constituents: lymphocytes (white blood cells), erythrocytes (red blood cells), and thrombocytes (platelets) and these are produced by hemopoietic or blood forming organs. Blood forming organs in adults include the spleen, thymus, lymph nodes, and the bone marrow; however, this chapter only includes codes for those diseases specific to the spleen and bone marrow.

Also included in this chapter are disorders that involve the immune mechanism. Examples of immune conditions that are reported using codes from this chapter include immunodeficiencies, sarcoidosis, and graft-versus-host disease.

> **Focus Point**
>
> *It is important to note that although HIV and AIDS are immune disorders, neither of these conditions is found in this chapter but rather in Chapter 1 Certain Infectious and Parasitic Diseases.*

The chapter is broken down into the following code blocks:

D5Ø-D53	Nutritional anemias
D55-D59	Hemolytic anemias
D6Ø-D64	Aplastic and other anemias and other bone marrow failure syndromes
D65-D69	Coagulation defects, purpura and other hemorrhagic conditions
D7Ø-D77	Other disorders of blood and blood-forming organs
D78	Intraoperative and postprocedural complications of the spleen
D8Ø-D89	Certain disorders involving the immune mechanism

Nutritional Anemias (D5Ø-D53)

Nutritional anemias are the result of inadequate intake or absorption of a vitamin or mineral that impacts the production of red blood cells or causes them to develop abnormally affecting the size and shape. The most common nutritional anemias are due to deficiencies in iron, vitamin B12, and folate.

> **Focus Point**
>
> *Documentation must identify a clear link between the anemia and the nutritional deficiency as some patients may have low levels of a particular nutrient and not develop anemia or have an anemia that is caused by another unrelated condition and not a nutrient deficiency that happens to be present at the same time.*

The categories in this code block are as follows:

D5Ø	Iron deficiency anemia
D51	Vitamin B12 deficiency anemia
D52	Folate deficiency anemia
D53	Other nutritional anemias

D5Ø.-   Iron deficiency anemia

Iron deficiency anemias are the result of low iron stores due to inadequate dietary intake, decreased iron absorption, or, the most common cause, blood loss. This condition is also known as hypoferric anemia, hypochromic or microcytic anemia, or chlorosis.

D5Ø.Ø   Iron deficiency anemia secondary to blood loss (chronic)

This condition is defined as insufficient circulating red blood cells due to iron deficiency caused by blood loss, usually indicated as chronic or prolonged. In adults, iron deficiency anemia is almost always due to blood loss most often from a chronically bleeding lesion in the gastrointestinal tract, such as a gastric ulcer or diverticulitis, or from a urologic or gynecologic site.

D5Ø.1   Sideropenic dysphagia

Sideropenic dysphagia is a syndrome that includes difficulty swallowing (dysphagia) due to partial obstruction of the upper esophagus with a thin web of mucosal tissue in combination with iron deficiency (sideropenia). This condition is rare occurring most commonly in postmenopausal women.

Focus Point

Sideropenic anemia without documentation of dysphagia is reported with D50.0 when the condition is documented as due to (chronic) blood loss, D62 if due to acute blood loss, or D50.9 if no qualifiers are present.

D50.8   Other iron deficiency anemias

Other iron deficiency anemias include anemia due to inadequate dietary intake of iron. A normal diet consists of 12 to 15 mg of iron daily, of which 0.6 to 1.5 mg are typically absorbed. When an inadequate amount of iron is consumed in food, the body is unable to make new red blood cells (RBCs) or makes RBCs that are smaller than normal resulting in anemia. Iron is also necessary for the formation of hemoglobin, which carries oxygen to organs, tissues, and cells. Neonates and young children may develop iron deficiency anemia due to new blood formation and increased iron utilization that exceeds dietary intake.

D51.-   Vitamin B12 deficiency anemia

Most anemias included in this category are the result of inadequate dietary intake, impaired absorption, or inadequate utilization of vitamin B12. Low vitamin B12 levels affect the cell cycle of red blood cells (RBC) causing the cells to grow without dividing, resulting in abnormally large and dysfunctional red blood cells called megaloblasts. Due to megaloblast formation, conditions included here may also be referred to as megaloblastic anemias.

D51.0   Vitamin B12 deficiency anemia due to intrinsic factor deficiency

More commonly called pernicious anemia, this condition is a chronic progressive anemia caused by an autoimmune disorder of the stomach. Parietal cells in the stomach produce a protein called intrinsic factor that is used by the intestines, primarily the ileum, to help with vitamin B12 absorption. In pernicious anemia, these parietal cells or the intrinsic factor itself are attacked by the body and destroyed resulting in a lower amount of intrinsic factor that in turn decreases the amount of vitamin B12 the intestines can absorb. Although the name pernicious means "deadly or fatal," this ominous description is really no longer relevant because the cause of the disease is now known and effective treatment regimens have been established. The term pernicious continues to be used more for historical reasons.

D51.1   Vitamin B12 deficiency anemia due to selective vitamin B12 malabsorption with proteinuria

This rare hereditary form of vitamin B12 deficiency anemia is caused by an autosomal recessive disorder that results in selective malabsorption of vitamin B12. The stomach produces a protein called intrinsic factor that binds to vitamin B12. Once bound, this vitamin-protein complex is absorbed by a receptor in the terminal ileum called the cubam, which is composed of two proteins: amnionless (AMN) and cubilin. This condition occurs when there is a defect in the AMN or the cubilin proteins preventing the absorption of vitamin B12 by the intestine. The condition typically appears in childhood and mild to moderate proteinuria (protein in the urine) may also be present despite normal kidney function.

D51.2   Transcobalamin II deficiency

Transcobalamin II (TCII) is a carrier protein found in plasma that binds with and facilitates uptake of vitamin B12 by cells. In order for vitamin B12 to be used by the body, the vitamin has to interact with many different proteins produced by the body so that it can be transported. This protein interaction with vitamin B12 starts in the mouth and continues through the digestive tract eventually ending at the cell level. At each stage, the specific protein that binds with vitamin B12 performs a different function, such as protection from acid erosion in the stomach or transport of the vitamin from one part of the body to another. TCII is a protein used to move vitamin B12 from the intestine into the cells throughout the body. Deficiency of TCII may be a result of inadequate amounts of TCII in the plasma or an abnormality in the TCII protein that causes it to fail to bind with vitamin B12 or leaves it with an inability to carry the vitamin into the cells. TCII deficiency causes nonspecific symptoms, such as vomiting and poor growth in infancy, as well as ulcers of the mouth and infections that typically begin around 1 to 2 months of age. In later stages of the disease, neurological symptoms can develop and if the deficiency is not corrected, neurologic impairments may become permanent.

D51.3   Other dietary vitamin B12 deficiency anemia

Dietary vitamin B12 deficiency anemia due to inadequate dietary intake of food rich in vitamin B12 is classified here. Foods rich in vitamin B12 include meat, poultry, fish and other seafood, eggs, and dairy products. Because a vegan diet does not include food naturally rich in vitamin B12, it is one of the more common causes of dietary vitamin B12 deficiency anemia.

D51.8   Other vitamin B12 deficiency anemias

This code includes other specified types of vitamin B12 deficiency anemia that are not due to decreased production of intrinsic factor, select vitamin B12 malabsorption, or other dietary causes.

D52.-   Folate deficiency anemia

Folate, also called folic acid, is a B complex vitamin that is needed for the production of healthy red blood cells. Folate deficiency anemia is typically caused by a poor diet with inadequate intake of folate. However, certain conditions may also affect absorption of folate from the digestive tract causing anemia that results in very large, immature nucleated erythrocytes called megaloblasts. Patients at risk for folate deficiency include pregnant women due to increased demand for folate especially in the first two months of pregnancy, patients with renal failure due to increased excretion, and patients who have Celiac disease or sprue that may reduce absorption of the mineral. Certain drugs can also affect how folate is absorbed or utilized.

D52.1 Drug-induced folate deficiency anemia

Folate deficiency anemia resulting from an adverse effect of a drug is classified here. Classes of therapeutic drugs most commonly associated with this condition include antineoplastic and immunosuppressant.

D52.8 Other folate deficiency anemias

Included here are those folate deficiency anemias that are caused by conditions such as Celiac disease or sprue, conditions that reduce absorption of the mineral from the gastrointestinal tract.

D53.- Other nutritional anemias

This category includes nutritional anemias due to other micronutrient deficiencies. Although low levels of folate and/or vitamin B12 may also be present, these nutritional anemias are unresponsive to vitamin B12 or folate therapy. Like vitamin B12 anemias, other nutritional anemias classified here result in very large, immature nucleated erythrocytes called megaloblasts.

D53.Ø Protein deficiency anemia

Protein deficiency anemia is due to the lack of protein in the diet and is often manifested in those whose diets are restricted, such as vegans, vegetarians, the elderly, athletes, or people with eating disorders. It may also manifest in conjunction with chronic kidney or liver disease or hypothyroidism. The decrease in protein consumption leads to sluggish metabolism, which decreases oxygen needed by the kidneys, thereby inhibiting the production of erythropoietin (EPO) hormones. These hormones aid in the production of red blood cells and when insufficient, lead to anemia.

D53.1 Other megaloblastic anemias, not elsewhere classified

Megaloblastic anemia, also referred to as megacystic anemia, occurs when the red blood cell count in the body is lower than normal and the size of the cells are larger than normal. This decrease in volume affects organ function since the body's organs and tissues require a certain amount of oxygen from the blood to operate effectively. The larger size of the cell inhibits its exit from the bone marrow, leading to the inadequate supply. Although most commonly caused by either vitamin B12 or folate deficiency, it can arise from a combination of deficiencies documented as dimorphic or diphasic anemia, all of which are categorized here. The symptoms vary by person but are typically

displayed with shortness of breath, fatigue, weakness, decrease in appetite, weight loss, nausea, diarrhea, or numbness/tingling of the extremities. Treatment depends on the underlying cause of the anemia as well as the age of the patient and whether or not other health conditions are present. In most cases, dietary modification and vitamin supplements can help to manage the condition.

> **Focus Point**
>
> *Code D53.1 Other megaloblastic anemias, not elsewhere classified, includes anemias caused by a combination of both vitamin B12 or folate deficiencies. However codes for anemia due to lack of vitamin B12 or folate alone are found in category D51 and category D52, respectively.*

D53.2 Scorbutic anemia

This anemia is a manifestation seen with the disease called scurvy when there is also a deficiency of folic acid in the diet. Scurvy is caused by a lack of vitamin C (ascorbic acid) consumption, which is needed for the production of collagen and for iron absorption. Without adequate iron absorption, the production of new red blood cells is reduced and anemia results. Scurvy in combination with folic acid deficiency causes a megaloblastic form of anemia.

> **Focus Point**
>
> *Scurvy alone, without folic acid deficiency and the resulting scorbutic anemia, is reported with E54.*

Hemolytic Anemias (D55-D59)

Hemolytic anemia occurs when there is premature destruction of red blood cells (RBC) resulting in reduced numbers of circulating healthy RBCs. When RBCs die before the end of their natural life cycle, roughly 110 to 120 days, the bone marrow must compensate for the early loss by increasing production. When the bone marrow cannot keep pace with RBC destruction, the result is hemolytic anemia. The cause of hemolysis development is divided into two groups: intrinsic and extrinsic. The intrinsic causes are most often hereditary due to a genetic defect of one or more of the components of the red blood cells. Extrinsic causes are usually acquired conditions where the red blood cells themselves are normal but there is targeted destruction of the red blood cells due to some external process.

The categories in this code block are as follows:

D55	Anemia due to enzyme disorders
D56	Thalassemia
D57	Sickle-cell disorders
D58	Other hereditary hemolytic anemias
D59	Acquired hemolytic anemia

D55.-   Anemia due to enzyme disorders

Red blood cells produce enzymes (proteins) to help protect them. When these enzymes are missing due to gene mutation, the red blood cells become fragile and susceptible to early damage or destruction.

D55.0   Anemia due to glucose-6-phosphate dehydrogenase [G6PD] deficiency

The most common enzyme deficiency in humans is glucose-6-phosphate dehydrogenase [G6PD] deficiency. The G6PD enzyme can be found in all types of cells but is particularly important in red blood cells because it provides RBCs protection from damage and destruction from oxidative forces. When oxidative forces cause premature destruction of the RBCs and the bone marrow cannot compensate, hemolytic anemia may result. The most common oxidative processes known to cause G6PD anemia in individuals with hereditary G6PD deficiency include infections, as well as the consumption of fava beans and other legumes.

Focus Point

Commons drugs such as sulfa and antimalarial drugs can also cause glucose-6-phosphate dehydrogenase deficiency through oxidative stress on the red blood cells. However, drug induced G6PD is not coded here but is included under code D59.2. This code captures all drug induced enzyme deficiency anemias.

D55.1   Anemia due to other disorders of glutathione metabolism

This form of anemia is an inherited condition affecting the red blood cells, specifically the enzymes of glutathione metabolism. The extent of this condition ranges from mild to severe based on the symptoms and the length of time it takes for red cells to break down in the blood. Premature death of red cells is problematic when the bone marrow cannot create new cells in a timely matter to make up for the loss. The mild form of this condition manifests as hemolytic anemia, but progression of the disorder may lead to an enlarged spleen and/or metabolic acidosis. Included in this code is anemia with documentation that notes that the anemia is due to a disorder of pentose phosphate pathway (PPP); a deficiency of 6 phosphogluconate dehydrogenase (6-PGD), erythrocytic glutathione, or glutathione reductase; or congenital nonspherocytic type 1. These are additional types of enzyme deficiencies and disorders that relate to the processing of sugars at the molecular level.

D55.2   Anemia due to disorders of glycolytic enzymes

This code includes the second most common enzyme deficiency, pyruvate kinase [PK] deficiency. The enzyme pyruvate kinase is needed by RBCs to breakdown glucose into a useable energy source called adenosine triphosphate or ATP. Without ATP the cell cannot maintain its cellular structure leading to premature cell destruction or death. Anemia occurs when RBCs cannot be replaced fast enough by the bone marrow to compensate for early loss of these RBCs. Although it can be found in patients of varying ethnic backgrounds, it is most prevalent in Pennsylvania Amish communities. Hereditary pyruvate kinase deficiency occurs when both parents pass the defective gene on to the child.

Focus Point

Acquired forms of pyruvate kinase deficiency can be associated with certain medical conditions including acute leukemia, preleukemia, and refractory sideroblastic anemia and are reported with D59.8.

D56.-   Thalassemia

Thalassemias are inherited disorders of the red blood cells caused by a genetic mutation or deletion of the genes needed for proper hemoglobin formation. An in-depth understanding of the genetic composition of the red blood cell is needed to distinguish between the different types of thalassemia. Hemoglobin is formed by two inherited proteins from both parents. These proteins are known as alpha globin and beta globin. There are four alpha (two from each parent) and two beta (one from each parent) globins that makeup hemoglobin. When one or more of the globins are missing or deformed, the incomplete hemoglobin causes misshapen and fragile red blood cells. The different types of thalassemia are divided by the type and number of missing or deformed globins. Due to their frail nature, the affected RBCs break apart and die quickly resulting in anemia. Symptoms vary depending on the specific genetic mutation or deletion, but some of the more common symptoms include jaundice, facial bone deformities, shortness of breath, and fatigue.

D56.Ø   Alpha thalassemia

Conditions represented under this code include those where at least three out of the four alpha genes have some sort of mutation or defect. Hemoglobin H disease is included here and is a moderate to severe form of alpha thalassemia that is a result of three mutated alpha genes. Symptoms include microcytic hypochromic hemolytic anemia, splenomegaly, jaundice, and skeletal changes. Diagnosis is usually made in infancy or early childhood, although some individuals are not diagnosed until adulthood. Alpha thalassemia major is the most severe form of alpha thalassemia and occurs when all four alpha genes have mutated. Also referred to as hydrops fetalis, death often occurs before or immediately after birth. Alpha thalassemia occurs most often in patients from southeast Africa, the Middle East, China, and those of African descent.

Focus Point

Hydrops fetalis has several etiologies. Only hydrops fetalis due to alpha thalassemia is reported here. Those causes that are not related to a defect in a hemoglobin gene are classified to Chapter 16 Certain Conditions Originating in the Perinatal Period.

D56.1   Beta thalassemia

This code represents subtypes of beta thalassemia that are the result of mutations to both beta globin genes. The most severe subtype is beta thalassemia major or Cooley's anemia. By 2 years of age, notable symptoms include severe often transfusion dependent anemia, skeletal deformities, and jaundice, as well as changes to the liver, spleen, and heart. Thalassemia intermedia, also classified here, is typically less severe in symptomology than its major cohort and often regular blood transfusions are not necessary. Diagnosis can occur early in childhood or later in life depending on the severity of symptoms, which can range from pallor alone to splenomegaly, skeletal abnormalities, and growth retardation. Beta thalassemia is most often seen in individuals of Mediterranean origin, those from China, and those of African descent.

D56.2   Delta-beta thalassemia

Delta-beta thalassemia is a rare form of thalassemia that results from a deletion of the delta and beta genes located on chromosome 11. These deletions result in increased production of gamma globulin and an increase of circulating fetal hemoglobin (HbF). Symptoms vary depending on whether the individual has inherited the defect from a single parent (heterozygote) or both parents (homozygote).

D56.3   Thalassemia minor

Included under this code are conditions that result when one or two alpha genes are mutated or one beta and/or one delta gene are mutated. When only one alpha gene has mutated, rarely do symptoms develop but instead patients are considered a carrier of alpha thalassemia, meaning they can pass on the genetic defect but they do not manifest symptoms themselves. Alpha thalassemia minor or alpha thalassemia trait occurs when two alpha genes are mutated. Symptoms vary with some individuals having no symptoms, similar to individuals who are carriers, while others have minor symptoms such as mild anemia. In both beta and delta-beta thalassemia minor or trait, only one of the beta and/or delta genes has mutated. Treatment is often not necessary as there are often only mild associated symptoms.

D56.4   Hereditary persistence of fetal hemoglobin [HPFH]

Hereditary persistence of fetal hemoglobin is an alteration in the blood caused by gene variants and is inherited by children from the parents. This alteration in the blood does not allow for the replacement of hemoglobin F in the infant with the adult form of hemoglobin. While this blood variant is present throughout a person's lifespan, it is a harmless anomaly.

D56.5   Hemoglobin E-beta thalassemia

Hemoglobin e-beta thalassemia disorder is due to an inherited hemoglobin E gene from one parent and a beta-thalassemia gene from the other parent, causing a reduction in the production of hemoglobin volume. This can lead to severe anemia depending on the level of beta-thalassemia and without medical attention may progress to heart failure, atrophy of the spleen and liver, and alterations of bone growth. Treatment may include recurrent blood transfusions.

D57.-   Sickle-cell disorders

Sickle-cell disorders are severe, chronic diseases caused by a genetic variation in the hemoglobin protein in the red blood cell. These are the most common types of inherited blood disorders in the United States and are found most predominantly in African Americans. A red blood cell is normally disc shaped, which allows it to move through the blood vessels easily. In sickle-cell disorders, the gene mutation causes the red blood cell to become hard, sticky, and crescent or sickle shaped. These changes make it harder for red blood cells to travel through the bloodstream disrupting blood flow and decreasing oxygen transport to tissues. Sickle-cell disorders are classified based on the specific type of sickle cell disease and whether the individual is experiencing a crisis. Crisis in sickle-cell disorders refers to recurring acute episodes of pain most often due to a vasoocclusive process that can involve any body system, but manifestations usually involve the chest, bones, or abdomen. The pain comes on without warning and can last hours or days. Specific forms of crises include:

- Acute chest syndrome: In young children this is characterized by chest pain, fever, cough, tachypnea, leukocytosis, and pulmonary infiltrates in the upper lobes. Adults are less symptomatic but may have dyspnea, severe chest pain, and multilobar or lower lobe disease.

- Splenic sequestration: This is characterized by rapid enlargement of the spleen and occurs most often during the first five years of life but can occur at any age.

- Unspecified or not otherwise specified crisis

D57.Ø- Hb-SS disease with crisis

This is the most common type of the sickle-cell disorder and occurs when both parents pass on a hemoglobin S gene. A code from this subcategory is assigned when the patient is currently experiencing a crisis.

D57.1 Sickle-cell disease without crisis

This is the most common type of the sickle-cell disorder and occurs when both parents pass on a hemoglobin S gene. This code is also used when the specific type of sickle-cell disease is not specified. This code is assigned when the patient is not currently experiencing a crisis.

D57.2- Sickle-cell/Hb-C disease

Sickle-cell/Hb-C diseases occur when one parent passes on a hemoglobin S gene and the other parent passes on a hemoglobin C gene. Symptoms may be similar to those seen in patients with Hb-SS disease but are usually less frequent and less severe.

D57.2Ø Sickle-cell/Hb-C disease without crisis

This code is used for patients with sickle-cell/Hb-C disease who are not currently experiencing a crisis.

D57.21- Sickle-cell/Hb-C disease with crisis

Codes in this subcategory are used when a patient with sickle-cell/Hb-C disease is currently in crisis with manifestations of acute chest syndrome or splenic sequestration, or with other or unspecified crisis manifestations.

D57.3 Sickle-cell trait

Sickle-cell trait occurs when only one parent passes on a hemoglobin S gene and the other parent passes on a normal hemoglobin gene. These individuals are most often carriers of the disease and rarely have symptoms.

D57.4- Sickle-cell thalassemia

Sickle-cell thalassemia occurs when one parent passes on a hemoglobin S gene and the other parent passes on a gene for beta thalassemia.

D57.4Ø Sickle-cell thalassemia without crisis

This code is used when a patient with sickle-cell thalassemia is not currently experiencing a crisis.

D57.41- Sickle-cell thalassemia with crisis

Codes in this subcategory are used when a patient with sickle-cell thalassemia is currently in crisis with manifestations of acute chest syndrome or splenic sequestration, or with other or unspecified crisis manifestations.

> **Focus Point**
>
> Thalassemia alone without an inherited hemoglobin S gene is classified under category D56 Thalassemia.

D58.- Other hereditary hemolytic anemias

Conditions under this category are genetic forms of hemolytic anemia but do not fall under the more specific categories for thalassemia and sickle-cell disorders. Most of these disorders occur because of a defect in the hemoglobin protein of the red blood cell, which usually results in asymptomatic anemia.

D58.Ø Hereditary spherocytosis

Hereditary spherocytosis is an inherited condition caused by a variety of mutations to genes responsible for the production of proteins that form the membranes of red blood cells. These mutations alter the shape and flexibility of the red blood cell membrane resulting in a decreased cell membrane surface area and a spherical shape. The more rounded or spherical shaped cells do not traverse the spleen easily and instead become trapped and destroyed by the spleen before the red blood cell has reached maturity. The severity of this condition varies and symptoms or manifestations may be mild, moderate, moderate-severe, or severe.

D58.1 Hereditary elliptocytosis

This inherited condition is due to a defect in the proteins necessary for maintaining the biconcave disc shape of a normal red blood cell. Most often the red blood cells will be oval or elliptical in shape. In most cases patients have only mild symptoms.

D58.2 Other hemoglobinopathies

Conditions included here represent other disorders of hemoglobin due to an alteration of the molecular structure of the red blood cell. Most of these disorders result in less severe forms of anemia and in some patients no symptoms may be present. Splenomegaly is almost always present but often is asymptomatic.

D58.8 Other specified hereditary hemolytic anemias

Included in this category is congenital stomatocytosis, which is a rare condition. Congenital stomatocytosis presents early in life and causes a severe form of hemolytic anemia.

D59.- Acquired hemolytic anemia

Conditions included under this category are nonhereditary anemias usually caused by an external process. One type classified here, paroxysmal nocturnal hemoglobinuria (PNH), is caused by a genetic mutation; however, in this case the genetic mutation is acquired rather than hereditary. Most of these disorders involve the breakdown of otherwise normal erythrocytes with a variety of etiologies including injury, infection, the use of certain drugs, or blood transfusions. Acquired hemolytic anemias are broadly differentiated as immune types or mechanical types. In immune hemolytic anemia, the patient's immune system inappropriately identifies its own erythrocytes as a pathogen, targeting and destroying the red blood cell. There are three types of immune hemolytic anemia: autoimmune, alloimmune, and drug-induced. In mechanical hemolytic anemia, the red blood cell membranes are physically damaged, which weakens the red blood cell (RBC) and results in premature destruction.

D59.3 Hemolytic-uremic syndrome

Hemolytic-uremic syndrome (HUS) is a condition that affects the blood and the kidneys. Hemolysis in this case refers to premature destruction of the red blood cells caused by a disease process that begins with abnormal blood clot formation in the capillaries of the kidneys. These blood clots partially obstruct the capillaries making it impossible for red blood cells to pass through these vessels intact. The damaged red blood cells further compromise kidney function preventing removal of urea and other waste products from the blood. Eventually acute kidney failure occurs. This condition is most common in children and very often is preceded by an episode of infectious,

sometimes bloody, diarrhea caused by certain types of *E. coli*, which is acquired as a foodborne illness. However, it may also occur in adults as a complication of *S. pneumoniae*, pregnancy, or AIDS.

> **Focus Point**
>
> *TTP or thrombotic thrombocytopenic purpura is a rare disorder that is often hard to differentiate from HUS as the mechanism of red blood cell destruction is the same in both diseases and both exhibit the same manifestations of hemolytic anemia, thrombocytopenia, and kidney involvement. HUS, however, predominantly affects children younger than 5 years of age, and exhibits more renal manifestations and fewer neurological manifestations. TTP is classified to Chapter 13 Diseases of the Musculoskeletal System and Connective Tissue.*

D59.5 Paroxysmal nocturnal hemoglobinuria [Marchiafava-Micheli]

Paroxysmal nocturnal hemoglobinuria (PNH) is the result of red blood cell destruction by the body's intrinsic immune system. In a normal red blood cell (RBC) there are surface proteins that help fortify the cell membrane and keep the RBC intact. With PNH, an essential component needed to form the surface membrane is missing leaving the membrane exposed to immune forces that breakdown the cell membrane, which in turn releases the cellular components, such as hemoglobin, into the circulation. As this is an acquired genetic mutation of stem cells, it not only affects the RBCs but also the white blood cells and platelets. As the description suggests, the most common symptom is hemoglobinuria, which is the presence of hemoglobin in the urine. Hemoglobin causes the urine to be dark in color, more so during the night when the urine is more concentrated. Patients with PNH are more susceptible to thrombosis (blood clot formation) in unusual sites such as the hepatic vein, veins of the abdomen and skin, and the cerebral vein. Thrombosis is the main cause of death in patients with PNH but can be managed if the disease is recognized early.

D59.6 Hemoglobinuria due to hemolysis from other external causes

Strenuous exercise can start the process of hemolysis of red blood cells. Direct trauma to the cell is the result of repetitive impact on the blood vessels, most often those found in the feet and hands. It can be seen in marathoners, soldiers, and bongo players.

Aplastic and Other Anemias and Other Bone Marrow Failure Syndromes (D60-D64)

Bone marrow is the production site of new blood cells. The bone marrow produces stem cells that change into red blood cells, white blood cells, or platelets. Conditions included in these categories report failure of the bone marrow to generate blood cells, typically resulting in a deficiency of all the formed elements of the blood (erythrocytes, platelets, and leukocytes).

The categories in this code block are as follows:

D60	Acquired pure red cell aplasia [erythroblastopenia]
D61	Other aplastic anemias and other bone marrow failure syndromes
D62	Acute posthemorrhagic anemia
D63	Anemia in chronic diseases classified elsewhere
D64	Other anemias

Focus Point

Myelodysplastic syndromes are neoplastic disorders that have similar characteristics and symptoms to aplastic anemia. In each disease process a lower than normal amount of healthy blood cells are present in the circulation. However, in aplastic anemias, even though the number of blood cells may be lower, the blood cells that are present are normal, whereas in myelodysplastic syndromes the blood cells do not develop and mature as they should. Myelodysplastic syndromes are categorized to the neoplasm chapter.

D60.- Acquired pure red cell aplasia [erythroblastopenia]

Acquired red cell aplasia is a form of anemia in which the bone marrow ceases to produce red blood cells. Unlike aplastic anemia where there are lowered numbers of all constituents of blood, pure red cell aplasia (PRCA) is characterized by nearly complete cessation of red blood cell production only. Normally the white blood cell and platelet levels are normal. PRCA may be due to chronic systemic disease, drugs, infection, radiation, or toxic materials. There are little to no signs of PRCA until anemia becomes severe. The first noticeable symptoms may present as reduced exercise tolerance and extreme pallor. Other symptoms that are present may not be related to the anemia but to the underlying disorder that triggered the PRCA.

D60.0 Chronic acquired pure red cell aplasia

The chronic form of acquired pure red cell aplasia may be associated with underlying disorders such as autoimmune diseases or a neoplasm of the thymus (thymoma). Although sometimes refractory to treatment, chronic acquired red cell aplasia usually responds to immunosuppressant drugs.

D60.9 Acquired pure red cell aplasia, unspecified

Included under this code are those PRCA conditions that are due to drugs. Common drugs associated with PRCA may include immunosuppressive agents such as azathioprine and mycophenolate and antiepileptic medications such as phenytoin.

D61.- Other aplastic anemias and other bone marrow failure syndromes

This category reports failure of bone marrow to generate blood cells, resulting in a deficiency of one or more of the formed elements of the blood (erythrocytes, platelets, and leukocytes). Signs and symptoms relate to which formed elements are deficient and the severity of the deficiency.

D61.0- Constitutional aplastic anemia

These are rare congenital (inherited) disorders of blood cell production in which the body fails to produce adequate amounts of healthy blood cells. Constitutional aplastic anemia is present at birth and symptoms generally manifest in infancy or early childhood.

D61.01 Constitutional (pure) red blood cell aplasia

Constitutional (pure) red blood cell aplasia (CPRCA) is a syndrome of failed erythropoiesis (formation of red blood cells), and is most often diagnosed within the first year of life. Also known as Blackfan-Diamond syndrome, this is a rare idiopathic blood disorder that is present at birth and distinguished by red blood cell deficiency. Other symptoms and physical findings vary greatly from case to case but may include slow growth, atypical weakness and fatigue, pallor, distinctive facial abnormalities, protruding scapulae, abnormal shortening or webbing of the neck caused by fusion of cervical vertebrae, hand malformations, and congenital heart defects. Blackfan-Diamond syndrome may be inherited as an autosomal dominant or recessive genetic trait.

D61.09 Other constitutional aplastic anemia

Other types of rare congenital (inherited) aplastic anemias including Fanconi's anemia (FA), which is the most frequently reported of the rare inherited bone marrow failure syndromes, are classified here. FA is present at birth and typically diagnosed in infancy. Symptoms of bone marrow failure, which is the major cause of death in FA, often present in childhood and include easy bruising, petechiae, fatigue, and pallor.

The majority of patients have characteristic birth defects such as hyper- or hypopigmented skin, short stature, musculoskeletal abnormalities, gonadal anomalies, microencephaly, eye and ear abnormalities, and systemic defects.

D61.3   Idiopathic aplastic anemia

In most cases of aplastic anemia, the source of the disease cannot be determined and these cases are classified as idiopathic aplastic anemia.

D61.8-   Other specified aplastic anemias and other bone marrow failure syndromes

This subcategory reports various types of pancytopenia and a condition called myelophthisis. Pancytopenia is characterized by a deficiency of all types of blood cells usually caused by dysfunction or suppression of stem cell development. Myelophthisis is a type of bone marrow failure syndrome.

D61.810 Antineoplastic chemotherapy induced pancytopenia

D61.811 Other drug-induced pancytopenia

D61.818 Other pancytopenia

Pancytopenia describes a deficiency of all types of blood cells, including white blood cells, red blood cells, and platelets. Pathogenesis is attributed to a dysfunction or suppression in the bone marrow stem cells as a result of existing disease, infection, hereditary predisposition, toxic exposures, and the adverse effects of certain medications. Pancytopenia is a common adverse effect of drugs used to treat cancer (antineoplastic chemotherapy). Other therapeutic drugs known to cause bone marrow depression and pancytopenia include chloramphenicol, sulfonamides, gold, and anti-inflammatory, antithyroid, psychotropic, and anticonvulsant/antidepressant drugs. Pancytopenia of other or unknown cause, including abnormal blood chemistry with a finding of pancytopenia not otherwise specified, is reported here with the code for other pancytopenia. If untreated or inadequately treated, pancytopenia can cause widespread damaging effects to multiple body systems, such as impaired oxygenation of tissues and immune system malfunction.

Focus Point

Pancytopenia and aplastic anemia are not synonymous terms. Aplastic anemia often presents with pancytopenia as a clinical indicator. If pancytopenia is present and documented but documentation also supports an aplastic anemia diagnosis, codes from this subcategory should not be used.

Pancytopenia due to other specified disease processes may have a more specific code. Review of the excludes1 notes is needed to ensure that the most specific code is assigned when pancytopenia is due to a specified disease process.

D61.82   Myelophthisis

Myelophthisis is also known as leukoerythroblastic anemia or myelophthisic anemia. This condition occurs when normal hematopoietic tissue in the bone marrow is replaced with abnormal tissue, such as fibrous tissue or tumors. The most common underlying causes of myelophthisis include metastatic carcinomas, with the primary site most often being the breast or prostate; lymphoma; granulomatous diseases such as miliary tuberculosis; and rare disorders such as Gaucher disease. Fungal infections, sarcoidosis, sickle cell disease, septicemia, and congenital osteopetrosis may also be causative factors. While myelophthisis is observed more frequently in countries where access to medical care is not readily available and diseases are more likely to progress to advanced stages, in the United States this disorder occurs most commonly during the advanced stages of cancer. Outcome is highly dependent upon the patient's access to medical care.

D62   Acute posthemorrhagic anemia

This condition is the result of frank, rapid blood loss. The etiology may be trauma, spontaneous rupture of a blood vessel, surgical procedures involving major blood vessels, bleeding from peptic ulcers or neoplasms, or extravasation secondary to a bleeding diathesis such as hemophilia. Symptoms include faintness, dizziness, thirst, weakness, rapid pulse, rapid respirations, orthostatic changes in blood pressure, and hypovolemic shock.

D63.-   Anemia in chronic diseases classified elsewhere

Certain chronic diseases can lead to reduced red blood cell production. When a low level of red blood cells persists it can result in anemia. As long as the chronic disease is compensated, the anemia will most likely be of little concern. It is when these chronic conditions become exacerbated that symptoms and signs of anemia may be present. Signs and symptoms may include weakness, headache, paleness, and shortness of breath.

Focus Point

All of the diagnosis codes under this category are considered manifestation codes. Documentation must clearly show a link between the anemia and the underlying disorder in order to assign a code from this category.

D64.-   Other anemias

This category reports other types of anemia such as sideroblastic anemia, congenital dyserythropoietic anemia, and anemia due to antineoplastic chemotherapy.

D64.0   Hereditary sideroblastic anemia

D64.1   Secondary sideroblastic anemia due to disease

D64.2   Secondary sideroblastic anemia due to drugs and toxins

D64.3   Other sideroblastic anemias

Sideroblastic anemia is a condition in which the red blood cells cannot effectively use iron, a nutrient needed to make hemoglobin. Although the iron can enter the red blood cell it does not get assimilated into the hemoglobin molecule. Instead the iron builds up in a ring around the nucleus of the cell, which is identified as ringed sideroblasts under microscopic examination. These ringed sideroblasts are the most telling sign of the disorder. Sideroblastic anemia is classified by etiology that may be hereditary (inherited) or secondary to a disease, drug, or toxin. Specific conditions that may cause secondary sideroblastic anemia include neoplastic states, chronic inflammatory states, preleukemia, and myeloid leukemia. Drug and toxin induced sideroblastic anemias may involve alcohol or lead poisoning, antibiotic drugs such as chloramphenicol, or antituberculosis drugs such as isoniazid and pyrazinamide.

D64.4   Congenital dyserythropoietic anemia

Congenital dyserythropoietic anemia (CDA) affects the development of red blood cells (RBC) resulting in a shortage of circulating RBCs. There are many variations of CDA, a majority of which have been grouped into three main subtypes: CDA type I, II and III. In some cases, the type of CDA can be diagnosed in utero but most patients experience the onset of the disease in childhood or early adulthood. Common symptoms include splenomegaly and/or hepatomegaly, jaundice, and symptomatic anemia. The primary concern with type I CDA is iron overload, which can lead to tissue and/or organ damage. Gallstones are common in CDA type II, which is the most common of the three subtypes of CDA. CDA III is rare and most patients are asymptomatic but this type of CDA can predispose the patient to other conditions such as monoclonal gammopathy, retinal angioid streaks, or myelomas, the presence of which may help in its diagnosis.

D64.81   Anemia due to antineoplastic chemotherapy

Chemotherapy-induced anemia affects approximately 20 percent to 60 percent of cancer patients, resulting in fatigue and inability to perform daily tasks. Cancer and cancer-related treatment often inhibits the production of bone marrow, resulting in decreased red blood cell production. Red blood cells carry oxygen throughout the body. When the production of red blood cells is too low, the body receives inadequate oxygen. Oxygen is of vital importance to the health of tissues and organs.

With insufficient oxygen supply, the heart works harder than normal in an attempt to oxygenate the body. As a result, the patient may feel weak, short of breath, dizzy, or fatigued. Anemia stresses the body, and may exacerbate other existing medical conditions. As a result, anemia can cause treatment delays and dosage adjustments that can decrease the effectiveness of cancer therapy.

D64.9   Anemia, unspecified

This code reports normochromic, normocytic anemia of unspecified type, including anemia described as atypical, essential, general, hemoglobin deficiency, idiopathic, infantile, normocytic, primary, profound, or progressive without more specific qualifying descriptors. This code is also used to report low hemoglobin or hematocrit levels that are not more specifically described.

Coagulation Defects, Purpura and Other Hemorrhagic Conditions (D65-D69)

Coagulation is the process by which the blood forms a clot. Clot formation is a complex process in which formed elements, such as platelets, and clotting factors, such as factor VIII, work together to manage bleeding. When there are a deficient amount of formed elements or clotting factors or there is a breakdown in the process itself, clot regulation is disrupted and abnormal bleeding results. Purpura, or what is more commonly called bruising, is an area of hemorrhage under the skin. The causes of purpura can range from insect bites to allergic reactions to thrombocytopenia and can occur spontaneously or result from very minor trauma.

The categories in this code block are as follows:

D65	Disseminated intravascular coagulation [defibrination syndrome]
D66	Hereditary factor VIII deficiency
D67	Hereditary factor IX deficiency
D68	Other coagulation defects
D69	Purpura and other hemorrhagic conditions

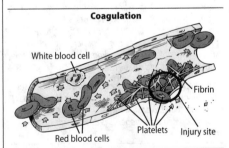

Coagulation

White blood cell

Fibrin

Red blood cells

Platelets

Injury site

D65 Disseminated intravascular coagulation [defibrination syndrome]

This disorder, also known as DIC, is not hereditary and is very rare. It is the result of a malfunction in the body's clotting factors in response to an external process. Normally when a patient is injured, a laceration to the finger for example, the clotting elements in the blood will go to work at the site of the injury to close off the area and prevent further blood loss. When a patient develops DIC, instead of the clotting factors responding to the site of the injury they begin to form clots in small blood vessels throughout the body, limiting blood flow in these areas while the site of the open wound continues to hemorrhage. Certain conditions can predispose a patient to DIC. These can include obstetrical complications, such as abruptio placentae or retained products of conception, infections, neoplasms, and shock. When DIC evolves slowly, conditions like deep venous thrombosis or pulmonary embolism may occur. When DIC evolves rapidly, severe bleeding in addition to thrombosis can occur, which can eventually lead to organ failure.

D66 Hereditary factor VIII deficiency

Hereditary factor VIII deficiency or as it is more commonly known, hemophilia A, is the most common of the coagulation disorders. Although most patients inherit the disease, some patients may develop factor VIII deficiency from a spontaneous gene mutation. The majority of patients with this disorder are males with females serving mostly as carriers, although in rare circumstances a female can inherit the disease as well. The severity of factor VIII deficiency is split into three levels: severe, moderate, and mild, based on the amount of factor VIII activity in the blood. Severe factor VIII deficiency is the most common. Patients frequently experience spontaneous bleeding into joints, muscles, or skin and trauma or surgery can be life-threatening as the hemorrhaging may be hard to control. Patients with moderate factor VIII deficiency may not have spontaneous bleeding but will have excessive bleeding from what are typically minor injuries.

D67 Hereditary factor IX deficiency

Commonly called Christmas disease, factor IX deficiency is part of the hemophilia family and is synonymous with hemophilia B. Factor IX deficiency has the same genetic susceptibility as factor VIII deficiency, in that it affects mostly males and is passed by a female carrier. Severity levels and development of antibodies to factor IX are similar to that of Factor VIII as well.

D68.- Other coagulation defects

This category comprises a range of inherited coagulation defects: hemorrhagic disorders due to intrinsic circulating anticoagulants, antibodies, or inhibitors; hemorrhagic disorders due to extrinsic circulating anticoagulants, which include drug induced hemorrhagic disorders; and acquired coagulation deficiencies such as those due to liver disease or vitamin K deficiencies. Also included in this category are some types of hypercoaguable states such as antiphospholipid syndrome and lupus anticoagulant syndrome. Coagulation defects of undetermined cause are also included here.

D68.0 Von Willebrand's disease

Von Willebrand's disease is the most common of the inherited bleeding disorders caused by low levels of the blood clotting protein called von Willebrand factor (vWF) or a flaw in the vWF protein. There are many variations to this disease but the underlying effect is essentially the same in that the bonding capability of the vWF protein is not as effective in eliciting clot formation. Clots take longer to form leaving the patient susceptible to excessive bleeding.

Focus Point

Factor VIII deficiency can occur in some variations of von Willebrand's disease. Factor VIII deficiency is also a clinical indicator of hemophilia A. Careful review of bleeding history and all lab tests is essential to ensure that vWF is not playing a role in the lowered factor VIII levels and to avoid a misdiagnosis of hemophilia A. The treatment for both conditions is also different; a patient with von Willebrand's disease does not typically respond to the usual hemophilia A treatments.

D68.1 Hereditary factor XI deficiency

Also known as hemophilia C, hereditary factor XI deficiency is different from hemophilia A (hereditary factor VIII deficiency) and hemophilia B (hereditary factor IX deficiency) in that patients rarely experience spontaneous bleeding and often there is no correlation between the severity of the deficiency and the symptoms.

D68.2 Hereditary deficiency of other clotting factors

This code includes several conditions for inherited clotting factor deficiencies hindering the normal functioning of the routine process. The conditions in this group occur rarely, unlike the more common clotting deficiencies such as von Willebrand or hemophilia A or B. The following list shows examples of disorders included in this group.

- AC globulin deficiency: Component of plasma imperative to the creation of thrombin, an enzyme assisting in the blood clotting process.

- Congenital afibrinogenemia: Occurs due to an anomaly within one of the genes FGA, FGB, or FGG, which tells the body how to create fibrinogen.

- Deficiency of factor I (fibrinogen): A protein in the blood that may be missing or malfunctioning causing problems in the clotting process.

- Deficiency of factor II (prothrombin): Another protein in the blood that aids the clotting process and is passed down to the child when both parents carry the gene.

- Deficiency of factor V (labile): Genetic anomaly in the F5 gene responsible for telling the body how to create the coagulation factor V protein.

- Deficiency of factor VII (stable): Factor VII, also referred to as proconvertin, is a protein that adheres to tissue, instigating the clotting process. It is passed down to a child when both parents carry the gene. Insufficient factor VII is also called Alexander's disease.

- Deficiency of factor X (Stuart-Prower): This protein has an important function in initiating enzymes for clot formation requiring vitamin K for formation.

- Deficiency of factor XII (Hageman): This deficiency prevents the development of thrombin needed to transition fibrinogen to fibrin, preventing the stabilization of platelets in clot formation.

- Deficiency of factor XIII (fibrin stabilizing): The rarest clotting factor deficiency responsible for keeping the blood clot in place. When the clot is not fixed to the needed location, it falls apart, leading to repetitive bleeding.

- Dysfibrinogenemia (congenital): Clotting disease that presents with structural anomalies within the fibrinogen molecule, preventing normal operation.

- Hypoproconvertinemia: This describes a seriously low amount of proconvertin within the blood, leading to extended prothrombin time.

- Owren's disease: Also referred to as factor V deficiency or parahemophilia.

- Proaccelerin deficiency: Essentially a factor V deficiency responsible for transitioning prothrombin into thrombin.

D68.3- Hemorrhagic disorder due to circulating anticoagulants

Coagulation is the process in which the blood forms clots and is a necessary mechanism used by the body to prevent blood loss and maintain hemostasis. The formation of a clot is complex with as many as 20 different clotting factors working together. Circulating anticoagulants alter the function of one or more of these clotting factors prolonging the time it takes to form a clot, which can result in a bleeding disorder.

D68.31- Hemorrhagic disorder due to intrinsic circulating anticoagulants, antibodies, or inhibitors

Intrinsic circulating anticoagulants are those made by the body usually as an autoimmune response.

D68.311 Acquired hemophilia

Acquired hemophilia is a spontaneous autoimmune disorder caused by the development of autoantibodies to coagulation factors in a patient with previously normal homeostasis. These autoantibodies attack and disable plasma coagulation factors, most commonly factor VIII. The underlying cause often cannot be identified, but the production of autoantibodies is sometimes associated with pregnancy, hepatitis, autoimmune disorders such as rheumatoid arthritis or MS, or it can result from a hematologic malignancy such as non-Hodgkin lymphoma or multiple myeloma.

D68.312 Antiphospholipid antibody with hemorrhagic disorder

Antiphospholipid antibodies are antibodies produced by the body that mistakenly attack protein phospholipid complexes in the blood cells. These protein phospholipid complexes are one of many chemical processes needed to form a blood clot. It would stand to reason that if these complexes were missing or damaged it would be hard for a patient to form blood clots but the opposite is true. Antiphospholipid antibodies actually elicit blood clot formation. Since clot formation is increased it would seem unlikely that a patient with antiphospholipid antibodies would also develop a bleeding disorder; however, in very rare cases these antibodies have been found to cause bleeding although the mechanism behind this phenomenon is not understood.

D68.32 Hemorrhagic disorder due to extrinsic circulating anticoagulants

Hemorrhagic disorders due to extrinsic circulating anticoagulants are caused by drugs, such as warfarin or heparin, which are administered to a patient specifically to prevent blood clots. Doses of these drugs are sometimes difficult to adjust and until the optimal dose is determined hemorrhagic disorders can occur. Maintaining optimal dosing in some patients also requires careful monitoring and ongoing dose adjustments.

D68.4 Acquired coagulation factor deficiency

Many coagulation factors are produced by the liver. When the liver does not function properly the number of coagulation factors that can be produced may be impacted. Coagulation factors also need certain substances in the body in order to initiate the chemical reaction needed to produce a blood clot. When these substances are deficient, the necessary chemical reactions may not occur resulting in limited clot formation. Conditions that can cause coagulation factor deficiency may include poor dietary intake of necessary nutrients, particularly vitamin K, various malabsorption disorders, and liver disease.

D68.5- Primary thrombophilia

Thrombophilia refers to an increased tendency of the blood to clot, which can lead to thrombus or embolus formation. Primary in this subcategory refers to thrombophilia that is inherited rather than acquired.

D68.51 Activated protein C resistance

Synonymous with factor V Leiden mutation, this disorder is a type of thrombophilia that results in the formation of abnormal blood clots (thrombosis). These blood clots most often form in the deep veins of the lower legs but can occur in other parts of the body. Blood clots have the potential to disengage and flow through the bloodstream eventually getting lodged in the lung, which can result in a pulmonary embolism. Activated protein C resistance is the most common of the inherited forms of thrombophilia.

D68.52 Prothrombin gene mutation

Prothrombin is a protein in blood that assists in the formation of fibrin, a key component needed to form a blood clot. A mutated prothrombin gene causes the body to produce too much prothrombin, which can result in blood clot formation when it really isn't needed. The increased risk of deep vein thrombosis (DVT) and/or pulmonary embolism (PE) is of primary concern.

D68.6- Other thrombophilia

Thrombophilia conditions covered in this subcategory are those that are acquired.

D68.61 Antiphospholipid syndrome

D68.62 Lupus anticoagulant syndrome

Both of these conditions are autoimmune disorders, meaning the body produces antibodies that attack components of the patient's own, normal blood cells, particularly phospholipid proteins. Although the specific cause is not quite understood, the significance of these syndromes is a propensity toward abnormal clot formation. The presence of antiphospholipid antibodies, alone, is not enough to diagnose a patient with these syndromes as the antibodies can be present without inciting a specific disease process. A patient will only be diagnosed with one of these syndromes if the presence of the antiphospholipid antibodies are related to blood clots or other conditions associated with these antibodies, such as cerebral vascular accident (stroke), myocardial infarction, pulmonary embolism, deep vein thrombosis, eclampsia, or miscarriage. Antiphospholipid syndrome and lupus anticoagulant syndrome may be used interchangeably; however, the two are distinct in the specific phospholipids they attack.

Focus Point

The presence of antiphospholipid antibodies or lupus anticoagulant antibodies does not preclude a diagnosis of systemic lupus erythematosus (SLE). A patient can have SLE in conjunction with the presence of these antibodies.

D69.- Purpura and other hemorrhagic conditions

Purpura refers to hemorrhage, or extravasation of blood, into the tissues or organs. When this occurs on the skin, the condition appears as bruises and small red patches. Depending on the size it may also be referred to as petechiae or ecchymosis. Purpura may be associated with thrombocytopenia, a decrease in the number of platelets circulating in the blood, but it can also occur in a nonthrombocytopenic form. The condition may be primary (hereditary or idiopathic) or secondary to a known cause. Purpura is in itself a symptom; any additional symptoms are related to the underlying etiology of the purpura. Other hemorrhagic conditions classified here include several primary types of thrombocytopenia such as Evans syndrome, secondary types of thrombocytopenia, and other specified and unspecified types of thrombocytopenia and hemorrhagic conditions.

D69.Ø Allergic purpura

This condition, also called Henoch-Schönlein purpura, most often occurs in young children. Allergic purpura (AP) occurs when antibodies bind with antigens (foreign proteins) in the blood. These large antibody-antigen complexes get lodged in the capillaries, the capillaries burst, and hemorrhage results. The skin, intestinal tract, and kidneys are the organs most affected. Although AP can be caused by a drug, other inciting events may include streptococcal infection, insect bites, food, or immunizations. Complications of the disease may include arthritis, usually of the knees and ankles, gastrointestinal problems, and kidney inflammation (nephritis).

D69.1 Qualitative platelet defects

Platelets that do not function properly or have an abnormality in their structure are considered to have a qualitative defect. Common qualitative defects may include failure of platelets to aggregate, which is a hallmark of Glanzmann's disease and Bernard-Soulier syndrome, or have failed platelet secretion following platelet activation, which is the cause of grey platelet syndrome. The important clinical feature when suspecting a qualitative platelet defect is that the number of platelets in circulation will be normal yet the patient still exhibits signs of platelet type bleeding such as purpura, mucous membrane bleeding, and generalized petechiae.

Focus Point

Glanzmann's disease and von Willebrand's disease are two inherited bleeding disorders characteristic of an inability of the blood to form a clot. Patients with either condition may present with frequent nose bleeds, easy bruising, abnormal or prolonged bleeding after surgery, and, in women, heavy menstrual bleeding. The dissimilarity occurs in the blood component that is defective. In Glanzmann's disease, the platelets cannot aggregate because of a defective protein in the platelet itself. Von Willebrand's disease occurs when cells of the vessel wall cannot bind to the platelet due to a missing or defective cell component called von Willebrand factor.

D69.2   Other nonthrombocytopenic purpura

Two common conditions included here are purpura simplex and senile purpura. Purpura simplex is more commonly found in women than men and is characterized by easy bruising without known trauma. It is a very common condition that does not result in serious bleeding. Senile purpura is most often seen in elderly patients and is a result of chronic sun exposure and aging. Dark purple ecchymoses, primarily located on the hands and forearms, is the defining characteristic. Brown discoloration may also be present after a particular lesion has healed, which may or may not be permanent.

D69.3   Immune thrombocytopenic purpura

Immune thrombocytopenic purpura is a condition where there are a decreased number of platelets in the circulating blood as a result of increased platelet destruction but without an identifiable exogenous cause or underlying disease. The condition, also known as idiopathic thrombocytopenic purpura (ITP) or hemorrhagic purpura, is characterized by a sudden onset of symptoms that may include petechiae, epistaxis, hematuria, or abnormal bleeding of the gums, vagina, and gastrointestinal tract. Tidal platelet dysgenesis, or periodic thrombocytopenia, which is also included here, is a rare condition in which platelet counts oscillate from normal to very low values between periods of 20 to 40 days. Many cases of this disorder involve the autoimmune destruction of circulating platelets.

D69.4-   Other primary thrombocytopenia

Types of thrombocytopenia included here are Evans syndrome, congenital and hereditary thrombocytopenia purpura, megalokaryocytic hypoplasia, and unspecified types of primary thrombocytopenia.

D69.41   Evans syndrome

This rare condition is the result of two different disorders, immune thrombocytopenia and autoimmune hemolytic anemia, occurring in the same individual. The two conditions may occur simultaneously or sequentially making the condition hard to diagnose. The disease is unpredictable in its course and how it affects each individual patient making treatment difficult.

D69.5-   Secondary thrombocytopenia

In thrombocytopenia, the blood has a decreased number of platelets, resulting in a coagulation dysfunction within the body. Secondary thrombocytopenia is a direct result of an exogenous cause or underlying condition, such as congestive splenomegaly, Felty's syndrome, Gaucher's disease, tuberculosis, sarcoidosis, myelofibrosis, lupus erythematosus, Wiskott-Aldrich syndrome, chronic alcoholism, or scurvy. It also may occur as a result of overhydration, blood transfusions, or drug therapy.

D69.51   Posttransfusion purpura

Posttransfusion purpura (PTP) is a potentially fatal blood transfusion complication characterized by the sudden onset of severe thrombocytopenia. Signs and symptoms may include fever, chills, bronchospasm, and cutaneous hemorrhaging. In the absence of prompt intervention, the patient may suffer fatal hemorrhage. Onset occurs approximately five to 12 days following transfusion of blood components (e.g., whole blood, RBCs, plasma, or platelets). This reaction is associated with the presence of antibodies produced by the body (alloantibodies) directed against the human platelet antigen (HPA) system (i.e., HPA-1a antigen), which destroys both the patient's platelets and donor platelets, resulting in a rapid decline in circulating platelets (i.e., blood-clotting cells). PTP occurs most commonly in HPA-sensitized patients, those with a history of blood transfusion, and women with a history of multiple pregnancies. Pregnancy contributes to the risk for PTP by increasing the likelihood of forming the platelet-specific antibody.

Other Disorders of Blood and Blood-forming Organs (D70-D77)

This code block includes disorders of the white blood cells, diseases of the spleen, methemoglobinemia, and other diseases of the blood and blood-forming organs that are not classified elsewhere including conditions affecting the bone marrow and lymphoreticular and reticulohistiocytic tissues.

White blood cells (leukocytes) play an important role in the body's immune system protecting the body from harmful pathogens like microorganisms that cause infection and cancer. Most leukocytes originate from stem cells in the bone marrow, circulate in the blood and lymph, and easily migrate to other tissues in the body. There are five different types of leukocytes each playing a specialized role in the immune response, these include:

- Neutrophils: This is the most numerous type of the leukocyte that primarily targets bacteria to protect against infection.

- Eosinophils: This type is most active during parasitic infections and allergic reactions.

- Basophils: This white blood cell contains histamine and heparin, important substances in the body's allergic response.

- Lymphocytes: There are several subtypes of lymphocytes, including T lymphocytes, B lymphocytes, and natural killer cells. These white blood cells are the key players in the body's immune system.

- Monocytes: These white blood cells assist other types of leukocytes in the removal of harmful substances and pathogens, as well as disposal of dead or damaged cells.

The spleen performs many functions including assisting the immune system in the fight against infection, recycling of red blood cells, and acting as a storage site for platelets and red blood cells. The spleen is located to the left of the stomach in the upper part of the abdomen.

Bone marrow is the production site of new blood cells and is located mostly in the flat bones and portions of the long bones. There are two types of bone marrow: red and yellow. Red bone marrow produces the majority of the new cells including red and white blood cells and platelets. The yellow marrow is mostly comprised of fat cells but does also assist in some white blood cell production.

The categories in this code block are as follows:

D70	Neutropenia
D71	Functional disorders of polymorphonuclear neutrophils
D72	Other disorders of white blood cells
D73	Diseases of the spleen
D74	Methemoglobinemia
D75	Other and unspecified diseases of blood and blood-forming organs
D76	Other specified diseases with participation of lymphoreticular and reticulohistiocytic tissue
D77	Other disorders of blood and blood-forming organs in diseases classified elsewhere

D70.-   Neutropenia

Neutropenia, also known as granulocytopenia or agranulocytosis, is an abnormally low number of neutrophils. Neutrophils are phagocytic, meaning they surround and consume harmful pathogens, primarily bacteria. When neutrophil counts decrease the risk of infection increases. Agranulocytosis is a severe form of neutropenia with almost complete absence of neutrophils. Neutropenia may be acute, occurring over a few days, often when the production of neutrophils is impaired, or chronic, most often arising from reduced neutrophil production or in instances in which the spleen sequesters too many neutrophils. Chronic neutropenia may last for months or years. Neutropenia may be caused by an intrinsic defect in the myeloid progenitors or it may be secondary to extrinsic factors. Neutropenia alone is asymptomatic; it is only when an associated infection is present that symptoms may be present. Fever is the most common symptom and in some cases the only presenting symptom.

D70.0   Congenital agranulocytosis

Congenital agranulocytosis is a severe type of neutropenia that is typically diagnosed at birth or shortly thereafter. Because neutrophils are needed to help fight infection, infants with congenital agranulocytosis have recurrent infections with common sites of infection being the sinuses, lungs, and liver. Congenital agranulocytosis is also linked to osteoporosis. The lack of bone density makes the bones prone to fracture and other bone disorders.

D70.1   Agranulocytosis secondary to cancer chemotherapy

Secondary neutropenia due to cancer chemotherapy is a common occurrence. Patients receiving chemotherapy for cancer are carefully monitored for lowered white blood cell counts and signs and symptoms of infection that result from destruction of white blood cells. Common infections indicative of secondary agranulocytosis include cutaneous cellulitis, liver abscess, pneumonia, septicemia, or furunculosis. Inflammation of the perirectal area, colon, mouth, ears, gums, and sinuses are also common symptoms.

D70.2   Other drug-induced agranulocytosis

One of the most common causes of secondary neutropenia is drugs. There are various forms of drug-induced neutropenia, including immune-mediated, toxic, idiosyncratic, or hypersensitivity.

D70.3   Neutropenia due to infection

Sometimes it is the infection that causes a patient's neutrophil counts to decrease. Some common infections that may cause neutropenia include tuberculosis, viral infections, bacterial sepsis, or malaria. In most cases, correction of the underlying infection brings the neutrophil count back to normal.

D70.4   Cyclic neutropenia

Cyclic neutropenia is an uncommon disorder often present at birth and manifested by recurring patterns of low neutrophil counts followed by normal levels of neutrophils. The neutropenic phase of the cycle in most individuals lasts roughly a week in which time the patient experiences recurrent bouts of infection. Signs and symptoms of cyclic neutropenia include ulcers of the mouth, stomatitis, or pharyngitis associated with enlargement of the lymph nodes. Pneumonia and chronic periodontitis are often seen. In rare instances, the condition can be acquired.

D71   Functional disorders of polymorphonuclear neutrophils

Polymorphonuclear neutrophils (PMN) are the most abundant circulating immune cells and are one of the first to respond to infection. PMNs are phagocytic cells that recognize, ingest, and destroy foreign invaders. When a mechanism in the phagocytic process is defective, foreign invaders are left to attack the host. This condition is characterized by recurrent infections from microorganisms such as staphylococci, fungi, and enterobacteria, as well as granuloma formation.

D72.-   Other disorders of white blood cells

This category of codes includes additional disorders of the white blood cells that may involve a decrease or increase in the white blood cell count or a genetic anomaly that is not defined by a more specific code.

D72.1   Eosinophilia

This condition is characterized by a higher than normal level of eosinophils in the peripheral blood or tissues. Eosinophilias described as allergic, idiopathic, or secondary are coded here.

D72.8-   Other specified disorders of white blood cells

This subcategory includes codes for decreased and increased levels of the five types of white blood cells and other abnormalities of white blood cells that are not classified elsewhere.

D72.81-   Decreased white blood cell count

A decrease in the white blood cell count may be manifested as leukocytopenia (reduction in the circulating leukocytes), lymphocytopenia (reduction in the lymphocytes in the blood), or as monocytopenia or plasmacytopenia (reduction in monocytes or plasma cells). The presence of these conditions may indicate an increased risk of infection, malignancy, myelofibrosis, or aplastic anemia, and further workup may need to be undertaken. Decreases in white blood cell counts can be detected by laboratory measurement of WBCs. Treatment is often dependent upon the underlying cause.

D72.82-   Elevated white blood cell count

An increase in white blood cell count may be manifested as elevated leukocytes (leukocytosis), elevated lymphocytes (lymphocytosis), or as elevations in monocytes, plasma cells, or basophils. A leukemoid reaction is a condition in which leukocytosis occurs as a physiologic response to stress or infection. The presence of these conditions may indicate acute infection, inflammation, hemorrhage, or other disease processes. Increases in white blood cell counts can be detected by laboratory measurement of WBCs. Treatment is often dependent upon the underlying cause.

D72.824 Basophilia

Basophilia is an increase in the basophils of the blood, a type of white blood cell, often seen in conjunction with neoplastic disorders. Testing for this condition should include a complete blood count (CBC) with manual differential in order to properly count the basophil population. Treatment is determined based on the underlying condition causing the increase of cell production within the bone marrow.

D72.825 Bandemia

Bandemia is a laboratory finding in which there is an increase in early neutrophil cells, also called band cells. Band cells get their name from the shape of their nucleus, which is band or rod shaped instead of segmented, as seen in mature neutrophils. An increase in the number of band cells is often an early response to an infection and can be present even before white blood cell numbers become elevated. Further testing or workup, such as a culture to confirm infection, may be performed.

D73.- Diseases of spleen

The spleen, a functionally diverse organ, not only is a blood-forming organ but also an important organ of the lymphatic system. Unlike other lymphatic organs, the spleen filters blood not lymph, removing old or damaged red blood cells. The spleen also functions in producing white blood cells important in fighting infection and also serves as a storage site for white blood cells and platelets.

D73.0 Hyposplenism

In hyposplenism the spleen is present but does not function normally. Hyposplenism may be indicative of an underlying disease and is commonly associated with sickle-cell disease and Celiac disease. The condition may be initially diagnosed based by peripheral blood smears that show Howell-Jolly bodies, monocytosis, lymphocytosis, and increased platelet counts. Confirmation typically involves radiological studies of the spleen using radiopharmaceutical agents. Patients with this disorder are more susceptible to bacterial infections, which must be diagnosed and treated promptly to prevent systemic infection and sepsis.

D73.1 Hypersplenism

Hypersplenism is a clinical syndrome characterized by splenic hyperactivity and enlargement of the spleen (splenomegaly). The condition results in a peripheral blood cell deficiency because the spleen traps and destroys the circulating peripheral blood cells. Signs and symptoms of hypersplenism include a history of frequent infection, bruising easily, and abnormal bleeding from the mucous membranes, genitourinary tract, or gastrointestinal tract. There may be fever, weakness, heart palpitations, and ulcers of the mouth, legs, or feet.

D73.2 Chronic congestive splenomegaly

Chronic congestive splenomegaly results from prolonged obstruction to venous outflow in the spleen. The underlying cause is due to conditions within the liver (intrahepatic) that prevent or slow down venous drainage from the portal vein or conditions external to the liver (extrahepatic) that compress the portal or splenic veins. Splenomegaly usually indicates that the spleen has increased from a normal weight of 150 grams to 400 to 500 grams. Symptoms may not always be present but if the spleen becomes enlarged the patient may experience discomfort or pain on the upper left side of the abdomen.

D73.5 Infarction of spleen

Splenic infarction is the result of occlusion of the splenic vascular supply, which can lead to necrosis (tissue death) in the spleen. Thromboembolic events and hematological disorders are most often found to be the underlying cause. Nontraumatic splenic rupture is included here.

D73.81 Neutropenic splenomegaly

Neutropenia is a very low amount of neutrophils, a type of white blood cell, within the body that are important in guarding against infections. When the body cannot fight infection, many associated conditions may arise, including enlargement of the spleen. Treatment and outcome rely on the underlying cause and fighting the infection. Typically neutropenia and splenomegaly are discovered during the course of treatment for another condition.

D74.- Methemoglobinemia

Methemoglobin is a form of hemoglobin but distinct in that it does not carry oxygen. It also can influence how oxygen is released by hemoglobin cells. When too much methemoglobin is produced, the amount of oxygen supplied to tissues is reduced because of a lower number of hemoglobin proteins and the inability of the hemoglobin proteins to release oxygen. The most common symptom is cyanosis or bluish coloring of the skin.

D75.- Other and unspecified diseases of blood and blood-forming organs

Conditions such as familial erythrocytosis, secondary polycythemia, myelofibrosis, and heparin induced thrombocytopenia (HIT) are included in this category.

D75.1 Secondary polycythemia

Polycythemia is an increase in the number of red blood cells. Secondary polycythemia is also known as secondary erythrocytosis, spurious polycythemia, and reactive polycythemia. Spurious polycythemia, which is characterized by increased hematocrit and normal or increased erythrocyte total mass, results from a decrease in plasma volume and hemoconcentration. Reactive polycythemia is a condition characterized by excessive production of circulating erythrocytes due to an identifiable secondary condition, such as hypoxia, or an underlying disease, such as a neoplasm.

D75.81 Myelofibrosis

Myelofibrosis is a rare disorder in which normal bone marrow is replaced by fibrous tissue. Myelofibrosis occurring as a secondary process may appear in various other disorders such as malignancies, infections, lipid storage disease, sarcoidosis, and osteoporosis or in individuals who have been exposed to certain toxic substances, such as benzene and radiation. Common symptoms include anemia, splenomegaly, and hepatomegaly. Patients may remain asymptomatic for years, but the anemia gradually worsens until its severity causes weakness, fatigue, weight loss, and general malaise.

D75.82 Heparin induced thrombocytopenia (HIT)

Heparin is one of the most frequently prescribed medications and is used to prevent blood clot formation. The use of heparin can lead to a particularly challenging adverse heparin induced thrombocytopenic (HIT) reaction. HIT is one of the three most common causes of iatrogenic thrombocytopenia, along with sepsis (with or without disseminated intravascular coagulation or DIC) and the adverse effects of other drugs. Fifty percent or more of those with HIT will have thrombotic complications. These thromboembolic events may be arterial or venous and can lead to limb amputation, pulmonary emboli, strokes, and myocardial infarction.

D76.- Other specified diseases with participation of lymphoreticular and reticulohistiocytic tissue

Reticular tissues are composed of a network of collagenous fibers that are associated with the reticular cells. Lymphoreticular tissue is composed of lymphatic tissue and reticular cells. Reticulohistiocytic tissue is composed of reticular cells and histiocytes. Histiocytes are a type of macrophage blood cell that undergoes final differentiation into more specific cell types in the tissues rather than in the bone marrow.

D76.1 Hemophagocytic lymphohistiocytosis

The primary form of hemophagocytic lymphohistiocytosis, familial hemophagocytic lymphohistiocytosis (FHL), is thought to be a genetically transmitted disease. Affecting infants and young children, symptoms of FHL include fever, enlargement of the liver and spleen, and pancytopenia. Another condition included here is macrophage activation syndrome (MAS), a hemophagocytic syndrome caused by excessive creation and production of T cells and macrophages. MAS can be a life-threatening complication of systemic-onset juvenile rheumatoid arthritis. Symptoms of MAS include prolonged fever, enlarged liver and spleen, bleeding, generalized adenomegaly, rash, and jaundice.

D76.2 Hemophagocytic syndrome, infection-associated

Hemophagocytic syndrome, also known as infection- or virus-associated hemophagocytic syndrome (VAHS), is a secondary form of hemophagocytic lymphohistiocytosis. It is an aggressive disorder associated with systemic viral infection and is manifested by the infiltration of hemophagocytic histiocytes into the lymphoreticular tissues of multiple organs. Associated viruses include Epstein-Barr, cytomegalovirus, adenovirus, and Herpes simplex virus. Association has also been made to various nonviral infections.

Intraoperative and Postprocedural Complications of the Spleen (D78)

This code block comprises a single category with codes that report complications of procedures resulting in injury to the spleen.

The category in this code block is as follows:

D78 Intraoperative and postprocedural complications of the spleen

D78.- Intraoperative and postprocedural complications of the spleen

Complications from medical care can sometimes result in an injury to an organ. The codes in this category classify splenic injuries that are the direct result of medical intervention with code selection based on the timing of the complication, the specific injury or complication involving the spleen, and whether the procedure was being performed on the spleen itself or on another organ or structure usually in close proximity to the spleen. The timing of the complication refers to whether the complication occurred intraoperatively, that is during the performance of the procedure, or postoperatively, that is following the procedure. There are classifications for five types of injury: hemorrhage, hematoma, seroma, laceration or puncture, and other specified injury or complication.

The descriptions of these injury types are as follows:

- Hemorrhage is considered rapid blood loss from vessels.

- Hematoma is a collection of blood clots within tissue or organs due to a broken blood vessel.

- Seroma is a fluid accumulation just under the skin surface, often developing after a surgery involving an incision or tissue extraction.

- Laceration is simply a torn wound.

- Puncture is a wound due to perforation or piercing.

Certain Disorders Involving the Immune Mechanism (D80-D89)

The immune system defends the body against foreign material called antigens. When the immune system is stimulated an immune response pathway is activated and responds based on the specific antigen that has invaded. An antigen is any substance that activates this immune response.

Primary immunodeficiencies are genetically determined, often presenting in infancy and childhood, and are classified based on the immune system component that is defective. These components include:

- B lymphocytes (B cells or Ig): Specialized white blood cells that produce antigen specific antibodies that target an antigen before it invades a healthy cell.

- T lymphocytes (T cells): Specialized white blood cells that recognize and kill cells that have been infected with specific antigens; T cells also stimulate B cell production and their respective antibodies.

- Natural killer (NK) cells: Specialized white blood cells that can attach to any cell in the body, healthy or infected. If the attached cell is normal, the killing mechanism will not be activated.

- Phagocytic cells: Specialized white blood cells that engulf and destroy antigens; includes neutrophils, eosinophils, basophils, and macrophages.

- Complement proteins: Proteins that assist the B cells in killing a specific antigen once the antibodies of the B cells bind to the antigen.

Secondary immunodeficiencies are the result of the immune response pathway being disrupted by another disease process. These may include diabetes, severe burns, prolonged or serious illness, or even chemotherapy.

The categories in this code block are as follows:

D80	Immunodeficiency with predominantly antibody defects
D81	Combined immunodeficiencies
D82	Immunodeficiency associated with other major defects
D83	Common variable immunodeficiency
D84	Other immunodeficiencies
D86	Sarcoidosis
D89	Other disorders involving the immune mechanism, not elsewhere classified

D80.- Immunodeficiency with predominantly antibody defects

An immunodeficiency is a condition that results from a defective immune mechanism, in this case an antibody defect. Antibodies are immunoglobulin molecules that are produced by B-cells in response to specific immunogens or antigens. Conditions classified here are characterized by the inability of B-cells to produce adequate amounts of healthy, mature antibodies that can respond effectively to pathogenic organisms.

D80.0 Hereditary hypogammaglobulinemia

This condition occurs when the B cells produced by the bone marrow do not develop into mature, antibody producing B cells; the result is lowered levels or complete absence of antibodies.

Focus Point

Hypogammaglobulinemia may often be used synonymously with common variable immunodeficiency (CVID). Although hypogammaglobulinemia is a clinical sign of CVID, CVID is much harder to diagnose. Common manifestations of CVID may include autoimmune disease, granulomatous disease, and, in some cases, malignancy. For a diagnosis of common variable immunodeficiency, review the codes in category D83.

D80.2 Selective deficiency of immunoglobulin A [IgA]

This is the most common of the antibody deficiency syndromes. IgA antibodies protect the body surfaces and are therefore found in places like the eyes, ears, nose, breathing passages, digestive tract, and vagina. Associated infections commonly involve the upper and lower respiratory tract and the gastrointestinal tract.

D80.3 Selective deficiency of immunoglobulin G [IgG] subclasses

Immunoglobulin G (IgG) is the most abundant immunoglobulin in the blood and is found in all body fluids. There are four subclassifications of IgG: IgG1, IgG2, IgG3, and IgG4. Just one of these subclasses can be deficient in order for the disease to present itself; however, it is often two subclasses that are jointly deficient.

D80.4 Selective deficiency of immunoglobulin M [IgM]

Immunoglobulin M (IgM) is the first antibody formed after exposure to a new antigen and is found in the blood and lymph fluid. IgM also influences other immune system cells to destroy foreign substances.

D80.5 Immunodeficiency with increased immunoglobulin M [IgM]

Also called hyper-IgM syndrome, this condition is characterized by normal or elevated levels of IgM with associated decrease in the levels of other immunoglobulins. As with other immunoglobulin disorders susceptibility to bacterial infection is high.

D80.7 Transient hypogammaglobulinemia of infancy

During pregnancy the mother provides antibodies to the fetus. These maternal antibodies remain in the blood for a period of time after birth, but are eventually removed. In a normal infant, production of its own antibodies has begun and is functioning by the time the mother's antibodies are gone. In this disorder the production of antibodies or immunoglobulins is delayed, leaving the infant without the necessary antibodies to ward off harmful microorganisms. Most often the child will begin producing antibodies by age 2 or 3 but antibody production can be delayed until as late as age 6. Recurrent upper respiratory tract infections are common in the first years of life in infants and young children with transient hypogammaglobulinemia, but these infections are rarely life-threatening.

D81.- Combined immunodeficiencies

Lymphocyte components of the immune system are primarily divided into B cells and T cells. The role of each cell type is important not only in how it functions by itself but also in how it may influence functions in the other cell type. T cell function in particular has a big impact on the way B cells respond to pathogens and in how they develop. In combined immunodeficiency disorders, both T cells and B cells are in some way deficient. Although pathologically it is the T cell that is abnormal, the B cell will be limited in its role in the immune response due to the T cell abnormality.

D81.Ø Severe combined immunodeficiency [SCID] with reticular dysgenesis

Reticular dysgenesis is the most severe form of severe combined immunodeficiency or SCID. It is characterized by bilateral sensorineural deafness and lack of immune function, which can lead to fatal septicemia within days after birth. The only curative treatment for the disease is allogenic hematopoietic stem cell transplant.

D81.3 Adenosine deaminase [ADA] deficiency

Adenosine deaminase (ADA) is an enzyme active in lymphocytes that helps remove toxic metabolites that are generated when DNA breaks down. These toxic metabolites block the development of T cells, B cells, and natural killer cells resulting in the near absence of these cells and the inability of the body to protect itself from foreign pathogens. Most often ADA presents and is diagnosed by six months of age; however, ADA can present later in life even into adulthood.

D81.4 Nezelof's syndrome

This condition is often diagnosed within the first six months of life. Infants born with this disorder have T cells and B cells that do not function properly although the exact cause for this is not yet understood. Common characteristics of the disorder are an underdeveloped thymus and persistent and often severe infections from organisms that usually do not cause severe infections in patients with a normal immune system.

D81.5 Purine nucleoside phosphorylase [PNP] deficiency

Purine nucleoside phosphorylase (PNP) is an enzyme active in lymphocytes that helps remove toxic metabolites that are generated when DNA breaks down. These toxic metabolites trigger the early destruction of immature T cells, lowering the number of mature T cells in the body and increasing the risk of infection.

> **Focus Point**
>
> *This disorder is similar to adenosine deaminase deficiency, however neurodevelopmental delays are more prevalent in PNP. Patients with PNP also have increased risk of developing autoimmune disorders.*

D81.6 Major histocompatibility complex class I deficiency

D81.7 Major histocompatibility complex class II deficiency

The immune system is constantly monitoring the body for foreign invaders. In order for the immune system to recognize foreign invaders it has to have a way of distinguishing between "self," cells that should be present in the body, and "nonself," cells or substances that are foreign. The major histocompatibility complex (MHC) assists the immune system with this process by displaying self and nonself proteins on the surface of each cell. Specialized T cells look at the protein complexes displayed and if the protein complex is identified as abnormal or foreign an immune response is triggered. MHC is divided into three basic groups: class I, class II, and class III. Each group has specific human leukocyte antigen (HLA) genes that produce proteins on the surface of a cell. The HLA genes are divided into the different classes based on how they function. HLA genes grouped under MHC class I can be found on almost all nucleated cell surfaces. These surface proteins are bound with peptides that are made in the cell and brought to the cell surface. The peptides are then displayed and analyzed by T cells, more specifically CD8+ T cells, which trigger a self-destruct mechanism within the cell if the peptides are considered foreign. HLA genes grouped under MHC class II present extracellular information to the surface of a cell to be analyzed by CD4+ T cells. If an immune response is triggered, the CD4 cells activate B cells and stimulate production of antibodies to rid the body of the foreign material before it invades normal cells.

D81.81- Biotin-dependent carboxylase deficiency

The biotinidase (BTD) gene provides instructions for making the enzyme biotinidase. This enzyme helps the body remove a B vitamin called biotin from foods such as egg yolks, liver, and milk. The resulting free form of biotin is then used to activate other enzymes important in critical cellular functions; these enzymes are called biotin-dependent carboxylases. Biotinidase can also recycle biotin within the body by breaking down the biotin-dependent carboxylase enzymes so that biotin can be reused. Biotinidase disorders can present as early as 1 week after birth to 1Ø years of age. Early symptoms often include seizures, hypotonia, and breathing problems. If left untreated the disorders can lead to hearing and vision loss, ataxia, skin rashes, alopecia, developmental delays, and immunological deficiencies. Newborn screening has been helpful in the early diagnosis of biotinidase disorders.

Focus Point

Biotin-dependent carboxylase deficiency can occur as a result of inadequate consumption of biotin (B vitamin) rich foods rather than a genetic defect. Refer to category E53 when low levels of biotin are due to dietary deficiencies.

D82.- Immunodeficiency associated with other major defects

An immunodeficiency is a condition that results from a defective immune mechanism. In this category, the immunodeficiency is associated with major defects in the immune mechanism that are not classified to other categories in this code block.

D82.Ø Wiskott-Aldrich syndrome

Wiskott-Aldrich syndrome is a genetic disorder in which mutations occur in the gene that encodes the Wiskott-Aldrich syndrome protein (WASP). WASP is an important protein for normal B and T cell signaling. When the protein is deficient, the B and T cells cannot respond to foreign invaders appropriately, which leads to increased susceptibility to infection. The lack of functional WASP also impairs the development of platelets, so reduced platelet counts (thrombocytopenia) will often be a clinical sign. Wiskott-Aldrich syndrome (WAS) primarily affects males and may present with what is known as the classic triad of WAS, which includes eczema, bloody diarrhea, and recurrent respiratory infections.

D82.1 Di George's syndrome

DiGeorge syndrome is the result of missing or mutated genes in the DiGeorge region of chromosome 22. The deletion of these genes results in disruption of embryonic development causing abnormal formation of certain tissues. The most common characteristics of Di George's syndrome include hypoparathyroidism with hypocalcemia, recurrent infections, abnormal facies (most often palatal abnormalities), congenital heart disorders, developmental delays, and behavioral and psychiatric problems.

D82.3 Immunodeficiency following hereditary defective response to Epstein-Barr virus

This genetic condition, also called X-linked lymphoproliferative syndrome, is caused by a mutation of T cells and natural killer cells resulting in a missing protein called SAP. The mutation of these cells does not in itself cause immunodeficiency but predisposes a patient to developing an impaired immune response when Epstein-Barr virus (EBV) is introduced to the body. EBV is a member of the herpes virus family and is one of the most common human viruses. Antibodies to EBV may be present without an individual ever having had symptoms to the virus. However, some patients develop infectious mononucleosis as a result of the virus. In a normal patient, when EBV is present the T cells and natural killer cells respond by multiplying and killing the infected cells. As the number of infected cells decrease, the need for T cells also diminishes and the body responds by reducing the proliferation of the T cells. However, without the SAP protein the T cells and natural killer cells lose their ability to kill infected cells. Still circulating in the body, the infected cells continue to stimulate the immune response and T cells multiply out of control resulting in an overstimulation of the immune system. The immune cells eventually build up in organs like the spleen and liver and their resulting chemical processes induce inflammation resulting in damage to these organs. EBV stimulated infectious mononucleosis is life-threatening in these patients. If patients survive the initial infection they are at risk of developing lymphoma and aplastic anemia.

D82.4 Hyperimmunoglobulin E [IgE] syndrome

Hyper-IgE syndrome is caused by a gene mutation and starts during infancy. Staphylococcal abscesses involving the skin, lungs, joints, and viscera are typical. A patient also may have recurrent fractures, pruritic eosinophilic dermatitis, coarse facial features, and osteopenia. Lifelong continuous antistaphylococcal antibiotics are the primary therapy.

D83.- Common variable immunodeficiency

Common variable immunodeficiency (CVID) is the result of mutations in genes that are involved in the development and function of B cells. Patients with CVID have insufficient numbers of B lymphocytes that are capable of producing antibodies, which results in low levels of most if not all immunoglobulin classes (i.e., IgA, IgG, IgM). Defects in how T lymphocytes function may also be a factor in patients with CVID. Recurrent bacterial infections are common, most often in the upper and lower respiratory tracts, and patients often present with otitis media, pneumonia, and/or sinusitis. Complications that commonly occur include an increased risk of lymphomas and autoimmune disorders, including rheumatoid arthritis, hemolytic anemia, thrombocytopenia (commonly ITP), neutropenia, and gastrointestinal autoimmune diseases.

D84.-   Other immunodeficiencies

An immunodeficiency is a condition that results from a defective immune mechanism. This category classifies a specific type of immunodeficiency called lymphocyte function antigen-1 defect, along with immunodeficiencies resulting from defects in the complement system, other specified types that do not have a more specific code, and unspecified immunodeficiency.

D84.Ø   Lymphocyte function antigen-1 [LFA-1] defect

Also called leukocyte adhesion deficiency, this genetic disorder is caused by a deficiency in a protein found on the surface of white blood cells. Without these proteins the cells cannot interact with other cellular components, attach to blood vessel walls, or assist in killing offending bacteria. Typical presentation includes delayed umbilical cord detachment, leukocytosis, recurrent soft-tissue infections, and poor wound healing.

D86.-   Sarcoidosis

In a normal immune response, specialized cells are sent to areas in the body where harmful substances are detected. These cells release chemicals to attract other cells to assist in isolating and destroying the harmful substance and also initiate an inflammatory response. When the threat is gone the cells and inflammation go away. In sarcoidosis, the cells and inflammation fail to dissipate once the harmful substance has been isolated and destroyed, and the immune cells then cluster together, resulting in granuloma formation. Sarcoidosis often affects the lungs and lymphatic system but can occur in any organ. This category is structured to identify the particular site the sarcoidosis is affecting.

D89.-   Other disorders involving the immune mechanism, not elsewhere classified

Disorders of the immune mechanism that do not fit well into more specific categories are classified here.

D89.1   Cryoglobulinemia

This condition occurs due to an abnormality in immunoglobulins that causes them to thicken in cold temperatures. This can reduce blood flow throughout the body and result in the development of vasculitis.

D89.3   Immune reconstitution syndrome

Sometimes patients that are being treated for certain immunodeficiency disorders deteriorate clinically despite an improvement in their immune system health. In most disease processes, the manifestations of the disease and/or the patient's clinical status

improve once treatment is initiated. With immunodeficiency disorders it is possible for covert infections or poorly treated infections to produce clinical manifestations only when the immune system is strong enough to mount an inflammatory response. When this occurs, it may appear as if the patient is getting sicker when really the patient's body is responding the way it should. However, these reactions can complicate the course of the patient's primary disease process as well as its treatment.

D89.4-   Mast cell activation syndrome and related disorders

Mast cell activation syndromes (MCAS) encompass a group of conditions involving hyperresponsive mast cells. Manifestations of the disease, although often non-specific, typically affect two or more body systems including skin, gastrointestinal, cardiovascular, respiratory and neurologic. The signs and symptoms are usually observed as an allergic response (anaphylaxis reaction) ranging from pruritic or urticarial type symptoms to more serious symptoms such as hypotension and syncope. There are three known types of MCAS—primary, secondary, and idiopathic.

> **Focus Point**
>
> *Mast cell activation syndromes (MCAS) should not be confused with another group of mast cell activation disorders, collectively categorized under the term mastocytosis. In patients with MCAS, the number of mast cells produced is normal but they are easily triggered, while patients with mastocytosis have an overproduction of mast cells by the body. The type of mastocytosis largely influences code selection: malignant mastocytosis, also called aggressive systemic mastocytosis, is coded to C96.21 Aggressive systemic mastocytosis; indolent systemic mastocytosis codes to D47.Ø2 Systemic mastocytosis. Mastocytosis that is documented as congenital cutaneous mastocytosis is coded to Q82.2.*

D89.41   Monoclonal mast cell activation syndrome

Monoclonal mast cell activation syndrome (MMAS), also called primary mast cell activation syndrome, is diagnosed when a consistent allergic cause cannot be definitively identified and the patient clearly does not have mastocytosis. Episodes are usually recurrent in nature and affect at least two organs, producing symptoms such as flushing, hypotension, and gastrointestinal cramping. Differentiation between MMAS and the remarkably similar systemic mastocytosis is based on the absence of urticarial pigmentosa in the patient as well as laboratory findings of normal or mildly elevated baseline serum tryptase. Having a previous diagnosis of idiopathic anaphylaxis or exercise-induced anaphylaxis is often typical in many of these patients.

D89.42 Idiopathic mast cell activation syndrome

Idiopathic mast cell activation syndrome is considered an appropriate diagnosis when no underlying cause—neither mast cell abnormality nor external stimulus—can be identified. Diagnosis of the idiopathic form of mast cell activation may evolve as additional genetic defects and/or external stimulants are identified and a more specific primary or secondary mast cell activation syndrome can be diagnosed.

D89.43 Secondary mast cell activation

In secondary mast cell activation syndrome (SMCAS), an external stimulus triggers a response in the mast cells. The stimulus may be in the form of an allergic disorder, such as to drugs, food, or plants; a physical or chronic autoimmune urticarial disorder; or a chronic inflammatory or neoplastic disorder. Laboratory findings show that the mast cells are normal in function and quality; however, other laboratory tests may be abnormal like IgE, IgG receptors, cytokines, and autoantibodies.

D89.81- Graft-versus-host disease

Graft-versus-host disease (GVHD) is a complication associated with the transplantation of bone marrow or stem cells from a donor (allogeneic transplant). The transplanted cells regard the patient's own cells as foreign and attack the host cells. Studying the donor's cells to see how closely they match the patient's is essential, as the closer the match the less likely the development of GVHD.

D89.810 Acute graft-versus-host disease

Acute graft-versus-host disease usually occurs within the first three months after transplant. Symptoms may include jaundice, abdominal pain, diarrhea, nausea, and vomiting.

D89.811 Chronic graft-versus-host disease

The chronic form of graft-versus-host disease most often presents three months after transplant. Most patients with chronic GVHD experience skin changes. Other symptoms may include hair loss, jaundice, and drying of the mouth, eyes, and vagina.

D89.812 Acute on chronic graft-versus-host disease

Acute on chronic GVHD describes an acute exacerbation of a chronic GVHD status, or an acute manifestation of a preexisting GVHD associated condition.

D89.82 Autoimmune lymphoproliferative syndrome [ALPS]

In autoimmune lymphoproliferative syndrome (ALPS), a rare inherited disorder, the body is unable to effectively regulate the production and elimination of lymphocytes. This results in production of an abnormally large number of lymphocytes that accumulate in the lymph nodes causing lymphadenopathy, in the liver causing hepatomegaly, and in the spleen causing splenomegaly. ALPS may present with different signs and symptoms; however, the most common set of symptoms is lymphoproliferation beginning in childhood with associated lymphadenopathy and splenomegaly followed by the development of other autoimmune disorders, particularly those affecting the blood. The majority of ALPS cases are due to a genetic alteration of a protein that is integral to the apoptosis process. Apoptosis refers to the normal process of programmed cell death, destruction of the dead cell, and removal of cell particles by phagocytosis. Apoptosis is essential in the postinfection period to ensure that the production of lymphocytes does not continue after the infection has been eradicated. When apoptosis does not occur, the result is twofold: lymphocytes accumulate in the lymph nodes, liver, and spleen causing enlargement of these organs and the increased number of B cells continue to make antibodies. Since the infection is resolved, the cells make antibodies against platelets, red blood cells, or other healthy cells destroying them. Individuals with ALPS are at increased risk of developing lymphoma and other cancers, as well as other autoimmune disorders, particularly those that target and destroy blood cells.

Chapter 4: Endocrine, Nutritional and Metabolic Diseases (E00-E89)

The endocrine system is a group of specialized organs and body tissues that produce, store, and secrete chemical substances known as hormones. Hormones provide information and instructions to regulate development, control the function of various tissues, support reproduction, and regulate metabolism.

The primary endocrine organs described in this chapter include:

- Adrenal gland
- Ovaries
- Pancreas
- Parathyroid gland
- Pituitary gland
- Testes
- Thymus
- Thyroid gland

Hormone production is stimulated by the nervous system or by chemical changes in the blood, such as glucose level. Hormones from the endocrine system are secreted into the blood, where proteins bind to them to keep them intact as the hormones are disbursed through the body. The hormones are carried via the bloodstream to the affected organs, where they react with target cells containing protein receptors. The proteins also regulate the release of hormones.

Usually, the changes a hormone produces also serve to regulate that hormone's secretion. For example, parathyroid hormone causes the body to increase the level of calcium in the blood. As calcium levels rise, the secretion of parathyroid hormone decreases. Other changes in the body also influence hormone secretions. For example, during illness, the adrenal glands increase the secretions of certain hormones to help the body overcome the stress of illness. The normal regulation of hormone secretion is suspended, allowing for a tolerance of higher levels of hormone in the blood until the illness is resolved.

This chapter also includes nutritional and metabolic disorders, including vitamin and other nutritional deficiencies, obesity, hyperalimentation and its related conditions, and fluid and electrolyte imbalances.

Nutritional deficiencies in this chapter cover deficiencies in vitamins, minerals, and protein-calorie malnutrition. Deficiencies of anemia are classified to Chapter 3 Diseases of the Blood and Blood-Forming Organs.

Metabolic diseases in this chapter cover a wide range of diseases, including problems with amino-acid transport, carbohydrate transport, lipoid metabolism, plasma protein metabolism, gout, mineral metabolism, and fluid, electrolyte, and acid-base imbalances. Also covered are cystic fibrosis, porphyria, disorders of purine and pyrimidine metabolism, and obesity.

The chapter is broken down into the following code blocks:

E00-E07	Disorders of the thyroid gland
E08-E13	Diabetes mellitus
E15-E16	Other disorders of glucose regulation and pancreatic internal secretion
E20-E35	Disorders of other endocrine glands
E36	Intraoperative complications of endocrine system
E40-E46	Malnutrition
E50-E64	Other nutritional deficiencies
E65-E68	Overweight, obesity and other hyperalimentation
E70-E88	Metabolic disorders
E89	Postprocedural endocrine and metabolic complications and disorders, not elsewhere classified

Disorders of Thyroid Gland (E00-E07)

The thyroid gland is located in the anterior aspect of the lower neck. It is attached to the trachea by loose connective tissue with the right and left lobes on each side of the trachea. It derives its blood supply from the superior and inferior thyroid arteries.

The function of the thyroid is to create, store, and secrete thyroxine and triiodothyronine. The thyroid gland secretes these hormones in response to stimulation by thyroid stimulating hormone (TSH) from the pituitary gland. The thyroid hormones regulate growth and metabolism and play a role in brain development during childhood.

The categories in this code block are as follows:

E00	Congenital iodine-deficiency syndrome
E01	Iodine-deficiency related thyroid disorders and allied conditions

E02	Subclinical iodine-deficiency hypothyroidism
E03	Other hypothyroidism
E04	Other nontoxic goiter
E05	Thyrotoxicosis (hyperthyroidism)
E06	Thyroiditis
E07	Other disorders of thyroid

Thyroid Gland

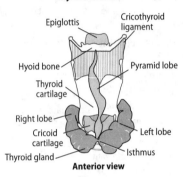

Anterior view

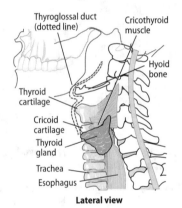

Lateral view

E00.- Congenital iodine-deficiency syndrome

Previously known as cretinism, this condition involves severely stunted mental and physical growth due to untreated congenital deficiency of thyroid hormones (congenital hypothyroidism) usually due to maternal hypothyroidism. The disorder has been nearly eliminated in the developed world.

E01.- Iodine-deficiency related thyroid disorders and allied conditions

This condition contains a constellation of symptoms from goiter (an abnormal enlargement of the thyroid gland) to developmental delays, most commonly caused by a lack of iodine in the diet. This form of the disease is not congenital, but can develop early in childhood.

E01.0 Iodine-deficiency related diffuse (endemic) goiter

Iodine deprivation leads to diminished production and secretion of thyroid hormone by the thyroid gland. This causes the characteristic thyroid gland swelling, which is called a diffuse goiter. Iodine-deficiency related diffuse goiter may occur in adolescents during puberty or in individuals living in geographic regions where a limited amount of iodine is present in the soil and thus not available in food.

E01.1 Iodine-deficiency related multinodular (endemic) goiter

Multinodular goiter is characterized by the presence of numerous nodules in the thyroid of differing consistencies separated by fibrous septa. Areas of hemorrhage and irregular calcification may also be seen.

E02 Subclinical iodine-deficiency hypothyroidism

This condition involves normal thyroid hormone levels, thyroxine (T4) and triiodothyronine (T3), with mild elevation of thyrotropin, thyroid-stimulating hormone (TSH). TSH is elevated but below the limit representing overt hypothyroidism. The condition is caused by iodine-deficiency in the diet. Early hypothyroidism is often asymptomatic and patients can have very mild symptoms, such as cold intolerance or increased sensitivity to cold, constipation, weight gain and water retention, bradycardia (low heartrate—fewer than sixty beats per minute), fatigue, decreased sweating, muscle cramps, and joint pain.

E03.- Other hypothyroidism

This condition involves a state in which the thyroid gland does not make enough thyroid hormone. Iodine deficiency is a common cause of hypothyroidism worldwide but it can be caused by many other factors. It can result from the lack of a thyroid gland or from iodine-131 treatment, and can also be associated with increased stress. Early hypothyroidism is often asymptomatic and patients can have very mild symptoms, such as cold intolerance or increased sensitivity to cold, constipation, weight gain and water retention, bradycardia (low heartrate—fewer than sixty beats per minute), fatigue, decreased sweating, muscle cramps, and joint pain.

E03.0   Congenital hypothyroidism with diffuse goiter

E03.1   Congenital hypothyroidism without goiter

Hypothyroidism is classified here when it is congenital, but does not involve the entire syndrome of iodine-deficiency disorders. Congenital hypothyroidism may occur with or without a diffuse goiter, which is a generalized swelling of the thyroid gland.

E03.2   Hypothyroidism due to medicaments and other exogenous substances

This code reports hypothyroidism that is due to a drug or toxic substance. The most common causes of drug-induced hypothyroidism include amiodarone (a cardiology drug), antithyroid drugs such as propylthiouracil and methimazole, lithium (psychiatric treatment), propranolol (beta blocker), and adrenal steroids, such as prednisone and hydrocortisone.

E03.4   Atrophy of thyroid (acquired)

Atrophy is a decrease in size or a wasting away of the thyroid gland.

E04.-   Other nontoxic goiter

This condition is a diffuse or nodular enlargement of the thyroid gland that isn't related to an inflammatory or neoplastic process and is not associated with abnormal thyroid function. The exact causes of nontoxic goiter are not known but heredity, medications, and foods that contain goitrogens (substances that inhibit thyroid hormone production) may all be factors. Nontoxic goiters usually grow very slowly and may not cause any symptoms or require treatment.

E04.0   Nontoxic diffuse goiter

A diffuse goiter involves enlargement of the entire thyroid gland.

E04.1   Nontoxic single thyroid nodule

E04.2   Nontoxic multinodular goiter

A nodular goiter is an enlargement associated with nodules or lumps on the thyroid gland. In some cases, only a single nodule is present, while in others cases multiple nodules or lumps are present.

E05.-   Thyrotoxicosis [hyperthyroidism]

This condition results from excessive concentrations of thyroid hormones (typically triiodothyronine (T3) and/or thyroxine (T4) in the body. There are several causes of hyperthyroidism. Commonly, the entire gland is overproducing thyroid hormone, but in some cases a single nodule is responsible for the excess hormone secretion, called a "hot" nodule. Thyroiditis (inflammation of the thyroid) can also cause hyperthyroidism. Thyrotoxic crisis (or thyroid storm) is a sudden, rare, but severe complication of hyperthyroidism, and can occur when a thyrotoxic patient becomes very ill, is postsurgical, or physically stressed. It's considered life-threatening and symptoms can include an increase in body temperature to more than 104 degrees Fahrenheit, tachycardia, arrhythmia, vomiting, diarrhea, and dehydration. It can progress to psychosis, heart complications, enlarged liver, coma, and death.

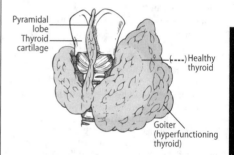

Goiter

Pyramidal lobe
Thyroid
Thyroid cartilage
(----) Healthy thyroid
Goiter (hyperfunctioning thyroid)

E05.0-   Thyrotoxicosis with diffuse goiter

This code reports oversecretion of thyroid hormone (hyperthyroidism), with generalized enlargement of the thyroid. Graves' disease, the most common form of hyperthyroidism, is classified here. This condition is often referred to as exophthalmic or toxic goiter or by several other names such as Basedow's disease, Marsh's disease, Parry's syndrome, and Parson's disease. This condition may occur with or without thyrotoxic crisis or storm.

E05.1-   Thyrotoxicosis with toxic single thyroid nodule

A nodular goiter is an enlargement caused by nodules or lumps on the thyroid gland. Assign one of the codes in this subcategory if only one nodule or lump is present.

E05.2-   Thyrotoxicosis with toxic multinodular goiter

A nodular goiter is an enlargement caused by nodules or lumps on the thyroid gland. Assign one of these codes only if multiple nodules or lumps are present.

E05.3- Thyrotoxicosis from ectopic thyroid tissue

Ectopic thyroid tissue refers to thyroid tissue that is not in the normal site of the thyroid in the anterior neck. In most cases, ectopic thyroid tissue is found in the region of the head and neck, such as along the path of the thyroglossal duct, in the lingual or sublingual regions of the pharynx, or in the trachea, submandibular, or lateral neck regions. However, ectopic thyroid tissue has been found at more remote sites as well. Ectopic thyroid tissue can cause hyperthyroidism and thyrotoxicosis that can occur with or without thyrotoxic crisis or storm.

E05.4- Thyrotoxicosis factitia

Thyrotoxicosis factitia is an uncommon form of hyperthyroidism ectopic thyroid tissue that is caused by the ingestion of exogenous (from outside the body) thyroid hormone. It can be the result of mistaken or intentional ingestion of excess drug, such as levothyroxine.

E06.- Thyroiditis

Thyroiditis is a group of disorders that all cause thyroidal inflammation. The condition is generally caused by an attack on the thyroid, resulting in inflammation and damage to the thyroid cells. Acute thyroiditis results from a bacterial infection while subacute is largely viral. Hashimoto's thyroiditis is the most common cause of hypothyroidism in the United States and can be considered an autoimmune disease because the body acts as if the thyroid gland is foreign tissue. Common hypothyroid symptoms that occur when thyroid cell damage is slow and chronic may include fatigue, weight gain, feeling "fuzzy headed," depression, dry skin, and constipation. Rarer symptoms include swelling of the legs, vague aches and pains, and decreased concentration.

E06.0 Acute thyroiditis

Acute thyroiditis, also referred to as infectious thyroiditis, involves invasion of the thyroid by bacteria, mycobacteria, fungi, or protozoa; it includes all forms of infection other than viral. It may be further qualified as suppurative (AST), nonsuppurative, or septic thyroiditis.

E06.1 Subacute thyroiditis

Subacute thyroiditis, also documented as de Quervain's thyroiditis, subacute nonsuppurative thyroiditis, migratory or creeping thyroiditis, and granulomatous, pseudotuberculous, pseudo-giant cell, or giant cell thyroiditis, most likely has a viral origin. It is self-limiting and goes through three clinical phases: hyperthyroidism, hypothyroidism, and a return to normal thyroid function.

E06.2 Chronic thyroiditis with transient thyrotoxicosis

The chronic form of this disease follows that of acute thyroiditis but assumes a chronic disease process.

E06.3 Autoimmune thyroiditis

Autoimmune thyroiditis is commonly referred to as chronic, Hashimoto's, or lymphocytic thyroiditis or lymphadenoid goiter and struma lymphomatosa. It usually persists for years and is the principal cause of non-iatrogenic primary hypothyroidism.

E06.4 Drug-induced thyroiditis

Drugs known to cause thyroiditis include amiodarone, lithium, interferons, and cytokines.

E06.5 Other chronic thyroiditis

Riedel's thyroiditis is classified here, which may be documented as Riedel's struma, ligneous thyroiditis, and invasive fibrous or chronic sclerosing thyroiditis. This condition is characterized by overgrowth of connective tissue that often extends into neighboring structures.

E07.- Other disorders of thyroid

There are a few additional disorders affecting the thyroid that are classified here.

E07.0 Hypersecretion of calcitonin

Calcitonin is a hormone produced in the thyroid gland that helps regulate calcium levels. When there is too much calcium in the blood (hypercalcemia), calcitonin is secreted and helps to move excessive calcium from the blood into the bones. Hypersecretion may be due to a medullary carcinoma of the thyroid (MTC). MTC is a tumor of the calcitonin producing C-cells of the thyroid gland.

E07.1 Dyshormogenetic goiter

Dyshormonogenetic goiters are genetically determined thyroid hyperplasias due to enzyme defects in thyroid-hormone synthesis. It is characterized by many solid nodular lesions with different patterns, a peculiar appearance of the surrounding nonnodular thyroid tissue, and the presence of features suspicious for carcinoma.

E07.81 Sick-euthyroid syndrome

Sick-euthyroid syndrome, also known as nonthyroidal illness syndrome, is characterized by abnormal levels of T3 and/or T4, but the thyroid gland does not appear to be dysfunctional. It is often associated with starvation and critical illness.

Diabetes Mellitus (E08-E13)

One of the most important endocrine organs is the pancreas, which secretes insulin and regulates glucose levels within the body. Diabetes mellitus describes conditions in which the body does not produce any insulin at all (Type 1) or it is unable to synthesize the insulin produced (Type 2). In addition, ICD-10-CM classifies several other distinct types of diabetes, depending upon underlying cause.

The categories in this code block are as follows:

E08	Diabetes mellitus due to underlying condition
E09	Drug or chemical induced diabetes mellitus
E10	Type 1 diabetes mellitus
E11	Type 2 diabetes mellitus
E13	Other specified diabetes mellitus

In addition to the expanded number of categories of diabetes codes, the subclassification of each type of diabetic disorder is much more detailed. Combination codes describe common associated conditions, along with severity classifications.

E08.- Diabetes mellitus due to underlying condition

Diabetes mellitus that is not specified as Type 1, Type 2, or due to a drug or chemical may be due to another underlying condition. Some of the underlying conditions that may cause diabetes include the following:

- Chronic pancreatitis or other chronic pancreatic disorders
- Cushing's disease
- Polycystic ovarian syndrome
- Cystic fibrosis
- Hemochromatosis

The major goal in treating diabetes is to minimize any elevation of blood glucose without causing abnormally low levels of blood sugar. For diabetics other than those classified as Type 1, treatment begins with weight reduction, a diabetic diet, and exercise. When these measures fail to control the elevated blood glucose, oral medications are used; if glucose levels are still elevated, treatment with insulin is considered.

E08.0- Diabetes mellitus due to underlying condition with hyperosmolarity

Hyperosmolarity, also known as hyperosmolar hyperglycemic state (HHS) and hyperosmolar hyperglycemic nonketotic syndrome (HHNS), is caused by extremely high levels of glucose in the blood.

Typically HHS is seen in older diabetics with a precipitating illness or infection. It is a potentially life-threatening complication. The extremely high blood glucose levels trigger a hyperosmolar response in which the body tries to filter the glucose from the blood by drawing fluid from the body into the kidneys so that the sugar can be excreted in the urine. However, this can cause severe dehydration that can result in coma and death. HHS is classified as with or without nonketotic hyperglycemic-hyperosmolar coma (NKHHC).

E08.1- Diabetes mellitus due to underlying condition with ketoacidosis

Diabetic ketoacidosis (DKA) is a potentially life-threatening complication due to a shortage of insulin in which the body switches to burning fatty acids and producing acidic ketone bodies that cause most of the symptoms and complications. DKA may be complicated by coma.

E08.2- Diabetes mellitus due to underlying condition with kidney complications

The two most common kidney complications associated with diabetes mellitus are diabetic nephropathy and diabetic chronic kidney disease.

E08.21 Diabetes mellitus due to underlying condition with diabetic nephropathy

Diabetic nephropathy is a progressive kidney disease caused by angiopathy of capillaries in the kidney glomeruli, where the blood is filtered. It is a prime indicator for kidney dialysis and/or kidney transplant.

E08.22 Diabetes mellitus due to underlying condition with diabetic chronic kidney disease

Generally, diabetic chronic kidney disease indicates kidney damage related to long-standing glomeruli damage, typically manifested by proteinuria, hypertension, and edema. CKD is classified in stages from 1 to 5 and end stage renal disease (ESRD).

E08.3- Diabetes mellitus due to underlying condition with ophthalmic complications

Complications of diabetes mellitus affecting the eye include diabetic retinopathy with or without macular edema and diabetic cataract.

E08.311 Diabetes mellitus due to underlying condition with unspecified diabetic retinopathy with macular edema

E08.319 Diabetes mellitus due to underlying condition with unspecified diabetic retinopathy without macular edema

E08.321- Diabetes mellitus due to underlying condition with mild nonproliferative diabetic retinopathy with macular edema

E08.329- Diabetes mellitus due to underlying condition with mild nonproliferative diabetic retinopathy without macular edema

E08.331- Diabetes mellitus due to underlying condition with moderate nonproliferative diabetic retinopathy with macular edema

E08.339- Diabetes mellitus due to underlying condition with moderate nonproliferative diabetic retinopathy without macular edema

E08.341- Diabetes mellitus due to underlying condition with severe nonproliferative diabetic retinopathy with macular edema

E08.349- Diabetes mellitus due to underlying condition with severe nonproliferative diabetic retinopathy without macular edema

Diabetic retinopathy is a common complication of diabetes affecting the vasculature of the retina. Leakage and scar tissue from damaged retinal blood vessels distort and blur vision. Diabetic retinopathy is the third most common cause of legal blindness in adults in the United States. Nonproliferative diabetic retinopathy describes the early stage of the disease. In the nonproliferative stage, microaneurysm formation, hemorrhages, and blind spots are characteristic. As the disease progresses, more vessel leakage occurs. The disease progresses from mild to moderate to severe nonproliferative retinopathy as follows: mild nonproliferative diabetic retinopathy is characterized by microaneurysm formation with small, balloon-like swelling of the retinal vessels; moderate nonproliferative diabetic retinopathy is characterized by microaneurysms becoming more pronounced with some vessel blockage occurring; severe nonproliferative diabetic retinopathy is characterized by vascular breakdown within the retina resulting in multiple blockages and numerous intraretinal hemorrhages in different quadrants. Nonproliferative diabetic retinopathy may be complicated by macular

edema. Macular edema occurs when damaged blood vessels leak fluid and lipids onto the macula, the part of the retina that allows detail recognition. The fluid makes the macula swell, which blurs vision.

E08.35- Diabetes mellitus due to underlying condition with proliferative diabetic retinopathy

Diabetic retinopathy is a common complication of diabetes affecting the vasculature of the retina. Leakage and scar tissue from damaged retinal blood vessels distort and blur vision. Diabetic retinopathy is the third most common cause of legal blindness in adults in the United States. In the first stages of diabetic retinopathy, nonproliferative changes occur; however, eventually the condition progresses to the proliferative stage in which new blood vessels proliferate. The lack of oxygen in the retina causes fragile, new blood vessels to grow along the retina and in the clear, gel-like vitreous humor that fills the inside of the eye. Without timely treatment, these new blood vessels can bleed, cloud vision, and destroy the retina.

E08.351- Diabetes mellitus due to underlying condition with proliferative diabetic retinopathy with macular edema

Proliferative diabetic retinopathy may be complicated by macular edema. Macular edema occurs when damaged blood vessels leak fluid and lipids onto the macula, the part of the retina that allows detail recognition. The fluid makes the macula swell, which blurs vision.

E08.352- Diabetes mellitus due to underlying condition with proliferative diabetic retinopathy with traction retinal detachment involving the macula

E08.353- Diabetes mellitus due to underlying condition with proliferative diabetic retinopathy with traction retinal detachment not involving the macula

E08.354- Diabetes mellitus due to underlying condition with proliferative diabetic retinopathy with combined traction retinal detachment and rhegmatogenous retinal detachment

Retinal detachment is the separation of what is known as the sensory retina from the retinal pigment epithelium (RPE). The RPE performs two primary functions: it keeps fluid from accumulating in the subretinal space, and it supplies nutrients to the retina.

The two most common forms of retinal detachment are rhegmatogenous retinal detachment and traction retinal detachment. In proliferative diabetic retinopathy, the proliferation of blood vessels within the retina and vitreous causes undue traction on these ocular layers. When the eye moves, the vessels pull on the retina causing it to either tear or detach from the

RPE layer. Traction that causes a tear in the retina, allowing fluid from the vitreous to accumulate between the retina and the RPE, is known as rhegmatogenous retinal detachment. Traction that does not cause an actual tear in the retina and instead only separates the retina away from the RPE is considered traction retinal detachment. The types and success of treatment and the extent of vision loss are proportionate to the extent of the retinal detachment. Those retinal detachments that involve the macula are the most severe, and although treatment can correct some of the visual loss, full recovery of the patient's vision is rare.

E08.355- Diabetes mellitus due to underlying condition with stable proliferative diabetic retinopathy

Vitrectomies, laser treatments, or intravitreal antivascular endothelial growth factor therapies are all current treatment options for proliferative diabetic retinopathy and/or its associated complications. When a patient's condition has quieted following any of these treatments, it is considered stable, allowing for greater intervals between follow-up visits.

E08.359- Diabetes mellitus due to underlying condition with proliferative diabetic retinopathy without macular edema

In some cases, a patient may have the proliferative form of diabetic retinopathy, characterized by extensive growth of new blood vessels along the retina and in the clear, gel-like vitreous humor that fills the inside of the eye without swelling of macular tissues.

E08.36   Diabetes mellitus due to underlying condition with diabetic cataract

As a result of a chemical imbalance and an intracellular accumulation of sorbitol, diabetic patients are at high risk of developing cataracts and also have a higher risk of complications after phacoemulsification cataract surgery compared to nondiabetics.

E08.37- Diabetes mellitus due to underlying condition with diabetic macular edema, resolved following treatment

Several modalities are available to treat diabetic macular edema, including different forms of laser photocoagulation, corticosteroids, anti-VEGF (vascular endothelial growth factor) therapy, and vitrectomy. While these methods have successfully resolved macular edema in some patients, they also carry a risk of complications like cataracts, hypertension, and scar tissue formation.

E08.39   Diabetes mellitus due to underlying condition with other diabetic ophthalmic complication

Diabetic glaucoma is reported with this code. Glaucoma is the failure of fluid in the eye to drain properly causing increased intraocular pressure that can result in damage to the optic nerve. When the optic nerve is damaged, vision becomes impaired; untreated glaucoma can lead to blindness.

E08.4-   Diabetes mellitus due to underlying condition with neurological complications

Diabetic neuropathy is a condition thought to be due to microvascular injury involving small blood vessels that supply nourishment to the nerves. It may affect all peripheral nerves including pain fibers, motor neurons, and the autonomic nervous system.

E08.41   Diabetes mellitus due to underlying condition with diabetic mononeuropathy

Diabetic mononeuropathy involves sudden onset damage to a single large nerve that may be due to infarction or other problems. Common manifestations of mononeuropathy include a wrist or foot drop, cranial nerve palsy, or a recurrent laryngeal nerve problem.

E08.42   Diabetes mellitus due to underlying condition with diabetic polyneuropathy

In diabetic polyneuropathy, decreased sensation and loss of reflexes occur first in the toes on each foot. As the disease progresses, the symptoms extend upward to involve the feet, lower legs, and finally the upper legs. The nerve damage eventually affects the fingers, hands, and arms as well. Patients with this condition cannot feel pain or other symptoms indicative of injury or complications and are consequently at high risk for ulcers and infections primarily affecting the legs and feet; the arms may be affected as well.

E08.43   Diabetes mellitus due to underlying condition with diabetic autonomic (poly)neuropathy

Autonomic neuropathy affects nerves of the autonomic body systems, such as the heart, lungs, blood vessels, bone, and gastrointestinal and genitourinary systems. One of the most commonly recognized autonomic dysfunctions in diabetics is orthostatic hypotension or fainting when standing up. Symptoms of autonomic neuropathy affecting the heart and vascular system can range from mild to life-threatening, such as those related to the heart and arteries failing to appropriately adjust the heartrate and vascular tone to keep blood continually and fully flowing to the brain. Another common diabetic autonomic neuropathy complication is diabetic gastroparesis. Gastroparesis results from damage to the vagus nerve, which controls the movement of food in the stomach and intestine. When vagus nerve damage occurs, the muscles of the stomach and digestive system cannot move food effectively along the digestive tract causing delayed emptying or an inability to empty the stomach contents. When food does not move along the digestive tract, bacterial overgrowth occurs causing bloating. A more serious complication of diabetic gastroparesis is the formation of hard masses of partially digested food called bezoars that can create stomach or intestinal obstructions.

E08.44 Diabetes mellitus due to underlying condition with diabetic amyotrophy

Diabetic amyotrophy, also called radiculoplexus neuropathy, femoral neuropathy, or proximal neuropathy, occurs when there is damage to the nerves of the thigh, hips, buttocks, and upper legs. Common symptoms include weakness followed by wasting of pelvic and femoral muscles, unilaterally or bilaterally, with associated pain. Sensory nerve damage (neuropathy) may also be present.

E08.5- Diabetes mellitus due to underlying condition with circulatory complications

Diabetes mellitus increases the risk of developing circulatory complications with the most common type being peripheral angiopathy.

E08.51 Diabetes mellitus due to underlying condition with diabetic peripheral angiopathy without gangrene

E08.52 Diabetes mellitus due to underlying condition with diabetic peripheral angiopathy with gangrene

There are two types of angiopathy: microangiopathy, which is a vascular malfunction due to hyperglycemia found in diabetes; and macroangiopathy, which is caused by diabetic conditions of insulin resistance and metabolic syndrome. In microangiopathy, walls of the smaller blood vessels become so thick and weak that they bleed, leak protein, and slow the flow of blood through the body. The decrease of blood flow through stenosis or clot formation impairs the flow of oxygen to cells and biological tissues and leads to cellular death and gangrene. For macroangiopathy, atherosclerosis and a resultant blood clot forms on the large blood vessels, sticks to the vessel walls, and blocks the flow of blood. Gangrene refers to dead or dying body tissue caused by inadequate blood supply. Dry gangrene typically results from conditions that reduce or block arterial blood flow such as diabetes.

E08.6- Diabetes mellitus due to underlying condition with other specified complications

Complications of diabetes mellitus that affect the joints, skin, and other sites are included here.

E08.61- Diabetes mellitus due to underlying condition with diabetic arthropathy

Diabetic arthropathy may be neuropathic or due to another disease process.

E08.610 Diabetes mellitus due to underlying condition with diabetic neuropathic arthropathy

Neuropathic arthropathy, also called Charcot's joint, involves progressive degeneration of a weight-bearing joint, a process marked by bony destruction, bone resorption, and eventual deformity.

E08.618 Diabetes mellitus due to underlying condition with other diabetic arthropathy

Diabetics are more likely to develop other types of arthropathy characterized by pain, inflammation, and articular cartilage damage to the joints.

E08.62- Diabetes mellitus due to underlying condition with skin complications

Diabetics are at risk of developing various skin complications, including skin inflammation (dermatitis) and skin and soft tissue ulcers.

E08.620 Diabetes mellitus due to underlying condition with diabetic dermatitis

One inflammatory skin condition affecting diabetics is necrobiosis lipoidica diabeticorum, which is a necrotizing skin condition that most frequently appears on the patient's shins, often on both legs. The lesions are often asymptomatic but may become tender and ulcerate when injured.

E08.621 Diabetes mellitus due to underlying condition with foot ulcer

E08.622 Diabetes mellitus due to underlying condition with other skin ulcer

The majority of diabetic skin ulcers occurs on the feet and lower legs and are due to one of two major underlying causes: damaged nerves and diseased blood vessels (vascular disease).

E08.63- Diabetes mellitus due to underlying condition with oral complications

Diabetes mellitus puts the patient at risk for developing periodontal disease and other oral complications.

E08.630 Diabetes mellitus due to underlying condition with periodontal disease

Diabetic patients may be at increased risk for periodontal disease due to capillary damage and decreased wound healing. Periodontal disease begins with inflammation of the gums (gingivitis) that progresses to involve deeper tissues and bone. Periodontal disease occurs when the gum pulls away from the underlying teeth leaving pockets where bacteria collect. The bacteria in the pockets prompt an immune system response to fight the infection. However, the enzymes created by the immune system to destroy the bacteria instead act with the toxins produced by the bacteria and end up destroying the connective tissue and bone around the teeth. Periodontal disease seen in diabetics may be acute or chronic. Chronic periodontitis signifies the progression of the inflammatory disease of the bony and ligamentous supporting tissues of the teeth over time as a result of failure to treat the disease in the acute stage. Patients with severe and widespread chronic periodontitis have a high risk for tooth loss.

E08.64- Diabetes mellitus due to underlying condition with hypoglycemia

Hypoglycemia refers to low blood sugar levels, typically defined as less than 70 mg/dl. When diabetic patients experience hypoglycemia, it is typically a complication of insulin or oral therapy diabetic treatment. Issues arise from an inadequate supply of glucose to the brain, resulting in impairment of function or neuroglycopenia. Effects can range from mild dysphoria to more serious issues such as seizures or unconsciousness. Diabetes mellitus complicated by hypoglycemia is differentiated as with or without coma.

E08.65 Diabetes mellitus due to underlying condition with hyperglycemia

Hyperglycemia in diabetes mellitus refers to blood glucose (sugar) levels that are too high. High blood glucose levels in diabetes mellitus are indicative of inadequate or poorly controlled diabetes.

E09.- Drug or chemical induced diabetes mellitus

Diabetes mellitus that is related to ingestion of a drug or chemical is classified as drug- or chemical-induced diabetes mellitus. These drugs may not, by themselves, cause diabetes but they may precipitate diabetes in patients with insulin resistance. Some of the most common drugs and chemicals that can cause diabetes include the following:

- Alpha- or beta-adrenergic agonists
- Atypical antipsychotic drugs
- Beta-blockers
- Calcineurin

- Corticosteroids in high doses
- Diazoxide
- Dilantin
- Glucocorticoids
- Interferon-alpha therapy
- Nicotinic acid
- Protease inhibitors
- Thiazide diuretics
- Thyroid hormone
- Vacor

E09.0- Drug or chemical induced diabetes mellitus with hyperosmolarity

Hyperosmolarity, also known as hyperosmolar hyperglycemic state (HHS) and hyperosmolar hyperglycemic nonketotic syndrome (HHNS), is caused by extremely high levels of glucose in the blood. Typically HHS is seen in older diabetics with a precipitating illness or infection. It is a potentially life-threatening complication. The extremely high blood glucose levels trigger a hyperosmolar response in which the body tries to filter the glucose from the blood by drawing fluid from the body into the kidneys so that the sugar can be excreted in the urine. However, this can cause severe dehydration that can result in coma and death. HHS is classified as with or without nonketotic hyperglycemic-hyperosmolar coma (NKHHC).

E09.1- Drug or chemical induced diabetes mellitus with ketoacidosis

Diabetic ketoacidosis (DKA) is a potentially life-threatening complication due to a shortage of insulin in which the body switches to burning fatty acids and producing acidic ketone bodies that cause most of the symptoms and complications. DKA may be complicated by coma.

E09.2- Drug or chemical induced diabetes mellitus with kidney complications

The two most common kidney complications associated with diabetes mellitus are diabetic nephropathy and diabetic chronic kidney disease.

E09.21 Drug or chemical induced diabetes mellitus with diabetic nephropathy

Diabetic nephropathy is a progressive kidney disease caused by angiopathy of capillaries in the kidney glomeruli, where the blood is filtered. It is a prime indicator for kidney dialysis and/or kidney transplant.

E09.22 Drug or chemical induced diabetes mellitus with diabetic chronic kidney disease

Generally, diabetic chronic kidney disease indicates kidney damage related to long-standing glomeruli damage, typically manifested by proteinuria, hypertension, and edema. CKD is classified in stages, from 1 to 5 and end stage renal disease (ESRD).

E09.3- Drug or chemical induced diabetes mellitus with ophthalmic complications

Complications of diabetes mellitus affecting the eye include diabetic retinopathy with or without macular edema and diabetic cataract.

E09.311 Drug or chemical induced diabetes mellitus with unspecified diabetic retinopathy with macular edema

E09.319 Drug or chemical induced diabetes mellitus with unspecified diabetic retinopathy without macular edema

E09.321- Drug or chemical induced diabetes mellitus with mild nonproliferative diabetic retinopathy with macular edema

E09.329- Drug or chemical induced diabetes mellitus with mild nonproliferative diabetic retinopathy without macular edema

E09.331- Drug or chemical induced diabetes mellitus with moderate nonproliferative diabetic retinopathy with macular edema

E09.339- Drug or chemical induced diabetes mellitus with moderate nonproliferative diabetic retinopathy without macular edema

E09.341- Drug or chemical induced diabetes mellitus with severe nonproliferative diabetic retinopathy with macular edema

E09.349- Drug or chemical induced diabetes mellitus with severe nonproliferative diabetic retinopathy without macular edema

Diabetic retinopathy is a common complication of diabetes affecting the vasculature of the retina. Leakage and scar tissue from damaged retinal blood vessels distort and blur vision. Diabetic retinopathy is the third most common cause of legal blindness in adults in the United States. Nonproliferative diabetic retinopathy describes the early stage of the disease. In the nonproliferative stage, microaneurysm formation,

hemorrhages, and blind spots are characteristic. As the disease progresses, more vessel leakage occurs. The disease progresses from mild to moderate to severe nonproliferative retinopathy as follows: mild nonproliferative diabetic retinopathy is characterized by microaneurysm formation with small, balloon-like swelling of retinal vessels; moderate nonproliferative diabetic retinopathy is characterized by microaneurysms becoming more pronounced with some vessel blockage occurring; severe nonproliferative diabetic retinopathy is characterized by vascular breakdown within the retina resulting in multiple blockages and numerous intraretinal hemorrhages in different quadrants. Nonproliferative diabetic retinopathy may be complicated by macular edema. Macular edema occurs when damaged blood vessels leak fluid and lipids onto the macula, the part of the retina that allows detail recognition. The fluid makes the macula swell, which blurs vision.

E09.35- Drug or chemical induced diabetes mellitus with proliferative diabetic retinopathy

Diabetic retinopathy is a common complication of diabetes affecting the vasculature of the retina. Leakage and scar tissue from damaged retinal blood vessels distort and blur vision. Diabetic retinopathy is the third most common cause of legal blindness in adults in the United States. In the first stages of diabetic retinopathy, nonproliferative changes occur; however, eventually the condition progresses to the proliferative stage in which new blood vessels proliferate. The lack of oxygen in the retina causes fragile, new blood vessels to grow along the retina and in the clear, gel-like vitreous humor that fills the inside of the eye. Without timely treatment, these new blood vessels can bleed, cloud vision, and destroy the retina.

E09.351- Drug or chemical induced diabetes mellitus with proliferative diabetic retinopathy with macular edema

Proliferative diabetic retinopathy may be complicated by macular edema. Macular edema occurs when damaged blood vessels leak fluid and lipids onto the macula, the part of the retina that allows detail recognition. The fluid makes the macula swell, which blurs vision.

E09.352- Drug or chemical induced diabetes mellitus with proliferative diabetic retinopathy with traction retinal detachment involving the macula

E09.353- Drug or chemical induced diabetes mellitus with proliferative diabetic retinopathy with traction retinal detachment not involving the macula

E09.354- Drug or chemical induced diabetes mellitus with proliferative diabetic retinopathy with combined traction retinal detachment and rhegmatogenous retinal detachment

Retinal detachment is the separation of what is known as the sensory retina from the retinal pigment epithelium (RPE). The RPE performs two primary functions: it keeps fluid from accumulating in the subretinal space, and it supplies nutrients to the retina.

The two most common forms of retinal detachment are rhegmatogenous retinal detachment and traction retinal detachment. In proliferative diabetic retinopathy, the proliferation of blood vessels within the retina and vitreous causes undue traction on these ocular layers. When the eye moves, the vessels pull on the retina causing it to either tear or detach from the RPE layer. Traction that causes a tear in the retina, allowing fluid from the vitreous to accumulate between the retina and the RPE, is known as rhegmatogenous retinal detachment. Traction that does not cause an actual tear in the retina and instead only separates the retina away from the RPE is considered traction retinal detachment. The types and success of treatment and the extent of vision loss are proportionate to the extent of the retinal detachment. Those retinal detachments that involve the macula are the most severe, and although treatment can correct some of the visual loss, full recovery of the patient's vision is rare.

E09.355- Drug or chemical induced diabetes mellitus with stable proliferative diabetic retinopathy

Vitrectomies, laser treatments, or intravitreal antivascular endothelial growth factor therapies are all current treatment options for proliferative diabetic retinopathy and/or its associated complications. When a patient's condition has quieted following any of these treatments, it is considered stable, allowing for greater intervals between follow-up visits.

E09.359- Drug or chemical induced diabetes mellitus with proliferative diabetic retinopathy without macular edema

In some cases, a patient may have the proliferative form of diabetic retinopathy, characterized by extensive growth of new blood vessels along the retina and in the clear, gel-like vitreous humor that fills the inside of the eye without swelling of macular tissues.

E09.36 Drug or chemical induced diabetes mellitus with diabetic cataract

As a result of a chemical imbalance and an intracellular accumulation of sorbitol, diabetic patients are at high risk of developing cataracts and also have a higher risk of complications after phacoemulsification cataract surgery compared to nondiabetics.

E09.37- Drug or chemical induced diabetes mellitus with diabetic macular edema, resolved following treatment

Several modalities are available to treat diabetic macular edema, including different forms of laser photocoagulation, corticosteroids, anti-VEGF (vascular endothelial growth factor) therapy, and vitrectomy. While these methods have successfully resolved macular edema in some patients, they also carry a risk of complications like cataracts, hypertension, and scar tissue formation.

E09.39 Drug or chemical induced diabetes mellitus with other diabetic ophthalmic complication

Diabetic glaucoma is reported with this code. Glaucoma is the failure of fluid in the eye to drain properly causing increased intraocular pressure that can result in damage to the optic nerve. When the optic nerve is damaged, vision becomes impaired; untreated glaucoma can lead to blindness.

E09.4- Drug or chemical induced diabetes mellitus with neurological complications

Diabetic neuropathy is a condition thought to be due to microvascular injury involving small blood vessels that supply nourishment to the nerves. It may affect all peripheral nerves including pain fibers, motor neurons, and the autonomic nervous system.

E09.41 Drug or chemical induced diabetes mellitus with neurological complications with diabetic mononeuropathy

Diabetic mononeuropathy involves sudden onset damage to a single large nerve that may be due to infarction or other problems. Common manifestations of mononeuropathy include a wrist or foot drop, cranial nerve palsy, or a recurrent laryngeal nerve problem.

E09.42 Drug or chemical induced diabetes mellitus with neurological complications with diabetic polyneuropathy

In diabetic polyneuropathy, decreased sensation and loss of reflexes occur first in the toes on each foot. As the disease progresses, the symptoms extend upward to involve the feet, lower legs, and finally the upper legs. The nerve damage eventually affects the fingers, hands, and arms as well. Patients with this condition cannot feel pain or other symptoms indicative of injury or complications and are consequently at high risk for ulcers and infections primarily affecting the legs and feet; the arms may be affected as well.

E09.43 Drug or chemical induced diabetes mellitus with neurological complications with diabetic autonomic (poly)neuropathy

Autonomic neuropathy affects nerves of the autonomic body systems, such as the heart, lungs, blood vessels, bone, and gastrointestinal and genitourinary systems. One of the most commonly recognized autonomic dysfunctions in diabetics is orthostatic hypotension or fainting when standing up. Symptoms of autonomic neuropathy affecting the heart and vascular system can range from mild to life-threatening, such as those related to the heart and arteries failing to appropriately adjust the heartrate and vascular tone to keep blood continually and fully flowing to the brain. Another common diabetic autonomic neuropathy complication is diabetic gastroparesis. Gastroparesis results from damage to the vagus nerve, which controls the movement of food in the stomach and intestine. When vagus nerve damage occurs, the muscles of the stomach and digestive system cannot move food effectively along the digestive tract causing delayed emptying or an inability to empty the stomach contents. When food does not move along the digestive tract, bacterial overgrowth occurs causing bloating. A more serious complication of diabetic gastroparesis is the formation of hard masses of partially digested food called bezoars that can create stomach or intestinal obstructions.

E09.44 Drug or chemical induced diabetes mellitus with neurological complications with diabetic amyotrophy

Diabetic amyotrophy, also called radiculoplexus neuropathy, femoral neuropathy, or proximal neuropathy, occurs when there is damage to the nerves of the thigh, hips, buttocks, and upper legs. Common symptoms include weakness followed by wasting of pelvic and femoral muscles, unilaterally or bilaterally, with associated pain. Sensory nerve damage (neuropathy) may also be present.

E09.5- Drug or chemical induced diabetes mellitus with circulatory complications

Diabetes mellitus increases the risk of developing circulatory complications with the most common type being peripheral angiopathy.

E09.51 Drug or chemical induced diabetes mellitus with diabetic peripheral angiopathy without gangrene

E09.52 Drug or chemical induced diabetes mellitus with diabetic peripheral angiopathy with gangrene

There are two types of angiopathy: microangiopathy, which is a vascular malfunction due to hyperglycemia found in diabetes; and macroangiopathy, which is caused by diabetic conditions of insulin resistance and metabolic syndrome. In microangiopathy, walls of the smaller blood vessels become so thick and weak that they bleed, leak protein, and slow the flow of blood through the body. The decrease of blood flow through stenosis or clot formation impairs the flow of oxygen to cells and biological tissues and leads to cellular death and gangrene. For macroangiopathy, atherosclerosis and a resultant blood clot forms on the large blood vessels, sticks to the vessel walls, and blocks the flow of blood. Gangrene refers to dead or dying body tissue caused by inadequate blood supply. Dry gangrene typically results from conditions that reduce or block arterial blood flow such as diabetes.

E09.6- Drug or chemical induced diabetes mellitus with other specified complications

Complications of diabetes mellitus that affect the joints, skin, and other sites are included here.

E09.61- Drug or chemical induced diabetes mellitus with diabetic arthropathy

Diabetic arthropathy may be neuropathic or due to another disease process.

E09.610 Drug or chemical induced diabetes mellitus with diabetic neuropathic arthropathy

Neuropathic arthropathy, also called Charcot's joint, involves progressive degeneration of a weight-bearing joint, a process marked by bony destruction, bone resorption, and eventual deformity.

E09.618 Drug or chemical induced diabetes mellitus with other diabetic arthropathy

Diabetics are more likely to develop other types of arthropathy characterized by pain, inflammation, and articular cartilage damage to the joints.

E09.62- Drug or chemical induced diabetes mellitus with skin complications

Diabetics are at risk of developing various skin complications, including skin inflammation (dermatitis) and skin and soft tissue ulcers.

E09.620 Drug or chemical induced diabetes mellitus with diabetic dermatitis

One inflammatory skin condition affecting diabetics is necrobiosis lipoidica diabeticorum, which is a necrotizing skin condition that most frequently appears on the patient's shins, often on both legs. The lesions are often asymptomatic but may become tender and ulcerate when injured.

E09.621 Drug or chemical induced diabetes mellitus with foot ulcer

E09.622 Drug or chemical induced diabetes mellitus with other skin ulcer

The majority of diabetic skin ulcers occur on the feet and lower legs and are due to one of two major underlying causes: damaged nerves and diseased blood vessels (vascular disease).

E09.63- Drug or chemical induced diabetes mellitus with oral complications

Diabetes mellitus puts the patient at risk for developing periodontal disease and other oral complications.

E09.630 Drug or chemical induced diabetes mellitus with periodontal disease

Diabetic patients may be at increased risk for periodontal disease due to capillary damage and decreased wound healing. Periodontal disease begins with inflammation of the gums (gingivitis) that progresses to involve deeper tissues and bone. Periodontal disease occurs when the gum pulls away from the underlying teeth leaving pockets where bacteria collect. The bacteria in the pockets prompt an immune system response to fight the infection. However, the enzymes created by the immune system to destroy the bacteria instead act with the toxins produced by the bacteria and end up destroying the connective tissue and bone around the teeth. Periodontal disease seen in diabetics may be acute or chronic. Chronic periodontitis signifies the progression of the inflammatory disease of the bony and ligamentous supporting tissues of the teeth over time as a result of failure to treat the disease in the acute stage. Patients with severe and widespread chronic periodontitis have a high risk for tooth loss.

E09.64- Drug or chemical induced diabetes mellitus with hypoglycemia

Hypoglycemia refers to low blood sugar levels, typically defined as less than 70 mg/dl. When diabetic patients experience hypoglycemia, it is typically a complication of insulin or oral therapy diabetic treatment. Issues arise from an inadequate supply of glucose to the brain, resulting in impairment of function or neuroglycopenia. Effects can range from mild dysphoria to more serious issues such as seizures or unconsciousness. Diabetes mellitus complicated by hypoglycemia is differentiated as with or without coma.

E09.65 Drug or chemical induced diabetes mellitus with hyperglycemia

Hyperglycemia in diabetes mellitus refers to blood glucose (sugar) levels that are too high. High blood glucose levels in diabetes mellitus are indicative of inadequate or poorly controlled diabetes.

E10.- Type 1 diabetes mellitus

Type 1 diabetes mellitus is a systemic disease that is the result of an inadequate secretion of insulin by the pancreas. Many patients with this type of diabetes are diagnosed at a young age, but this type of diabetes only accounts for approximately 10 percent of total cases. Treatment requires regular injections of insulin due to the autoimmune destruction of pancreatic beta cells, which cease to produce insulin.

E10.1- Type 1 diabetes mellitus with ketoacidosis

Diabetic ketoacidosis (DKA) is a potentially life-threatening complication due to a shortage of insulin in which the body switches to burning fatty acids and producing acidic ketone bodies that cause most of the symptoms and complications. It predominantly affects Type 1 diabetics. DKA may occur with or without coma.

E10.2- Type 1 diabetes mellitus with kidney complications

The two most common kidney complications associated with diabetes mellitus are diabetic nephropathy and diabetic chronic kidney disease.

E10.21 Type 1 diabetes mellitus with diabetic nephropathy

Diabetic nephropathy is a progressive kidney disease caused by angiopathy of capillaries in the kidney glomeruli where the blood is filtered. It is a prime indicator for kidney dialysis and/or kidney transplant.

E10.22 Type 1 diabetes mellitus with diabetic chronic kidney disease

Generally, diabetic chronic kidney disease indicates kidney damage related to long-standing glomeruli damage, typically manifested by proteinuria, hypertension, and edema. CKD is classified in stages, from 1 to 5 and end stage renal disease (ESRD).

E10.3- Type 1 diabetes mellitus with ophthalmic complications

Complications of diabetes mellitus affecting the eye include diabetic retinopathy with or without macular edema and diabetic cataract.

E10.311 Type 1 diabetes mellitus with unspecified diabetic retinopathy with macular edema

E10.319 Type 1 diabetes mellitus with unspecified diabetic retinopathy without macular edema

E10.321- Type 1 diabetes mellitus with mild nonproliferative diabetic retinopathy with macular edema

E10.329- Type 1 diabetes mellitus with mild nonproliferative diabetic retinopathy without macular edema

E10.331- Type 1 diabetes mellitus with moderate nonproliferative diabetic retinopathy with macular edema

E10.339- Type 1 diabetes mellitus with moderate nonproliferative diabetic retinopathy without macular edema

E10.341- Type 1 diabetes mellitus with severe nonproliferative diabetic retinopathy with macular edema

E10.349- Type 1 diabetes mellitus with severe nonproliferative diabetic retinopathy without macular edema

Diabetic retinopathy is a common complication of diabetes affecting the vasculature of the retina. Leakage and scar tissue from damaged retinal blood vessels distort and blur vision. Diabetic retinopathy is the third most common cause of legal blindness in adults in the United States. Nonproliferative diabetic retinopathy describes the early stage of the disease. In the nonproliferative stage, microaneurysm formation, hemorrhages, and blind spots are characteristic. As the disease progresses, more vessel leakage occurs. The disease progresses from mild to moderate to severe nonproliferative retinopathy as follows: mild nonproliferative diabetic retinopathy is characterized by microaneurysm formation with small, balloon-like swelling of retinal vessels; moderate nonproliferative diabetic retinopathy is characterized by microaneurysms becoming more pronounced with some vessel blockage occurring; severe nonproliferative diabetic retinopathy is characterized by vascular breakdown within the retina resulting in multiple blockages and numerous intraretinal hemorrhages in different quadrants. Nonproliferative diabetic retinopathy may be complicated by macular edema. Macular edema occurs when damaged blood vessels leak fluid and lipids onto the macula, the part of the retina that allows detail recognition. The fluid makes the macula swell, which blurs vision.

E10.35- Type 1 diabetes mellitus with proliferative diabetic retinopathy

Diabetic retinopathy is a common complication of diabetes affecting the vasculature of the retina. Leakage and scar tissue from damaged retinal blood vessels distort and blur vision. Diabetic retinopathy is the third most common cause of legal blindness in adults in the United States. In the first stages of diabetic retinopathy, nonproliferative changes occur; however, eventually the condition progresses to the proliferative stage in which new blood vessels proliferate. The lack of oxygen in the retina causes fragile, new blood vessels to grow along the retina and in the clear, gel-like vitreous humor that fills the inside of the eye. Without timely treatment, these new blood vessels can bleed, cloud vision, and destroy the retina.

E10.351- Type 1 diabetes mellitus with proliferative diabetic retinopathy with macular edema

Proliferative diabetic retinopathy may be complicated by macular edema. Macular edema occurs when damaged blood vessels leak fluid and lipids onto the macula, the part of the retina that allows detail recognition. The fluid makes the macula swell, which blurs vision.

E10.352- Type 1 diabetes mellitus with proliferative diabetic retinopathy with traction retinal detachment involving the macula

E10.353- Type 1 diabetes mellitus with proliferative diabetic retinopathy with traction retinal detachment not involving the macula

E10.354- Type 1 diabetes mellitus with proliferative diabetic retinopathy with combined traction retinal detachment and rhegmatogenous retinal detachment

Retinal detachment is the separation of what is known as the sensory retina from the retinal pigment epithelium (RPE). The RPE performs two primary functions: it keeps fluid from accumulating in the subretinal space, and it supplies nutrients to the retina.

The two most common forms of retinal detachment are rhegmatogenous retinal detachment and traction retinal detachment. In proliferative diabetic retinopathy, the proliferation of blood vessels within the retina and vitreous causes undue traction on these ocular layers. When the eye moves, the vessels pull on the retina causing it to either tear or detach from the RPE layer. Traction that causes a tear in the retina, allowing fluid from the vitreous to accumulate between the retina and the RPE, is known as rhegmatogenous retinal detachment. Traction that does not cause an actual tear in the retina and instead only separates the retina away from the RPE is considered traction retinal detachment. The types and success of treatment and the extent of vision loss are proportionate to the extent of the retinal detachment. Those retinal detachments that involve the macula are the most severe, and although treatment can correct some of the visual loss, full recovery of the patient's vision is rare.

E10.355- Type 1 diabetes mellitus with stable proliferative diabetic retinopathy

Vitrectomies, laser treatments, or intravitreal antivascular endothelial growth factor therapies are all current treatment options for proliferative diabetic retinopathy and/or its associated complications. When a patient's condition has quieted following any of these treatments, it is considered stable, allowing for greater intervals between follow-up visits.

E10.359- Type 1 diabetes mellitus with proliferative diabetic retinopathy without macular edema

In some cases, a patient may have the proliferative form of diabetic retinopathy, characterized by extensive growth of new blood vessels along the retina and in the clear, gel-like vitreous humor that fills the inside of the eye without swelling of macular tissues.

E10.36 Type 1 diabetes mellitus with diabetic cataract

As a result of a chemical imbalance and an intracellular accumulation of sorbitol, diabetic patients are at high risk of developing cataracts and also have a higher risk of complications after phacoemulsification cataract surgery compared to nondiabetics.

E10.37- Type 1 diabetes mellitus with diabetic macular edema, resolved following treatment

Several modalities are available to treat diabetic macular edema, including different forms of laser photocoagulation, corticosteroids, anti-VEGF (vascular endothelial growth factor) therapy, and vitrectomy. While these methods have successfully resolved macular edema in some patients, they also carry a risk of complications like cataracts, hypertension, and scar tissue formation.

E10.39 Type 1 diabetes mellitus with other diabetic ophthalmic complication

Diabetic glaucoma is reported with this code. Glaucoma is the failure of fluid in the eye to drain properly causing increased intraocular pressure that can result in damage to the optic nerve. When the optic nerve is damaged, vision becomes impaired; untreated glaucoma can lead to blindness.

E10.4- Type 1 diabetes mellitus with neurological complications

Diabetic neuropathy is a condition thought to be due to microvascular injury involving small blood vessels that supply nourishment to the nerves. It may affect all peripheral nerves including pain fibers, motor neurons, and the autonomic nervous system.

E10.41 Type 1 diabetes mellitus with diabetic mononeuropathy

Diabetic mononeuropathy involves sudden onset damage to a single large nerve that may be due to infarction or other problems. Common manifestations of mononeuropathy include a wrist or foot drop, cranial nerve palsy, or a recurrent laryngeal nerve problem.

E10.42 Type 1 diabetes mellitus with diabetic polyneuropathy

In diabetic polyneuropathy, decreased sensation and loss of reflexes occur first in the toes on each foot. As the disease progresses, the symptoms extend upward to involve the feet, lower legs, and finally the upper legs. The nerve damage eventually affects the fingers, hands, and arms as well. Patients with this condition cannot feel pain or other symptoms indicative of injury or complications and are consequently at high risk for ulcers and infections primarily affecting the legs and feet; the arms may be affected as well.

E10.43 Type 1 diabetes mellitus with diabetic autonomic (poly)neuropathy

Autonomic neuropathy affects nerves of the autonomic body systems, such as the heart, lungs, blood vessels, bone, and gastrointestinal and genitourinary systems. One of the most commonly recognized autonomic dysfunctions in diabetics is orthostatic hypotension or fainting when standing up. Symptoms of autonomic neuropathy affecting the heart and vascular system can range from mild to life-threatening, such as those related to the heart and arteries failing to appropriately adjust the heartrate and vascular tone to keep blood continually and fully flowing to the brain.

Another common diabetic autonomic neuropathy complication is diabetic gastroparesis. Gastroparesis results from damage to the vagus nerve, which controls the movement of food in the stomach and intestine. When vagus nerve damage occurs, the muscles of the stomach and digestive system cannot move food effectively along the digestive tract causing delayed emptying or an inability to empty the stomach contents. When food does not move along the digestive tract bacterial overgrowth occurs causing bloating. A more serious complication of diabetic gastroparesis is the formation of hard masses of partially digested food called bezoars that can create stomach or intestinal obstructions.

E10.44 Type 1 diabetes mellitus with diabetic amyotrophy

Diabetic amyotrophy, also called radiculoplexus neuropathy, femoral neuropathy, or proximal neuropathy, occurs when there is damage to the nerves of the thigh, hips, buttocks, and upper legs. Common symptoms include weakness followed by wasting of pelvic and femoral muscles, unilaterally or bilaterally, with associated pain. Sensory nerve damage (neuropathy) may also be present.

E10.5- Type 1 diabetes mellitus with circulatory complications

Diabetes mellitus increases the risk of developing circulatory complications with the most common type being peripheral angiopathy.

E10.51 Type 1 diabetes mellitus with diabetic peripheral angiopathy without gangrene

E10.52 Type 1 diabetes mellitus with diabetic peripheral angiopathy with gangrene

There are two types of angiopathy: microangiopathy, which is a vascular malfunction due to hyperglycemia found in diabetes; and macroangiopathy, which is caused by diabetic conditions of insulin resistance and metabolic syndrome. In microangiopathy, walls of the smaller blood vessels become so thick and weak that they bleed, leak protein, and slow the flow of blood through the body. The decrease of blood flow through stenosis or clot formation impairs the flow of oxygen to cells and biological tissues and leads to cellular death and gangrene. For macroangiopathy, atherosclerosis and a resultant blood clot forms on the large blood vessels, sticks to the vessel walls, and blocks the flow of blood. Gangrene refers to dead or dying body tissue caused by inadequate blood supply. Dry gangrene typically results from conditions that reduce or block arterial blood flow such as diabetes.

E10.6- Type 1 diabetes mellitus with other specified complications

Complications of diabetes mellitus that affect the joints, skin, and other sites are included here.

E10.61- Type 1 diabetes mellitus with diabetic arthropathy

Diabetic arthropathy may be neuropathic or due to another disease process.

E10.610 Type 1 diabetes mellitus with diabetic neuropathic arthropathy

Neuropathic arthropathy, also called Charcot's joint, involves progressive degeneration of a weight-bearing joint, a process marked by bony destruction, bone resorption, and eventual deformity.

E10.618 Type 1 diabetes mellitus with other diabetic arthropathy

Diabetics are more likely to develop other types of arthropathy characterized by pain, inflammation, and articular cartilage damage to the joints.

E10.62- Type 1 diabetes mellitus with skin complications

Diabetics are at risk of developing various skin complications, including skin inflammation (dermatitis) and skin and soft tissue ulcers.

E10.620 Type 1 diabetes mellitus with diabetic dermatitis

One inflammatory skin condition affecting diabetics is necrobiosis lipoidica diabeticorum, which is a necrotizing skin condition that most frequently appears on the patient's shins, often on both legs. The lesions are often asymptomatic but may become tender and ulcerate when injured.

E10.621 Type 1 diabetes mellitus with foot ulcer

E10.622 Type 1 diabetes mellitus with other skin ulcer

The majority of diabetic skin ulcers occur on the feet and lower legs and are due to one of two major underlying causes: damaged nerves and diseased blood vessels (vascular disease).

E10.63- Type 1 diabetes mellitus with oral complications

Diabetes mellitus puts the patient at risk for developing periodontal disease and other oral complications.

E10.630 Type 1 diabetes mellitus with periodontal disease

Diabetic patients may be at increased risk for periodontal disease due to capillary damage and decreased wound healing. Periodontal disease begins with inflammation of the gums (gingivitis) that progresses to involve deeper tissues and bone. Periodontal disease occurs when the gum pulls away from the underlying teeth leaving pockets where bacteria collect. The bacteria in the pockets prompt an immune system response to fight the infection. However, the enzymes created by the immune system to destroy the bacteria instead act with the toxins produced by the bacteria and end up destroying the connective tissue and bone around the teeth. Periodontal disease seen in diabetics may be acute or chronic. Chronic periodontitis signifies the progression of the inflammatory disease of the bony and ligamentous supporting tissues of the teeth over time as a result of failure to treat the disease in the acute stage. Patients with severe and widespread chronic periodontitis have a high risk for tooth loss.

E10.64- Type 1 diabetes mellitus with hypoglycemia

Hypoglycemia refers to low blood sugar levels, typically defined as less than 70 mg/dl. When diabetic patients experience hypoglycemia, it is typically a complication of insulin or oral therapy diabetic treatment. Issues arise from an inadequate supply of glucose to the brain, resulting in impairment of function or neuroglycopenia. Effects can range from mild dysphoria to more serious issues such as seizures or unconsciousness. Diabetes mellitus complicated by hypoglycemia is differentiated as with or without coma.

E10.65 Type 1 diabetes mellitus with hyperglycemia

Hyperglycemia in diabetes mellitus refers to blood glucose (sugar) levels that are too high. High blood glucose levels in diabetes mellitus are indicative of inadequate or poorly controlled diabetes.

E11.- Type 2 diabetes mellitus

Type 2 diabetes mellitus is a systemic disease whose causes are multifactorial. It comprises between 90 to 95 percent of diabetes cases in the United States, and while the pancreas of a Type 2 diabetic produces insulin, the insulin secreted is not enough or the body is unable to recognize the insulin and use it properly (insulin resistance).

E11.0- Type 2 diabetes mellitus with hyperosmolarity

Hyperosmolarity, also known as hyperosmolar hyperglycemic state (HHS) and hyperosmolar hyperglycemic nonketotic syndrome (HHNS), is caused by extremely high levels of glucose in the blood. Typically HHS is seen in older diabetics with a precipitating illness or infection. It is a potentially life-threatening complication. The extremely high blood glucose levels trigger a hyperosmolar response in which the body tries to filter the glucose from the blood by drawing fluid from the body into the kidneys so that the sugar can be excreted in the urine. However, this can cause severe dehydration that can result in coma and death. HHS is classified as with or without nonketotic hyperglycemic-hyperosmolar coma (NKHHC).

E11.1- Type 2 diabetes mellitus with ketoacidosis

Diabetic ketoacidosis (DKA) is a potentially life-threatening complication due to a shortage of insulin in which the body switches to burning fatty acids and producing acidic ketone bodies that cause most of the symptoms and complications. DKA may be complicated by coma.

E11.2- Type 2 diabetes mellitus with kidney complications

The two most common kidney complications associated with diabetes mellitus are diabetic nephropathy and diabetic chronic kidney disease.

E11.21 Type 2 diabetes mellitus with diabetic nephropathy

Diabetic nephropathy is a progressive kidney disease caused by angiopathy of capillaries in the kidney glomeruli where the blood is filtered. It is a prime indicator for kidney dialysis and/or kidney transplant.

E11.22 Type 2 diabetes mellitus with diabetic chronic kidney disease

Generally, diabetic chronic kidney disease indicates kidney damage related to long-standing glomeruli damage, typically manifested by proteinuria, hypertension, and edema. CKD is classified in stages, from 1 to 5 and end stage renal disease (ESRD).

E11.3- Type 2 diabetes mellitus with ophthalmic complications

Complications of diabetes mellitus affecting the eye include diabetic retinopathy with or without macular edema and diabetic cataract.

E11.311 Type 2 diabetes mellitus with unspecified diabetic retinopathy with macular edema

E11.319 Type 2 diabetes mellitus with unspecified diabetic retinopathy without macular edema

E11.321- Type 2 diabetes mellitus with mild nonproliferative diabetic retinopathy with macular edema

E11.329- Type 2 diabetes mellitus with mild nonproliferative diabetic retinopathy without macular edema

E11.331- Type 2 diabetes mellitus with moderate nonproliferative diabetic retinopathy with macular edema

E11.339- Type 2 diabetes mellitus with moderate nonproliferative diabetic retinopathy without macular edema

E11.341- Type 2 diabetes mellitus with severe nonproliferative diabetic retinopathy with macular edema

E11.349- Type 2 diabetes mellitus with severe nonproliferative diabetic retinopathy without macular edema

Diabetic retinopathy is a common complication of diabetes affecting the vasculature of the retina. Leakage and scar tissue from damaged retinal blood vessels distort and blur vision. Diabetic retinopathy is the third most common cause of legal blindness in adults in the United States. Nonproliferative diabetic retinopathy describes the early stage of the disease. In the nonproliferative stage, microaneurysm formation, hemorrhages, and blind spots are characteristic. As the disease progresses, more vessel leakage occurs. The disease progresses from mild to moderate to severe nonproliferative retinopathy as follows: mild nonproliferative diabetic retinopathy is characterized by microaneurysm formation with small, balloon-like swelling of retinal vessels; moderate nonproliferative diabetic retinopathy is characterized by microaneurysms becoming more pronounced with some vessel blockage occurring; severe nonproliferative diabetic retinopathy is characterized by vascular breakdown within the retina resulting in multiple blockages and numerous intraretinal hemorrhages in different quadrants. Nonproliferative diabetic retinopathy may be complicated by macular edema. Macular edema occurs when damaged blood vessels leak fluid and lipids onto the macula, the part of the retina that allows detail recognition. The fluid makes the macula swell, which blurs vision.

E11.35- Type 2 diabetes mellitus with proliferative diabetic retinopathy

Diabetic retinopathy is a common complication of diabetes affecting the vasculature of the retina. Leakage and scar tissue from damaged retinal blood vessels distort and blur vision. Diabetic retinopathy is the third most common cause of legal blindness in adults in the United States. In the first stages of diabetic retinopathy, nonproliferative changes occur; however, eventually the condition progresses to the proliferative stage in which new blood vessels proliferate. The lack of oxygen in the retina causes fragile, new blood vessels to grow along the retina and in the clear, gel-like vitreous humor that fills the inside of the eye. Without timely treatment, these new blood vessels can bleed, cloud vision, and destroy the retina.

E11.351- Type 2 diabetes mellitus with proliferative diabetic retinopathy with macular edema

Proliferative diabetic retinopathy may be complicated by macular edema. Macular edema occurs when damaged blood vessels leak fluid and lipids onto the macula, the part of the retina that allows detail recognition. The fluid makes the macula swell, which blurs vision.

E11.352- Type 2 diabetes mellitus with proliferative diabetic retinopathy with traction retinal detachment involving the macula

E11.353- Type 2 diabetes mellitus with proliferative diabetic retinopathy with traction retinal detachment not involving the macula

E11.354- Type 2 diabetes mellitus with proliferative diabetic retinopathy with combined traction retinal detachment and rhegmatogenous retinal detachment

Retinal detachment is the separation of what is known as the sensory retina from the retinal pigment epithelium (RPE). The RPE performs two primary functions: it keeps fluid from accumulating in the subretinal space, and it supplies nutrients to the retina.

The two most common forms of retinal detachment are rhegmatogenous retinal detachment and traction retinal detachment. In proliferative diabetic retinopathy, the proliferation of blood vessels within the retina and vitreous causes undue traction on these ocular layers. When the eye moves, the vessels pull on the retina causing it to either tear or detach from the RPE layer. Traction that causes a tear in the retina, allowing fluid from the vitreous to accumulate between the retina and the RPE, is known as rhegmatogenous retinal detachment. Traction that does not cause an actual tear in the retina and instead only separates the retina away from the RPE is considered traction retinal detachment. The types and success of treatment and the extent of vision loss are proportionate to the extent of the retinal detachment. Those retinal detachments that involve the macula are the most severe, and although treatment can correct some of the visual loss, full recovery of the patient's vision is rare.

E11.355- Type 2 diabetes mellitus with stable proliferative diabetic retinopathy

Vitrectomies, laser treatments, or intravitreal antivascular endothelial growth factor therapies are all current treatment options for proliferative diabetic retinopathy and/or its associated complications. When a patient's condition has quieted following any of these treatments, it is considered stable, allowing for greater intervals between follow-up visits.

E11.359- Type 2 diabetes mellitus with proliferative diabetic retinopathy without macular edema

In some cases, a patient may have the proliferative form of diabetic retinopathy, characterized by extensive growth of new blood vessels along the retina and in the clear, gel-like vitreous humor that fills the inside of the eye without swelling of macular tissues.

E11.36 Type 2 diabetes mellitus with diabetic cataract

As a result of a chemical imbalance and an intracellular accumulation of sorbitol, diabetic patients are at high risk of developing cataracts and also have a higher risk of complications after phacoemulsification cataract surgery compared to nondiabetics.

E11.37- Type 2 diabetes mellitus with diabetic macular edema, resolved following treatment

Several modalities are available to treat diabetic macular edema, including different forms of laser photocoagulation, corticosteroids, anti-VEGF (vascular endothelial growth factor) therapy, and vitrectomy. While these methods have successfully resolved macular edema in some patients, they also carry a risk of complications like cataracts, hypertension, and scar tissue formation.

E11.39 Type 2 diabetes mellitus with other diabetic ophthalmic complication

Diabetic glaucoma is reported with this code. Glaucoma is the failure of fluid in the eye to drain properly causing increased intraocular pressure that can result in damage to the optic nerve. When the optic nerve is damaged, vision becomes impaired; untreated glaucoma can lead to blindness.

E11.4- Type 2 diabetes mellitus with neurological complications

Diabetic neuropathy is a condition thought to be due to microvascular injury involving small blood vessels that supply nourishment to the nerves. It may affect all peripheral nerves including pain fibers, motor neurons, and the autonomic nervous system.

E11.41 Type 2 diabetes mellitus with diabetic mononeuropathy

Diabetic mononeuropathy involves sudden onset damage to a single large nerve that may be due to infarction or other problems. Common manifestations of mononeuropathy include a wrist or foot drop, cranial nerve palsy, or a recurrent laryngeal nerve problem.

E11.42 Type 2 diabetes mellitus with diabetic polyneuropathy

In diabetic polyneuropathy, decreased sensation and loss of reflexes occur first in the toes on each foot. As the disease progresses, the symptoms extend upward to involve the feet, lower legs, and finally the upper legs. The nerve damage eventually affects the fingers, hands, and arms as well. Patients with this condition cannot feel pain or other symptoms indicative of injury or complications and are consequently at high risk for ulcers and infections primarily affecting the legs and feet; the arms may be affected as well.

E11.43 Type 2 diabetes mellitus with diabetic autonomic (poly)neuropathy

Autonomic neuropathy affects nerves of the autonomic body systems, such as the heart, lungs, blood vessels, bone, and gastrointestinal and genitourinary systems. One of the most commonly recognized autonomic dysfunctions in diabetics is orthostatic hypotension or fainting when standing up. Symptoms of autonomic neuropathy affecting the heart and vascular system can range from mild to life-threatening, such as those related to the heart and arteries failing to appropriately adjust the heartrate and vascular tone to keep blood continually and fully flowing to the brain. Another common diabetic autonomic neuropathy complication is diabetic gastroparesis. Gastroparesis results from damage to the vagus nerve, which controls the movement of food in the stomach and intestine. When vagus nerve damage occurs, the muscles of the stomach and digestive system cannot move food effectively along the digestive tract causing delayed emptying or an inability to empty the stomach contents. When food does not move along the digestive tract bacterial overgrowth occurs causing bloating. A more serious complication of diabetic gastroparesis is the formation of hard masses of partially digested food called bezoars that can create stomach or intestinal obstructions.

E11.44 Type 2 diabetes mellitus with diabetic amyotrophy

Diabetic amyotrophy, also called radiculoplexus neuropathy, femoral neuropathy, or proximal neuropathy, occurs when there is damage to the nerves of the thigh, hips, buttocks, and upper legs. Common symptoms include weakness followed by wasting of pelvic and femoral muscles, unilaterally or bilaterally, with associated pain. Sensory nerve damage (neuropathy) may also be present.

E11.5- Type 2 diabetes mellitus with circulatory complications

Diabetes mellitus increases the risk of developing circulatory complications with the most common type being peripheral angiopathy.

E11.51 Type 2 diabetes mellitus with diabetic peripheral angiopathy without gangrene

E11.52 Type 2 diabetes mellitus with diabetic peripheral angiopathy with gangrene

There are two types of angiopathy: microangiopathy, which is a vascular malfunction due to hyperglycemia found in diabetes; and macroangiopathy, which is caused by diabetic conditions of insulin resistance and metabolic syndrome. In microangiopathy, walls of the smaller blood vessels become so thick and weak that they bleed, leak protein, and slow the flow of blood through the body. The decrease of blood flow through stenosis or clot formation impairs the flow of oxygen to cells and biological tissues and leads to cellular death and gangrene. For macroangiopathy, atherosclerosis and a resultant blood clot forms on the large blood vessels, sticks to the vessel walls, and blocks the flow of blood. Gangrene refers to dead or dying body tissue caused by inadequate blood supply. Dry gangrene typically results from conditions that reduce or block arterial blood flow such as diabetes.

E11.6- Type 2 diabetes mellitus with other specified complications

Complications of diabetes mellitus that affect the joints, skin, and other sites are included here.

E11.61- Type 2 diabetes mellitus with diabetic arthropathy

Diabetic arthropathy may be neuropathic or due to another disease process.

E11.610 Type 2 diabetes mellitus with diabetic neuropathic arthropathy

Neuropathic arthropathy, also called Charcot's joint, involves progressive degeneration of a weight-bearing joint, a process marked by bony destruction, bone resorption, and eventual deformity.

E11.618 Type 2 diabetes mellitus with other diabetic arthropathy

Diabetics are more likely to develop other types of arthropathy characterized by pain, inflammation, and articular cartilage damage to the joints.

E11.62- Type 2 diabetes mellitus with skin complications

Diabetics are at risk of developing various skin complications, including skin inflammation (dermatitis) and skin and soft tissue ulcers.

E11.620 Type 2 diabetes mellitus with diabetic dermatitis

One inflammatory skin condition affecting diabetics is necrobiosis lipoidica diabeticorum, which is a necrotizing skin condition that most frequently appears on the patient's shins, often on both legs. The lesions are often asymptomatic but may become tender and ulcerate when injured.

E11.621 Type 2 diabetes mellitus with foot ulcer

E11.622 Type 2 diabetes mellitus with other skin ulcer

The majority of diabetic skin ulcers occur on the feet and lower legs and are due to one of two major underlying causes: damaged nerves and diseased blood vessels (vascular disease).

E11.63- Type 2 diabetes mellitus with oral complications

Diabetes mellitus puts the patient at risk for developing periodontal disease and other oral complications.

E11.630 Type 2 diabetes mellitus with periodontal disease

Diabetic patients may be at increased risk for periodontal disease due to capillary damage and decreased wound healing. Periodontal disease begins with inflammation of the gums (gingivitis) that progresses to involve deeper tissues and bone. Periodontal disease occurs when the gum pulls away from the underlying teeth leaving pockets where bacteria collect. The bacteria in the pockets prompt an immune system response to fight the infection. However, the enzymes created by the immune system to destroy the bacteria instead act with the toxins produced by the bacteria and end up destroying the connective tissue and bone around the teeth. Periodontal disease seen in diabetics may be acute or chronic. Chronic periodontitis signifies the progression of the inflammatory disease of the bony and ligamentous supporting tissues of the teeth over time as a result of failure to treat the disease in the acute stage. Patients with severe and widespread chronic periodontitis have a high risk for tooth loss.

E11.64- Type 2 diabetes mellitus with hypoglycemia

Hypoglycemia refers to low blood sugar levels, typically defined as less than 70 mg/dl. When diabetic patients experience hypoglycemia, it is typically a complication of insulin or oral therapy diabetic treatment. Issues arise from an inadequate supply of glucose to the brain, resulting in impairment of function or neuroglycopenia. Effects can range from mild dysphoria to more serious issues such as seizures or unconsciousness. Diabetes mellitus complicated by hypoglycemia is differentiated as with or without coma.

E11.65 Type 2 diabetes mellitus with hyperglycemia

Hyperglycemia in diabetes mellitus refers to blood glucose (sugar) levels that are too high. High blood glucose levels in diabetes mellitus are indicative of inadequate or poorly controlled diabetes.

E13.- Other specified diabetes mellitus

Some types of diabetes mellitus are due to other rare conditions, such as those related to genetic defects of beta-cell function or to genetic insulin action disorders. In addition, some patients develop diabetes after a pancreatectomy or other procedure.

E13.0-   Other specified diabetes mellitus with hyperosmolarity

Hyperosmolarity, also known as hyperosmolar hyperglycemic state (HHS) and hyperosmolar hyperglycemic nonketotic syndrome (HHNS), is caused by extremely high levels of glucose in the blood. Typically HHS is seen in older diabetics with a precipitating illness or infection. It is a potentially life-threatening complication. The extremely high blood glucose levels trigger a hyperosmolar response in which the body tries to filter the glucose from the blood by drawing fluid from the body into the kidneys so that the sugar can be excreted in the urine. However, this can cause severe dehydration that can result in coma and death. HHS is classified as with or without nonketotic hyperglycemic-hyperosmolar coma (NKHHC).

E13.1-   Other specified diabetes mellitus with ketoacidosis

Diabetic ketoacidosis (DKA) is a potentially life-threatening complication due to a shortage of insulin in which the body switches to burning fatty acids and producing acidic ketone bodies that cause most of the symptoms and complications. DKA may occur with or without coma.

E13.2-   Other specified diabetes mellitus with kidney complications

The two most common kidney complications associated with diabetes mellitus are diabetic nephropathy and diabetic chronic kidney disease.

E13.21   Other specified diabetes mellitus with diabetic nephropathy

Diabetic nephropathy is a progressive kidney disease caused by angiopathy of capillaries in the kidney glomeruli, where the blood is filtered. It is a prime indicator for kidney dialysis and/or kidney transplant.

E13.22   Other specified diabetes mellitus with diabetic chronic kidney disease

Generally, diabetic chronic kidney disease indicates kidney damage related to long-standing glomeruli damage, typically manifested by proteinuria, hypertension, and edema. CKD is classified in stages, from 1 to 5 and end stage renal disease (ESRD).

E13.3-   Other specified diabetes mellitus with ophthalmic complications

Complications of diabetes mellitus affecting the eye include diabetic retinopathy with or without macular edema and diabetic cataract.

E13.311   Other specified diabetes mellitus with unspecified diabetic retinopathy with macular edema

E13.319   Other specified diabetes mellitus with unspecified diabetic retinopathy without macular edema

E13.321- Other specified diabetes mellitus with mild nonproliferative diabetic retinopathy with macular edema

E13.329- Other specified diabetes mellitus with mild nonproliferative diabetic retinopathy without macular edema

E13.331- Other specified diabetes mellitus with moderate nonproliferative diabetic retinopathy with macular edema

E13.339- Other specified diabetes mellitus with moderate nonproliferative diabetic retinopathy without macular edema

E13.341- Other specified diabetes mellitus with severe nonproliferative diabetic retinopathy with macular edema

E13.349- Other specified diabetes mellitus with severe nonproliferative diabetic retinopathy without macular edema

Diabetic retinopathy is a common complication of diabetes affecting the vasculature of the retina. Leakage and scar tissue from damaged retinal blood vessels distort and blur vision. Diabetic retinopathy is the third most common cause of legal blindness in adults in the United States. Nonproliferative diabetic retinopathy describes the early stage of the disease. In the nonproliferative stage, microaneurysm formation, hemorrhages, and blind spots are characteristic. As the disease progresses, more vessel leakage occurs. The disease progresses from mild to moderate to severe nonproliferative retinopathy as follows: mild nonproliferative diabetic retinopathy is characterized by microaneurysm formation with small, balloon-like swelling of retinal vessels; moderate nonproliferative diabetic retinopathy is characterized by microaneurysms becoming more pronounced with some vessel blockage occurring; severe nonproliferative diabetic retinopathy is characterized by vascular breakdown within the retina resulting in multiple blockages and numerous intraretinal hemorrhages in different quadrants. Nonproliferative diabetic retinopathy may be complicated by macular edema. Macular edema occurs when damaged vessels leak fluid and lipids onto the macula, the part of the retina that allows detail recognition. The fluid makes the macula swell, which blurs vision.

E13.35- Other specified diabetes mellitus with proliferative diabetic retinopathy

Diabetic retinopathy is a common complication of diabetes affecting the vasculature of the retina. Leakage and scar tissue from damaged retinal blood vessels distort and blur vision. Diabetic retinopathy is the third most common cause of legal blindness in adults in the United States. In the first stages of diabetic retinopathy, nonproliferative changes occur; however, eventually the condition progresses to the proliferative stage in which new blood vessels proliferate. The lack of oxygen in the retina causes fragile, new blood vessels to grow along the retina and in the clear, gel-like vitreous humor that fills the inside of the eye. Without timely treatment, these new blood vessels can bleed, cloud vision, and destroy the retina.

E13.351- Other specified diabetes mellitus with proliferative diabetic retinopathy with macular edema

Proliferative diabetic retinopathy may be complicated by macular edema. Macular edema occurs when damaged blood vessels leak fluid and lipids onto the macula, the part of the retina that allows detail recognition. The fluid makes the macula swell, which blurs vision.

E13.352- Other specified diabetes mellitus with proliferative diabetic retinopathy with traction retinal detachment involving the macula

E13.353- Other specified diabetes mellitus with proliferative diabetic retinopathy with traction retinal detachment not involving the macula

E13.354- Other specified diabetes mellitus with proliferative diabetic retinopathy with combined traction retinal detachment and rhegmatogenous retinal detachment

Retinal detachment is the separation of what is known as the sensory retina from the retinal pigment epithelium (RPE). The RPE performs two primary functions: it keeps fluid from accumulating in the subretinal space, and it supplies nutrients to the retina.

The two most common forms of retinal detachment are rhegmatogenous retinal detachment and traction retinal detachment. In proliferative diabetic retinopathy, the proliferation of blood vessels within the retina and vitreous causes undue traction on these ocular layers. When the eye moves, the vessels pull on the retina causing it to either tear or detach from the RPE layer. Traction that causes a tear in the retina, allowing fluid from the vitreous to accumulate between the retina and the RPE, is known as rhegmatogenous retinal detachment. Traction that does not cause an actual tear in the retina and instead only separates the retina away from the RPE is

considered traction retinal detachment. The types and success of treatment and the extent of vision loss are proportionate to the extent of the retinal detachment. Those retinal detachments that involve the macula are the most severe, and although treatment can correct some of the visual loss, full recovery of the patient's vision is rare.

E13.355- Other specified diabetes mellitus with stable proliferative diabetic retinopathy

Vitrectomies, laser treatments, or intravitreal anti-vascular endothelial growth factor therapies are all currently used treatment options for proliferative diabetic retinopathy and/or its associated complications. When a patient's condition has quietened following any of these treatments, it is considered stable allowing for greater intervals between follow-up visits.

E13.359- Other specified diabetes mellitus with proliferative diabetic retinopathy without macular edema

In some cases, a patient may have the proliferative form of diabetic retinopathy, characterized by extensive growth of new blood vessels along the retina and in the clear, gel-like vitreous humor that fills the inside of the eye without swelling of macular tissues.

E13.36 Other specified diabetes mellitus with diabetic cataract

As a result of a chemical imbalance and an intracellular accumulation of sorbitol, diabetic patients are at high risk of developing cataracts and also have a higher risk of complications after phacoemulsification cataract surgery compared to nondiabetics.

E13.37- Other specified diabetes mellitus with diabetic macular edema, resolved following treatment

Several modalities are available to treat diabetic macular edema, including different forms of laser photocoagulation, corticosteroids, anti-VEGF (vascular endothelial growth factor) therapy, and vitrectomy. While these methods have successfully resolved macular edema in some patients, they also carry a risk of complications like cataracts, hypertension, and scar tissue formation.

E13.39 Other specified diabetes mellitus with other diabetic ophthalmic complication

Diabetic glaucoma is reported with this code. Glaucoma is the failure of fluid in the eye to drain properly causing increased intraocular pressure that can result in damage to the optic nerve. When the optic nerve is damaged, vision becomes impaired; untreated glaucoma can lead to blindness.

E13.4-   Other specified diabetes mellitus with neurological complications

Diabetic neuropathy is a condition thought to be due to microvascular injury involving small blood vessels that supply nourishment to the nerves. It may affect all peripheral nerves including pain fibers, motor neurons, and the autonomic nervous system.

E13.41   Other specified diabetes mellitus with diabetic mononeuropathy

Diabetic mononeuropathy involves sudden onset damage to a single large nerve that may be due to infarction or other problem. Common manifestations of mononeuropathy include a wrist or foot drop, cranial nerve palsy, or a recurrent laryngeal nerve problem.

E13.42   Other specified diabetes mellitus with diabetic polyneuropathy

In diabetic polyneuropathy decreased sensation and loss of reflexes occur first in the toes on each foot. As the disease progresses, the symptoms extend upward to involve the feet, lower legs, and finally the upper legs. The nerve damage eventually affects the fingers, hands, and arms as well. Patients with this condition cannot feel pain or other symptoms indicative of injury or complications and are consequently at high risk for ulcers and infections primarily affecting the legs and feet; the arms may be affected as well.

E13.43   Other specified diabetes mellitus with diabetic autonomic (poly)neuropathy

Autonomic neuropathy affects nerves of the autonomic body systems, such as the heart, lungs, blood vessels, bone, and gastrointestinal and genitourinary systems. One of the most commonly recognized autonomic dysfunctions in diabetics is orthostatic hypotension or fainting when standing up. Symptoms of autonomic neuropathy affecting the heart and vascular system can range from mild to life-threatening, such as those related to the heart and arteries failing to appropriately adjust the heartrate and vascular tone to keep blood continually and fully flowing to the brain. Another common diabetic autonomic neuropathy complication is diabetic gastroparesis. Gastroparesis results from damage to the vagus nerve, which controls the movement of food in the stomach and intestine. When vagus nerve damage occurs, the muscles of the stomach and digestive system cannot move food effectively along the digestive tract causing delayed emptying or an inability to empty the stomach contents. When food does not move along the digestive tract bacterial overgrowth occurs causing bloating. A more serious complication of diabetic gastroparesis is the formation of hard masses of partially digested food called bezoars that can create stomach or intestinal obstructions.

E13.44   Other specified diabetes mellitus with diabetic amyotrophy

Diabetic amyotrophy, also called radiculoplexus neuropathy, femoral neuropathy, or proximal neuropathy, occurs when there is damage to the nerves of the thigh, hips, buttocks, and upper legs. Common symptoms include weakness followed by wasting of pelvic and femoral muscles, unilaterally or bilaterally, with associated pain. Sensory nerve damage (neuropathy) may also be present.

E13.5-   Other specified diabetes mellitus with circulatory complications

Diabetes mellitus increases the risk of developing circulatory complications with the most common type being peripheral angiopathy.

E13.51   Other specified diabetes mellitus with diabetic peripheral angiopathy without gangrene

E13.52   Other specified diabetes mellitus with diabetic peripheral angiopathy with gangrene

There are two types of angiopathy: microangiopathy, which is a vascular malfunction due to hyperglycemia found in diabetes; and macroangiopathy, which is caused by diabetic conditions of insulin resistance and metabolic syndrome. In microangiopathy, walls of the smaller blood vessels become so thick and weak that they bleed, leak protein, and slow the flow of blood through the body. The decrease of blood flow through stenosis or clot formation impairs the flow of oxygen to cells and biological tissues and leads to cellular death and gangrene. For macroangiopathy, atherosclerosis and a resultant blood clot forms on the large blood vessels, sticks to the vessel walls, and blocks the flow of blood. Gangrene refers to dead or dying body tissue caused by inadequate blood supply. Dry gangrene typically results from conditions that reduce or block arterial blood flow such as diabetes.

E13.6-   Other specified diabetes mellitus with other specified complications

Complications of diabetes mellitus that affect the joints, skin, and other sites are included here.

E13.61-   Other specified diabetes mellitus with diabetic arthropathy

Diabetic arthropathy may be neuropathic or due to another disease process.

E13.610   Other specified diabetes mellitus with diabetic neuropathic arthropathy

Neuropathic arthropathy, also called Charcot's joint, involves progressive degeneration of a weight-bearing joint, a process marked by bony destruction, bone resorption, and eventual deformity.

E13.618 Other specified diabetes mellitus with other diabetic arthropathy

Diabetics are more likely to develop other types of arthropathy characterized by pain, inflammation, and articular cartilage damage to the joints.

E13.62- Other specified diabetes mellitus with skin complications

Diabetics are at risk of developing various skin complications, including skin inflammation (dermatitis) and skin and soft tissue ulcers.

E13.620 Other specified diabetes mellitus with diabetic dermatitis

One inflammatory skin condition affecting diabetics is necrobiosis lipoidica diabeticorum, which is a necrotizing skin condition that most frequently appears on the patient's shins, often on both legs. The lesions are often asymptomatic but may become tender and ulcerate when injured.

E13.621 Other specified diabetes mellitus with foot ulcer

E13.622 Other specified diabetes mellitus with other skin ulcer

The majority of diabetic skin ulcers occur on the feet and lower legs and are due to one of two major underlying causes: damaged nerves and diseased blood vessels (vascular disease).

E13.63- Other specified diabetes mellitus with oral complications

Diabetes mellitus puts the patient at risk for developing periodontal disease and other oral complications.

E13.630 Other specified diabetes mellitus with periodontal disease

Diabetic patients may be at increased risk for periodontal disease due to capillary damage and decreased wound healing. Periodontal disease begins with inflammation of the gums (gingivitis) that progresses to involve deeper tissues and bone. Periodontal disease occurs when the gum pulls away from the underlying teeth leaving pockets where bacteria collect. The bacteria in the pockets prompt an immune system response to fight the infection. However, the enzymes created by the immune system to destroy the bacteria instead act with the toxins produced by the bacteria and end up destroying the connective tissue and bone around the teeth. Periodontal disease seen in diabetics may be acute or chronic. Chronic periodontitis signifies the progression of the inflammatory disease of the bony and ligamentous supporting tissues of the teeth over time as a result of failure to treat the disease in the acute stage. Patients with severe and widespread chronic periodontitis have a high risk for tooth loss.

E13.64- Other specified diabetes mellitus with hypoglycemia

Hypoglycemia refers to low blood sugar levels, typically defined as less than 70 mg/dl. When diabetic patients experience hypoglycemia, it is typically a complication of insulin or oral therapy diabetic treatment. Issues arise from an inadequate supply of glucose to the brain, resulting in impairment of function or neuroglycopenia. Effects can range from mild dysphoria to more serious issues such as seizures or unconsciousness. Diabetes mellitus complicated by hypoglycemia is differentiated as with or without coma.

E13.65 Other specified diabetes mellitus with hyperglycemia

Hyperglycemia in diabetes mellitus refers to blood glucose (sugar) levels that are too high. High blood glucose levels in diabetes mellitus are indicative of inadequate or poorly controlled diabetes.

Other Disorders of Glucose Regulation and Pancreatic Internal Secretion (E15-E16)

Insulin causes cells in the liver, skeletal muscles, and fat tissue to take up glucose from the blood. In the liver and skeletal muscles, glucose is stored as glycogen, and in fat cells (adipocytes) it is stored as triglycerides. Any disorder affecting this production and secretion can have far-reaching effects in the endocrine and other body systems.

The categories in this code block are as follows:

E15   Nondiabetic hypoglycemic coma

E16   Other disorders of pancreatic internal secretion

E15   Nondiabetic hypoglycemic coma

Hypoglycemia is an abnormally diminished content of glucose in the blood that may occur in a nondiabetic patient as a result of excessive insulin produced in the body (hyperinsulinemia), inborn error of metabolism, medications and poisons, alcohol, hormone deficiencies, prolonged starvation, alterations of metabolism associated with infection, or organ failure. Prolonged extreme hypoglycemia may lead to stupor and coma.

E16.-   Other disorders of pancreatic internal secretion

Hypoglycemia secondary to medications or due to other causes is included here, along with other increased secretion of glucagon, gastrin, and other hormones secreted by the pancreas.

E16.0 Drug-induced hypoglycemia without coma

This condition is defined as low blood sugar that results from medication, particularly if in combination with other activities such as alcohol consumption, excessive physical activity, or missing meals or from intentional or unintentional overdose of diabetes medications.

E16.3 Increased secretion of glucagon

Glucagon is a peptide hormone secreted by the pancreas that raises blood glucose levels. Its effect is opposite that of insulin, which lowers blood glucose levels. The pancreas releases glucagon when glucose levels fall too low. Glucagon causes the liver to convert stored glycogen into glucose, which is then released into the bloodstream.

E16.4 Increased secretion of gastrin

Gastrin is a peptide hormone that stimulates secretion of gastric acid (HCl) by the parietal cells of the stomach and aids in gastric motility. In Zollinger-Ellison syndrome, gastrin is produced at excessive levels, often by a gastrinoma (gastrin-producing tumor, mostly benign) of the duodenum or the pancreas.

Disorders of Other Endocrine Glands (E20-E36)

This section of ICD-10-CM includes the classification of the following endocrine glands: parathyroid, pituitary, adrenal, thymus, ovaries, and testes.

The parathyroid glands are four pea-sized glands located at the four corners of the thyroid gland. They secrete the parathyroid hormone, which regulates the level of calcium in the blood.

The pituitary gland has two lobes that secrete hormones that regulate a variety of functions, including those related to the regulation of the thyroid and adrenal and reproductive glands and those related to water balance control within the body.

The adrenal glands are located on the kidneys and are divided into two sections. The adrenal cortex produces corticosteroids, which help regulate metabolic rates, salt and water balance, and interact with the immune system. The adrenal medulla produces catecholamines, such as epinephrine or adrenaline, which increase the blood pressure and heartrate during times of stress.

The thymus is located in the anterior superior mediastinum, and is comprised of lymphatic and epithelial tissue. It processes white blood cells (WBCs), which kill foreign cells and stimulates other immune cells to produce antibodies.

The ovaries are the female gonads that secrete sex hormones in response to the pituitary gland. Besides producing eggs, the ovaries produce estrogen and progesterone, two hormones that regulate development of the reproductive organs, female sex characteristics, menstruation, and pregnancy.

The testes (testicles) are the male gonads and produce and secrete testosterone. This hormone regulates development of the reproductive organs, male secondary sex characteristics, and muscle.

The categories in this code block are as follows:

E20	Hypoparathyroidism
E21	Hyperparathyroidism and other disorders of parathyroid gland
E22	Hyperfunction of pituitary gland
E23	Hypofunction and other disorders of the pituitary gland
E24	Cushing's syndrome
E25	Adrenogenital disorders
E26	Hyperaldosteronism
E27	Other disorders of adrenal gland
E28	Ovarian dysfunction
E29	Testicular dysfunction
E30	Disorders of puberty, not elsewhere classified
E31	Polyglandular dysfunction
E32	Diseases of thymus
E34	Other endocrine disorders
E35	Disorders of endocrine glands in diseases classified elsewhere

E20.- Hypoparathyroidism

Hypoparathyroidism is a disorder in which there is not enough parathyroid hormone (PTH) secreted from one or more of the parathyroid glands, which are four pea-sized glands located at the four corners of the thyroid gland. The parathyroid hormone regulates the level of calcium in the blood. In hypoparathyroidism, blood calcium levels fall and phosphorus levels rise. The most common cause of hypoparathyroidism is injury to the parathyroid glands during thyroid and neck surgery, but the condition may also be due to low blood magnesium levels or metabolic alkalosis.

> **Focus Point**
>
> *The code for postprocedural hypoparathyroidism is located later in this chapter at code E89.2. Familial hypoparathyroidism is located at E20.8 Other hypoparathyroidism.*

E20.0 Idiopathic hypoparathyroidism

This condition is one of the rarer abnormalities of endocrine function in childhood. It may be documented as autoimmune hypoparathyroidism and is typically diagnosed in the first 10 years of life. Hypocalcemia is the most serious effect and must be treated before the condition progresses to cardiac involvement.

E20.1 Pseudohypoparathyroidism

Pseudohypoparathyroidism is a genetic disorder in which the body fails to respond to parathyroid hormone (PTH) even though the parathyroid glands secrete it. The three types of pseudohypoparathyroidism are Type Ia, Type Ib, and Type II; all three are rare. The three variants are characterized by decreased levels of calcium in the blood, increased levels of phosphates, and increased levels of serum PTH with a lack of response to PTH. Pseudohypoparathyroidism causes developmental and musculoskeletal defects, including short stature, shortened bones of the hands and feet, and soft tissue calcifications and ossifications. Other characteristics include a rounded face, obesity, and dental anomalies.

E21.- Hyperparathyroidism and other disorders of parathyroid gland

Hyperparathyroidism is as an excessive secretion of the parathyroid hormone (PTH) from one or more of the parathyroid glands, which are four pea-sized glands located at the four corners of the thyroid gland. The parathyroid hormone regulates the level of calcium in the blood. When calcium levels are too low, the body responds by making more parathyroid hormone. This hormone causes calcium levels in the blood to rise, as more calcium is taken from the bone and reabsorbed by the intestines and kidney.

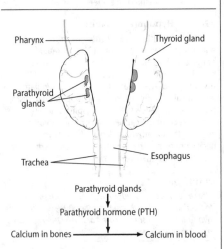

Pharynx

Thyroid gland

Parathyroid glands

Trachea

Esophagus

Parathyroid glands
↓
Parathyroid hormone (PTH)

Calcium in bones ⟶ Calcium in blood

E21.0 Primary hyperparathyroidism

The primary form of hyperparathyroidism is due to an inborn overproduction or oversecretion of parathyroid hormone (PTH). Von Recklinghausen's disease is classified here, which includes fibrous degeneration, cyst formation, and fibrous nodules in bone, due to hyperparathyroidism.

E21.1 Secondary hyperparathyroidism, not elsewhere classified

The secondary form of hyperparathyroidism reported with this code is a result of another disease that is not classified to a more specific code.

E21.2 Other hyperparathyroidism

Tertiary hyperparathyroidism is classified here and is usually seen in patients who have undergone a kidney transplant for renal failure. Instead of the parathyroid gland function returning to normal after the kidney transplant, the parathyroid glands fail to respond to the normal signals for PTH secretion and regulation of calcium levels.

E22.- Hyperfunction of pituitary gland

The pituitary gland has two lobes, anterior and posterior, that provide a variety of functions, including those related to the regulation of the thyroid and adrenal and reproductive glands and those related to water balance control within the body. Hyperfunction of this gland can cause various disorders and may require different treatments. The most common cause of pituitary hyperfunction is a pituitary adenoma.

E22.0 Acromegaly and pituitary gigantism

Pituitary gigantism is a rare condition in growing children due to growth hormone (GH) excess. When the hormone excess occurs before fusion of the epiphyseal growth plates, elevated levels of serum GH and IGF-I cause rapid, excessive linear growth and, if unchecked, extremely tall adult stature. Acromegaly patients have the same hormone excess but when it occurs in adults, although there is no change in stature, certain bones may increase in size, particularly the bones in the hands, feet, and face.

E22.1 Hyperprolactinemia

This condition is characterized by excess secretion of the hormone prolactin, the hormone responsible for milk production in a woman's breasts. Potential causes include a prolactin-secreting tumor (prolactinoma), pregnancy, or the use of numerous medications, particularly psychiatric medications or to a large pituitary tumor that compresses the rest of the gland.

E22.2 Syndrome of inappropriate secretion of antidiuretic hormone

This condition is characterized by the hyponatremia and hypoosmolality that result from an inappropriate, continued secretion or action of the antidiuretic hormone despite normal or increased plasma volume, which results in impaired water excretion. An important clinical indicator of this syndrome is that the hyponatremia is a result of an excess of water rather than a deficiency of sodium.

E23.- Hypofunction and other disorders of the pituitary gland

As a two-sectioned gland, the pituitary's anterior and posterior lobes provide a variety of functions, including those related to the regulation of the thyroid and adrenal and reproductive glands and those related to water balance control within the body. Hypofunction of this gland can cause various disorders and may require different treatments. Underlying causes of pituitary hypofunction relate to dysfunction of the pituitary itself and/or to the hypothalamus gland. Conditions are classified to this category whether they are related to pituitary or hypothalamus disorders.

E23.0 Hypopituitarism

Hypopituitarism is a condition in which the pituitary gland does not produce normal amounts of some or all of its hormones, which may include one or more of the following:

- Adrenocorticotropic hormone (ACTH): Stimulates the adrenal gland to release cortisol; cortisol helps to maintain blood pressure and blood sugar

- Antidiuretic hormone (ADH): Controls water loss by the kidneys

- Follicle stimulating hormone (FSH): Controls sexual function and fertility in males and females

- Growth hormone (GH): Stimulates growth of tissues and bone

- Luteinizing hormone (LH): Controls sexual function and fertility in males and females

- Oxytocin: Stimulates the uterus to contract during labor and the breasts to release milk

- Prolactin: Stimulates female breast development and milk production

- Thyroid stimulating hormone (TSH): Stimulates the thyroid gland to release hormones that affect the body's metabolism.

E23.1 Drug-induced hypopituitarism

Assign an additional code from category range T36-T50 with 5th or 6th character 5 when the drug causing the condition is specified.

E23.2 Diabetes insipidus

Diabetes insipidus (DI) is the passage of large volumes of diluted urine due to a decreased secretion of antidiuretic hormone (ADH), which results in polyuria and polydipsia by diminishing the person's ability to concentrate urine. It is also known as central diabetes insipidus.

E24.- Cushing's syndrome

Cushing's syndrome is a rare disorder that results from too much of the hormone cortisol. If not treated adequately, it can lead to serious problems, such as diabetes, high blood pressure, depression, and osteoporosis. Common indicators of Cushing's disease are a fatty hump between the shoulders, a round (moon) face, or pink stretch marks on the skin.

E24.0 Pituitary-dependent Cushing's disease

The underlying cause of this disorder is typically a pituitary adenoma, which causes the gland to create an abnormally large amount of pituitary adrenocorticotropic hormone (ACTH). In turn, the ACTH hormone causes overproduction of cortisol.

E24.1 Nelson's syndrome

Nelson syndrome refers to a spectrum of signs and symptoms arising from an adrenocorticotropin (ACTH)–secreting pituitary macroadenoma after a therapeutic bilateral adrenalectomy.

E24.2 Drug-induced Cushing's syndrome

Drug-induced Cushing's syndrome may be caused by long-term use of corticosteroid medications.

E24.3 Ectopic ACTH syndrome

This rare syndrome accounts for less than 1 percent of cases of Cushing's syndrome. It involves a tumor lying outside of the pituitary gland that is overproducing ACTH. The most common sites are in the lung and thymus and, more rarely, the thyroid, ovary, adrenal gland, and liver. These ACTH-producing tumors produce too much ACTH and in turn cause the adrenal glands to make too much cortisol.

E24.4 Alcohol-induced pseudo-Cushing's syndrome

This is a disorder with clinical and/or biochemical features similar to those seen in Cushing's syndrome, but these features are related to alcohol abuse. The symptoms may be transient and typically resolve following abstinence from alcohol.

E25.- Adrenogenital disorders

Adrenogenital disorders are a group of conditions caused by a family of autosomal recessive disorders of steroid hormone production in the adrenal glands leading to a deficiency of cortisol, the stress fighting hormone. When the pituitary senses the deficiency, it secretes massive amounts of the stimulating hormone corticotropin to bring the cortisol levels up to normal. This hormone in turn causes the adrenal glands to overproduce certain intermediary hormones which have testosterone-like effects on the fetus and child, leading to so-called "virilization."

Females with adrenogenital disorders have an enlarged clitoris at birth with the urethral opening at the base and ambiguous genitalia. In females, there is also masculinization of features as the child grows, such as deepening of the voice, facial hair, and failure to menstruate or abnormal periods at puberty. However, internal structures of the reproductive tract, including the ovaries, uterus, and fallopian tubes, are normal. In males, genitals are normal at birth, but the child becomes muscular, the penis enlarges, pubic hair appears, and the voice deepens long before normal puberty, sometimes as early as 2 to 3 years of age. At puberty, the testes are small. Treatment is aimed at returning androgen levels to normal. This is usually accomplished through drug therapy, although surgery may be an alternative for children with little or no enzyme activity. Lifelong treatment is required.

E25.Ø   Congenital adrenogenital disorders associated with enzyme deficiency

Deficiency of 21-hydroxylase is classified here. This condition is related to a gene located on the short arm of chromosome 6 and leads to a hyperfunction and increased size (hyperplasia) of the adrenals. In the severe salt-wasting form of CAH, newborns may develop symptoms shortly after birth, including vomiting, dehydration, electrolyte changes, and cardiac arrhythmias. If not treated, this form of CAH can result in death within one to six weeks after birth.

E26.-   Hyperaldosteronism

Hyperaldosteronism is a disease caused by an excess production of the normal adrenal hormone aldosterone. This hormone is responsible for sodium and potassium balance, which then directly controls water balance to maintain appropriate blood pressure and blood volume. Aldosterone also causes the tubules of the kidneys to retain sodium and water, which increases the volume of fluid in the body and drives up blood pressure. Treatment depends on the cause. If bilateral hyperplasia is the cause of hyperaldosteronism, it is treated with specific medications that block the effect of aldosterone.

E26.Ø-   Primary hyperaldosteronism

In primary hyperaldosteronism, the condition is typically due to one of three causes: a tumor of the adrenal gland, usually a benign adrenal adenoma; an inherited condition; or overgrowth of the adrenal glands.

E26.Ø1   Conn's syndrome

When the cause is a single adrenal tumor, this disorder is classified as Conn's syndrome. Surgical removal of the tumor can cure the disease.

E26.Ø2   Glucocorticoid-remediable aldosteronism

This condition is also known as familial hyperaldosteronism Type I. Its unique distinguishing feature is the complete and rapid suppression of aldosterone by exogenous glucocorticoid (dexamethasone) administration.

E26.1   Secondary hyperaldosteronism

In secondary hyperaldosteronism, the excess aldosterone is caused by something outside the adrenal gland that mimics the primary condition. Underlying causes may include cirrhosis of the liver, heart failure, or nephrotic syndrome.

E26.81   Bartter's syndrome

Patients with Bartter's syndrome primarily lose too much sodium through the urine, which causes a rise in the level of aldosterone and causes the kidneys to excrete too much potassium, known as potassium wasting. Other symptoms include high levels of potassium, calcium, and chloride in the urine; high levels of the hormones renin and aldosterone in the blood; low blood chloride; and metabolic alkalosis.

E27.-   Other disorders of adrenal gland

Other disorders of the adrenal gland may involve the adrenal cortex or the adrenal medulla. The adrenal cortex produces corticosteroids that help regulate metabolic rates, salt and water balance, and interact with the immune system. The adrenal medulla produces catecholamines, such as epinephrine or adrenaline, which increase the blood pressure and heartrate during times of stress.

E27.1   Primary adrenocortical insufficiency

This code is assigned for Addison's disease, in which the adrenal glands produce too little cortisol and often insufficient levels of aldosterone as well.

E27.2   Addisonian crisis

Acute Addisonian crisis is a life-threatening condition that occurs when there is not enough cortisol excreted from the adrenal glands. This may be due to injury to the adrenal glands or to the pituitary gland, which controls adrenal hormone secretion. It also may occur when a patient stops hydrocortisone treatment too quickly or too early.

E27.3   Drug-induced adrenocortical insufficiency

Glucocorticoids (such as prednisone, hydrocortisone, and dexamethasone) can slow down the production of adrenal hormones by acting on the pituitary gland, which controls the adrenal glands. If glucocorticoids are stopped or decreased too quickly, the adrenal glands may not begin making cortisol fast enough to meet the body's needs and adrenal insufficiency may result.

E27.5   Adrenomedullary hyperfunction

The adrenal medulla is the inner layer of the adrenal gland, which produces two hormones that are involved in the body's response to stress: epinephrine and norepinephrine. Hyperfunction of the adrenal medulla is most often the result of a medullary tumor, which causes overactivity and production of excess amounts of hormone, resulting in hypertension.

E28.-   Ovarian dysfunction

The ovary secretes female sex hormones in response to the pituitary gland. Besides producing eggs, the ovaries produce the hormones estrogen and progesterone, which regulate development of the reproductive organs, female sex characteristics, menstruation, and pregnancy. Most symptoms of ovarian dysfunction before menopause are related to improper ratios of estrogen as compared with progesterone. Treatment depends upon the specific disorder.

E28.0   Estrogen excess

Estrogen excess can be due to a number of different underlying causes, including an intrinsic hormonal imbalance, but the most common causes of estrogen excess are oral contraceptives and postmenopausal hormone replacement therapy (HRT). Estrogen excess can also be due to adrenal insufficiency with ovarian overcompensation or from liver overload preventing estrogen breakdown.

E28.1   Androgen excess

Androgens, so-called "male" hormones, normally circulate in women's bloodstreams, but excessive levels can cause a variety of symptoms, including acne, weight gain, excessive hair growth (hirsutism), menstrual dysfunction, and infertility.

E28.2   Polycystic ovarian syndrome

Polycystic ovarian syndrome (PCOS) is a common hormonal disorder among women of reproductive age, which involves enlarged ovaries with numerous small cysts located along the outer ovarian edge. One of the major symptoms is increased levels of androgens.

E28.3-   Primary ovarian failure

Primary ovarian failure, also known as premature ovarian failure, may result from premature menopause or it may be due to other conditions such as resistant ovary syndrome.

E28.31-   Premature menopause

Menopause that occurs before the age of 40, whether natural or induced, is classified as premature menopause. When making a diagnosis, the most important test utilized is the lab test that measures follicle stimulating hormone (FSH), which causes the ovaries to produce estrogen. When estrogen levels decrease, the levels of FSH increase, and when these levels rise above 40 mIU/mL, it usually indicates menopause. Premature menopause is classified based on whether or not it is accompanied by symptoms. Some of the more common symptoms include hot flashes, flushing, sleeplessness, headache, lack of concentration, bladder irritability, emotional changes, and vaginal dryness.

E28.39   Other primary ovarian failure

Resistant ovary syndrome is classified here. While the symptoms are the same as those seen in premature menopause, including the cessation of menstruation that may occur with or without systemic menopausal symptoms, the cause is different. In resistant ovary syndrome, the ovary still has a normal supply of eggs, but they are not released because the ovary is not responding to the hormones that would normally trigger development and release of the egg.

E29.-   Testicular dysfunction

The testicles are the male gonads that produce and secrete testosterone. This hormone regulates development of the reproductive organs, male secondary sex characteristics, and muscle. Testicular diseases are typically classified as endocrine disorders or as disorders of the reproductive system.

E29.0   Testicular hyperfunction

This condition is extremely rare and is usually caused by a tumor. Treatment primarily involves treatment of the tumor itself.

E29.1   Testicular hypofunction

Hypofunction typically presents as male infertility and is treated with gonadotrophic hormones.

E30.-   Disorders of puberty, not elsewhere classified

Disorders of pubertal development should be recognized early and correctly diagnosed by a pediatric endocrinologist. Treatment is directed at the acute and long-term consequences of precocious, markedly delayed, or absent pubertal development.

E30.0   Delayed puberty

Delayed puberty is the failure to begin sexual maturation within the expected timeframe. There are wide variations in the age range at which most individuals begin to show evidence of sexual maturation, but most medical references identify age 13 as the age by which secondary sexual characteristics should being to appear. In boys, this is evidenced by lack of testicular development by the age of 13 and in girls it is lack of breast development by age 13 or lack of menstruation by age 16.

E30.1   Precocious puberty

Precocious puberty occurs when secondary sexual characteristics appear earlier than expected. For girls precocious puberty is designated when any of the following develop before age 8: armpit or pubic hair, faster growth, breasts, first period (menstruation), or mature outer genitals. In boys, precocious puberty is when any of the following develop before age 9: armpit or pubic hair, growth of the testes and penis, facial hair, muscle growth, or voice change (deepening). In some cases, the early development may represent a variation of normal development; diagnosis by an endocrinologist should be performed.

E31.-   Polyglandular dysfunction

Polyglandular deficiency syndromes (PDS) are characterized by sequential or simultaneous deficiencies in the function of several endocrine glands that have a common cause. Etiology is typically autoimmune and symptoms depend on the combination of deficiencies. Diagnosis requires measurement of hormone levels and autoantibodies against the affected endocrine glands. Treatment includes replacement of missing or deficient hormones and sometimes immunosuppressant treatment as well.

E31.0   Autoimmune polyglandular failure

Schmidt's syndrome is classified here, which includes adrenal insufficiency, hypo- or hyperthyroidism, and Type 1 diabetes mellitus of autoimmune etiology.

E31.2-   Multiple endocrine neoplasia [MEN] syndromes

Multiple endocrine neoplasia [MEN] syndromes are a group of conditions in which several endocrine glands grow excessively (such as in adenomatous hyperplasia) and/or develop benign or malignant tumors. Tumors and hyperplasia associated with MEN often produce excess hormones, which impede normal physiology. Many of these syndromes are inherited. They can be diagnosed as early as infancy or remain in quiescence until advanced age. Genetic testing is advised for persons with a family history of the disease or conditions that may be associated with MEN.

E31.21   Multiple endocrine neoplasia [MEN] type I

Type I MEN is characterized by tumors of the parathyroid glands, pancreas, or pituitary gland. As a result, hyperparathyroidism, secondary diabetes mellitus, and possibly adrenocorticosteroid abnormalities are common complications. Thyroid and adrenal tumors may coexist. This condition may be documented as Wermer's syndrome.

E31.22   Multiple endocrine neoplasia [MEN] type IIA

Type IIA MEN is closely associated with certain types of medullary thyroid cancer, and pheochromocytomas with resultant hypertension and hyperthyroidism. Adrenal and parathyroid glands can also be affected. Hypercalcemia and kidney stones are common complications. MEN type IIA is inherited in an autosomal dominant fashion, which affects roughly 50 percent of all children of a parent with the defective gene. This condition may be documented as Sipple's syndrome.

E31.23   Multiple endocrine neoplasia [MEN] type IIB

MEN type IIB is similar to MEN type IIA, but with the distinction of the presence of mucosal neuromas. These neuromas present as bumps around the lips, tongue, buccal lining, eyelids, and surfaces of the eyes. As a result, eyelids and lips may appear thickened or hypertrophied. Digestive tract abnormalities are characteristic of MEN type IIB disease and may manifest as constipation or diarrhea. Megacolon is a complication of this abnormal growth and is attributed to intestinal neuromas. Patients may also have spinal abnormalities as well, such as scoliosis. The condition is often diagnosed in infants and has a more rapid growth and progression than type IIA disease. Treatment is directed at the hyperplasia or tumors in each individual gland, along with hormonal injections used to correct hormonal imbalances.

E32.-   Diseases of thymus

Located in the anterior superior mediastinum, the thymus gland is comprised of lymphatic and epithelial tissue. It processes white blood cells (WBC), which kill foreign cells and stimulates other immune cells to produce antibodies.

E32.0   Persistent hyperplasia of thymus

True thymic hyperplasia is defined as an increase in the size and weight of the gland while maintaining normal architecture. It can be idiopathic, which is extremely rare, and may be due to a rebound phenomenon during recovery from a stressful event, such as steroid therapy or chemotherapy for malignant tumor. It can also present in association with endocrine abnormalities, sarcoidosis, and Beckwith-Wiedemann syndrome.

Focus Point

Beckwith-Wiedemann syndrome is reported with code Q87.3 in Chapter 17 Congenital Malformations, Deformations and Chromosomal Abnormalities. It is classified as a genetic overgrowth syndrome that affects many parts of the body. Infants are larger than normal and continue to gain height and weight at an abnormally fast rate through childhood. After the growth slows, the adults are generally not abnormally tall.

E32.1   Abscess of thymus

An abscess of the thymus may present with chest pain behind the sternum and is one of many possible causes of cysts in the mediastinum.

Focus Point

Even though it is a type of thymus abscess, if the documentation states Dubois' abscesses, it is included in code A50.59 Other late congenital syphilis symptomatic.

E34.-   Other endocrine disorders

This category contains codes representing endocrine disorders affecting multiple body systems, as well as those for which the specific etiology is not well defined.

E34.0   Carcinoid syndrome

Carcinoid syndrome is the set of symptoms that may occur in patients who have carcinoid tumors, which most commonly arise in the mucosa of the gastrointestinal tract. An overproduction of serotonin and other hormones causes the symptoms, which include flushing, diarrhea, heart valve lesions, cramping, telangiectasia, and peripheral edema.

E34.2   Ectopic hormone secretion, not elsewhere classified

An ectopic hormone is defined as one released from a neoplasm or cells outside the usual gland or tissue that produces the hormone. This most commonly occurs in patients with nonendocrine tumors.

E34.4   Constitutional tall stature

Tall stature is defined as height in excess of two standard deviations above the mean for the person's gender and age. There may be a family history of tallness.

E34.5-   Androgen insensitivity syndrome

Androgen insensitivity syndrome (AIS) is a more accurate term for the condition formally known as testicular feminization, or Goldberg Maxwell syndrome. It is a genetic disorder that affects the development of the reproductive organs and may be diagnosed at any stage of life.

E34.51   Complete androgen insensitivity syndrome

In complete androgen insensitivity syndrome (AIS), the external genitalia development appears characteristically female. Internally, the patient may have a short vagina but no internal female organs. Diagnosis may be delayed until amenorrhea is recognized during the teen years, at which time the absence of a uterus and other reproductive organs is discovered.

E34.52   Partial androgen insensitivity syndrome

In partial androgen insensitivity syndrome (AIS), the external genitalia may be characteristically male or female, or a degree of both. People with this condition may identify as male, female, or intergendered. Treatment options include decisions for surgical modification that are sensitive to the individual's circumstances, hormone replacement therapies, and psychological support.

E35   Disorders of endocrine glands in diseases classified elsewhere

Endocrine disorders may occur as a result of underlying conditions that are multisystemic or relate to other body systems.

Malnutrition (E40-E46)

Malnutrition results from an insufficient total intake of energizing nutrients and proteins. Vitamin or mineral deficiencies are the result of insufficient intake of very specific nutrients. While patients with malnutrition may also commonly have vitamin or mineral deficiencies, it is also possible to develop a vitamin or mineral deficiency without malnutrition.

The primary form of malnutrition results from a diet that lacks sufficient sources of protein and/or energy. The secondary type is more common in the United States, where it usually occurs as a complication of AIDS, malignancies, chronic kidney failure, inflammatory bowel disease, and other illnesses that impair the body's ability to absorb or use nutrients or to compensate for nutrient losses.

Malnutrition is typically diagnosed when providers identify at least two or more of the following six characteristics:

- Insufficient energy (calorie) intake
- Weight loss
- Loss of muscle mass
- Loss of subcutaneous fat
- Localized or generalized fluid accumulation that may sometimes mask weight loss
- Diminished functional status as measured by hand grip strength

Providers must assess these six characteristics in the context of an acute illness or injury, a chronic illness, or social or environmental circumstances to determine if malnutrition is present and whether it is severe or nonsevere (moderate).

The categories in this code block are as follows:

E40	Kwashiorkor
E41	Nutritional marasmus
E42	Marasmic kwashiorkor
E43	Unspecified severe protein-calorie malnutrition

E40   Kwashiorkor

Kwashiorkor is a severe form of malnutrition that occurs when there is not enough protein in the diet and is most common in areas where there is famine or limited food supply. Kwashiorkor is considered a third-degree malnutrition disorder and is rarely seen in the United States.

E41   Nutritional marasmus

Marasmus results from near starvation with a deficit in protein and nonprotein intake. Typically marasmus is a childhood disease in underdeveloped countries and occurs when the mother is unable to breastfeed. The child is very thin, with little muscle or body fat. Marasmus is considered a third-degree malnutrition disorder.

E42   Marasmic kwashiorkor

Marasmic-kwashiorkor is a mixed form of marasmus and kwashiorkor and is characterized by the presence of wasting and bilateral pitting edema of the extremities.

E43   Unspecified severe protein-calorie malnutrition

Protein-calorie malnutrition that is severe is classified as third degree and occurs when an individual does not receive adequate protein or calories for normal growth, body maintenance, and the energy necessary for ordinary activities. Elderly patients are most likely to develop malnutrition and are therefore more susceptible to health problems related to an inadequate diet.

E44.-   Protein-calorie malnutrition of moderate and mild degree

Protein-calorie malnutrition occurs when an individual does not receive adequate protein or calories for normal growth, body maintenance, and the energy necessary for ordinary activities. Moderate malnutrition is classified as second degree and is characterized by superimposed biochemical changes in electrolytes, lipids, and blood plasma. Mild malnutrition is classified as first degree and is characterized by tissue wasting in an adult or growth failure in a child, but few or no biochemical changes.

E45   Retarded development following protein-calorie malnutrition

When inadequate nutrition occurs over an extended period of time, physical effects may appear, including nutritional short stature, stunting, or systemic physical retardation.

E46   Unspecified protein-calorie malnutrition

Protein-calorie malnutrition occurs when an individual does not receive adequate protein or calories for normal growth, body maintenance, and the energy necessary for ordinary activities. This code is reported when the severity of the protein-calorie malnutrition has not been documented.

Other Nutritional Deficiencies (E50-E64)

There are a variety of vitamins and minerals that are essential to good health; deficiencies of these substances can cause complications ranging from mild to life-threatening. Treatment usually consists of replacing missing nutrients and treating any associated or underlying causes.

The categories in this code block are as follows:

E50	Vitamin A deficiency
E51	Thiamine deficiency
E52	Niacin deficiency [pellagra]
E53	Deficiency of other B group vitamins
E54	Ascorbic acid deficiency
E55	Vitamin D deficiency
E56	Other vitamin deficiencies
E58	Dietary calcium deficiency
E59	Dietary selenium deficiency
E60	Dietary zinc deficiency
E61	Deficiency of other nutrient elements
E63	Other nutritional deficiencies

Focus Point

Anemia that is a result of a nutritional deficiency is not classified to a code from range E50-E64, but instead to a code in range D50-D53.

E50.-   Vitamin A deficiency

Vitamin A is found in green leafy vegetables, fish, and dairy products, and serious deficiencies can cause growth retardation in children, blindness, and increased susceptibility to infection. Vitamin A deficiency is common in kwashiorkor and is endemic to areas in which rice is the diet staple.

E50.0   Vitamin A deficiency with conjunctival xerosis

Conjunctival xerosis is dryness of the eye surfaces caused by deficiency of tears or conjunctival secretions; one of most common causes is vitamin A deficiency.

E50.1   Vitamin A deficiency with Bitot's spot and conjunctival xerosis

Bitot spots are triangular, perilimbal, gray plaques of keratinized conjunctival debris overlying an area of conjunctival xerosis (dryness of the eye surfaces).

E50.2   Vitamin A deficiency with corneal xerosis

Corneal xerosis is pathologic dryness and keratinization of the cornea.

E50.3   Vitamin A deficiency with corneal ulceration and xerosis

A corneal ulcer is an open sore on the cornea, which is complicated by xerosis (pathologic dryness and keratinization of the cornea).

E50.4   Vitamin A deficiency with keratomalacia

Keratomalacia is a softening and necrosis of the cornea associated with vitamin A deficiency.

E50.5   Vitamin A deficiency with night blindness

Night blindness is poor vision at night or in dim light. Vitamin A deficiency is a rare cause, but can be treated with supplements. Vitamin A is an essential component of rhodopsin, the pigment responsible for optimal rod function and necessary for night vision.

E50.6   Vitamin A deficiency with xerophthalmic scars of cornea

If the cornea becomes damaged, the resulting scars can interfere with vision by blocking or distorting light as it enters the eye. Depending on the degree of scarring, vision can range from a blur to total blindness. Deep abrasions and ulcerations/lacerations result in a loss of corneal tissue, which is replaced by scar tissue.

E50.7   Other ocular manifestations of vitamin A deficiency

Xerophthalmia may be documented in the medical record and although it literally means "dry eye," it denotes the entire spectrum of ocular abnormalities arising from vitamin A deficiency.

E50.8   Other manifestations of vitamin A deficiency

Conditions classified to this code include follicular keratosis and xeroderma. Follicular keratosis is an inflammation on the skin (typically the face) that occurs in or near a hair follicle; it looks like a papule and it usually has a pinkish color. Xeroderma is excessive or abnormal dryness of the skin.

E51.-   Thiamine deficiency

Alcohol is the primary cause of thiamine deficiency in the United States. In other countries it can result from eating a diet of highly polished rice. Infants can develop a thiamine deficiency when breast-fed by a thiamine-deficient mother. The condition can lead to metabolic coma and death if untreated.

E51.1-   Beriberi

There are two types of beriberi: dry and wet. Beriberi is treated by increasing dietary intake of foods rich in thiamine and by dietary supplements.

E51.11   Dry beriberi

This condition is characterized primarily by peripheral neuropathy, which is symmetric impairment of sensory, motor, and reflex functions. It affects distal more than proximal limb segments and causes calf muscle tenderness.

E51.12   Wet beriberi

In addition to peripheral neuropathy, this form of the disease is associated with mental confusion, muscular atrophy, edema, tachycardia, cardiomegaly, and congestive heart failure.

E51.2   Wernicke's encephalopathy

This condition is characterized as a triad of acute mental confusion, ataxia, and ophthalmoplegia. The vast majority of affected patients are alcoholic.

E52   Niacin deficiency [pellagra]

Also known as vitamin B3 or nicotinic acid, niacin is one of eight B vitamins and plays a role in converting carbohydrates into glucose, metabolizes fats and proteins, and keeps the nervous system in balance. Niacin also assists in making sex- and stress-related hormones and improves circulation and cholesterol levels. Symptoms of mild niacin deficiency include indigestion, fatigue, canker sores, vomiting, and depression. Severe deficiency, called pellagra, can cause symptoms related to the skin, digestive system, and nervous system, including thick, scaly pigmented rash on skin exposed to sunlight, swollen mouth and bright red tongue, vomiting and diarrhea, headache, apathy, fatigue, depression, disorientation, and memory loss.

E53.-   Deficiency of other B group vitamins

B vitamins are a group of eight water-soluble vitamins that play important roles in cell metabolism. Deficiencies in the different B vitamins can cause a variety of disorders.

E53.0   Riboflavin deficiency

Riboflavin, also known as vitamin B2, is important for energy production, enzyme function, and normal fatty acid and amino acid synthesis and is also necessary for the reproduction of glutathione, a free radical scavenger. Primarily found in milk and other dairy products, riboflavin is also found in cereals, meats, and dark green vegetables. Dermatologic manifestations of riboflavin deficiency include cheilosis, or chapping and fissuring of the lips; a sore, red tongue; and oily, scaly skin rashes on the scrotum, vulva, and philtrum.

E53.1   Pyridoxine deficiency

Vitamin B6 (Pyridoxine) plays a role in more than 100 different biochemical processes as a coenzyme. Vitamin B6 helps the body to metabolize proteins and carbohydrates for energy, and helps to promote a healthy immune system and maintain proper immune system function. The risk of Vitamin B6 deficiency is very low due to the fact that nearly all foods contain at least some of the vitamin. Vitamin B6 deficiency most often results from a problem with the absorption of nutrients in the intestines. A deficiency of vitamin B6 can result in disruption in the normal functioning of the central nervous system. This can result in a variety of symptoms, including weakness, tingling sensations, loss of coordination, confusion, seizures, depression, and insomnia.

E54   Ascorbic acid deficiency

A deficiency of ascorbic acid (vitamin C) causes weak skin, poor wound healing, and weak blood vessels. It is seen most often in those with poor diet, and if left untreated can lead to a diagnosis of scurvy. Symptoms include bleeding gums, weight loss, and myalgias. The major sources of vitamin C include vegetables and fresh fruit, especially citrus.

E55.-   Vitamin D deficiency

Vitamin D is produced by the body in response to sunlight and also occurs naturally in some foods, including some fish, fish liver oils, and egg yolks, and in fortified dairy and grain products. This vitamin is essential for strong bones because it helps the body use calcium from the diet. Symptoms typically consist of bone pain and muscle weakness.

E55.0   Rickets, active

Vitamin D helps the body control calcium and phosphate levels. If the blood levels of these minerals become too low, the body may produce hormones that cause calcium and phosphate to be released from the bones. This potentially leads to weak and soft bones and a diagnosis of rickets. Rickets is rare in the United States. It is most likely to occur in children during periods of rapid growth, when the body needs high levels of calcium and phosphate.

E56.-   Other vitamin deficiencies

Vitamin deficiencies may cause significant disorders and should be classified as specifically as possible.

E56.0   Deficiency of vitamin E

This condition causes neurological problems due to poor nerve conduction and typically arises from fat malabsorption. Frank vitamin E deficiency is rare and overt deficiency symptoms have not been found in healthy people who obtain little vitamin E from their diets. Food sources of vitamin E are nuts, seeds, egg yolks, whole grains, and green leafy vegetables. Peanuts, soybean, corn oil, wheat germ oil, and sunflower seeds also contain vitamin E.

E56.1   Deficiency of vitamin K

Vitamin K is a fat-soluble vitamin and is known as the clotting vitamin, because without it blood would not clot. Vitamin K deficiency is very rare and primarily occurs when the body can't properly absorb the vitamin from the intestinal tract. Vitamin K deficiency can also occur after long-term treatment with antibiotics.

E58   Dietary calcium deficiency

Calcium deficiency is a condition in which the body has an inadequate amount of calcium. It is a mineral that is essential for the health of bones and teeth and a normal heart rhythm. It is also required for muscle contractions and relaxation, nerve and hormone function, and blood pressure regulation. Foods that naturally contain calcium include milk and other dairy products, green leafy vegetables, seafood, nuts, and dried beans. Calcium is also added to orange juice, breakfast cereals, breads, and other fortified food products.

Focus Point

Hypocalcemia is a low level of calcium in the blood. If this condition is documented it should not be classified in category E58. Refer instead to subcategory E83.5-.

E59   Dietary selenium deficiency

Selenium is a trace mineral that is essential to good health but required only in small amounts. The antioxidant properties of selenoproteins help prevent cellular damage from free radicals. Severe gastrointestinal disorders may decrease the absorption of selenium, resulting in selenium depletion or deficiency. Plant foods are the major dietary sources of selenium in most countries throughout the world. The content of selenium in food depends on the selenium content of the soil where plants are grown. Selenium deficiency is rare in the United States but is seen in other countries, most notably China, where soil concentration of selenium is low. Keshan disease, which results in an enlarged heart and poor heart function, occurs in selenium deficient children.

E60   Dietary zinc deficiency

Zinc is an essential trace element that plays an essential role in numerous biochemical pathways. Zinc deficiency results in dysfunction of humoral and cell-mediated immunity and increases the susceptibility to infection. Many organ systems are affected by severe zinc deficiency, including the integumentary, gastrointestinal, central nervous, immune, skeletal, and reproductive systems.

E61.-   Deficiency of other nutrient elements

Besides vitamins and minerals, there are other nutrient elements that should be kept in balance in the body for optimal health.

Focus Point

Codes in category E61 can be used when the nutrient deficiency is due to an adverse effect of a drug but require an additional code from category range T36-T50 with 5th or 6th character 5 to capture the adverse effect.

E61.0   Copper deficiency

Copper is an essential cofactor in many enzymatic reactions vital to the normal function of the hematologic, vascular, skeletal, antioxidant, and neurologic systems. Although rare in the United States, it has been found in the setting of zinc supplementation, myelodysplastic syndrome, use of parenteral nutrition and chronic tube feeding, and in various malabsorptive syndromes.

E61.1   Iron deficiency

Iron deficiency is the most common nutritional deficiency in the United States and can be caused by an increased need for iron (e.g., by a pregnant woman) or from an inability to absorb the mineral appropriately. Iron from meat, poultry, and fish (i.e., heme iron) is absorbed most efficiently.

Focus Point

If the condition is documented as iron deficiency anemia, refer to category D50.

E61.2   Magnesium deficiency

Magnesium is the fourth most abundant mineral in the body and is essential to good health and is needed for more than 300 biochemical reactions in the body. It helps maintain normal muscle and nerve function, keeps heart rhythm steady, supports a healthy immune system, and keeps bones strong. Magnesium also helps regulate blood sugar levels, promotes normal blood pressure, and is known to be involved in energy metabolism and protein synthesis. Green vegetables such as spinach are good sources of magnesium as are some legumes (beans and peas), nuts and seeds, and whole, unrefined grains are also good sources of magnesium.

E61.3   Manganese deficiency

Manganese is a component of some enzymes and stimulates the development and activity of other enzymes. It is a vital element of nutrition in very small quantities, but in greater amounts manganese, like most metals, is poisonous when eaten or inhaled. Manganese is found in leafy green vegetables, fruits, nuts, and whole grains.

E61.4 Chromium deficiency

Chromium is a mineral that humans require in trace amounts, although its mechanisms of action in the body and the amounts needed for optimal health are not well defined. It is thought that few Americans are chromium deficient, although a few clear cases of deficiency have been observed in hospital patients who were fed defined liquid diets intravenously for long periods of time. It is widely distributed in the food supply, but most foods provide only small amounts (less than 2 micrograms [mcg] per serving). Meat and whole-grain products, as well as some fruits, vegetables, and spices, are relatively good sources.

E61.5 Molybdenum deficiency

Molybdenum is an essential trace element that contributes to the functions of the nervous system and kidneys. Because the amount of molybdenum that the body requires for healthy function is very small, and the mineral occurs in many foods (such as beans, peas, lentils, nuts, leafy vegetables, and liver), deficiency is rare in humans.

E61.6 Vanadium deficiency

Vanadium is an essential trace mineral that is required in the diet in very small amounts and is rare in humans. The best sources of vanadium are mushrooms, shellfish, eggs, black pepper, parsley, dill seed, strawberries, radishes, vegetable oils, olives, root vegetables, lettuces, soybeans, nuts, grain, and whole grain products.

E63.- Other nutritional deficiencies

Besides vitamins and minerals, there are other nutrient elements that should be kept in balance in the body for optimal health.

E63.0 Essential fatty acid [EFA] deficiency

EFAs are fatty acids that humans and other animals must ingest because the body requires them for good health but cannot synthesize them. Only two EFAs are known for humans: alpha-linolenic acid (an omega-3 fatty acid) and linoleic acid (an omega-6 fatty acid). Other fatty acids that are only "conditionally essential" include gamma-linolenic acid (an omega-6 fatty acid), lauric acid (a saturated fatty acid), and palmitoleic acid (a monounsaturated fatty acid). Essential fatty acid (EFA) deficiency has become a clinical problem since the advent of fat-free total parenteral nutrition (TPN).

E63.1 Imbalance of constituents of food intake

Constituents are substances that provide nourishment essential for the maintenance of life and for growth and are classified into the major groups, which includes proteins, carbohydrates, fats, vitamins, and minerals. A balanced diet refers to the intake of edibles that can provide all the essential constituents necessary for growth and maintenance of the body in definite amount in which they are required by the body.

E64.- Sequelae of malnutrition and other nutritional deficiencies

Malnutrition and some of the other nutritional deficiencies may cause other late effect disorders or sequelae, even after the deficiency itself has been corrected. In some cases the sequela may be transient but in others it may have long-term effects.

E64.0 Sequelae of protein-calorie malnutrition

Early malnutrition, particularly if severe in nature, can cause several long-term late effects, including growth failure and delayed wound healing.

Overweight, Obesity and Other Hyperalimentation (E65-E68)

Excessive calorie intake leading to overweight and obesity and other causes of obesity are classified here. Also included in here are conditions caused by hyperalimentation, which is the ingestion of excessive amounts of certain nutrients, such as megadoses of certain vitamins.

Overweight and obesity are defined based on whether the patient is an adult or a child. An adult is generally considered overweight if he or she has a body mass index (BMI) between 25 and 29.9 kg/m2. Obesity is defined as a BMI of 30 or higher. Obesity is epidemic in the United States. It is more common among women than men and more common among African-Americans than Caucasians. Obesity occurs when caloric intake chronically outpaces the energy required. Obesity puts patients at risk for diabetes, hypertension, and coronary artery disease.

The CDC provides four weight classifications for children:

- "Underweight" refers to a weight that is under the fifth percentile for the child's age.

- "Healthy" refers to a weight between the fifth and 85th percentile.

- "At risk" refers to a weight between the 85th and 95th percentile for the child's age. This corresponds to a BMI of 25, which is considered overweight for an adult.

- "Overweight" refers to a weight ranking above the 95th percentile for the child's age. This is the most severe level of childhood obesity, corresponding to a BMI of at least 30, which is the same indicator used to classify adult obesity.

The categories in this code block are as follows:

E65   Localized adiposity

E66   Overweight and obesity

E67   Other hyperalimentation

E68   Sequelae of hyperalimentation

E66.-   Overweight and obesity

The most common causes of overweight and obesity is consuming too many calories along with a sedentary lifestyle, although certain drugs can also increase the potential for overweight.

E66.0-   Obesity due to excess calories

This subcategory classifies obesity due to excess calories based on the severity of the condition.

E66.01   Morbid (severe) obesity due to excess calories

Morbid obesity is defined as greater than 100 pounds overweight. Risk for comorbidities is extremely high.

E66.09   Other obesity due to excess calories

Obesity is defined as a BMI of 30 or higher.

E66.1   Drug-induced obesity

Drugs that can cause rapid weight gain and obesity include antipsychotic drugs used to treat schizophrenia, Tricyclic antidepressants, lithium, valproate, and glucocorticoids. These drugs are associated with persistent weight gain affecting more than 50 percent of the patients depending on dose and duration of exposure.

E66.2   Morbid (severe) obesity with alveolar hypoventilation

Obesity hypoventilation syndrome (OHS) is a chronic condition involving poor breathing characterized by a combination of inadequate oxygen intake and an accumulation of carbon dioxide in the blood. Associated conditions may include right-sided heart failure with pitting edema, hypertension, and cor pulmonale. If inadequately treated or if weight loss attempts are unsuccessful, the condition can progress to debilitating cardiovascular disease.

E66.3   Overweight

Overweight is defined for an adult as a body mass index between 25 and 29.9 kg/m2.

E67.-   Other hyperalimentation

Hyperalimentation is broadly defined as the ingestion or administration of a greater than optimal amount of nutrients. It can refer to the total nutrient intake or to single components.

> **Focus Point**
>
> *When hyperalimentation refers to excessive eating or is listed as NOS, it should be classified to code R63.2 Polyphagia.*

E67.0   Hypervitaminosis A

Vitamin A hypervitaminosis may be acute or chronic. The acute is caused by taking too much vitamin A over a short period of time. The chronic form occurs when too much of the vitamin is present over a longer period.

E67.1   Hypercarotinemia

Hypercarotenemia is defined as excessive carotene in the blood, often with yellowing of the skin (carotenosis). It may follow overeating of such carotenoid-rich foods as carrots, sweet potatoes, or oranges.

E67.2   Megavitamin-B6 syndrome

Overdosage of vitamin B6 has been found to have a profound effect on the nervous system, including difficulty walking and leg numbness.

E67.3   Hypervitaminosis D

An excess of vitamin D causes abnormally high levels of calcium in the blood. This can severely damage the bones, soft tissues, and kidneys over time.

Chapter 4, Endocrine, Nutritional and Metabolic Diseases (E00-E89)

Metabolic Disorders (E70-E88)

Metabolism is the processes the body uses to break down chemicals, convert them to other substances, and transport the new substances to sites where they can be used by the body or excreted. Enzymes and proteins are the substances responsible for initiating metabolic processes that are necessary to maintain homeostasis.

Metabolic disorders occur when the necessary enzymes and proteins are not present or are present in a genetically altered form that cannot be used by the body. Inherited genetic abnormalities are the cause of most metabolic disorders and usually result from the absence of an enzyme needed for a specific metabolic process or the presence of a defective enzyme.

The categories in this code block are as follows:

E70	Disorders of aromatic amino-acid metabolism
E71	Disorders of branched-chain amino-acid metabolism and fatty-acid metabolism
E72	Other disorders of amino-acid metabolism
E73	Lactose intolerance
E74	Other disorders of carbohydrate metabolism
E75	Disorders of sphingolipid metabolism and other lipid storage disorders
E76	Disorders of glycosaminoglycan metabolism
E77	Disorders of glycoprotein metabolism
E78	Disorders of lipoprotein metabolism and other lipidemias
E79	Disorders of purine and pyrimidine metabolism
E80	Disorders of porphyrin and bilirubin metabolism
E83	Disorders of mineral metabolism
E84	Cystic fibrosis
E85	Amyloidosis
E86	Volume depletion
E87	Other disorders of fluid, electrolyte and acid-base balance
E88	Other and unspecified metabolic disorders

E70.- Disorders of aromatic amino-acid metabolism

Amino-acids are classified based on certain characteristics of their molecular structures with aromatic being one type of molecular structure. Disorders of aromatic amino-acid metabolism manifest in a variety of ways causing phenylketonuria, albinism, and other conditions.

E70.0 Classical phenylketonuria

Phenylketonuria (PKU) is an inherited metabolic disorder that is caused by a mutation of the phenylalanine hydroxylase (PAH) gene that is responsible for synthesis of the phenylalanine hydroxylase, an enzyme that allows the body to process and use the amino-acid phenylalanine. When this enzyme is not present the body cannot effectively process phenylalanine causing increased levels to circulate in the blood. The brain is particularly sensitive to elevated levels of phenylalanine, which is why PKU causes intellectual, developmental, and behavioral health problems. Symptoms vary depending on the specific mutation of the PAH gene. Classical PKU is the most severe form of the disorder and without treatment beginning in infancy this amino-acid disorder causes brain damage. Treatment involves a low phenylalanine diet.

E71.- Disorders of branched-chain amino-acid metabolism and fatty-acid metabolism

Amino-acids are classified based on certain characteristics of their molecular structures with branched-chain being one type of molecular structure. Fatty acids are carboxylic acids with long hydrocarbon chains. Conditions classified here involve the inability to break down and use branched chain amino-acids and fatty acids.

E71.31- Disorders of fatty-acid oxidation

Disorders of fatty acid oxidation are genetic metabolic disorders that render the body incapable of breaking down fatty acids to make that energy available. Different types of specific enzyme deficiencies, in which one may be missing or improperly functioning, may manifest themselves as the cause. If undiagnosed, fatty acid oxidation disorders can result in serious complications of the liver, heart, eyes, and muscle development, and may lead to coma and possibly death, especially if metabolic crisis arises after a fasting period, such as during an infection or flu. Other signs include chronic bouts of low blood sugar, vomiting, diarrhea, lethargy, and even seizures.

E71.311 Medium chain acyl CoA dehydrogenase deficiency

Medium-chain acyl-CoA dehydrogenase deficiency (MCAD) is a disorder of the enzyme involved in mitochondrial fatty acid B-oxidation. This is usually diagnosed when a child is between 3 and 24 months of age, but may present later. Once the diagnosis is made, the child requires increased feedings to prevent long periods of fasting.

E71.5- Peroxisomal disorders

Peroxisomal disorders are problems at the subcellular level involving the improper formation or functioning of peroxisomes. These are special compartments within cells, called organelles, that are bound by their own membrane and contain certain enzymes. These peroxisomes help to do a number of jobs that are needed for digestion, producing certain hormones, and making the nervous system work properly. Peroxisomal disorders occur when a defect in the assembly of the peroxisome happens, such as when necessary proteins fail to transport inside the peroxisome membrane or a defect in a specific, single function of the peroxisome arises.

E73.- Lactose intolerance

Lactose is a sugar found in dairy products. Lactose intolerance is the inability to break down this sugar due to a deficiency in the enzyme lactase.

E78.- Disorders of lipoprotein metabolism and other lipidemias

This category includes some common lipoprotein metabolic disorders including hypercholesterolemia, hyperglyceridemia, and hyperlipidemia. Cholesterol is a waxy fat that is present in the human body. Two sources contribute to the amount of cholesterol in the human body. First, the liver manufactures about 80 percent of it. Second, people consume it by eating animal products such as meat, eggs, and dairy products. Cholesterol is carried through the bloodstream by certain proteins (apolipoproteins). When these proteins wrap around cholesterol and other types of fats (lipids) to transport them through the bloodstream, they combine and are called lipoproteins. There are three different types of lipoproteins that carry cholesterol through the bloodstream. High-density lipoproteins (HDL) are associated with "good" cholesterol. Low-density lipoproteins (LDL) are associated with "bad" cholesterol. Very low-density lipoproteins (VLDL) are associated with "very bad" cholesterol. High levels of LDL cholesterol have been associated with arteriosclerosis (hardening of the arteries) and coronary artery disease. In contrast, high levels of HDL cholesterol have been shown to reduce some of the harmful effects of LDL cholesterol. Hyperlipidemia (hyperlipemia) is a condition where an overabundance of fat or lipid is found in the bloodstream.

E78.0- Pure hypercholesterolemia

Hypercholesterolemia, also called high cholesterol, affects millions of patients in the United States. Although considered a chronic condition, hypercholesterolemia can often go unrecognized, as it usually does not present any symptoms. Without symptoms, diagnosis can be determined only via a blood test. The longer the cholesterol is present in the blood, the more likely plaque is to form along arterial walls. This can lead to symptoms such as chest pain or more serious conditions such as a heart attack or stroke. Causative reasons for hypercholesterolemia are heredity (familial), diets high in saturated fat and cholesterol, as well as other disorders, such as diabetes mellitus, Cushing's syndrome, and hypothyroidism. Risk factors include poor diet, obesity, large waist circumference, lack of exercise, and smoking.

E78.01 Familial hypercholesterolemia

Familial hypercholesterolemia (FH) is classified as a genetic disorder that is demonstrated as a chromosomal 19 defect. As a result of this defect, the low-density lipoprotein (LDL) cholesterol, or bad cholesterol, cannot be removed from the body, resulting in a high level of LDL in the bloodstream. Familial hypercholesterolemia is believed to affect over 600,000 people in the United States, even though most of this population has not officially been diagnosed, and is present in all racial and ethnic groups. Fatty skin deposits, also known as xanthomas, occurring on hands, elbows, knees, ankles, and around the cornea of the eye, are hallmark signs. A patient may also experience chest pain or other signs of coronary artery disease, cramping in the legs while walking, or symptoms of stroke including trouble speaking, facial droop, and weakness in an extremity and/or loss of balance.

E78.2 Mixed hyperlipidemia

Hyperlipidemia is an elevated level of lipids or lipoproteins in the blood. Mixed hyperlipidemia indicates multiple types of lipoproteins are elevated, including triglycerides, cholesterol, phospholipids, and special proteins within the lipoproteins.

E78.3 Hyperchylomicronemia

Hyperchylomicronemia is an excessive amount of chylomicrons, lipoproteins saturated with triglycerides, found in the bloodstream.

E78.6 Lipoprotein deficiency

A lipoprotein deficiency is a condition where there are abnormally low levels of fats and proteins in the blood. Although a familial etiology is rare it does occur and while infants appear healthy at birth, within the first month of life they develop signs of this disorder. Common symptoms for this inherited lipoprotein metabolic condition include abdominal distention, failure to thrive, retinitis pigmentosa, progressive ataxia, and death by the time the individual reaches 30 years of age. Acquired cases of lipoprotein deficiencies typically include a secondary condition such as coronary heart disease or peripheral artery disease. In acquired cases, it is often the high density lipoproteins or "good" cholesterol that is too low and is a risk factor of coronary artery disease.

E83.-   Disorders of mineral metabolism

There are many minerals that are essential to health. Disorders of mineral metabolism cause a variety of conditions, depending on which mineral is not being effectively metabolized.

E83.1-   Disorders of iron metabolism

A few types of iron metabolism disorders classified here include disorders of iron storage, excessive absorption of iron from the intestine due to a genetic mutation, and acquired iron overload due to repeated red blood cell transfusions.

E83.11-   Hemochromatosis

Hereditary, acquired, and other types of hemochromatosis, an excessive accumulation of iron in the blood, are included here. Signs and symptoms include darkening or "bronzing" of the skin, weakness and fatigue, heart palpitations, joint or abdominal pain, infertility, impotence, or cessation of menstruation. Early detection is essential in preventing potentially serious complications of prolonged hemochromatosis, including liver damage, endocrine (e.g., pituitary, adrenal, thyroid) suppression, arthritis, secondary diabetes, heart failure, and increased risk for opportunistic infections. Treatment includes therapeutic phlebotomy or chelation therapy to remove excess serum iron, as indicated by monitoring hemoglobin and serum ferritin concentrations.

Focus Point

Hemochromatosis that is documented as gestational or neonatal is coded to P78.84 Gestational Alloimmune Liver disease.

E83.110   Hereditary hemochromatosis

Hereditary forms are caused by a genetic mutation of the gene responsible for iron absorption. Normally iron is absorbed from the intestine during the digestive process. When the body has adequate amounts of iron in the blood the amount absorbed from the intestine is decreased, and when the body requires more iron more is absorbed. In hereditary hemochromatosis iron continues to be absorbed from the intestine even when blood levels are adequate causing an overload of iron in the blood.

E83.111   Hemochromatosis due to repeated red blood cell transfusions

Excessive levels of iron in the blood can result from repeated red blood cell transfusions. Associated conditions that require serial transfusions include myelodysplasia and certain anemias (e.g., sickle cell anemia).

E83.5-   Disorders of calcium metabolism

Disorders of calcium metabolism include decreased or elevated levels of calcium in the blood.

E83.51   Hypocalcemia

Hypocalcemia is the result of too much calcium being lost from the blood or too little entering the blood from the digestive tract despite adequate dietary intake of calcium or from the bones when dietary intake is low.

E83.52   Hypercalcemia

Hypercalcemia is an excessive amount of calcium in the blood. It is caused by too much calcium in the extracellular fluid or failure of the kidneys to excrete the excess calcium. The most common causes are hyperparathyroidism or malignant neoplasms.

E83.81   Hungry bone syndrome

Hungry bone syndrome (HBS) describes a state of severe or long-standing hypocalcemia, most commonly due to primary or secondary (including postsurgical) hypoparathyroidism. Elevated levels of parathyroid hormone and bone demineralization cause the bone to sequester calcium. This results in increased bone formation (density) and decreased bone resorption, characterized by a rapid fall in plasma calcium, phosphorus, and magnesium levels. The hypocalcemia may resolve within weeks, but in some cases, can persist for years. The resultant metabolic imbalance may precede osteoporosis and associated pathological fracture, tetany, or seizures. Other causal conditions for HBS include neoplasm or associated therapies, systemic metabolic acidosis, or other chronic disease (e.g., chronic renal disease).

E84.-   Cystic fibrosis

Cystic fibrosis is a hereditary disorder in which the body secretes thick, sticky mucus that clogs organs and leads to problems with breathing and digestion. It is caused by a defect in the manufacture of cystic fibrosis transmembrane conductance regulator (CFTR). Normally, CFTR forms a channel through which chloride ions traverse the cells lining the lungs, pancreas, sweat glands, and small intestine. With cystic fibrosis, malfunctioning CFTR precludes chloride from entering or leaving cells, resulting in production of thick, sticky mucus. In the lungs, this mucus blocks airways. In the digestive system, the mucus prevents enzymes produced in the pancreas from reaching the intestines, impairing digestion. In addition, the malfunctioning CFTR causes excessive amounts of salt to escape in the sweat. Cystic fibrosis is an autosomal recessive genetic disorder. To have cystic fibrosis, both parents must carry the disease. Cystic fibrosis symptoms may be apparent soon after birth, or the symptoms may go undiagnosed for years. In 20 percent of cases, the first symptom is meconium ileus, intestinal blockage in newborns, which may require surgery. Cystic fibrosis is classified based on manifestations, which include pulmonary, intestinal, or other manifestations.

E85.- Amyloidosis

Amyloidosis is a condition in which abnormal proteins, called amyloid, deposit in various tissues, such as heart and brain tissue. These proteins, or fibrils, are produced in excess and deposited in different organs and slowly replace normal tissue. The deposits damage the tissues and interfere with the function of the involved organ. Amyloidosis occurs in multiple forms: spontaneous, hereditary, secondary to hemodialysis, and resulting from a cancer of the blood cells called myeloma. Hereditary amyloidosis is an inherited form that is transmitted as an autosomal dominant trait.

E85.0 Non-neuropathic heredofamilial amyloidosis

This particular type of inherited amyloidosis targets tissue that is not of neuropathic origin. This may include the heart, kidneys, or gastrointestinal tract.

> **Focus Point**
>
> *Familial Mediterranean fever (FMF), once an inclusion term under code E85.0, has now been reclassified to code M04.1 Periodic fever syndromes. Familial Mediterranean fever is considered an autoinflammatory syndrome manifested by a rash on the legs, episodic fever, and serositis. Although amyloidosis may also manifest in some individuals with FMF, it is not always present.*

E85.1 Neuropathic heredofamilial amyloidosis

This hereditary form of amyloidosis is the result of a mutation of transthyretin (TTR) gene and causes a variety of sensory, motor, and autonomic neurological symptoms, which is dependent on the specific mutation. Sensory symptoms typically manifest first as paresthesia, pain, and loss of temperature sensation. Autonomic manifestations include postural hypotension and other cardiac symptoms, gastrointestinal disorders, and genitourinary disorders. Loss of motor function typically occurs later.

E85.4 Organ-limited amyloidosis

Cerebral amyloid angiopathy (CAA) is an organ-limited (localized) amyloidosis. This relatively asymptomatic condition is characterized by deposits of amyloid protein in the cerebral vasculature. The amyloid deposits predispose the patient to stroke, brain hemorrhage, or dementia. The most common form of CAA is the sporadic type, typically associated with aging, affecting patients 45 to 65 year of age. There are also other inherited autosomal dominant forms.

E85.81 Light chain (AL) amyloidosis

Immunoglobulin light chain (AL) amyloidosis, previously known as primary amyloidosis, or light chain deposition disease (LCDD), is caused when antibody-producing cells malfunction and produce abnormal protein fibers made of components of antibodies (immunoglobins) called light chains. These light chain fibers form amyloid deposits, which can cause damage affecting the kidneys, liver, heart, spleen, lungs, tongue, skin, ligaments, peripheral nerves, adrenal glands, bladder, intestines, and bone marrow. AL amyloidosis is the most common type of systemic amyloidosis.

E85.82 Wild-type transthyretin-related (ATTR) amyloidosis

Wild-type transthyretin amyloidosis (WTTA), also known as senile systemic amyloidosis (SSA), is a nonhereditary disease that typically affects the heart and carpal tendons of elderly people, almost exclusively in men over 60 years of age. The natural, normal, "wild-type" transthyretin (TTR) proteins without genetic mutations clump together and form amyloid deposits, mainly in the heart. These amyloid deposits can cause arrhythmias and heart failure. It is often not diagnosed as an amyloid disease because so many elderly patients develop heart problems.

E86.- Volume depletion

Dehydration and hypovolemia are often used interchangeably although both are different conditions. Dehydration is the loss of total body water and contraction of the total intravascular plasma while hypovolemia is the depletion of the volume of plasma or total blood volume.

E86.0 Dehydration

Dehydration is characterized by excessive free water loss and plasma volume contraction disproportionate to the loss of sodium. Solutes become imbalanced resulting in hypernatremia (increased concentration of serum sodium) as an indicator for true dehydration. Blood volume can be replaced, but the plasma solutes must be correctly balanced as well. Gradual volume restoration is imperative to restore optimal fluid balance slowly. Dehydration may follow bouts of diarrhea, vomiting, or profuse sweating. It is often a manifestation of the patient's illness (e.g., gastroenteritis), and in such cases the code for dehydration would not be sequenced first. However, if the patient's dehydration becomes significant enough to warrant separate treatment for rehydration, the dehydration code would be sequenced first.

E87.- Other disorders of fluid, electrolyte and acid-base balance

A variety of fluid, electrolyte, and acid-base balance disorders are classified here, including sodium overload or deficiency; acidosis, potassium overload or deficiency; alkalosis, and mixed disorders; and fluid overload.

E87.2 Acidosis

Acidosis occurs when there is a decrease of pH (hydrogen ion) concentration in the blood and cellular tissues caused by an increase in acid and decrease in bicarbonate. Respiratory acidosis happens when the body is unable to remove carbon dioxide through exhaling completely causing an excess usually due to chest deformities, chest muscle weakness or injury, lung disease, or sedation drug overuse. When the kidneys can't remove enough acid from the body or too much acid is being produced, it is referred to as metabolic acidosis. Some causes of metabolic acidosis include kidney disease, dehydration, overdose of aspirin, or antifreeze ingestion. Lactic acidosis is an excess of lactic acid that can be due to cancer, alcohol overuse, vigorous exercise, liver failure, hypoglycemia, lack of oxygen, seizures, or certain medications.

E87.3 Alkalosis

Alkalosis is the opposite of acidosis in that the body fluids have an excess of base or alkali. The proper pH balance of acids and base is maintained by the kidneys and lungs. Respiratory alkalosis is a decrease in carbon dioxide levels in the blood that can be due to several causes, including fever, salicylate poisoning, lung or liver disease, hyperventilation, or lack of oxygen. Metabolic alkalosis occurs when there is an excess of bicarbonate in the blood, which can occur with kidney disease.

E87.71 Transfusion associated circulatory overload

Transfusion-associated circulatory overload (TACO) is a volume overload that occurs several hours after initiation of transfusion due to a rapid rate of transfusion or massive volumes of blood or blood products. Underlying cardiac or pulmonary pathology may exacerbate overload. Due to their relative physiologic sensitivity, infants and the elderly are at an increased risk for TACO, even though the transfusion volumes may be small in comparison with those of other patients. Incidences of TACO have been historically underreported due to differential diagnoses that present in a similar manner with posttransfusion respiratory distress (e.g., TRALI, anaphylaxis). TACO may be differentiated from TRALI (transfusion related acute lung injury) by blood pressure effects. TACO patients become hypertensive, whereas TRALI is associated with hypotension. Signs and symptoms of TACO include acute respiratory distress (e.g., dyspnea, orthopnea), increased blood pressure, peripheral edema, and pulmonary edema secondary to congestive heart failure during or within six hours of transfusion. Preventative identification of patients at risk for TACO is essential to ensure therapeutic administration of controlled rates of reduced volumes of required blood components.

E88.- Other and unspecified metabolic disorders

A variety of metabolic disorders are classified here, including disorders of plasma-protein metabolism, tumor lysis syndrome, mitochondrial metabolism disorders, and metabolic syndrome.

E88.01 Alpha-1-antitrypsin deficiency

Alpha-1 antitrypsin deficiency is one of the most common and serious hereditary diseases involving plasma protein metabolism. A person with Alpha-1-antitrypsin deficiency carries a gene that produces an abnormal AAT protein that cannot be secreted by the liver. This results in a severe reduction of the circulating levels of the protein, as well as damaging accumulation within the liver. The deficiency also results in lung disease, since the protein is designed to protect the lungs from destructive enzymatic activity. Since Alpha-1 begins in the liver and is a hereditary problem, liver involvement is often seen in children more than in adults, although chronic liver disease can occur at any time in life. Alpha-1 deficiency is the leading genetic cause of liver transplantation in children. This disease is also a major cause of lung transplantation. Lung disease is usually seen in adults, often striking in the prime of life with debilitating lung damage.

E88.3 Tumor lysis syndrome

Tumor lysis syndrome (TLS) is a potentially fatal metabolic complication of spontaneous or treatment-related tumor necrosis. It comprises a constellation of metabolic conditions caused by intracellular byproducts of dying cancer cells. When intracellular waste products are not effectively eliminated from the body, metabolic and electrolyte disturbances occur causing the characteristic symptoms of TLS. Symptoms may include nausea and vomiting, shortness of breath, an irregular heartbeat, abnormal urine, fatigue, and joint pain. With delayed treatment, symptoms may progress to acute kidney failure, arrhythmias, seizures, dyskinesia, and cardiorespiratory failure. Metabolic disturbances include hyperkalemia, hyperphosphatemia, and hyperuricemia often associated with acute renal failure. Although tumor lysis occurs most commonly after treatment of leukemia and lymphoma, it can occur spontaneously in the absence of antineoplastic therapy. Spontaneous tumor lysis syndrome that occurs prior to the initiation of chemotherapy may also be referred to as "pretreatment" TLS. This type of TLS, characterized by acute renal failure due to uric acid nephropathy, is differentiated from post-therapeutic TLS in that the "spontaneous" or "pretreatment" forms are not associated with hyperphosphatemia.

E88.4-   Mitochondrial metabolism disorders

Mitochondria are another of the subcellular compartment organelles separated from the rest of the cell by its own membrane and containing its own DNA. The mitochondrion is responsible for handling the energy considerations of the cell. Many different clinical problems can present with mitochondrial metabolism disorders, especially involving neurological problems, such as mitochondrial encephalopathies and myoclonus with epilepsy.

Postprocedural Endocrine and Metabolic Complications and Disorders, Not Elsewhere Classified (E89)

Surgery and other procedures such as radiation therapy can impact the ability of the affected endocrine gland to produce hormones in sufficient quantities. Procedures on or near an endocrine gland can comprise function leading to hypofunction or failure of the gland. This results in lowered levels of hormone secretion from the affected gland or failure of the gland to secrete any hormones.

E89.8-   Other postprocedural endocrine and metabolic complications and disorders

This group of codes pertains to a postprocedural hemorrhage or hematoma and seroma following an endocrine system procedure or other procedure. The descriptions of these terms are as follows:

- Hemorrhage is rapid blood loss from vessels.

- Hematoma is a collection of blood clots within tissue or organs due to a broken blood vessel.

- Seroma is a fluid accumulation just under the skin surface often developing after a surgery involving an incision and/or tissue extraction.

Code assignment is based on the complication type and whether the complication occurs following an endocrine or other procedure.

Chapter 5: Mental, Behavioral, and Neurodevelopmental Disorders (FØ1-F99)

Mental, behavioral, and neurodevelopmental disorders encompass a broad and diverse group of illnesses that affect a patient's mood, thinking, behavior, and/or development. On occasion, mental health concerns may be experienced by any person, but when the symptoms and signs persist and inhibit a person's ability to function, a mental disorder may be diagnosed. The exact causes for mental illness are not known, but just as in diseases affecting other parts of the body, mental disorders can be attributed to genetic, biological, and/or environmental factors. These may include:

- Inherited traits
- Environmental exposure to toxic chemicals or viruses
- Brain chemistry
- Negative life experiences
- Injury
- Other disease processes
- Substance use

Conditions in this chapter are classified into 11 code blocks based on whether conditions are primarily mental, behavioral, or neurodevelopmental.

The chapter is broken down into the following code blocks:

FØ1-FØ9	Mental disorders due to known physiological conditions
F1Ø-F19	Mental and behavioral disorders due to psychoactive substance use
F2Ø-F29	Schizophrenia, schizotypal, delusional, and other non-mood psychotic disorders
F3Ø-F39	Mood [affective] disorders
F4Ø-F48	Anxiety, dissociative, stress-related, somatoform and other nonpsychotic mental disorders
F5Ø-F59	Behavioral syndromes associated with physiological disturbances and physical factors
F6Ø-F69	Disorders of adult personality and behavior
F7Ø-F79	Intellectual disabilities
F8Ø-F89	Pervasive and specific developmental disorders
F9Ø-F98	Behavioral and emotional disorders with onset usually occurring in childhood and adolescence
F99	Unspecified mental disorder

Mental disorders are diseases that predominantly impact the mind. These conditions comprise the majority of the chapter with specific code blocks that integrate codes related to anxiety disorders, mood disorders, non-mood disorders, and mental disorders that are the direct result of a medical condition.

The largest code block in the chapter classifies mental and behavioral disorder due to psychoactive substance use. This section has had a complete overhaul and better represents the relationship between the substances used and the consequential mental or behavioral disorder.

Code blocks that represent behavioral disorders include those specific to time of onset—childhood or adulthood—and those that are related to physiological disturbances, such as eating or sleeping disorders.

There are two sections devoted to developmental disorders, the intellectual disabilities section and the pervasive and specific developmental disorders section, which includes conditions related to speech, math, or motor function problems, as well as autism.

Mental Disorders Due to Known Physiological Conditions (FØ1-FØ9)

The conditions outlined in this code block comprise a collection of mental disorders that are a consequence of a medical condition. Just like other organs in the body, the brain is susceptible to the effects of certain disease processes. The disease process may impact the brain directly as is seen with cancer or injury or it can be a secondary process as seen in systemic diseases like multiple sclerosis.

The categories in this code block are as follows:

FØ1	Vascular dementia
FØ2	Dementia in other diseases classified elsewhere

F03	Unspecified dementia
F04	Amnestic disorder due to known physiological condition
F05	Delirium due to known physiological condition
F06	Other mental disorder due to known physiological condition
F07	Personality and behavioral disorders due to know physiological condition
F09	Unspecified mental disorder due to known physiological condition

F01.-   Vascular dementia

Vascular dementia is the second most common form of dementia after Alzheimer's dementia. It can also coexist with dementia in Alzheimer's disease, dementia with Lewy bodies, or other forms of dementia making differentiating between the types very difficult.

F01.5-   Vascular dementia

Vascular dementia, also referred to as arteriosclerotic dementia or multi-infarct dementia (MID), has varying etiologies but is largely attributed to three vascular related mechanisms: small vessel disease, multiple cortical infarcts, or single strategic infarcts. Measured by the severity of cognitive function, the type of insult and the area in the brain that is involved impacts how the disease manifests in each patient. In small vessel disease, cognitive decline may progress slowly and may only impact memory and not daily functioning, while a single strategic infarct can cause immediate and substantial cognitive decline and drastic changes in activities of daily living.

F01.50   Vascular dementia without behavioral disturbance

F01.51   Vascular dementia with behavioral disturbance

Vascular dementia is classified based on the presence or absence of behavioral disturbances. Agitation is the most common behavioral disturbance often exhibited in the form of aggression, combativeness, pacing, and wandering. Hallucinations and paranoia are also common. Behavioral disturbances occur typically in the evening, and may be referred to as sundowning.

F02.-   Dementia in other diseases classified elsewhere

Dementia is the deterioration of cognition, usually of a progressive nature and serious enough to impact daily life functions. This category reports dementia that is a consequence of a separate physiological condition, the most common of which is Alzheimer's disease.

F02.8-   Dementia in other diseases classified elsewhere

The list of diseases that can cause dementia is extensive, ranging from nutritional deficiencies to systemic disorders. The onset and severity of the dementia symptoms can vary greatly depending on the underlying cause. In some cases, the dementia can be reversible. Treatment is typically directed at the underlying disorder, which can hinder the development of the dementia and reduce the symptoms.

F02.80   Dementia in other diseases classified elsewhere without behavioral disturbance

F02.81   Dementia in other diseases classified elsewhere with behavioral disturbance

Dementia in other diseases classified elsewhere is coded based on the presence or absence of behavioral disturbances. In some patients, the behavioral disturbances can be more challenging to manage than the cognitive losses. Hallucinations and paranoia, aggression and agitation, and depression are common behavioral and/or psychological symptoms that can affect a dementia patient.

F03.-   Unspecified dementia

Dementia refers to a decline in cognitive functioning to the point where it interferes with daily life. Dementia is a nonspecific diagnosis that includes a large range of symptoms and manifestations. When there is no documented cause or associated underlying disease process, the dementia is classified here.

F03.9-   Unspecified dementia

The terms senile dementia and presenile dementia are outdated but were used in the past to classify dementia when it was thought that mental decline was a normal part of aging. Senile dementia was typically used for mental decline occurring after age 65 and presenile dementia was used to describe mental decline occurring at or before age 65.

F03.90   Unspecified dementia without behavioral disturbance

F03.91   Unspecified dementia with behavioral disturbance

The two codes used to report unspecified dementia identify the presence or absence of behavioral disturbances. Behavioral disturbances can manifest as mood disorders, sleep disorders, psychotic disorders, or agitation, and most individuals with dementia exhibit one or more of these. Mood disorders may be marked by depression, mania, or simple apathy. Insomnia, hypersomnia, and reversal of sleep patterns (sleeping during the day, awake at night) are common sleep disorders. Psychotic disorders include conditions such as delusions and hallucinations. Agitation may manifest as aggression, combative behavior, pacing, or wandering.

F04   Amnestic disorder due to known physiological condition

Amnesia is the loss of facts, information, and experiences and can be temporary or, in very rare cases, permanent. Amnesia is characterized by prominent and lasting reduction of memory span, including striking loss of recent memory, disordered time appreciation, and confabulation.

There are two main types of amnesia: retrograde and anterograde. Retrograde is the result of damage to the retrieval process in the brain, which makes it difficult for the patient to recall preexisting memories. Anterograde is the more common of the two and results in the patient's inability to memorize new things. The patient's brain is unable to take the new data and transfer it into a long-term memory.

The most common cause of amnesia is a lesion to the brain, which may be due to direct trauma or a neurological disease. Physiologic conditions affecting the brain such as encephalitis, other inflammatory and degenerative diseases in which there is bilateral involvement of the temporal lobes, and certain temporal lobe tumors may also be responsible for amnesiac disorder. Other causes include severe acute and chronic illnesses and diseases, severe malnutrition, intense stress, and oxygen deprivation.

Focus Point

Classified here is nonalcoholic Korsakov's (Korsakoff's) psychosis or syndrome, a neurological disorder that is caused by a deprivation in thiamine, which is essential in biochemical processes in the brain. Patient's with Korsakov's experience retrograde and anterograde amnesia, hallucinations, and tend to confabulate or make up stories.

F05   Delirium due to known physiological condition

Delirium is a severe disturbance in an individual's mental functioning brought on by temporary impairment in brain activity. It is not a disease but rather a clinical set of symptoms that is the result of another underlying condition. Key diagnostic features include an acute or rapid onset of confused thinking and a decreased awareness of one's environment. It may also be characterized by extreme disturbances of arousal, attention, orientation, perception, intellectual functions, and affect, often accompanied by fear and agitation.

Underlying etiologies are extensive, but delirium is commonly seen in dementia, infection, high fever, dehydration, and terminal illnesses. Age also plays an important role as the risk of delirium increases as patients age.

Focus Point

It often can be difficult to differentiate between a diagnosis of dementia vs. delirium; this is especially true in the later stages of dementia. Determining a patient's baseline mental status is critical through review of past history and interviews with family and/or other caregivers. With a careful look at timing and type of symptoms in relation to the patient's baseline mental function, a physician may notice the following indicators that can help differentiate between the two syndromes.

Dementia Indicators

- Onset is gradual, with cognitive impairment declining as the disease progresses.

- Symptoms do not fluctuate much during the course of a day.

- Staying focused or maintaining attention is not usually a problem in a patient in early stage dementia.

Delirium Indicators

- Onset occurs very rapidly, within hours or days.

- Symptoms fluctuate significantly and often several times a day.

- Patients are unable to maintain focus and attention span is short.

F06.-   Other mental disorders due to known physiological condition

Mental disorders may have their origin in a physiological condition, such as diseases of the brain, endocrine disorders, or systemic diseases. These may be exhibited as psychotic disorders with schizophrenia-like symptoms, including paranoia, catatonia, and hallucinations, or as mental disorders with changes in mood, anxiety, and other types of psychosis. Early recognition of symptoms, diagnosis of the underlying cause, and management of the contributing factors are essential in preventing progression of and reducing the severity of mental disorders caused by physiological conditions.

F06.0   Psychotic disorder with hallucinations due to known physiological condition

Hallucinations are the perception of an event involving sight (visual hallucination), hearing (auditory hallucination), smell, taste, or touch (tactile hallucination) in the absence of an actual event. Hallucinations are caused by irritation or activation of neural pathways responsible for all of the senses.

Chapter 5. Mental and Behavioral Disorders (F01-F99)

Physiological conditions that may cause hallucinations include diseases of the brain, such as infection or inflammation, vascular disease, brain tumors, or epilepsy, as well as exposure to toxic substances and other acute or chronic diseases affecting other body systems.

F06.1   Catatonic disorder due to known physiological condition

Catatonia caused by a physiological medical condition is a neuromuscular disorder that may manifest as stupor, immobility, or agitated and purposeless movements. In stuporous catatonia, the patient appears to be unaware of people and surroundings, may move slowly or be immobile, does not speak, and may stare into space. In the immobile type, the patient remains motionless, often in what appears to be an uncomfortable position, for what may be a significant amount of time (hours, days, weeks, or longer). In the excited type, the patient is agitated or hyperactive and may exhibit impulsive or combative behavior.

Parkinson's disease and encephalitis are two medical conditions that may cause a catatonic-type disorder. Catatonia may also be a consequence of infection, metabolic disorders, vascular disease, and diseases of the brain, such as a tumor or inflammation.

F06.2   Psychotic disorder with delusions due to known physiological condition

A delusion is a strongly held belief in something that can be proven not to be true or can be proven to be greatly exaggerated even though the belief may have some basis in reality. Delusions vary greatly in structure from poorly organized, to not fixed but loosely organized, to fixed and well organized. There are a variety of themes to which the delusions may manifest themselves, such as persecution, plots, threats, being controlled by an external force, or grandiose beliefs related to power, wealth, or importance. Delusions may also relate to personal interactions, such as a belief that someone is not who they say they are, or a place, such as a belief that one is not really in their own home. Hallucinations may also be present.

Delusions are a consequence of certain brain conditions, epilepsy, Alzheimer's disease, and brain tumors. Conditions affecting other body systems such as endocrine or metabolic disorders can also provoke a delusional psychotic disorder.

F06.3-   Mood disorder due to known physiological condition

A mood disorder, such as depressive or bipolar disorder, is a disturbance in an individual's emotional state that also affects thought and behavior. Other terms used may include organic depressive disorder, organic depressive syndrome, and transient organic depressive type psychosis. Parkinson's disease,

Alzheimer's disease, multiple sclerosis, cerebrovascular disease, stroke, and brain tumors are a few known physiological conditions that can elicit a mood disorder.

F06.31   Mood disorder due to known physiological condition with depressive features

Sadness, diminished interest in activities, fatigue, insomnia or hypersomnia, and change in weight are a few of the classic depressive features.

F06.32   Mood disorder due to known physiological condition with major depressive-like episode

A major depressive-like episode is when a patient has severely depressed mood and loss of interest in their usual activities that lasts for weeks or longer. The patient displays one or more of the depressive features above as well as physical symptoms such as pain, fatigue, or digestive problems.

F06.33   Mood disorder due to known physiological condition with manic features

Mania is a state of uncharacteristically elevated mood and/or energy level. It may be exhibited as elation, excitement, rapid thought process, increased psychomotor activity, and emotional instability.

F06.34   Mood disorder due to known physiological condition with mixed features

In a mixed type mood disorder, symptoms related to depression and mania may be present or the patient may cycle between episodes of depression and mania.

F06.8   Other specified mental disorders due to known physiological condition

An inclusion term found under this code is epileptic psychosis NOS. Patients with epilepsy may experience hallucinations, delusions, or disorganized thoughts that can be interictal, in between seizures or postictal, after a seizure. In particular, those patients with temporal lobe epilepsy or those that experience complex partial or tonic-clonic seizures are at increased risk of related psychosis.

F07.-   Personality and behavioral disorders due to known physiological condition

Patients with a personality disorder find it hard to relate to other people or situations and behave in a way that deviates from the normal culture of that individual. Thoughts and behaviors are often unhealthy and inflexible. A person with a personality disorder may not realize they have a disorder because to them their behavior and thoughts seem normal and the problem is in the people around them.

F07.0 Personality change due to known physiological condition

Personality changes are sudden and drastic alterations in a patient's behavior or thinking in comparison to how he or she normally behaves. How the behavior is altered depends on the area of the brain that is damaged and can include an array of symptoms from inappropriate social behavior to depression to perseveration.

A condition included here is frontal lobe syndrome where changes in behavior follow damage to the frontal areas of the brain or follow interference with the connections of those areas. There is a general diminution of self-control, foresight, creativity, and spontaneity, which may be manifest as increased irritability, selfishness, restlessness, and lack of concern for others. Conscientiousness and powers of concentration are often diminished, but measurable deterioration of intellect or memory is not necessarily present. The overall picture is often one of emotional dullness, lack of drive, and slowness, but, particularly in persons previously with energetic, restless, or aggressive characteristics, there may be a change toward impulsiveness, boastfulness, temper outbursts, silly fatuous humor, and the development of unrealistic ambitions. The direction of change usually depends upon the previous personality.

F07.8- Other personality and behavioral disorders due to known physiological condition

This subcategory captures the more obscure personality or behavioral changes that may arise secondary to another medical condition.

F07.81 Postconcussional syndrome

This syndrome refers to a compilation of mental and behavioral changes, along with physical symptoms that emerge following a head injury. The timeline of onset is usually around seven to 10 days after the initial injury and is usually short term, a few weeks to months, but can last longer. Headache, dizziness, fatigue, and sensitivity to light and sound are among the usual physical symptoms. Specific emotional or behavioral changes can include:

- Anxiety
- Irritability
- Loss of concentration
- Depressed mood
- Memory problems

Mood may fluctuate and ordinary stress may produce exaggerated fear and apprehension. There may be marked intolerance of mental and physical exertion, undue sensitivity to noise, and hypochondriacal preoccupation. The symptoms are more common in persons who have previously suffered from neurotic or personality disorders. This syndrome is particularly associated with the closed type of head injury when signs of localized brain damage are slight or absent, but it may also occur in other conditions.

F07.89 Other personality and behavioral disorders due to known physiological condition

Postencephalitic syndrome and Klüver-Bucy syndrome are two conditions included here. Postencephalitic syndrome occurs in patients that have recovered from bacterial or viral encephalitis. Symptoms may include apathy, irritability, altered sleep or eating patterns, learning difficulties, and changes in social judgment.

Mental and Behavioral Disorders due to Psychoactive Substance Use (F10-F19)

Psychoactive substances are chemical substances that alter brain function, temporarily changing a person's mood, perception, behavior, and/or consciousness. In some cases, this may be a beneficial response needed to treat a particular disease or disorder. However, even substances with beneficial uses can be misused. Mental and behavioral disorders due to psychoactive substance use, abuse, and dependence are negative effects and complications related to misuse of these substances.

The categories in this code block are as follows:

F10	Alcohol related disorders
F11	Opioid related disorders
F12	Cannabis related disorders
F13	Sedative, hypnotic, or anxiolytic related disorders
F14	Cocaine related disorders
F15	Other stimulant related disorders
F16	Hallucinogen related disorders
F17	Nicotine dependence
F18	Inhalant related disorders
F19	Other psychoactive substance related disorders

Categories and codes are organized based on the psychoactive substance, pattern of use, and associated mental or behavioral disorder.

The type of psychoactive substance involved sets up the framework for this code block. Once the psychoactive substance has been identified, the pattern of use must be identified as use, abuse, or dependence. There is one exception to pattern use and that is for nicotine. Dependence is the only pattern of use that is recognized for the nicotine. For all other categories, the following patterns of use apply and are defined as follows:

- Use is irregular or low frequency use of a substance that is not habitual.

- Abuse is habitual use of a substance that negatively impacts a patient's health or social functioning but has not arrived at the point of physical and/or mental dependency.

- Dependence is a chronic mental and physical state where the patient has to use a substance in order to function normally; generally these patients experience signs of withdrawal upon cessation of the substance.

- In the subcategories for dependence there are codes available for "in remission" to indicate that the clinical criteria for dependence on a psychoactive substance are no longer met. Assignment of a code for "in remission" requires physician judgment that the patient is in remission.

Focus Point

Diagnosing a mental or behavioral disorder is very complex but it becomes even more so when a psychoactive substance is involved. The provider needs to establish whether the presenting mental or behavioral disturbances are:

- *Due to a primary mental disorder*

- *Part of the intoxication or withdrawal phase of a specific psychoactive substance*

- *Due to a substance but beyond the scope of what would be exhibited during intoxication or withdrawal of the substance alone and needs independent clinical consideration*

Codes for disorders related to psychoactive substance use are assigned based on any complications associated with the use of the psychoactive substance. While not all psychoactive substances or patterns of use are associated with the same complications, there are a number of complications that can occur regardless of the psychoactive substance and the pattern of use. A basic description of the most common complications is included below.

Amnestic disorder: Memory disorder characterized by loss of facts, information, and experiences. Amnesia is characterized by prominent and lasting reduction of memory span, including striking loss of recent memory, disordered time appreciation, and confabulation.

Anxiety disorder: Array of symptoms with the most common being relentless and often debilitating feelings of worry and/or fear. Other symptoms include hysteria, obsession, compulsion, feelings of worthlessness, or phobias. Behavior may be greatly affected although it usually remains within socially acceptable limits.

Delirium: Severe disturbance in mental functioning brought on by temporary impairment in brain activity. Key diagnostic features include an acute or rapid onset of confused thinking and a decreased awareness of physical environment. It may also be characterized by extreme disturbances of arousal, attention, orientation, perception, intellectual functions, and affect that are often accompanied by fear and agitation.

Delusions: False beliefs or altered perception of a real stimulus.

Dementia: Decline in cognitive functioning to the point where it interferes with daily life. Dementia includes a large range of symptoms and manifestations.

Hallucinations: False perceptions involving the senses that occur in the absence of an apparent stimulus. Hallucinations may involve sight (visual hallucination), hearing (auditory hallucination), smell, taste, or touch (tactile hallucination).

Intoxication: Acute but reversible effects of a psychoactive substance on the user. Manifestations of intoxication are dependent on the type and dose of the substance and the tolerance level of the user, as well as other factors.

Mood disorder: Disturbance of emotions manifested by prolonged periods of abnormally depressed (low), elated (high), or alternating mood.

Perceptual disturbance: Disturbance related to how sensory stimuli are interpreted or understood.

Psychotic disorder: Gross impairment of reality that may include schizophrenia-like symptoms, including delusions, paranoia, hallucinations, and catatonia.

Sexual dysfunction: Problems with sexual dysfunction that may include loss of desire, inability to become aroused or achieve orgasm, and/or pain during sex.

Sleep disorder: Disruption of normal sleep patterns. Insomnia, hypersomnia, and reversal of sleep patterns (sleeping during the day, awake at night) are common sleep disorders.

Withdrawal: Physical and/or emotional symptoms that occur with sudden cessation or reduction of a psychoactive substance by an individual with a physical or mental dependence on the substance. Withdrawal is usually the result of heavy or prolonged use. Withdrawal manifestations are specific to the psychoactive substance.

F10.- Alcohol related disorders

Alcohol is one of the oldest recreational, psychoactive substances used by humans. In chemistry, the term "alcohol" refers to a large group of organic chemical compounds of which there are many types. Alcohol, without further qualification, usually refers to ethyl alcohol or ethanol, which is the type used to make alcoholic beverages such as beer, wine, and spirits. Alcohol affects the central nervous system by slowing down brain activity and is considered a depressant. Alcohol related mental disorders are organic psychotic states due mainly to excessive consumption of alcohol. Defects of nutrition are also thought to play an important role in alcoholic mental disorders. Alcoholic mental disorders are classified according to the documented severity, which is differentiated as abuse, dependence, or use, and the complex of presenting symptoms.

F10.1- Alcohol abuse

Alcohol abuse is a pattern of drinking that is harmful to health, adversely affects interpersonal relationships, or impairs the ability to work. Abuse of alcohol may be evidenced by failure to assume necessary responsibilities at home, school, or work; drinking in dangerous situations such as drinking and driving; legal issues related to alcohol such as a drunk driving arrest or assault of another person while under the influence of alcohol; and interpersonal relationship problems directly related to excessive alcohol consumption.

> **Focus Point**
>
> *Alcohol abuse codes should only be assigned based on provider documentation. Codes from this subcategory that describe a mental or behavioral disorder should be used only when the relationship between alcohol abuse and the documented mental or behavioral disorder has been clearly established in the provider documentation.*

F10.10 Alcohol abuse, uncomplicated

Uncomplicated alcohol abuse refers to documented alcohol abuse without documentation of a coexisting alcohol-induced mental or behavioral health problem.

F10.11 Alcohol abuse, in remission

When a patient who has previously been diagnosed with alcohol abuse or mild use disorder has stopped consuming alcohol recently or over an extended period of time it is considered as remission. The use of this code is based on provider documentation of remission.

F10.12- Alcohol abuse with intoxication

This subcategory classifies documented alcohol abuse in combination with a current acute intoxicated state as evidenced by mental and physical impairment directly related to the current episode of alcohol consumption. Common symptoms of mental impairment due to alcohol intoxication include euphoria, loss of social inhibitions, poor judgment, memory loss, confusion, and disorientation. Common symptoms of physical impairment due to alcohol intoxication include loss of muscle coordination, slurred speech, lethargy, nausea, and vomiting.

F10.120 Alcohol abuse with intoxication, uncomplicated

This code is reported for documented alcohol abuse in combination with a current acute intoxicated state as evidenced by mental and physical impairment directly related to the consumption of alcohol but described as uncomplicated.

F10.121 Alcohol abuse with intoxication delirium

This code is reported for documented alcohol abuse in combination with a current acute intoxicated state as evidenced by mental and physical impairment directly related to the consumption of alcohol and complicated by intoxication delirium. Alcohol intoxication delirium is characterized by a level of mental disorientation in excess of the level that one would typically see in an individual using alcohol. Symptoms of alcohol intoxication delirium vary but typically include extreme shifts in mental alertness, mental excitability, and physical mobility. There may also be extreme and alternating levels of anger, agitation, anxiety, confusion, depression, euphoria, and irritability.

F10.14 Alcohol abuse with alcohol-induced mood disorder

In an alcohol-induced mood disorder, all or most of the disordered mood is the direct result of alcohol abuse. Alcohol-induced mood disorders may present as depression, mania, or a combination of the two. Depression is characterized by a marked loss of interest or pleasure in most activities that would typically engage a person who was not depressed. A manic state is characterized by an elevated, elated, expansive, or irritable mood. Alternating depressed and manic mood swings may also indicate a mood disorder related to the alcohol abuse.

F10.15- Alcohol abuse with alcohol-induced psychotic disorder

In an alcohol-induced psychotic disorder, all or most of the psychotic symptoms are the direct result of alcohol abuse. Alcohol-induced psychotic disorders often present with delusions or hallucinations. Delusions are false beliefs or altered perceptions. Hallucinations are false perceptions involving the senses that occur in the absence of an apparent stimulus. Hallucinations may involve sight (visual hallucination), hearing (auditory hallucination), smell, taste, or touch (tactile hallucination).

F10.2- Alcohol dependence

Alcohol dependence is a chronic disease characterized by a strong craving for alcohol and the inability to limit drinking even when continued use of alcohol results in physical or psychological health issues; the inability to fulfill personal responsibilities at home, school, or work; legal problems; or interpersonal relationship problems. Dependence is also exhibited by a tolerance to alcohol and the need to drink larger amounts to achieve the desired effect. In addition, the patient may suffer from withdrawal symptoms when alcohol consumption ceases. Alcohol dependence may also be referred to as alcohol addiction or alcoholism.

Focus Point

Alcohol dependence codes should only be assigned based on provider documentation. Codes from this subcategory that describe a mental or behavioral disorder should be used only when the relationship between and alcohol dependence and the documented mental or behavioral disorder has been clearly established in the provider documentation.

F10.20 Alcohol dependence, uncomplicated

Alcohol dependence may present with or without mental or behavioral disorders. Use this code when dependence on alcohol is documented but the patient has no documented mental or behavioral disorders associated with the dependence.

F10.21 Alcohol dependence, in remission

Because alcohol dependence is a chronic disease, even after an alcoholic has successfully stopped drinking for a period of time or has changed the pattern of use to one that does not meet the criteria of dependence, a diagnosis of alcohol dependence may still apply but the condition will be classified as in remission. The code for in remission is assigned only when the clinical criteria for alcohol dependence are no longer met and the physician documentation indicates that the patient is in remission.

F10.22- Alcohol dependence with intoxication

Excessive alcohol consumption can lead to intoxication with depression of central nervous system function characterized by mood changes, impaired motor function, and impaired mental capacity. Symptoms of mood changes include anger, agitation, anxiety, depression, euphoria, and irritability. Symptoms of mental impairment include loss of social inhibitions, poor judgment, memory loss, confusion, and disorientation. Common symptoms of physical impairment due to alcohol intoxication include loss of muscle coordination, slurred speech, lethargy, nausea, and vomiting.

F10.220 Alcohol dependence with intoxication, uncomplicated

Use this code for alcohol dependence with uncomplicated intoxication.

F10.221 Alcohol dependence with intoxication delirium

Alcohol intoxication delirium is characterized by a level of mental disorientation in excess of the level that one would typically see in an individual using alcohol. Symptoms of alcohol intoxication delirium vary but typically include extreme shifts in mental alertness, mental excitability, and physical mobility. There may also be extreme and alternating levels of anger, agitation, anxiety, confusion, depression, euphoria, and irritability.

F10.23- Alcohol dependence with withdrawal

The phenomenon of alcohol withdrawal begins when an individual greatly reduces or ceases consumption of alcohol after a period of prolonged and heavy use. Acute alcohol withdrawal refers to a cluster of symptoms; however, these symptoms vary individually and may range from mild to severe. Uncomplicated acute alcohol withdrawal includes two or more of the following symptoms when these symptoms are not related to another medical condition: hand tremor, anxiety, psychomotor agitation (excessive restlessness), nausea or vomiting, insomnia, and autonomic symptoms (low-grade fever, rapid breathing, and profuse sweating). The symptoms must also severely impair the ability of individual to function at home, at work, or in social settings. Acute alcohol withdrawal may be complicated by seizures, delirium tremens, and perceptual disturbances. Typically withdrawal symptoms peak on the second day and improve markedly by the fourth day. However, symptoms of anxiety, insomnia, and autonomic dysfunction can linger for as long as six months.

F10.230 Alcohol dependence with withdrawal, uncomplicated

Use this code for alcohol dependence with uncomplicated withdrawal.

F10.231 Alcohol dependence with withdrawal delirium

Alcohol dependence withdrawal delirium, also called delirium tremens (DT), is an acute or subacute organic psychotic state in alcoholics in which the individual experiences extreme hyperactivity of the autonomic system (low-grade fever, rapid breathing, and profuse sweating), along with hallucinations of any kind, but most notably visual and tactile. Other symptoms commonly present with delirium tremens include clouded consciousness, disorientation, fear, illusions, delusions, psychomotor agitation, and tremor.

F10.232 Alcohol dependence with withdrawal with perceptual disturbance

Perceptual disturbance occurs in the absence of delirium in up to 10 percent of alcohol dependent patients experiencing withdrawal symptoms. Perceptual disturbance refers to visual, auditory, and/or tactile hallucinations that may occur from 12 hours to several days following cessation or reduction in alcohol consumption. Other symptoms of acute alcohol withdrawal may also be present, such as hand tremor, anxiety, psychomotor agitation (excessive restlessness), nausea or vomiting, and insomnia.

F10.24 Alcohol dependence with alcohol-induced mood disorder

Alcohol induced mood or affective disorders are significant disturbances of mood caused by alcohol consumption. Alcohol induced mood disorders may present as depression or a marked loss of interest or pleasure in most activities that would typically engage a person who was not depressed, a manic state characterized by an elevated, elated, expansive, or irritable mood, or alternating depressed and manic mood swings.

Focus Point

Code F10.24 is reported for any condition classified as a mood or affective disorder in code block F30-F39 when the mood or affective disorder is due to or caused by alcohol dependence. Do not use code F10.24 when the patient has an independent mood disorder that is unrelated to alcohol dependence.

If the documentation is unclear as to whether the mood disorder is alcohol-induced or an independent mood disorder unrelated to alcohol dependence, query the provider.

Alcohol induced anxiety disorder is not classified as a mood disorder. For alcohol dependence with alcohol induced anxiety disorder, use code F10.280.

F10.26 Alcohol dependence with alcohol-induced persisting amnestic disorder

Alcohol-induced persisting amnestic disorder is a syndrome of prominent and lasting reduction of memory span, including striking loss of recent memory, disordered time appreciation, and confabulation, occurring in alcoholics as the sequel to an acute alcoholic psychosis (especially delirium tremens) or, more rarely, in the course of chronic alcoholism. It is usually accompanied by peripheral neuritis and may be associated with Wernicke's encephalopathy. Korsakov's syndrome is included here and is the result of deficient thiamine in the blood due to excessive use of alcohol. Most often the memory disturbance is manifested as an inability to learn new information or anterograde amnesia. Another

important feature of Korsakov's is confabulation. Often the patient makes up stories to fill in gaps of memory that are very convincing, especially to the patient, even though the information is not based on fact.

F11.- Opioid related disorders

Opioids are psychoactive chemicals that bind to opioid receptors found in the brain and other sites in the central nervous system and the gastrointestinal tract. Medicinally they have been used for thousands of years to relieve pain but additional uses include cough suppression, anesthesia, antidiarrheal, and weaning addicted patients off other opioid type drugs. The most frequently abused opioids are heroin and methadone. Other common opioids with the potential for abuse include morphine, codeine, hydrocodone, oxycodone (Oxycontin®), hydromorphone (Dilaudid®), meperidine (Demerol®), tramadol, and fentanyl.

F11.1- Opioid abuse

Opioid abuse is a pattern of use that is harmful to health, adversely affects interpersonal relationships, or impairs the ability to work. Abuse of opioids may be evidenced by failure to assume necessary responsibilities at home, school, or work; legal issues related to opioid use; and interpersonal relationship problems directly related to opioid consumption.

F11.10 Opioid abuse, uncomplicated

Uncomplicated opioid abuse refers to documented opioid abuse without documentation of a coexisting opioid-induced mental or behavioral health problem.

F11.11 Opioid abuse, in remission

When a patient who has previously been diagnosed with opioid abuse or mild use disorder has stopped abusing opioid recently or over an extended period of time it is considered as remission. The use of this code is based on provider documentation of remission.

F11.12- Opioid abuse with intoxication

Opioid intoxication refers to the acute but reversible physical, mental, and psychological effects of a psychoactive substance on the user. Symptoms of opioid intoxication may include euphoria, slurred speech, indifference to pain, small pupils, extreme sleepiness, and respiratory depression.

F11.2- Opioid dependence

Dependence on opioids is characterized by a set of psychological and behavioral changes that include drug craving, compulsive use, and a tendency to relapse following detoxification and rehabilitation. In addition, the dependent person is unable to limit use of the substance even when continued use results in physical or psychological health issues; the inability to fulfill personal responsibilities at home, school, or work; legal problems; or interpersonal relationship problems.

F11.23   Opioid dependence with withdrawal

Unless the patient has an underlying medical condition, withdrawal from opioids is usually not life-threatening. Common withdrawal symptoms include negative mood, watery eyes, yawning, muscle aches, restlessness, insomnia, goose bumps, sweating, and elevated blood pressure. Withdrawal symptoms can manifest as soon as six hours after last use and usually peak around day two. Symptoms typically resolve in seven to 10 days but some may persist as long as six months or more.

F12.-   Cannabis related disorders

Cannabis or marijuana is a plant that produces a psychoactive chemical compound or cannabinoid called delta-9-tetrahydrocannabinol or THC. It is most often smoked but can also be consumed by mixing in food or brewed as tea. Cannabis affects the brain by overstimulating cannabinoid receptors found in brain cells. The areas of the brain that have the highest concentration of cannabinoid receptors are the areas that influence memory, thinking, pleasure, concentration, and coordinated movement. When these receptor pathways are overstimulated, it can cause memory and learning difficulties, impaired coordination, thinking and problem solving difficulties, and distorted perceptions.

F12.1-   Cannabis abuse

Cannabis abuse is a pattern of use that is harmful to health, adversely affects interpersonal relationships, or impairs the ability to work. Abuse of cannabis may be evidenced by failure to assume necessary responsibilities at home, school, or work; use of cannabis in dangerous situations such as when driving; legal issues related to use; and interpersonal relationship problems directly related to cannabis use.

F12.10   Cannabis abuse, uncomplicated

Uncomplicated cannabis abuse refers to documented abuse without documentation of a coexisting cannabis-induced mental or behavioral health problem.

F12.11   Cannabis abuse, in remission

When a patient who has previously been diagnosed with cannabis abuse or mild use disorder has stopped abusing cannabis recently or over an extended period of time it is considered as remission. The use of this code is based on provider documentation of remission.

F12.12-   Cannabis abuse with intoxication

The intoxicating effects of cannabis vary from person to person and the amount of the drug used. Younger individuals whose brains have not fully developed typically experience more problems in relation to cannabis use than those who begin use later in life. Generally cannabis use produces a relaxing or euphoric

effect but negative effects can also result. Symptoms may include reduced motivation, slow thinking, slow reflexes, difficulty concentrating, dilated pupils, bloodshot eyes, and mouth dryness.

F13.-   Sedative, hypnotic, or anxiolytic related disorders

A sedative is a drug that depresses the activity of the central nervous system. A hypnotic drug induces sleep. An anxiolytic drug inhibits anxiety. Sedative, hypnotic, or anxiolytic drugs alter the speed of nerve impulses that are regulated by neurotransmitters in the brain by increasing a chemical called gamma-aminobutyric acid (GABA). When GABA levels increase, the nerve impulse speed decreases and the nervous system slows down. Although sedative, hypnotic, and anxiolytic drugs are distinct in how they affect the mind and body, it is rare to find drugs in these three classes that exhibit affects in only one area. For example, a sedative that depresses the central nervous system, in most cases, also induces hypnotic and/or anxiolytic effects.

F13.1-   Sedative, hypnotic or anxiolytic-related abuse

Abuse of sedative, hypnotic, or anxiolytic substances is a pattern of use that is harmful to health, adversely affects interpersonal relationships, or impairs the ability to work. Abuse of these substances may be evidenced by failure to assume necessary responsibilities at home, school, or work; legal issues related to use; and interpersonal relationship problems directly related to excessive use of these substances.

F13.10   Sedative, hypnotic or anxiolytic abuse, uncomplicated

Uncomplicated abuse of sedatives, hypnotics, or anxiolytics refers to documented abuse without documentation of a coexisting mental or behavioral health problem resulting from the use of these substances.

F13.11   Sedative, hypnotic or anxiolytic abuse, in remission

When a patient who has previously been diagnosed with abuse or mild use disorder of a sedative, hypnotic, or anxiolytic has stopped abusing the substance recently or over an extended period of time it is considered as remission. The use of this code is based on provider documentation of remission.

F13.12-   Sedative, hypnotic or anxiolytic abuse with intoxication

Intoxication is the acute but reversible effects of a psychoactive substance on the user. Manifestations of intoxication are dependent on the type and dose of the substance and the tolerance level of the user, as well as other factors. Physical symptoms of intoxication due to sedative, hypnotic, or anxiolytic abuse can include hypothermia, respiratory depression, hypotension, nystagmus, ataxia, and stupor. Mental or behavioral symptoms may include aggression, memory problems, paranoia, illusions, hallucinations, and mood lability.

F13.2- Sedative, hypnotic or anxiolytic-related dependence

Dependence on sedatives, hypnotics, or anxiolytic substances is characterized by a set of psychological and behavioral changes that include drug craving, compulsive use, and a tendency to relapse following detoxification and rehabilitation. In addition, the dependent person is unable to limit use of the substance even when continued use results in physical or psychological health issues; the inability to fulfill personal responsibilities at home, school, or work; legal problems; or interpersonal relationship problems.

F13.23- Sedative, hypnotic or anxiolytic dependence with withdrawal

Withdrawal is a set of physical and/or emotional symptoms that occur with sudden cessation or reduction of a psychoactive substance by an individual with a physical or mental dependence on the substance. Withdrawal is usually the result of heavy or prolonged use. Withdrawal manifestations are specific to the psychoactive substance and in the case of sedatives, hypnotics, or anxiolytics include tachycardia, palpitations, ataxia, tachypnea, anxiety, tremors, fever, and seizures. Some individuals may experience symptom rebound when withdrawing from these drugs. Symptom rebound is the recurrence of the symptoms that were being treated with a prescribed sedative, hypnotic, or anxiolytic, often with increased intensity of the symptoms after stopping the drug. However, the symptoms do usually subside with time.

F14.- Cocaine related disorders

Obtained from the leaves of the coca plant, cocaine is a central nervous system stimulant. There are two forms of the drug: powdered, which is snorted or injected, and crack, which is smoked. Cocaine interrupts communication between neurons in the brain by blocking reabsorption of certain biochemicals by the neuron cells. These biochemicals, such as dopamine, build up in the junction between neurons and produce the euphoric feeling or "high" that the user feels. Along with psychiatric disorders, cocaine increases the risk of heart attack, stroke, seizures, and respiratory failure. Sudden death can result from cocaine use even with first-time users.

F14.1- Cocaine abuse

Cocaine abuse is a pattern of cocaine use that is harmful to health, adversely affects interpersonal relationships, or impairs the ability to work. Abuse of cocaine may be evidenced by failure to assume necessary responsibilities at home, school, or work; legal issues related to cocaine use; and interpersonal relationship problems directly related to the use of cocaine.

F14.10 Cocaine abuse, uncomplicated

Uncomplicated cocaine abuse refers to documented abuse without documentation of a coexisting cocaine-induced mental or behavioral health problem.

F14.11 Cocaine abuse, in remission

When a patient who has previously been diagnosed with cocaine abuse or mild use disorder has stopped abusing cocaine recently or over an extended period of time it is considered as remission. The use of this code is based on provider documentation of remission.

F14.12- Cocaine abuse with intoxication

The "high" experienced by cocaine users can include feelings of euphoria, increased energy, and decreased sensation of pain, just to name a few. However, there are many undesirable effects that may also be associated with cocaine intoxication, such as anxiety, agitation, restlessness, headache, tremors, paranoia, cold sweats, and elevated body temperature and blood pressure.

F14.2- Cocaine dependence

Dependence on cocaine is characterized by a set of psychological and behavioral changes that include drug craving, compulsive use, and a tendency to relapse following detoxification and rehabilitation. In addition, the dependent person is unable to limit use of cocaine even when continued use results in physical or psychological health issues; the inability to fulfill personal responsibilities at home, school, or work; legal problems; or interpersonal relationship problems.

F15.- Other stimulant related disorders

Stimulants, as the name implies, speed up or stimulate the central and peripheral nervous systems. There are many medicinal uses for stimulant drugs, including treatment of attention deficit hyperactivity disorder (ADHD), relief of nasal and sinus congestion, and treatment of narcolepsy. Stimulants interrupt communication between neurons by increasing the "feel-good" chemicals in the brain. The body eventually decreases its natural production of these same chemicals to compensate for the increase imposed by the drug. The user ends up needing a higher dose of the drug to feel the same euphoric effects because the natural production of these chemicals by the body is reduced. If use of the stimulant drug is stopped events that normally make the patient "feel good" do not incite the same response. In fact, the low or "crash" may be so intense that the need for the drug is also intensified just to feel better. Common stimulant drugs include Adderall®, Ritalin®, methamphetamine, pseudoephedrine, mephedrone (drone, MCAT), and methylenedioxymethamphetamine (MDMA, Ecstasy). Caffeine, although not commonly thought of as a psychoactive substance, is the most widely used stimulant in the world and is included in this category.

Focus Point

Cocaine is a common stimulant that is not included here. See category F14 for cocaine-related mental and behavioral disorders.

F15.1-   Other stimulant abuse

Stimulant abuse is a pattern of use that is harmful to health, adversely affects interpersonal relationships, or impairs the ability to work. Abuse of stimulants may be evidenced by failure to assume necessary responsibilities at home, school, or work; legal issues related to stimulant use; and interpersonal relationship problems directly related to the use of stimulants.

F15.10   Other stimulant abuse, uncomplicated

Uncomplicated stimulant abuse refers to documented abuse without documentation of a coexisting stimulant-induced mental or behavioral health problem.

F15.11   Other stimulant abuse, in remission

When a patient who has previously been diagnosed with abuse or mild use disorder of another type of stimulant and has stopped abusing that substance recently or over an extended period of time, it is considered as remission. The use of this code is based on provider documentation of remission.

F15.12-   Other stimulant abuse with intoxication

Intoxication is the acute but reversible effects of a psychoactive substance on the user. Manifestations of intoxication are dependent on the type and dose of the substance and the tolerance level of the user, as well as other factors. Intoxication due to stimulant abuse may resemble a manic state with symptoms that include increased psychomotor activity, hyperawareness, hypersexuality, hypervigilance and paranoia, and impaired judgment or insight. Other signs of stimulant intoxication include increased blood pressure and heart rate, dilated pupils, anxiousness, and restlessness.

F15.2-   Other stimulant dependence

Dependence on other stimulants is characterized by a set of psychological and behavioral changes that include drug craving, compulsive use, and a tendency to relapse following detoxification and rehabilitation. In addition, the dependent person is unable to limit use of the substance even when continued use results in physical or psychological health issues; the inability to fulfill personal responsibilities at home, school, or work; legal problems; or interpersonal relationship problems.

F15.23   Other stimulant dependence with withdrawal

Withdrawal is a set of physical and/or emotional symptoms that occur with sudden cessation or reduction of a psychoactive substance by an individual with a physical or mental dependence on the substance. Withdrawal is usually the result of heavy or prolonged use. Withdrawal manifestations are specific to the psychoactive substance. In the case of stimulants, withdrawal from the manic state associated with these drugs may initially result in a crash state with symptoms of depression, anxiety, agitation, and intense drug craving. These initial withdrawal symptoms may be followed by fatigue, decreased attention, and decreased physical and mental energy. Withdrawal from stimulants may also be accompanied by periods of intense drug craving even after the physical and mental withdrawal symptoms have subsided.

F16.-   Hallucinogen related disorders

Hallucinogens are a broad grouping of drugs that distort the way a person perceives reality. Similar to other drugs in this section, hallucinogens disrupt chemical signals in the brain altering normal brain function. Hallucinogens have a very unpredictable nature, much more so than other psychoactive drugs, with significant variations in subjective experience, not only between users but between ingestions.

F16.1-   Hallucinogen abuse

Hallucinogen abuse is a pattern of use that is harmful to health, adversely affects interpersonal relationships, or impairs the ability to work. Abuse of hallucinogens may be evidenced by failure to assume necessary responsibilities at home, school, or work; legal issues related to use; and interpersonal relationship problems directly related to the use of hallucinogens.

F16.10   Hallucinogen abuse, uncomplicated

Uncomplicated hallucinogen abuse refers to documented abuse without documentation of a coexisting hallucinogen-induced mental or behavioral health problem.

F16.11   Hallucinogen abuse, in remission

When a patient who has previously been diagnosed with hallucinogen abuse or mild use disorder has stopped abusing hallucinogens recently or over an extended period of time it is considered as remission. The use of this code is based on provider documentation of remission.

F16.12-   Hallucinogen abuse with intoxication

Intoxication is the acute but reversible effects of a psychoactive substance on the user. Manifestations of intoxication are dependent on the type and dose of the substance and the tolerance level of the user, as well as other factors. Symptoms due to hallucinogen intoxication are extremely varied. Some of the more common physical symptoms may include dilated pupils, hyperthermia, sweating, increased heart rate and blood pressure, tremors, blurred vision, and lack of coordination. The psychological symptoms of intoxication range from euphoria and/or enlightenment to panic and/or anxiety. "Set" and "setting" are often key factors in how a hallucinogenic drug impacts a user. "Set" is the state of mind a person is in at the time of the drug use. The "setting" is the environment in which the drug use takes place.

F16.2-   Hallucinogen dependence

Dependence on hallucinogen substances is characterized by a set of psychological and behavioral changes that include drug craving, compulsive use, and a tendency to relapse following rehabilitation. In addition, the dependent person is unable to limit use of the substance even when continued use results in physical or psychological health issues; the inability to fulfill personal responsibilities at home, school, or work; legal problems; or interpersonal relationship problems.

F17.-   Nicotine dependence

This code is used when the patient is known to be dependent on nicotine or tobacco. This is essentially an addiction as nicotine may be classified as a drug. Nicotine dependence indicates the patient's inability to stop using, even knowing the harmful effects. The adverse cycle involves the patient's temporary feeling of overall well-being during use but anxiety, inability to concentrate, depression, difficulty sleeping, digestive problems, and irritable behavior during withdrawal. Nicotine dependence leads to several related diseases, including heart disease, stroke, and cancer. This category includes dependence on, use disorder of, and remission of: cigarettes, chewing tobacco, and other tobacco products.

Schizophrenia, Schizotypal, Delusional, and Other Non-mood Psychotic Disorders (F20-F29)

Diagnostic criteria for psychotic disorders grouped to this code block incorporate the following symptoms:

- Delusions: A false belief that cannot be changed regardless of contradictory evidence

- Disorganized speech: Rambling, derailment, incoherency

- Motor behavior abnormalities/disorganized behavior: Catatonia, childlike silliness, agitation

- Hallucinations: Perception of the senses that only the individual can perceive; auditory is the most common

- Negative symptoms: Anhedonia, lack of motivation, blunted affect

Diagnostic assessment is based on how many of the above symptoms are exhibited and whether these symptoms have altered the individual's daily functioning.

The categories in this code block are as follows:

F20	Schizophrenia
F21	Schizotypal disorder
F22	Delusional disorders
F23	Brief psychotic disorder
F24	Shared psychotic disorder
F25	Schizoaffective disorders
F28	Other psychotic disorder not due to a substance or known physiological condition
F29	Unspecified psychosis not due to a substance or known physiological condition

F20.-   Schizophrenia

Schizophrenia is a group or spectrum of severe, chronic brain disorders that manifest as disturbances of thought, perception, mood, conduct or behavior, and personality. Symptoms of schizophrenia are grouped into three categories: positive, negative, and cognitive symptoms. Positive symptoms are those that are not seen in individuals with normal brain functioning and include hallucinations, delusions, disturbances in thought content or thought processes, and motion disorders ranging from agitation and repetitive movements to catatonia. Negative symptoms are associated with changes in mood or emotions and conduct or behavior and may include the inability to plan or carry out daily activities, the inability to interact with others, and lack of emotion as exhibited by a flat affect. Cognitive symptoms are those related to thought, problem solving ability, and memory and include the inability to process information and make decisions, the inability to focus, and the inability to remember or to retrieve information. Schizophrenia is classified based on the predominant manifestations of the brain disorder and include the following types: paranoid, disorganized, catatonic, undifferentiated, residual, schizophreniform disorder, and other types.

F20.0   Paranoid schizophrenia

Paranoid schizophrenia's main feature is delusions often accompanied by auditory hallucinations. The delusions and hallucinations typically revolve around a specific theme, usually relating to persecution or conspiracy that does not change over time. Behavioral changes are reflective of the content of the delusions and hallucinations. Paranoid schizophrenics may be distrustful and suspicious of others. They may believe that others are lying to them, exploiting them, or planning to harm them. They may misinterpret benign actions or remarks as threatening, insulting, or as attacks on their character or reputation.

F20.1   Disorganized schizophrenia

Disorganized schizophrenia is considered to be one of the more severe forms of schizophrenia because individuals with this subtype often cannot communicate intelligibly with others or perform daily activities needed to care for themselves. It is characterized by disorganized thought processes, behaviors with no meaningful purpose, and inappropriate or lack of emotional responses.

Disorganized thought processes are most evident in speech. Speech may be rambling, jumping from one topic to another, or garbled and unintelligible and the individual may have a tendency to make up words, which are referred to as neologisms.

Disorganized behavior typically manifests as the inability to start and/or complete a seemingly simple task, such as taking a shower. Bizarre dress, unprovoked agitation, and inappropriate behaviors may also be exhibited. Lack of and inappropriate emotional responses, such as flat affect or hysterical laughter for no apparent reason, are common. Rarely are delusions or visual and/or auditory hallucinations seen with disorganized schizophrenia but, when present, they typically are not theme oriented.

F20.2   Catatonic schizophrenia

Catatonic schizophrenia is a rare subtype of schizophrenia with features predominantly related to disturbances in movement. It is typically manifested in three forms: stuporous, immobile, and excited. In stuporous catatonia, the patient appears to be unaware of people and surroundings, may move slowly or be immobile, does not speak, and may stare into space. In the immobile form, the patient remains motionless often in what appears to be an uncomfortable position, which may be held for hours, days, weeks, or longer. Agitated or hyperactive movements, impulsive or combative behavior, and purposeless activities generally characterize the excited form of catatonia.

Symptoms of catatonic schizophrenia typically begin to appear in late adolescence often after a stressor, such as leaving home or the death of a family member or close friend. Catatonic schizophrenia is a lifelong illness with periods of worsening of symptoms alternating with periods of remission or less severe symptoms.

F20.3   Undifferentiated schizophrenia

When the symptoms or manifestations of schizophrenia do not fit one of the more specific subtypes, a diagnosis of undifferentiated schizophrenia is made. The patient's symptomology may fluctuate, exhibiting symptoms of each subtype at different points in time, or the patient's symptomology may be stable but lack definitive characteristics of a specific subtype. In the undifferentiated type, there is typically an absence of delusions and hallucinations.

F20.5   Residual schizophrenia

Residual schizophrenia is diagnosed based on documentation of at least one psychotic episode associated with schizophrenia; a waning of the frequency and/or severity of positive symptoms, such as hallucination and delusions; and the continued presence of negative symptoms. Negative symptoms seen in residual schizophrenia include lack of activity, lack of initiative, lack of emotion, inability to communicate, absence of facial expressions, lack of social skills, and an inability to take care of daily needs.

F21   Schizotypal disorder

Schizotypal disorder is characterized by the inability to establish and maintain close relationships with others. The condition is sometimes called latent or borderline schizophrenia as there is potential for developing schizophrenia under emotional distress; however, these two terms are not recommended for patient diagnosis because a general consensus of their definitions has not been reached.

F22   Delusional disorders

A delusion is a strongly held belief in something that can be proven not to be true or can be proven to be greatly exaggerated even though the belief may have some basis in reality. Delusions may revolve around a variety of themes, paranoia being the most prominent.

Paranoia is a condition in which patients show persistent distrust and suspiciousness of others. They typically present with four or more of the following:

- Suspicion that others are exploiting, harming, or deceiving him or her; preoccupied with unjustified doubts about the loyalty or trustworthiness of friends or associates.

- Unwillingness to confide in others because of an unwarranted fear that the information will be used maliciously against him or her; reads hidden unbecoming or threatening meanings into benign remarks or events.

- Persistently bears grudges (e.g., is unforgiving of insults, injuries, or slights).

- Perceives attacks on character or reputation that are not apparent to others and is quick to react angrily or counterattacks.

- Suspicions, without justification, regarding fidelity of spouse or sexual partner.

Other themes may include grandiose beliefs related to power, wealth, or importance; erotomanic beliefs in which the patient believes another person is infatuated with them; and mixed, where more than one theme may manifest but one is not more predominant than the other.

F25.-   Schizoaffective disorders

Diagnostic criteria for schizoaffective disorders are the presence of at least one of the following schizophrenia spectrum symptoms: delusions, hallucinations, negative symptoms (e.g., lack of motivation), disorganized thinking and speech, and disorganized behavior (including motor behavior) in conjunction with concurrent major depressive or manic mood episodes. These major mood episodes should not be sporadic or brief, but should be observed throughout the course of the psychotic illness.

Mood [Affective] Disorders (F30-F39)

A mood or affective disorder is a disturbance in an individual's emotional state that also affects thought and behavior.

The categories in this code block are as follows:

F30   Manic episode

F31   Bipolar disorder

F32   Major depressive disorder, single episode

F33   Major depressive disorder, recurrent

F34   Persistent mood [affective] disorders

F39   Unspecified mood [affective] disorder

F30.-   Manic episode

A manic episode may be elevated, expansive, or irritable in nature. Manic episode mood changes typically last for at least a week or, if less than a week, are severe enough to require hospitalization. Symptoms that characterize a manic episode include elation, excitement, elevated self-esteem, grandiose ideas, rapid thought process, rapid or frenzied speech pattern, distractibility, flight of ideas, increased goal directed activity, increased psychomotor activity, and pleasure seeking behaviors without concern for risk or adverse consequences. Emotional instability may also be present and is characterized by euphoria alternating with irritability.

F30.1-   Manic episode without psychotic symptoms

Manic episodes may vary significantly in severity and are subclassified as mild, moderate, or severe.

F30.11   Manic episode without psychotic symptoms, mild

During a mild manic episode there may be only a mildly elevated or expansive mood change or minimally increased level of irritability and the individual may act out of character, saying or doing things that he or she would not normally do.

F30.12   Manic episode without psychotic symptoms, moderate

Related manic symptoms are extremely out of proportion to how the patient typically acts and impaired judgement may be observed.

F30.13   Manic episode, severe, without psychotic symptoms

During a severe manic episode the potential for the patient to cause harm to themselves or others is high and often the patient needs constant supervision.

F30.2   Manic episode, severe with psychotic symptoms

Psychotic symptoms in a manic episode usually present as delusions and/or hallucinations. As with other manic episodes, the patient is experiencing higher energy levels, elevated mood, irritability, and distractibility. Delusions and hallucinations can exacerbate the manic symptoms or the manic symptoms can feed into the delusions creating an extremely volatile experience for the patient that in most cases requires hospitalization in order to keep the patient safe.

F32.-   Major depressive disorder, single episode

Depression goes beyond the occasional sad or down feelings. The feelings that occur in depression do not pass within a couple days but last weeks or longer and severely interfere with work, sleep, personal relationships, and the overall ability of the patient to enjoy life.

Major depressive disorder is a severe form of depression where in addition to a depressed mood and loss of interest in doing any activity, the patient also experiences changes in weight or appetite, too much or too little sleep, slowed motor function, loss of energy, indecisiveness, and feelings of worthlessness that may be accompanied by suicidal thoughts.

A single episode of a major depressive disorder lasts a minimum of two weeks with persistent symptoms throughout the day, every day. An individual can experience only one single depressive episode during his or her lifetime; however, in most cases, the depressive episodes continue, although the timing of the episodes for each patient varies.

F32.8-   Other depressive episodes

This subcategory includes conditions that exhibit depressive symptoms that are isolated in nature, i.e., episodic, but are not of the nature or severity typically classified as a major depressive disorder.

F32.81   Premenstrual dysphoric disorder

Premenstrual dysphoric disorder (PMDD) is a severe manifestation of premenstrual syndrome (PMS) affecting 3 percent to 8 percent of women experiencing monthly menstrual cycles. The disorder occurs during the luteal phase of the menstrual cycle (ovulation through the first two days of menstruation) and can be disabling and destructive to day-to-day activities. Pre-existing emotional disorders like depression and anxiety are commonly present and exacerbated with PMDD. Besides feeling anxious or depressed, those with PMDD may experience additional emotional attributes such as feelings of loss of control, fatigue, and irritability. Physical attributes, such as headaches, breast tenderness and abdominal bloating may also be present. Diagnosis is based on the presence of five or more physical and/or emotional symptoms prior to or during the majority of the patient's menstrual cycles over the course of a year. The symptoms must not be related to other medical conditions and significant enough to alter how the patient functions in daily life. Treatment is directed towards the physical and emotional symptoms exhibited. Some researchers believe that PMDD is caused by a combination of genetics (predisposition to hormone sensitivity) and environmental stress, but no clear cause has been established.

F33.-   Major depressive disorder, recurrent

Depression goes beyond the occasional sad or down feelings. The feelings that occur in depression do not pass within a couple days but last weeks or longer and severely interfere with work, sleep, personal relationships, and the patient's overall ability to enjoy life.

Major depressive disorder is a severe form of depression where, in addition to a depressed mood and loss of interest in doing any activity, the patient also experiences changes in weight or appetite, too much or too little sleep, slowed motor function, loss of energy, indecisiveness, and feelings of worthlessness that may be accompanied by suicidal thoughts.

A single episode of a major depressive disorder lasts a minimum of two weeks with persistent symptoms through the day, every day. Although an individual may experience only one single depressive episode during his or her lifetime in most cases the depressive episodes will recur, although the timing of the episodes for each patient will vary.

F34.-   Persistent mood [affective] disorders

This category is used to classify conditions whose primary feature is a disturbance in mood but whose symptoms do not meet the severity of those categorized to major depressive, manic, or bipolar disorders. Conditions categorized here include cyclothymia, dysthymia, and disruptive mood dysregulation disorder.

F34.81   Disruptive mood dysregulation disorder

Disruptive mood dysregulation disorder (DMDD) is a newly recognized childhood psychiatric disorder characterized by severe, frequent temper tantrums. Although tantrums are, to an extent, normal in childhood development, tantrums exhibited in DMDD are inappropriate for the given situation and tend to be destructive in nature causing an inability for the child to function either at home or in social settings. Although the hallmark attribute of DMDD is severe and frequent tantrums, it is how the child acts between tantrums that is the most characteristic feature of this condition: the child remains irritable, as if in a constant state of anger. A comprehensive evaluation is needed by a qualified professional since the symptoms of DMDD are similar to those of other psychiatric disorders in children, like depression, attention deficit hyperactivity disorder, and oppositional defiant disorder. Specific criteria have been developed to properly diagnosis DMDD, which incorporates duration, setting, and onset of the disorder. Individualized therapeutic treatment is recommended and, in some cases, medication is used to treat symptoms.

Anxiety, Dissociative, Stress-related, Somatoform and Other Nonpsychotic Mental Disorders (F40-F48)

Nonpsychotic mental disorders have no obvious evidence of an organic etiology, and there is no lost sense of reality or disorganized personality. Symptoms may include excessive worrying, hysteria, obsession, compulsion, feelings of worthlessness, or phobias. Behavior may be greatly affected although usually remaining within socially acceptable limits.

The categories in this code block are as follows:

F40	Phobic anxiety disorders
F41	Other anxiety disorders
F42	Obsessive-compulsive disorder
F43	Reaction to severe stress, and adjustment disorders
F44	Dissociative and conversion disorders
F45	Somatoform disorders
F48	Other nonpsychotic mental disorders

F40.- Phobic anxiety disorders

In phobic anxiety disorders, the patient experiences abnormal, intense dread of certain objects or specific situations. The fear and anxiety experienced by the individual are out of proportion to typical societal responses to the stimulus and the individual exhibits "active avoidance" to ensure he or she is not subjected to the situation or object. This active avoidance behavior is typically very obvious to those around the individual.

F40.0- Agoraphobia

Agoraphobia is profound anxiety or fear of leaving familiar settings like home, being in unfamiliar enclosed or open space locations, or being with strangers or crowds. Those with agoraphobia avoid locations or situations where they feel like they cannot get out of the situation without embarrassing consequences.

F40.01 Agoraphobia with panic disorder

F40.02 Agoraphobia without panic disorder

Agoraphobia codes reflect whether or not a concomitant panic disorder is also present. Panic attacks are unpredictable and include intense feelings of fear. The symptoms that occur are physical and can include feelings of weakness, faintness, chest pain, apparent loss of control and even fear of death. Individuals with a panic disorder experience these attacks frequently and the fear of an attack can severely debilitate the person.

F41.- Other anxiety disorders

Anxiety is a physical and/or emotional response to something that might happen in the future. The feelings of fear or worry in an anxiety disorder are overwhelming but not appropriate to the current situation and may be so prominent that they can prevent the patient from performing daily activities.

F41.0 Panic disorder [episodic paroxysmal anxiety]

Panic disorder is characterized by recurrent panic attacks. Panic attacks are described as a sudden feeling of fear, an intense desire to escape, and/or a sense of doom, dread, or impending danger. Physical symptoms may include heart palpitations, trembling and dizziness, shortness of breath, a choking sensation, chest pain, nausea, abdominal distress, and lightheadedness. Sometimes symptoms are so severe patients think they are experiencing a heart attack. These attacks occur without warning, leaving the patient constantly worrying about when another attack will occur.

F41.1 Generalized anxiety disorder

Generalized anxiety disorder (GAD) causes constant, severe worry that interferes with daily tasks. Individuals with GAD feel unable to control worries about family issues, social acceptance, upcoming events, personal abilities, and/or school or work performance. GAD may cause trouble sleeping and irritability, which often leads to problems being attentive and functioning efficiently. Many individuals also report feeling "keyed up" or "on edge" most or all of the time. Individuals may have difficulty concentrating or may describe having their minds go blank. All individuals experience some level of anxiety at some period in their lives, but when anxiety is constant and interferes with normal activities, GAD may be diagnosed.

F42.- Obsessive-compulsive disorder

Obsession is a recurrent urge or thought that is unwanted and significantly distressing. Compulsion is a behavior or action that a person is driven to perform. Although the two can occur independently, they most often occur simultaneously with the compulsive action being performed as a type of coping mechanism, designed to relieve the anxiety associated with the obsession.

F42.2 Mixed obsessional thoughts and acts

Obsessive-compulsive disorders (OCD) can manifest in two ways: via thoughts or actions. Obsessive thoughts are distressing mental images or ideas that continuously plague the patient. Obsessive actions are physical urges that compel the patient to perform certain ritualistic movements. In mixed obsessional thought and acts, a patient has both obsessive thoughts and actions. This is the more common type of OCD.

F42.3   Hoarding disorder

Hoarding disorder was first defined as a mental disorder in 2013, and although it is seen as its own individual disorder it can also be a symptom of obsessive-compulsive disorder (OCD). The diagnosis of hoarding disorder is most often made in adulthood, but behavior starts exhibiting itself during childhood or adolescence. A hoarder possesses an enormous number of items that other people may consider useless; however, they tend not to perceive the accumulated items as an issue and strongly believe that the hoarded items need to be saved. In its most severe form, hoarding can cause health and safety concerns such as fire hazards, pest infestations, and an increased risk of falling. As research continues into hoarding disorders, three common types are emerging: pure hoarding, hoarding plus OCD, and OCD-based hoarding. Treatment is difficult as people who hoard do not typically see an issue with their behavior. Psychotherapy is the first line of treatment.

Focus Point

Hoarding disorder is not to be confused with people who collect a single item like stamps, clocks, etc. Hoarding behavior does not single out a certain object and/or variations of that object. Individuals who hoard accumulate large amounts of different items.

F42.4   Excoriation (skin-picking) disorder

Excoriation disorder, categorized as an impulse control disorder, is picking at one's own skin usually to the extent of tissue damage. The behavior is exhibited by the repeated urge to pick at sores, cuticles, or imperfections on the skin to the point that those with the disorder are embarrassed at their need to pick, so much so that the behavior interferes with normal daily activities. There is no particular age of onset and the trigger is different for each individual. In some the picking may start as an act of boredom, while highly stressful situations can be the catalyst in others.

F43.-   Reaction to severe stress, and adjustment disorders

There are many events and situations a person might see or be involved in that are so terrible that the brain cannot cope with what happened. Stress reactions and adjustment disorders are how the body and mind react to these stressful events.

F43.0   Acute stress reaction

An acute stress reaction is the rapid development and resolution of stress-related emotional and physical symptoms in response to a specific stressful event. Emotional symptoms may include anxiety, depressed mood, poor concentration, an inability to be alone, recurrent dreams or flashbacks, emotional numbness, anger, and aggression. Physical symptoms may include heart palpitations, chest pain, shortness of breath, abdominal pain, nausea, and headache. There may also be avoidance behaviors designed to prevent recall of the event. The symptoms usually develop within minutes to hours of the event and then lessen in intensity and eventually resolve over days or at most a few weeks.

F43.1-   Post-traumatic stress disorder (PTSD)

Post-traumatic stress disorder (PTSD) is a severe stress reaction resulting from an exceptionally terrifying event involving physical harm or the threat of physical harm to oneself or another person. In PTSD, the symptoms do not diminish or resolve and cause major disruptions to daily activities. PTSD sufferers exhibit three types of symptoms: re-experiencing symptoms, avoidance symptoms, and hyperarousal symptoms. Re-experiencing symptoms include flashbacks, nightmares, and terrifying memories. Avoidance symptoms involve avoiding people, places, events, or objects that are reminders of the event or situation. Avoidance symptoms may also manifest as depression, emotional numbness, or the inability to recall the triggering event. Hyperarousal symptoms include anger accompanied by outbursts, feeling unusually tense or "wound up," and being "jumpy," or easily startled. A person with PTSD experiences symptoms from all three categories, and the symptoms typically last more than one month. PTSD is further classified as acute, with symptoms resolving within three months, and chronic, with symptoms persisting for longer than three months.

F43.2-   Adjustment disorders

An adjustment or adaptation reaction is a mild or transient disorder lasting longer than acute stress reactions and occurring in individuals of any age without any apparent preexisting mental disorder. Such disorders are often relatively circumscribed or situation-specific, are generally reversible, and usually last only a few months. They are usually closely related in time and content to stressors such as bereavement, migration, or other experiences. Reactions to major stress that last longer than a few days are also included. In children, such disorders are associated with no significant distortion of development. Each individual reacts differently to the inciting stimulus and, as such, codes in this category are classified by predominant symptoms (e.g., sad or depressed mood, changes in normal conduct, and so on).

F44.-   Dissociative and conversion disorders

In order to cope with a stressful or traumatic situation, some individuals disconnect themselves from reality, distancing their memory, consciousness, or identity to the adverse event. These are known as dissociative disorders.

Conversion disorder is diagnosed when physical signs and symptoms are present but workup cannot identify an underlying medical or neurological condition. The symptoms themselves are often brought on or exacerbated by a stressor or other associated conflict and the symptoms are not intentionally produced.

F44.0   Dissociative amnesia

In dissociative amnesia, also called psychogenic or hysterical amnesia, there is a temporary disturbance in the ability to recall important personal information that has already been registered and stored in memory. The sudden onset of this disturbance in the absence of an underlying organic mental disorder, and the extent of the disturbance being too great to be explained by ordinary forgetfulness, are the essential features.

F44.1   Dissociative fugue

Dissociative fugue is where a trauma or stressor triggers an amnesic effect on an individual; this person suddenly and completely forgets who they are and leaves his or her current environment for another completely separate environment. In most cases, these are short-lived episodes, hours or days, but they can last much longer. During the fugue, the person does not realize the change and it is not until the fugue ends that the person realizes he or she is not living his or her customary life.

F44.2   Dissociative stupor

This disorder occurs when a stressful or traumatic event causes the patient to not be able to move, speak, or respond to external stimuli, while at the same time being fully conscious and awake.

F48.-   Other nonpsychotic mental disorders

With nonpsychotic mental disorders there is no lost sense of reality (psychosis). In general, the attributes of nonpsychotic mental disorders are centered on mood, emotions, and behavior and compared to psychotic disorders, are usually less severe.

F48.2   Pseudobulbar affect

Pseudobulbar affect (PBA) is a neurologic condition caused by underlying structural damage in the brain that triggers frequent, involuntary outbursts of disruptive crying or laughing. PBA episodes are exhibited as an exaggerated or disproportionate response that belies the patient's underlying emotional state. The pathophysiology of PBA is widely believed to involve impairment of neurologic pathways that regulate the emotions. Causal factors may include neurological disease or traumatic injury. Associated conditions include amyotrophic lateral sclerosis (ALS), multiple sclerosis (MS), stroke, and traumatic brain injury (TBI). Although PBA is highly prevalent among persons with underlying neurologic conditions, it has remained underdiagnosed and

undertreated in neurological, psychiatric, and general medical settings, where it is often misdiagnosed as a psychiatric illness (e.g., anxiety, depression, bipolar disorder, schizophrenia).

Pseudobulbar affect is a recent change in terminology to what was previously referred to as pathological laughter and crying, emotional lability, emotionalism, emotional dysregulation, or, more recently, involuntary emotional expression disorder (IEED). PBA can have a significantly negative impact on the patient's social functioning and relationships. The patient's inappropriate laughter may cause embarrassment in social situations, and the crying may be misinterpreted as depression.

Behavioral Syndromes Associated with Physiological Disturbances and Physical Factors (F50-F59)

The conditions found in this code block relate deviations in behavior that affect the healthy and normal functioning of an individual.

The categories in this code block are as follows:

F50	Eating disorders
F51	Sleep disorders not due to a substance or known physiological condition
F52	Sexual dysfunction not due to a substance or known physiological condition
F53	Puerperal psychosis
F54	Psychological and behavioral factors associated with disorders or diseases classified elsewhere
F55	Abuse of non-psychoactive substances
F59	Unspecified behavioral syndromes associated with physiological disturbances and physical factors

F50.-   Eating disorders

Eating disorders have become more common in recent years. Anorexia nervosa is the third most frequent chronic disease in the United States, with 95 percent of cases occurring in females. There is an increased occurrence of anorexia nervosa and bulimia in adolescence between the ages of 15 and 19. Certain sports and activities, such as cheerleading, ballet, gymnastics, and wrestling, may put some adolescents at increased risk for eating disorders. With these disorders, adolescents often have an extreme fear of gaining weight and a distorted view of body size and shape. In addition, they may also have low self-esteem and their focus on weight can be an attempt to gain a sense of control at a time when their lives feel out of control. Once adolescents are afraid of gaining weight and begin starving themselves, binging and purging, and/or over-exercising, they are considered to have an eating disorder.

Eating disorders are dangerous, causing multiple complications, and can sometimes be fatal. Early diagnosis and treatment are imperative for best outcome.

F50.0- Anorexia nervosa

The symptoms of anorexia nervosa include restriction of caloric intake resulting in an exceptionally low and unhealthy body weight. This is directly related to an intense fear of gaining weight and a disturbed self-evaluation on what the individual perceives as the appropriate body weight or shape. Anorexia nervosa generally begins with an innocent diet and progresses into self-starvation, by severely restricting the amount of food consumed or by periodic eating with subsequent purging. Compulsive exercise is also common. Amenorrhea in women is common and in advanced cases slowed pulse and respiration, low body temperature, dependent edema, and heart rhythm abnormalities can arise. Early diagnosis and treatment are vital as this condition can be fatal. Typically the disorder begins in teenage girls but it may begin before puberty and rarely does it occur in males.

F50.01 Anorexia nervosa, restricting type

In the restricting type of anorexia nervosa the individual severely restricts the amount of food consumed or restricts food altogether extending over a period of three months or longer.

F50.02 Anorexia nervosa, binge eating/ purging type

One of the most dangerous eating disorders is the binge and/or purge type of anorexia nervosa. In binge/purge, the person periodically eats but the fear of gaining weight compels him or her to expel the food, even if the calories consumed were minimal. Purging may be in the form of self-induced vomiting or laxative, diuretic, or enema use. Similar to the restricting type, the binge/purge behavior must transpire over a three month or longer time period.

F50.2 Bulimia nervosa

Poor self-evaluation of body shape and/or weight is the driving force behind bulimia nervosa. Bulimia is characterized by periods of uncontrollable binging followed by compensating measures used to remove excess calories from the body, including purging and nonpurging. Purging includes self-induced vomiting and the use of laxatives or enemas and nonpurging includes excessive exercise or fasting methods. When a person binges, large amounts of food are consumed within a short period of time (usually less than two

hours). Typically eating binges take place at least twice a week for three months and may occur as often as several times a day. An individual with bulimia may undergo weight fluctuations, but rarely experiences the low weight associated with anorexia.

Patients with bulimia nervosa may experience dizziness, palpitations, edema, and, in females, amenorrhea. In patients who induce vomiting, pharyngeal and dental damage from gastric juices may be present. Cutaneous manifestations are also common, presenting as dry skin, hair loss, and even self-induced trauma.

F50.8- Other eating disorders

This subcategory captures conditions such as binge eating disorder, pica in adults, and psychogenic loss of appetite.

F50.81 Binge eating disorder

Binge eating disorder, although not officially recognized as a formal medical condition until just recently, is the most common eating disorder in the United States. Individuals with binge eating disorder follow a certain pattern that involves at least three of the following: eating large amounts of food in a relatively short period of time even if not hungry and even if feeling full, a tendency to hide the excessive eating, and along with that, feeling very upset with the behavior. People with this disorder binge eat at least once a week for an average of three months but do not feel the need to reverse the effects of the overeating by exercising more, using laxatives, or throwing up as is seen in other eating disorders. While the cause is not known, certain chemical imbalances in the brain, life experiences, and a family history of eating disorders may play important roles.

F50.82 Avoidant/restrictive food intake disorder

Avoidant/restrictive food intake disorder (ARFID), previously known as selective eating disorder (SED), is an eating and/or feeding disorder characterized by selective inability to eat or avoidance of consumption of certain foods or food groups. It is often based on the sensory properties of food, such as the appearance, color, smell, taste, texture, temperature, brand, preparation technique, presentation, or negative consequences of consumption such as bloating or discomfort. Patients with ARFID may experience adverse reactions to foods like gagging, choking, or vomiting. ARFID may result in delayed growth/gain in children and cause significant nutritional deficiencies, requiring nutritional supplements.

F50.89 Other specified eating disorder

This code captures the adult form of pica disorder. Pica is the persistent consumption of substances that have no nutritive or caloric benefit (nonfood substances) continuously, for at least a month in duration.

Cigarette butts, newspaper, hair, ash, ice, and chalk are just a few nonfood substances that may be eaten. Often a concomitant intellectual or mental disorder is also present, especially in adults.

F51.- Sleep disorders not due to a substance or known physiological condition

Sleep disorders classified here have a nonorganic origin. Nonorganic conditions may be of psychophysiological origin, due to disturbance in sleep environment, paradoxical conditions that exhibit seemingly contradictable aspects, and/or idiopathic conditions that are self-originated or of unknown etiology.

F51.0- Insomnia not due to a substance or known physiological condition

Insomnia is the inability to fall or stay asleep. Daytime signs and symptoms may include tired or sleepiness, irritability, and concentration and/or memory problems.

F51.01 Primary insomnia

When no direct health condition or physiological problem is identified as a causative factor for the inability to sleep it is considered primary insomnia.

F51.02 Adjustment insomnia

Adjustment insomnia is directly related to some sort of stressor, most often related to a significant life change, such as a new job, divorce, shift work, or death of a loved one.

F51.03 Paradoxical insomnia

In paradoxical insomnia, the patient has a perception that he or she is not getting adequate sleep but is not evidenced by daytime impairment. Subjectively, the patient feels like he or she did not sleep well and were awake most the night. Objectively it is observed that the patient is in an active state of sleep but the brain rarely reaches a deep sleep stage but instead is staying in a lighter stage of sleep where cognitive activity is still occurring.

F51.04 Psychophysiologic insomnia

Psychophysiologic insomnia is a conditioned response to a perceived inability to sleep. The patient becomes so preoccupied with thoughts on whether or not he or she will be able to sleep that the body and mind cannot relax enough to allow sleep. This sleep pattern is often triggered by a stressful event but continues after the stress has resolved.

F53 Puerperal psychosis

This mental health condition occurs in women hours to weeks after having a baby. Obstetric patients with a history of bipolar disorder or who have experienced psychosis after previous births are found to be more susceptible to this condition. It is exhibited by extreme changes in thought, mood, and behavior, ranging from depression to confusion to hallucinations. Symptoms can change rapidly, cycling through many different symptoms. Depending on how the psychosis manifests, the patient may pose a threat to herself, her new baby, and, if present, other children in the household.

Puerperal psychosis is not synonymous with postpartum depression, which is also coded here. Postpartum depression is much more common than postpartum psychosis and is generally less severe. Symptoms are typical of nonobstetric related depression, such as low mood and energy and sadness. Diagnosis for postpartum depression is based on depressive symptoms being present for at least two weeks.

Disorders of Adult Personality and Behavior (F60-F69)

Personality is defined as thinking, behaving, and feeling patterns that are characteristic to a certain individual.

Behavior is how an individual reacts (whether via action or inaction) toward certain environmental stimulus, external or internal.

Personality and behavioral disorders occur when extreme deviations in an individual's personality or behavior are not typical to that individual's normal environment or culture.

The categories in this code block are as follows:

F60	Specific personality disorders
F63	Impulse disorders
F64	Gender identity disorders
F65	Paraphilias
F66	Other sexual disorders
F68	Other disorders of adult personality and behavior
F69	Unspecified disorder of adult personality and behavior

F60.- Specific personality disorders

A personality disorder is a pattern of unhealthy and inflexible behaviors and/or thoughts that although stable are far removed from what is typically experienced in that individual's culture, leading to severe impairment and distress.

F60.0   Paranoid personality disorder

This disorder is characterized by excessive distrust and suspicion of others, even those he or she is very close to, to such an extreme that he or she finds it hard to form close relationships and tends to withdraw from others.

F60.5   Obsessive-compulsive personality disorder

This disorder correlates with a preoccupation of being perfect and in control; every rule and schedule is followed and everything is organized down to the smallest detail. Although these individuals are devoted to work and productivity, the need for perfection can prevent tasks from being completed. In addition to their own need for perfection, they also demand the same from others and as such often have strained interpersonal relationships.

F60.7   Dependent personality disorder

Lack of self-confidence, fear of abandonment, and an obsessive need to be taken care of characterize dependent personality disorder. Patients with this condition often permit another individual to take control of his or her life, allowing the needs of that person to supersede personal needs.

F63.-   Impulse disorders

Impulse disorders are the result of an impaired ability to effectively inhibit or control an impulse or urge. Disorders included in this category are classified together based on the commonality between their initiation and progression. Although performing the act itself is pleasurable or brings a sense of relief, it is often followed by intense feelings of guilt or regret. However, the remorse that is felt does not outweigh the compulsive need to perform the act again.

F63.3   Trichotillomania

This condition is the compulsive need to pull one's hair out. Hair plucking can occur on any part of the body that has hair and can be so extreme that bald patches may result.

F64.-   Gender identity disorders

Gender identity disorder encompasses several conditions that are characterized by a disparity between the individual's biological sex and their perceived sexual identity. To be classified as a gender identity disorder, this mismatch between biological and perceived gender must be accompanied by significant emotional distress and impair the individual's ability to function in daily life. The term "gender identity disorder" is now more commonly referred to as gender dysphoria. Another term for this condition is gender incongruity.

F64.0   Transsexualism

Transsexualism, also referred to as transgender, is a type of gender dysphoria that can manifest as early as 2 years of age. A transsexual person experiences a gender identity that is not consistent with their biological sex, causing the transsexual person significant distress that impairs their ability to function. In adults and adolescents there are a number of common feelings or desires that are characteristic of transsexualism. Individuals may experience some or all of the following feelings or desires:

- A desire to be the gender that they perceive themselves to be as opposed to being the gender that conforms with their biological gender

- Discomfort with and a desire to change their primary and/or secondary sex characteristics

- The desire to be recognized as and treated as their perceived gender

- The belief that their emotions, feelings, and reactions align with their perceived gender

A person with transsexualism may feel so strongly that they belong to the opposite sex that they will undergo sexual reassignment therapy. Sexual reassignment almost always involves surgery in addition to hormone therapy.

F64.1   Dual role transvestism

Also referred to as cross-dressing, dual-role transvestism has three distinct criteria: an individual wants to dress like the opposite sex, the motivation is not a sexual desire to be the opposite sex, and the individual does not wish to permanently change their assigned sex. A dual-role transvestite lives in both worlds, the gender to which their physical sex coincides and the gender opposite of their physical sex. Although the latter is what the individual identifies with more, the need to be this sex is not a debilitating obsession.

Focus Point

Do not confuse dual-role transvestism and transvestic fetishism. The clear distinction between the two is that there is not a sexual component for a dual-role transvestite to dress or act like the opposite sex, but there is a clear sexual influence for the fetishistic transvestite. ICD-10-CM categorizes transvestic fetishism as a paraphilia and is coded to F65.1.

F68.-   Other disorders of adult personality and behavior

Personality and behavioral disorders occur when extreme deviations in an individual's personality or behavior are not typical to that individual's normal environment or culture.

F68.1- Factitious disorder

In factitious illness, there are physical or psychological symptoms that are not real, genuine, or natural, but are produced by the individual and are under voluntary control. The presentation of physical symptoms may be fabricated, self-inflicted, an exaggeration or exacerbation of a preexisting physical condition, or any combination or variation of these.

Intellectual Disabilities (F70-F79)

Intellectual disabilities is defined as general intellectual functioning at least two standard deviations below the norm as measured in a standardized intelligence test and accompanied by significant limitation in communication, self-care, home living, interpersonal skills, self-direction, work, leisure, health, or safety. The onset must occur before adulthood.

The categories in this code block are as follows:

F70	Mild intellectual disabilities
F71	Moderate intellectual disabilities
F72	Severe intellectual disabilities
F73	Profound intellectual disabilities
F78	Other intellectual disabilities
F79	Unspecified intellectual disabilities

F70 Mild intellectual disabilities

In mild intellectual disabilities, the patient has an IQ of 50 to 70. Individuals with this level of retardation are usually educable. During the preschool period, they can develop social and communication skills, have minimal delay in sensorimotor areas, and often are not distinguished from children with higher intellectual function until a later age. During the school age period, they can learn academic skills up to approximately the sixth-grade level. During the adult years, they can usually achieve social and vocational skills adequate for minimum self-support, but may need guidance and assistance when under social or economic stress.

F71 Moderate intellectual disabilities

In moderate intellectual disabilities, the patient has an IQ of 35 to 49. Individuals with this level of disability are usually trainable. During the preschool period, they can talk or learn to communicate but have poor social awareness and only fair motor development. During the school age period, they can profit from training in social and occupational skills, but they are unlikely to progress beyond the second-grade level in academic

subjects. During their adult years, they may achieve self-maintenance in unskilled or semiskilled work under sheltered conditions. They need supervision and guidance when under mild social or economic stress.

F72 Severe intellectual disabilities

In severe intellectual disabilities, the patient has an IQ of 20 to 34. Individuals with this level of retardation evidence poor motor development, minimal speech, and are generally unable to profit from training and self-help during the preschool period. During the school age period, they can talk or learn to communicate, can be trained in elementary health habits, and respond to systematic habit training. During the adult years, they may contribute partially to self-maintenance under complete supervision.

F73 Profound intellectual disabilities

In profound intellectual disabilities, the patient has an IQ less than 20. Individuals with this level of retardation evidence minimal capacity for sensorimotor functioning and need nursing care during the preschool period. Typically physical and congenital abnormalities are also obvious. During the school age period, some further motor development may occur and they may respond to minimal or limited training in self-help. During the adult years, some motor and speech development may occur but achieve very limited self-care functioning. Nursing care is essential.

Pervasive and Specific Developmental Disorders (F80-F89)

This code block classifies a group of disorders in which a specific delay in development is the main feature. For many, the delay is not explicable in terms of general intellectual delay or of inadequate schooling. In each case, development is related to biological maturation, but it is also influenced by nonbiological factors. A diagnosis of a specific developmental delay carries no etiological implications. A diagnosis of specific delay in development should not be made if it is due to a known neurological disorder.

The categories in this code block are as follows:

F80	Specific developmental disorders of speech and language
F81	Specific developmental disorders of scholastic skills
F82	Specific developmental disorders of motor function
F84	Pervasive developmental disorders
F88	Other disorders of psychological development

F89   Unspecified disorder of psychological
          development

F80.-   Specific developmental disorders of speech and language

A speech disorder is when an individual cannot produce correct or fluent sounds from their mouths.

Language disorders are an inability to express what you want or feel in a coherent or complete way or it is a problem understanding what others are trying to express.

Deficits in speech and language, from stuttering and lisping to the inability to form coherent sentences, can adversely affect social, academic, and behavior skills in children. Early identification and intervention is critical.

F80.1   Expressive language disorder

Developmental expressive language disorder is a condition where there is decreased vocabulary, the inability to produce complex sentences, and the inability to remember words. Children with this disorder usually understand language better than they are able to communicate. Developmental expressive language disorder usually becomes evident when a child is starting to talk. Although the cause is unknown, in some cases it may be linked to malnutrition or damage to the cerebrum of the brain. Signs and symptoms vary considerably from child to child.

F80.2   Mixed receptive-expressive language disorder

In this mixed type language disorder, the individual has trouble conveying what he or she is thinking or feeling in spoken language (expressive) and in understanding something that is spoken to him or her (receptive). If related to a developmental issue, it's typically apparent around the time the child begins to talk. Acquired forms may also occur, often seen after stroke or traumatic brain injuries.

> **Focus Point**
>
> Auditory processing disorder (APD) has been reclassified to Chapter 8 Diseases of the Ear and Mastoid Processes, and is reported with code H93.25 Central auditory processing disorder. ADP can be the result of neurological problems, as well as infection or trauma. ADP is one of the underlying causes of learning disability.

F80.8-   Other developmental disorders of speech and language

A speech disorder is one where the individual cannot be easily understood by others due the inability to produce speech sounds. Language disorder is the inability to understand spoken words or express spoken words in a coherent way.

F80.81   Childhood onset fluency disorder

Stuttering is a common fluency disorder characterized by uncontrolled interruption of the normal rate and pattern of speech. Onset typically occurs in early to mid-childhood and may persist well into adolescence or adulthood in the absence of therapeutic intervention. Persistent stuttering is a potentially handicapping and disabling condition with significant educational, social, and vocational consequences. Causal conditions may include environmental or emotional factors, genetic predisposition, or trauma. The majority of preschool age children who stutter spontaneously recover by 3.5 years of age; however, if stuttering persists until 6 years of age, the child is unlikely to recover without speech therapy. Male children who stutter outnumber female children by a ratio of four to one. It is unknown whether the neurological abnormalities identified by diagnostic imaging of adult stutterers are present in children who stutter.

Cluttering is a fluency disorder characterized by rapid speech in which certain sounds are omitted and, as a result, speech becomes unintelligible. It is often associated with other expressive or language organizational disorders. Although both conditions disrupt normal speech patterns, patients who clutter also experience disorganization of thoughts during speaking. These disruptive thought patterns commonly affect the ability to express thoughts in writing and conversation, whereas patients who stutter have a clear and coherent pattern of thought but have difficulty expressing those thoughts.

F80.82   Social pragmatic communication disorder

The specific criteria for diagnosing social communication disorders include, but are not limited to, difficulty in greetings and sharing information, inability to change the conversation based on the listener or the environment (going from a classroom setting to a play setting), not understanding inferences and ambiguous meanings of conversation, and sometimes not knowing how to handle the give and take of conversation. Persons with this communication disorder have limitations in their academic achievement and social relationships that can ultimately affect occupational performances. Manifestations of this disorder are not always recognized early since the behavior cannot be observed until situations involving continued conversation occur. Play-based therapies are widely used with parents, therapists, and peers and have had some success in helping mitigate the challenges of this communication disorder.

Focus Point

Social pragmatic communication disorder can also be observed as a symptom in other mental disorders, such as autism spectrum disorder, as well as in developmental delays. When the disorder is identified as a component of another condition, F80.82 is not usually coded as a secondary diagnosis.

F80.89   Other developmental disorders of speech and language

Semantic pragmatic disorder (SPD) is a communication disorder that typically manifests in childhood with delayed language development and difficulty understanding others in a nonliteral or social context.

Focus Point

Semantic pragmatic disorder (SPD) that occurs in conjunction with autism is included in the autistic disorder code F84.0.

F84.-   Pervasive developmental disorders

Pervasive developmental disorders (PDD) are a group of developmental conditions that involve children and include delays in normal development, as well as impaired communication skills, social skills, cognitive skills, and behavior. Autism is the most familiar of the disorders, so PDDs are also known as autism spectrum disorders. Children diagnosed with spectrum disorders can have relatively few symptoms or be developmentally devastated. Thus, it is possible for one individual to be intelligent and verbal while another individual suffers from intellectual deficits and is unable to communicate.

F84.0   Autistic disorder

Autism is a syndrome present from birth or beginning almost invariably in the first 30 months of life. Responses to auditory and sometimes to visual stimuli are abnormal, and there are usually severe problems in the understanding of spoken language. Speech is delayed and, if it develops, is characterized by echolalia, the reversal of pronouns, immature grammatical structure, and an inability to use abstract terms. There is generally an impaired social use of verbal and gestural language. Problems in social relationships are most severe before the age of 5 years and include an impaired development of eye-to-eye gaze, social attachments, and cooperative play. Ritualistic behavior is usual and may include abnormal routines, resistance to change, attachment to odd objects, and stereotyped patterns of play. Individuals with autism may demonstrate repetitive movements such as rocking and twirling or self-abusive behavior such as biting or head-banging. Another characteristic

of autism is a diminished capacity for abstract or symbolic thought and for imaginative play. Intelligence ranges from severely subnormal to normal or above. Performance is usually better on tasks involving rote memory or visuospatial skills than on those requiring symbolic or linguistic skills.

F84.3   Other childhood disintegrative disorder

Childhood disintegrative disorder, a condition that is synonymous with dementia infantalis, disintegrative or symbiotic psychosis, and Heller's syndrome, is a rare disorder in which a child typically develops normally until age 2 and then suddenly loses the capability to communicate. Emotional and social behaviors regress and these children become less likely to interact with others, including parents. Motor skills are also affected.

F84.5   Asperger's syndrome

Asperger's syndrome (AS) is a high-functioning form of autism. Children with AS usually develop speech on schedule, are generally very intelligent, and communicate well, but they have considerable social shortcomings. Asperger's syndrome has a higher prevalence in male children. Diagnosis of AS is much later than other pervasive developmental disorders, with children commonly diagnosed between the ages of 5 and 9.

Behavioral and Emotional Disorders with Onset Usually Occurring in Childhood and Adolescence (F90-F98)

Emotional and/or behavioral disorders are typically diagnosed based on one or more of the following:

- Failure to build interpersonal relationships

- Failure to learn despite adequate intellect or health factors

- Consistent inappropriate feelings and/or behavior in relation to environment

- Physical symptoms that occur with stress

- Generally unhappy or depressed mood

The frequency and intensity of the above features are often way beyond what should typically be experienced for other children or adolescents of the same age and development level with notable disturbances in personal, academic, and other functioning.

The categories in this code block are as follows:

F90   Attention-deficit hyperactivity disorders

F91   Conduct disorders

F93	Emotional disorders with onset specific to childhood
F94	Disorders of social functioning with onset specific to childhood and adolescence
F95	Tic disorder
F98	Other behavioral and emotional disorders with onset usually occurring in childhood and adolescence

F90.- Attention-deficit hyperactivity disorders

Attention deficit disorder, commonly referred to as ADD or ADHD, is an organic, brain-based disorder that is characterized by inattention, impulsive behaviors, and/or hyperactivity. Symptoms can be severe enough to interfere with learning, interacting with peers, participating in extracurricular activities (including sports), or functioning at home. To meet the diagnostic criteria, symptoms must be present prior to the age of 7, present for at least six months duration, and present in two or more settings (e.g., school, work, home). ADHD is one of the most common mental disorders in children. Symptoms can continue into adolescence and adulthood. ADHD frequently is a genetic condition, with many parents of children with ADHD reporting similar symptoms when they were younger. ADHD is frequently also found in siblings.

F90.0 Attention-deficit hyperactivity disorder, predominantly inattentive type

ADHD predominantly inattentive type describes children that have ADHD without hyperactivity or impulsive behavior. Children typically have symptoms of inattentiveness and are easily distracted. They have trouble paying attention, following directions, completing assignments, and are disorganized. Children with inattentive ADHD are inclined to be sluggish and slow to process information. They seem as if they are daydreaming or in a fog. Sometimes children appear shy or withdrawn. Symptoms are not as apparent as with hyperactivity and impulsive behavior, and oftentimes this type goes undiagnosed.

F90.1 Attention-deficit hyperactivity disorder, predominantly hyperactive type

The predominantly hyperactive type of ADHD describes children that have ADHD with primary symptoms of hyperactivity and/or impulsive behavior. These children have trouble focusing. They understand the instructions they are to follow but they are unable to concentrate or sit in one place long enough to complete a task. They tend to be fidgety, restless, and talk excessively. They often act and speak without thinking, frequently interrupt others in conversation, and blurt out answers in class settings. They have these problems regardless of their setting (e.g., school, work, home). The hyperactivity and impulsiveness interferes with the ability to function academically, socially, and at home.

F91.- Conduct disorders

Conduct disorders mainly involve aggressive and destructive behavior and delinquency. While conduct disorders typically present in childhood or adolescence, codes in this category may be used for abnormal behavior in individuals of any age and that give rise to social disapproval when the behavior is not part of any other psychiatric condition. Minor emotional disturbances may also be present. To be included, the behavior, as judged by its frequency, severity, and type of associations with other symptoms, must be abnormal in its context.

Focus Point

Disturbances of conduct are distinguished from an adjustment reaction by a longer duration and by a lack of close relationship in time and content to some stressor. They differ from a personality disorder by the absence of deeply ingrained maladaptive patterns of behavior present from adolescence or earlier.

F91.3 Oppositional defiant disorder

Oppositional defiant disorder (ODD) is an illness where a child, for at least a six-month period, exhibits frequent loss of his or her temper, refuses or defies compliance with rules, argues with adults, blames others for misbehavior, is angry, spiteful, and/or vindictive. These behaviors are out of proportion in frequency and severity than what is normally seen in a particular age and development level and greatly impacts how the patient functions in social and academic environments.

F95.- Tic disorder

Tics are sudden, recurrent involuntary motor activity or sounds that appear out of context. Tics may be simple with brief, insignificant movements, such as eye blinking, facial grimacing, head jerks, or shoulder shrugs. They are usually very brief, lasting less than one second. A child may also have complex motor tics, which involve movements of several muscle groups. The movements are slower, longer, and more purposeful movements like sustained looks, facial gestures, biting, banging, whirling or twisting around, or the use of obscene gestures. Tics are fairly common in childhood. In the vast majority of cases, they are temporary conditions that resolve on their own. In some cases, the tics continue over time and become more severe. Symptoms may worsen during periods of stress, anxiety, fatigue, illness, recent head injury, or excitement. The exact cause of tics is unknown, although children with a family history of tic disorders may be more likely to develop it. Males are about three to four times more likely than females to develop these disorders.

F95.2   Tourette's disorder

Tourette's disorder is a familial neuropsychiatric disorder of variable expression that is characterized by multiple recurrent involuntary tics involving body movements (e.g., eye blinks, grimaces, or knee bends) and vocalizations (e.g., grunts, snorts, or utterance of inappropriate words). This syndrome often has one or more associated behavioral or psychiatric conditions (e.g., attention deficit disorder or obsessive-compulsive behavior) and is more common in males than females. It usually has an onset in childhood and often stabilizes or ameliorates in adulthood.

F98.-   Other behavioral and emotional disorders with onset usually occurring in childhood and adolescence

Emotional and/or behavioral disorders are often hard to define and are a diagnosis of exclusion, in that the symptoms are emotionally based but cannot be better defined by an intellectual or cultural factor or that cannot be explained by a general health condition.

F98.3   Pica of infancy and childhood

Pica is an eating disorder characterized by the persistent and compulsive cravings to eat nonfood items, including dirt, stones, and wood. This disorder is common in infants and toddlers, with as many as 25 to 30 percent of kids affected by it. Generally most children outgrow pica by the time they are about 3 years old. For a true diagnosis of pica, the child should be craving and eating these things for at least a month. Pica is commonly seen with other disorders, such as mental retardation, autism, and other developmental disabilities, as well as children who have suffered a brain injury. While consumption of some items may not be detrimental, pica is considered to be a serious eating disorder that can cause serious health problems. Accidental ingestion of poisons such as lead, life-threatening toxicities such as hyperkalemia from burnt match head ingestion, and soil borne parasite infections from consuming soil and clay are just a few of the potential consequences of pica. Other conditions secondary to pica include iron deficiency anemia and gastrointestinal complications, such as obstructions, constipation, ulcerations, and perforations.

Chapter 6: Diseases of the Nervous System (G00-G99)

The nervous system is a complex network of specialized organs, tissues, and cells that coordinate the body's actions and functions. It consists of two main subdivisions: the central nervous system and the peripheral nervous system. The central nervous system includes the brain, the spinal cord, and the membranes that cover these structures. The peripheral nervous system includes the sense organs and the nerves that link the organs, muscles, and glands to the central nervous system.

The central nervous system (CNS) is the control center for almost all functions of the body and comprises two major structures: the brain and the spinal cord. The brain resides in and is protected by the cranial bones and the spinal cord extends from the base of the brain, residing in and protected by the spinal column.

The brain can be subdivided into several regions:

- The cerebral hemispheres form the largest part of the brain, occupying the anterior and middle cranial fossae in the skull.

- The diencephalon includes the thalamus, hypothalamus, epithalamus, and subthalamus, and forms the central core of the brain.

- The midbrain is located at the junction of the middle and posterior cranial fossae.

- The pons is in the anterior part of the posterior cranial fossa; fibers within the pons connect one cerebral hemisphere with its opposite cerebellar hemisphere.

- The medulla oblongata is continuous with the spinal cord and controls the respiratory and cardiovascular systems.

- The cerebellum overlies the pons and medulla and controls motor functions that regulate muscle tone, coordination, and posture.

The spinal column, which encloses the spinal cord, consists of vertebrae linked by intervertebral discs and held together by ligaments. The spinal cord extends from the medulla at the base of the brain to the first lumbar vertebra. The outer layer of the spinal cord consists of nerve fibers enclosed in a myelin-sheath that conduct impulses triggered by pressure, pain, heat, and other sensory stimuli or conduct motor impulses activating muscles and glands. The inner layer, or gray matter, is primarily composed of nerve cell bodies. The central canal, within the gray matter, circulates the cerebrospinal fluid.

The brain and spinal cord are covered by three membranes: the dura mater, arachnoid, and pia mater, collectively defined as the meninges. The dura mater lies closest to the skull and functions as a protective layer and as a collection area for cerebral spinal fluid (CSF) and blood that needs to be returned to general circulation. The arachnoid is the middle layer that is a loose sac surrounding the brain. Arteries and veins of the brain, as well as CSF, can be found in the space below the arachnoid membrane or subarachnoid space. The layer closest to the brain is the pia mater. This layer adheres very closely to the surface of the brain and spinal cord and contains small blood vessels.

There are 31 pairs of spinal nerves that deliver sensory impulses from the peripheral nervous system to the spinal cord, which in turn relays them to the brain. Conversely, motor impulses generated in the brain are relayed by the spinal cord to the spinal nerves, which pass the impulses to peripheral nerves in the muscles and glands.

The chapter is broken down into the following code blocks:

G00-G09	Inflammatory diseases of the central nervous system
G10-G14	Systemic atrophies primarily affecting the central nervous system
G20-G26	Extrapyramidal and movement disorders
G30-G32	Other degenerative diseases of the nervous system
G35-G37	Demyelinating diseases of the central nervous system
G40-G47	Episodic and paroxysmal disorders
G50-G59	Nerve, nerve root and plexus disorders
G60-G65	Polyneuropathies and other disorders of the peripheral nervous system
G70-G73	Diseases of myoneural junction and muscle
G80-G83	Cerebral palsy and other paralytic syndromes
G89-G99	Other disorders of the nervous system

Inflammatory Diseases of the Central Nervous System (G00-G09)

Inflammatory diseases are the result of an invasion of organisms spreading from a nearby infection (e.g., a chronic sinus or middle ear infection). The bloodstream may carry the organism from other sites to the CNS or, in rare cases, head trauma or surgical procedures may introduce the organism directly into the CNS.

Bacterial infection of the CNS can result in abscesses and empyemas. CNS infections are classified according to the location where they occur. For example, a spinal epidural abscess is located above the dura mater and a cranial subdural empyema occurs between the dura mater and the arachnoid. As pus and other material from an infection accumulate, pressure is exerted on the brain or spinal cord. This pressure can damage the nervous system tissue and, without treatment, the infection can be fatal. Specific symptoms of CNS infections depend on location, but may include severe headache or back pain, weakness, sensory loss, and a fever. An individual may complain of a stiff neck, nausea or vomiting, and tiredness or disorientation. There is a potential for seizures, paralysis, or coma. The fatality rate associated with CNS infections ranges from 10 to 40 percent, and those surviving an infection may experience permanent damage, such as partial paralysis, speech problems, or seizures.

The categories in this code block are as follows:

G00	Bacterial meningitis, not elsewhere classified
G01	Meningitis in bacterial diseases classified elsewhere
G02	Meningitis in other infectious and parasitic diseases classified elsewhere
G03	Meningitis due to other and unspecified causes
G04	Encephalitis, myelitis and encephalomyelitis
G05	Encephalitis, myelitis and encephalomyelitis in diseases classified elsewhere
G06	Intracranial and intraspinal abscess and granuloma
G07	Intracranial and intraspinal abscess and granuloma in diseases classified elsewhere
G08	Intracranial and intraspinal phlebitis and thrombophlebitis
G09	Sequelae of inflammatory diseases of central nervous system

Categories in this code block report inflammatory conditions that are primarily infectious in etiology. However, many infections and inflammatory conditions of the central nervous system are classified in Chapter 1 Certain Infectious and Parasitic Diseases, so careful review of excludes notes is required to ensure that the correct code is assigned. In addition, some inflammatory conditions of the central nervous system with noninfectious etiologies are found in other categories within the nervous system chapter.

G00.- Bacterial meningitis, not elsewhere classified

Meningitis occurs when one or more of the three meningeal membranes or the space between the membranes becomes inflamed, in this case due to a bacterial infection. Initial symptoms of bacterial meningitis are common to all types of meningitis and may include stiff neck, headache, fever, nausea and vomiting, positive Kernig's and Brudzinski's signs, and rash. Bacterial meningitis usually progresses rapidly resulting in more serious symptoms, such as drowsiness, alterations in sensorium, seizures, and coma. Morbidity and mortality rates from bacterial meningitis are high if the condition is not diagnosed and treated promptly.

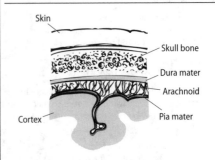

The meninges constitute the three layers that cover the brain and spinal cord: the dura mater, pia mater, and arachnoid

> **Focus Point**
>
> *Bacterial meningitis codes are also found in Chapter 1 Certain Infectious and Parasitic Diseases, so use of the alphabetic index and review of excludes notes are required to ensure that the correct code is assigned.*

G00.0 Hemophilus meningitis

Haemophilus influenzae type b (Hib) is the most common type of bacteria in this genus to cause meningitis, most often occurring in young children. Immunizations have been effective in reducing the incidence of meningitis due to this organism.

G00.1   Pneumococcal meningitis

The most common type of pneumococcal bacteria seen in meningitis is *Streptococcus* pneumoniae. Healthy adults and children can have colonization of this organism in the nasopharynx without developing meningitis. These bacteria may spread to the meninges from local infections of the ear or sinus or when the immune mechanism needed to destroy these bacteria is compromised.

G00.2   Streptococcal meningitis

Streptococci organisms are commonly found in the gastrointestinal tract and female genital tract. Due to the prevalence of this organism in the female genital tract, streptococcal meningitis is often seen in neonates.

G00.3   Staphylococcal meningitis

Meningitis associated with staphylococci species primarily occurs as a result of surgical intervention; *Staphylococcus aureus* and *Staphylococcus epidermidis* being the most prevalent.

G00.9   Bacterial meningitis, unspecified

A diagnosis of gram-negative meningitis without documentation of the specific gram-negative bacterium is reported here.

Focus Point

The terms "gram-negative" and "gram-positive" refer to a method of differential staining of bacteria for bacterial taxonomy and identification. Gram-positive bacteria retain the basic dye crystal violet and gram-negative bacteria lose the crystal violet dye to become colorless. Counterstains color gram-negative bacteria pink to red and leave gram-positive bacteria dark purple.

G01   Meningitis in bacterial diseases classified elsewhere

G02   Meningitis in other infectious and parasitic diseases classified elsewhere

Meningitis that develops as a manifestation of separate and distinct disease processes is classified in these two categories based on whether the infectious organism is bacterial or due to other infectious or parasitic organisms. Although the inciting disease is due to an infection, the infection does not initially present in the meninges but spreads to the meninges from a remote site.

Focus Point

Review the index carefully to ensure proper use of the above manifestation codes. Many meningitis conditions code to the infectious and parasitic disease chapter as the meningitis is part of the code description or an inclusion term under that specific code. In these cases, no additional manifestation code of G01 or G02 is needed from the nervous system chapter.

G03.-   Meningitis due to other and unspecified causes

This category reports inflammations of the meninges that are aseptic or nonbacterial in nature, are chronic, have etiologies other than infectious organisms, or are due to an unknown etiology.

G03.0   Nonpyogenic meningitis

Noninfectious meningitis is another term used to describe this condition, meaning there is no bacterial, viral, or other infectious source that explains the meningitis symptomology. The symptoms experienced are similar to those of infectious meningitis although less severe and often resolve quickly and cerebral spinal fluid is often nondiagnostic.

Focus Point

In most of the literature, aseptic meningitis is often equated to a viral source (i.e., nonbacterial). However, it is not classified that way in ICD-10-CM. When a viral source is documented along with a diagnosis of nonpyogenic or aseptic meningitis, the appropriate code in most cases comes from Chapter 1 Certain Infectious and Parasitic Diseases.

G03.1   Chronic meningitis

This condition is defined by prolonged inflammation of the brain or spinal cord meninges lasting longer than four weeks. It often is slow to develop and with only mild symptoms.

G03.2   Benign recurrent meningitis [Mollaret]

Benign recurrent meningitis is an aseptic or noninfectious inflammation of the meninges that is also called Mollaret meningitis due to the presence of Mollaret cells in the spinal fluid. In Mollaret meningitis, the patient experiences recurrent bouts of inflammation, lasting anywhere from two to five days, with typical meningitis symptoms of stiff neck, fever, and headache. These symptoms are sudden in onset but tend to resolve without any long-term neurologic damage, except in very rare cases where there may be hearing or vision loss and/or seizures. The time interval between episodes of inflammation may range from weeks to months to years.

Focus Point

Although the underlying etiology of benign recurrent meningitis is not fully understood, studies have shown that herpes simplex virus type 2 (HSV-2) may, in most cases, be the culprit. If HSV-2 is documented as the underlying cause, a herpes virus meningitis code is used instead of Mollaret.

G03.8   Meningitis due to other specified causes

Noninfectious causes of meningitis that are in some way linked to a noninfectious underlying etiology are classified here, including meningitis due to preventive immunization, inoculation, or vaccination and meningitis due to other specified causes not elsewhere classified. The underlying etiology can range from drugs such as NSAIDS or intravenous immunoglobulins or systemic diseases such as systemic lupus erythematosus (SLE), Behçet's disease, and rheumatoid arthritis.

Focus Point

Sarcoidosis is a systemic disease that is caused by granuloma formation in an organ. When the granuloma formation occurs in the meninges it is considered sarcoid meningitis. Sarcoid meningitis is not classified in the nervous system chapter but is instead classified with the other sarcoidosis codes found in Chapter 3 – Diseases of the Blood and Blood-forming Organs under category D86.

G04.-   Encephalitis, myelitis and encephalomyelitis

Encephalitis, myelitis, and encephalomyelitis are inflammations of the central nervous system that alter the function of various portions of the brain (encephalitis), spinal cord (myelitis), or both (encephalomyelitis). In some instances the meninges may also be concurrently involved along with the brain (meningoencephalitis) or the spinal cord (meningomyelitis). Signs and symptoms of encephalitis, myelitis, and encephalomyelitis depend on the cause. With mild benign forms, symptoms include malaise, fever, headache, dizziness, apathy, neck stiffness, nausea and vomiting, ataxia, tremors, hyperactivity, and speech difficulties. With severe central nervous system involvement, there is high fever, stupor, seizures, disorientation, ocular palsies, paralysis, spasticity, and coma that may proceed to death.

G04.0-   Acute disseminated encephalitis and encephalomyelitis (ADEM)

ADEM is a condition caused by inflammatory lesions within the brain and/or spinal cord. The inflammation causes demyelination or breakdown of the myelin sheath surrounding a nerve fiber, interrupting the conduction of impulses along that nerve fiber. Typical ADEM symptoms include fever, headache, and drowsiness usually with rapid onset. Neurological symptoms can include difficulty with voluntary muscle control, vision loss, paresis, and/or coma. This condition is most often seen after a viral or bacterial infection or following certain immunizations, with symptoms typically appearing a week to two weeks postinfection or postimmunization.

Focus Point

Differentiating ADEM from multiple sclerosis (MS), another demyelinating disease, can be difficult as both present with similar symptoms and white matter appearance. Unlike multiple sclerosis, ADEM is most often seen in children and is most often a singular event with no imaging suggesting older inflammatory brain lesions. Symptom onset is very rapid and can include loss of consciousness.

G04.1   Tropical spastic paraplegia

This condition is almost always caused by a virus called human T-cell lymphotrophic virus type 1 (HTLV-1). It is a chronic disease with slow progression of muscle weakness in the legs resulting in sensory disturbances, difficulty walking, and urinary incontinence.

Focus Point

A code from the infectious and parasitic diseases chapter identifying the HTLV-1 virus may also be reported to give greater specificity as to the cause of the tropical spastic paraplegia.

G04.3-   Acute necrotizing hemorrhagic encephalopathy

This condition is very rare and presents similarly to ADEM. However, acute necrotizing hemorrhagic encephalopathy is distinct in that along with demyelination, hemorrhaging in the white matter and edema is also apparent within the brain. The rapid progression of the disease and the severity of the symptoms also distinguish this condition from its milder form, ADEM. This condition primarily affects young adults and is often secondary to an upper respiratory infection.

G05.-   Encephalitis, myelitis and encephalomyelitis in diseases classified elsewhere

Encephalitis, myelitis, and encephalomyelitis are inflammations of the central nervous system that alter the function of various portions of the brain (encephalitis), spinal cord (myelitis), or both (encephalomyelitis). In some instances, the meninges may also be concurrently involved along with the brain (meningoencephalitis) or the spinal cord (meningomyelitis). Signs and symptoms of encephalitis, myelitis, and encephalomyelitis depend on the cause. With mild benign forms symptoms include malaise, fever, headache, dizziness, apathy, neck stiffness, nausea and vomiting, ataxia, tremors, hyperactivity, and speech difficulties. With severe central nervous system involvement, there is high fever, stupor, seizures, disorientation, ocular palsies, paralysis, spasticity, and coma that may proceed to death. For the two codes in this category, the inflammation of the brain and/or spinal cord is a direct result of a separate disease process. Although the underlying disease process may in fact be due to a virus or other infectious agent, unlike postinfectious encephalitis, myelitis, or encephalomyelitis, the underlying disease is still present and active.

G06.- Intracranial and intraspinal abscess and granuloma

Intracranial and intraspinal abscess is the localized collection of pus in a cavity or pocket in the brain or spinal regions. Infectious granulomas are tumor-like masses that form as a result of the infectious process. Both intracranial and intraspinal abscesses are usually caused by bacterium with the most common organisms being streptococci, pneumococci, and staphylococci.

G06.0 Intracranial abscess and granuloma

Intracranial abscess is the localized collection of purulent material and liquified brain tissue that may be located in the epidural (extradural) or subdural spaces or within the substance of the brain itself. The etiology is usually bacterial and occurs through direct extension from a contiguous focus, blood-borne metastases, or by penetrating injury. Signs and symptoms of intracranial abscess, with brain abscess, include headache, altered sensorium (lethargy, irritability, confusion, or coma), nausea and vomiting, fever, seizures, multiple alternation nerve palsies, and other neurologic deficits. Signs and symptoms of intracranial abscess, with subdural abscess, include headache, sinusitis, altered sensorium (lethargy, obtundation, or coma), seizures, fever and chills, hemiparesis, and aphasia. Signs and symptoms of intracranial abscess, with cerebral epidural abscess, involve limited localized symptoms.

G06.1 Intraspinal abscess and granuloma

The definition of intraspinal abscess is the localized collection of pus in a cavity involving the layers of the spinal cord, including epidural (extradural) and subdural regions. The etiology is usually due to blood-borne spread, direct extension from contiguous sites, or as a consequence of an invasive procedure.

Most spinal abscesses are epidural. Signs and symptoms of intraspinal abscess include spinal ache, root pain, weakness, paresthesias, and eventually paralysis.

G07 Intracranial and intraspinal abscess and granuloma in diseases classified elsewhere

Intracranial and intraspinal abscess is the localized collection of pus in a cavity or pocket in the brain or spinal regions. In this category, the abscess or granuloma develops as a manifestation of a separate and distinct disease process.

G08 Intracranial and intraspinal phlebitis and thrombophlebitis

Phlebitis is defined as inflammation of a vein. Thrombophlebitis is when inflammation in a vein is a consequence of a blood clot or thrombus. The principal veins in the cranial cavity are incorporated into the dura mater, which is closely bound to the inner bone of the cavity. The venous sinuses of the brain (e.g., the sagittal, cavernous, petrosal, sphenoparietal, sigmoid, and transverse sinuses) are held in an open position and generally occur where there is a wide separation between major anatomical entities. The sinuses contain an endothelial lining continuous into the veins connected to them. There are no valves in the sinuses or in the veins and the majority of the venous blood in the sinus drains from the cranium via the internal jugular vein. Venous thrombosis and thrombophlebitis occur as complications of intracranial or intraspinal infections. When the blood clot and inflammation occur in the brain, symptoms such as headaches, focal seizures, and focal neurologic signs affecting the legs more than the arm occur. Massive venous infarction, due to thrombosis, may be fatal. Septic intracranial thrombophlebitis is an extremely serious complication that even with appropriate therapy is fatal in more than one-third of cases. Deep or superficial septic phlebitis can occur by direct invasion from adjacent nonvascular infections associated with a long-term intravenous cannula being used for chronic administration of fluids or medications. The etiologic agent usually can be cultured from blood and from any metastatic sites of infection.

Systemic Atrophies Primarily Affecting the Central Nervous System (G10–G14)

Atrophy is a reduction in the size or activity of an anatomic structure, due to wasting away from disease or other factors. In this case, atrophy occurs in structures in the brain or spinal cord. Manifestations of systemic atrophies are dependent on the specific central nervous system structures that are affected by the disease process.

The categories in this code block are as follows:

G10   Huntington's disease

G11   Hereditary ataxia

G12   Spinal muscular atrophy and related syndromes

G13   Systemic atrophies primarily affecting the central nervous system in diseases classified elsewhere

G14   Postpolio syndrome

G10   Huntington's disease

Huntington's disease, also called Huntington's chorea, is a fatal hereditary disease affecting the basal ganglia and cerebral cortex. The onset varies but usually begins in the fourth decade of life. Death usually follows within 15 years. Signs and symptoms of Huntington's chorea include family history of Huntington's chorea; weight loss; facial grimacing; ceaseless rapid, complex, jerky movements; personality changes, including irritability and indifference; mental deterioration until dementia is reached; and, in children, rigid rather than choreic movements and seizures.

G12.-   Spinal muscular atrophy and related syndromes

Motor neurons are specialized nerve cells found in the brainstem and spinal cord that stimulate the muscles. Atrophy is a reduction in the size or activity of an anatomic structure, due to wasting away from disease or other factors. When motor neurons are damaged or degenerate it can lead to atrophy and weakness of muscles.

G12.0   Infantile spinal muscular atrophy, type I [Werdnig-Hoffman]

Of all the types of spinal muscular atrophy, the Werdnig-Hoffman type is the most severe. A diagnosis can be made anywhere from a few days after birth to 6 months of age. Infants may not be able to sit up or hold their head up on their own and often have problems swallowing. Prognosis is poor due to the effects on the respiratory muscles causing breathing difficulties and eventually respiratory failure.

G12.1   Other inherited spinal muscular atrophy

Except for the most severe form, infantile spinal muscular atrophy, the other types of spinal muscular atrophy are categorized here. Type II, III, and IV or adult spinal muscular atrophy is defined based on the age of symptomology and severity of the muscle wasting. The older the patient is when diagnosed the more likely the symptoms will be less severe and the disease process less fatal.

G12.2-   Motor neuron disease

Motor neuron diseases cause degeneration of motor neurons or motor nerves and are classified based on whether the upper motor neurons originating in the primary motor cortex of the cerebrum, the lower motor neurons originating in the brainstem and spinal cord, or both are affected. When motor neurons in these areas degenerate, the communication between the brain and the muscle is lost and the muscle cannot be stimulated. Without stimulation the muscle becomes weak and atrophies.

G12.21   Amyotrophic lateral sclerosis

The most common motor neuron disease is amyotrophic lateral sclerosis or ALS, also known as Lou Gehrig disease. ALS is typically classified into two types: sporadic and familial. The familial types are linked to specific gene mutations known to be passed down through generations. Sporadic types can, in some cases, be linked to a genetic mutation but most often the etiology is unknown. Because the death of motor neurons in ALS is progressive, this condition is rarely diagnosed before the age of 40. Initial symptoms include muscle weakness, cramping, and twitching. Continued muscle atrophy can lead to dysphagia and walking and breathing difficulties. Prognosis varies between patients but rarely do patients live more than five years after the first notable symptoms.

G12.22   Progressive bulbar palsy

This motor neuron disease primarily affects the nerves found in the medulla causing problems with the muscles involved in speech, swallowing, and chewing. Aspiration of food or saliva is common due to dysphagia leading to pneumonia, the most common cause of death.

Focus Point

Progressive bulbar palsies of childhood including two rare progressive bulbar palsy conditions, Brown-Vialetto-Van Laere syndrome and Fazio-Londe disease, are reported with G12.1.

G12.23   Primary lateral sclerosis

Primary lateral sclerosis (PLS) is a rare, slowly progressive degenerative motor neuron disease characterized by spasticity, usually affecting first the lower extremities, then the trunk, upper extremities, and finally the muscles that control speech, swallowing, and chewing. The diagnosis of PLS may require following the clinical course for 3 to 4 years and extensive testing to exclude other diseases. Because of the similarity in presentation and symptoms, PLS may be mistaken for the more common amyotrophic lateral sclerosis (ALS). However, the disease progression in PLS is more gradual than in ALS, progressing over many years, and survival rates are longer. Unlike ALS, PLS in most cases is not fatal. PLS is more common in men than in women and can happen at any age, but onset generally occurs between ages 40 and 60.

G12.24   Familial motor neuron disease

Familial motor neuron disease is caused by an inherited mutated gene. The familial type is rare representing only 10 percent of all cases of motor neuron disease. The age at which symptoms of this type of motor neuron disease present can vary widely—as early as the 20s and as late as the 80s. The average age of onset is about 45 years. The first symptoms can appear at different ages and in different areas of the body, even within the same family.

Carriers of the mutated gene have a fifty percent chance of passing it on to their children. Only one copy of the mutated gene is required to cause the disease, but not all people with the mutation develop motor neuron disease. Genetic testing may be performed for patients who have symptoms of motor neuron disease, or are planning a family, and have a family member with the disease.

G12.25   Progressive spinal muscle atrophy

Progressive spinal muscle atrophy (PSMA), or spinal muscular atrophy (SMA), is a genetic motor neuron disease involving the loss of lower motor neurons in the spinal cord causing atrophy and affecting the control of voluntary muscle movement. PSMA most often affects the muscles of the shoulders, hips, thighs, and upper back. The muscles used for breathing and swallowing may be affected, and spinal curvatures can develop. Age of onset, symptoms, and rate of progression vary, but generally the earlier the age of onset, the greater degree of impact on motor function.

Extrapyramidal and Movement Disorders (G20-G26)

There are two primary pathways within the central nervous system, known as extrapyramidal and pyramidal, used to control and coordinate muscle movement. A movement disorder develops when one or more of the constituents in the extrapyramidal or pyramidal pathway are compromised. Extrapyramidal disorders usually invoke involuntary muscle movements due to damage to basal ganglia while pyramidal disorders cause loss of voluntary muscle control.

The categories in this code block are as follows:

G20	Parkinson's disease
G21	Secondary parkinsonism
G23	Other degenerative diseases of basal ganglia
G24	Dystonia
G25	Other extrapyramidal and movement disorders
G26	Extrapyramidal and movement disorders in diseases classified elsewhere

G20   Parkinson's disease

Parkinson's disease (paralysis agitans) is an idiopathic neurological condition marked by degeneration and dysfunction within the basal ganglia, clusters of nerve cells (neurons) at the base of the cerebrum located on both sides of the thalamus, above the brainstem. The basal ganglia may also be referred to as separate structures that include the caudate nucleus, putamen, and globus pallidus. This disease involves the degeneration of the nigral neurons, a group of specialized cells in the midbrain that contain neuromelanin and manufacture the neurotransmitter dopamine. When 75 to 80 percent of the dopamine innervation is destroyed, signs and symptoms of parkinsonism begin to manifest. These symptoms include tremor, rigidity, shuffling gait, drooling, "pill rolling" hand movement, and impaired control of facial muscles.

> **Focus Point**
>
> *Parkinson's disease is associated with mental disorders such as dementia, depression, and delirium. True dementia affects 20 to 30 percent of patients. Dementia with parkinsonism is excluded from this category and is instead reported with code G31.83.*

G21.-   Secondary parkinsonism

The same symptoms seen in Parkinson's disease are also seen in secondary parkinsonism. The differentiating factor is that secondary parkinsonism is the result of another condition or inciting event.

Specific causes may include the use of certain drugs or toxic chemicals, stroke, trauma, and infectious or inflammatory diseases such as encephalitis or meningitis.

G21.0   Malignant neuroleptic syndrome

This syndrome, also referred to as neuroleptic malignant syndrome (NMS) is a parkinsonism reaction brought on by exposure to antipsychotic or neuroleptic drugs. Signature symptoms include fever, severe muscle rigidity, autonomic dysfunction and alteration in consciousness.

G21.11   Neuroleptic induced parkinsonism

This secondary Parkinsonism condition is due to an adverse effect from antipsychotic or neuroleptic drugs. The distinguishing factor between this condition and neuroleptic malignant syndrome (NMS) is neuroleptic induced parkinsonism typically presents with classic Parkinson's disease symptoms and without the severity seen in NMS.

G24.-   Dystonia

Dystonia is a disorder of abnormal muscle tone, excessive or inadequate. Involuntary movements and prolonged muscle contractions result in tremors, abnormalities in posture, and twisting body motions that affect an isolated area or the whole body. Multiple forms of dystonia exist and may be genetic or acquired.

G24.01   Drug induced subacute dyskinesia

Subacute dyskinesia due to drugs is often characterized by rapid, jerking motions that can include blepharospasm (a focal dystonia characterized by increased blinking and involuntary eye closure) or orofacial dyskinesia (involuntary, repetitive movements of the mouth and face). Symptoms may develop after weeks or years of drug exposure.

G24.3   Spasmodic torticollis

Also known as cervical dystonia, this condition is characterized by a twisted, unnatural position of the neck due to involuntary cervical muscle contractions that pull the head to one side. It is diagnosed in women more than men and can occur at any age although it is often seen in patients 25 and older.

G24.5   Blepharospasm

This condition is the continuous, tonic spasm of the orbicularis oculi muscle that can ultimately result in the eyelids being involuntarily kept closed. Blepharospasm can be classified as essential, in which there is no abnormality of the eye or of the trigeminal nerve, or symptomatic, in which there is an associated eye lesion or trigeminal nerve abnormality.

G25.-   Other extrapyramidal and movement disorders

Extrapyramidal disorders usually invoke involuntary muscle movements, such as tremors or muscle contractions, due to damage to basal ganglia.

G25.0   Essential tremor

An essential tremor is characterized by involuntary shaking usually worse with movement. It most often affects the upper extremities but can also be seen in the head. Considered to be monosymptomatic, it rarely is associated with other neurological symptoms.

G25.3   Myoclonus

There are many forms of myoclonus or quick, involuntary muscle contractions. This code is used to describe myoclonus that is due to an undetermined etiology, is drug-induced, or is a specific type (i.e., Friedreich's myoclonia).

> **Focus Point**
>
> *In most instances, a myoclonus code would not be used when the myoclonia is described as epileptic; instead the epileptic disorder, a code from category G40, would be coded. This is not true in the case of familial (progressive) epilepsy, a benign form of epilepsy that can be associated with tonic-clonic seizures but is most often only characterized by myoclonic jerks and cortical hand tremors.*

G25.81   Restless legs syndrome

Restless legs syndrome (RLS) is a common but often misdiagnosed neurologic movement disorder whose characteristics include unpleasant sensations deep within the legs that take place at rest and worsen at bedtime or during sleep. An irresistible urge to move the legs, which may temporarily relieve the symptoms, is accompanied by motor restlessness and sensations of pain, burning, prickling, or tingling. Dopaminergic dysfunction is thought to be a factor since RLS has a favorable response to antiparkinsonian medications such as levodopa and dopamine agonists. Symptoms may occur as a result of other underlying conditions, such as pregnancy, end-stage renal disease, various polyneuropathies, or deficiencies in iron, vitamin B12, folate, or magnesium. Restless legs syndrome can occur at any age but is more prevalent in women than men and those who are middle aged and older.

> **Focus Point**
>
> *The symptoms of restless legs syndrome may worsen at bedtime or during sleep. This syndrome should not be confused with organic sleep disorders that manifest as abnormal movements during sleep, such as periodic limb movement disorder (G47.61) or sleep related leg cramps (G47.62). RLS is a syndrome and definitive diagnosis, not a symptom.*

Other Degenerative Diseases of the Nervous System (G30-G32)

Degenerative diseases of the nervous system are associated with loss of neurons and secondary scarring, but these conditions do not involve inflammation or necrosis of nervous system tissues or organs. Some conditions classified here are relatively common, such as Alzheimer's disease, while others are quite rare.

The categories in this code block are as follows:

G30	Alzheimer's disease
G31	Other degenerative diseases of the nervous system, not elsewhere classified
G32	Other degenerative diseases of the nervous system in diseases classified elsewhere

G30.- Alzheimer's disease

Alzheimer's disease, the most common form of dementia, is caused by the destruction of the subcortical white matter of the brain through the development of neurofibrillary tangles and amyloid plaques that eventually lead to death of the nerve cells. It is characterized by increasing loss of intellectual functioning beginning with minor memory loss and eventually resulting in total loss of ability to function.

G30.0 Alzheimer's disease with early onset

This is a rare form of Alzheimer's with clinical presentation of symptoms as early as 30 years old but most often presenting between 40 and 50 years old. Myoclonus may also be a distinguishing factor as it is often seen in early onset and not late onset Alzheimer's.

G30.1 Alzheimer's disease with late onset

This is the most common form with clinical presentation of symptoms usually occurring after the age of 65. Causes of late onset Alzheimer's have not specifically been identified although it is thought that a combination of environmental and genetic factors may play a role in its development.

G30.8 Other Alzheimer's disease

This code includes any specified type of Alzheimer's that is not documented as early onset or late onset.

G30.9 Alzheimer's disease, unspecified

The etiology cannot be identified or the type of Alzheimer's is not stated in the documentation.

G31.- Other degenerative diseases of nervous system, not elsewhere classified

The etiology of many degenerative diseases of the nervous system is not fully understood. Corticobasal degeneration, which is classified here, is an example of a degenerative disease with an unknown etiology. Two other types also included in this category, Alpers' disease and Leigh's disease, are known to be inherited.

G31.81 Alpers disease

Alpers' disease is an inherited autosomal recessive disorder caused by mutations in the mtDNA, specifically identified as the POLG gene. Initial symptoms in infancy include developmental delay, hypotonia, and spasticity. Disease progression is marked by progressive paralysis, dementia, and mental retardation. Myoclonic seizures are characteristic of Alpers' disease. Diagnostic imaging of the central nervous system often displays status spongiosis degeneration of the cerebrum. Prognosis is poor. Patients often expire within the first decade of life.

G31.82 Leigh's disease

Leigh's disease is an inherited neurometabolic disorder of the central nervous system that occurs due to mutations of the mitochondrial DNA (mtDNA). These mutations impair the growth and development of essential brainstem cells, which inhibits motor skills. The disease is characterized by the patient's inability to control movement. In infants, early symptoms include poor sucking ability, inability to control head movements, and seizure. As the disease progresses, organ function and development are delayed or regress, resulting in failure to thrive. Prognosis varies widely in accordance with age of onset and severity.

G31.83 Dementia with Lewy bodies

Lewy bodies are protein deposits that form in the nerve cells of the brain causing the nerve cells to die. Lewy bodies can be found in patients with Parkinson's disease and Alzheimer's disease making diagnosis difficult. Certain characteristics of Lewy body dementia not associated with Alzheimer's disease may include the inability to copy or draw; fluctuation between coherency and incoherency, especially in the early stages; visual hallucinations; and minimal issues with memory upon initial onset.

> **Focus Point**
>
> *Any form of dementia associated with Alzheimer's is coded to category G30 Alzheimer's disease. Parkinson's disease with dementia, however, is not coded to the Parkinson's category, G20, but is instead classified to Lewy bodies.*

G31.84   Mild cognitive impairment, so stated

Mild cognitive impairment (MCI), also known as age-associated memory impairment (AAMI) or benign senescent forgetfulness, is considered to be a strong early predictor of Alzheimer's disease and is described as "the transitional stage between normal aging and dementia." This disorder is widespread among the elderly. These patients do not meet established criteria for dementia but demonstrate impairment beyond that which is normal for age in one or more cognitive areas. Patients with MCI may otherwise function normally in society but may exhibit deficiencies in one or more of the following areas:

- Language: Recall of words may be slower than previously; frequent repetition of statements may occur

- Visuospatial ability: Time or space relationships may pose difficulty, such as the ability to draw a box with the correct proportions

- Executive function: Decision-making ability may be challenged

- Memory: Decrease in recent recall may be present; details of conversations, events, and appointments may be impaired

There is no single test to diagnose MCI. Rather, diagnosis is made by excluding other conditions and disorders that could be responsible for the signs and symptoms. No cure for MCI currently exists.

G31.85   Corticobasal degeneration

Corticobasal degeneration (CBD) is a progressive condition characterized by degeneration of multiple areas of the brain, including the cerebral cortex and basal ganglia. Causation is unknown. The pathological atrophy of tissue in multiple areas of the brain correlates with the nature and onset of symptoms. Typically, onset occurs around the age of 60. An initial unilateral presentation of symptoms commonly progresses to affect both sides of the body. Symptoms include progressive impairment of cognitive, motor, visuospatial, and sensory functions. Cognitive manifestations resemble those of certain frontotemporal dementias, with marked loss of executive function, visuospatial and number processing, and language impairment. The characteristic decline in motor function mimics those of Parkinson's disease in which the patient demonstrates progressive impaired balance, poor coordination, akinesia, myoclonus, rigidity, dystonia, and dysphagia. Greater than half of the patients diagnosed with CBD experience alien hand syndrome, which is failure to control the movements of (usually) one or both hands.

Demyelinating Diseases of the Central Nervous System (G35-G37)

Demyelinating diseases affect the central and peripheral nervous systems. Pathogenesis of demyelination may be summarized as the abnormal loss of myelin, the protective white matter substance that insulates nerve endings and facilitates neuroreception and neurotransmission. When this substance is damaged, nerve function is short-circuited, resulting in impaired or loss of function. As a result, patches of scar tissue (sclerosis) develop where the protective myelin has been damaged at the nerve endings. Although healing remyelination can occur in certain disease processes, there could be permanent damage in the form of sequelae and long-term effects. The anatomic location of demyelination may be associated with certain types or manifestations of disease. Causal factors include genetic predisposition, certain infections, autoimmune disease, and exposures to certain drugs or chemicals.

The categories in this code block are as follows:

G35	Multiple sclerosis
G36	Other acute disseminated demyelination
G37	Other demyelinating diseases of the central nervous system

Multiple sclerosis is a chronic demyelinating disease affecting the white matter of the spinal cord and brain. Multiple sclerosis is characterized by the breaking down of the myelin fibers of the nervous system; patches of scarred nervous fibers develop at these sites. The etiology is unknown, but recent studies suggest the condition may be a cell-mediated autoimmune disease due to an inherited disorder of immune regulation. The disease affects adults usually between ages 20 and 40 and occurs more often in women. Signs and symptoms of multiple sclerosis include acute optic neuritis, diplopia, internuclear ophthalmoplegia, frequent dropping of articles, stumbling or falling for no reason, Lhermitte's phenomenon (flexion of the neck producing tingling and paresthesias of legs), and mental changes. Evoked-potential testing of the visual evoked response, brainstem auditory evoked response, and somatosensory evoked response is abnormally delayed.

G35   Multiple sclerosis

Multiple sclerosis is a chronic demyelinating disease affecting the white matter of the spinal cord and brain. Multiple sclerosis is characterized by the breaking down of the myelin fibers of the nervous system; patches of scarred nervous fibers develop at these sites. The etiology is unknown, but recent studies suggest the condition may be a cell-mediated autoimmune disease due to an inherited disorder of immune regulation. The disease affects adults usually between ages 20 and 40 and occurs more often in women. Signs and symptoms of multiple sclerosis include acute optic neuritis, diplopia, internuclear ophthalmoplegia, frequent dropping of articles, stumbling or falling for no reason, Lhermitte's phenomenon (flexion of the neck producing tingling and paresthesias of legs), and mental changes. Evoked-potential testing of the visual evoked response, brainstem auditory evoked response, and somatosensory evoked response is abnormally delayed.

G37.- Other demyelinating diseases of central nervous system

Demyelinating diseases may be diffuse, affecting multiple sites of the central nervous system, or focal, affecting a specific site.

G37.3 Acute transverse myelitis in demyelinating disease of central nervous system

Acute (transverse) myelitis is a focal inflammatory condition of the spinal cord resulting in motor, sensory, and autonomic dysfunction. "Transverse" indicates dysfunction at a specific level across the spinal cord, with altered function below it and normal function above it. Sixty percent of ATM cases are idiopathic. Other cases can be linked to known, underlying diseases. The most optimal treatment of ATM is dependent upon a timely and accurate diagnosis. Rapid symptom progression, back pain, and spinal shock predict a poor recovery. ATM tends to peak between the ages of 10 and 19 and 30 and 39 years. The classic symptoms of transverse myelitis are weakness of the extremities causing stumbling, dragging of one foot, or legs feeling heavier than normal; altered sensation manifesting as numbness, tingling, coldness, or burning, and a heightened, painful sensitivity to touch; pain in the back or intense, shooting sensations that radiate down the legs, arms, or around the torso; loss of the ability to feel pain or temperature sensitivity; and bowel or bladder dysfunction.

> **Focus Point**
>
> *Although similar to multiple sclerosis (MS) in pathology and symptomology, there are often distinct differences in the appearance and location of lesions associated with acute transverse myelitis when compared to MS lesions. In acute transverse myelitis, demyelination occurs most often at the thoracic spine level, with associated lower extremity, bowel, and bladder impairments.*

Episodic and Paroxysmal Disorders (G40-G47)

Episodic disorders occur at intervals and paroxysmal conditions are those that occur suddenly or with varying levels of severity or intensity.

The categories in this code block are as follows:

G40	Epilepsy and recurrent seizures
G43	Migraine
G44	Other headache syndromes
G45	Transient cerebral ischemic attacks and related syndromes
G46	Vascular syndromes of brain in cerebrovascular diseases
G47	Sleep disorders

G40.- Epilepsy and recurrent seizures

Epilepsy is a disorder characterized by recurrent transient disturbances of the cerebral function. An abnormal paroxysmal neuronal discharge in the brain usually results in convulsive seizures, but may result in loss of consciousness, abnormal behavior, and sensory disturbances in any combination. Epilepsy may be secondary to prior trauma, hemorrhage, intoxication (toxins), chemical imbalances, anoxia, infections, neoplasms, or congenital defects. Signs and symptoms of epilepsy include momentary interruption of activity, staring, and mental blankness. More severe symptoms include complete loss of consciousness, sudden momentary loss or contracture of muscle tone, rolling of the eyes, stiffness, violent jerking movements, and incontinence of urine and feces. Most of the codes in this category are classified based on the type of epilepsy/seizure, whether it is intractable or not intractable, and whether it is associated with status epilepticus. Intractable epilepsy should only be coded if it is documented. Documentation of recurrence does not substantiate intractable epilepsy because all seizures in an epileptic patient are recurrent. Status epilepticus is a series of seizures at intervals too brief to allow consciousness between attacks and can result in death.

G40.0- **Localization-related (focal) (partial) idiopathic epilepsy and epileptic syndromes with seizures of localized onset**

G40.1- **Localization-related (focal) (partial) symptomatic epilepsy and epileptic syndromes with simple partial seizures**

G40.2- **Localization-related (focal) (partial) symptomatic epilepsy and epileptic syndromes with complex partial seizures**

Localized seizures involve one part of the brain and are classified based on the extent to which consciousness is affected: localized onset, simple or complex partial seizures. With simple partial seizures consciousness is unaffected and in complex partial seizures consciousness is impaired.

G40.3- Generalized idiopathic epilepsy and epileptic syndromes

Generalized forms of epilepsy occur throughout multiple areas of the brain. All types of generalized epilepsy lead to impairment or loss of consciousness.

G40.81- Lennox-Gastaut syndrome

Lennox-Gastaut syndrome is a severe form of epilepsy with usual onset in early childhood. Seizures are difficult to treat, varying in type and occurring frequently, causing falls and injuries.

G40.82- Epileptic spasms

Epileptic spasms, also called infantile spasms or West's syndrome, is a rare form of epilepsy, affecting about one infant in 2,500 and begins between 3 and 12 months of age. The spasms or seizures commonly occur during sleep or upon awakening. They are characterized by a series or cluster of spasms. The head nods forward, the arms are outstretched and up, the legs may or may not lift up toward the abdomen, muscles become stiff and then relax, eyes look to the side or up, and breathing changes. These movements may be accompanied by a small cry or the child may cry after the spasm. The spasms do not cause pain, but the baby may cry from being startled. Seizures last a few seconds and recur many times a day. A brain disorder or brain injury, such as lack of oxygen to the baby during delivery, precedes the seizures in 60 percent of these infants. However, in the other 40 percent no cause can be determined, and development is normal prior to the onset of seizures. Typically the spasms only occur during the first five years of life and then are replaced by other types of seizures. With the onset of the spasms, a child may regress developmentally. The child may stop smiling, rolling over, or sitting. Spasms can be serious and have long-term complications.

G43.- Migraine

Migraine is a common type of vascular headache. Migraine headaches appear to be caused by blood vessels that overreact to various triggers, such as stress, or an allergic reaction that creates vasoconstrictive spasm. The spasm reduces blood flow and therefore oxygen supply to the brain. In response, vasodilation occurs, triggering the release of pain-producing substances called prostaglandins. The result is a throbbing pain in the head. Diagnosis of migraine may be made based on clinical presentation. Migraine pain can last three to four days. Migraines affect both males and females, and most often the disorder begins between the ages of 5 and 35. No medical test exists for migraine, so the diagnosis is based on having some or all of the following symptoms:

- Moderate to severe throbbing pain for up to 72 hours; pain may be localized to a specific part or region of the head

- Nausea, with or without vomiting

- Sensitivity to light and sound

- Visual or auditory hallucinations

Most of the codes in this category are classified based on the type of migraine, whether it is intractable or not intractable, and whether it is associated with status migrainosus. Intractable migraine describes frequently occurring, continuous, unremitting, or other migraine recalcitrant to conventional medical therapy that often requires acute care to resolve. Status migrainosus describes a severe, debilitating migraine lasting more than 72 hours, with pain and nausea so intense that the patient must be hospitalized. This is a relatively rare, but life-threatening migraine complication that could result in a potentially fatal ischemic stroke.

G43.0- Migraine without aura

Migraine without an aura, also called common migraine, is the most frequent type of migraine seen in younger children and adolescents. This type of headache is frequently bilateral and around the eyes and temples. No preceding motor or sensory disturbance (aura) occurs. Associated symptoms may include irritability, paleness, dark circles under the eyes, and severe stomach symptoms.

G43.1- Migraine with aura

Migraine with aura, also called classical migraine is characterized by a sharply defined headache that is preceded by blurred vision, transient muscle weakness, or floaters crossing the visual field. About 20 percent of migraine sufferers experience visual and other disturbances about 15 minutes before the head pain. These symptoms, collectively known as "aura," may include flashing lights, bright spots, loss of part of one's field of vision, or numbness or tingling in the hand, tongue, or side of the face. Other symptoms may include mental fuzziness, mood changes, fatigue, and unusual retention of fluids. Basilar migraine, also known as basilar artery migraine or Bickerstaff syndrome, is a form of migraine with aura that involves a disturbance of the basilar artery, a major brain artery. A basilar migraine causes an occipital headache in addition to ataxia, diplopia, tinnitus, or vertigo.

G43.4- Hemiplegic migraine

Hemiplegic migraine is characterized by the feeling of numbness on one side of the body. It may be familial or sporadic in nature. Familial hemiplegic migraine (FHM) has been linked to mutations of specific genes on chromosomes 1 and 19. Sporadic hemiplegic migraine (SHM) is FHM without the familial connection and that particular genetic mutation.

G43.B- Ophthalmoplegic migraine

An ophthalmoplegic migraine presents with a unilateral frontal headache associated with pain around the eye, paralysis of the extraocular muscles, double vision, and other sight problems. While this type of migraine may be intractable, meaning that it has not responded to treatment, status migrainosus is not a component of the condition.

G43.D- Abdominal migraine

Abdominal migraine is characterized by recurrent bouts of stomach pain with nausea and vomiting. No headache is present. As the child gets older, this type of migraine develops into classic migraine. While this type of migraine may be intractable, meaning that it has not responded to treatment, status migrainosus is not a component of the condition.

G43.82- Menstrual migraine, not intractable

G43.83- Menstrual migraine, intractable

Menstrual migraine is associated with hormonal changes that occur during the menstrual cycle. "Menstrual headache" and "menstrual migraine" are synonymous and all forms of menstrually related headache are classified to these two subcategories.

G44.- Other headache syndromes

A wide range of headache syndromes are included under this category, including cluster, tension-type, post-traumatic and drug-induced headaches. Most of the codes in this category are classified based on the chronicity of the condition and whether or not the condition is intractable to medical or pharmacological therapies.

G44.0- Cluster headaches and other trigeminal autonomic cephalgias (TAC)

Cluster headaches get their name from the cyclical pattern of frequent and very painful headache attacks followed by remission periods. Headaches can occur once a day to several times a day but most often attack at night, usually within two hours of falling asleep or with onset of rapid eye movement (REM) sleep. The most common symptoms are one sided pain in or around the eye and most patients become extremely restless. Trigeminal autonomic cephalgia (TAC) is a group of primary headache disorders characterized by unilateral distribution of pain along the fifth cranial nerve occurring in association with characteristic autonomic ipsilateral cranial features.

Focus Point

Diagnostic differentiation between the various types of headache, such as cluster headache and migraine, can be difficult. To further complicate matters, patients may experience overlapping types of headache, such as a migraine and cluster headache combination. However, cluster headaches can be differentiated from migraine in that:

- *There are no discernible phases (i.e., prodrome, aura, headache, and postdrome).*

- *They typically occur spontaneously, while migraine headaches are often precipitated by sentinel symptoms such as aura or other warning.*

- *Gastrointestinal symptoms are rarely reported, while 40 percent of migraine patients report nausea or vomiting symptoms.*

- *Cluster headaches are comparatively short in duration.*

- *Cluster headaches may go into remission for an extended period of time when the patient is pain-free.*

- *Cluster headaches are commonly nocturnal occurrences, and may wake the patient from sleep.*

- *Patients generally prefer to remain upright during a cluster headache. During migraine attacks, movement is often reported to worsen the pain.*

- *Cluster headaches are more common in men than women. Migraines are more common in women than men.*

G44.2- Tension-type headache

Tension-type headaches are the most common type of headaches among adults. Tension headaches are idiopathic, but may be triggered by or associated with various factors including stress, sleep habits, and emotional state. Tension headaches may be episodic or chronic and may or may not respond to medical or pharmaceutical therapy.

G44.3- Post-traumatic headache

Post-traumatic headache is a common occurrence following head trauma. Although it has the potential to persist for months or even years, frequency and severity of post-traumatic headache usually resolves within six to 12 months of injury. Associated symptoms may include dizziness, insomnia, difficulties in concentration, and mood and personality changes. Chronic headache after trauma is commonly caused by sustained muscle contractions of the neck and scalp or by vascular changes caused by previous injury. Emotional stress and reactions to the headache occurrences and initial injury can complicate treatment by creating a situational anxiety cycle.

G44.4- Drug-induced headache, not elsewhere classified

Drug-induced headaches are those caused by the frequent use of certain over the counter (OTC) or prescription drugs. When the effect of one dose wears off, a withdrawal effect occurs, triggering the next headache and another round of medication, perpetuating the cycle.

G44.5- Complicated headache syndromes

Each headache syndrome has its own defining characteristics. These complicated headache syndromes differ from more common headache syndromes like migraine and often do not respond well to traditional medical therapies for headaches.

G44.51 Hemicrania continua

Hemicrania continua is a persistent primary unilateral headache of unknown causation. It is characteristically responsive to indomethacin, differentiating hemicrania continua from migraine or cluster headache. Other medications, including Triptans, are not effective. Additional diagnostic criteria includes headache for more than three months, unilateral daily and continuous pain of moderate intensity with severe exacerbations, and autonomic features on the same side (ipsilateral) as the pain, such as lacrimation (tearing), rhinorrhea (runny nose), and ptosis (drooping of the eyelids).

G44.52 New daily persistent headache (NDPH)

New daily persistent headache (NDPH) is defined as rapid development (over less than three days) of a new, unrelenting headache that occurs daily at the same time. NDPH is not a continuum of a migraine or tension headache, but may present with similar features. The cause is unknown, but it may be associated with viral infection. NDPH is typically unresponsive to traditional medical therapies.

G45.- Transient cerebral ischemic attacks and related syndromes

Cerebral ischemia occurs when the blood supply to tissues in the brain is restricted, resulting in insufficient oxygen supply to the affected area. Previously classified in the circulatory system, this category was reclassified into the nervous system chapter due to the associated neurological dysfunction that results from these attacks.

G45.4 Transient global amnesia

This type of amnesia refers to an episode of short-term memory loss, not often recurrent and not due to psychological factors. The pathogenesis is not known and rarely are there signs or symptoms of a neurological disorder.

G45.8 Other transient cerebral ischemic attacks and related syndromes

A condition that has been reclassified here is subclavian steal syndrome. Subclavian steal syndrome occurs when the subclavian artery occludes causing backflow (retrograde) blood flow into the vertebral artery. The most prominent diagnostic factor is the occurrence of cerebral ischemic symptoms upon movement of the ipsilateral (same side) arm.

G45.9 Transient cerebral ischemic attack, unspecified

Transient cerebral ischemia or attack (TIA) describes sudden but often brief episodes of focal neurological symptoms that result in little to no permanent brain damage. A typical transient ischemic event may last between two and 15 minutes, yet resolve within 24 hours. The most common cause of a TIA-type event is embolization due to cardiovascular causes, including rheumatic heart disease, arrhythmia, valve disease, endocarditis, and myocardial infarction.

G46.- Vascular syndromes of brain in cerebrovascular diseases

Vascular syndromes are the result of decreased blood flow to certain portions in the brain. The type and severity of symptoms will depend on the part of the brain that is affected.

G46.0 Middle cerebral artery syndrome

The middle cerebral artery supplies the corona radiata; lateral aspects of the frontal, temporal, and parietal lobes; the globus pallidus; caudate; and putamen. Facial hemiparesis or hemiplegia of the contralateral side is the most common presentation.

G46.1 Anterior cerebral artery syndrome

The anterior cerebral artery supplies the basal ganglia, anterior fornix, anterior corpus callosum, and the medial aspects of the frontal and parietal lobes. The most common symptom is lower limb and pelvic floor hemiparesis or hemiplegia of the contralateral side.

G46.2 Posterior cerebral artery syndrome

The posterior cerebral artery supplies the midbrain, upper brainstem, occipital lobe, the inferomedial temporal lobe, and a part of the thalamus. Symptoms usually involve visual field defects affecting the contralateral side.

G46.3   Brain stem stroke syndrome

Multiple clinical variations of brainstem stroke syndrome have been identified that may be differentiated by the pattern of deficits caused by the interruption of specific affected cranial nerves. A brainstem stroke may be potentially life-threatening if the cranial nerves that control respiration and cardiac function are disrupted. Similarly, certain brainstem strokes may cause double vision, ataxia, impaired speech, and gastrointestinal symptoms.

Brain stem stroke syndromes include the following:

- Benedikt's, Foville's, Weber, Millard-Gubler, and Claude syndrome, characterized by oculomotor nerve palsy, contralateral hemiparesis, ataxia, and hemiplegia of the face and upper extremities

- Paraplegia and anesthesia over part of the body caused by lesions in the brain or spinal cord

- Wallenberg syndrome, characterized by dysphagia, hoarseness, loss of taste, and paralysis of the ipsilateral vocal cord and tongue due to lesions of the glossopharyngeal (IX) and vagus (X) nerves

G46.5   Pure motor lacunar syndrome

Lacunar syndromes described as "pure motor" are a common type of transient cerebrovascular disease characterized by hemiparesis, weakness on one side of the body that may include the face and/or the extremities. Speech, vision, and other sensory symptoms may also be present, though are often relatively minor and transient. Anatomic sites affected in lacunar cerebrovascular disease with motor manifestations may include the vasculature of the internal capsule or the basis pontis or the anterior portion of the pons.

G46.6   Pure sensory lacunar syndrome

Cerebrovascular syndromes described as "pure sensory" are characterized by sensory abnormalities that may include visual or auditory disturbances, numbness, and variations in the perceptions of pain, temperature, and pressure. These sensory syndromes typically arise from pathology affecting the thalamus.

G47.-   Sleep disorders

Organic sleep disorders listed in this section include various types of specified sleep disorders that are, by definition, the result of a demonstrable anatomic or physiologic abnormality or any pathologic (disease) process, as opposed to a psychological, behavioral, or substance-induced disorder.

Focus Point

Sleep disorders or conditions that are not due to any known physiological condition cannot be classified as organic and should be coded elsewhere, most often in Chapter 5 Mental, Behavioral, and Neurodevelopmental Disorders, or Chapter 18 Symptoms, Signs and Abnormal Clinical and Laboratory Findings, Not Elsewhere Classified.

G47.0-   Insomnia

Insomnia conditions classified here refer to difficulty in initiating or maintaining sleep due to a known physiologic disturbance or pathogenic condition. Insomnia with an undetermined or unspecified etiology would also be coded under this subcategory.

G47.1-   Hypersomnia

Hypersomnia conditions classified here include excessive sleepiness (somnolence) or excessive time spent in a sleep state due to a known physiologic disturbance or pathogenic origin, as well as hypersomnia due to an unspecified cause.

G47.2-   Circadian rhythm sleep disorders

Circadian rhythm sleep disorders are disturbances in the normal sleep-wake cycle rhythm or schedule that have a known physiological or pathogenic origin or are due to such conditions as jet lag or shift work. Also included here is unspecified circadian rhythm or sleep wake schedule disorder.

G47.3-   Sleep apnea

Sleep apnea conditions are transient periods when breathing ceases during sleep. Sleep apnea may cause hypoxemia and result in severely fragmented sleep with arousal occurring many times in any given sleep period. Sleep apnea conditions classified here are those that are due to a known physiologic disturbance or pathogenic origin. Other types included here are primary central, obstructive, congenital central, and idiopathic sleep apneas.

G47.4-   Narcolepsy and cataplexy

Cataplexy is a neurologic condition, often confused with epilepsy. Patients with cataplexy experience sudden loss of muscle tone and fall to the floor because of laughter, stress, or frightening experiences. The cataplectic patient does not lose consciousness but lies without moving for a few minutes until normal body tone returns. Cataplexy can exist by itself, or more commonly, as a feature of narcolepsy.

Narcolepsy is a disorder characterized by sudden attacks of irrepressible REM sleep. It is sometimes associated with cataplexy. Narcolepsy may also be associated with frightening and recurring visual hallucinations when falling to or arousing from sleep and paralysis of voluntary musculature while falling asleep. Narcolepsy rarely begins before adolescence. Patients with narcolepsy are easily aroused and become spontaneously alert and are often treated by stimulants such as caffeine, amphetamines, and methylphenidate. These same stimulants are not useful in treating cataplexy, which can be controlled with imipramine or desipramine, given in gradually increasing doses.

G47.5- Parasomnia

Parasomnia refers to abnormal behavioral events and falsely timed activation of physiological systems that disrupt sleep. Parasomnias can occur at any time during the sleep cycle including during the falling asleep phase. Manifestations of parasomnia may differ depending on the period of the sleep cycle in which they occur. During the falling asleep phase the most common manifestations are hallucinations and sleep paralysis.

G47.52 REM sleep behavior disorder

This parasomnia condition occurs during the rapid eye movement (REM) sleep phase, which is the phase where dreaming occurs. Normally dreaming is a purely mental activity, but people with REM sleep behavior disorder act out their dreams, which may cause them to shout, scream, thrash about, or get out of bed and move about performing various actions or activities. If the dream is of a violent nature, punching or hitting may be involved with the potential to injure or harm self or others. Men are more often affected than women and the condition most often occurs after the age of 50. Clonazepam is used to treat the condition.

G47.6- Sleep related movement disorders

Codes found under this subcategory address movement disorders occurring during sleep, such as teeth grinding, muscle cramping, and limb movement.

G47.61 Periodic limb movement disorder

This sleep related movement disorder is characterized by repetitive limb movements most often in the lower extremities that only occur during sleep. The movements are fast and of a short duration but are significant enough that it can wake a patient up, causing poor sleep and daytime somnolence.

> **Focus Point**
>
> *Periodic limb movement disorder (PLMD) and restless leg syndrome (RLS) are not synonymous. Periodic limb movement disorder occurs during sleep, while RLS usually manifests itself during wakefulness often just after a person lies down to go to sleep. RLS is also accompanied by other manifestations such as unpleasant sensations in the lower limbs that are exacerbated when the patient is inactive. Often the only manifestation to PLMD is an unexplained daytime somnolence. RLS is coded within the nervous system chapter under category G25.*

Nerve, Nerve Root and Plexus Disorders (G50-G59)

A nerve root is the starting point of a nerve from the central nervous system. Nerve roots may originate in the brain or the spinal cord. A nerve plexus is a network of nerve fibers connecting one or more centrally located nerve to peripheral body parts or organs. Nerves, which are bundles of nerve cells that transmit electrical impulses, are the terminal aspects of the nervous system. Peripheral nerves may be motor or sensory. Motor nerves transmit motor impulses from the brain to the muscles and glands while sensory nerves transmit sensory impulses back to the spinal cord and brain.

The categories in this code block are as follows:

G50	Disorders of the trigeminal nerve
G51	Facial nerve disorders
G52	Disorders of other cranial nerves
G53	Cranial nerve disorders in diseases classified elsewhere
G54	Nerve root and plexus disorders
G55	Nerve root and plexus compressions in diseases classified elsewhere
G56	Mononeuropathies of upper limb
G57	Mononeuropathies of lower limb
G58	Other mononeuropathies
G59	Mononeuropathy in diseases classified elsewhere

G50.- Disorders of trigeminal nerve

This category identifies disorders of the trigeminal (V) nerve, which is a mixed (motor/sensory) cranial nerve and the largest of the cranial nerves. The trigeminal nerve has three branches: ophthalmic, maxillary, and mandibular.

G50.0   Trigeminal neuralgia

Trigeminal neuralgia is characterized by intermittent, shooting pain in the gums, teeth, and lower face initiated by shaving, chewing, or a particular jaw motion. The pain may present for weeks or months and then cease spontaneously for a variable period of time. Diagnosis is based on medical history and an exam that rules out other conditions. An enlarged looping artery or vein pressing the trigeminal nerve is the most common cause. A brain tumor identified by magnetic resonance imaging (MRI) may also cause the disorder. Trigeminal neuralgia can occur at any age, though onset is generally 50 years of age or older.

G51.-   Facial nerve disorders

This category identifies disorders of the facial (VII) nerve, which is a mixed (motor/sensory) cranial nerve. Its motor fibers originate from the pons and are distributed to facial, scalp, and neck muscles. The sensory fibers convey sensations from the face, scalp, and taste buds of the tongue.

G51.0   Bell's palsy

Bell's palsy describes paralysis of muscles on one side of the face that results from temporary damage to the facial nerve. Abnormal tearing from the eye may result when the weakened eyelid can no longer funnel tears into the lacrimal ducts. Severity depends on the extent of nerve damage and although the cause is unknown, a viral infection is suspected. The disorder occurs at all ages, but is most frequent between ages 30 and 60. Ninety percent of patients with Bell's palsy recover without treatment. A cortisone substance may be prescribed to reduce inflammation if the diagnosis is made within the first 48 hours. If eyelid function is compromised, the eye must be covered to prevent drying or injury. Electrophysiologic testing of facial nerve function, though not diagnostic of Bell's palsy, may locate a lesion.

G51.2   Melkersson's syndrome

Melkersson (-Rosenthal) syndrome is a genetic condition with onset in childhood or adolescence. It is characterized by chronic facial swelling, localized particularly to the lips, and recurrent facial palsy. Recurrent attacks may become permanent, with a hardening, discoloration, and cracking of labial tissue. Associated conditions include fissured tongue and ophthalmic symptoms, including lagophthalmos, blepharochalasis, corneal opacities, retrobulbar neuritis, and exophthalmos.

G51.3   Clonic hemifacial spasm

Clonic facial spasm is an idiopathic disorder with onset in the fifth or sixth decade of life. Presentation is most commonly unilateral, although bilateral presentations have been observed in severe cases. Characteristic clonic facial muscle spasm occurs on one side of the face, with abnormally rapid periods of alternating muscular contractions and relaxations. Facial muscles typically affected include the corrugator, frontalis, orbicularis oris, platysma, and zygomaticus. Sustained tonic contractions can result in chronic irritation of the facial nerve, hyperexcitability, and disruptions in neurotransmission. Causal conditions include compressive lesions (e.g., tumor), stroke, multiple sclerosis, and infection.

G51.4   Facial myokymia

Facial myokymia may be described as a form of involuntary movement, or "quivering," in which the affected muscle appears to spasm in continuous, rippling motions. Causal conditions include neoplasm (typically a brainstem glioma), demyelinating diseases (e.g., multiple sclerosis), or certain polyneuropathies (e.g., Guillain Barré syndrome).

G52.-   Disorders of other cranial nerves

Ten of the 12 pairs of cranial nerves originate from the brain stem, but all leave the skull through the foramina of the skull. The nerves are designated by Roman numerals that indicate the order in which the nerves arise from the brain (anterior to posterior), while the name of each pair indicates the function—sensory, motor, or mixed motor/sensory. The name and order of each cranial nerve are as follows: olfactory (I) nerve, optic (II) nerve, oculomotor (III) nerve, trochlear (IV) nerve, trigeminal (V) nerve, abducens (VI) nerve, facial (VII) nerve, vestibulocochlear (VIII) nerve, glossopharyngeal (IX) nerve, vagus (X) nerve, accessory (XI) nerve, and hypoglossal (XII) nerve.

> **Focus Point**
>
> Category G52 does not capture disorders of the following cranial nerves:
>
> - Optic nerve (cranial nerve II)—see category H47
>
> - Oculomotor nerve (cranial nerve III)—see subcategory H49.0-
>
> - Trochlear nerve (cranial nerve IV)—see subcategory H49.1-
>
> - Trigeminal nerve (cranial nerve V)—see category G50
>
> - Abducens nerve (cranial nerve VI)—see subcategory H49.2-
>
> - Facial nerve (cranial nerve VII)—see category G51
>
> - Vestibulocochlear nerve (cranial nerve VIII), also known as the acoustic nerve—see subcategory H93.3-

G54.-   Nerve root and plexus disorders

A nerve plexus is a network of nerve fibers connecting one or more centrally located nerves to peripheral body parts or organs. The two major plexuses included under this category are the brachial plexus, distributing nerves to the arms and the lumbosacral plexus, which distributes nerves to the legs and pelvis.

The nerve root is the starting point of a nerve from the central nervous system. There are eight cranial nerves, 12 thoracic nerves, five lumbar nerves, five sacral nerves, and one coccygeal nerve.

G54.Ø   Brachial plexus disorders

The brachial plexus is a network of nerves formed by fibers located between the shoulder and the neck. One type of brachial plexus disorder is thoracic outlet syndrome, a group of symptoms arising from the upper extremity, the chest, neck, shoulders, and head. The Selmonosky Triad test (e.g., tenderness in the supraclavicular area, tingling and burning sensations in the hand on elevation, and adduction and abduction weakness of fingers) during physical examination may be used for diagnosis.

G54.5   Neuralgic amyotrophy

Sudden, severe shoulder and upper arm pain followed by marked upper arm weakness characterizes Parsonage-Turner syndrome, also known as brachial plexus neuritis or neuralgic amyotrophy. This condition is thought to be due to an autoimmune reaction causing inflammation of the brachial plexus rather than a specific injury or lesion (i.e., cancer).

G54.6   Phantom limb syndrome with pain

G54.7   Phantom limb syndrome without pain

Phantom limb syndrome is a side effect of the brain's attempt to reorganize following a serious disruption in the sensory information processed in the cerebral cortex, thalamus, and brainstem. Those who have lost limbs through amputation are not the only people who have phantom sensations; those with spinal cord injuries, peripheral nerve injury, diabetic neuropathy, and stroke survivors all report similar feelings

G56.-   Mononeuropathies of upper limb

Mononeuropathy occurs when there is damage to a single nerve or nerve group located outside the brain and spinal cord (peripheral neuropathy), in this case affecting the upper extremities. Common etiologies may include injury, inflammation, pressure, and entrapment. The damage to the nerve may cause loss of or abnormal sensations, weakness, and pain.

Upper Limb Nerves

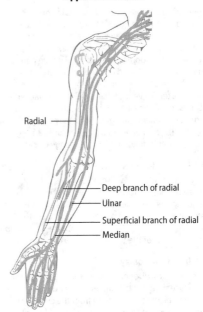

Radial

Deep branch of radial
Ulnar
Superficial branch of radial
Median

G56.Ø-   Carpal tunnel syndrome

The carpal tunnel is a tight canal or "tunnel" at the base of the palm through which tendons and nerves must pass on their way from the forearm to the hand and fingers. The median nerve passes through this narrow tunnel to reach the hand. If anything takes extra room in the canal, such as an inflammation of the tendons, things become too tight and the nerve in the canal becomes constricted or "pinched." This pinching of the nerve causes numbness and tingling in the area of the hand that the nerve travels to. The most common cause of carpal tunnel syndrome is repetitive strain injuries (RSI). This is caused by long periods of steady hand movement. RSIs tend to come with work that demands repeated grasping, turning, and twisting, such as hammering nails or operating a power tool.

G56.4-   Causalgia of upper limb

Causalgia, also called complex regional pain syndrome II (CRPS II), is a chronic progressive pain condition characterized by intense pain out of proportion to the severity of the injury with swelling and changes in the skin, including color and temperature. The skin over the affected limb exhibits symptoms of intense burning pain, skin sensitivity, sweating, and swelling. CRPS II most often affects one of the arms, legs, hands, or feet. In causalgia there is evidence of obvious nerve damage.

G57.- Mononeuropathies of lower limb

Mononeuropathy occurs when there is damage to a single nerve or nerve group located outside the brain and spinal cord (i.e., the peripheral nerves), in this case affecting the lower extremities. Common etiologies may include injury, inflammation, pressure, and entrapment. The damage to the nerve may cause loss of or abnormal sensations, weakness, and pain.

Lower Limb Nerves

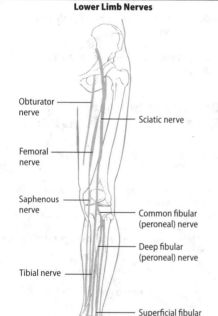

Obturator nerve

Sciatic nerve

Femoral nerve

Saphenous nerve

Common fibular (peroneal) nerve

Deep fibular (peroneal) nerve

Tibial nerve

Superficial fibular (peroneal) nerve

G57.1- Meralgia paresthetica

This condition is the result of compression on the lateral femoral cutaneous nerve of the thigh resulting in often painful paresthesia. Causes may include tight clothing, obesity, and pregnancy.

G57.7- Causalgia of lower limb

Causalgia, also called complex regional pain syndrome II (CRPS II), is a chronic progressive pain condition characterized by intense pain out of proportion to the severity of the injury with swelling and changes in the skin, including color and temperature. The skin over the affected limb exhibits symptoms of intense burning pain, skin sensitivity, sweating, and swelling. CRPS II most often affects one of the arms, legs, hands, or feet. In causalgia there is evidence of obvious nerve damage.

Polyneuropathies and Other Disorders of the Peripheral Nervous System (G60-G65)

Polyneuropathy occurs when there is simultaneous damage to many nerves located outside the brain and spinal cord (i.e., the peripheral nerves). Common etiologies may include infection, drug or toxic substances, or as a result of another disease process such as neoplastic disease.

The categories in this code block are as follows:

G60	Hereditary and idiopathic neuropathy
G61	Inflammatory polyneuropathy
G62	Other and unspecified polyneuropathies
G63	Polyneuropathy in diseases classified elsewhere
G64	Other disorders of peripheral nervous system
G65	Sequelae of inflammatory and toxic polyneuropathies

G61.- Inflammatory polyneuropathy

Inflammatory neuropathy is pain, swelling, and loss of function of the peripheral nerves in response to another disease process, injury, or unknown etiology.

G61.0 Guillain-Barre syndrome

Guillain-Barré syndrome or acute inflammatory demyelinating polyneuropathy is characterized by rapid development of symmetrical weakness or flaccid paralysis beginning in the legs and progressing up to the arms and head or, in rare cases, beginning in the arms or head and progressing down to the legs. It is considered to be an autoimmune reaction, in most cases triggered by a mild viral infection, surgery, or following an immunization. In severe cases, ventilation and/or feeding tubes may be necessary because muscle weakness makes it difficult for the patient to breathe and/or swallow. Acute infective polyneuritis, also coded here, is an inflammatory polyneuropathy due to an infective organism, usually viral or bacterial. Signs and symptoms include history of recent herpes virus infection or immunization (cytomegalovirus, Epstein-Barr virus), paresthesia and tingling, depressed respirations in severe disease, weakness of hands and feet, and inability to perform fine movements.

Focus Point

Symptoms related to Guillain-Barré syndrome usually peak around week three or four. When symptoms continue to worsen beyond the three- to four-week timeframe, the condition is considered chronic inflammatory demyelinating polyneuropathy (CIDP) and is coded to G61.81.

G61.81 Chronic inflammatory demyelinating polyneuritis

CIDP occurs when an autoimmune reaction causes the body to attack the nerves. Symptoms include weakness and abnormal sensations although these may not affect both sides of the body in the same way and can be more irregular and slow to progress. Diagnosis is primarily based on whether the symptoms, which are similar to Guillain-Barre syndrome, continue to progress after eight weeks.

G61.82 Multifocal motor neuropathy

Multifocal motor neuropathy (MMN) is considered an autoimmune disease in which the immune system sees the nerve cells as invaders and attacks them. The nerve cells attacked are the motor nerves, which control the muscles by sending electrical signals to the brain. MMN affects adults usually in their 40s and 50s; however, cases have been seen as early as the 20s and late as the 80s. The severity level of MMN ranges from mild to severe, with little to no change in activity levels and little to no treatment, to interference with daily tasks, like dressing. Initial symptoms of cramping and/or twitching as well as weakness are usually concentrated in the hands and lower arms. Eventual progression to the lower extremities is also possible. It is important to note that MMN is not a painful condition as the sensory nerves are not affected, only the motor nerves. Ruling out other disease processes is the first course of action when diagnosing MMN since the symptoms (such as twitching) are very similar to other diseases like amyotrophic lateral sclerosis (ALS), Lou Gehrig's disease, and chronic inflammatory demyelinating polyneuropathy (CIDP).

G62.- Other and unspecified polyneuropathies

Polyneuropathy occurs when there is simultaneous damage to many peripheral nerves.

G62.0 Drug-induced polyneuropathy

Drug-induced polyneuropathy is pain, swelling, and loss of function of the peripheral nerves in response to a drug or biological substance.

G62.1 Alcoholic polyneuropathy

Alcoholic polyneuropathy, also called polyneuritis potatorum, is due to thiamine and other vitamin deficiency caused by chronic alcohol abuse. In addition, alcohol is believed to be neurotoxic. Signs and symptoms of alcoholic polyneuropathy are pain, particularly in the midcalf and soles of the feet, tingling, loss of sensation, weakness of hands and feet, inability to perform fine movements, diminished tendon reflexes, excessive perspiration, and atrophy of lower limbs.

G62.2 Polyneuropathy due to other toxic agents

Toxic neuropathy is pain, swelling, and loss of function of the peripheral nerves in response to a toxic substance.

Diseases of the Myoneural Junction and Muscle (G70-G73)

The myoneural or neuromuscular junction is the connection point at which a nerve fiber innervates a muscle. When a signal is sent from the nerve via a chemical messenger called acetylcholine, the neuromuscular junction is "stimulated" and sends an electrical pulse through the muscle. A disease of the myoneural junction can be the result of faulty receptors at the neuromuscular junction, interference with the chemical messenger, or damage to the nerves themselves.

The categories in this code block are as follows:

G70	Myasthenia gravis and other myoneural disorders
G71	Primary disorders of muscles
G72	Other and unspecified myopathies
G73	Disorders of myoneural junction and muscle in diseases classified elsewhere

G70.- Myasthenia gravis and other myoneural disorders

Myasthenia gravis and other myoneural disorders are due to disorders of neuromuscular transmission of nerve impulses.

G70.00   Myasthenia gravis without (acute) exacerbation

G70.01   Myasthenia gravis with (acute) exacerbation

Myasthenia gravis is a disorder of neuromuscular transmission due to the presence of autoimmune antibodies at the neuromuscular junction. Signs and symptoms of myasthenia gravis include skeletal muscle weakness and fatigability, dysarthria, chewing fatigue, dysphagia, fever, respiratory distress, ptosis, and ocular muscle weakness.

Symptoms may come and go episodically; classification is based on the presence or absence of these exacerbated symptoms.

G70.80   Lambert-Eaton syndrome, unspecified

G70.81   Lambert-Eaton syndrome in disease classified elsewhere

Lambert-Eaton myasthenic syndrome (LEMS) (a.k.a., Lambert-Eaton syndrome; LES) is an autoimmune disorder of the neuromuscular junction that occurs when antibodies disrupt the release of acetylcholine and subsequent neurotransmission of impulses from nerves to the muscle, causing muscle weakness. Causation is often linked to an underlying disease process resulting in immunosuppression. Initial onset of symptoms may include a persistent tingling sensation in the affected areas, fatigue, and dry mouth, progressing in type and severity. In general, symptoms are similar to myasthenia gravis, with the exception of a Lambert's sign on neurological examination, a short-term increase in hand-grip muscle strength that occurs as the acetylcholine accumulates in the muscle. When at rest, reflexes are reduced; however, with muscle use, reflex strength increases. As a result, LEMS is characterized by muscle weakness in the head, neck, and limbs, with additional autonomic nervous system disturbances. These disturbances may manifest as diplopia, dysphagia, orthostatic hypotension, and difficulty breathing. Complications include respiratory failure, pneumonia, malnutrition, and injury due to impairment of coordination and increased risk for falls.

G71.-   Primary disorders of muscles

When the muscle itself is impaired due to varying types of pathologies and not the nerve or neuromuscular junction, it is considered a primary muscle disorder.

G71.0   Muscular dystrophy

Muscular dystrophy is a group of progressive muscle disorders that are genetic in origin and cause degeneration of muscles. Progressive muscle weakness is common to all types of muscular dystrophy leading to difficulties with walking, breathing, and/or swallowing. The type of gene mutation determines the age of onset, what muscle groups are affected, and the severity of the condition. Classified here are any of the inherited types of dystrophy such as Duchenne's, Emery-Dreifuss, Landouzy-Dejerine disease, or the limb-girdle form.

G71.1-   Myotonic disorders

Myotonia, a neuromuscular disorder characterized by the slow relaxation of the muscles following contraction, may be inherited or acquired. Caused by an abnormality in the muscle membrane, it can affect all muscle groups.

G71.11   Myotonic muscular dystrophy

The most common form of myotonic disorders is myotonic muscular dystrophy (MMD, Steinert disease), which is often manifested by weakness and wasting of the voluntary muscles of the face, neck, and lower arms and legs.

G71.12   Myotonia congenita

Myotonia congenita is inherited and typically first noticed at the age of 2 to 3 years. Muscle stiffness, especially in the legs, may be brought on by sudden activity after rest. Muscle enlargement may occur and muscle strength may be increased.

G71.13   Myotonic chondrodystrophy

Myotonic chondrodystrophy is a rare genetic disorder characterized by joint contractures, bone dysplasia, myotonic myopathy, and growth delays resulting in dwarfism.

G72.-   Other and unspecified myopathies

Myopathies that are due to alcohol, drugs, or other toxic substances are a few of the conditions classified to this category. Also included here are inflammatory and immune myopathies that do not have more specific codes listed elsewhere and other specified myopathies such as critical illness myopathy.

G72.41   Inclusion body myositis [IBM]

Inclusion body myositis (IBM) is a progressive, debilitating inflammatory muscle disease characterized by chronic muscle swelling, weakness, and atrophy (wasting). It most commonly affects men older than 50 years of age, but can occur decades earlier. Onset is usually gradual, progressing over a period of months or years. Initial symptoms include excessive muscle weakness or falling and tripping. As the disease progresses, individuals commonly experience weakness and atrophy of the muscles of the extremities and difficulty with fine motor skills. Approximately half of patients with IBM experience difficulty swallowing. Muscle biopsy is essential to diagnosis.

G73.- Disorders of myoneural junction and muscle in diseases classified elsewhere

Codes in this category are manifestation codes that are reported secondarily. The inciting disease that has caused the myoneural junction or muscle disease must be coded first.

G73.1 Lambert-Eaton syndrome in neoplastic disease

Lambert-Eaton myasthenic syndrome (LEMS) (a.k.a., Lambert-Eaton syndrome; LES) is an autoimmune disorder of the neuromuscular junction that occurs when antibodies disrupt the release of acetylcholine and subsequent neurotransmission of impulses from nerves to the muscle, causing muscle weakness. Causation is often linked to an underlying disease process, in this case cancer, resulting in immunosuppression. It is estimated that more than half of LEMS patients have an underlying malignancy, most often associated with lung cancer. Initial onset of symptoms may include a persistent tingling sensation in the affected areas, fatigue, and dry mouth, progressing in type and severity. In general, symptoms are similar to myasthenia gravis, with the exception of a Lambert's sign on neurological examination, a short-term increase in hand-grip muscle strength that occurs as the acetylcholine accumulates in the muscle. When at rest, reflexes are reduced; however, with muscle use, reflex strength increases. As a result, LEMS is characterized by muscle weakness in the head, neck, and limbs, with additional autonomic nervous system disturbances. These disturbances may manifest as diplopia, dysphagia, orthostatic hypotension, and difficulty breathing. Complications include respiratory failure, pneumonia, malnutrition, and injury due to impairment of coordination and increased risk for falls.

Cerebral Palsy and Other Paralytic Syndromes (G80-G83)

Cerebral palsy (CP) is a group of disorders, in which chronic but nonprogressive brain lesions cause damage to the motor function of the brain.

The categories in this code block are as follows:

G80	Cerebral palsy
G81	Hemiplegia and hemiparesis
G82	Paraplegia (paraparesis) and quadriplegia (quadriparesis)
G83	Other paralytic syndromes

G80.- Cerebral palsy

Cerebral palsy (CP) is a group of disorders in which chronic but nonprogressive brain lesions cause damage to the motor function of the brain. These lesions can develop early in pregnancy while the brain is still developing or they may occur later in pregnancy, during delivery, or early in a baby's life. CP affects muscle control, movement, and motor skills (the ability to move in a coordinated and purposeful way). The functional impairment may range from disorders of movement or coordination to paresis. Vital functions such as bladder and bowel control, breathing, eating, and learning may be affected. Cerebral palsy can also cause other health issues, including hearing, vision, speech problems, and learning disabilities. Premature babies with low birth weight (less than 3.3 pounds) have a higher risk of CP than full-term babies, as do multiple births, such as twins and triplets. There are four main types of CP: spastic, ataxic, athetoid, and mixed. Spastic cerebral palsy is the most commonly diagnosed variety of CP, affecting 70 to 80 percent of patients with CP. Spastic CP causes a child's muscles to be rigid and jerky, making it difficult to get around. Symptoms generally appear in the first few years of life and once they appear, they generally do not progress with age. Spastic cerebral palsy is classified as quadriplegic, diplegic, and hemiplegic.

G80.0 Spastic quadriplegic cerebral palsy

Spastic quadriplegia or tetraplegia is when lesions in the brain cause all four limbs to have muscle stiffness (spasticity) to an equal extent. This is the most severe type of spastic CP and is often associated with intellectual disability. Due to extensive brain damage or considerable brain malformations, children are unable to walk, speech is difficult to comprehend, and seizures are frequent. Occasionally a child may have a milder form of spastic quadriplegia and be able to sit, lift him or herself into a wheelchair without help, be able to feed him or herself, and walk short distances with a walker.

G80.1 Spastic diplegic cerebral palsy

Spastic diplegia is when lesions in the brain cause both arms or both legs to have muscle stiffness. In addition to spasticity, most children may also have difficulty with balance and coordination. Limbs may not develop appropriately due to poor muscle development and consequently the joints may become stiff and have limited range of motion. The rigidity of the muscles of the legs and hips cause the legs to cross at the knees, a movement often called "scissoring." As a result, walking is delayed and the child may require a walker or leg braces. Children generally have normal intelligence and minimal chance of seizures. Spastic monoplegia is also coded here and occurs when a single limb or a single group of muscles is affected.

G80.2 Spastic hemiplegic cerebral palsy

Spastic hemiplegia affects one side of the child's body, including both the arm and leg. One limb may be affected more than another. Children with spastic hemiplegia generally are delayed in walking and develop "tip-toe" walking because of the tight heel tendons. The limbs may not develop correctly and are frequently shorter and thinner than the unaffected side. Depending upon the amount and location of brain damage, the child may suffer from delayed speech and seizures.

G80.3   Athetoid cerebral palsy

Athetoid, or dyskinetic, cerebral palsy is manifested by abnormal, uncontrolled, slow, and writhing movements, usually affecting the extremities. The muscles of the tongue and face may also be affected, resulting in drooling or grimacing. Symptoms may be exacerbated during times of stress and often disappear during sleep.

G80.8   Other cerebral palsy

This code includes mixed types of cerebral palsy and those hemiplegic, diplegic, and monoplegic forms that are not considered spastic. The most commonly seen mixed type is a combination of spastic and athetoid.

G81.-   Hemiplegia and hemiparesis

Hemiplegia is defined as paralysis of one vertical side of the body, total or partial, due to damage to the part of the brain that controls muscle movements. Hemiparesis is defined as weakness of one vertical side of the body due to brain damage.

Focus Point

Hemiplegia is not inherent to acute cerebrovascular accident (CVA) and should be coded in addition to CVA, regardless of whether the hemiplegia resolves before discharge. Hemiplegia affects the care patients receive and coders are instructed to report any neurological deficits caused by a CVA. However, hemiplegia due to sequela of cerebrovascular disease is not reported here, but is instead reported with a code from category I69.

G81.0-   Flaccid hemiplegia

Flaccid hemiplegia is the loss of muscle tone in paralyzed body parts with absence of tendon reflex. It may be caused by disease or trauma affecting the nerves associated with the involved muscles.

G81.1-   Spastic hemiplegia

Spastic hemiplegia is a muscle spasm within the paralyzed parts of the body with increased tendon reflexes. It may be caused by disease or trauma affecting the nerves associated with the involved muscles.

G82.-   Paraplegia (paraparesis) and quadriplegia (quadriparesis)

Paraplegia is defined as paralysis of both lower limbs and is often due to injury or a disease process at or below the chest. Quadriplegia is defined as paralysis of all four limbs and is due to injury or disease process at the level of the neck.

G82.2-   Paraplegia

This subcategory is classified based on whether the paraplegia is complete, incomplete, or unspecified. Complete paraplegia is described as permanent loss of motor or sensory functions in the lower limbs. In incomplete paraplegia there is only partial damage to the spinal cord. Motor and sensory functions in the lower limbs will vary from patient to patient depending on the extent of the spinal cord damage and the area and level the damage occurred.

G82.5-   Quadriplegia

This subcategory is classified based on the level of the spinal cord damage, C1-C4 or C5-C7, and whether the damage is considered complete or incomplete. Complete quadriplegia occurs when the spinal cord is so severely damaged that there is permanent loss of motor and sensory functions in all four limbs. In incomplete quadriplegia there is only partial damage to the spinal cord. Functionality of all four limbs will vary from patient to patient depending on where along the cervical spinal cord the damage occurred.

G83.-   Other paralytic syndromes

Codes classified under other paralytic syndromes are to be used only when there is not enough detail in the documentation to assign a more specific code or when the condition is of longstanding but undocumented cause.

G83.4   Cauda equina syndrome

Cauda equina syndrome is due to a compression of the lumbosacral nerve roots. Symptoms include a dull aching pain in the sacral region and/or pain in the legs. There is weakness or paralysis of the muscles. These symptoms slowly progress and a loss of bladder control referred to as neurogenic bladder syndrome may eventually occur.

G83.8-   Other specified paralytic syndromes

Codes from this subcategory are for use when the cause of the paralytic syndrome is not documented or the paralytic syndrome is longstanding without a documented cause.

G83.82   Anterior cord syndrome

This condition results from damage to the front of the spinal cord. Sensations such as touch and pain may be lost or impaired.

G83.83   Posterior cord syndrome

This condition is the result of damage to the back of the spinal cord; coordinating limb movements may be difficult, while other sensations, such as pain and temperature, are preserved.

Other Disorders of the Nervous System (G89-G99)

Conditions classified here are generalized in nature, such as pain, or conditions that do not fit well into a more specific code block.

The categories in this code block are as follows:

G89   Pain, not elsewhere classified

G90   Disorders of autonomic nervous system

G91   Hydrocephalus

G92   Toxic encephalopathy

G93   Other disorders of brain

G94   Other disorders of brain in diseases classified elsewhere

G95   Other and unspecified diseases of spinal cord

G96   Other disorders of central nervous system

G97   Intraoperative and postprocedural complications and disorders of nervous system, not elsewhere classified

G98   Other disorders of nervous system not elsewhere classified

G99   Other disorders of nervous system in diseases classified elsewhere

G89.-   Pain, not elsewhere classified

Pain that is not classified elsewhere and pain that is not a symptom of a documented disease process is classified here. Pain conditions in this category that are described as due to trauma, post-thoracotomy, or postprocedural are typically more severe and more intractable than would normally be expected. Expected levels of pain following trauma or surgery should not be reported with codes in this category.

G89.0   Central pain syndrome

Central pain syndrome is a neurological condition caused by injury to or dysfunction of the central nervous system and has multiple etiologies, including stroke, tumors, epilepsy, brain or spinal cord trauma, multiple sclerosis, or Parkinson's disease. Central pain syndrome may affect a smaller area, such as the hands or feet, or a large portion of the body. Pain is characteristically constant, moderate to severe in intensity, and is frequently made worse by touch, movement, strong emotions, and changes in temperature. Pain sensations vary from "pins and needles" type sensations to a pressing, lacerating, or aching type of pain or brief, excruciating bursts of sharp pain. Central pain syndrome often starts soon after the causative injury or damage, but may also be delayed by months or years, particularly if it is related to a previous stroke.

G89.1-   Acute pain, not elsewhere classified

Acute pain is a sensation generated in the nervous system that may be an alert to possible injury, as a response to trauma or postoperative sequelae. Analgesics are often prescribed to treat acute pain. Other treatment options include heat and cold applications, massage, therapeutic touch, transcutaneous electrical nerve stimulation (TENS), relaxation techniques, guided imagery, hypnosis, music distraction, or cognitive therapies such as art and activity therapy.

G89.2-   Chronic pain, not elsewhere classified

Chronic pain is a persistent condition in which the nervous system generates pain signals that may be ongoing for weeks to years. Often occurring as a result of past injuries, infections, or surgical interventions, chronic pain may also be due to ongoing disease processes, such as arthritis, or recurrent infections. Some patients suffer chronic pain in the absence of past injury or physical damage. A variety of chronic pain conditions affect older adults. Treatment options for chronic pain include medications, acupuncture, local electrical stimulation, surgery, psychotherapy, relaxation, medication therapies, biofeedback, and behavior modification.

G89.3   Neoplasm related pain (acute) (chronic)

Neoplasm-related pain on a scale from moderate to severe affects approximately 50 percent of cancer patients and continually requires complex management due to the various types of pain as well as the patient's personal history. Neoplasm pain can be related to several issues, such as inflammation, neuropathy, and ischemia or compression by tumors. Acute versus chronic is determined by onset of symptoms and how long they last. Acute pain comes on suddenly with specific time frame onset and determinable cause and may improve with treatment. Chronic pain is less specific in terms of specific onset or cause, duration, and anticipated course. To identify the most beneficial treatment of neoplasm-related pain, the provider must perform a detailed evaluation of the patient to include any historical pain factors in order to properly treat/manage the pain.

G89.4   Chronic pain syndrome

Chronic pain syndrome includes a plethora of symptoms that continually require further investigation by the medical community and providers in general. It is often diagnosed when the chronic pain causes secondary symptoms, which in turn exacerbate the chronic pain. Treatment for this condition can be challenging due to the often vague history and less-than-favorable response to previous therapies. Opinions also differ on what qualifies as indicating this syndrome, with some providers indicating that pain lasting over six months is sufficient for diagnosis and others holding that a three-month time frame is adequate. Often, treating chronic pain requires several providers to work together since the condition may be traced to various body systems. As of 2017, reports indicate about 35 percent of Americans have some form of chronic pain while about 50 million people have some variation of disability due to chronic pain.

G90.-   Disorders of autonomic nervous system

The nervous system consists of the central nervous system (the brain and the spinal cord) and the peripheral nervous system (the sense organs and the nerves linking the sense organs, muscles, and glands to the central nervous system). The structures of the peripheral nervous system are subdivided into the autonomic nervous system and the somatic nervous system. The autonomic nervous system conveys sensory impulses from the blood vessels, the heart, and all of the organs in the chest, abdomen, and pelvis through nerves to other parts of the brain (mainly the medulla, pons, and hypothalamus). These impulses are largely automatic or reflex responses through the efferent autonomic nerves, and cause reactions of the heart, the vascular system, and all the organs of the body to variations in environmental temperature, posture, food intake, stressful experiences, and other

changes to which all individuals are exposed. There are two major components of the autonomic nervous system: the sympathetic and the parasympathetic systems. The parasympathetic division of the autonomic nervous system controls anabolism (energy storage); an anabolic activity occurs in normal, nonstressful situations, such as initiating digestion after eating. In general, sympathetic processes reverse parasympathetic responses. The sympathetic division operates for defense or in response to stress. In defensive situations, catabolism (energy use) produces an increased heart rate, an expansion of the lungs to hold more energy, dilated pupils, and blood flow to the muscles.

G90.0-   Idiopathic peripheral autonomic neuropathy

Idiopathic conditions are those that do not have a known cause; in this case it refers to autonomic nervous system disorders with an unknown cause.

G90.01   Carotid sinus syncope

Carotid sinus syndrome (e.g., carotid sinus syncope, carotid sinus hypersensitivity) is an exaggerated vagal response to carotid sinus baroreceptor stimulation characterized by dizziness and syncope. Specialized nerve cells called baroreceptors detect changes in pressure and tension in the large vessels of the body, such as the carotid arteries. The carotid sinus reflex plays an integral part in regulating normal blood pressure. This vagal response is a result of transient diminished cerebral perfusion resulting in dizziness or syncope. CSS attributes to 0.5 to 9 percent of patients with recurrent syncope and is associated with an increased risk of falls, drop attacks, bodily injuries, and fractures in elderly patients. CSS is more common in males than in females, is predominantly a disease of elderly people, and is rarely identified in patients younger than 50 years of age. Symptoms of CSS may include recurrent dizziness, syncope or near syncope, unexplained falls, symptoms associated with head turning or constriction of the neck, and possible amnesia related to the event. Physical signs observed with CSS include hypotension, bradycardia, and asystole.

G90.2   Horner's syndrome

Horner's syndrome, also called oculosympathetic palsy, results from disruption of the sympathetic nerve pathway from the brain to one side of the face affecting the eye on the affected side. Horner's syndrome results from another medical condition such as a stroke, trauma, or intracranial neoplasm, although sometimes the cause is undetermined. Signs and symptoms of Horner's syndrome include small pupil size, ptosis (drooping) of the eyelid on the same side, and occasionally loss of sweat formation on the skin on the affected side. The pupil will still react to light stimulus and accommodate to distant vision, but will not enlarge in the dark.

G90.5- Complex regional pain syndrome I (CRPS I)

Complex regional pain syndrome (CRPS) is a chronic progressive pain condition characterized by intense pain out of proportion to the severity of the injury, swelling, and changes in the skin, including color and temperature. The skin over the affected limb exhibits symptoms of intense burning pain, skin sensitivity, sweating, and swelling. CRPS most often affects one of the arms, legs, hands, or feet. Type I, also known as reflex sympathetic dystrophy (RSD), Sudeck's atrophy, reflex neurovascular dystrophy (RND), or algoneurodystrophy, does not have demonstrable nerve lesions. Precipitating factors include illness, injury, and surgery, although there are cases that have no documentable injury to the original site.

Focus Point

Complex regional pain syndrome II (CRPS II), also known as causalgia, has evidence of obvious nerve damage, and is reported with codes in subcategory G56.4- when the upper limb is affected or G57.7- when the lower limb is affected.

G91.- Hydrocephalus

The definition of hydrocephalus is an excessive accumulation of cerebrospinal fluid (CSF) in the brain. There must be a constant balance between the CSF being produced and that which is being absorbed. If absorption is compromised in some way, through a disease process or injury, and the CSF builds up in one of the ventricles in the brain, the undue pressure can cause damage to the surrounding brain tissue.

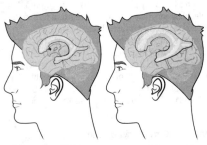

Normal ventricles   Hydrocephalic ventricles

G91.2 (Idiopathic) normal pressure hydrocephalus

Idiopathic normal pressure hydrocephalus (INPH), an abnormal increase of cerebrospinal fluid in the brain's ventricles of unknown cause, is most often diagnosed during the sixth or seventh decade of a patient's life. INPH is typically manifested by a triad of symptoms that includes dementia and progressive mental impairment, gait disturbance, and impaired bladder control.

G93.- Other disorders of brain

Disorders of the brain that are classified here are those that do not fit well into another more specific category. Some conditions classified here are cerebral cysts, encephalopathy of unknown cause, anoxic brain damage that cannot be classified elsewhere, and cerebral edema.

G93.2 Benign intracranial hypertension

This condition is the result of elevated pressure in the brain due to fluid retention in the brain cavities. Obese women of childbearing age are the most likely to be affected. The most common symptoms are headache and papilledema, or optic disc swelling, with the latter being the most important due to the fact that if left untreated the papilledema can lead to permanent vision loss.

G93.7 Reye's syndrome

An extremely rare but serious condition of childhood, Reye's syndrome is comprised of five stages of increasing severity. Untreated, it is characterized by inflammation in the brain and hepatic failure. The blood sugar levels typically drop at the same time the level of ammonia and acidity in the blood rises. Simultaneously, the liver swells and develops fatty deposits. Symptoms also include brain swelling, convulsions, disturbances of consciousness, seizures, and recurrent vomiting. The onset of this illness is usually preceded by a viral illness, in particular an upper respiratory tract infection (URTI), influenza B, varicella, or gastroenteritis. This syndrome rarely occurs in newborns or in children older than 18 years of age. It usually affects children between the ages of 4 and 12, and is most common at age 6. The length of the illness varies with the severity of the disease, which can range from mild and self-limiting to, in rare cases, death within hours. All cases of Reye's syndrome should be treated as potentially life-threatening and medical treatment should be sought. When the condition is detected early and treatment is initiated, children have the best chances of full recovery. Reye's syndrome appears to occur when children use aspirin to treat a viral illness or infection. Since this discovery, incidence of Reye's syndrome has dropped dramatically. Parents have been advised not to give aspirin to children unless otherwise instructed.

G93.8- Other specified disorders of brain

Only three codes are included here: temporal sclerosis, brain death, and other specified disorders of the brain, which includes postradiation encephalopathy.

G93.81 Temporal sclerosis

Temporal sclerosis (a.k.a., mesial temporal sclerosis, hippocampal sclerosis) is a condition associated with certain brain injuries that is caused by scarring or hardening of the tissues of the temporal lobe of the brain with resultant loss of functional neurons. Additional contributing factors include structural changes in the brain due to conditions such as tumors, vascular or cortical malformations, and hypoxic or traumatic injury, which has affected the temporal or hippocampus area of the brain. These structures include the amygdale, hippocampus, and parahippocampal gyrus. The physical changes diagnostic of temporal sclerosis are readily identifiable on magnetic resonance imaging (MRI) scan. As the sclerosis progresses, the resultant brain damage is demonstrated radiographically by neuronal loss, fibrillary gliosis (scarring), and hippocampal atrophy (shrinkage).

Focus Point

Epilepsy is closely associated with temporal sclerosis. Approximately 70 percent of patients with temporal lobe epilepsy also have mesial temporal sclerosis. Temporal lobe epilepsy is thought to be one of the most common forms of epilepsy in adults, with onset of seizures in childhood or adolescence. Treatment is focused on suppression of the seizures with antiepileptic medications. However, as scar formation progresses and seizures persist, surgical measures may be indicated, such as temporal lobectomy, which involves removing the scarred tissue from the temporal lobe of the brain. Mesial temporal sclerosis is considered integral to a temporal lobe seizure and as such should only be coded to the localization-related epilepsies in category G40.

G93.82   Brain death

Brain death is defined as the irreversible end of all brain activity upon physical examination, the absence of pain response, negative reflexes, and absence of spontaneous respiration. Toxicology tests are often performed to rule out the presence of medications that would suppress the reflexes. A "flat" EEG is not required for certification of death, yet it may serve as confirmatory support. Similarly, a negative cerebral blood flow study (CBF) provides solid evidence of a brain death. Pathogenesis of brain death typically includes death of the nerve cells and tissues within the brain (necrosis) due to a lack of oxygen (anoxia). The cessations of certain bodily functions, primarily respiration and heartbeat, have been the traditional medicolegal indicators in determining death. However, the advent of life support, organ transplantation, and advancing abilities to sustain bodily functions to prolong external signs of life necessitated consideration of the central nervous system criteria in refining the definition of death. In 1981, the Uniform Determination of Death Act was enacted into law, allowing the definition of "brain death" as a basis for the declaration of legal death, regardless of life support status. The next of kin, or families of a patient declared brain dead, are provided the option of organ donation by law. If consent is secured, the regional organ procurement organization is involved. If organ donation is refused, or otherwise contraindicated, life support is discontinued. Organs are harvested for

donation in the setting of brain death, with the vital functioning of the body maintained on life support until cardiac death is allowed to occur. A positive exam for brain death includes:

- No response to command (e.g., verbal, visual)
- Flaccid extremities with absent reflexes
- Unreactive (fixed) pupils
- Negative oculocephalic reflex
- Negative bilateral corneal reflexes
- Negative oculovestibular reflex
- Negative gag reflex
- No spontaneous respiration

G97.-   Intraoperative and postprocedural complications and disorders of nervous system, not elsewhere classified

Some conditions included in this category are cerebrospinal fluid leak (CSF) from spinal puncture, accidental puncture or laceration of a nervous system organ during a procedure, and hemorrhage or hematoma, during a procedure or occurring after a procedure. These conditions are a direct result of medical or surgical intervention for which documentation should reflect a cause and effect relationship.

G97.0   Cerebrospinal fluid leak from spinal puncture

This code describes cerebrospinal fluid (CSF) leak due to accidental puncture of the dura during the course of a diagnostic or therapeutic procedure performed along the spine. The leak at the site of the initial puncture. Typical procedures performed that may lead to this complication may include:

- Lumbar puncture
- Spine anesthesia
- Steroid injections

Spinal Puncture

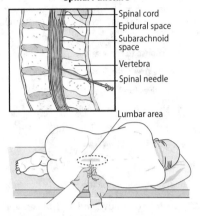

G97.3- **Intraoperative hemorrhage and hematoma of a nervous system organ or structure complicating a procedure**

G97.4- **Accidental puncture and laceration of a nervous system organ or structure during a procedure**

G97.5- **Postprocedural hemorrhage of a nervous system organ or structure following a procedure**

G97.6- **Postprocedural hematoma and seroma of a nervous system organ or structure following a procedure**

These four subcategories are further classified based on whether the nervous system organ or structure was damaged during a procedure on the nervous system itself or during a procedure on an organ or structure other than the nervous system. The descriptions of the complication terms are as follows:

- Hemorrhage is considered rapid blood loss from vessels.

- Hematoma is a collection of blood clots within tissue or organs due to a broken blood vessel.

- Seroma is a fluid accumulation just under the skin surface often after surgery involving an incision and/or tissue extraction.

- Laceration is simply a torn wound.

- Puncture is a wound due to perforation or piercing.

> **Focus Point**
>
> *There is a hierarchy of sorts for subcategories G97.3- and G97.4-; both codes would not be reported if an accidental puncture/laceration and intraoperative hemorrhage were documented, only a code from subcategory G97.4- Accidental puncture or laceration of a nervous system organ or structure during a procedure, would be assigned.*

G99.- **Other disorders of nervous system in diseases classified elsewhere**

Codes in this category are manifestation codes that are reported secondarily. The inciting disease that has caused the nervous system disorder must be listed first.

G99.0 **Autonomic neuropathy in diseases classified elsewhere**

The autonomic nervous system is composed of peripheral nerves that supply the internal organs and help regulate the body processes of these organs. These body processes range from controlling blood pressure, to digestion, to tear production and occur automatically, without conscious effort from an individual. Signs and symptoms of peripheral autonomic nerve damage depend on which body process is affected. This code identifies autonomic neuropathy as part of another disease process such as amyloidosis or gout.

> **Focus Point**
>
> *Damage to peripheral autonomic nerves as a result of diabetes can be found in the diabetes categories of E08-E13 in Chapter 4 Endocrine, Nutritional and Metabolic Diseases, as combination codes; therefore, a secondary G99.0 code is not necessary*

Chapter 7: Diseases of the Eye and Adnexa (H00-H59)

The eye is the organ of sight and has a complex anatomy and physiology. The structures of the eye, which include structures of the ball or globe, are differentiated from its supporting structures, which are ocular adnexa and bony orbit. The globe can be divided into two segments: the anterior segment, which includes the lens and all tissue anterior to the lens, and the posterior segment, which includes everything in the eyeball that is situated behind the lens. The structures of the anterior and posterior segments are surrounded by fluid: aqueous humor in the anterior segment and vitreous humor in the posterior segment. The fluid within the globe is what gives the eye its shape and it is also essential to the health of the internal structures of the eye. The globe of the eye rests in fatty tissue in the bony orbit of the skull where it is protected from jarring actions. The external structures of the eye, which include the eyelids, lacrimal system, and ocular muscles, together make up the ocular adnexa. These structures provide further protection of the globe and are also responsible for essential functions such as eye movement.

A thin, vascular mucous membrane covers the inner eyelids and the white outer shell of the eye (sclera). This membrane is called the conjunctiva. The cornea is the bulging "window" through which we see and the retina is the light-sensitive "viewing screen" at the back of the eye. The choroid is a vascular layer of the inside of the eyeball.

The chapter is broken down into the following code blocks:

H00-H05	Disorders of eyelid, lacrimal system and orbit
H10-H11	Disorders of conjunctiva
H15-H22	Disorders of sclera, cornea, iris and ciliary body
H25-H28	Disorders of lens
H30-H36	Disorders of choroid and retina
H40-H42	Glaucoma
H43-H44	Disorders of vitreous body and globe
H46-H47	Disorders of optic nerve and visual pathways
H49-H52	Disorders of ocular muscles, binocular movement, accommodation and refraction
H53-H54	Visual disturbances and blindness
H55-H57	Other disorders of eye and adnexa

H59	Intraoperative and postprocedural complications and disorders of eye and adnexa, not elsewhere classified

Disorders of Eyelid, Lacrimal System and Orbit (H00-H05)

The lacrimal system of each eye, also called the lacrimal apparatus, consists of the lacrimal gland, ducts, canaliculi, and the nasolacrimal sac. The lacrimal gland produces the watery component of tears, which mixes with an oil component produced by the meibomian glands that line the edge of the eyelids and a mucous component produced by the goblet cells in the conjunctiva. The lacrimal glands consist of superior and inferior lobes and are located above and at the outer aspect of the eye behind the eyebrow bilaterally. The lacrimal ducts are connected to the inferior lobes of the lacrimal glands and carry the tears to the eye where this watery tear film is distributed over the surface of the eye by blinking of the eyelids. Any excess tear film leaves the eyes via two small openings called the lacrimal puncta, located at the inner corner of the eye, and drain into the superior and inferior lacrimal canaliculi. From there, the fluid enters the lacrimal sac and then the nasolacrimal duct where it drains into the nose.

The categories in this code block are as follows:

H00	Hordeolum and chalazion
H01	Other inflammation of eyelid
H02	Other disorders of eyelid
H04	Disorders of lacrimal system
H05	Disorders of orbit

Focus Point

The majority of codes in this code block have laterality as a component of the code and most conditions that affect the eyelid also identify the site as the upper or lower eyelid.

H00.- Hordeolum and chalazion

A hordeolum is a purulent, localized infection of the sebaceous or meibomian glands of the eyelid, resulting in swelling. A hordeolum may be preceded by a chalazion, which is a chronic, inflammatory, noninfectious lesion. A hordeolum is characterized by a sudden and rapidly progressive (acute) presentation. Due to the nature of the infection, a hordeolum is often tender to palpation, reddened, and painful. The most common causal organism is *Staphylococcus*.

H00.0- Hordeolum (externum) (internum) of eyelid

A hordeolum is an infection or inflammation of the eyelid involving the hair follicles of the external eyelid or the meibomian glands of the internal eyelid.

H00.01- Hordeolum externum

Hordeolum externum, or stye, may present as a small, superficial lump due to infection involving the Moll (oil) gland (also termed glands of Zeis), which arise from the eyelash follicle along the lid margins. It is typically painful and is located at the external skin side of the eyelid margin.

H00.02- Hordeolum internum

Hordeolum internum is usually a larger lump affecting the meibomian gland and arises from the internal eyelid margin toward the conjunctiva.

H00.03- Abscess of eyelid

Abscess of eyelid is an inflamed pocket of pus on the eyelid, possibly with an unknown point of origin.

H00.1- Chalazion

A chalazion is a chronic inflammation of the meibomian gland resulting in an eyelid mass. The meibomian gland is a tiny excretory gland in the eyelid that produces sebum to lubricate the eye. The sebum is discharged through tiny openings along the edges of the eyelids. The sebum secreted from the meibomian gland is an oily substance that also serves to prevent the tear film from evaporating and creates a protective barrier. When the glands become obstructed due to inflammation, a mass (chalazion) forms as a result of the blockage.

H01.- Other inflammation of eyelid

Four specific inflammatory conditions of the eyelid are included in this category: blepharitis, noninfectious dermatoses, eczematous dermatitis, and xeroderma.

H01.0- Blepharitis

Blepharitis is an inflammation of the eyelids. It is a common condition linked to bacterial infections and/or skin diseases. Blepharitis appears in two locations: anterior and posterior. Anterior blepharitis involves the outer-front portion of the eyelid margins, where the eyelashes are located. Posterior blepharitis involves the inner portion of the eyelid that makes contact with the eyes. It is not typically contagious, but recurrence can result in complications such as styes, hordeola, and chalazia.

H01.01- Ulcerative blepharitis

Ulcerative blepharitis is a severe presentation characterized by marked swelling and erosive, purulent ulcer formation along the lid margins, resulting in loss of eyelashes. It is typically caused by an infectious organism such as a virus or bacteria. Symptoms include crust formation in and around the eyelash area that often becomes matted during sleep, making it difficult to open the eyes. Also, bleeding from the eyelash follicle can occur, which can lead to loss of eyelashes, scar formation on the eyelid, and corneal inflammation.

H01.02- Squamous blepharitis

Squamous blepharitis is a milder presentation, causing redness and scales on the eyelid, usually along the margin. It is intensified by extended use of the eyes and prolonged exposure to light. Factors contributing to this condition include poor hygiene, seborrheic dermatitis, and occupational exposures in which the hands are often dirty.

H01.1- Noninfectious dermatoses of eyelid

Dermatosis is a general term that refers to any skin inflammation, lesion, or defect. Only dermatoses of the eyelid that are not due to an infectious process are included in this subcategory.

H01.12- Discoid lupus erythematosus of eyelid

Discoid lupus erythematosus (DLE) is an autoimmune skin disorder. DLE lesions are characteristically raised erythematous lesions. They are often scaling, progressive, and plaque-forming. Failure to establish diagnosis and initiate treatment can result in tissue atrophy, permanent scarring, and disfigurement. Lacrimal gland involvement may cause proptosis. Certain infections, exposures, hormones, and medications may trigger or exacerbate DLE lesions. The exact etiology is unknown, although genetic predisposition is suspected. The relationship between discoid lupus erythematosus and systemic lupus erythematosus (SLE) is unclear. Although skin involvement is characteristic of 90 percent of SLE patients, only approximately 20 to 30 percent of SLE patients manifest lesions that are classified as DLE lesions. Although the majority of patients with DLE do not manifest the same serological abnormalities as SLE patients, approximately 10 percent of patients with discoid lupus progress to SLE.

H02.- Other disorders of eyelid

Some of the common disorders affecting the eyelid are classified here. Types of conditions seen in this category include abnormal inversion (entropion) or eversion (ectropion) of the eyelid, the inability to completely close the eyelid (lagophthalmos), drooping of the skin over the eyelid (blepharochalasis), or the entire eyelid (ptosis) causing obstruction of vision.

H02.0- Entropion and trichiasis of eyelid

Entropion is a condition where the eyelids are inverted toward the eyeball (globe), resulting in irritation to the cornea or scleral surface by friction from the eyelashes. This eyelid instability is commonly due to a laxity or other abnormality of the lower eyelid retractor muscles. Corrective surgical procedures employ a variety of surgical techniques to repair the instability of the eyelid. Multiple associated causal conditions exist for entropion, including a lack of muscle tone as part of the normal aging process. Trichiasis is ingrown or impinged eyelashes on the corneal surface resulting in irritation.

H02.01- Cicatricial entropion of eyelid
Cicatricial entropion is caused by scar tissue of the conjunctiva due to trauma, trachoma, chronic infection, or burns.

H02.02- Mechanical entropion of eyelid
Mechanical entropion is caused by insufficient support of the globe to the eyelids. This is often due to tumors, ptosis, or chemosis of conjunctiva.

H02.03- Senile entropion of eyelid
Senile entropion is associated with loss of elasticity of the skin and muscle of the eyelid as part of the aging process. It is the most common type of entropion. It is caused by a lag of the eyelid in a horizontal manner.

H02.04- Spastic entropion of eyelid
Spastic entropion occurs as a result of spasm of the extraocular muscles inhibiting closure of the eye. It is often a sequela of neurologic or inflammatory eye disorders.

H02.05- Trichiasis without entropion
Trichiasis is ingrown or impinged eyelashes on the corneal surface resulting in irritation. It can be preceded by chronic lid disorders such as blepharitis, which results in scar tissue of the eyelash follicles and causes misdirected growth. In these instances, treatment is focused on correcting the causal condition.

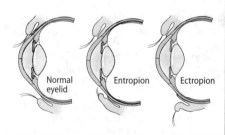

Normal eyelid   Entropion   Ectropion

H02.1- Ectropion of eyelid
Ectropion is the sagging or turning outward (eversion) of the lower eyelid, pulling it away from the eye surface and exposing the cornea. It is typically due to decreased muscle tone. The most common occurrence is seen in patients older than age 60, as it is part of the normal aging process.

H02.11- Cicatricial ectropion of eyelid
Cicatricial ectropion is caused by scarring or burns of the eyelid. It can occur as a postsurgical complication associated with blepharoplasty or eyelid reconstruction. Other causal conditions include infections or skin disorders such as herpes and acne rosacea.

H02.12- Mechanical ectropion of eyelid
Mechanical ectropion is a rare condition that typically accompanies a mass in or around the eyelid. Causal conditions include masses caused by neurofibromatosis.

H02.13- Senile ectropion of eyelid
Senile ectropion is caused by sagging muscle and skin due to the normal aging process. It is not related to a separate underlying disease.

H02.14- Spastic ectropion of eyelid
Spastic ectropion can result from irritation within the eye or spasms of the muscle surrounding the eye.

H02.2- Lagophthalmos
Lagophthalmos is a condition of incomplete closure of the eyelids. When the eyelids close, tears cover the surface of the eye providing lubrication and removing foreign matter. In lagophthalmos, eyelid function is disrupted. This can lead to several complications, including corneal drying, increased risk of injury, corneal ulceration, varying degrees of visual loss, and distorted appearance. There are three specific types classified here: cicatricial, mechanical, and paralytic, and an additional code for unspecified lagophthalmos. Cicatricial lagophthalmos is caused by scarring from aging, sun exposure, dermatitis, or other skin diseases (e.g., ichthyosis, scleroderma). Mechanical lagophthalmos is caused by outside factors, such as other diseases or conditions of the eye or eyelid, muscle disorders, or a post-blepharoplasty complication. Paralytic lagophthalmos is due to paralysis of the extraocular muscle that encircles the orbit. Causal conditions include facial nerve paralysis.

H02.3- Blepharochalasis
Blepharochalasis is characterized by eyelid skin that is abnormally thickened or indurated or has lost elasticity. It is associated with recurrent episodes of idiopathic edema causing intracellular tissue atrophy. It is a degenerative condition of the eyelid characterized by the onset of rapid swelling with periods of remission. Over time this condition contributes to the stretching of the eyelid and eventual destruction or atrophy. It typically affects a younger population of patients. Although the cause is largely unknown, it may be linked to angioedema, autoimmune mechanisms, or other systemic diseases. Treatment includes surgical interventions such as levator myoplasty, blepharoplasty, canthoplasty, or dermal grafts.

H02.4-   Ptosis of eyelid

Ptosis is a drooping or sagging of the eyelid. It may be due to weakness within the muscle, nerve damage to the muscle, or other laxity of the eyelid tissues. Causal conditions include the normal aging process, congenital anomalies, injury, systemic illness, or other ophthalmic conditions.

H02.41- Mechanical ptosis of eyelid

Mechanical ptosis occurs when the weight of the eyelid is too great for the muscles to raise it. Causal conditions include tumors or excess skin in the eyelid area.

H02.42- Myogenic ptosis of eyelid

Myogenic ptosis is related to a congenital or acquired muscle disorder in which the muscles of the eyelid are weakened or functionally impaired. Causal conditions include muscle disorders such as myasthenia gravis. In congenital presentations, the muscle tissue can become progressively scarred or nonfunctioning as part of a multisystemic syndrome or genetic defect.

H02.43- Paralytic ptosis of eyelid

Paralytic ptosis occurs when the muscle that elevates the eyelid is not working properly due to a nerve disorder. The nerve that controls muscle function of the eyelid is also responsible for pupillary function and rotation of the eyeball. In certain cases of paralytic ptosis, the patient has other nerve-disorder conditions affecting control of these ocular functions.

H02.5-   Other disorders affecting eyelid function

Eyelid function disorders included here are abnormal innervation syndrome, narrowing of the eyelid opening, and eyelid retraction.

H02.51- Abnormal innervation syndrome

Also referred to as jaw-winking syndrome, abnormal innervation syndrome occurs when a rapid abnormal motion of the eyelid resembling a wink is triggered by movement in the jaw, such as opening the mouth, smiling, or chewing. Although generally unilateral, it can be bilateral. It is often discovered in infancy during bottle or breastfeeding.

H02.52- Blepharophimosis

Blepharophimosis is an abnormal narrowing of the eyelid aperture (opening). It is caused by congenital or acquired lateral displacement of the inner canthi. It may be accompanied by bilateral ptosis or smaller-than-normal eyelids. This code reports the acquired form. Ankyloblepharon is also included here. Ankyloblepharon is the abnormal clinging (fusion) of all or part of the eyelids to each other, usually along the margins. It can occur as a congenital or acquired condition. This code reports the acquired form. Acquired ankyloblepharon is associated with certain autoimmune disorders (e.g., cicatricial pemphigoid) or skin disorders (e.g., Stevens-Johnson syndrome). Complications include corneal scarring and neovascularization.

> **Focus Point**
>
> *The code for congenital blepharophimosis can be found at Q10.0 Congenital ptosis. Additionally, the correct code for congenital ankyloblepharon is located at Q10.3 Other congenital malformations of eyelid.*

H02.53- Eyelid retraction

Lid retraction occurs when the eyelid migrates apart abnormally (scleral show) and cannot perform adequate closure. As such, it cannot perform the natural functions of cleaning and moisturizing the surface of the eye. It can be caused by insufficient support or decreased tissue (e.g., skin and muscle) due to the aging process, hormonal imbalances, or neuromuscular disease. Other causal factors include an imbalance in thyroid hormones, Bell's palsy, postsurgical complications, or scar formation. Lid retraction may cause significant discomfort, such as dry eye or corneal irritation. Treatment includes injection procedures or surgical correction.

H02.6-   Xanthelasma of eyelid

Xanthelasma refers to a condition in which there are small yellow tumors that occur on the eyelid, usually appearing near the nose. The condition is seen in patients with high blood-fat levels and in the elderly.

H02.8-   Other specified disorders of eyelid

Some conditions classified here include retained foreign body, cysts, connective tissue disorders, edema, vascular anomalies, and hemorrhage affecting the eyelid.

H02.82- Cysts of eyelid

A cyst is an enclosed cavity that contains fluid or other material. A sebaceous cyst is a cavity comprised of fatty or oily material (sebum). The primary function of sebum is to lubricate the skin. A cyst occurs due to an abnormal accumulation of sebum within a cutaneous cavity. It is often associated with obstruction, inflammatory process, or infection (abscess). The skin in the eyelids contains sebaceous glands and a sebaceous cyst may form when the glands become obstructed. If the cyst becomes reddened, swollen, or painful, an abscess may be present. Infection may require treatment with antibiotics. The cyst may require incision and drainage or excision to relieve the obstruction.

H02.83- Dermatochalasis of eyelid

Dermatochalasis is an acquired form of a connective tissue disorder commonly associated with the aging process. It is characterized by sagging of the skin, muscle, or connective tissues of the eyelids. It is due primarily to loss of elasticity, forces of gravity, and progressive weakness of the skin and connective tissues. Dermatochalasis of the lower eyelids is associated with excessive skin and wrinkles. Although this condition is usually considered cosmetic, the wrinkling, sagging, or excess skin can obstruct the superior visual field. Additionally, some patients complain of irritation, blepharitis, dermatitis, entropion, or ectropion. A herniation of orbital fat (i.e., steatoblepharon) is frequently associated with dermatochalasis.

H04.- Disorders of lacrimal system

The lacrimal glands are located above the orbit just below the eyebrow.

H04.0- Dacryoadenitis

Dacryoadenitis is an inflammation of the tear-producing lacrimal glands. The lacrimal glands are located above the orbit just below the eyebrow. The fifth character provides separate classifications for acute and chronic presentations. Acute dacryoadenitis is commonly due to viral, bacterial, or fungal infection (e.g., Epstein-Barr, mumps, gonococcus). Symptoms include rapid onset of swelling and erythema of the upper-outer eyelid associated with pain. Additionally, fever, chemosis, purulent discharge, excess tearing, or preauricular lymphadenopathy may be present. Chronic dacryoadenitis is often a secondary effect of chronic systemic inflammatory disorders, including sarcoidosis, thyroid disease, and Sjogren's syndrome. Symptoms include long-standing nontender swelling of the upper-outer eyelid with preserved ocular motility. Chronic inflammation may cause ptosis and dry eye. Treatment is most effectively directed at the underlying cause. Infections may require antibiotic therapy. Viral infections may require only palliative treatment, with rest and warm compresses. Chronic inflammations may be treated with steroid therapy.

H04.3- Acute and unspecified inflammation of lacrimal passages

This subcategory classifies acute or unspecified inflammation of the lacrimal passages. In acute presentations, symptoms occur suddenly and run a short course. Two conditions are included here: dacryocystitis and canaliculitis. Canaliculitis is an inflammation of the lacrimal duct while dacryocystitis is an inflammation of the lacrimal sac. Dacryocystitis is further subclassified by type, which includes phlegmonous and acute.

H04.31- Phlegmonous dacryocystitis

Phlegmonous dacryocystitis is an infection of the tear sac characterized by the formation of pockets of pus. Antibiotics are often effective in treating infection, but surgical intervention may be necessary to irrigate ductal structures, incise and drain pockets of infection, or relieve obstructions.

H04.32- Acute dacryocystitis

In dacryocystitis, the punctum and canaliculus appear normal, with a tender, red mass involving only the lacrimal sac. Dacryocystitis is an inflammatory condition of the lacrimal sac that is typically caused by infection.

H04.33- Acute lacrimal canaliculitis

Canaliculitis can be differentiated from dacryocystitis by the presenting clinical signs and symptoms. Canaliculitis is commonly characterized by redness, sensitivity, and swelling of the punctum and canaliculus. It is an infection of the lacrimal duct that causes increased tearing or drainage from the eye.

H04.4- Chronic inflammation of lacrimal passages

This subcategory classifies chronic inflammation of the lacrimal passages, indicating the symptoms develop over time and have extensive duration and regular recurrence. Canaliculitis can be differentiated from dacryocystitis by the presenting clinical signs and symptoms. Canaliculitis is commonly characterized by redness and swelling of the punctum and canaliculus. In dacryocystitis, the punctum and canaliculus appear normal, with a tender, red mass involving only the lacrimal sac. Conditions classifiable to this subcategory are often interrelated or associated with other eye conditions. For example, causation of dacryocystitis includes ductile stenosis or obstruction, resulting in stagnation of tears and bacterial overgrowth.

H04.41- Chronic dacryocystitis

Chronic dacryocystitis describes any ongoing or recurrent inflammatory condition of the lacrimal sac. It is typically caused by an untreated, partially treated, or ineffectively treated infection.

H04.42- Chronic lacrimal canaliculitis

Chronic canaliculitis is an infection of the lacrimal duct that causes increased tearing or drainage from the eye. It can be accompanied by localized redness and/or sensitivity. Chronic canaliculitis may be linked with the *Actinomyces israelii* pathogen or other bacteria, fungi, and viruses (e.g., herpes simplex).

H04.43- Chronic lacrimal mucocele

Lacrimal mucocele is a cyst within the lacrimal system. It is caused by blockage of the excretory duct, which results in the formation of a pocket of retained secretions.

H04.5- Stenosis and insufficiency of lacrimal passages

The lacrimal passages are part of a system designed to protect and lubricate the eyes. This set of codes describes conditions where the lacrimal passages are blocked and/or functioning inefficiently due to obstruction or narrowing of the passageway.

H04.51- Dacryolith

A dacryolith is a calcified stone or mass in the lacrimal system, which can lodge in a duct and cause obstruction.

H04.52- Eversion of lacrimal punctum

Eversion of lacrimal punctum is a condition characterized by the circular opening of the tear duct abnormally turned inside out.

H04.53- Neonatal obstruction of nasolacrimal duct

Obstruction of the nasolacrimal duct is a blocked tear duct, in this case occurring in a newborn. Tears normally drain from the surface of the eye into small openings, called puncta, at the inner aspects of the upper and lower eyelids. From the puncta, tears enter canals, called canaliculi, drain into the nasolacrimal ducts, and are excreted into the nose. When the nasolacrimal puncta are obstructed, tears overflow from the eye. In newborns, the most common cause of obstruction is failure of the membrane at the end of the tear duct to open prior to or shortly after birth. Generally this condition resolves spontaneously within the first year of life. Occasionally surgical treatment is required, including tear duct probing, balloon dilatation, and/or tube placement.

H04.54- Stenosis of lacrimal canaliculi

H04.55- Acquired stenosis of nasolacrimal duct

H04.56- Stenosis of lacrimal punctum

H04.57- Stenosis of lacrimal sac

Stenosis is a narrowing or stricture of an opening or tubular structure. Stenosis can occur in any region of the lacrimal passages and codes are specific to site. Stenosis of the lacrimal canaliculi is an abnormal narrowing or stricture of the tubes in the inner corner of the eyelid through which tears travel. Stenosis of the nasolacrimal duct, acquired, also documented as dacryostenosis, excludes a congenital condition and defines a narrowing in this area. Blockage of the tear duct and/or canalicular system can be a side effect of chemotherapy using docetaxel. Stenosis of the lacrimal punctum occurs when there is narrowing within the lacrimal passage. Radiation therapy directed at the canthal area can lead to punctual stenosis. Stenosis of the lacrimal sac is an abnormal narrowing of the tear sac.

H05.- Disorders of orbit

This category identifies disorders of the orbit, which is the bony housing for the globe, also called the eyeball. Conditions classified here include the orbital bones, as well as connective and soft tissues within the bony walls of the orbit, that cover and protect the globe. Between the bony housing and the eyeball are other structures such as fat, muscle, blood vessels, and glands. The orbital fat cushioning each globe is divided into central and peripheral compartments. The central space contains the optic, oculomotor, abducent, and nasociliary nerves. The peripheral space contains the trochlear, lacrimal, frontal, and infraorbital nerves. Disorders of the orbit covered here include inflammatory disorders, with subcategories for acute and chronic inflammations, exophthalmic conditions, deformity of the orbit, enophthalmos, retained foreign bodies, other specified disorders, and unspecified disorders. Exophthalmic conditions are those that cause the globe to protrude from the orbit and enophthalmic conditions are those that cause the eye to recede into the orbit.

H05.0- Acute inflammation of orbit

Acute inflammation of the orbit is classified by the tissues involved. Acute inflammation is often due to bacterial or other infection, but may also be caused by a noninfectious disease process. In orbital cellulitis, the tissues posterior to the orbital septum are affected. In osteomyelitis, the orbital bones are involved. In periostitis, the periosteum, a thin layer of connective tissue covering the bone, is inflamed or infected. In tenonitis, there is inflammation or infection of the Tenon's capsule, the thin membrane covering the sclera. There is also a code for unspecified acute inflammation of the orbit.

H05.00 Unspecified acute inflammation of orbit

This code classifies acute inflammation or infection of an unspecified part of the orbit. Acute inflammation or infection that is not documented as affecting a specific site or tissue (e.g., soft tissue, bone, periosteum, or Tenon's capsule) that comprise the orbit is reported with this code.

H05.01- Cellulitis of orbit

In orbital cellulitis, the infection is between the orbital bone and the globe. Orbital cellulitis is inflammation of the orbital tissues posterior to the orbital septum. Symptoms include proptosis, also called exophthalmos, which is a protrusion of the globe; ophthalmoplegia, which is paralysis of one or more eye muscles; pain on eye movement; and loss of vision. Orbital cellulitis may be caused by bacteria introduced by trauma, by infection that originates in the nasal sinuses or teeth and extends into the eye region, or by migration of infection from elsewhere in the body.

> **Focus Point**
>
> *A second code from Chapter 1 Infectious and Parasitic Diseases, should be reported when the infectious agent is documented.*
>
> *Orbital cellulitis does not include preseptal cellulitis of the eyelid. Report cellulitis of the eyelid with a code from subcategory H00.03- Abscess of eyelid.*

H05.02- Osteomyelitis of orbit

In orbital osteomyelitis, the bone is infected. Osteomyelitis of the orbit is typically the result of one of three processes: hematogenous infection, direct inoculation, or contiguous infection. In children, the most common type is hematogenous orbital osteomyelitis resulting from a remote infection that spreads via the bloodstream to the orbital bones. In adults, orbital osteomyelitis is most often the result of direct inoculation from an open traumatic or surgical wound or by an acute infection of the sinuses with contiguous spread to the orbital bone. Osteomyelitis of the orbit is characterized by pain and swelling around the eye and restricted movement of the eye along with systemic symptoms such as fever and chills.

H05.03- Periostitis of orbit

In orbital periostitis, the inflammation or infection is in the periosteum, which is the connective tissue covering the orbital bones. The periosteum contains blood vessels that provide nutrients to the bone, as well as sensory nerves.

H05.04- Tenonitis of orbit

In tenonitis, the inflammation or infection is in the Tenon's capsule, the thin fibroelastic membrane that envelops the sclera, extending from the optic nerve in the posterior aspect of the globe to the ciliary muscles in the anterior aspect.

Disorders of Conjunctiva (H10-H11)

The conjunctiva is the thin, translucent, mucous membrane covering the anterior surface of the globe and inner aspect of eyelids. The portion that covers the globe is called the bulbar conjunctiva and the portion that covers the eyelids is called the palpebral conjunctiva. Disorders of the conjunctiva are divided into two categories: one for conjunctivitis, which covers both acute and chronic inflammatory conditions of the conjunctiva, and one for all other disorders of the conjunctiva.

The categories in this code block are as follows:

H10	Conjunctivitis
H11	Other disorders of the conjunctiva

Focus Point

Laterality is a component of most codes in this code block.

H10.- Conjunctivitis

Conjunctivitis is an inflammation of the mucous membrane covering the anterior surface of the eyeball and the lining of the eyelids. Conjunctivitis may be acute or chronic. Acute conjunctivitis includes mucopurulent types, which are usually due to bacterial infections, allergens, exposure to chemicals, pseudomembranous, and serous. Chronic conjunctivitis includes simple, giant papillary, follicular, and vernal types. There is also a subcategory for blepharoconjunctivitis, which is used for inflammation of the palpebral conjunctiva and eyelids, and for pingueculitis, which is a raised area of conjunctival tissue that is often associated with sunlight damage. Signs and symptoms vary depending on whether the condition is acute or chronic and on the etiology of the inflammation.

Focus Point

Not all conjunctivitis codes are found in this chapter. When conjunctivitis has a known infectious etiology, the code may be located in Chapter 1 Infectious and Parasitic Diseases. For example, chlamydial conjunctivitis is reported with code A74.0.

H10.0- Mucopurulent conjunctivitis

Bacterial infections of the conjunctiva cause a mucopurulent form of acute conjunctivitis, characterized by a thick, sticky purulent discharge from the conjunctiva and redness, pain, and itching of the conjunctiva. Common infectious organisms include *Staphylococcus aureus*, *Staphylococcus epidermidis*, *Streptococcus pneumoniae*, *Streptococcus pyogenes*, and *Moraxella lacunata*. Diagnostic tests include culture and sensitivity of discharge to identify the infective organism. Treatment involves topical antibiotics applied as drops or a salve to the conjunctiva. Mucopurulent conjunctivitis is differentiated as acute follicular or other mucopurulent type. Acute follicular conjunctivitis is characterized by severe conjunctival inflammation with dense infiltrations of lymphoid tissues of the inner eyelids that resemble small, white masses along with purulent discharge.

H10.1- Acute atopic conjunctivitis

Acute atopic conjunctivitis is a sudden and severe onset of conjunctival inflammation as an autoimmune response to exposure to allergens.

H10.2- Other acute conjunctivitis

Acute conjunctivitis is an inflammation of the mucous membrane covering the anterior surface of the eyeball and the lining of the eyelids. It is commonly due to exposure of the conjunctiva to contaminants or irritants. In acute presentation, symptoms develop suddenly and typically run a short course. Other types of acute conjunctivitis classified here include acute toxic conjunctivitis caused by exposure of the conjunctiva to chemicals. Chemical conjunctivitis is an inflammatory condition of the eye associated with redness, pain, and excess tearing (i.e., pink eye) in milder presentations. Acute chemical conjunctivitis may progress to include a worsening of swelling, pain, and redness, with blurring of vision. It is due to ocular exposure to various irritating substances such as detergents, airborne chemicals or solvents, smoke, industrial pollutants, and chlorine in swimming pools. There is also a pseudomembranous type of conjunctivitis where a thin membrane that can easily be removed forms over the conjunctiva and a serous type characterized by inflammation and a watery discharge from the eye.

H10.4-   Chronic conjunctivitis

Chronic conjunctivitis is chronic inflammation of the conjunctiva characterized by acute exacerbations and remissions occurring over months or years. It often has an allergic etiology. Degenerative changes or damage may occur from repeated acute attacks. The clinical presentation is similar in most respects to acute conjunctivitis except that it is more innocuous at the onset and runs a more protracted course.

H10.41- Chronic giant papillary conjunctivitis

Chronic giant papillary conjunctivitis is a relatively new classification of conjunctivitis characterized by enlarged papillae particularly on the conjunctiva of the upper eyelid and allergic symptoms usually resulting from long-term contact lens use. The inflammation and enlargement of the papillae are caused by an immunoglobulin E (IgE) hypersensitivity response to the presence of contact lens. Because this condition is seen most frequently in contact lens wearers, the condition is also called contact lens–induced papillary conjunctivitis (CLPC). Less common causes are other ocular devices including scleral buckles, ocular sutures, and raised corneal scars. Symptoms include itching, redness, blurred vision, and the inability to tolerate contact lenses. Treatment involves discontinuation of contact lens use for two to four weeks and replacing the offending lens type with another type that may be less irritating.

H10.42- Simple chronic conjunctivitis

Simple chronic conjunctivitis presents with congested conjunctival vessels, papillary hypertrophy, and a sticky appearance at the eyelid margin. It is often due to continuous exposure to medications, contact eye solution with irritant preservatives, or other chronic environmental factors.

H10.43- Chronic follicular conjunctivitis

Chronic follicular conjunctivitis presents with localized infiltrations of lymphoid tissues. These appear as small, pale masses in the folds of the conjunctiva in the inner eyelid, and are often located in the passage of the globe onto the eyelid. It may be caused by chronic infection or as a reactive inflammatory response to topical medications.

H10.44   Vernal conjunctivitis

Vernal conjunctivitis is inflammation of the outer eyelid lining caused by an allergic reaction. This form of conjunctivitis can be severe in that it can lead to corneal complications such as scarring and decreased vision. It is often characterized by rough bumps that form on the underside of the eyelids, accompanied by a mucus discharge. The cornea may have a rough and swollen appearance.

H11.-   Other disorders of conjunctiva

This category classifies noninflammatory conditions affecting the conjunctiva.

H11.0-   Pterygium of eye

Pterygium is an external growth that starts in the conjunctiva and invades the cornea. This growth is fed by capillaries supplying blood to the tissue. The growths range from small, inclusive masses to large, excessive growths. These masses are benign, but in some cases progress into the field of vision, obstructing sight. Causal factors include excessive environmental exposure to sun, dust, and wind, or other chronic eye irritants. Pterygiums are classified by site and other distinctive characteristics. Amyloids are proteins that are sometimes deposited in body tissues. An amyloid pterygium is characterized by the presence of these protein depositions. Central pterygium is a centrally located lesion that may or may not affect vision. Peripheral pterygium is located on the medial or lateral side of the eye. Peripheral pterygiums may be stationary meaning that the outer portion does not extend into the visual field or progressive meaning that the pterygium is growing rapidly and invading the visual field. Double pterygium refers to two lesions in the same eye. Recurrent indicates that a pterygium that has been removed is now growing back.

H11.15- Pinguecula

A pinguecula is a raised area of conjunctival tissue that is often associated with sunlight damage. Pingueculae are characterized by yellowish, slightly raised, lipid-like deposits in the nasal and temporal limbal conjunctiva and are most commonly seen in middle-aged patients with chronic sun exposure. Normally pingueculae are asymptomatic and an incidental finding; however, pingueculae can lead to the formation of pterygia. Both pingueculae and pterygia can become vascularized and inflamed, causing corneal thinning secondary to dryness.

Focus Point

Pinguecultis describes pinguecula that has become acutely vascularized, red, irritated, and highly symptomatic and is reported with a code from subcategory H10.81-.

Disorders of the Sclera, Cornea, Iris and Ciliary Body (H15-H22)

The sclera is the white, fibrous outer wall of the eye. It is covered by conjunctiva and joins with the cornea anteriorly and the optic nerve sheath posteriorly.

The cornea is the transparent tissue that covers the front of the eye. It has three layers: epithelium, stroma, and endothelium. The epithelium blocks the passage of foreign material and provides a smooth surface that absorbs oxygen and other needed cell nutrients that are contained in tears. The stroma gives the cornea its strength and elasticity, and the protein fibers of the stroma produce the cornea's light-conducting transparency. The endothelium pumps excess water out of the stroma.

Unlike most tissues in the body, the cornea contains no blood vessels to protect it against infection. The cornea serves as a physical barrier that shields the inside of the eye from germs, dust, and other foreign objects. It also acts as the eye's outermost lens. When light strikes the cornea, it refracts the incoming light onto the crystalline lens. The lens focuses the light onto the retina. Although much thinner than the lens, the cornea provides about 65 percent of the eye's power to bend light. Most of this power resides in the center of the cornea, which is rounder and thinner than the outer part of the tissue and is better suited to bend lightwaves.

The iris, which extends partly over the lens, is composed of the two layers forming the edge of the optic cup and a layer of vascularized connective tissue containing the pupillary muscle. The iris muscles can make the pupil larger or smaller and the pigmented layer is responsible for eye color. The iris is continuous with the ring-shaped ciliary body behind it. The iris, ciliary body, and choroid ensure that light only enters the eye through the pupil, and blood vessels in the choroid help to nourish the retina.

The ciliary body is formed from the two layers composing the rim of the optic cup, which undergo folding to form the ciliary processes. The ciliary body produces the clear fluid within the eye that goes through the pupil and drains back into the bloodstream through a tissue in front of the periphery of the iris. The ciliary body also contains the muscle that attaches to the outside of the lens of the eye and alters the focus of the eye. In turn, the ciliary body is continuous with a pigmented layer, the choroid, which lines the back of the eye outside the light sensitive retina.

The categories in this code block are as follows:

H15	Disorders of sclera
H16	Keratitis
H17	Corneal scars and opacities
H18	Other disorders of cornea
H20	Iridocyclitis
H21	Other disorders of iris and ciliary body
H22	Disorders of iris and ciliary body in diseases classified elsewhere

> **Focus Point**
>
> *Laterality is a component of most codes in this code block.*

H15.- Disorders of sclera

The sclera, like other structures of the eye, can become inflamed. Depending on the tissue affected, the condition is classified as scleritis or episcleritis. Another condition affecting the sclera is staphyloma, which refers to a weakening or thinning of the fibrous wall of the sclera with protrusion of the underlying uveal tissue.

H15.0- Scleritis

Scleritis is the inflammation of the sclera (the white, outer wall of the eye) that can be superficial or deep. In addition to redness, some patients experience pain. Visual acuity is often reduced and intraocular pressures may be elevated. Dilation of the vasculature often leads to characteristic discoloration of the sclera or episclera, which can be observed upon slit lamp examination. It is often associated with systemic diseases, particularly those with an autoimmune component, infections, or chemical injuries, but sometimes the cause is unknown. It occurs most often in people between the ages of 30 and 60 and is rare in children. Scleritis is classified by the site and/or other characteristics.

H15.01- Anterior scleritis

Anterior scleritis is any inflammatory condition focused on the anterior portion of the sclera. Widespread inflammation in this area is often associated with rheumatoid arthritis.

H15.02- Brawny scleritis

Brawny scleritis symptoms appear as gelatinous swelling and thickening of the peripheral scleral margins. Scleral abscess is the collection of pus in the sclera and typically includes swelling.

H15.03- Posterior scleritis

Posterior scleritis is less common, but can occur in conjunction with anterior scleritis.

H15.05- Scleromalacia perforans

Scleromalacia perforans is a degenerative inflammatory condition of the sclera characterized by tissue thinning and degeneration. Similar to anterior scleritis, it is often associated with rheumatoid arthritis.

H15.1-   Episcleritis

Episcleritis is typically a nonthreatening condition affecting the vascularized layer of connective tissue between the cornea and sclera. It presents as redness in one or both eyes, is short-lived, and requires minimal treatment unless associated with a systemic disorder, in which specific therapy may be indicated. Two specific types are classified here. Episcleritis periodica fugax is a typically self-limiting inflammation that tends to run its course within a few hours to a few days, but may recur. Nodular episcleritis is a form of anterior scleritis that presents with tender, inflamed erythematous nodules.

H16.-   Keratitis

Keratitis is inflammation of the cornea, the transparent membrane at the front of the eye. It may occur with or without conjunctivitis. When both the cornea and conjunctiva are inflamed, the condition is referred to as keratoconjunctivitis. Signs and symptoms of keratitis include impaired vision (early) or blindness (late), opacity of the cornea, irritation and tearing, and photophobia.

> **Focus Point**
>
> *Not all inflammations of the cornea are reported here. When the etiology is infectious and the infectious agent is known, the correct code may be listed in Chapter 1 Infectious and Parasitic Diseases.*

H16.24- Ophthalmia nodosa

Ophthalmia nodosa is the presence of nodular swellings on the cornea and conjunctiva, due to penetration of ocular tissues by embedded hairs. The name derives from the inflammatory response observed after exposure to certain insect or vegetable hairs. Transmission often occurs after handling objects such as vegetables or pets (particularly insects, tarantulas, caterpillars, moths) with fine hairs. These hairs can be introduced through hand-eye contact or via airborne transmission. The hairs embed in the conjunctiva, causing foreign body reaction such as pain and conjunctival injection (redness). Treatment with topical corticosteroids can be effective in reducing inflammation. Diagnosis may be established by slit-lamp examination.

H20.-   Iridocyclitis

Iridocyclitis is a combination of inflammation of the iris and inflammation of the ciliary body. When the iris is inflamed, its blood vessels dilate and the blood vessels of the white of the eye make it reddened. The dilated vessels leak proteins and blood cells into the clear eye fluid, which tends to prevent fluid from going through the pupil. The iris tissue and the ciliary body are richly supplied with sensory nerves so that the inflamed tissue causes pain especially when it moves in bright light or when focusing on near objects.

H21.-   Other disorders of iris and ciliary body

Conditions classified here include hyphema, vascular conditions, degenerative disorders, cystic lesions, and adhesions, as well as two conditions associated with eye surgery: floppy iris syndrome and plateau iris syndrome.

H21.0-   Hyphema

Hyphema is bleeding into the anterior chamber of the eye. It occurs when blood vessels in the iris bleed and leak into the clear aqueous fluid, and the eyes appear reddened or bloodshot. Hyphema can partially or completely impair vision. Symptoms include visible pool of blood in the anterior chamber and elevated intraocular pressure.

Hyphema

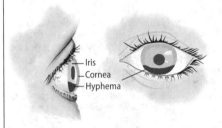

Iris
Cornea
Hyphema

> **Focus Point**
>
> *Hyphema is often associated with head injury or direct trauma to the eye; however, traumatic hyphema is not included here. See subcategory S05.1- when trauma is documented as the cause.*

H21.1-   Other vascular disorders of iris and ciliary body

One condition classified here is rubeosis iridis, which involves an abnormal formation of new blood vessels (neovascularization) and connective tissue on the surface of the iris. It is often associated with diabetic retinopathy, central retinal vein occlusion, and retinal detachment. Pathogenesis involves retinal ischemia resulting in compensatory formation of new blood vessels. If untreated, the new vessels swell, causing an increase in intraocular pressure (neovascular glaucoma).

H21.81   Floppy iris syndrome

Floppy iris syndrome is a complication that may occur intraoperatively during cataract extractions in certain patients, specifically those who have taken alpha-blockers for urinary symptoms such as benign prostatic hypertrophy. The iris is typically dilated using medication during cataract surgery. However, certain alpha-blockers relax the iris dilator muscle, resulting in a flaccid iris that does not remain properly dilated, but instead may billow or flap. Intraoperative floppy iris syndrome may also be linked to other causes of small pupils, such as adhesions or synechiae, white, flaky deposits known as pseudoexfoliation, or medications for other conditions such as hypertension, glaucoma, or diabetes.

H21.82 Plateau iris syndrome (post-iridectomy) (postprocedural)

Plateau iris syndrome is a rare postoperative condition that may occur after removal of a pupillary block by iridectomy to treat closed angle glaucoma. Plateau iris syndrome is diagnosed when angle closure recurs without plateauing or shallowing of the anterior chamber angle axially. Recurrence of angle closure typically manifests in the early postprocedural period, but it may manifest much later following spontaneous dilation of the pupil or dilation in response to eyedrops that dilate the pupil. It is treated with pilocarpine drops, a medication that reduces the amount of fluid in the eye thereby reducing eye pressure.

Focus Point

Do not confuse plateau iris configuration with plateau iris syndrome. Plateau iris configuration is a preoperative condition associated with closed angle glaucoma. Eye exam shows a flat iris plane with an anterior chamber that is not shallow axially. Plateau iris configuration with glaucoma is reported with a code from subcategory H40.22-.

Disorders of Lens (H25-H28)

The lens of the eye is a nearly transparent (crystalline) biconvex structure that is suspended behind the iris. The function of the lens of the eye is to focus rays of light onto the retina. The most common condition affecting the lens is the development of cataracts. Cataracts are opacities that form within the lens and obscure vision. A far less common condition affecting the lens is dislocation or displacement.

The categories in this code block are as follows:

H25	Age-related cataract
H26	Other cataract
H27	Other disorders of lens
H28	Cataract in diseases classified elsewhere

Focus Point

Laterality is a component of most codes in this code block.

H25.- Age-related cataract

An age-related or senile cataract is characterized by partial or total opacity of the lens due to degenerative changes that occur with age. Typically patients diagnosed with age-related cataract are older than 55 years of age. Senile cataracts are identified by increased opacity of the lens followed by its softening

and shrinkage associated with degeneration. Signs and symptoms of age-related cataract include slowly progressing and painless loss of vision, leukocoria, altered color perception, strabismus, and difficulty in night driving.

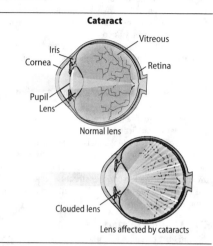

Cataract

Vitreous
Iris
Cornea
Retina
Pupil
Lens
Normal lens

Clouded lens

Lens affected by cataracts

H25.0- Age-related incipient cataract

An incipient cataract is an incomplete cataract occurring when the lens is only slightly opaque and the cortex is clear. Cataracts can be classified by the zones of the lens involved in the opacity such as cortical, anterior subcapsular, or more commonly posterior subcapsular polar.

H25.01- Cortical age-related cataract

A cortical cataract affects the lens cortex, which is the peripheral edge of the lens. It often begins with sharp, limited, clear fluid clefts, causing opaque spokes or clear lamellar separations with cuneiform opacities. The clefts can cause light that enters the eye to abnormally manifest as blurred vision, glare, contrast, and depth perception.

H25.03- Anterior subcapsular polar age-related cataract

An anterior subcapsular polar cataract occurs as an acquired, senile cataract and may be secondary to late effects of uveitis or trauma resulting in anterior subcapsular opacities.

H25.04- Posterior subcapsular polar age-related cataract

A posterior subcapsular cataract is an opacification in the rear of the lens capsule that begins as a small opaque or cloudy area and spreads throughout the back of the lens, with associated visual impairment.

H25.1- Age-related nuclear cataract

A nuclear cataract, the most common type, is an opacity that forms at the center or nucleus of the eye typically caused by degenerative hardening and discoloration of the lens over time. The lens can turn yellow and eventually brown. When light enters the eye and focuses on the retina by the cornea and lens, the lens becomes opaque or cloudy and gradually loses the ability to keep images focused on the retina leading to clouded vision and trouble with color distinction.

H25.2- Age-related cataract, morgagnian type

This is referred to as a hypermature senile cataract and involves lens opacification characterized by a soft liquefied or flattened lens that is prone to cortical matter leak through the capsule. The nucleus shifts to the bottom of the lens capsule, which may cause swelling and irritation of other structures in the eye. This type of cataract has been encountered less often in modern times.

H26.- Other cataract

This category classifies infantile and juvenile cataracts, traumatic cataracts, drug-induced cataracts, and cataracts due to other secondary causes.

H26.0- Infantile and juvenile cataract

The definition of infantile and juvenile cataract is the partial or total opacity of the lens occurring in an infant, a young child, or a young adult. Signs and symptoms of infantile and juvenile cataract include slowly progressing and painless loss of vision, leukocoria, behavioral problems indicative of vision problems, and strabismus.

> **Focus Point**
>
> *Codes for infantile and juvenile cataract do not include congenital cataract, which is reported with code Q12.0 located in Chapter 17 Congenital Malformation, Deformations and Chromosomal Abnormalities.*

H26.3- Drug-induced cataract

Drug-induced cataracts are also called "toxic" cataracts. The most common cause of drug-induced cataracts is long-term use of steroids.

> **Focus Point**
>
> *Drug-induced cataracts are considered adverse effects and require an additional code from categories T36-T50 to identify the drug. If the drug-induced cataract is due to long-term use of a medication, a code from category Z79 should also be assigned.*

Disorders of the Choroid and Retina (H30-H36)

The choroid is the layer of blood vessels and connective tissue between the sclera and the retina. The choroid is heavily pigmented, which prevents stray light from reaching the retina. It supplies oxygen and nutrients to the inner parts of the eye and acts to exchange heat generated by retinal metabolism. Part of the choroid develops into the cores of the ciliary processes. At the posterior end of the optic cup, the choroid forms a sheath around the optic nerve. The choroid, iris, and ciliary body are also referred to as the uvea.

The retina is sensitive nervous tissue that sends messages via the optic nerve to the brain. The retina begins just posterior to the iris, behind the area called the pars plana, and lines the inner wall of the eye. The central portion of the retina is the macula, which is roughly the area inside of the arcade vessels that extends from the optic nerve and around the macula. The macula is the area of the retina where central vision is the clearest for color and reading vision. The true focal point of the eye is the foveal avascular zone (FAZ), which is only 400 microns wide (0.4mm). The single-layer retinal pigment epithelium (RPE) outside the retina provides nutrients to the photoreceptors; it is also dark with melanin, which decreases light scatter within the eye. The rod and cone are photoreceptors: the cone system dominates vision in daytime, whereas the rod system dominates night vision. Below the RPE is a multilayered membrane called Bruch's membrane, which separates the RPE and retina from the choroid. The vitreous is a clear gel-like substance that fills up most of the inner space of the eyeball. It lies behind the lens and is in contact with the retina.

The categories in this code block are as follows:

H30	Chorioretinal inflammation
H31	Other disorders of choroid
H32	Chorioretinal disorders in diseases classified elsewhere
H34	Retinal vascular occlusions
H35	Other retinal disorders
H36	Retinal disorders in diseases classified elsewhere

> **Focus Point**
>
> *Laterality is a component of most codes in this code block.*

H33.- Retinal detachments and breaks

Retinal detachment is the separation of the retina from the underlying retinal pigment epithelium (RPE). Retinal detachment can occur gradually due to a degenerative process or suddenly, causing total vision loss in the affected eye. There are often precipitous retinal defects or tears with risk of vitreous hemorrhage and visual impairment. Detachments can also occur without retinal defects or tears and these are classified as serous retinal detachments. Conversely, retinal defects or breaks can occur without retinal detachment and these are classified as retinal breaks without detachment. Traction retinal detachments are another type seen in patients with diabetic retinopathy, retinopathy of prematurity, and in traumatic eye injuries.

Retinal Detachment

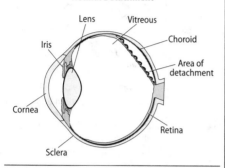

H33.0-   Retinal detachment with retinal break

Retinal detachments with retinal breaks are classified by severity as partial or total. Partial retinal detachments are further differentiated by the number and type of breaks or defects. Patients with severe, high, or degenerative forms of myopia (near-sightedness) are at greater risk for retinal detachment. Rhegmatogenous retinal detachment is classified here and is characterized by a full-thickness break or tear of the retina. Vitreous hemorrhage is commonly associated with rhegmatogenous retinal detachment.

H33.03-   Retinal detachment with giant retinal tear

Giant retinal tear is a sight-threatening, large retinal break involving at least a fourth of the retinal circumference. If the retinal tear is one quarter of the retina or more, it is called a "giant retinal tear." The tear may be so large that the retina folds over on itself. Postoperative prognosis is positive for most patients; yet some develop scar tissue (proliferative vitreoretinopathy) that adversely affects visual acuity on a long-term basis.

H33.04-   Retinal detachment with retinal dialysis

Retinal dialysis describes separation of the sensory retinal layer from the pigment layer at the ora ciliaris retinae. It is often a precursory condition to retinal detachment. The most common cause of retinal dialysis is direct trauma to the eye.

H33.1-   Retinoschisis and retinal cysts

Retinoschisis is a condition in which a portion of the retina separates into two layers resulting in impaired vision at the site of the separation. Retinal cysts also involve the splitting of the retina into two layers with development of fluid-filled sacs on the retina at the site of the split. There are two primary causes of retinoschisis and formation of cysts, one is congenital and the other is degenerative. Only the degenerative form is reported here. Degenerative retinoschisis is typically seen in the elderly as a result of aging. A third type of retinoschisis with retinal cyst formation is caused by parasitic infestation, but this type is rarely seen in the United States. Vision impairment due to retinoschisis or retinal cyst formation is the result of damage to the retina and is permanent.

H33.11-   Cyst of ora serrata

The ora serrata is the region of the eye where the retina and ciliary body join. The ora serrata gets its name from its serrated or notched appearance. It marks the point where the photosensitive area of the retina ends. A cyst of the ora serrata is a fluid-filled sac that develops in this region.

H33.12-   Parasitic cyst of retina

A parasitic cyst of the retina results when a parasite, such as a helminth (worm), migrates through the bloodstream from the primary site of infestation such as the digestive tract to another site, such as the eye, and forms a cystic lesion. Parasitic cysts of the retina are rarely seen in the United States.

H33.19-   Other retinoschisis and retinal cysts

All other degenerative types of retinoschisis and retinal cyst formation are classified here including pseudocyst of the retina. Pseudocysts are empty spaces or microscopic holes between the layers of the retina. A pseudocyst has no wall as a true cyst does and the empty space does not contain fluid.

H33.2-   Serous retinal detachment

Serous retinal detachment is separation of the retina from the choroid without breaks or tears in the retina. Usually spontaneous, although it may be due to a trauma, this condition usually occurs in patients 50 years of age or older. This condition is primarily due to fluid accumulation beneath the retina due to neovascularization or other diseases of the retina, or as a secondary effect of inflammation, injury, or other vascular abnormality. Causal inflammatory conditions include uveitis and neoplasm. In pathogenesis, small, blister-like accumulations of fluid develop as a secondary effect of other disease processes, which causes areas of raised, elevated retinal detachment. Signs and symptoms of serous retinal detachment include reduced vision, flashing lights (photopsia), vitreous floaters, and no light perception. Use this code for retinal detachment NOS or retinal detachment without retinal break.

H33.3- Retinal breaks without detachment

Included in this subcategory are retinal defects such as tears, holes, and breaks that are not associated with detachment. A retinal defect is a pathological imperfection of the retina. Although retinal defects can precipitate retinal detachments, these codes report retinal defects that are not associated with retinal detachment at the time the patient seeks medical care. The pathogenesis of retinal holes and breaks classified to this subcategory include tension or traction on the retina by the vitreous, resulting in a weakening of the tissues and thus the retinal defect. Some retinal defects, such as horseshoe tears, are described in accordance with their appearance upon physical exam.

H33.31- Horseshoe tear of retina without detachment

A horseshoe tear occurs when a flap of retina separates from the posterior vitreous retina creating a crescent-shaped defect. Horseshoe tears are large retinal defects that can cause significant disruption of sight. Horseshoe defects that are identified early may be corrected to prevent impending retinal detachment. Untreated, the horseshoe tear may progress to a retinal detachment.

H33.32- Round hole of retina without detachment

A round or oval hole appears as a deep reddish spot with an overlying retinal defect. Round hole defects allow passage of fluid between the sensory retina and the retinal pigmented epithelium. Retinal detachments may occur anywhere in the retina where a hole or tear is located.

H33.4- Traction detachment of retinas

Traction detachment of the retina is caused by scar tissue formation or other abnormal tissue growth on the retina that pulls the retina away from the underlying retinal pigment epithelium (RPE) by tractional (gravitational) forces. Traction retinal detachment is characteristically localized along the vasculature and typically does not extend to the ora serrata, the front edge of the retina. However, traction detachment can occur at any location including the macula. Mild traction detachment may not affect vision and may not need immediate repair, but those involving the macula require immediate repair to

restore central vision. Traction detachment is a frequent complication of proliferative diabetic retinopathy, ocular trauma, and retinopathy of prematurity.

H34.- Retinal vascular occlusions

Retinal vascular occlusion occurs when a blood vessel supplying the retina becomes blocked, limiting the supply of nutrients delivered and waste removal from the area. When this happens, the retina does not adequately filter light, leading to vision loss. The level of vision loss depends on where the blockage is located. This condition can lead to serious complications, particularly if atherosclerosis is present. The symptoms may present as blurred vision or partial to complete vision loss that typically affects one eye with limited or permanent duration depending on the length of time before treatment in addition to any contributing conditions.

H34.0- Transient retinal artery occlusion

While transient indicates a temporary condition with no permanent deficiency, the condition requires medical attention to prevent possible future complications or visual emergencies. The codes reported from this subcategory apply to the retinal artery.

H34.1- Central retinal artery occlusion

Central artery occlusion causes permanent, and often significant, vision loss in most patients. The codes from this subcategory apply when the occlusion is within the main artery leading to the retina.

H34.21- Partial retinal artery occlusion

Partial retinal artery occlusion, also referred to as Hollenhorst's plaque or retinal microembolism, is essentially a small stroke within the retinal artery from emboli leading to vision loss in only a portion of the visual field. Immediate medical intervention is required; however only 21 percent to 35 percent of patients are able to retain optimal vision. This condition tends to be a precursor to other systemic conditions, which require quick evaluation.

H34.23- Retinal artery branch occlusion

A branch retinal artery occlusion (BRAO) occurs when the blockage is located within one of the branches split off from the ophthalmic artery after it runs through the optic disc and enters the inner layers of the retina. This is generally seen as a secondary condition to an embolus that has moved from an original, larger vessel and gets lodged in the retinal artery branch. The occlusion often occurs at the bifurcation point due to the narrowing of the lumen in that area. These occlusions are reported within the temporal retinal vessels for 90 percent of the incidents and present with a painless and more focal vision impairment. Patients with these types of retinal artery branch occlusions are at a higher risk for mortality due to the primary condition of cardiovascular or cerebrovascular disease. Vasospasm from migraines, drug use, or certain infectious or inflammatory conditions is also a known cause of BRAO.

H34.81- Central retinal vein occlusion

Central retinal vein occlusion (CRVO) indicates a blockage within the main vein for the retina, weakening the walls of the vein and allowing blood and fluid to spill over into the retina. Blurry vision occurs with fluid accumulation in the macula. There are two types of CRVO: nonischemic is less serious and is most often the case with this diagnosis; or ischemic, which is the more serious condition because of more complications such as macular edema, vision loss, and potentially the loss of the entire eye itself.

Focus Point

This subcategory of codes requires a seventh character to indicate if macular edema or retinal neovascularization is present or if the condition is stable and/or related to an old central vein occlusion. Macular edema is fluid buildup in the retina that is common to this condition; retinal neovascularization refers to the formation of new, abnormal vessels within the retina.

H34.82- Venous engorgement

Venous engorgement is when the vessels become congested with fluid, such as blood. This subcategory includes incipient, or partial, retinal vein occlusion, which can indicate a risk for developing central retinal vein occlusion (CRVO). Some studies refer to venous engorgement as impending central retinal vein occlusion; however, this symptom has not been proven to be directly related to developing the more serious condition.

H34.83- Tributary (branch) retinal vein occlusion

Branch retinal vein occlusion (BRVO) is diagnosed when the blockage is located within a smaller vein of the retina. This typically happens when atherosclerosis of the retinal arteries increase the pressure on a retinal vein. Pressure that progresses to occlusion of a retinal vein can lead to necrosis of the nerve cells in the eye.

Focus Point

This subcategory of codes requires a seventh character to indicate if macular edema or retinal neovascularization is present or if the condition is stable and/or related to an old branch occlusion. Macular edema is fluid buildup in the retina that is common to this condition; retinal neovascularization refers to the formation of new, abnormal vessels within the retina.

H35.- Other retinal disorders

This category includes retinopathy, which is any noninflammatory degenerative disease of the retina, retinopathy of prematurity, and other retinal vascular and degenerative disorders.

H35.0- Background retinopathy and retinal vascular changes

Background retinopathy is characterized by the formation of microaneurysms, hemorrhages, and hard exudates. Microaneurysms represent weakened blood vessels that are prone to rupture and hemorrhage. Exudates are areas of hardened protein and lipid deposits caused by damaged retinal vasculature. Although background retinopathy is most commonly associated with early diabetic ophthalmic complications, it may be idiopathic in nature or due to other causal conditions.

H35.00 Unspecified background retinopathy

This code includes retinal sclerosis, which is described as a "hardening" of the retinal vessels.

Focus Point

Diabetic background retinopathy is not included in this category. Codes for diabetic retinal disorders are located in Chapter 4 Endocrine, Nutritional and Metabolic Diseases.

H35.02- Exudative retinopathy

Exudative retinopathy is a degenerative condition characterized by masses of white or yellowish exudate (lipid or protein deposits) in the posterior part of the fundus oculi. It is often associated with areas of retinal hemorrhage and progressive vision loss. Coat's disease is a progressive familial form of exudative retinopathy that primarily affects the retinal capillaries, causing progressive loss of central vision. Incidence is most common among male children or young male adults.

H35.03- Hypertensive retinopathy

Hypertensive retinopathy is a condition in which retinal irregularities occur as a result of systemic hypertensive disease. Retinal manifestations of hypertension are usually attributed to severe, long-standing, or poorly controlled hypertension. Initial signs include swelling or dilation of retinal arterioles accompanied by retrovenous irregularities. Patients with malignant or accelerated hypertension can exhibit extensive retinopathy with hemorrhage, infarction, optic disk edema, and retinal detachment. Precipitous blood pressure reduction can have a negative impact, resulting in further damage.

H35.04- Retinal micro-aneurysms, unspecified

Retinal microaneurysms are microscopic dilations of the retinal vessels. On exam, they appear as small, darkened red spots on the retinal surface. They are commonly associated with capillary occlusion and retinal ischemia, which are contributing factors in the progression of retinopathy.

H35.05- Retinal neovascularization, unspecified

Retinal neovascularization is the process in which new abnormal vascular growth occurs in the retina. These new vessels may spontaneously grow and proliferate in the retina improving the blood flow in tissue compromised due to other disease processes. However, where neovascularization bleeds into the vitreous, severe vision loss can occur.

H35.06- Retinal vasculitis

Retinal vasculitis is inflammation of the retinal blood vessels. It may be associated with primary ocular conditions or inflammatory or infectious diseases in other parts of the body.

H35.07- Retinal telangiectasis

Retinal telangiectasia is the dilation of retinal blood vessels. Although dilation of retinal vasculature may be idiopathic in origin, it is usually caused by an underlying disease process or represents a progression of a separate, primary ophthalmic disease.

H35.09 Other intraretinal microvascular abnormalities

This code includes retinal varices, which often heralds the presence of an underlying ocular or systemic disease process. Retinal varices are varicose veins of the retina characterized by dilation and tortuosity. This condition can result in impaired retinovascular circulation and precede complications such as hemorrhage and thrombosis.

H35.1- Retinopathy of prematurity

Retinopathy of prematurity (ROP) is a serious vasoproliferative disorder involving the developing retina in premature infants and is a leading cause of blindness in children. In ROP, the ocular vessels fail to grow or develop normally, resulting in fragile, weak, abnormal vasculature that is prone to bleeding. Preemies that are routinely treated with supplemental oxygen therapy for hypoxemia associated with delayed lung maturation and breathing gas mixtures containing high levels of oxygen for a prolonged period are at risk for injury to the retina. O_2 therapy is a significant risk factor for the development of ROP. While mild forms may regress without affecting visual function, severe forms of ROP can lead to progressive vision loss due to retinal scarring and damage. When ROP becomes severe it usually requires intervention, such as retinal photocoagulation. Retinal detachment is a common complication of late-stage ROP, which can

result in blindness. Early detection and treatment can improve outcomes; however, many preterm infants, especially those with extreme prematurity, will develop some level of ROP. ROP is classified by severity, from stage 0 to stage 5 as follows:

Stage 0:	Immature vasculature of the retina
Stage I:	Mildly abnormal blood vessel growth
Stage II:	Moderately abnormal blood vessel growth
Stage III:	Severely abnormal blood vessel growth
Stage IV:	Severely abnormal blood vessel growth with a partially detached retina
Stage V:	Total retinal detachment

H35.17- Retrolental fibroplasia

Retrolental fibroplasia is a disease of fibrous tissue in the vitreous, from retinal to lens, causing blindness. It is associated with premature infants requiring high amounts of oxygen. This code represents cicatricial end-stage retinopathy of prematurity in which the damaged retina is irreversibly scarred.

H35.3- Degeneration of macula and posterior pole

The macula is part of the posterior pole of the globe and is the central part of the retina that provides the sharp, central vision. This acute central vision is integral in discerning fine detail and color. The macula is located on the central portion of the retina surrounding the fovea.

H35.30 Unspecified macular degeneration

Macular degeneration results in the loss of central (sharp-focus) vision. It is the most common cause of visual acuity loss in people older than age 50. Symptoms include blurring (usually in central visual field), dimming of color, and difficulty focusing on close objects and fine detail.

H35.31- Nonexudative age-related macular degeneration

Macular degeneration may be classified as wet (exudative, neovascular) or dry (nonexudative, non-neovascular). The dry form, which is classified here, is the most common. It is the result of a deterioration of the retinal pigment epithelium (RPE) as part of the aging process. The cellular regeneration process of the RPE deteriorates over time. As a result, waste products accumulate and impair vision. The damaged cells become malnourished and fail to send transmit signals effectively to the optic nerve, resulting in blurred vision and blind spots in the central visual field.

H35.32- Exudative age-related macular degeneration

Macular degeneration may be classified as wet (exudative, neovascular) or dry (nonexudative, non-neovascular). The wet form, which is classified here, refers to the leakage caused by fragile, new blood vessels that form beneath the retina. Wet macular degeneration may initially present as the dry form of the disease and progress to the wet form if neovascularization occurs.

H35.34- Macular cyst, hole, or pseudohole

Macular hole is a defect associated with the aging process in which the vitreous thins and separates from the retina, creating tension that causes a hole to form in the central portion of the retina (macula). Although age-related degenerative effects are the most common cause, certain inflammatory eye diseases, infections, or injuries can precipitate creation of a macular defect.

H35.35- Cystoid macular degeneration

Cystoid macular degeneration (CME) is characterized by fluid-filled cyst formation in the macular region with resultant loss of visual acuity. CME is often associated with diabetes, infection (e.g., uveitis), or retinal vein occlusion.

H35.36- Drusen (degenerative) of macula

Drusen (degenerative) consist of white, hyaline deposits on the Bruch's membrane associated with macular degeneration. They are typically the result of accumulation of lipid and protein waste products as part of the aging process.

H35.37- Puckering of macula

Macular puckering of the retina is a wrinkling of the maculae (central vision area) caused by contraction of scar tissue due to damage or injury to the eye, causing distorted vision.

Glaucoma (H40-H42)

Glaucoma is a group of eye diseases that share several common traits. In most cases there is increased intraocular pressure (IOP) that when left untreated, results in optic nerve damage with subsequent vision loss. The optic nerve delivers images from the retina to the brain. When optic nerve fibers become damaged, visual field defects consisting of blind spots develop. As more damage occurs to the optic nerve, more visual field defects develop and the glaucoma can lead to blindness.

The categories in this code block are as follows:

| H40 | Glaucoma |
| H42 | Glaucoma in diseases classified elsewhere |

H40.- Glaucoma

Glaucoma is a group of eye diseases that share several common traits. In most cases, there is increased intraocular pressure (IOP) that causes optic nerve damage with subsequent vision loss. The optic nerve delivers images from the retina to the brain. When optic nerve fibers become damaged, visual field defects consisting of blind spots develop. As more damage occurs to the optic nerve, more visual field defects develop and, left untreated, can lead to blindness. Glaucoma is classified into glaucoma suspect; open angle, which includes primary open angle glaucoma; primary angle-closure glaucoma; secondary glaucoma, which includes specific codes for glaucoma secondary to eye trauma, eye inflammations, eye disorders, and drugs; and other glaucoma. Glaucoma suspect, primary glaucoma, and other glaucoma are classified into multiple subtypes.

Focus Point

Most, although not all, glaucoma codes in category H40 specify laterality (right eye, left eye, bilateral eyes), as well as glaucoma stage (unspecified, mild, moderate, severe, indeterminate).

Stage captures the extent of visual field loss and changes in the optic disc, which is the intraocular portion of the optic nerve that is visible on eye exam. Optic disc changes seen in glaucoma are thinning of the neuroretinal rim (outer aspect of the optic nerve containing nerve fiber/neuroretinal tissue) with corresponding enlargement of the cup (inner aspect of the optic nerve that contains no nerve fiber/neuroretinal tissue). Stages are defined as follows:

0	stage unspecified: Stage is not documented
1	mild stage: Early visual field defects but no changes in the optic disc
2	moderate stage: Increased visual field loss with an arc-shaped blind spot (arcuate scotoma) and evidence of neuroretinal thinning
3	severe stage: Marked visual field loss including loss of central vision with extensive neuroretinal thinning
4	indeterminate stage: Stage cannot be determined

More than one glaucoma code may be required to accurately identify the type of glaucoma, the eye affected, and the glaucoma stage. Refer to the Official Guidelines for Coding and Reporting in the ICD-10-CM code book for rules related to glaucoma diagnoses.

H40.0-   Glaucoma suspect

A diagnosis of glaucoma suspect indicates that an individual has risk factors for glaucoma but does not currently have optic nerve damage or visual field defects normally associated with glaucoma. The individual may have an open angle with borderline findings, an anatomical narrow angle, elevated intraocular pressure (IOP) without associated optic nerve damage (ocular hypertension), elevated IOP due to steroid use (steroid responder), or angle closure without associated optic nerve damage.

H40.00-   Preglaucoma, unspecified

Preglaucoma is synonymous with the terms glaucoma suspect and borderline glaucoma. A diagnosis of preglaucoma indicates that the individual has risk factors for glaucoma but does not currently have optic nerve damage or visual field defects normally associated with glaucoma. Use this code only when the specific risk factor associated with a diagnosis of preglaucoma is not documented.

> **Focus Point**
>
> *The Alphabetic Index directs the coder to subcategory H40.00- for a diagnosis of open angle with borderline intraocular pressure (IOP). For elevated IOP or ocular hypertension, see subcategory H40.05-.*

H40.01-   Open angle with borderline findings, low risk

H40.02-   Open angle with borderline findings, high risk

In a glaucoma suspect, open angle with borderline findings means that the angle between the iris and cornea through which aqueous humor flows is open but that the intraocular pressure is elevated because of overproduction of aqueous humor or an obstruction in the trabecular meshwork through which the aqueous humor passes before it leaves the eye and enters the bloodstream. Indicators evaluated to determine risk include intraocular pressure (IOP), age, family history, ocular perfusion pressure, blood pressure, central cornea thickness, optic disc changes, cup-to-disc ratio, and visual field tests. The level of risk is determined by the number of risk factors present, as well as the strength of each risk factor.

> **Focus Point**
>
> *The only exception to physician documentation specifically indicating low risk is a diagnosis of open angle glaucoma suspect with cupping of discs without documentation of any additional borderline findings or glaucoma risk factors.*

H40.03-   Anatomical narrow angle

An anatomically narrow angle between the iris and cornea is a risk factor for the development of acute or chronic angle closure glaucoma. In a glaucoma suspect, the anatomically narrow angle is not currently affecting the flow of aqueous humor from the anterior chamber through the angle and trabecular meshwork and into the bloodstream. However, since anatomically narrow angles predispose an individual to the development of glaucoma, these individuals require careful monitoring of intraocular pressure and any other signs or symptoms that might indicate that the flow of aqueous is obstructed. Primary angle closure suspect is also included in this subcategory.

H40.04-   Steroid responder

Glaucoma suspects who are steroid responders experience significant increases in intraocular pressure (IOP) when steroid medications are used. Steroids, also called corticosteroids, are commonly prescribed as antiinflammatory medications for ophthalmic inflammatory conditions, as well as for other types of inflammation, such as asthma. Up to 30 percent of individuals prescribed local or systemic steroids experience increased IOP, which is likely a genetically determined response, although the increase in pressure varies significantly from one individual to the next. The increase in IOP appears to be due to a decrease in outflow of aqueous humor. Once it is determined that IOP has risen significantly due to steroid therapy, steroids are typically discontinued unless the risk of not treating the inflammatory condition outweighs the risk of optic nerve damage from the steroid medication. If the steroid medication cannot be discontinued, the increase in IOP is treated with eye drops for glaucoma or, in rare cases, surgery may be performed. When the steroid medication is discontinued, IOP typically returns to normal in a steroid responder, although it may take several weeks during which time eye drops for glaucoma are typically administered to reduce IOP.

> **Focus Point**
>
> *A diagnosis of steroid responder in preglaucoma or a glaucoma suspect differs from a diagnosis of glaucoma due to steroids. A steroid responder does not have a diagnosis of glaucoma or evidence of optic nerve damage due to the elevated IOP. For a diagnosis of glaucoma due to steroids, see subcategory H40.6- Glaucoma secondary to drugs.*

H40.05-   Ocular hypertension

Intraocular pressure above 21 mm Hg is the definitive characteristic of ocular hypertension, which may also be called intraocular hypertension. A glaucoma suspect with ocular hypertension shows no evidence of optic nerve damage and no visual field abnormalities. The optic disc and optic nerve fibers appear normal on eye exam and special testing reveals a normal appearing open angle between the iris and the cornea. In addition, there are no other eye conditions that could contribute to the elevated intraocular pressure, such as neovascular disease or inflammation of the uvea. Ocular hypertension may be present in only one eye or may be bilateral.

Focus Point

Other terms indicating ocular hypertension in preglaucoma or glaucoma suspect include increased intraocular pressure (IOP) or elevated IOP. For open angle with borderline intraocular pressure, use a code from subcategory H40.00-.

H40.06- Primary angle closure without glaucoma damage

In primary angle closure without glaucoma damage there is typically an anatomic narrow angle with evidence of trabecular obstruction at the peripheral aspect of the iris, but no evidence of damage to the optic nerve. Along with elevation of intraocular pressure (IOP), there is typically evidence of trabecular obstruction, which may include the presence of adhesions, also called synechiae, in the peripheral aspect of the iris; a characteristic whorled or spiral pattern in the iris indicative of obstruction; atrophy of the iris; and/or increased pigmentation of the trabecular surface.

H40.1- Open-angle glaucoma

Open angle glaucoma is the most common type of glaucoma. It is characterized by a normal open angle between the iris and cornea, but there is overproduction of aqueous humor or an obstruction in the trabecular meshwork through which the aqueous humor passes before it leaves the eye and enters the bloodstream causing an increase in intraocular pressure with damage to the optic nerve. The subtypes of open angle glaucoma include primary open angle, low tension, pigmentary, capsular with pseudoexfoliation of the lens, and residual stage.

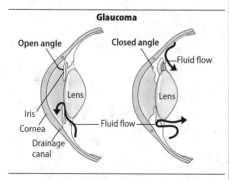

Glaucoma

Open angle — Closed angle

Fluid flow

Lens — Lens

Iris
Cornea — Fluid flow
Drainage canal

H40.11- Primary open-angle glaucoma

Open angle glaucoma is the most common type of glaucoma and primary open angle glaucoma (POAG) is the most common of all the subtypes accounting for about 70 percent of all glaucoma cases. POAG is characterized by high IOP and damage to the optic nerve despite a normal open angle between the iris and cornea. Damage to the optic nerve is believed to occur due to loss of function in the trabecular meshwork through which the aqueous humor passes before it leaves the eye and enters the bloodstream. There is typically no identifiable damage to the trabecular meshwork evident on examination of the eyes, and it is believed that the changes responsible for the impaired drainage of aqueous humor occur at the cellular level possibly due to structural changes or an enzyme disorder. Symptoms include gradual, progressive loss of peripheral vision, blurred or foggy vision, reduced night vision, and halo visual effects. Pain, especially during the initial stages, is rare. POAG is a chronic eye disease that requires lifelong treatment to prevent additional optic nerve damage and preserve sight.

H40.12- Low-tension glaucoma

In low-tension glaucoma, also called normal tension or normal pressure glaucoma, damage to the optic nerve occurs in the absence of elevated intraocular pressure (IOP). The reasons for susceptibility of the optic nerve to damage even with normal IOP, is not well understood. Risk factors for low-tension glaucoma include a family history of low-tension glaucoma, Japanese ancestry, and certain heart conditions, such as arrhythmias. Low-tension glaucoma is diagnosed based on visualization of the optic nerve and visual field testing. The optic nerve shows evidence of damage such as thinning of the neuroretinal rim and cupping of the optic disc and the visual field examination shows loss of peripheral vision. Treatment involves topical measures to lower eye pressure using medicated eye drops, glaucoma surgery, or both.

H40.2- Primary angle-closure glaucoma

Primary angle closure glaucoma is a progressive optic disease associated with high intraocular pressure that can lead to irreversible vision loss. The aqueous humor is the clear fluid filling the chambers of the eye that is continually drained and renewed, produced by the ciliary body and passing out through the pupil and trabecular meshwork. Angle closure glaucoma causes an increase in intraocular pressure due to an impairment of aqueous outflow caused by a narrowing or closing of the anterior chamber angle as the iris comes into contact with the trabecular meshwork.

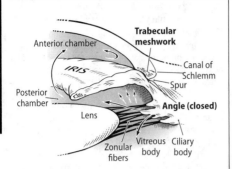

H40.21- Acute angle-closure glaucoma

Acute angle closure glaucoma is a rare form of glaucoma characterized by sudden onset of narrowing of the angle between the iris and cornea resulting in obstruction of the flow of aqueous humor, rapid increase in intraocular pressure, and high risk of blindness that can occur in as little as three to five days.

H40.22- Chronic angle-closure glaucoma

Plateau iris associated with glaucoma is classified here. Plateau iris is an important cause of chronic angle closure glaucoma that most commonly affects patients younger than 50 years of age. The cause and effect mechanism is due to a large or anteriorly positioned ciliary body that alters the position of the peripheral iris, pushing it forward against the trabecular meshwork. Some degree of pupillary block is usually present, whereby the edges of the iris that form the pupil push against the lens, obstructing the flow of aqueous humor from the posterior chamber to the anterior chamber. The increased intraocular pressure between the anterior and posterior chambers results in acute angle closure glaucoma.

> **Focus Point**
>
> *Plateau iris syndrome is a postoperative condition that increases the risk of glaucoma and is reported with code H21.82.*

Disorders of the Vitreous Body and Globe (H43-H44)

The globe of the eye refers to the hollow wall that forms the eyeball. The vitreous body is the clear fluid behind the eye lens that contains collagen fibers.

The categories in this code block are as follows:

H43	Disorders of the vitreous body
H44	Disorders of the globe

> **Focus Point**
>
> *Laterality is a component of most codes in this code block.*

H43.- Disorders of vitreous body

The vitreous body is the clear fluid behind the eye lens that contains collagen fibers. Its primary functions include supporting the architecture of the eye and its contents and providing an unobstructed path for light to reach the retina.

H43.1- Vitreous hemorrhage

Vitreous hemorrhage occurs when blood escapes into the vitreous area, typically from surrounding blood vessels within the eye. This usually accompanies an underlying condition such as proliferative diabetic retinopathy, but can be the result of trauma to the eye.

H43.3- Other vitreous opacities

Floaters, strands, and vitreous membranes are included here. Strands and vitreous membranes have a specific code while floaters are included in the other specified subcategory. Vitreous opacities are common findings that occur over time, causing visual disturbances that appear as specks or strands in the visual field. These may be caused by condensations of collagen due to aging, blood from a retinal tear, or even glial tissue tear near the optic nerve.

H43.81- Vitreous degeneration

Vitreous degeneration (detachment) is a normal condition associated with the aging process. The vitreous shrinks over time and pulls away from the retina. It commonly occurs in people older than age 50. Those who are nearsighted have an increased risk. It typically does not affect sight; however, there are cases where significant changes in symptoms warrant additional testing.

H43.82- Vitreomacular adhesion

Vitreomacular adhesion (VMA) is a potentially sight-threatening condition affecting the macula, the small portion of the retina that contains the fovea, an avascular area responsible for visual acuity. It is commonly associated with age-related macular degeneration and diabetic retinopathy. As a natural result of the aging process, the vitreous gel pulls or collapses away from the retina, resulting in posterior vitreous detachment (PVD). Subsequently, the collagen fibers that comprise the vitreous cavity condense and form bands of dense, fibrous tissue (adhesions). These adhesions cause the vitreous gel to pull on the retina, distorting vision and damaging the retinal tissue.

H44.- Disorders of globe

Disorders classified here affect multiple structures of the eye and include inflammatory conditions such as endophthalmitis, degenerative conditions such as degenerative myopia, atrophy, and retained foreign bodies.

H44.0- Purulent endophthalmitis

Purulent endophthalmitis is an inflammation of the tissues and internal structures of the eye due to an infectious process. The infection may be acute, subacute, or chronic. It is separated into two distinct types: endogenous (internal cause) and exogenous (external cause). Endogenous endophthalmitis results from the hematogenous spread of organisms from a distant source of infection such as endocarditis. Exogenous endophthalmitis results from direct inoculation, such as foreign bodies and/or ocular trauma. Necrosis of intraocular tumors, retained intraocular foreign bodies, and fungi can also cause purulent endophthalmitis. Purulent endophthalmitis is characterized by white nodules on the lens capsule, iris, retina, or choroid, with inflammation of all of the ocular tissues, resulting in a globe of full, purulent exudates. Inflammation can spread to the orbital soft tissue. Symptoms may include acute pain, redness, lid swelling, decreased visual acuity, headache, photophobia, and ocular discharge.

> **Focus Point**
>
> Postoperative endophthalmitis is not included here. For postoperative purulent panophthalmitis, see code T81.4- Infection following a procedure. For noninfectious (sterile) endophthalmitis resulting from retained native lens material after an operation, see subcategory H59.02- Cataract lens fragments in eye following cataract eye surgery. For infection of postprocedural bleb, see subcategory H59.4- Inflammation (infection) postprocedural bleb.

H44.01- Panophthalmitis (acute)

Panophthalmitis is acute inflammation or infection of the inner structures of the eye with necrosis of the sclera, which may extend into the orbit. It is often accompanied by severe ocular pain, with risk of globe rupture. It often originates as an inflammation of the inner eye that affects all layers of the eye. Etiologies include penetrating eye injury or an extension of a systemic or other generalized infection.

H44.02- Vitreous abscess (chronic)

Vitreous abscess is an abscess of the vitreous humor (the transparent, colorless, soft gelatinous material filling the eyeball behind the lens) of the eye due to infection, trauma, or foreign body. Vitreous abscess is confined to the vitreous body. It may result from intraocular infection or foreign body reaction.

H44.1- Other endophthalmitis

Endophthalmitis is inflammation of the tissues and internal structures of the eye and, in this case, the inflammation is not due to an infection. Panuveitis, parasitic endophthalmitis, and sympathetic uveitis are conditions included in this subcategory that have specific codes.

> **Focus Point**
>
> For endophthalmitis that is due to cysticercosis, see code B69.1; onchocerciasis, see B73.01, or toxocariasis, see B83.0.

H44.11- Panuveitis

Uveitis is an inflammation (swelling and irritation) of the uvea. The uvea extends toward the front of the eye and consists of the iris, choroid layer, and ciliary body. Panuveitis is inflammation of the entire vascular layer of the eye, which includes the retina and vitreous humor along with the uvea. It is a vision-threatening disease. The inflammation may be due to a chronic inflammatory disease, such as a systemic rheumatologic disorder. However, the cause is often unknown.

H44.12- Parasitic endophthalmitis, unspecified

Parasitic endophthalmitis is an infection of the eye due to invasion by a parasitic microorganism. Parasitic infections of the eye arise from direct exposure to the parasite by contamination or following blood-borne transportation to the eye or adjacent structures. There are multiple possible parasites that can invade the eye. Only parasitic endophthalmitis where the specific parasitic organism is not known or not documented is reported here.

H44.13- Sympathetic uveitis

Uveitis is an inflammation (swelling and irritation) of the uvea and can lead to permanent vision loss. The uvea extends toward the front of the eye and consists of the iris, choroid layer, and ciliary body. Sympathetic uveitis, also called sympathetic ophthalmia, is a rare form of uveitis that occurs in the uninjured eye following a penetrating injury, surgery, or irradiation to the opposite eye. It is potentially a vision-threatening disease. The onset of sympathetic ophthalmia is usually two weeks to three months following ocular injury or interventional surgical or other procedure.

H44.2- Degenerative myopia

Myopia (near-sightedness) is a type of refractive error in which objects can be readily seen when close to the eye, but out of focus when distant. Degenerative myopia is a rare type of severe myopia that has progressed to such an extent that it causes degenerative changes in the eye, such as retinal damage and staphyloma formation. Central vision loss occurs most commonly in degenerative myopia, with the peripheral vision less affected. The degenerative component is a result of the associated stretching and thinning of the structures of the eye, particularly in the macula (central retina), retinal epithelium, and choroid. Thinning causes the structures to weaken (e.g., degenerate), increasing susceptibility to damage. Degenerative myopia may also be described as progressive high, malignant, pathological, or pernicious. Other descriptors for degenerative myopia include Fuchs' black (myopic) spots, Terry's syndrome, myopic changes in retina, and progressive myopic chorioretinitis.

H44.2A- Degenerative myopia with choroidal neovascularization

This code reports degenerative myopia that also includes a process called choroidal neovascularization. This occurs when new abnormal vascular growth occurs beneath the retina. These new vessels may spontaneously grow and proliferate in the retina improving the blood flow in tissue compromised due to other disease processes. However, where neovascularization bleeds into the vitreous, severe vision loss can occur.

H44.2B- Degenerative myopia with macular hole

This code is used when the progression of degenerative myopia includes a defect in which the vitreous thins and separates from the retina, creating tension that causes a hole to form in the central portion of the retina (macula).

H44.2C- Degenerative myopia with retinal detachment

Degenerative myopia which includes retinal detachment is reported with this combination code. This retinal detachment is the separation of the retina from the underlying retinal pigment epithelium (RPE) which progressed over time due to the degenerative process.

H44.2D- Degenerative myopia with foveoschisis

This excessive progression of high myopia causes foveoschisis, which is the accumulation of fluid in the macula from the stretching and tearing of the retinal layers. This is often difficult to detect until vision loss occurs.

H44.4- Hypotony of eye

Hypotony of the eye is a functional defect of low intraocular pressure (IOP) that can occur as a primary condition or secondary to other ophthalmic disease or injury. Normal IOP is between 10 and 20 mm Hg (millimeters of mercury). Hypotony of the eye is an IOP of 10 mm Hg, although it may not be considered problematic until the pressure drops below 6 mm Hg. Prolonged low pressure can result in distortion and degeneration of the chorioretinal vascular, cornea, and optic disc. Causal factors for hypotony include postsurgical wound leak, inflammatory eye diseases, and chorioretinal detachments. In the past, hypotony was a common complication of trabeculectomy procedures used to treat glaucoma. However, advances in surgical technique have rendered incidence to minimal, although leakage around the scleral flap incision occasionally occurs. Certain eye conditions, such as chronic inflammations and retinal defects, may alter the osmotic state of the eye, resulting in hypotony. Stabilization of IOP on secondary hypotony requires treatment of the underlying condition.

H44.41- Flat anterior chamber hypotony of eye

Flat anterior chamber hypotony is low intraocular pressure in the anterior chamber of the eye, which is the region behind the cornea, causing compression of anterior structures.

H44.42- Hypotony of eye due to ocular fistula

Low intraocular pressure can result from a leak due to fistula development following surgery or injury to the eye.

H44.43- Hypotony of eye due to other ocular disorders

Certain eye conditions, such as chronic inflammations and retinal defects, may alter the osmotic state of the eye, resulting in hypotony.

H44.44- Primary hypotony of eye

Primary hypotony of the eye is low intraocular pressure without an apparent underlying cause.

H44.5- Degenerated conditions of globe

Degenerative conditions classified here include absolute glaucoma, atrophy of the globe, and leucocoria (leukocoria).

H44.51- Absolute glaucoma

Absolute glaucoma is the final stage of glaucoma in which there is complete vision loss. A predisposing factor to the development of absolute glaucoma is untreated ocular hypertension, which is why the term blind hypertensive eye was used to describe the condition, although that term is now outdated. Ocular hypertension may be defined as an IOP greater than 24 mm Hg, with absolute glaucoma representing vision loss due to the severity and progression of ocular hypertension. It is associated with eye pain and is characterized by a stone-like appearance of the eye. Blind hypertensive eye represents the end stage of intraocular hypertensive disease, whereby the ocular structures have sustained irreparable damage.

H44.52- Atrophy of globe

Atrophy of the globe, also called phthisis bulbi, describes vision loss due to extremely low intraocular pressure (IOP). Atrophy of the globe occurs when disease or damage causes the ciliary body to cease producing aqueous fluid, resulting in a loss of IOP (hypotony). Prolonged low pressure can result in distortion and degeneration of the chorioretinal vascular layer, cornea, and optic disc. Characteristics of the atrophy of the globe include a small, shrunken globe with marked thickening of the sclera, metaplasia of the retinal pigment epithelium, displacement or atrophy of the intraocular contents, and ossification. Atrophy of the globe is an end-stage severity presentation of ocular hypotony characterized by a soft, atrophic, and nonfunctional eye.

H44.53- Leucocoria

Leucocoria is an abnormal reflection from the retina that causes the pupil to appear white instead of black. The condition may be obvious on casual observation or may only be detected under certain circumstances, such as when the pupil is dilated in a darkened room. In some cases, the condition is only noted on photographs, when instead of both eyes reflecting back red as seen in "red eye," one reflects back red and the other white. One or both eyes may be affected. Leucocoria can indicate the presence of congenital cataracts, neoplasm, retrolental fibroplasia, retinal detachment, infection, or other congenital or acquired eye disorders. Leucocoria is a significant finding in retinoblastoma, a potentially life-threatening malignancy and the most common ocular malignancy in childhood. Treatment is dependent upon the nature of the underlying condition.

H44.6- Retained (old) intraocular foreign body, magnetic

H44.7- Retained (old) intraocular foreign body, nonmagnetic

A retained intraocular foreign body is the result of an old penetrating injury to the eye where a foreign body remains in the intraocular structures. The presence of an intraocular foreign body may not be readily apparent following initial trauma. Some injuries are self-sealing, concealing the foreign body from clinical detection. Retained foreign bodies may remain relatively asymptomatic depending on location, size, composition, and nature of the initial injury. However, some foreign bodies develop late sequelae or complicating conditions over time. The greatest risk for retained foreign body is the development of potentially sight-threatening infections (e.g., uveitis,

endophthalmitis). Other complications include aqueous leakage, hypotony, impaired visual acuity, scarring, and vitreous hemorrhage. Retained intraocular foreign bodies are classified based on whether they are magnetic or nonmagnetic and then by site. Retained foreign bodies are subclassified first by type as magnetic (e.g., metal fragments) or nonmagnetic (e.g. plastic, wood, glass, or stone) and then by site. Laterality is also a component of the code.

H44.8- Other disorders of globe

Only two conditions are classified in this subcategory: hemophthalmos and luxation of the globe.

H44.82- Luxation of globe

Luxation of the globe (eyeball) is displacement or dislocation of the eye from its normal anatomic position. The mechanism of luxation occurs when the midline of the globe protrudes beyond the eyelids. The orbicularis muscle may contract, often causing further anterior displacement. This code reports only nontraumatic luxation. Spontaneous globe luxation occurring without conscious effort or precipitating factor is rare. More often luxation is precipitated by eyelid manipulation (e.g., contact lens insertion, foreign body removal). Nontraumatic luxation may also occur in patients with exophthalmos, space-occupying orbital lesions or conditions, and anomalous shallow orbits. Another type of nontraumatic luxation can occur voluntarily. Voluntary luxation describes an individual's ability to dislocate the globe at will. Medical care may be sought, however, if the individual is unable to successfully reduce the dislocation, due to blepharospasm or other involuntary muscle response.

Disorders of Optic Nerve and Visual Pathways (H46-H47)

The optic nerve is the extent of the visual system pathway from the back of the eyeball up to the optic chiasm. It contains axons of ganglion cells in the retina of the ipsilateral (i.e., same side) eye. Each optic nerve splits and half of its fibers cross over to the other side at the optic chiasm. If the optic nerve is damaged between an eyeball and the optic chiasm, the person may become blind in that eye. If the problem lies farther back in the optic nerve pathway, both eyes may lose half of the visual fields, a condition called hemianopia. If both eyes lose peripheral vision, the cause may be damage at the optic chiasm. If both eyes lose half of the visual field on the same side, the cause is usually damage to the optic nerve pathway on the opposite side of the brain caused by a stroke, hemorrhage, or tumor. Dysfunction of the optic nerve may be congenital or acquired. If congenital, it is usually hereditary. The acquired type may be due to vascular disturbances, secondary to degenerative retinal disease (e.g., papilledema or optic neuritis), a result of pressure against the optic nerve, or related to metabolic diseases (e.g., diabetes), trauma, glaucoma, or toxicity (e.g., alcohol, tobacco, or other poisons).

The categories in this code block are as follows:

H46	Optic neuritis
H47	Other disorders of optic nerve [2nd] nerve and visual pathways

Focus Point

Laterality is a component of most codes in this code block.

H47.- Other disorders of optic [2nd] nerve and visual pathways

This category covers primarily noninflammatory conditions affecting the optic nerve and visual pathways, including ischemia, hemorrhage, papilledema, optic atrophy, disorders of the optic disc, and chiasm. Also included are disorders of the visual pathways and cortex that include conditions due to inflammation, neoplasm, and vascular disorders.

H47.Ø3- Optic nerve hypoplasia

Optic nerve hypoplasia (ONH) is a condition present at birth in which the optic nerve is not fully developed. Bilateral occurrence is more common than unilateral and is one of the three most common causes of impaired vision in children. ONH is not progressive, nor is it inherited, and it cannot be cured. In the majority of cases, there is no known cause, although studies have indicated that maternal factors such as diabetes, alcohol abuse, use of antiseizure drugs, and young maternal age (2Ø years of age or younger) may be associated with the condition. Characteristics include photophobia, depressed visual fields, impaired depth perception, and nystagmus. Visual function may range from normal visual acuity to the absence of light perception. There may be generalized loss of detailed vision in central and peripheral visual fields, or there may be only subtle peripheral field loss. Visual function may improve minimally as the brain undergoes the maturation process. Diagnosis is made by examination of the optic nerve and observation of its size together with that of the nerve head. Neuroimaging techniques are helpful in diagnosing ONH. There is currently no cure and treatment is generally directed toward the visual difficulties associated with this disorder.

H47.1- Papilledema

Papilledema is swelling of the optic papilla, the raised area connected to the optic disk made up of nerves that enter the eyeball. It may be caused by increased intracranial pressure, decreased ocular pressure, or a retinal disorder. Another cause is Foster-Kennedy syndrome.

H47.11 Papilledema associated with increased intracranial pressure

This condition is caused by pressure within the brain that causes swelling and engorgement of the optic disc and its blood vessels. It may herald a potentially life-threatening condition, although intracranial hypertension can present in the absence of associated papilledema. It usually affects both eyes and may develop over hours or weeks. This code is not to be used in cases documented as disc swelling caused by other underlying conditions such as infection or inflammation.

H47.12 Papilledema associated with decreased ocular pressure

This type of papilledema occurs when the aqueous humor production is out of balance with regular excretions. This condition usually presents as a complication or side effect of another ocular disorder.

H47.13 Papilledema associated with retinal disorder

Papilledema associated with retinal disorders is reserved for use when swelling accompanies a specific condition affecting the retina.

H47.14- Foster-Kennedy syndrome

Foster Kennedy syndrome is a constellation of findings characterized by symptoms of central scotoma, optic disc atrophy in one eye, with papilledema of the other eye due to optic nerve compression and increased intracranial pressure due to associated CNS mass or neoplasm. The condition may occur in one or both eyes.

Disorders of Ocular Muscles, Binocular Movement, Accommodation and Refraction (H49-H52)

There are six ocular muscles including the superior rectus, responsible for upward eye motion; inferior rectus, responsible for downward eye movement; lateral rectus, responsible for eye movement away from the center of the body; medial rectus, responsible for eye movement toward the center of the body; superior oblique, responsible for upward and medial movement of the eye; and inferior oblique, responsible for upward and lateral movement of the eye. These muscles all work together to provide the complex coordinated eye movement of both the eyes.

Binocular movement and fixation is necessary to see three-dimensionally and to aid in depth perception. A visual defect in which the two eyes fail to work together results in a partial or total loss of binocular depth perception and stereoscopic vision. At least 12 percent of the population has some type of binocular vision disability, of which amblyopia and strabismus are the most common.

Accommodation refers to the ability of the eye to alter focus and see objects clearly when switching from seeing things at a distance to seeing things that are closer. Accommodation also includes the ability of both eyes to adjust to change in the printed word at various distances and to different print sizes. Presbyopia, an age-related condition affecting near focus, is a type of accommodation disorder.

Refraction is the ability of the lens of the eye to deflect, reflect, bend, and absorb light rays off objects to create a clear and precise point of focus. Disorders of refraction include myopia (near-sightedness), hypermetropia (far-sightedness), and astigmatism.

The categories in this code block are as follows:

H49	Paralytic strabismus
H50	Other strabismus
H51	Other disorders of binocular movement
H52	Disorders of refraction and accommodation

Focus Point

Laterality is a component of most codes in this code block.

H49.- Paralytic strabismus

Strabismus disorders relate to the eyes inability to coordinate focus in the same direction due to conditions affecting the muscles controlling this function. These disorders are often inherited, but some cases are a result of paresis or due to underlying anomalies, classified as paralytic strabismus. Paralytic strabismus originates in the three cranial nerves (III, IV, VI) responsible for eye movement, which can be weak or palsied. Paralytic strabismus codes caused by single nerve palsy are specific to the affected nerve. Other specific types in this category include total external ophthalmoplegia, progressive external ophthalmoplegia, and Kearns-Sayre syndrome.

H49.0- Third [oculomotor] nerve palsy

H49.1- Fourth [trochlear] nerve palsy

H49.2- Sixth [abducent] nerve palsy

The third cranial nerve is responsible for the majority of eye motion. Only two eye motions are generated by other cranial nerves. Lateral abduction eye motion controlled by the lateral rectus eye muscle is generated by the sixth cranial nerve. Downward and inward eye motion controlled by the superior oblique eye muscle is generated by the fourth cranial nerve. Codes in this range are specific to the cranial nerve affected by the nerve palsy. One or both eyes may be affected.

H50.- Other strabismus

Strabismus disorders classified under other strabismus relate to the eyes inability to coordinate movement and focus in the same direction due to conditions affecting the muscles controlling these functions. The strabismus disorders classified here are often inherited and include esotropia, exotropia, vertical strabismus, as well as others.

H50.0- Esotropia

Esotropia is a form of strabismus, also described as convergent concomitant, in which the eye turns inward toward the nose. Convergent refers to eye movement inward toward the nose. Concomitant means the inequality between the eyes remains the same no matter which direction the eyes are focused. Tropias are visually noticeable misalignments that the brain cannot correct.

H50.01- Monocular esotropia

H50.02- Monocular esotropia with A pattern

H50.03- Monocular esotropia with V pattern

H50.04- Monocular esotropia with other noncomitancies

In monocular esotropia, only one eye is affected or deviates from the norm. Monocular esotropia with A pattern describes the inward deviation of the eye, which is more prominent when looking down as opposed to looking up. It is believed to be due to a superior oblique overaction. Monocular esotropia with V pattern describes the inward deviation of the eye, which is more prominent when looking up as opposed to looking down. It is believed to be due to an inferior oblique overaction. Monocular esotropia that refers to other noncomitancies, such as the X pattern, is an increase in deviation both in an upward and downward direction. This is possibly due to overaction of all four oblique muscles. In the Y pattern, the inward deviation is more prominent in the upward gaze, with conflicting opinions as to which, if any, oblique muscle is responsible for this condition.

H50.05   Alternating esotropia

H50.06   Alternating esotropia with A pattern

H50.07   Alternating esotropia with V pattern

H50.08   Alternating esotropia with other noncomitancies

In alternating esotropia, the affected eye varies or changes depending on the direction of focus. Alternating esotropia is classified based on the pattern of the eye deviation. A pattern describes the inward deviation of the eye, which is more prominent when looking down as opposed to looking up. It is believed to be due to a superior oblique overaction. V pattern describes the inward deviation of the eye, which is more prominent when looking up as opposed to looking down. It is believed to be due to an inferior oblique overaction. Other noncomitancies include X pattern and Y pattern. X pattern is an increase in deviation in an upward and downward direction, possibly due to overaction of all four oblique muscles. In Y pattern, the inward deviation is more prominent in the upward gaze, with conflicting opinions as to which, if any, oblique muscle is responsible for this condition.

H50.1-   Exotropia

Exotropia is a form of strabismus, also described as divergent concomitant, in which the eye turns outward away from the nose. Divergent refers to eye movement outward and away from the nose. Concomitant means the inequality between the eyes remains the same no matter which direction the eyes are focused. Tropias are visually noticeable misalignments that the brain cannot correct.

H50.11-   Monocular exotropia

H50.12-   Monocular exotropia with A pattern

H50.13-   Monocular exotropia with V pattern

H50.14-   Monocular exotropia with other noncomitancies

In monocular exotropia, only one eye is affected or deviates from the norm. A pattern describes outward deviation of the eye, which is more prominent when looking down as opposed to looking up. It is believed to be due to a superior oblique overaction. V pattern describes outward deviation of the eye, which is more prominent when looking up as opposed to looking down. It is believe to be due to an inferior oblique overaction. Other noncomitancies include X pattern and Y pattern. X pattern is an increase in deviation in an upward and downward direction, possibly due to overaction of all four oblique muscles. In Y pattern, the outward deviation is more prominent in the upward gaze, with conflicting opinions as to which, if any, oblique muscle is responsible for this condition.

H50.15   Alternating exotropia

H50.16   Alternating exotropia with A pattern

H50.17   Alternating exotropia with V pattern

H50.18   Alternating exotropia with other noncomitancies

In alternating exotropia, the affected eye varies or changes depending on the direction of focus. Alternating exotropia is classified based on the pattern of the eye deviation. A pattern describes outward deviation of the eye, which is more prominent when looking down as opposed to looking up. It is believed to be due to a superior oblique overaction. V pattern describes outward deviation of the eye, which is more prominent when looking up as opposed to looking down. It is believe to be due to an inferior oblique overaction. Other noncomitancies include X pattern and Y pattern. X pattern is an increase in deviation in an upward and downward direction, possibly due to overaction of all four oblique muscles. In Y pattern, the outward deviation is more prominent in the upward gaze, with conflicting opinions as to which, if any, oblique muscle is responsible for this condition.

H52.-   Disorders of refraction and accommodation

A refractive error occurs due to a disorder among the optical components of the eye (i.e., the curvatures, refractive indices, and distances between the cornea, aqueous, crystalline lens, and vitreous) and the overall axial length of the eye. An accommodation disorder refers to an inability of the eye to alter focus and see objects clearly when switching from seeing things at a distance to seeing things that are closer. Accommodation also includes the ability of both eyes to adjust to change in the printed word at various distances and to different print sizes.

H52.0-   Hypermetropia

In hypermetropia, also called hyperopia, parallel rays of light entering the eye reach a focal point behind the plane of the retina, while accommodation is maintained in a state of relaxation. The additional dioptric power of the converging lenses required to advance the focusing of light rays onto the retina determines the degree of impairment. Corrective lenses may be spherical or spherocylindrical, depending on the nature of the hyperopia and the amount of astigmatic refractive error present.

H52.1-   Myopia

In myopia, parallel light rays from an object are focused in front of the retina, with accommodation relaxed. The term nearsightedness comes from the manifestation, which is blurred distance vision. Correction includes concave spectacle or contact lenses or corneal modification to decrease refractive power. In some cases of pseudomyopia, unaided distance vision can be improved with vision therapy. Myopia can increase the risk for more severe conditions, such as retinal breaks or detachment and glaucoma.

H52.2-   Astigmatism

Astigmatism is due to an elliptically shaped cornea, rather than the normal spherical shape. A point of light, going through an astigmatic cornea, has two points of focus, instead of one sharp image on the retina, resulting in blurred vision. The degree of impairment depends upon the amount and the direction of the astigmatism. A person with myopia or hyperopia may see a dot as a blurred circle, while a person with astigmatism may see the same dot as a blurred oval-shape. Astigmatism is classified as regular or irregular based on measurements that are performed using meridians, which measure the curvature of the cornea. Two meridians, called the principal meridians, determine the steepest and flattest lines passing through the cornea. The principal meridians are used to determine whether the curvature is regular or irregular. In regular astigmatism, the two meridians are perpendicular, meaning that they create a 90-degree angle. In irregular astigmatism, the lines are not perpendicular and do not create a 90-degree angle.

H52.4   Presbyopia

Presbyopia is an age-related condition of near focus. It is caused by loss of ciliary muscle function and/or crystalline lens elasticity due to the aging process, resulting in errors of accommodation. Consequently, the lens loses its ability to focus on nearby objects. Normally the lens is flexible and can change shape with the help of a circular muscle (ciliary muscle) that surrounds it. When focusing on distant objects, the ciliary muscle relaxes. When looking at something nearby, the muscle constricts. This enables the lens to curve, making accommodations as necessary to achieve focus. Presbyopia is caused by a loss of elasticity of the lens and/or loss of ciliary muscle function as a natural part of the aging process. Onset occurs at approximately 40 to 45 years of age. For patients without previous refractive error, the first noticeable symptom is the inability to read small print or focus on close objects.

Visual Disturbances and Blindness (H53-H54)

Visual disturbances encompass a wide variety of conditions including amblyopia, diplopia (double vision), visual field defects, color vision abnormalities, and night blindness. Low vision and blindness codes have very specific definitions and correct code assignment requires use of the parameters defined in the ICD-10-CM coding book.

The categories in this code block are as follows:

| H53 | Visual disturbances |
| H54 | Blindness and low vision |

Focus Point

Laterality is a component of most codes in this code block.

H53.-   Visual disturbances

Visual disturbances encompass a wide variety of conditions including amblyopia, diplopia (double vision), visual field defects, color vision abnormalities, and night blindness.

H53.0-   Amblyopia ex anopsia

Amblyopia is a visual impairment without any detectable organic lesion, anomaly, or damage. Amblyopia, also known as "lazy eye," is usually a unilateral condition of idiopathic poor vision due to failure of the neurotransmission of images to the brain. As a result, the brain favors one eye, causing weakening of the other eye. Onset of functional amblyopia usually occurs in children from 6 to 8 years of age, although it may persist for life once established. Amblyopia is the leading cause of monocular vision loss in adults from 20 to 70 years of age and affects about two to three of every 100 children. Causation includes prolonged visual deprivation due to anomaly or eye disorder (e.g., congenital cataract, optic nerve hypoplasia), strabismus, and unequal refractive error. It may be attributed to a single etiology or multiple overlapping etiologies.

H53.01-   Deprivation amblyopia

Deprivation amblyopia is the most severe form of amblyopia in terms of vision loss, and occurs because the retina does not receive a clear image. The eye loses visual acuity after central fixation. This may occur due to corneal or vitreous opacity, cataract formation, excessive patching, or severe ptosis (droopy eyelid). It usually affects children with unilateral or bilateral congenital cataracts.

H53.02-   Refractive amblyopia

Refractive amblyopia occurs in children when there is a large or unequal amount of refractive error in the eyes due to myopia or astigmatism. The brain does not process visual signals from the eye with the highest degree of myopia or astigmatism, effectively turning off vision in that eye. The better eye or "good eye" retains vision, so the child is able to see clearly, but the condition must be treated or the child will permanently lose vision in the "bad eye."

H53.03- Strabismic amblyopia

Strabismic amblyopia, also known as squint, lazy eye, crossed eyes, or deviating eyes, occurs in approximately 5 percent of children and is associated with prematurity and cerebral palsy. Strabismus causes abnormal vision in the deviating or strabismic eye due to the difference between the images projecting to the brain from both eyes. Normally the images from each eye are fused into one, but with strabismus, the images from the two eyes are so different the central nervous system cannot fuse the images, so the central vision in one eye is suppressed.

H53.04- Amblyopia suspect

Amblyopia is a common condition found in two to three out of every 100 children. As a correctable condition, early detection and treatment is essential to avoid permanent damage to the child's vision. In the absence of obvious underlying etiologies, such as strabismus, cataract, or other vision abnormalities or a family history of these, it may be difficult to determine whether amblyopia is present, especially in a young child. Early childhood eye exams may be abnormal but not conclusive enough to make a full amblyopia diagnosis. A diagnosis of amblyopia suspect provides physicians a way to track patients to ensure that if and when amblyopia is confirmed, treatment is conducted in a timely manner.

H53.2 Diplopia

Diplopia is double vision that may be the result of a refractive error, light splitting objects into two images by a defect in the eye's optical system, or it may result from failure of both eyes to point at the object being viewed, a condition referred to as ocular misalignment. If the eyes do not point at the same object, the image seen by each eye is different and cannot be fused. This results in double vision.

H53.5- Color vision deficiencies

Also called color blindness, this condition refers to a lack of perceptual sensitivity to certain colors. There are three types of color receptors in our eyes—red, green, and blue—in addition to black and white receptors. Color vision deficiencies result from a lack of one or more color receptors in the eye. Most color vision deficiencies are inherited disorders and codes for achromatopsia, deuteranomaly, protanomaly, and tritanomaly all refer to inherited forms of the color vision deficiencies. Acquired color vision deficiencies, regardless of the type or cause, are reported with the code for acquired forms.

H53.51 Achromatopsia

Individuals with achromatopsia, also called monochromatism or complete color blindness, lack all three color receptors resulting in black-and-white vision only. Usually with this condition, the patient also has severe light sensitivity, poor vision, and nystagmus (jerky eye movements).

H53.52 Acquired color vision deficiency

Acquired color vision deficiency may be due to a disease process, injury, or an adverse effect of a drug. Common causes of yellow-blue (deutan defect) are retinal detachment, central nervous system disease, and adverse drug reactions.

H53.53 Deuteranomaly

Deuteranomaly, also called deuteranopsia, is a sex-linked, male-only, red-green color blindness without shortened spectrum that is caused by a lack of red receptors.

H53.54 Protanomaly

Protanomaly, also called protanopia, is red-green color blindness with shortened spectrum. It is often sex-linked, affecting approximately 1 percent of males, but the condition also affects a smaller percentage of females.

H53.55 Tritanomaly

Tritanomaly, also called tritanopia, is yellow-blue color blindness. This inherited type of color vision deficiency can affect both sexes, but is very rare.

H53.6- Night blindness

Night blindness is an eye disorder in which vision is abnormally impaired in dim light or at night due to a deficiency in rhodopsin (visual purple) in the rods, which is responsible for light sensitivity and the degree of dark adaptation. Night blindness most commonly occurs as a result of retinitis pigmentosa, a degenerative condition of the retina. Visual purple may also decrease if there is a dietary deficiency of its principal component vitamin A.

H54.- Blindness and low vision

Blindness typically refers to vision loss that is not correctable with eyeglasses or contact lenses, and some people who are considered blind may perceive slowly moving lights or colors. Low vision refers to moderately impaired vision. People with low vision may have a visual impairment that affects only central vision or peripheral vision. Visual acuity and visual field are the two measurements used to assess vision. Visual acuity is the ability to see details (normal vision is 20/20) and visual field refers to peripheral vision (normal visual field is 180 degrees in diameter). Cataract, trachoma, macular degeneration, and glaucoma account for more than 70 percent of all blindness and low vision. Cataracts are not a disease, but a condition affecting the eye. Cataracts usually start as a slight cloudiness that grows more opaque. Light that does reach the retina becomes increasingly blurred and distorted. If left untreated, cataracts can cause blindness. Trachoma is caused by the bacterium *Chlamydia trachomatis*. It begins in childhood and repeated infections into adulthood irritate and scar the inside of the eyelid and, eventually, the cornea. Scarring on the cornea leads to vision loss. Macular degeneration is a disturbance of the retina and the leading cause of legal blindness in people older than 55 years of age. Glaucoma is a group of conditions related by optic nerve damage, predominantly as a result of elevated intraocular pressure (IOP). The pressure on the optic nerve affects peripheral vision and with glaucoma, central vision is affected as the disease progresses. Levels of blindness and low vision are classified by five different visual impairment categories:

Category	Maximum less than, with best possible correction	Minimum equal or better than, with best possible correction	Classified as
1	20/70	20/200	Low vision
2	20/200	20/400	Low vision
3	20/400	20/1200 (5/300)	Blindness
4	20/1200 (5/300)	Only light perception	Blindness
5	No light perception		Blindness
9	Undetermined or unspecified		

Other Disorders of Eye and Adnexa (H55-H57)

This code block classifies nystagmus and a small number of other disorders of the eye and adnexa that cannot be classified to a specific part of the eye.

The categories in this code block are as follows:

H55   Nystagmus and other irregular eye movements

H57   Other disorders of eye and adnexa

Focus Point

Laterality is a component of many codes in this code block.

Intraoperative and Postprocedural Complications and Disorders of Eye and Adnexa, Not Elsewhere Classified (H59)

Intraoperative and postoperative complications affecting the eye and adnexa are also included in this code block.

The categories in this code block are as follows:

H59   Intraoperative and postoperative complications and disorders of the eye and adnexa, not elsewhere classified

H59.-   Intraoperative and postprocedural complications and disorders of eye and adnexa, not elsewhere classified

Complications and disorders affecting the eye and adnexa may be directly related to a procedure on the eye. In particular, cataract surgery is associated with a number of specific complications that are classified here, including keratopathy, cystoid macular edema, and cataract fragments remaining in the eye postoperatively. Also classified here are more general complications, such as hemorrhage and hematoma and accidental puncture and laceration.

H59.4-   Inflammation (infection) of postprocedural bleb

Inflammation of postprocedural blebs is a complication of certain ophthalmologic procedures now occurring on a more frequent basis due to the increased use of antimetabolites in these procedures over the past decade. During certain procedures, an auxiliary drain on the outside of the eyeball, known as a filtering bleb, is created. Most often associated with trabeculectomy for the treatment of glaucoma, filtering blebs may also be created with other procedures, such as full-thickness filtration surgery. Antimetabolites are applied locally to retard healing so that scar formation will be decreased. In addition to producing extensive thin-walled filtration blebs that may be easily invaded by bacteria, antimetabolites such as mitomycin-C and 5-fluorouracil may also create low pressure or ocular hypotony and inflammation or infection can occur. Postprocedural bleb inflammation has three stages of severity.

H59.41   Inflammation (infection) of postprocedural bleb, stage 1

In stage 1, bleb purulence is present with or without mild inflammation of the anterior segment. Treatment usually consists of topical antibiotics.

H59.42 Inflammation (infection) of postprocedural bleb, stage 2

In stage 2, moderate inflammation of the anterior segment is present in addition to bleb purulence. Treatment consists of topical drugs and oral antibiotics; however, subconjunctival antibiotic injection may be required if improvement is not noted within 24 to 48 hours.

H59.43 Inflammation (infection) of postprocedural bleb, stage 3

Stage 3 is characterized by severe pain, vitreitis, and obvious anterior chamber reaction. Bleb-related endophthalmitis and acute visual loss may occur. Repeat subconjunctival antibiotic injections may be required and surgical revision of the bleb may be needed following resolution of the infection.

Chapter 8: Diseases of the Ear and Mastoid Process (H60-H95)

The ear is a sense organ primarily responsible for the detection of sound but also functions to facilitate equilibrium of balance and body position. The ear is divided into three parts: the outer or external ear, the middle ear, and the inner ear.

The external ear includes the auricle (pinna), which is the visible part of the ear, the external ear canal, and the outer surface of the tympanic membrane (eardrum). The auricle is composed of cartilage that gives the ear its shape and is covered with skin. The auricle acts as a funnel for sound waves, which travel through the pinna into the external auditory canal, a short tube that terminates at the tympanic membrane.

The middle ear is an air-filled cavity behind the tympanic membrane. Three small bones, called ossicles, vibrate in response to sound waves. These bones include the malleus (hammer), incus (anvil), and stapes (stirrup), which vibrate and strike against the tympanic membrane to amplify sound waves. Also within the middle ear is the eustachian tube (auditory tube), which drains fluid from the middle ear into the pharynx and equalizes pressure between the outer and middle ears.

Structures of the inner ear include the oval window, cochlea, semicircular ducts, and vestibule. These structures are encased within the temporal bone of the skull. The middle ear and the inner ear connect at the oval window. The cochlea is a spiral-shaped (snail-like) structure that takes sound and transforms it into signals for the brain. The semicircular canals (labyrinths) contain receptor cells to facilitate balance together with the vestibular apparatus.

The mastoid process is a bony protuberance at the base of the skull that lies behind each ear. This process serves several functions, including as an attachment for muscles of the neck. The mastoid process is also filled with air cells that communicate with the middle ear.

The chapter is broken down into the following code blocks:

H60-H62   Diseases of external ear

H65-H75   Diseases of middle ear and mastoid

H80-H83   Diseases of inner ear

H90-H9   Other disorders of ear

H95   Intraoperative and postprocedural complications and disorders of ear and mastoid process, not elsewhere classified

Diseases of External Ear (H60-H62)

Disorders of the external ear include those of the auricle (pinna) and external auditory meatus. The auricle consists of the helix, anthelix, scapha, concha, tragus, antitragus, intertragic notch, and lobule. The auricle is a single, elastic cartilage covered in skin and normal adnexal features (hair follicles, sweat glands, and sebaceous glands). The ridged nature of the auricle is to channel sounds into the acoustic meatus. The semicircular depression leading to the ear is named the concha, Latin for shell. The external auditory meatus consists of cartilaginous and osseous portions with the canal lined with epidermis, hair, and ceruminous glands that extend to the tympanic membrane.

The primary functions of the ear canal are to funnel sound into the middle and inner ear and to shield the ear from infection and foreign objects. The outer portion of the ear canal has naturally occurring defenses to protect the ear. Cerumen is produced, creating an acidic environment in the ear canal that reduces bacterial and fungal growth and provides a barrier against debris. The hair in the ear canal provides a further barrier against debris entering the ear. Any break down in the skin lining can result in infection, allowing bacteria or fungi to invade the external ear.

The categories in this code block are as follows:

H60   Otitis externa

H61   Other disorders of external ear

H62   Disorders of external ear in diseases classified elsewhere

H60.-   Otitis externa

Otitis externa is an inflammation of the auricle and/or external auditory canal. Although infection with bacteria, such as *Pseudomonas*, *Proteus vulgaris*, *Streptococcus*, and *Staphylococcus aureus*, are classic causative agents of inflammation, there are also noninfectious agents such as allergens or chemicals that can cause inflammation. Some systemic diseases also manifest as inflammation. Signs and symptoms of otitis externa include redness and swelling that can obstruct the meatus, serous or purulent drainage, external ear tenderness, and enlarged regional lymph nodes. Whether the otitis externa is from an infectious or noninfectious source, related signs and symptoms are often very similar, sometimes making diagnosis difficult.

Focus Point

Codes for otitis externa documented as due to aspergillosis, candidiasis, herpes zoster, or simplex include the inflammatory and infectious disease processes and do not require a separate code from category H60.

H60.2-   Malignant otitis externa

Malignant or necrotizing otitis externa is a severe infection starting in the outer ear canal that rapidly progresses to nearby tissue causing necrosis and damage to bone, nerves, and even the brain. It is more prevalent in older patients, especially those with diabetes, although rare cases do occur in children. Malignant otitis externa may lead to cellulitis and osteomyelitis of adjacent soft tissue and bone.

H60.5-   Acute noninfective otitis externa

Noninfectious forms of otitis externa may be secondary to a systemic disease or contact with some external irritant. Acute forms of otitis externa manifest with rapid onset of symptoms that typically resolve in a short period of time.

H60.54-   Acute eczematoid otitis externa

Susceptibility to otitis externa is largely dependent upon the condition of the skin in the external ear and ear canal. Healthy skin keeps pathogens out. Chronic skin conditions such as eczema and psoriasis may damage the skin of the external ear resulting in inflammation or allow normal but usually harmless pathogens of the ear to infect the skin.

H61.-   Other disorders of external ear

This category contains codes for infectious and noninfectious inflammatory disease processes such as chondritis and perichondritis, other conditions of the pinna such as acquired deformity, impacted cerumen, and narrowing or stenosis of the external ear canal.

H61.0-   Chondritis and perichondritis of external ear

This subcategory captures infection of the skin and cartilage layers of the external ear.

H61.00-   Unspecified perichondritis of external ear

H61.01-   Acute perichondritis of external ear

H61.02-   Chronic perichondritis of external ear

The perichondrium is the skin and tissue layer surrounding the cartilage of the external ear. Inflammation of the perichondrium may occur from an infectious or noninfectious disease process. Acute perichondritis is characterized by rapid onset and more severe symptoms and resolves in a short period of time. Chronic perichondritis occurs over a longer period of time and initially may produce few symptoms.

H61.03-   Chondritis of external ear

Chondritis is an infection that has progressed into the cartilage itself. Though not a common infection, the recent increase in ear piercing through the cartilage around the outside of the ear has increased this risk. It is also a serious complication following surgery or injury as the damage can be severe, progressing to necrosis, requiring removal and reconstruction of the pinna.

Diseases of Middle Ear and Mastoid (H65-H75)

The middle ear starts at the tympanic membrane and ends at the oval window. This air-filled cavity, also called the tympanic cavity, contains the eardrum, the auditory ossicles, and the eustachian (auditory) tube.

The tympanic membrane (eardrum), which separates the outer ear from the middle ear, is a three-layer structure consisting of a cutaneous outer layer, a fibrous middle layer, and an inner layer of mucous membrane. Sound waves entering the ear strike the tympanic membrane causing it to vibrate.

Attached to the tympanic membrane are three ear bones (auditory ossicles) known as the malleus, incus, and stapes. When sound waves strike the eardrum, it vibrates and sets the bones into motion—the malleus pushing the incus, the incus pushing the stapes, which transmit these sound waves to the inner ear, generating nerve impulses that are sent to the brain. The muscles of the middle ear modify the performance of the middle ear bones and act as safety devices to protect the ear against excessively strong vibrations from loud noises.

The eustachian tube is a small tubular structure that attaches the middle ear to the back of the nose and nasopharynx. Its most important function is to ventilate the middle ear space by equalizing the air pressure in the middle ear with the pressure outside it. Another function of the eustachian tube is to drain any accumulated secretions, infection, or debris from the middle ear space.

The bone that sits behind the ear is called the mastoid and is part of the temporal bone. It is atypical to most bones in that it is composed of air spaces, called mastoid cells, which allow drainage from the middle ear.

The categories in this code block are as follows:

H65	Nonsuppurative otitis media
H66	Suppurative and unspecified otitis media
H67	Otitis media in diseases classified elsewhere
H68	Eustachian salpingitis and obstruction
H69	Other and unspecified disorders of Eustachian tube
H70	Mastoiditis and related conditions
H71	Cholesteatoma of middle ear
H72	Perforation of tympanic membrane
H73	Other disorders of tympanic membrane
H74	Other disorders of middle ear mastoid
H75	Other disorders of middle ear and mastoid in diseases classified elsewhere

H65.-   Nonsuppurative otitis media

Otitis media is primarily a consequence of a dysfunctional eustachian tube (ET). Normally, the eustachian tube is closed, which helps prevent the unintentional contamination of the middle ear space by the normal secretions found in the back of the nose. Swallowing or yawning opens the eustachian tube and allows air to flow into or out of the middle ear, keeping the air pressure on both sides of the eardrum equal and ventilating the middle ear so the cavity stays dry and clean. If the tube is blocked, due to an obstruction or developmental abnormality, differences in pressure can occur between the two sides of the eardrum. The lining of the middle ear absorbs the trapped air and creates a negative pressure that pulls the eardrum inward and causes fluid from surrounding tissues to leak into the cavity. The accumulation of fluid in the middle ear space alone causes pressure and hearing loss and the newly created moist and warm environment allows pathogens, either native to the ear or coming from the nasopharynx, to infect the fluid. Nonsuppurative otitis media, also referred to as otitis media with effusion, is an inflammation of the middle ear with fluid that is not infected. The fluid may be described as serous or mucoid, but the defining characteristic is that the fluid is nonpurulent, meaning that it does not contain pus.

H65.0-   Acute serous otitis media

Serous otitis media is inflammation with a collection of fluid in the middle ear. The condition is often due to a viral infection and is generally painless, although the fluid can impair hearing, which in turn may impact speech, language development, and learning. Serous otitis media may also occur in the absence of an infection as a result of an obstruction of the eustachian tube caused by inflammation or enlarged adenoids. Once the obstruction or blockage resolves, the fluid is once again able to drain down the eustachian tube into the throat. Acute serous otitis media is classified based on whether the condition is recurrent or not recurrent.

H65.1-   Other acute nonsuppurative otitis media

Acute or subacute forms of otitis media described as mucoid, sanguinous, or serous, regardless if related to an allergy or not, are coded to this subcategory. Mucoid effusion is simply an accumulation of mucus in the middle ear. Sanguinous fluid is bloody or blood-tinged. Serous fluid is watery and clear.

H65.11- Acute and subacute allergic otitis media (mucoid) (sanguinous) (serous)

Allergies cause an inflammatory response in the body that may result in an acute inflammation of the middle ear. Dust, mold, pollen, and food are some of the more common allergens suspected in allergic otitis media. Middle ear effusion associated with allergies may be mucoid, sanguinous, or serous. Allergic otitis media is classified based on whether the condition is recurrent or not recurrent.

H65.2-   Chronic serous otitis media

Chronic serous otitis media results from long-standing eustachian tube dysfunction resulting in fluid in the ear for a prolonged period of time. Chronic serous otitis media is typically associated with hearing impairment and can cause delays in speech, language development, and learning.

H65.3-   Chronic mucoid otitis media

Chronic mucoid otitis media occurs when mucus becomes trapped in the middle ear for a prolonged period of time. The mucus can become very thick preventing absorption and drainage. A major concern with chronic mucoid otitis media is that it impairs hearing because sound cannot be effectively conducted through the thickened mucus in the middle ear.

H65.4-   Other chronic nonsuppurative otitis media

This subcategory classifies chronic forms of otitis media with middle ear fluid not described as serous or mucoid.

H65.41- Chronic allergic otitis media

Allergies cause an inflammatory response in the body that may result in chronic inflammation of the middle ear, particularly if the allergen is not identified and removed from the environment or the patient is not desensitized to the allergen. Inflammation in the middle ear may be triggered by many allergens, with dust, mold, pollen, and food being some of the more common.

H66.- Suppurative and unspecified otitis media

Eustachian tube (ET) dysfunction is the principal etiology behind otitis media. If the ET is not functioning properly, air pressure builds in the middle ear causing surrounding tissues to leak fluid into the cavity. The fluid provides a breeding site for pathogens, bacterial and viral alike. Bacteria can enter through the external ear itself or because the ET is connected to the upper respiratory tract, pathogens associated with certain respiratory tract infections can find their way to the middle ear.

H66.0- Acute suppurative otitis media

The definitive characteristic of suppurative otitis media is the presence of purulent fluid (pus) in the middle ear. Infections with *Streptococcus pneumoniae*, *Haemophilus* influenza, and *Moraxella catarrhalis* are the most common causes of acute suppurative otitis media. Most complications of otitis media are associated with chronic or subacute disease. The classic signs of acute otitis media are pain, redness, and bulging of the tympanic membrane due to the presence of purulent fluid in the middle ear. Acute suppurative otitis is classified based on whether the condition is recurrent or not recurrent.

H66.00- Acute suppurative otitis media without spontaneous rupture of ear drum

The accumulation of pus in the middle ear that occurs with suppurative otitis media can cause tremendous pressure buildup behind the eardrum. Intense pain in the middle ear is common due to this increased pressure and also a good indicator that the eardrum has not spontaneously ruptured.

H66.01- Acute suppurative otitis media with spontaneous rupture of ear drum

Acute suppurative otitis media with spontaneous rupture of the eardrum occurs when the buildup of pus within the middle ear causes a perforation in the eardrum. This releases the pus that has accumulated, allowing it to drain out through the external ear canal. In most instances, any associated ear pain ceases after the rupture. A perforated eardrum generally heals after the infection resolves.

H68.- Eustachian salpingitis and obstruction

Obstruction or inflammation of the eustachian tube that does not result in the accumulation of fluid in the middle ear would be coded to this category.

H68.0- Eustachian salpingitis

Salpingitis is inflammation of a tubular structure, in this case the eustachian tube that runs from the middle ear to the back of the nose and upper throat. Further classification in this subcategory identifies whether the condition is acute or chronic.

H68.1- Obstruction of Eustachian tube

About one third of the eustachian tube is bone and the other two thirds of the tube is cartilage. The bony (osseous) portion is always open and the cartilaginous portion is usually closed, opening only when swallowing or yawning. Obstruction codes identify which portion of the tube is obstructed: the osseous or the cartilaginous portion.

H68.11- Osseous obstruction of Eustachian tube

An osseous obstruction is one where there is blockage affecting the bony portion of the eustachian tube.

H68.12- Intrinsic cartilagenous obstruction of Eustachian tube

Intrinsic cartilaginous obstruction is one that originates from the cartilage portion of the eustachian tube itself. Typically this is due to cartilage overgrowth reducing the size of or completely blocking the eustachian tube.

H68.13- Extrinsic cartilagenous obstruction of Eustachian tube

Extrinsic refers to an external cause, which in the case of obstruction of the cartilaginous portion of the eustachian tube means that the obstruction is external to the eustachian tube itself. The cartilaginous portion of the eustachian tube is flexible tissue so when an extrinsic force is applied it can collapse the walls of the tube, compressing or blocking the passage of air. Outside forces that may compress the tube include tumors or enlarged adenoids.

H69.- Other and unspecified disorders of Eustachian tube

Dysfunction and/or disorders of the eustachian tube specifically described as distortion or patency, or that does not have an etiology related to obstruction, infection, or inflammation, are included in this category.

H69.0- Patulous Eustachian tube

Normally the eustachian tube is closed, opening only for a few brief seconds when swallowing or yawning. A eustachian tube that is patulous is one that remains open, intermittently or permanently. Autophonia, described as hearing one's own voice, respiration, or heartbeat inside the ear, is the most common symptom. Although typically idiopathic in causality, patent eustachian tube has been linked to pregnancy and weight loss.

H69.9- Unspecified Eustachian tube disorder

Eustachian tube dysfunction or disorder without documentation of a specific etiology (e.g., blockage, infection, and distortion) is classified here. Dysfunction of the eustachian tube can cause sensations of clicking, popping, ear fullness, and sometimes moderate to severe ear pain. Children may identify the sensation as a tickle in their ear. Children are at increased risk for eustachian tube dysfunction due to the fact that they have very narrow eustachian tubes.

H70.- Mastoiditis and related conditions

The mastoid is a part of the temporal bone of the skull. It is a bony bump just behind and slightly above the level of the external ear that is connected with the middle ear. In adults, the mastoid portion of the temporal bone contains air cells that are separated from the brain by thin bony partitions. When there is a collection of fluid in the middle ear, there is usually also a slight collection of fluid within the airspaces of the mastoid.

H70.0- Acute mastoiditis

Mastoiditis is inflammation and/or infection of the mastoid bone or an abscess in the mastoid antrum. The infections usually are due to *Streptococcus pneumoniae*, *Haemophilus influenzae*, beta-hemolytic *Streptococcus*, and gram-negative organisms. Signs and symptoms of mastoiditis include dull ache and tenderness over the mastoid process, low-grade fever, thick and purulent discharge, postauricular edema, erythema, and conductive hearing loss. Typically mastoiditis is a complication of otitis media and symptoms often overlap.

H70.2- Petrositis

The petrous bone is actually a pyramid-shaped piece of temporal bone found between the sphenoid and occipital bones in the base of the skull. Like the mastoid bone, the petrous bone is porous with air cells that communicate with the eustachian tube. Although it is rare for inflammation and/or infection to affect this part of the temporal bone, it sometimes occurs as an extension of infection in the mastoid and/or middle ear.

H71.- Cholesteatoma of middle ear

Cholesteatoma of the middle ear is an abnormal buildup of squamous epithelial cells from the external ear canal. Any introduction of skin into the middle ear can result in cholesteatoma formation but it is typically caused by negative pressure in the middle ear. When pressure in the middle ear is not regulated due to a dysfunctional eustachian tube, a pocket in the middle ear is created and dead epithelial tissue, which is

usually forced to the exterior of the ear with the movement of the earwax, instead builds up in the pocket. Continuous skin accumulation and related enzyme secretions facilitate erosion of nearby structures, including the mastoid, the ossicles, facial nerves, and other parts of the temporal bone. In some cases, the brain may become exposed leading to infection or abscess of the brain. Although rare, cholesteatomas may occur as a congenital disorder, but in most cases they are a consequence of chronic ear infections. Persistent otorrhea is the most prominent sign of cholesteatoma often accompanied by an abnormal odor. Hearing loss, paralysis, and balance issues can also occur with severity dependent on the structures in the ear being eroded.

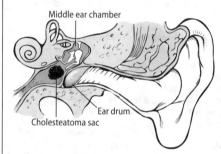

Cholesteatoma

Middle ear chamber

Ear drum

Cholesteatoma sac

H72.- Perforation of tympanic membrane

A perforated eardrum is a hole or rupture in the eardrum, of which there are several causes, such as a skull fracture, a foreign object, or barotrauma. Middle ear infections are also a common cause of perforation. Most eardrum perforations heal spontaneously within weeks after rupture, during which time the ear must be protected from water. However, some perforations do not heal. Complications from persistent tympanic membrane perforation and treatment are dependent on the site of the perforation.

H72.0- Central perforation of tympanic membrane

Any perforation that does not extend to the margin of the eardrum and does not involve separation of the tympanic membrane from the bony canal is classified as a central perforation. In a central perforation, a rim of tympanic membrane is present around the entire perforation and this rim of tympanic membrane remains attached to the bony canal.

H72.1- Attic perforation of tympanic membrane

An attic perforation is a type of marginal perforation that occurs in the superior aspect of the eardrum. This type of perforation involves the upper edge of the tympanic membrane and the perforation extends to the bony canal.

H72.2- Other marginal perforations of tympanic membrane

Marginal perforation involves the edge of the eardrum (tympanic annulus), where the eardrum and bony ear canal meet. Any marginal perforation that does not involve the attic of the tympanum is classified here.

H72.8- Other perforations of tympanic membrane

Holes or ruptures in the eardrum described as total or multiple are coded to this subcategory.

H72.82- Total perforations of tympanic membrane

A total perforation is the complete acquired absence of the tympanic membrane, frequently a result of recurrent and chronic suppurative otitis media due to *Streptococcus*. When the entire tympanic membrane is absent, there is often simultaneous moderate conductive hearing loss.

H73.- Other disorders of tympanic membrane

The tympanic membrane, also referred to as the eardrum, is a thin, flexible membrane separating the external part of the ear from the middle ear.

H73.0- Acute myringitis

Myringitis, an inflammation of the tympanic membrane, may occur due to the presence of a foreign body in the ear, from trauma, or from infection. Hearing may be compromised and pain and congestion may also be present. The first three weeks of inflammation is considered the acute state; subacute lasts no longer than three months.

H73.01- Bullous myringitis

Bullous myringitis is an inflammatory and contagious disorder of the eardrum or tympanum caused by infection resulting in painful blisters on the eardrum. Viral infections, such as influenza and *Streptococcus pneumoniae*, a common bacterial infection, are associated with bullous myringitis.

H73.1- Chronic myringitis

Chronic myringitis is an inflammation of the tympanic membrane lasting three months or longer.

H74.- Other disorders of middle ear mastoid

This category captures disorders of the middle ear and mastoid, several of which involve disorders of the ossicles. Conditions that affect the ossicles impair the conduction of sound through the middle ear.

H74.0- Tympanosclerosis

Tympanosclerosis involves abnormal deposits on the layers of the eardrum, generally as a manifestation of chronic ear infection. The pathological calcified plaques resemble scar tissue and cause the eardrum to lose flexibility and stiffen resulting in hearing impairment. In advanced stages of tympanosclerosis, the plaques spread to the ossicles (bones of the middle ear) causing more severe or even permanent hearing damage.

H74.1- Adhesive middle ear disease

Adhesive middle ear disease is thickening of the eardrum with fibrous bands of tissue that cause the eardrum to retract into the middle ear space. This impedes the ability of the ossicles (bones) to move freely resulting in conductive hearing impairment.

Diseases of Inner Ear (H80-H83)

The inner ear consists of a system of fluid-filled tubes and sacs called the labyrinth and also contains the nerves that connect the labyrinth to the brain. The labyrinth, which rests inside the bone of the skull, contains the cochlea for hearing and the vestibule for balance and equilibrium.

The categories in this code block are as follows:

H80	Otosclerosis
H81	Disorders of vestibular function
H82	Vertiginous syndromes in diseases classified elsewhere
H83	Other diseases of inner ear

H80.- Otosclerosis

Otosclerosis is the abnormal growth of spongy bone in the middle and inner ear. It typically affects the ossicles of the middle ear but also occurs in the otic capsule, which is the bone surrounding the inner ear, the cochlea, and the oval window. The abnormal bony growth fixates the bones in the middle or inner ear inhibiting vibration within the ear and resulting in hearing loss. Depending on the site of the bone growth, the hearing loss may be conductive, sensory, or mixed type. Conductive hearing loss occurs when the otosclerosis involves the ossicles and/or the oval window. Sensory hearing loss more often occurs with otosclerosis of the otic capsule. When the ossicles and the cochlea are affected, it results in a mixed type of hearing loss.

H80.0- Otosclerosis involving oval window, nonobliterative

In nonobliterative otosclerosis of the oval window, only a portion of the oval window and its margins are affected by the spongy bone growth.

H80.1- Otosclerosis involving oval window, obliterative

In obliterative otosclerosis, the entire oval window and its margins are obscured by spongy bone growth.

H81.- Disorders of vestibular function

The vestibular system is responsible for the maintenance of balance, spatial orientation, and equilibrium. The first part of the vestibular system is made up of three semicircular canals and the cupula, a sensory receptor. Rotational or angular movements are detected when the movement of fluid in one or more semicircular canals pushes against the cupula. Hair cells within the cupula translate the movements and the cupula then sends a signal to the brain. In order for angular movement to be successfully detected, the semicircular canals work in pairs: one side stimulating the cupula receptor and the other inhibiting the cupula receptor. The second part consists of otolithic organs known as the utricle and the saccule. These organs contain receptors called macula (hair cells) that when stimulated help to recognize vertical orientation (body position in respect to gravity) and linear movement. These organs are also paired, one of each on either side of the head. Dizziness, unsteadiness or imbalance when walking, and nausea are the most common symptoms of vestibular disorders. Because the vestibular system interacts with other parts of the nervous system, there may be problems with vision, muscles, thinking, and memory.

H81.0- Meniere's disease

Meniere's disease, also referred to as idiopathic endolymphatic hydrops, is a disorder of the inner ear that causes episodes of vertigo, tinnitus, a feeling of fullness or pressure in the ear, and fluctuating hearing loss, which may last for several hours. Meniere's disease episodes may occur in clusters or weeks, months, or years may pass between episodes. Between the acute attacks, most people are free of symptoms or note only mild imbalance and tinnitus. Often this disease is a diagnosis of exclusion as many other conditions can produce the hallmark symptoms.

H81.1- Benign paroxysmal vertigo

Benign paroxysmal vertigo is a type of vertigo that occurs after head movement. It occurs when small pieces of calcium, normally found in the utricle and saccule, are displaced into the semicircular canals of the inner ear. These calcium pieces easily stimulate hair cells in the semicircular canals due to their density, triggering a signal to the brain and a perception of head motion even when the head has stopped moving. Diagnosis is through the Dix Halpike maneuver, which involves moving the patient rapidly from a sitting position, to the head hanging position below horizontal, such as with a head hanging off the end of an examining table, which triggers an attack of vertigo. This maneuver disperses the calcium pieces so that they are not clumped together and reduces their density, thereby stimulating the hair cells, which results in the characteristic symptoms of dizziness and nystagmus (rapid eye movements).

H81.2- Vestibular neuronitis

The vestibulocochlear nerve (eighth cranial nerve) is a nerve in the inner ear that relays to the brain information on balance (vestibular nerve) and hearing (cochlear nerve). Inflammation (neuronitis) of the vestibular part of the nerve disrupts the balance signals being sent to the brain, resulting in a sudden loss of balance, nausea and vomiting, and concentration difficulties. Initially these symptoms are so severe that they impact the daily functioning of the patient. Within a few days, the severity of the symptoms lessens but often continues to be present, in some cases for several months. Viral neuronitis or a blood clot in the arterial system may precipitate the disorder.

H83.- Other diseases of inner ear

The inner ear is composed of the labyrinth, which rests inside the petrous portion of the temporal bone, and contains the following sensory organs: the cochlea for hearing and the vestibule, which is composed of the utricle, saccule, and semicircular canals, for balance and equilibrium. Nerves connect the labyrinth sensory organs to the brain.

H83.0- Labyrinthitis

Labyrinthitis is an inflammation of the labyrinth or inner ear. Inflammation is usually caused by a bacterial or viral infection, although sometimes the causal factor in labyrinthitis is an autoimmune process.

Other Disorders of Ear (H90-H94)

The ear consists of three parts: the outer ear, middle ear, and inner ear. The outer ear is the visible part plus the ear canal. The ear canal funnels sound to the eardrum, the structure that separates the outer ear from the middle ear. The eardrum is attached to the ossicles; the eardrum vibrates causing the ossicles to move and these amplify and conduct sound to the inner ear. The inner ear consists of the cochlea, which contains hair cells that vibrate when a sound is conducted to them by the eardrum and ossicles. The movement of the hair cells transmits electrical impulses down the auditory nerve to the brain, translating the sound waves.

Codes included in this code block identify problems related to hearing loss, ear pain, auditory nerve function, and other specified disorders of the ear not classified to another code block in this chapter.

The categories in this code block are as follows:

H90	Conductive and sensorineural hearing loss
H91	Other and unspecified hearing loss
H92	Otalgia and effusion of ear
H93	Other disorders of ear, not elsewhere classified
H94	Other disorders of ear in diseases classified elsewhere

H90.- Conductive and sensorineural hearing loss

Conductive hearing loss results from external or middle ear problems, which are often mechanical in nature. Sensorineural hearing loss is caused by damage to the inner ear or the nerve pathways to the brain. When both middle ear and inner ear problems occur, it results in what is known as mixed hearing loss.

H90.0 Conductive hearing loss, bilateral

H90.1- Conductive hearing loss, unilateral with unrestricted hearing on the contralateral side

H90.2 Conductive hearing loss, unspecified

Conductive hearing loss is the inability of sound waves to move from the outer (external ear) to the inner ear. This may be due to things like a blocked external auditory canal, fluid or abnormal bone growth in the middle ear, or a rupture of the eardrum. Each of these conditions in some way limits the movement of the structures in the middle ear, inhibiting transmission of the sound wave from the middle ear to the inner ear. Although the sound is typically not distorted, the sounds are much quieter. The most common cause of conductive hearing loss in children and adults is otitis media infection and otosclerosis respectively.

H90.3 Sensorineural hearing loss, bilateral

H90.4- Sensorineural hearing loss, unilateral with unrestricted hearing on the contralateral side

H90.5 Unspecified sensorineural hearing loss

The terms sensory, neural, cochlear, and inner ear hearing loss are all synonymous with sensorineural hearing loss. This hearing disorder is a consequence of damage to inner ear structures, including the cochlea and/or the auditory nerve. Sensory hearing loss is due to damaged hair cells within the cochlea. Neural hearing loss is due to damage to the auditory nerves.

Identifying the specific culprit for the loss of hearing is not always possible and as such the two are typically listed together. Sensorineural hearing loss can result from exposure to extremely loud noise, infections, injuries, genetic predisposition, and, in some cases, age may also play a role. Damage to the auditory nerve may be secondary to benign tumors, trauma, or infection. Sensorineural hearing loss is usually a permanent loss of hearing sensitivity, often occurring more in the high frequencies than in the lower frequencies. It also can affect speech, cognition, and the ability to hear clearly and understand conversations.

Focus Point

Presbycusis is a form of sensorineural hearing loss related to the natural effects of aging. This condition however, is not reported to the sensorineural hearing loss codes but instead has its own set of codes in category H91.

H90.6 Mixed conductive and sensorineural hearing loss, bilateral

H90.7- Mixed conductive and sensorineural hearing loss, unilateral with unrestricted hearing on the contralateral side

H90.8 Mixed conductive and sensorineural hearing loss, unspecified

Occasionally, conductive hearing loss occurs in combination with sensorineural hearing loss due to damage in the outer or middle ear, as well as in the inner ear (cochlea) or auditory nerve. This type of hearing loss is referred to as mixed hearing loss.

H90.A1- Conductive hearing loss, unilateral, with restricted hearing on the contralateral side

Conductive hearing loss occurs when there is an obstruction or impairment in the outer or middle ear, and sometimes both locations, which decreases the volume of what one hears. The severity of the hearing loss may vary based on cause, but it is unlikely to lead to complete loss of hearing and can be treated with medical/surgical intervention. This subcategory further indicates that the loss occurred in only one ear with restricted hearing on the contralateral side.

H90.A2- Sensorineural hearing loss, unilateral, with restricted hearing on the contralateral side

Sensorineural hearing loss is seen when impairment of the cochlea or nerve decreases the volume of what one hears as well as clarity of sound. There are several causes of this kind of hearing loss: aging, repetitive loud noise, as well disease like Meniere's and/or viruses like the mumps. There is no curative treatment for this kind of hearing loss, which is permanent, and symptoms are managed with hearing aids. This subcategory further indicates that the loss occurred in only one ear with restricted hearing on the contralateral side.

H90.A3- Mixed conductive and sensorineural hearing loss, unilateral with restricted hearing on the contralateral side

Mixed hearing loss is seen when there is impairment in both the outer/middle ear as well as the nerves of the ear, possibly as a result of a perforated eardrum in conjunction with aging, among other examples. This subcategory further indicates that the loss occurred in only one ear with restricted hearing on the contralateral side.

H91.- Other and unspecified hearing loss

Hearing loss can impact learning and development in young children and can have negative effects on work and social interactions in adults. This category classifies hearing loss due to drugs, aging, sudden and unexplained etiology, and conditions that cannot be better captured in other categories in this chapter.

H91.1- Presbycusis

Deterioration of the structures in the cochlea and/or the acoustic nerve occurs naturally as a person ages. This results in the gradual loss of hearing of higher frequencies, which is typically symmetrical, affecting both ears simultaneously.

H92.- Otalgia and effusion of ear

Ear pain is the definition of otalgia while effusion is defined as fluid in the ear.

H92.0- Otalgia

Ear pain may be of the ear itself (intrinsic), often occurring in relation to another condition such as otitis media or mastoiditis. Ear pain may also be a referred pain (extrinsic), with the origin of the pain occurring at a separate anatomical site, such as from the sinuses, neck, or mouth, but is also felt or referred to the ear.

H92.1- Otorrhea

Otorrhea is drainage from the ear. The natural state of the ear is clean and dry; therefore, drainage from the ear beyond the typical cerumen discharge indicates that the natural environment of the ear has been compromised. The type, duration, amount, and onset of the drainage assist the physician in determining the etiology behind the otorrhea.

H92.2- Otorrhagia

Bleeding from the ear is called otorrhagia.

H93.- Other disorders of ear, not elsewhere classified

Disorders classified to this category range from vascular disorders to problems with auditory perceptions to nerve disorders.

H93.1- Tinnitus

Tinnitus is when a patient observes ringing, swooshing, clicking, and sometimes even music in their ears but in the absence of external noise. A majority of tinnitus cases are subjective, where only the patient can hear the sound. Objective tinnitus, a much rarer condition, is when the ear noises can be heard also by other individuals. Tinnitus is very rarely cured, but there are treatments that can lessen the noise.

H93.A- Pulsatile tinnitus

Pulsatile tinnitus, sometimes referred to as vascular tinnitus, is a condition in which the patient hears a rhythmic pulsing, whooshing, or thumping sound that in many cases coincides with the heartbeat. The condition is usually not serious but can be a symptom of hypertension, arteriosclerosis of the vessels of the head and neck, intracranial vascular lesions, or aneurysms of the internal carotid or vertebral artery. Unlike nonpulsatile tinnitus, the underlying cause is usually determined in the majority of cases.

H93.2- Other abnormal auditory perceptions

Auditory perception begins at the ear and ends in the brain. Sound waves move into the ear and cause the internal ear structures—the eardrum, ossicles, and cochlea—to vibrate. This stimulates hair cells in the cochlea, which then communicate with auditory nerve fibers. The nerve fibers send an impulse to the brain where the sound wave is translated into something meaningful and useful. Problems in auditory perception revolve around the brains inability to segregate, organize, or translate audible signals.

H93.21- Auditory recruitment

Auditory recruitment, the perception that sounds get too loud too fast, is directly related to sensorineural hearing loss. Within the cochlea there are groups of hair cells and each group is responsible for transmitting a unit of sound. When hair cells in a particular group are damaged or die, as occurs in sensorineural hearing loss, the impaired group of hair cells recruits hair cells from adjacent groups to help transmit the units of sound from the damaged region. The adjacent groups of hair cells must send sound for their own group in addition to sending sounds for the impaired groups. Because more than one unit of sound is simultaneously being sent to the brain, the sound is perceived as being much louder than the actual noise level. The result is a very narrow range of sound volume that is loud enough for the hearing impaired person to hear, but not so loud that it causes discomfort.

H93.25 Central auditory processing disorder

Central auditory processing disorder is a neurological defect of the brain. In this disorder, the brain fails to interpret or filter auditory information. Spoken language, in particular, is hard to understand with a central auditory processing disorder, especially when significant background noise is present. The ability to hear is not compromised but the person is unable to receive, use, understand, or remember auditory information, which can cause various communication and learning difficulties.

Focus Point

Because central processing disorder is a disorder of the brain and not the ear structures, there are no laterality options for this code.

Intraoperative and Postprocedural Complications and Disorders of Ear and Mastoid Process, Not Elsewhere Classified (H95)

Conditions that may arise during or as a result of a procedure include, but are not limited to, granulation or cholesteatoma formation after mastoidectomy, hemorrhage and hematoma of the ear or mastoid, and stenosis of the external ear canal.

The categories in this code block are as follows:

H95 Intraoperative and postprocedural complications and disorders of ear and mastoid process, not elsewhere classified

H95.- **Intraoperative and postprocedural complications and disorders of ear and mastoid process, not elsewhere classified**

Intraoperative and postoperative complications related to the external, middle, or inner ear or of the mastoid bone are included in this category.

H95.0- **Recurrent cholesteatoma of postmastoidectomy cavity**

Cholesteatoma is an abnormal buildup of squamous epithelial cells from the external ear canal in the middle ear. Any introduction of skin into the middle ear can result in cholesteatoma formation, but it is typically caused by negative pressure in the middle ear. In order to ensure that a surgically removed cholesteatoma will not return, it is necessary to remove all of the disease present within the ear, which is performed through a mastoidectomy. However, removing all cholesteatoma tissue can be difficult as the preservation of hearing is also an important goal. Cholesteatoma formation of the hearing structures in the ear, the ossicles in particular, can be extremely difficult to remove from these tiny bones without compromising their function. Unfortunately, if any residual disease is left behind, the cholesteatoma reforms in the middle ear and mastoid cavity.

Chapter 9: Diseases of the Circulatory System (I00-I99)

The cardiovascular system houses some of the most important components needed for day-to-day survival. The heart and the approximately 60,000 miles of blood vessels in the circulatory system provide oxygen-rich blood, nutrients such as amino acids and electrolytes, and important hormones to all of the body's cells and carry off carbon dioxide and other waste products of metabolism. In addition, the cardiovascular system stabilizes body temperature and pH. This chapter includes disease processes affecting all areas of the circulatory system, including the heart and all of its systems and functions; the coronary, cerebral, and peripheral veins, arteries, arterioles and capillaries; and the lymphatic vessels and nodes.

The chapter is broken down into the following code blocks:

I00-I02	Acute rheumatic fever
I05-I09	Chronic rheumatic heart diseases
I10-I16	Hypertensive diseases
I20-I25	Ischemic heart diseases
I26-I28	Pulmonary heart disease and diseases of pulmonary circulation
I30-I52	Other forms of heart disease
I60-I69	Cerebrovascular diseases
I70-I79	Diseases of arteries, arterioles and capillaries
I80-I89	Diseases of veins, lymphatic vessels and lymph nodes, not elsewhere classified
I95-I99	Other and unspecified disorders of the circulatory system

Acute Rheumatic Fever (I00-I02)

Acute rheumatic fever is a systemic disease with a nonsuppurative acute complication that generally affects the joints (arthritis), subcutaneous tissue (nodules), skin (erythema marginatum), heart (carditis), or brain (chorea). The fever usually follows a throat infection by *Group A streptococci*. Therapies comprise medications such as antibiotics including antistreptococcal prophylaxis following the acute infection, analgesics, and antiinflammatory agents. Rheumatic fever is classified according to the site of inflammation. In acute rheumatic fever, the infection is active.

The categories in this code block are as follows:

I00	Rheumatic fever without heart involvement
I01	Rheumatic fever with heart involvement
I02	Rheumatic chorea

I00   Rheumatic fever without heart involvement

This code is limited to rheumatic fever that may have acute or subacute arthritis, but no heart involvement.

I01.-   Rheumatic fever with heart involvement

Acute rheumatic fever, a complication of strep pharyngitis in children, results in various cardiac conditions in more than a third of patients affected. Depending on the extent of heart inflammation involved, patients with the acute form of the disease may develop heart failure, pericarditis, myocarditis, or endocarditis. Endocarditis typically manifests as insufficiency of the mitral valve and/or aortic valve. In adults, acute rheumatic fever is the most common cause of mitral valve stenosis and the leading cause for valvular replacement surgery. Although the mitral valve is most commonly affected, the aortic and tricuspid valves may also be involved. Chronic manifestations due to protracted disease and continued valve deformity also occur in some adults with previous rheumatic heart disease. Two to 10 years after an acute episode of rheumatic fever, the valve apparatus may fuse, with resulting stenosis or stenosis with insufficiency.

I01.0   Acute rheumatic pericarditis

Acute rheumatic pericarditis is acute rheumatic fever with inflammation of the lining surrounding the heart muscle. It is uncommon in adults.

I01.1   Acute rheumatic endocarditis

Acute rheumatic endocarditis is an acute rheumatic fever with inflammation of the interior lining of the heart and/or heart valves. A common finding in acute rheumatic endocarditis is the presence of large, friable vegetations on the heart valves or chordae tendineae.

I01.2   Acute rheumatic myocarditis

Acute rheumatic myocarditis is an acute rheumatic fever with inflammation of the heart muscle. While this manifestation has minor initial symptoms, it can quickly lead to heart failure and death. Initial signs and symptoms may include tachycardia out of proportion to fever, cardiac manifestations such as heart blocks and arrhythmias, and a history of recent upper respiratory infection, pharyngitis, or tonsillitis. In addition to heart block and arrhythmias, the condition may be complicated by congestive heart failure, thromboembolism, and pericarditis.

I02.-   Rheumatic chorea

Rheumatic chorea is an inflammatory complication of *Group A streptococcal* infection or rheumatic fever involving the central nervous system that may occur with or without cardiac involvement. Also known as chorea minor, chorea dance, Sydenham's chorea, and Saint Vitus dance, it generally affects children and young adults. Signs and symptoms include involuntary, irregular, jerky movements of the face (excluding eyes), neck, or limbs. This condition is classified based on whether or not there is heart involvement.

Chronic Rheumatic Heart Diseases (I05-I09)

Chronic rheumatic heart disease results from single or repeated episodes of acute rheumatic fever that alter the structure of the heart, usually the endocardium. Sequelae include rigidity and deformity of the valvular cusps, fusion of the commissures, or shortening and fusion of the chordae tendinea. Damage also may occur in the myocardium following severe bouts of acute rheumatic myocarditis affecting cardiac performance.

The categories in this code block are as follows:

I05	Rheumatic mitral valve diseases
I06	Rheumatic aortic valve diseases
I07	Rheumatic tricuspid valve diseases
I08	Multiple valve diseases
I09	Other rheumatic heart diseases

I05.-   Rheumatic mitral valve diseases

Depending on the extent of heart inflammation, patients with the acute form of the rheumatic heart disease may develop chronic heart conditions, including mitral valve disease. The mitral valve is also called the bicuspid valve because it has dual cusps. Blood passes through the mitral valve from the left atrium to the left ventricle.

I05.0   Rheumatic mitral stenosis

I05.1   Rheumatic mitral insufficiency

I05.2   Rheumatic mitral stenosis with insufficiency

Mitral stenosis is a narrowing of the orifice of the mitral valve, between the left atrium and left ventricle, due to rheumatic heart disease that impedes left ventricular filling. Signs and symptoms include left or combined left and right heart failure, hemoptysis, systematic embolism, hoarseness, atrial fibrillation, or pulmonary rales and increased S1/S2 heart sounds. Rheumatic mitral insufficiency is a reflux of a portion of blood back into the left atrium instead of forward into the aorta, resulting in increased atrial pressure and decreased forward cardiac output. Signs and symptoms may include dyspnea due to left ventricular failure (which may be combined with right heart failure in severe cases), pulmonary hypertension, holosystolic apical murmur, S3 heart sound, or brisk carotid upstroke.

Focus Point

Mitral stenosis, mitral valve disease (unspecified), and mitral valve failure are presumed to be rheumatic in origin for classification purposes and need not be stated as rheumatic. Other manifestations, such as insufficiency, incompetence, or regurgitation (without stenosis) must be specified as due to rheumatic heart disease or the default is the code for the nonrheumatic condition.

I06.-   Rheumatic aortic valve diseases

Depending on the extent of heart inflammation, patients with the acute form of the rheumatic heart disease may develop chronic heart conditions, including aortic valve disease. Blood flows from the left ventricle into the aorta through the aortic valve.

I06.0   Rheumatic aortic stenosis

I06.1   Rheumatic aortic insufficiency

I06.2   Rheumatic aortic stenosis with insufficiency

Rheumatic aortic stenosis is a pathological narrowing of the aortic valve orifice due to fibrosis of the commissures and/or degenerative distortion of the aortic valve cusps. Commissural fusion and scarring may be present early in the progression of the disease, and calcification of the valve is often a late complication. The resulting stenosis produces a pressure overload on the left ventricle due to the increased pressure needed to force the blood through the narrowed aortic valve orifice. Signs and symptoms of rheumatic aortic stenosis include angina, syncope, heart failure, delayed carotid upstroke, and/or a sustained forceful apex beat, systolic ejection murmur, or softened singular S2 heart sound with S4 heart sound. Rheumatic aortic insufficiency is the reflux of blood into the left ventricle during diastole due to an incompetent aortic valve. Chronic aortic insufficiency eventually leads to left ventricular dysfunction and failure. The condition is also known as rheumatic aortic regurgitation and rheumatic aortic incompetence. Signs and symptoms include left ventricular failure, syncope, angina, diastolic murmur along the left sternal border or an Austin Fling murmur, and/or stroke volume increase.

I07.- Rheumatic tricuspid valve diseases

Although the mitral valve is most commonly affected in rheumatic heart disease, the tricuspid valves may also be involved. The tricuspid valve lies between the right atrium and the right ventricle.

I07.0 Rheumatic tricuspid stenosis

I07.1 Rheumatic tricuspid insufficiency

I07.2 Rheumatic tricuspid stenosis and insufficiency

Rheumatic diseases of the tricuspid valve include stenosis (obstruction) and insufficiency (incompetence, regurgitation), presenting alone or together. Tricuspid valve disorders occur when there is a malfunction of the valve between the right atrium and right ventricle due to functional or structural conditions. Tricuspid regurgitation may occur secondary to right ventricular pressure overload from left-sided lesions or it may occur as a result of primary rheumatic heart disease of the tricuspid valve itself. Tricuspid stenosis is a mechanical obstruction blocking the return of blood to the right ventricle of the heart. Tricuspid stenosis usually means the leaflets have become thicker than normal, causing narrowing, as opposed to the buildup of the actual valve itself.

Focus Point

Tricuspid valve disease is presumed to be rheumatic in origin for classification purposes when the cause is not specified. If specified as nonrheumatic, the code is located in category I36. If mitral or aortic valves are also included, the appropriate code is located in category I08.

I08.- Multiple valve diseases

This category is used when multiple combinations of mitral, aortic, and tricuspid valve disease is present. The fourth character indicates which valves are involved.

I09.- Other rheumatic heart diseases

This subcategory includes sequela of rheumatic fever that affect the heart wall and the protective layers that surround the heart, including the myocardium, endocardium, and pericardium.

I09.0 Rheumatic myocarditis

Chronic inflammation of the muscular walls of the heart (myocarditis) specified as due to or a late effect of rheumatic heart disease is reported here.

Focus Point

Code rheumatic myocarditis, in addition to rheumatic valve disease, when both conditions are documented.

I09.2 Chronic rheumatic pericarditis

Chronic rheumatic pericarditis is a set of conditions such as adhesive pericarditis and constrictive pericarditis that may occur following an acute rheumatic infection. Adhesive pericarditis occurs when adhesions develop between the two-pericardial layers or between the pericardium and the heart or other neighboring structures. Constrictive pericarditis is a thickening of the pericardial membrane with constriction of the cardiac chambers.

I09.81 Rheumatic heart failure

Congestive rheumatic heart failure is a common complication of rheumatic valvular disease. Heart failure occurs when there is a malfunction in the rate the blood is being pumped or a malfunction in the filling pressure and leads to circulatory failure.

Focus Point

When heart failure is present with rheumatic aortic and mitral valve insufficiency, the heart failure is always classified as rheumatic.

I09.89 Other specified rheumatic heart diseases

Rheumatic diseases of pulmonary valves are classified here and include pulmonary valve insufficiency and stenosis. Pulmonary valve insufficiency is a reflux of blood back into the right ventricle through an incompetent pulmonary valve and may be associated with pulmonary hypertension. Pulmonary valve stenosis is narrowing of the pulmonary valve orifice causing an obstruction of blood flow through the pulmonary valve.

Hypertensive Diseases (I10-I16)

Hypertension occurs when the arterioles narrow, causing the blood to exert excessive pressure against the vessel wall and the heart to work harder to maintain the higher pressure. The World Health Organization (WHO) defines hypertension as pressures exceeding 140/90 mm Hg, but studies have shown that increased morbidity and mortality are associated with diastolic pressures of just 85 mm Hg. Hypertension is generally asymptomatic until complications develop. Complications may include retinal changes, loud aortic sounds and an early systolic ejection click heard on auscultation, headache, tinnitus, and palpitations. Over time, damage to the heart and kidneys can result and codes are available to capture hypertensive heart and/or chronic kidney disease.

Focus Point

In ICD-9-CM, all hypertension diagnoses were subclassified as benign or malignant with an unspecified code available if documentation did not support a more specific code. In ICD-10-CM, hypertension is no longer subclassified as benign or malignant.

The categories in this code block are as follows:

I10	Essential (primary) hypertension
I11	Hypertensive heart disease
I12	Hypertensive chronic kidney disease
I13	Hypertensive heart and chronic kidney disease
I15	Secondary hypertension
I16	Hypertensive crisis

I10   Essential (primary) hypertension

Essential (primary) hypertension accounts for the majority of hypertension diagnoses. Essential or primary hypertension means that there is no underlying condition that is causing the blood pressure to increase. Essential hypertension is typically defined as a systolic pressure higher that 140 mm Hg and a diastolic pressure of less than 90 mm Hg.

I11.-   Hypertensive heart disease

This category reports heart disease due to complications of hypertension. When hypertension is uncontrolled, it can eventually cause changes to the heart including the conduction system, the coronary vessels, and the myocardium itself. In addition to arrhythmias, infarction, and angina, these changes may also result in hypertrophy of the left ventricle that can progress to heart failure. Hypertension causes the heart to work harder in order to pump blood throughout the body. When this happens for long periods of time, the heart muscle begins to thicken and the volume of blood pumped by the heart decreases.

Hypertensive heart disease is the most common cause of illness and death resulting from high blood pressure. Hypertensive heart disease is classified based on the presence or absence of heart failure, which is captured by the fourth character.

I12.-   Hypertensive chronic kidney disease

Hypertensive chronic kidney disease, also known as arteriolar nephrosclerosis, is characterized by intimal thickening of the afferent arteriole of the glomerulus due to long-standing or poorly controlled hypertension. In severe nephrosclerosis, the nephron is deprived of its blood supply, and areas of infarction occur with subsequent scar tissue formation. Renal insufficiency occurs when the kidney is scarred and contracted. In most cases, the patient eventually develops kidney failure. The stage of hypertensive chronic kidney disease is identified by the fourth character.

Focus Point

An additional code should be assigned from category N18 to more specifically describe the stage of chronic kidney disease.

I13.-   Hypertensive heart and chronic kidney disease

This category is used for combined forms of heart and renal disease. Hypertension causes the heart to work harder in order to pump blood throughout the body. When this happens for long periods of time, the heart muscle begins to thicken and the volume of blood pumped by the heart decreases. Chronic kidney disease occurs when there is damage to the kidneys from heart disease and high blood pressure. Fourth and fifth characters identify the presence or absence of heart failure plus indicate the stage of chronic kidney disease.

I15.-   Secondary hypertension

Secondary hypertension is caused by renovascular or other diseases, such as renal parenchymal diseases, oral contraceptives, primary aldosteronism, Cushing's syndrome, pheochromocytoma, hyperparathyroidism, hyperthyroidism, and acromegaly.

Focus Point

Codes in category I15 do not include any reference to chronic kidney disease or renal failure. If chronic kidney disease is documented, an additional code from category N18 should be assigned.

I15.0   Renovascular hypertension

Renovascular hypertension is caused by obstruction of renal blood flow at the level of the renal artery. The obstruction stimulates the renin-angiotensin system causing an increase in systemic angiotensin, which in turn causes the retention of sodium and water resulting in hypertension.

I15.1 Hypertension secondary to other renal disorders

This classification includes hypertension due to renal parenchymal diseases. Renal parenchymal diseases are conditions that reduce kidney function by affecting the kidney's ability to excrete water and sodium.

I16.- Hypertensive crisis

Hypertensive crisis is a life-threatening rapid increase in a patient's blood pressure. The presence or absence of associated organ damage further classifies the type of hypertensive crisis as urgent or emergent.

I16.0 Hypertensive urgency

When a patient has a systolic blood pressure equal to or greater than 180 or a diastolic pressure greater than 110 in the absence of associated organ damage or dysfunction, he or she is said to be in hypertensive urgency. Immediate blood pressure reduction is often not necessary and acute complications are unlikely, but the patient will need his or her medication adjusted and blood pressure monitored more closely to ensure it continues to stay at a suitable level.

I16.1 Hypertensive emergency

A patient is experiencing a hypertensive emergency when blood pressure levels exceed 180 systolic over 120 diastolic and organ damage is present. The organ systems typically affected include cardiac, renal, and neurologic, manifested as coronary ischemia, disturbed cerebral function, renal failure, cerebrovascular events, and pulmonary edema. These cases require intensive care hospital admission for immediate but controlled blood pressure reduction via IV medications. Complete work-up and evaluation should be completed to determine the underlying cause or trigger of the hypertensive emergency.

Ischemic Heart Diseases (I20-I25)

Ischemic heart disease is an inadequate flow of blood through the coronary arteries to the tissue of the heart. The predominant etiology of the ischemia is arteriosclerosis. Partially obstructed coronary artery blood flow can manifest in angina pectoris; complete obstruction results in an infarction of the myocardium.

The categories in this code block are as follows:

I20	Angina pectoris
I21	Acute myocardial infarction
I22	Subsequent ST elevation (STEMI) and non-ST elevation (NSTEMI) myocardial infarction
I23	Certain current complications following ST elevation (STEMI) and non-ST elevation (NSTEMI) myocardial infarction (within the 28 day period)
I24	Other acute ischemic heart diseases
I25	Chronic ischemic heart disease

I20.- Angina pectoris

Angina pectoris is chest pain due to myocardial ischemia, most often caused by atherosclerotic heart disease, but it may be due to coronary artery spasm, severe aortic stenosis or insufficiency, syphilitic aortitis, vasculitis, marked anemia, paroxysmal tachycardia with rapid ventricular rates, or any disease or disorder that markedly increases metabolic demands on the heart. Symptoms result from decreased oxygen supply to the heart muscle due to narrowed vessels.

I20.0 Unstable angina

Unstable angina is an intermediate state between angina pectoris of effort and acute myocardial infarction. The patient's pain is more acute, longer lasting, and more frequent then angina, and more resistant to antianginal treatment. Unstable angina, with its increased likelihood of impending myocardial infarction, is a medical emergency and requires acute care hospitalization. Unstable angina may be documented as accelerated, crescendo, preinfarction, or intermediate coronary syndrome.

> **Focus Point**
>
> The term "Class III" and "Class IV" describing the functional classification of patients with heart disease may be used in conjunction with unstable angina. However, do not assume every patient with Class III or Class IV angina or heart disease has unstable angina. Code I20.0 cannot be assigned when the condition evolves into an acute myocardial infarction during the same encounter. See categories I21 and I22 for acute myocardial infarction classifications.

I20.1 Angina pectoris with documented spasm

This type of angina is caused by a temporary spasm of a coronary artery that constricts the artery partially or completely, blocking blood flow. When the coronary artery spasms the region of the heart muscle supplied by the coronary artery does not receive the necessary oxygen and other nutrients from the blood. Prolonged spasm has the potential to cause heart damage and may lead to myocardial infarction. Angina due to coronary artery spasm is characterized by chest pain at rest and by sinus tachycardia (ST) segment elevation, rather than depression, during the attack.

I20.8 Other forms of angina pectoris

Angina equivalent is classified here and describes other symptoms of interrupted blood flow to the heart muscle that do not include the more characteristic chest pain symptoms. Angina equivalent symptoms may include pain characterized as indigestion, shortness of breath, and generalized weakness or malaise. Chest pain that occurs on exertion, which is called angina of effort, is also classified here. Angina of effort is caused by partially blocked coronary arteries that are unable to deliver the increased amount of blood to the heart that is necessary during periods of exertion. Coronary slow flow syndrome is characterized by slow flow of contrast through the coronary arteries during diagnostic radiographic studies. These patients may not have obvious obstruction but they do present with recurrent chest pain, which is typically the symptom that leads to the diagnostic studies. Stenocardia is another term used to describe chest pain associated with slow flow of blood through the coronary arteries. Stable angina is also classified here.

I20.9 Angina pectoris, unspecified

This is the appropriate code for unspecified angina and anginal syndrome. Ischemic chest pain is also included in this code.

I21.- Acute myocardial infarction

Acute myocardial infarction (AMI) can be defined as showing evidence of myocardial necrosis with clinical criteria that support the diagnosis. Some of the clinical criteria include elevation of biomarkers (troponins), ECG changes, blood tests, imaging, and symptoms of ischemia. AMI may be due to coronary artery embolism, occlusion, thrombosis, or rupture. ST-elevation (STEMI) myocardial infarction is generally due to plaque rupture with complete obstruction of one or more coronary arteries causing full-thickness heart damage. Non-ST elevation (NSTEMI) myocardial infarction occurs with the development of partial occlusion causing partial-thickness heart muscle damage. The following are myocardial infarction (MI)

clinical classifications type 1-5, as defined by the Task Force for the Universal Definition of Myocardial Infarction, which have been added as inclusion notes to codes in this category.

Type 1 MI: Refers to a spontaneous myocardial infarction event caused by an intraluminal thrombus that occurs due to atherosclerotic plaque disruption such as a rupture, ulceration, or erosion. This obstruction of one or more coronary arteries causes decreased blood flow (ischemia) and necrosis of myocardial muscle cells. Type 1 can be associated with either a STEMI or NSTEMI.

Type 2 MI: Refers to a myocardial infarction due to ischemia and necrosis resulting from an oxygen imbalance to the heart. This mismatch between oxygen decreased supply and increased demand is caused by conditions other than coronary artery disease such as vasospasm, embolism, anemia, hypertension, hypotension, or arrhythmias.

Type 3 MI: Refers to a myocardial infarction that causes sudden cardiac death. This occurs with symptoms or ECG changes that suggest myocardial infarction although blood tests and biomarkers have not yet been taken or identified.

Type 4 and 5: These refer to an MI that is related to the performance of a current or prior revascularization procedure such as a percutaneous coronary intervention (4a), in-stent thrombosis (4b), or CABG (5). This can occur intraoperatively or postoperatively, and it is necessary to review the instructional codes at I21.A9 to accurately reflect this information. Complication codes may also be required.

> **Focus Point**
>
> *Any STEMI or NSTEMI that is documented as acute or has a stated duration of four weeks (28 days) from onset is coded in category I21.-. For encounters occurring during the four-week duration, including transfers or continuing care, the codes from I21.- may continue to be reported if the condition meets the definition of a reportable secondary diagnosis as outlined in section III of the ICD-10-CM Official Guidelines for Coding and Reporting. For care related to the MI after the four-week timeframe, the appropriate aftercare code is assigned and not one from I21.-. Code I25.2 Old myocardial infarction, is assigned when care is no longer needed for an old or healed MI.*

I21.0- ST elevation (STEMI) myocardial infarction of anterior wall

This subcategory includes STEMI occurring toward the front side of the heart. Anterior infarcts are likely to be larger and have a poorer prognosis than do inferoposterior infarcts. They are most often due to obstruction of the left coronary artery, particularly the anterior descending artery. Codes for anterior wall STEMI identify the affected coronary artery as the left main coronary artery, the left anterior descending coronary artery, or other coronary arteries affecting the anteroapical, anterolateral, or anteroseptal walls and involving a transmural (Q wave) infarction. Type 1 MI of the anterior wall is included in this code and refers to a spontaneous myocardial infarction event caused by an intraluminal thrombus that occurs due to atherosclerotic plaque disruption such as a rupture, ulceration, or erosion. This obstruction of one or more coronary arteries causes decreased blood flow (ischemia) and necrosis of myocardial muscle cells.

I21.1-   ST elevation (STEMI) myocardial infarction of inferior wall

This subcategory includes STEMI occurring toward the bottom of the heart. Codes for inferior wall STEMI identify the specific site involved as the right or inferoposterior transmural coronary artery or other sites of the inferior wall, such as inferolateral transmural (Q wave). Type 1 MI of the inferior wall is included in this code and refers to a spontaneous myocardial infarction event caused by an intraluminal thrombus that occurs due to atherosclerotic plaque disruption such as a rupture, ulceration, or erosion. This obstruction of one or more coronary arteries causes decreased blood flow (ischemia) and necrosis of myocardial muscle cells.

I21.2-   ST elevation (STEMI) myocardial infarction of other sites

This subcategory reports STEMI involving other sites. Codes for STEMI involving other sites include a specific code for the left circumflex or oblique marginal coronary artery and a second code for all other sites such as lateral, apical-lateral, basal-lateral, high lateral, posterior, posterobasal, posterolateral, posteroseptal, and septal transmural (Q wave) infarctions. Type 1 MI of the other sites reported with this code refers to a spontaneous myocardial infarction event caused by an intraluminal thrombus that occurs due to atherosclerotic plaque disruption such as a rupture, ulceration, or erosion. This obstruction of one or more coronary arteries causes decreased blood flow (ischemia) and necrosis of myocardial muscle cells.

I21.4   Non-ST elevation (NSTEMI) myocardial infarction

Even though the clinical presentations are similar in STEMI and NSTEMI, they are very different conditions. Non-ST elevation MI (NSTEMI), also referred to as non-Q wave myocardial infarction, tends to occur mainly in a subendocardial or midmyocardial site. Because it does not extend through the entire ventricular wall, it does not display the usual ST elevations or progress to Q wave patterns seen in STEMIs. Other terms that describe NSTEMI include subendocardial infarction, which is an MI involving the pericardium instead of the endocardium, and nontransmural, which is an MI that fails to extend through the entire heart wall from the endocardium to

the epicardium and instead extends only part way through the heart wall. Type 1 NSTEMI is included in this code and refers to a myocardial infarction caused by an intraluminal thrombus that occurs due to atherosclerotic plaque rupture. This partial obstruction of one or more coronary arteries causes decreased blood flow (ischemia) and may cause partial thickness necrosis of myocardial muscle cells.

Focus Point

NSTEMI typically involves a total occlusion of a minor coronary artery or a partial occlusion of a major coronary artery with only partial thickness heart muscle damage. In distinction, full thickness damage is normally incurred by a STEMI because of the occurrence of a major coronary artery occlusion. Complications such as cardiogenic shock, heart failure, and cardiac tamponade are more prevalent in STEMI. Short-term mortality is lower in NSTEMI vs. STEMI, but reinfarction rate is higher in NSTEMI than STEMI, with long-term mortality that is equal to STEMI.

I21.A1   Myocardial infarction type 2

This type 2 MI is often referred to as due to demand ischemia. It refers to a myocardial infarction due to ischemia and necrosis resulting from an oxygen imbalance to the heart. This mismatch between oxygen decreased supply and increased demand is caused by conditions other than coronary artery disease such as vasospasm, embolism, anemia, hypertension, hypotension, or arrhythmias.

I21.A9   Other myocardial infarction type

This code includes MI classified as types 3, 4, and 5. Type 3 is used to reflect a myocardial infarction that causes sudden cardiac death. This occurs with symptoms or ECG changes that suggest myocardial infarction although blood tests and biomarkers have not yet been taken or identified.

Types 4 and 5 refer to an MI that is related to the performance of a current or prior revascularization procedure such as a percutaneous coronary intervention (4a), in-stent thrombosis (4b), or CABG (5). This can occur intraoperatively or postoperatively, and it is necessary to review the instructional notes at I21.A9 to accurately reflect this information. Complication codes may also be required.

I22.-   Subsequent ST elevation (STEMI) and non-ST elevation (NSTEMI) myocardial infarction

This category reports a subsequent acute myocardial infarction (AMI) that occurs during the recovery phase following the first AMI. The recovery phase of an AMI is currently defined as four weeks (28 days) and is the period during which the heart damage undergoes the process of healing following the myocardial infarction. A subsequent AMI during the recovery phase following previous AMI increases the complexity of medical care and also increases the risk of mortality. There are codes for both STEMI and NSTEMI. Subsequent STEMI codes identify only the general region of the infarction as anterior wall, inferior wall, or other site rather than the specific artery or more specific sites.

I23.-   Certain current complications following ST elevation (STEMI) and non-ST elevation (NSTEMI) myocardial infarction (within the 28 day period)

There are a number of complications affecting the heart that may occur during the acute phase of care following a myocardial infarction, such as rupture of the cardiac wall, chordae tendineae, or papillary muscle; hemopericardium; or thrombosis within one of the heart chambers.

I23.1   Atrial septal defect as current complication following acute myocardial infarction

Atrial septal defect occurs as a rare complication of acute myocardial infarction (AMI) and typically manifests within a few days to three weeks after an AMI. An atrial septal defect is an opening or hole in the interatrial septum between the two upper chambers of the heart. This complication causes shunting of blood from the left to the right atrium, which in turn causes blood to back up into the right ventricle with resultant right ventricular overload and increased pulmonary artery pressure. An untreated atrial septal defect can cause right heart failure.

I23.4   Rupture of chordae tendineae as current complication following acute myocardial infarction

The chordae tendineae are thin fibrous cords of connective tissue that extend from the papillary muscles in the right or left ventricle wall to the leaflets in the tricuspid (right ventricle) and mitral (left ventricle) heart valves. The chordae tendineae keep the closed leaflets from prolapsing into the atria as the heart muscle in the ventricles contracts and propels blood into the pulmonary and systemic circulation. Rupture of the chordae tendineae is an acute injury to

these structures and acute myocardial infarction is the most common cause of this type of injury. When the chordae tendineae rupture the closed leaflets in the affected valve prolapse into the atrium as the ventricle walls contract to propel blood into the pulmonary arteries or aorta. The prolapsed leaflets allow blood to regurgitate (flow backward) into the atrium causing increased blood volume on the affected side of the heart.

I23.5   Rupture of papillary muscle as current complication following acute myocardial infarction

In the normal heart, the papillary muscles are attached to the lower segment of the inside ventricular walls. They connect to the chordae tendineae, which are the cord-shaped tendons attached to the tricuspid valve (right ventricle) and the mitral valve (left ventricle). When the papillary muscles contract, the valves open and when they relax, the valves close. Injury caused by an acute myocardial infarction (AMI) can cause the papillary muscle to rupture. When the papillary muscles rupture the affected valve no longer opens and closes properly allowing blood to regurgitate (flow backward) from the ventricle into the atrium. Rupture of the papillary muscles of the tricuspid or mitral valve is a rare complication of AMI that can lead to pulmonary edema, cardiogenic shock, and death. The most common AMI site resulting in papillary muscle rupture is an inferior AMI of the left ventricle with occlusion of the posterior descending artery. The posterior descending artery is the only blood supply to the posteromedial papillary muscle of the mitral valve, and rupture of that papillary muscle can result even when only a small region is affected by the infarction.

I23.7   Postinfarction angina

Some patients experience postinfarction angina pectoris after a recent acute myocardial infarction (AMI) because of persistent coronary artery disease and obstructed blood flow to the heart muscle. Postinfarction angina occurs more frequently following non-ST elevation myocardial infarction (NSTEMI) as compared with ST elevation myocardial infarction (STEMI). Postinfarction angina is a risk factor for recurrent AMI and other acute cardiac disorders, as well as for sudden death.

I24.-   Other acute ischemic heart diseases

Acute forms of ischemia include conditions with a relatively short and severe course, and subacute forms of ischemia denote a course of ischemic disease that falls in between acute and chronic disease.

I24.0   Acute coronary thrombosis not resulting in myocardial infarction

Coronary occlusion without myocardial infarction or tissue death is reported here. This code classifies patients with an acute or subacute, complete or incomplete, occlusion of the coronary artery, not associated with acute myocardial infarction. The occlusion may be embolic, thrombotic, other, or unspecified and is usually associated with some form of angina.

I24.1   Dressler's syndrome

Dressler's syndrome, also known as postmyocardial infarction syndrome, postpericardiotomy syndrome, or postcardiac injury syndrome, is a complication occurring several days to several weeks following an acute myocardial infarction. It is characterized by inflammation of the pericardium. Symptoms include chest pain similar to that experienced during a myocardial infarction and fever. This condition is believed to be due to an antibody antigen reaction that takes place in the myocardial tissue during the healing phase of an infarction.

Focus Point

Some patients experience postinfarction angina pectoris after a recent myocardial infarction because of persistent coronary artery disease. Do not confuse postinfarction angina with postmyocardial infarction syndrome. Report code I23.7 for postinfarction angina.

I24.9   Acute ischemic heart disease, unspecified

Acute coronary syndrome (ACS) not otherwise specified is reported as unspecified acute ischemic heart disease. It is included here because the term acute coronary syndrome is nonspecific and may refer to a wide range of ischemic heart conditions from unstable angina to myocardial infarction.

Focus Point

For intermediate coronary syndrome or insufficiency, report the code for unstable angina I20.0. For coronary syndrome with slow flow, report the code for other angina I20.8.

I25.-   Chronic ischemic heart disease

This category reports prolonged or ongoing obstruction of blood flow to the heart. Chronic ischemia is the most common form of ischemic heart disease and coronary atherosclerosis is the most common cause. Coronary atherosclerosis results from accumulation of fatty and fibrous tissue within the blood vessels. In time, the fatty and fibrous tissue accumulations calcify, which is why this condition is commonly referred to as "hardening of the arteries."

I25.1-   Atherosclerotic heart disease of native coronary artery

Coronary atherosclerosis is localized, subintimal accumulations of fatty and fibrous tissue in a native coronary artery caused by proliferation of smooth muscle cells in combination with a disorder of lipid metabolism. Atherosclerotic heart disease (ASHD) eventually leads to acute and subacute forms of ischemic heart disease, such as unstable angina and myocardial infarction. Subcategory combination codes identify whether the atherosclerosis of the native artery is accompanied by specific types of angina pectoris or whether there is no angina pectoris present.

I25.10   Atherosclerotic heart disease of native coronary artery without angina pectoris

Arteriosclerotic heart disease (ASHD) without any chest pain symptoms is reported with this code.

I25.11-   Atherosclerotic heart disease of native coronary artery with angina pectoris

Angina pectoris is a common symptom of arteriosclerotic heart disease (ASHD).

I25.110   Atherosclerotic heart disease of native coronary artery with unstable angina pectoris

ASHD may be accompanied by unstable angina. Unstable angina is an intermediate state between angina pectoris of effort and acute myocardial infarction. The patient's pain is more acute, longer lasting, and more frequent then angina, and more resistant to antianginal treatment. Unstable angina, with its increased likelihood of impending myocardial infarction, is a medical emergency and requires acute care hospitalization. Unstable angina may be documented as accelerated, crescendo, preinfarction, or intermediate coronary syndrome.

I25.111   Atherosclerotic heart disease of native coronary artery with angina pectoris with documented spasm

ASHD may be accompanied by angina due to coronary artery spasm. This type of angina is caused by a temporary spasm of a coronary artery that constricts the artery partially or completely blocking blood flow. When the coronary artery spasms the region of the heart muscle supplied by the coronary artery does not receive the necessary oxygen and other nutrients from the blood. Prolonged spasm has the potential to cause heart damage and may lead to myocardial infarction. Angina due to coronary artery spasm is characterized by chest pain at rest and by sinus tachycardia (ST) segment elevation, rather than depression, during the attack.

I25.118   Atherosclerotic heart disease of native coronary artery with other forms of angina pectoris

ASHD with angina equivalent is classified here. The term angina equivalent is used to describe other symptoms of interrupted blood flow to the heart muscle that do not include the more characteristic chest pain symptoms. Angina equivalent symptoms may include pain characterized as indigestion, shortness of breath, and generalized weakness or malaise. Chest pain that occurs on exertion, which is called angina of effort, is also classified here. Angina of effort is caused by partially blocked coronary arteries that are unable to deliver the increased amount of blood to the heart that is necessary during periods of exertion. Coronary slow flow syndrome is characterized by slow flow of contrast through the coronary arteries during diagnostic radiographic studies. These patients may not have obvious obstruction but they do present with recurrent chest pain, which is typically the symptom that leads to the diagnostic studies. Stenocardia is another term used to describe chest pain associated slow flow of blood through the coronary arteries. When documentation states that the ASHD is accompanied by stable angina, it is also classified here.

I25.119 Atherosclerotic heart disease of native coronary artery with unspecified angina pectoris

This is the appropriate code when ASHD is accompanied by unspecified angina. ASHD with ischemic chest pain is also included in this code.

I25.2 Old myocardial infarction

This code represents a healed myocardial infarction and is reported for any myocardial infarction described as older than four weeks (28 days). This code may also be used when patients have evidence of a healed myocardial infarction that is observed via clinical testing such as an ECG. In these cases, the patient is generally asymptomatic and may require no medical intervention. A history of a myocardial infarction typically requires ongoing monitoring of the patient to address any long-term complications or new symptoms that can arise as a result of the damage caused by the previous myocardial infarction.

I25.3 Aneurysm of heart

Aneurysm of the heart is a dilatation, stretching, weakening, or bulging of the tissue of the heart. An aneurysm of the heart wall is an aneurysm of heart muscle, known as a cardiac, mural, or ventricular wall aneurysm, which is usually a consequence of myocardial infarction.

I25.41 Coronary artery aneurysm

Aneurysm of the coronary vessels is a circumscribed dilatation of a coronary artery or a blood-containing mass connecting directly with the lumen of a coronary artery. Also reported here is a coronary arteriovenous fistula. This type of abnormal communication between a coronary artery and vein results in the formation of an arteriovenous aneurysm and is usually the result of a previous myocardial infarction.

I25.42 Coronary artery dissection

Dissection happens when the layers within the coronary artery tear and blood infiltrates those layers causing further separation. This inhibits the blood flow that may lead to a burst vessel.

I25.5 Ischemic cardiomyopathy

Ischemic cardiomyopathy is ischemic heart disease with diffuse fibrosis or multiple infarctions, resulting in heart failure with left ventricular dilation.

I25.7- Atherosclerosis of coronary artery bypass graft(s) and coronary artery of transplanted heart with angina pectoris

Atherosclerosis is the accumulation of fatty deposits and plaque formation in a native artery or bypass graft that narrows the lumen of the artery or graft and obstructs blood flow. Atherosclerosis may occur in coronary artery bypass grafts or in native or bypassed coronary arteries of a transplanted heart. Codes in this subcategory are used when atherosclerosis of autologous, nonautologous, or other types of coronary artery bypass grafts occurs or when the native or bypassed coronary arteries of a transplanted heart is present along with chest pain or other symptoms related to angina pectoris.

I25.81- Atherosclerosis of other coronary vessels without angina pectoris

Atherosclerosis is the accumulation of fatty deposits and plaque formation in a native artery or bypass graft that narrows the lumen of the artery or graft and obstructs blood flow. Atherosclerosis may occur in coronary artery bypass grafts or in native or bypassed coronary arteries of a transplanted heart. Codes in this subcategory are used when atherosclerosis of these structures is not associated with chest pain or other symptoms related to angina pectoris.

I25.82 Chronic total occlusion of coronary artery

Chronic total occlusion of a coronary artery is a complete blockage of the artery that has been present for an extended duration (typically longer than three months). In these cases, myocardial infarction may be avoided by a collateral flow process. Collateral flow, or vessels that "re-route" blood flow, do not function as efficiently and often result in symptoms of ischemic heart disease. In addition, vascular "re-routing" places stress on the vasculature of the heart and puts the patient at significant risk for myocardial infarction while increasing the risk of other morbidity and/or mortality. Due to the difficulty in passing a guidewire through a chronic total occlusion, treatment of this form of blockage is often more challenging than for other types of coronary stenosis.

I25.83   Coronary atherosclerosis due to lipid rich plaque

Lipid-rich atherosclerotic plaques are particularly unstable and vulnerable to rupture, increasing the risk of acute coronary events such as thrombosis, arrhythmia, and myocardial infarction. Atherosclerotic plaques containing lipid-rich cores have been identified as a cause of arterial filling defects during angiography procedures. In atherogenesis, plaque stability depends on multiple factors including plaque composition, size and location of the core, arterial wall stress, and the relationship of plaque to blood flow. Vulnerable or high-risk lipid rich plaques must be evaluated and monitored more closely to determine the optimal course of treatment based on the nature and composition of the patient's coronary artery plaques.

Focus Point

Lipid-rich plaque of coronary vessels cannot be present without coronary atherosclerosis. Therefore, the appropriate coronary atherosclerosis code from subcategory I25.- should be sequenced first, followed by code I25.83.

I25.84   Coronary atherosclerosis due to calcified coronary lesion

In the treatment of coronary atherosclerosis, calcified lesions present significant treatment challenges. Calcified coronary artery lesions are less amenable to angioplasty and stenting procedures due to the recalcitrant blockages caused by the hardened calcium deposits in the arteries. Additional time and skill are often required of physicians when treating these lesions. If the calcified plaques prove impassable by catheter or are resistant to treatment, coronary artery bypass may be indicated to restore circulation. Research has indicated that calcified lesions are associated with a higher incidence of major adverse cardiac events than noncalcified lesions, including those comprised of lipid-rich plaque. Calcium deposits in the coronary arteries can be detected by x-ray during coronary angiography and with intravascular ultrasound.

Pulmonary Heart Disease and Diseases of Pulmonary Circulation (I26-I28)

In the circulatory pathway, the blood leaves the right ventricle via the pulmonary trunk, which splits into the right and left pulmonary arteries to be reoxygenated. Ultimately four (two left, two right) pulmonary veins return oxygen-rich blood to the left atrium, then the left ventricle, where the oxygenated blood is pumped into the systemic circulation. This chapter includes diseases of these pulmonary vessels.

The categories in this code block are as follows:

I26	Pulmonary embolism
I27	Other pulmonary heart diseases
I28	Other diseases of pulmonary vessels

I26.-   Pulmonary embolism

Pulmonary embolism occurs when a thrombus, usually forming in the veins of the lower extremities or pelvis or less often in the right atrium secondary to atrial fibrillation or flutter, travels through the right-sided circulation of the heart and becomes lodged in the pulmonary artery. This blocks blood flow to the lungs. Complications that can arise from blocked pulmonary circulation include damage to the blocked portion of the lung, reduced oxygenation of blood in the systemic circulation, and damage to other organs and tissues due to the lack of oxygen in the blood. Pulmonary infarction may also occur and is the consequential hemorrhagic consolidation and necrosis of the lung parenchyma due to pulmonary embolus. Pulmonary embolism is classified based on the type of embolus, which includes septic, saddle, or other or unspecified type.

I26.0-   Pulmonary embolism with acute cor pulmonale

Acute cor pulmonale is a dilation and failure of the right side of the heart due to increased blood pressure (hypertension) in the pulmonary arteries. In this case, the pulmonary hypertension is due to a pulmonary embolism. The acute form is usually reversible once the obstruction due to the pulmonary embolism is treated.

I26.01   Septic pulmonary embolism with acute cor pulmonale

Septic pulmonary embolism is a rare disorder that usually presents with a subtle onset of fever, respiratory symptoms, and lung infiltrates. Infarction in the pulmonary vasculature is caused by an embolic blood clot, which in the case of septic pulmonary embolism also contains microorganisms that provoke a focal abscess. Because of the nonspecific clinical and radiologic features on presentation, diagnosis of this disorder is often delayed. Although septic pulmonary embolism has historically been associated with such risk factors as IV drug use, pelvic thrombophlebitis, or suppurative processes in the head and neck, the increasing use of indwelling catheters and devices have changed the clinical signs and symptoms. Epidemiology has also been altered by the increased numbers of immunocompromised patients. When acute cor pulmonale is present there is also pulmonary hypertension and right heart failure.

I26.02 Saddle embolus of pulmonary artery with acute cor pulmonale

Saddle embolus is so named because this type of embolism straddles the bifurcation of a blood vessel. A pulmonary saddle embolus is often large in diameter and may cause catastrophic circulatory obstructions and pulmonary infarctions. In the pulmonary artery, a saddle embolus is often fatal. This is particularly true if it occurs in the main pulmonary artery and extends into the right and left main pulmonary artery branches obstructing blood flow to a large area of the lungs with resultant pulmonary infarction and respiratory failure. When acute cor pulmonale is present there is also pulmonary hypertension and right heart failure. Other complications include spontaneous fragmentation with multiple distal arterial obstructions and sudden cardiac arrest.

I27.- Other pulmonary heart diseases

This category includes diseases such as pulmonary hypertension, kyphoscoliotic heart disease, cor pulmonale, and chronic pulmonary embolism of the pulmonary arteries that adversely affect heart function.

I27.0 Primary pulmonary hypertension

Primary pulmonary hypertension occurs when pressure within the pulmonary artery is elevated and vascular resistance is observed in the lungs, in the absence of any other disease of the lungs or heart. It is marked by diffuse narrowing of the pulmonary arterioles and, in moderate to severe cases, formation of pulmonary thrombi and emboli. The clinical picture is similar to pulmonary hypertension from any other cause, and has a poor prognosis with patients developing severe right heart failure within two to three years.

I27.1 Kyphoscoliotic heart disease

Kyphoscoliotic heart disease arises from a forward and lateral deformity of the spine. When the spine deformity is severe, it restricts the growth and size of the chest cavity leading to secondary pulmonary artery hypertension and eventually to right-sided heart failure.

I27.2- Other secondary pulmonary hypertension

Secondary pulmonary hypertension (PH) occurs when pressure within the pulmonary arteries is elevated and vascular resistance is observed in the lungs. PH is clinically classified into five groups based on categories that share similar pathological findings, hemodynamic characteristics, and management. Group 1 is pulmonary arterial hypertension (PAH), which can be idiopathic, heritable, due to drugs and toxins, or associated with conditions such as connective tissue diseases, congenital heart disease, portal hypertension, and others. Group 2 is left-heart related PH; Group 3 is PH due to chronic respiratory disorders; Group 4 is chronic thromboembolic PH; Group 5 is PH with unclear multifactorial mechanisms, including hematologic disorders such as myeloproliferative disorders and splenectomy; systemic disorders such as sarcoidosis and pulmonary Langerhans cell histiocytosis; metabolic disorders such as glycogen storage disease, Gaucher disease and thyroid disorders; and other conditions that lead to PH.

I27.21 Secondary pulmonary arterial hypertension

Secondary pulmonary hypertension occurs when pressure within the pulmonary arteries is elevated and vascular resistance is observed in the lungs. This code includes secondary pulmonary arterial hypertension (PAH) due to drugs or toxins, or underlying conditions such as congenital heart disease, HIV, lupus polymyositis, portal hypertension due to advanced liver disease, rheumatoid arthritis, schistosomiasis, sickle cell disease, Sjögren syndrome, and systemic sclerosis. Treatment consists of management of the underlying condition. The most important treatment for pulmonary hypertension related to drugs or toxins is to stop the drug or toxic substance. PAH leads to progressive increase in pulmonary vascular resistance (PVR) and eventually a decrease in cardiac output, leading to right heart failure and death.

I27.22 Pulmonary hypertension due to left heart disease

Pulmonary hypertension (PH) is a common complication of left heart disease and is due mainly to increased left ventricular and pulmonary venous pressures. Left heart failure is the most common cause of PH and is diagnosed by right and/or left heart catheterization. Treatment is with aggressive management of the underlying cardiac or valvular disease, with diuretics for fluid control and relief of congestion in heart failure, and/or repair of valvular heart disease. Treatment also includes that for any associated comorbidities, as well as risk factor modification. Patients may be evaluated for heart transplantation or implantation of ventricular assist devices to support cardiac output, either as a bridge to transplant or as destination therapy.

I27.23 Pulmonary hypertension due to lung diseases and hypoxia

Pulmonary hypertension due to chronic lung diseases and/or hypoxia is caused by an increase in pulmonary vascular resistance (PVR) from chronic pulmonary vascular changes in response to inflammation of lung tissue and airways, fibrotic lung changes, or hypoxic vasoconstriction with poor gas exchange. It may be caused by chronic lung diseases such as chronic obstructive pulmonary disease (COPD), interstitial lung disease (ILD), other pulmonary diseases with mixed restrictive and obstructive patterns, or conditions that cause hypoxemia such as obstructive sleep apnea (OSA), alveolar hypoventilation disorders, chronic exposure to high altitude, and developmental lung diseases. Treatment of the associated underlying condition is indicated to prevent progression with consideration of lung transplant depending on the extent of loss of pulmonary function.

I27.24 Chronic thromboembolic pulmonary hypertension

In some patients, thromboembolisms can become organized and form scar-like tissue that narrows or blocks the pulmonary arteries, leading to chronic thromboembolic pulmonary hypertension (CTEPH) due to increased resistance to blood flow through the arteries. Months or years may pass after the acute thromboembolic event before clinically significant pulmonary hypertension manifests. The main symptoms include fatigue, shortness of breath, chest discomfort, peripheral edema, hemoptysis, and dyspnea, dizziness, or syncope on exertion. CTEPH is potentially curable without a lung transplant if the chronic thromboembolic material can be removed by pulmonary thromboendarterectomy (PTE). If surgical correction is not possible, in some patients, medications and balloon pulmonary angioplasty can improve the symptoms.

I27.82 Chronic pulmonary embolism

Pulmonary embolism (PE) may present as an acute event (generally within two weeks of onset) or as a chronic condition—one which is longstanding over many weeks, months, or years. In chronic PE, small blood clots travel to the lungs repeatedly over a period of years. Chronic PE is often closely associated with pulmonary hypertension. The embolus blocks pulmonary circulation from the right side of the heart to the left, causing an increase in pulmonary arterial pressure. Pulmonary hypertension may initially be asymptomatic, but common early symptoms include dizziness or syncope resulting from impairment in the cardiopulmonary circulation. As the right heart is forced to work harder in order to pump blood through the lungs and into the left heart, right heart failure occurs. As a result, the patient is likely to experience ischemic chest pain (angina) accompanied by peripheral edema or ascites.

I27.83 Eisenmenger's syndrome

Eisenmenger's syndrome is a life-threatening condition that develops from a congenital heart defect such as a ventricular septal defect (VSD), atrial septal defect (ASD), or patent ductus arteriosus (PDA). Eisenmenger's syndrome results from pulmonary arterial hypertension (PAH) due to congenital heart disease with defects that cause a left-to-right shunt. The previous long-standing left-to-right cardiac shunt reverses into a right-to-left shunt secondary to increased pressure of the blood flow from elevated pulmonary artery pressures and associated pulmonary vascular disease. The defect causes reduced oxygen saturation in the arterial blood, leading to cyanosis and organ damage. Eisenmenger's syndrome, once it develops, is irreversible, and a heart–lung transplant or a lung transplant with repair of the heart defect is the only treatment option.

I28.- Other diseases of pulmonary vessels

This category represents disorders of the pulmonary vessels including arteriovenous fistula, aneurysm, stenosis, stricture, rupture, and arteritis of the vessels.

I28.0 Arteriovenous fistula of pulmonary vessels

An arteriovenous fistula occurs when an abnormal communication between a pulmonary artery and vein is established within the lungs. When this happens, the blood that flows through the lungs is deficient of essential oxygen. Acquired arteriovenous fistula can result as a complication of pulmonary infarction.

I28.1 Aneurysm of pulmonary artery

Acquired aneurysm of the pulmonary artery is a rare condition characterized by a focal enlargement of a pulmonary artery affecting all three layers of the artery: intima (inner layer), media (middle muscular layer), and adventitia (outer connective tissue layer). Acquired aneurysm may be caused by chronic pulmonary emboli, pulmonary hypertension, pulmonary atherosclerosis, vasculitis, infection, neoplasm, and trauma, including intraoperative or iatrogenic trauma.

Other Forms of Heart Disease (I30-I52)

Heart disease can encompass a number of complex conditions that can affect the function of the heart. Diseases of the protective outer covering or pericardium, the endocardium and myocardium (heart walls), valves, and conduction system are all included in this code block.

The categories in this code block are as follows:

I30	Acute pericarditis
I31	Other diseases of pericardium
I32	Pericarditis in diseases classified elsewhere
I33	Acute and subacute endocarditis
I34	Nonrheumatic mitral valve disorders
I35	Nonrheumatic aortic valve disorders
I36	Nonrheumatic tricuspid valve disorders
I37	Nonrheumatic pulmonary valve disorders
I38	Endocarditis, valve unspecified
I39	Endocarditis and heart valve disorders in diseases classified elsewhere
I40	Acute myocarditis
I41	Myocarditis in diseases classified elsewhere
I42	Cardiomyopathy
I43	Cardiomyopathy in diseases classified elsewhere
I44	Atrioventricular and left bundle-branch block
I45	Other conduction disorders
I46	Cardiac arrest
I47	Paroxysmal tachycardia
I48	Atrial fibrillation and flutter
I49	Other cardiac arrhythmias
I50	Heart failure
I51	Complications and ill-defined descriptions of heart disease
I52	Other heart disorders in diseases classified elsewhere

Focus Point

This code block only includes conditions that are not caused by rheumatic fever. Conditions caused by rheumatic fever are located in code block I00–I09.

I30.- Acute pericarditis

Acute pericarditis is inflammation of the fibroserous membrane that surrounds the heart. Typically this membrane contains small amounts of fluid that provide lubrication. When inflammation occurs, there is little room for this lubrication, which causes friction against the outer layer of the heart. The inflammation may be described as fibrinous, serous, sanguineous, hemorrhagic, or purulent. Etiologies for acute pericarditis include viral and bacterial infections, collagen vascular disease, adverse reaction to drugs (such as procainamide, hydralazine, and isoniazid), and metastatic disease.

Focus Point

Uremic pericarditis is reported with code N18.9 Chronic kidney disease, unspecified, sequenced first to identify the etiology and code I32 Pericarditis in diseases classified elsewhere, sequenced additionally to describe the manifestation.

I31.- Other diseases of pericardium

The pericardium is the protective, two-layer membrane that surrounds the heart. The outer layer, the fibrous pericardium, is made up of dense connective tissue. The serous pericardium is double layered, with the outermost parietal layer adherent to the fibrous pericardium and the inner visceral layer (epicardium) adherent to the heart's surface. Between these two layers, the pericardial cavity contains lubricating pericardial fluid that decreases friction caused by the beating of the heart. This category includes pericarditis (inflammation), hemopericardium, effusion, and other conditions affecting the pericardium.

I31.0 Chronic adhesive pericarditis

Chronic adhesive pericarditis may result from adhesions between the two pericardial layers, between the heart and the pericardium, or between the pericardium and other contiguous structures in the chest. Other terms that describe chronic adhesive pericarditis are fibrosis of pericardium, plastic pericarditis, milk spots, obliterative pericarditis, and soldiers' patches.

I31.1 Chronic constrictive pericarditis

Chronic constrictive pericarditis is a diffuse thickening of the pericardium as a late effect of inflammation. Cardiac output is limited due to the reduced distensibility of the cardiac chambers, and filling pressures are increased in response to the external constrictive force placed on the heart by the pericardium. This condition may be associated with congestive heart failure.

I31.2 Hemopericardium, not elsewhere classified

Hemopericardium is the presence of blood in the pericardial sac. Emergency pericardiocentesis is usually performed.

I31.4 Cardiac tamponade

Cardiac tamponade is a life-threatening condition in which fluid or blood accumulates in the space between the muscle of the heart (myocardium) and the outer sac that covers the heart (pericardium), resulting in compression of the heart. The ventricles are unable to fully expand, therefore hampering the ability to adequately fill and pump blood. Often associated with bacterial or viral pericarditis, other factors that can lead to cardiac tamponade may include heart surgery, dissecting thoracic aortic aneurysm, injuries to the heart, end-stage lung cancer, and acute myocardial infarction. Treatment often involves draining the fluid around the heart by pericardiocentesis or the creation of a pericardial window by removing a portion of the pericardium.

I33.- Acute and subacute endocarditis

The endocardium is the innermost layer covering the four chambers of the heart, the valves, and the lining of large blood vessels connected to the heart.

I33.0 Acute and subacute infective endocarditis

I33.9 Acute and subacute endocarditis, unspecified

Endocarditis is an inflammation of the inner layer of the heart and may affect the lining of the heart chambers and the cardiac valves. Acute or subacute endocarditis is usually due to bacterial infection. A variety of organisms may cause endocarditis, but *Staphylococcus aureus* is the most common pathogen. Infection of previously damaged valves is often due to *Viridans streptococci* or other organisms comprising normal oral flora and may be secondary to a dental procedure. Infection of a prosthetic valve may be due to staphylococci, which typically occurs within the first two months of surgery or streptococci, which is more common when more than two months have elapsed since the surgery. Infection of normal valves is rare and is usually associated with intravenous drug abuse.

I34.- Nonrheumatic mitral valve disorders

Mitral valve disorders constitute any condition that weakens or damages the function of the valve. These conditions cause blood to back up into the left atrium of the heart, requiring the heart to work harder in order to pump blood into the body.

I34.0 Nonrheumatic mitral (valve) insufficiency

Insufficiency of the mitral valve, also referred to as regurgitation or incompetence, occurs when the valve does not completely close. This allows some of the blood in the left ventricle to flow backward through the mitral valve into the left atrium instead of forward into the aorta, resulting in increased atrial pressure and decreased forward cardiac output.

I34.1 Nonrheumatic mitral (valve) prolapse

Mitral valve prolapse occurs when the leaflets of the mitral valve, which is the valve between the left atrium and left ventricle, bulge (prolapse) up and back into the left atrium during systole preventing proper closure. Systole is the period when the heart muscle contracts and heart chambers expel blood. This allows blood to leak back into the left atrium and causes a characteristic heart sound known as click-murmur, so the condition is sometimes referred to as click-murmur syndrome or Barlow's syndrome.

I34.2 Nonrheumatic mitral (valve) stenosis

This condition identifies mitral valve orifice narrowing that restricts the flow of blood from the left atrium into the left ventricle in diastole. Diastole is the period when the heart muscle relaxes and the heart chambers fill with blood.

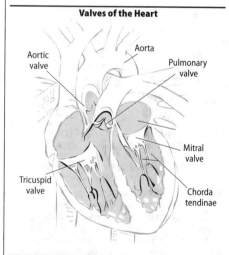

Valves of the Heart

Aortic valve · Aorta · Pulmonary valve · Mitral valve · Tricuspid valve · Chorda tendinae

---

Focus Point

Because most mitral valve stenosis is caused by rheumatic fever, when the cause is not specified code I05.0 for rheumatic mitral stenosis should be assigned. Mitral valve stenosis documented as congenital is reported with a code from category Q23.

I35.-   Nonrheumatic aortic valve disorders

The aortic valve regulates blood flow from the left ventricle to aorta. The aortic valve has three leaflets (cusps). Factors contributing to aortic valve disorders include acquired abnormalities of the valve leaflets, which are attached to the ascending aorta.

I35.0   Nonrheumatic aortic (valve) stenosis

I35.1   Nonrheumatic aortic (valve) insufficiency

I35.2   Nonrheumatic aortic (valve) stenosis with insufficiency

Insufficiency is a malfunction in the operation of the aortic valve leaflets, which results in failure of the valve to close properly allowing regurgitation of blood from the aorta back into the left ventricle. Stenosis is narrowing of the aortic valve, which may block blood flow into the aorta. These two conditions can occur alone or together. A common cause of aortic valve disorders in people older than age 65 is calcium deposits on the leaflets, causing stenosis and reducing the leaflet mobility. In severe cases of aortic stenosis and insufficiency, backflow of blood can accumulate in the lungs and prevent the necessary flow of blood to the brain or extremities.

I36.-   Nonrheumatic tricuspid valve disorders

The tricuspid valve regulates blood flow from the right atrium to the right ventricle. Tricuspid disorders of a nonrheumatic nature can be caused by conditions such as infective endocarditis, carcinoid tumors, or chronic pulmonary diseases such as emphysema, pulmonary hypertension, or stenosis.

I36.0   Nonrheumatic tricuspid (valve) stenosis

I36.1   Nonrheumatic tricuspid (valve) insufficiency

I36.2   Nonrheumatic tricuspid (valve) stenosis with insufficiency

Tricuspid insufficiency, also called regurgitation, results from improper closure of the tricuspid valve causing blood in the right ventricle to back up into the right atrium. It is typically caused by inflammation of the right ventricle and may be a complication of various disorders. Tricuspid stenosis affects the same location, but the primary problem results in narrowing or blockage.

I37.-   Nonrheumatic pulmonary valve disorders

The pulmonary valve separates the right ventricle from the pulmonary artery, which delivers blood to the lungs.

I37.0   Nonrheumatic pulmonary valve stenosis

I37.1   Nonrheumatic pulmonary valve insufficiency

I37.2   Nonrheumatic pulmonary valve stenosis with insufficiency

Stenosis of the pulmonary valve is characterized by thickening or fusion of the valve leaflets causing narrowing or constriction of the valve opening. Stenosis reduces the flow of oxygen-depleted blood from the right ventricle through the pulmonary arteries and into lungs. Mild pulmonary valve stenosis may be asymptomatic and may not require treatment. However, moderate to severe stenosis is usually symptomatic with cyanosis, shortness of breath, chest pain, fainting, and fatigue being some of the more common symptoms. Without treatment the condition typically worsens and may be complicated by right heart enlargement, as the right ventricle works harder to force blood through the stenosed valve and into the pulmonary artery. Insufficiency occurs when the valve does not completely close allowing blood to flow backward from the pulmonary artery into the right ventricle.

I38   Endocarditis, valve unspecified

Endocarditis is inflammation of the lining within the heart chambers and heart valves. These codes are reported when the specific valve is not documented or when the underlying cause of the inflammation is not known. Typically patients diagnosed with endocarditis have heart disease affecting the valves and, in some cases, the cause may be difficult to determine.

I40.-   Acute myocarditis

Myocarditis is inflammation of the middle layer of the heart, which is composed of muscle tissue. In severe manifestations, myocarditis impairs the heart's ability to pump effectively, resulting in decreased oxygen supply to the rest of the body. In milder manifestations, there may be no apparent symptoms or mild, general symptoms often related to a viral infection, and spontaneous recovery can occur. Myocarditis typically affects previously healthy people and can progress at a rapid pace leading to fatal heart failure and/or arrhythmias. In addition, blood clots may be caused by the decreased ability of the pumping function within the heart, resulting in a stroke or heart attack.

I40.0   Infective myocarditis

Infective myocarditis may be caused by viral, bacterial, rickettsial, fungal, or parasitic disease. Two of the more common infectious organisms responsible for acute infections of the heart muscle are *staphylococcus* and *Group A streptococcus*.

Focus Point

There are more specific codes for some infections complicated by acute infective myocarditis, including myocarditis due to influenza, toxoplasmosis, meningococcus, as well as others. Only acute infective myocarditis without a more specific code is reported here.

I40.1   Isolated myocarditis

Isolated myocarditis is inflammation of the heart muscle usually due to an unknown cause, which is why it is also referred to as idiopathic myocarditis. Isolated myocarditis is a rare and particularly devastating form of myocarditis that rapidly leads to heart failure and death often within a few weeks or months following the first symptoms. The only definitive treatment is heart transplant. Giant cell myocarditis is a form of isolated myocarditis. While the cause of giant cell myocarditis is unknown, it has been linked to autoimmune disorders. Fielder's myocarditis is another form of isolated myocarditis that causes granulomatous lesions of the heart.

I42.-   Cardiomyopathy

Cardiomyopathy is a complex and heterogenous group of diseases of the heart muscle. Inflammation or abnormal thickening occurs in all of these diseases. In some cases, scar tissue forms in the place of normal heart muscle tissue. Many factors may contribute to cardiomyopathy, such as myocardial infarction, hypertension, infection, or genetic causes.

Focus Point

Hypertensive cardiomyopathy is not coded here as it is actually considered to be a form of hypertensive heart disease and is reported with code from category I11 Hypertensive heart disease.

I42.0   Dilated cardiomyopathy

Dilated cardiomyopathy is characterized by enlargement of the left ventricle with thinning of the myocardium. Due to thinning of the heart muscle, the left ventricle cannot contract with enough force to expel enough oxygen rich blood and deliver it to the systemic circulation. This results in too much blood remaining in the left ventricle, which causes volume overload and congestive heart failure.

Focus Point

Becker's cardiomyopathy is related to a form of muscular dystrophy called Becker's muscular dystrophy. It is characterized by skeletal and cardiac muscle wasting. The cardiac muscle wasting in Becker's muscular dystrophy causes dilated cardiomyopathy; however, Becker's cardiomyopathy is reported with code I42.8.

I42.1   Obstructive hypertrophic cardiomyopathy

I42.2   Other hypertrophic cardiomyopathy

Hypertrophic cardiomyopathy (HCM) is clinically differentiated as obstructive or nonobstructive. The presence of obstruction indicates an increased severity of disease, with indications for a different level of treatment than disease without obstruction. HCM may be attributed to inherited, acquired, or idiopathic causation. HCM is characterized by a thickening and stiffening of the myocardium, ventricles, and mitral valve. The thickening of these structures narrows the passage for circulating blood as the myocardial muscle loses the ability to relax and contract normally. When the blood flow from the ventricle to the aorta is significantly reduced, or when the left ventricular outflow disrupts the functioning of the mitral valve, an "outflow obstruction" occurs. Circulation is decreased and the heart is forced to work harder than normal to maintain circulation. Mitral valve impairment can cause the blood to backflow into the atrium. Many people with HCM are asymptomatic, whereas others with HCM develop heart conditions that are life-threatening or decrease quality of life. HCM is associated with sudden cardiac death, ventricular tachycardia, atrial fibrillation, and heart failure. In addition, HCM patients have an increased risk of developing bacterial or infective endocarditis and, as a result, are often prescribed preventative antibiotic therapy.

Focus Point

Note that inherited obstructive cardiomyopathy is considered a congenital anomaly and is reported with code Q24.8.

I42.3   Endomyocardial (eosinophilic) disease

Endomyocardial eosinophilic disease, also called endomyocardial tropical fibrosis or Loffler's endocarditis, is a thickening of the ventricular endocardium due to fibrosis that results in restrictive cardiomyopathy. The condition occurs in tropical and subtropical regions, primarily in East, Central, and West Africa. The areas of fibrosis typically begin in the apical regions of the right and left ventricles. Occasionally, the tricuspid and mitral valves are also involved resulting in tricuspid and mitral regurgitation. The disease process begins with infiltration of the myocardium with eosinophils, a white blood cell associated with allergic reactions. This initial phase usually occurs within the first 5 weeks of the disease process. This is followed by the second phase involving tissue death (necrosis) of the subendocardium. The subendocardium consists of three layers of connective tissue. The outer subendocardium is composed of connective tissue, the middle layer of connective tissue and some muscle fibers, and an outer layer that fuses with the muscle tissue of the myocardium. The conductive tissue of the heart is also found within the subendocardium. The final stage of endomyocardial eosinophilic disease is fibrosis of the endocardium. Symptoms differ depending on which ventricle is primarily involved. If the right ventricle is the focus of the disease process, patients experience abdominal and lower extremity edema. If the left ventricle is the primary focus, symptoms include difficulty breathing (dyspnea) and fatigue. Treatment typically involves measures to reduce symptoms of the disease.

Focus Point

South African cardiomyopathy, also called obscure cardiomyopathy of Africa, is reported with code I42.8.

I42.4   Endocardial fibroelastosis

Endocardial fibroelastosis is a congenital condition characterized by thickening of the endocardium and subendocardium, with malformation of the cardiac valves, hypertrophy of the heart, and proliferation of elastic tissue in the myocardium. Also called elastomyofibrosis, many patients with this condition do not survive infancy.

I42.8   Other cardiomyopathies

Becker's cardiomyopathy and South African cardiomyopathy, also called obscure cardiomyopathy of Africa, are reported here. Cardiomyopathy, a disease affecting the heart muscle, is a rare condition in most countries; however, it is endemic in Africa. It is believed to be caused by a combination of inherited and environmental factors. Obscure cardiomyopathy of Africa is a dilated form of cardiomyopathy that causes congestive heart failure that progresses rapidly and is nearly always fatal. Becker's cardiomyopathy is related to a form of muscular dystrophy called Becker's

muscular dystrophy. It is characterized by skeletal and cardiac muscle wasting. The cardiac muscle wasting in Becker's muscular dystrophy causes dilated cardiomyopathy.

Focus Point

Endomyocardial tropical fibrosis, which is another form of cardiomyopathy found predominantly in Africa, is limited to the subtropical and tropical regions of East, Central, and West Africa and is reported with code I42.3.

I44.-   Atrioventricular and left bundle-branch block

In the normal heart, the electrical impulse that initiates a heartbeat originates from the sinus node (also called the sinoatrial node or the SA node) in the top right atrium. This pulse passes to the lower chambers of the heart (ventricles) via the atrioventricular (AV) node, where it is sent to the bundle of His. The bundle of His further divides into right and left Purkinje fibers that form the right and left bundle branches, which control the rhythm of the right and left ventricles. Atrioventricular and left bundle branch blocks occur when transmission of these electrical signals becomes disrupted at or below the AV node.

I44.0   Atrioventricular block, first degree

First-degree atrioventricular block typically involves a delay in conduction at the AV node. All electrical impulses from the sinus node in the atrium reach the AV node and are conducted to the ventricles; the impulses are slowed at the AV node. First-degree blocks are usually asymptomatic and do not require treatment.

I44.1   Atrioventricular block, second degree

Second-degree atrioventricular (AV) block involves an interruption of electrical impulses below the AV node in the His bundle or further along the conduction system in the Purkinje fibers. In second-degree block, not all electrical impulses conducted from the sinus node reach the ventricles. Most often the electrical impulses are interrupted at the AV node but the interruption may also occur below the AV node. There are several ways that electrical impulses may be interrupted in second-degree AV block and each has distinctive effects on heart rhythm, as well as distinctive ECG characteristics. In Mobitz I AV block, also called Wenckebach's block, the PR interval becomes progressively longer causing a pause and failure to conduct a single P-wave causing a missed beat. Mobitz II AV block is characterized by a constant PR interval, but an occasional failure of conduction of a P-wave (dropped P-wave) or a regular pattern of transmitted and dropped P-waves, such as 3:1 (3 transmitted, 1 blocked) or 2:1 (2 transmitted, 1 blocked). Mobitz II AV block results in a heart rhythm with intermittent missed beats or a regular irregularity in heart rhythm.

I44.2   Atrioventricular block, complete

Complete atrioventricular block, also called third-degree bundle branch block, is the most advanced form of heart block. In complete atrioventricular block, there is a lesion distal to the bundle of His, which blocks the electrical impulse bilaterally, causing a right and left bundle branch block. This prevents electrical signals from traveling along their normal pathways to reach the ventricles. Instead the electrical impulses are conducted along an alternate pathway that stimulates the ventricles to contract but at a slower rate resulting in bradycardia. This condition is typically treated by insertion of an artificial pacemaker.

I44.4   Left anterior fascicular block

The left bundle branch of the electrical conduction system of the heart divides into anterior and posterior fascicles that transmit the electrical impulses throughout the left ventricle. When the anterior fascicle is blocked, the electrical impulses travel only along the left posterior fascicle, which inserts into the inferior septal wall in the subendocardial tissue. Electrical impulses travel through the left ventricle but because of the block in the left anterior fascicle, the impulses are initially distributed in a downward and rightward direction followed by an upward and leftward direction. Because there is no transmission of electrical impulses through the anterior fascicles, it takes the impulses longer to travel to the upper left side of the ventricle and these changes are seen on ECG. Left anterior fascicular block, also called left anterior hemiblock, is typically asymptomatic. However, the condition is significant in that it indicates that there is fibrosis in the left anterior region of the left ventricle and this is a risk factor for the development of other cardiac arrhythmias and congestive heart failure.

Focus Point

Left anterior fascicular block is more common than left posterior fascicular block because the anterior fascicles are arranged in a narrow single tract so a small area of fibrosis can interrupt anterior electrical impulses. In comparison, left posterior fascicles are broadly distributed making it more difficult for a single area of fibrosis to interrupt the electrical impulses.

I44.5   Left posterior fascicular block

The left bundle branch of the electrical conduction system of the heart divides into anterior and posterior fascicles that transmit the electrical impulses throughout the left ventricle. When the posterior fascicle is blocked, the electrical impulses travel only along the left anterior fascicle, which inserts into the upper lateral wall of the left ventricle in the subendocardial tissue. Electrical impulses travel through the left ventricle but because of the block in the left posterior fascicle, the impulses are initially distributed in an upward and leftward direction followed by a downward and rightward direction. Because there is no transmission of electrical impulses through the posterior fascicles, it takes the impulses longer to travel to the lower right side of the ventricle and these changes are reflected on ECG. Left posterior fascicular block, also called left posterior hemiblock, is relatively rare because the fibers are arranged in a broad pattern making them more resistant to damage.

I45.-   Other conduction disorders

Other cardiac conduction disorders include a group of conditions in which the transmission of cardiac electrical impulses controlling heart rhythm is abnormal, slowed, or interrupted.

I45.2   Bifascicular block

I45.3   Trifascicular block

Fascicles are specialized muscle fibers in the heart that conduct electrical impulses that cause the heart muscle to contract. There is a single fascicle in the right side of the heart and there are two fascicles in the left heart—an anterior fascicle and a posterior fascicle. A bifascicular block occurs when the right fascicle and the left anterior or left posterior fascicle are blocked with conduction to the ventricles running through the one remaining fascicle. Bifascicular block is usually asymptomatic. Trifascicular block indicates that electrical impulses in the right fascicle, left anterior fascicle, and left posterior fascicle are partially or completely blocked. Incomplete or partial trifascicular block is indicated by complete block of one or two fascicles with delayed conduction or intermittent blockage of the remaining fascicles as evidenced by changes on ECG. Trifascicular block is usually asymptomatic, but it is a risk factor for complete heart block and must be monitored.

I45.6   Pre-excitation syndrome

Pre-excitation syndrome, also known as Wolff-Parkinson-White syndrome (WPW), occurs when impulses from the atria circumvent the normal pathway and activate the ventricle via an accessory pathway. The normal delay that occurs at the AV node doesn't take place, and the patient is prone to developing episodes of extremely rapid and irregular heart rhythm called tachyarrhythmias. Pre-excitation syndrome is classified as a congenital anomaly. Symptoms may occur in infancy or childhood or may not present until adulthood. Symptoms vary in severity from mild chest discomfort or occasional heart palpitations to life-threatening tachycardia or cardiac arrest. Pre-excitation syndrome may be treated medically with antiarrhythmia or atrioventricular node blocking drugs or surgically by ablation of the accessory conduction pathway.

I45.81   Long QT syndrome

Long QT syndrome is a serious and potentially fatal condition that can be precipitated by vigorous exertion, emotional upset, or startling moments. The QT interval is the time it takes for the duration of electrical activity that controls the pumping action of the heart's ventricles, measured in fractions of a second. When the interval is longer than normal, it is identified as long QT syndrome. The condition may be genetic, due to specific medications, or due to low levels of potassium, magnesium, or calcium in the blood as seen in patients with anorexia nervosa. This imbalance in electrical timing makes the patient susceptible to recurrent episodes of syncope and rapid arrhythmias that can become malignant, leading to sudden death. However, in most cases, the patient has no signs or symptoms of the condition. Other names for long QT syndrome include Jervell-Lang-Nielsen syndrome and Romano-Ward syndrome.

I46.-   Cardiac arrest

Cardiac arrest is an abrupt loss of heart function, breathing capacity, and consciousness. In cardiac arrest, the heart stops beating, causing an electrical impulse malfunction within the heart that halts the pumping of the blood to the rest of the body. Cardiac arrest may also be referred to as pulseless electrical activity (PEA). PEA indicates the presence of electrical cardiac activity, although too insufficient to coordinate myocardial contractions to produce a detectable pulse. Cardiorespiratory arrest is also included in this category. The fourth character in this code identifies whether or not the cause of the cardiac arrest was due to an underlying cardiac condition.

Focus Point

Sequence cardiac arrest first only when the underlying cause of the event is unknown or not established before the patient expires and only when it meets the definition of principal diagnosis. Cardiac arrest is a reportable secondary diagnosis when the cause is known (sequencing underlying cause first), regardless of the success of resuscitation attempts. Report also resuscitative and life support procedures.

I47.-   Paroxysmal tachycardia

Typically the heart beats in a regular pattern coordinated within the atria and ventricles due to the electrical impulses originating in the sinoatrial node. These signals tell the heart when to contract. A malfunction in these electrical impulses causes the heart to beat irregularly. Paroxysmal tachycardia is a cardiac dysrhythmia characterized by periods of rapid heartbeats that start and stop abruptly. People at increased risk for these conditions include those who consume alcohol, caffeine, drugs, and smoke. Symptoms may be sporadic with varying lengths of duration. Cardiac dysrhythmias are disturbances in cardiac rate and rhythm, including abnormalities in the rate, regularity, and sequence of atrial and/or ventricular contractions.

I47.1   Supraventricular tachycardia

Supraventricular tachycardia (SVT) is a very rapid heart rate (160 to 220 beats per minute) that does not originate in the ventricles. Also called paroxysmal supraventricular tachycardia (PSVT), this condition has several causes. It may be caused by two electrical conduction pathways in the atrioventricular node and this type of SVT may be referred to as atrioventricular nodal re-entrant supraventricular tachycardia. A second cause is an abnormal conduction pathway between the atria and the ventricles and this type is also called atrioventricular reciprocating supraventricular tachycardia. A third cause is abnormal rapid or circling impulses originating in the atria, which may be referred to as paroxysmal atrial tachycardia (PAT).

I47.2   Ventricular tachycardia

Paroxysmal ventricular tachycardia (PVT) is a rapid heart rate (more than 120 beats per minute) that originates in the ventricles. While less common than other types of paroxysmal tachycardia, PVT requires emergency care, including monitoring with cardioversion and/or drug therapy because prolonged PVT can be fatal.

I47.9   Paroxysmal tachycardia, unspecified

Unspecified paroxysmal tachycardia refers to a rapid heart rate that starts and ends abruptly, but for which the specific type is not specified or does not have a more specific code. Bouveret-Hoffmann syndrome is one type of paroxysmal tachycardia that is reported here. Bouveret-Hoffman syndrome is a type of junctional tachycardia meaning that the rapid heart rate does not originate in the atria or the ventricles, but instead originates in the atrioventricular node. It is characterized by rapid heart rate and sudden onset of palpitations; it primarily affects children. In most instances, Bouveret-Hoffman syndrome resolves on its own without treatment.

I48.-   Atrial fibrillation and flutter

Cardiac dysrhythmia is essentially a disturbance in heart rate and rhythm, including rate, regularity, and sequence of atrial and/or ventricular contractions. Atrial fibrillation and flutter are classified as cardiac dysrhythmias, where a rapid heart rate occurs due to the atria contracting in an uncoordinated pattern.

I48.0   Paroxysmal atrial fibrillation

I48.1   Persistent atrial fibrillation

I48.2   Chronic atrial fibrillation

Atrial fibrillation is the most common dysrhythmia. It occurs when the two upper chambers of the heart lose their normal rate and rhythm and beat chaotically. Paroxysmal atrial fibrillation refers to intermittent episodes of atrial fibrillation that resolve on their own. Episodes may last minutes, hours, or days. Persistent atrial fibrillation does not resolve on its own. It requires medical intervention to return to a normal rate and rhythm, which may include antiarrhythmic drugs and/ or electrical cardioversion. Chronic atrial fibrillation is resistant to treatment and cannot be converted to a normal rate and rhythm even with medication and attempts at electrical cardioversion.

I48.3   Typical atrial flutter

I48.4   Atypical atrial flutter

Atrial flutter, another common dysrhythmia, occurs when one or both atria beat too fast. The rapid muscle contractions in the atria are not matched by the ventricles and so the upper and lower heart rhythms lose their synchronization. It is caused by disruption of the normal electrical pathways originating in the atria. The defining characteristic of atrial flutter is that the electrical impulses follow an electrical circuit around the tricuspid annulus moving in a clockwise or counterclockwise direction. Typical atrial flutter (Type I) affects the right atrium only and results in organized, although more rapid than normal, atrial contractions. In atypical atrial flutter (Type II), the electrical impulses do not travel around the tricuspid annulus but instead follow one of a number of atypical pathways that may originate in the right or left atrium or in pathways that follow surgical scars. Types of atypical atrial flutter that originate in the right atrium include lower loop re-entry, fossa ovalis flutter, superior vena cava flutter, and upper loop re-entry. Types that originate in the left atrium include peri-mitral flutter, peri-pulmonary vein flutter, and those that follow re-entry pathways in the septum, roof, or posterior wall of the left atrium. Atypical flutter may also occur when the electrical impulses follow surgical scars that result from correction of congenital heart defects referred to as incisional flutter. Both typical and atypical flutters are diagnosed based on characteristic ECG patterns.

I49.-   Other cardiac arrhythmias

Cardiac arrhythmias are disturbances in cardiac rate and rhythm, including abnormalities in the rate, regularity, and sequence of atrial and/or ventricular contractions. Cardiac dysrhythmias can take many forms, the clinical significance of each depends on the extent to which they lower blood pressure and reduce cardiac output with resulting hypoperfusion of vital organs such as the brain, kidneys, and the heart.

Cardiac dysrhythmias may be benign or malignant, depending on the severity of the dysrhythmia and the patient's ability to tolerate it. This category identifies various arrhythmias not captured in tachycardia, atrial fibrillation, or flutter categories. Some of these conditions include ventricular fibrillation and flutter, premature depolarization (premature beats), and sick sinus syndrome.

> **Focus Point**
>
> *Holiday heart syndrome is a condition noted in patients with no known heart disease who develop cardiac arrhythmias due to acute alcohol consumption. The condition may appear in patients who are alcohol dependent or nondependent. Two codes are necessary to identify this condition: one for the specific type of arrhythmia (e.g., atrial fibrillation, atrial flutter) and the other for the acute ingestion of alcohol. If the specific arrhythmia is not known, use code I49.9 Cardiac arrhythmia, unspecified. Holiday heart syndrome may also be noted in patients with a diagnosis of chronic alcohol consumption with associated congestive cardiomyopathy. In this situation, three codes are required to accurately report the patient's diagnoses. Code the type of arrhythmia, the alcoholic cardiomyopathy with code I42.6, and the appropriate alcohol dependence code.*

I49.0-   Ventricular fibrillation and flutter

Ventricular fibrillation and flutter are classified as cardiac dysrhythmias, where a rapid heart rate occurs due to the ventricles contracting in an uncoordinated pattern. When this happens, blood is not completely expelled from the heart and pumped out to the body and the result can be sudden death. Ventricular fibrillation can be caused by a lack of oxygen in the blood, as well as underlying heart conditions. Ventricular fibrillation and ventricular flutter are both emergent medical conditions. Death may result within minutes or days. Immediate care is necessary for defibrillation. Medication and implantable cardioverter defibrillators are suggested for those who survive the initial attack in order to decrease risk of another.

I49.01   Ventricular fibrillation

Ventricular fibrillation is complete disorganization of the electrical activity of the heart, and the ventricles cease to function effectively. Rather than beating, the ventricles just quiver. Causes of this condition include myocardial infarction, electrolyte imbalances, weakness of the heart muscle, poisoning, and drug overdoses. Emergent treatment is required.

I49.02   Ventricular flutter

Ventricular flutter is rapid ventricular contractions at a regular pace. In this condition, the ventricles continue to beat, but emergent treatment is required to avoid the deterioration of the condition to ventricular fibrillation.

I49.1   Atrial premature depolarization

I49.2   Junctional premature depolarization

I49.3   Ventricular premature depolarization

These three conditions cause premature heartbeats. Premature heartbeats result from an irregularity in the rate and rhythm of the heart's contraction and pumping function. This may be felt as extra or missed heartbeats. Just about anyone may occasionally experience this and may not even notice when this occurs without cause. Most often premature beats are not treated and cause no damage or concern. Premature depolarization is classified based on the region in which it occurs, which may be in the atrium, ventricle, or AV junction. When this extra contraction occurs in the atrium, a signal is sent to the heart to beat before it is quite ready based on the regular pattern. Premature atrial beats are also referred to as premature atrial contractions or PACS. Supraventricular premature beats are also included in the premature atrial depolarization code since they are initiated in the atria or in another site above the bundle branch. Similarly, the ventricle may contract prematurely when there is not the typical amount of blood within the heart for the ventricle to pump out. Junctional premature depolarization occurs with the premature beat arising from an ectopic focus within the AV junction.

I49.5   Sick sinus syndrome

Sick sinus syndrome, also referred to as sinoatrial node dysfunction or tachycardia-bradycardia syndrome, refers to dysrhythmias related to a malfunction of the sinoatrial node. This rhythm disorder is the alternation between slow and fast beats and is typically seen in patient's age 50 years and older or in those who have underlying heart conditions. As with other arrhythmias, the electrical impulses of the heart are disrupted causing an irregular heart rhythm.

I50.-   Heart failure

Heart failure is a mechanical inability of the heart to pump blood efficiently, thus compromising circulation and causing systemic complications due to congestion and edema of fluids in the tissues.

I50.1   Left ventricular failure, unspecified

Left ventricular failure is the most common type of heart failure and occurs when there is a malfunction in the pumping mechanism of the left ventricle that limits the amount of blood that can be pumped from the left ventricle into the systemic circulation to supply the body with oxygen-rich blood. Typical causes of left-sided heart failure include end stage coronary arteriosclerosis, history of myocardial infarction, hypertension, excessive alcohol consumption, and any disorder that may damage or infect the heart muscle.

I50.20   Unspecified systolic (congestive) heart failure

I50.21   Acute systolic (congestive) heart failure

I50.22   Chronic systolic (congestive) heart failure

I50.23   Acute on chronic systolic (congestive) heart failure

The normal heart is able to stretch as it fills with blood (diastole) and then contract to pump blood to the body (systole). Systolic heart failure, which is more common than diastolic heart failure, occurs when the ventricle cannot contract normally and there is not enough power to push the blood out to the body. Contractile function of the heart decreases when the myocardium has been damaged as in myocardial infarction or coronary artery disease, which reduces the ventricle's ability to contract forcefully. This causes the blood to remain in the heart and collect in the lungs and veins, which results in symptoms of congestive heart failure that include fluid accumulation particularly in the lower extremities and in the lungs. Acute systolic heart failure indicates a sudden onset of the condition. Chronic systolic heart failure indicates a condition with a long duration or manifestations that occur over a period of time as opposed to suddenly. Acute on chronic systolic heart failure refers to an acute flare up or exacerbation of systolic heart failure in a patient with chronic systolic heart failure.

I50.30   Unspecified diastolic (congestive) heart failure

I50.31   Acute diastolic (congestive) heart failure

I50.32   Chronic diastolic (congestive) heart failure

I50.33   Acute on chronic diastolic (congestive) heart failure

The normal heart is able to stretch as it fills with blood (diastole) and then contract to pump blood to the body (systole). In diastolic failure, the ventricle does not relax adequately between heartbeats and the heart does not fill to capacity. The stiffness of the heart muscle causes blood to back up into the left atrium, as well as the blood vessels of the lung. Acute diastolic heart failure is a sudden onset of the condition. Chronic diastolic heart failure indicates a condition with a long duration or manifestations that occur over a period of time as opposed to suddenly. Acute on chronic diastolic heart failure refers to an acute flare up or exacerbation of diastolic heart failure in a patient with chronic heart failure.

I50.40   Unspecified combined systolic (congestive) and diastolic (congestive) heart failure

I50.41   Acute combined systolic (congestive) and diastolic (congestive) heart failure

I50.42   Chronic combined systolic (congestive) and diastolic (congestive) heart failure

I50.43   Acute on chronic combined systolic (congestive) and diastolic (congestive) heart failure

The normal heart is able to stretch as it fills with blood (diastole) and then contract to pump blood to the body (systole). Heart failure is an abnormality of heart function that renders it unable to pump blood at a rate adequate for tissue metabolism. In systolic failure, the ventricle does not contract normally and there is not enough power to push the blood out to the body. In diastolic failure, the ventricle does not stretch as it should and the heart does not fill appropriately during the period between heartbeats. These heart dysfunctions may occur together. Acute combined systolic and diastolic heart failure indicates a sudden onset of the condition. Chronic combined systolic and diastolic heart failure indicates a condition with a long duration or manifestations that occur over a period of time as opposed to suddenly. Acute on chronic combined systolic and diastolic heart failure is acute flare up or exacerbation of combined systolic and diastolic heart failure in a patient with chronic combined heart failure.

I50.8-   Other heart failure

This subcategory is used to report heart failure other than the types documented as left ventricular, diastolic, systolic, or combined. The symptoms and causes of the various types of heart failure can be diverse, but there also may be an overlap, and different types of heart failure may coexist.

I50.81-   Right heart failure

Right heart failure or right ventricular (RV) heart failure is a condition in which the right side of the heart loses its ability to efficiently pump blood to the lungs. It usually occurs because of left-sided failure. When the left ventricle fails, increased fluid pressure is transferred back through the lungs, ultimately damaging the right ventricle. When the right ventricle loses pumping power, blood backs up in the veins, causing peripheral edema and abdominal ascites.

Right heart failure may also be caused by pulmonary heart disease (cor pulmonale), chronic lung disease, coronary artery disease, pulmonic stenosis, tricuspid regurgitation or stenosis, pericardial constriction, and left-to-right shunt. The right ventricle eventually weakens and begins to fail, even without problems with the left ventricle.

Acute right heart failure indicates a sudden onset of the condition. Chronic right heart failure indicates a condition with a long duration or manifestations that occur over a period of time as opposed to suddenly. Acute on chronic right heart failure refers to an acute flare up or exacerbation of right heart failure in a patient with chronic right heart failure. Right heart failure is most commonly due to left heart failure.

I50.82   Biventricular heart failure

Biventricular heart failure occurs when both sides of the heart are affected. Right heart failure is characterized by peripheral edema and left heart failure by pulmonary congestion. Both are present in patients with biventricular heart failure. Many different conditions can cause biventricular heart failure, but high blood pressure is one of the most common causes.

I50.83   High output heart failure

High output heart failure occurs when the high demand for blood exceeds the capacity of a normally functioning heart to meet the demand. This type of heart failure may occur in patients with severe anemia, arteriovenous fistula with shunting of blood, hyperthyroidism, Paget's disease, and pregnancy. The symptoms of high output heart failure are similar to other forms of heart failure, and include fatigue and shortness of breath.

I50.84   End stage heart failure

End stage or advanced heart failure (American Heart Association class D, New York Heart Association Class 4) has progressed to the point where conventional heart therapies and symptom management no longer work. Patients are severely limited and unable to perform any physical activity without discomfort. Patients also experience symptoms such as shortness of breath even at rest.

I50.9   Heart failure, unspecified

Congestive heart failure is the mechanical inability of the heart to pump blood efficiently, thus compromising circulation and causing systemic complications due to congestion and edema. This becomes a life-threatening condition due to the backup of blood into other organs and an inadequate supply of oxygen and nutrients to the rest of the body, causing damage and malfunction to those organs as well. When heart failure is not documented as left ventricular, diastolic, systolic, combined, right ventricular, biventricular, high output, or end stage, it is reported with this unspecified code.

I51.- Complications and ill-defined descriptions of heart disease

This category captures miscellaneous disorders—some rare and some common—that are not classified in the other categories. Some of these conditions include septal defect, chordae tendineae or papillary muscle rupture, intracardiac (not intracoronary) thrombosis, Takotsubo syndrome, and cardiomegaly.

I51.0 Cardiac septal defect, acquired

Cardiac septal defect is an acquired abnormal communication between opposite heart chambers.

Focus Point

Acquired cardiac septal defects classified here are not present at birth (congenital) and are not a current complication related to an acute myocardial infarction.

I51.1 Rupture of chordae tendineae, not elsewhere classified

The chordae tendineae are thin fibrous cords of connective tissue that extend from the papillary muscles in the right or left ventricle wall to the leaflets in the tricuspid (right) and mitral (left) valves. The chordae tendineae keep the closed leaflets from prolapsing into the atria as the heart muscle in the ventricles contracts and propels blood into the pulmonary and systemic circulation. Rupture of the chordae tendineae is an acute injury to these structures that may be caused by acute or subacute endocarditis, rheumatic heart disease, or myxomatous heart degeneration. When the chordae tendineae rupture the leaflets in the affected valve prolapse into the atrium as the ventricle walls contract to propel blood into the pulmonary arteries or aorta. The prolapsed leaflets allow blood to regurgitate (flow backward) into the atrium causing increased blood volume on the affected side of the heart.

Focus Point

The most common cause of chordae tendineae rupture is acute myocardial infarction, which is reported with code I23.4.

I51.2 Rupture of papillary muscle, not elsewhere classified

In the normal heart, the papillary muscles are attached to the lower segment of the inside ventricular walls. They connect to the chordae tendineae, which are the cord-shaped tendons attached to the tricuspid valve (right ventricle) and the mitral valve (left ventricle). When the papillary muscles contract, the valves open

and when they relax, the valves close. Injury caused by acute or subacute endocarditis, rheumatic heart disease, or myxomatous degenerative heart disease can cause the papillary muscle to rupture. When the papillary muscle ruptures the affected valve no longer opens and closes properly, allowing blood to regurgitate (flow backward) into the atrium and causing increased blood volume on the affected side of the heart and fluid overload.

I51.3 Intracardiac thrombosis, not elsewhere classified

Intracardiac thrombosis describes a clot that is in one of the heart chambers, not the coronary vessels. It includes left atrial appendage thrombus.

I51.5 Myocardial degeneration

Myocardial degeneration is breakdown of the heart muscle leading to functional impairment. Myocardial degeneration is typically a complication of heart disease. It can indicate that arteriosclerosis is present and may be the cause of the degeneration. Continued degeneration of the heart muscle leads to more severe problems depending on the underlying condition causing the breakdown. As in arteriosclerosis, untreated blockage of blood vessels can lead to heart attack and stroke.

I51.7 Cardiomegaly

Cardiomegaly, also referred to as cardiac hypertrophy, is an enlarged heart. This is typically not a disease itself, but a symptom of a more serious condition. Most often the muscles of the heart become thickened due to excessive work caused by an underlying disease. The underlying condition may be cardiovascular (e.g., hypertension, congenital anomalies of the heart, arrhythmias, or cardiomyopathy) or it may be related to conditions such as amyloidosis, thyroid disease, or anemia.

I51.81 Takotsubo syndrome

Takotsubo syndrome is a form of stress cardiomyopathy, also known as broken heart syndrome and left ventricular apical balloon syndrome. The majority of cases are diagnosed in women. Heart muscles are temporarily weakened in patients without a known history of coronary artery disease, and the symptoms can easily be confused with a heart attack. A sudden, massive surge of adrenalin stuns the heart, greatly reducing the ability to pump blood. The common treatment of administering adrenalin to support blood pressure during a heart attack is therefore not appropriate for this condition. It is a reversible left ventricular dysfunction in patients without coronary disease, precipitated by emotional or physiological stress. The word "takotsubo" refers to a Japanese fishing pot used for trapping octopus. The shape of this pot mimics that of the heart abnormalities characteristic in the syndrome. Clinical signs and symptoms include chest pain that mimics acute myocardial infarction, ST-segment elevation in the precordial leads similar to AMI, slight elevation of cardiac enzyme and biomarker levels, and transient apical systolic left ventricular dysfunction or failure. An intense takotsubo episode is usually transient though severe, but it can become lethal if not properly treated because it can progress to cardiogenic shock.

Cerebrovascular Diseases (I60-I69)

This code block classifies the acute, organic conditions of the cerebrovascular system. Conditions coded to this section are nontraumatic in origin and include hemorrhages, thromboses, embolisms, transient cerebral ischemia, other ill-defined cerebrovascular diseases, and the late effects of cerebrovascular disease.

The categories in this code block are as follows:

I60	Nontraumatic subarachnoid hemorrhage
I61	Nontraumatic intracerebral hemorrhage
I62	Other and unspecified nontraumatic intracranial hemorrhage
I63	Cerebral infarction
I65	Occlusion and stenosis of precerebral arteries, not resulting in cerebral infarction
I66	Occlusion and stenosis of cerebral arteries, not resulting in cerebral infarction
I67	Other cerebrovascular diseases
I68	Cerebrovascular disorders in diseases classified elsewhere
I69	Sequelae of cerebrovascular disease

I60.- Nontraumatic subarachnoid hemorrhage

A subarachnoid hemorrhage is an extravasation of blood into the subarachnoid space. Nontraumatic subarachnoid hemorrhage is due to primary disease such as arteriovenous malformation, or hemorrhagic diathesis. The episodes usually are sudden in nature and account for 5 to 10 percent of all cerebrovascular accidents. Nontraumatic subarachnoid hemorrhage is classified by site and requires identification of the specific precerebral or cerebral artery involved and laterality except in the case of the basilar artery, which is a single blood vessel that joins the vertebral arteries and is located at the base of the skull, or when the code for other intracranial arteries applies. Laterality is also not applicable to subarachnoid hemorrhage occurring in the meninges or due to rupture of a cerebral arteriovenous malformation or when the blood vessel or site is not specified.

Focus Point

When subarachnoid hemorrhage is secondary to head trauma the condition is classified to the injury chapter.

I61.- Nontraumatic intracerebral hemorrhage

A nontraumatic intracerebral hemorrhage is a spontaneous extravasation of blood within the brain. Etiologies include hypertension with microaneurysmal formation, bleeding diathesis (leukemia, thrombocytopenia, and hemophilia), disseminated intravascular coagulation, anticoagulant therapy, liver disease, cerebral amyloid angiopathy, AV malformation, and brain neoplasms. Also referred to as intraparenchymal hemorrhage, nontraumatic intracerebral hemorrhage is classified by the site involved, such as the cerebrum (hemisphere), brainstem, cerebellum, intraventricular, multiple sites, other, or unspecified site.

Focus Point

Patients with intracerebral hemorrhage may develop cerebral vasogenic edema, an accumulation of fluid in the brain. If the provider documents clinically significant cerebral vasogenic edema, assign code G93.6 in addition to a code from category I61, since cerebral vasogenic edema is not inherent to cerebral hemorrhage. A coma is not inherent to an intracerebral hemorrhage. When coma is documented it is reported additionally with codes from subcategory R40.2-.

I63.- Cerebral infarction

Cerebral infarction can result from a blocked blood vessel due to a thrombus, embolus, or a constriction or narrowing of an artery in the head or neck (stenosis). A thrombus is a mass of platelets, fibrin, and other blood components that form within the precerebral or cerebral vessels that supply blood to the brain. An embolism is a clot or thrombus that travels from a remote site to another site; in this case, the embolus travels to the precerebral or cerebral arteries. Thrombi and emboli can obstruct the cerebral arteries causing damage from the lack of blood supply reaching the brain. Cerebral infarction is classified based on the type of occlusion—thrombosis, embolism, or stenosis—the site of the occlusion, which requires identification of the specific precerebral or cerebral artery, and laterality. Laterality does not apply to the basilar artery because it is a single blood vessel that joins the vertebral arteries and is located at the base of the skull.

Focus Point

Although a code exists for stroke, unspecified (I63.9), it is appropriate to use imaging reports to assist in establishing a more specific site location so that a more specific code for the cerebral infarction can be assigned.

I65.- Occlusion and stenosis of precerebral arteries, not resulting in cerebral infarction

These codes describe narrowing and occlusion of the precerebral arteries that do not result in a cerebral infarction or stroke. The precerebral arteries—basilar, carotid, and vertebral—extend from the aortic arch. Blood is supplied to the brain by the internal carotid arteries and vertebral arteries. The right and left vertebral arteries come together at the base of the brain to form the basilar artery. The right common carotid originates in the innominate artery and the left common carotid is normally the second branch from the aortic arch. The common carotids have no branches until their terminal bifurcation where they divide into the internal and external carotid arteries. The internal carotid artery ascends through the base of the skull to give rise to the anterior and middle cerebral arteries. The external carotid artery supplies blood to the face and scalp. The vertebral arteries arise from the subclavian arteries and emerge from the posterior base of the skull to form the basilar artery. Occasionally, the basilar artery splits into two vessels that reunite. The vertebral artery takes blood to the basilar artery, and from there the blood goes to the circle of Willis, which controls blood pressure in the brain and allows a continued supply of oxygenated blood to the brain in the event that a vessel becomes occluded. Occlusion and stenosis of the precerebral arteries is classified based on site, which requires identification of the specific precerebral artery, and laterality. Laterality does not apply to the basilar artery because it is a single blood vessel that joins the vertebral arteries and is located at the base of the skull.

I67.- Other cerebrovascular diseases

This category represents varied diseases and disorders of the cerebral vasculature, including nonruptured dissection or aneurysm of the cerebral arteries, atherosclerosis, hypertensive encephalopathy, arteritis, vasospasm, ischemia, and other conditions.

Focus Point

Transient cerebral ischemia (TIA) is excluded from this chapter and is located in Chapter 6 Diseases of the Nervous System in category G45.

I67.3 Progressive vascular leukoencephalopathy

Leukoencephalopathy is a disorder that affects the white matter of the brain and, in this case, is caused by an underlying vascular disease. This code includes Binswanger's disease, also called subcortical vascular dementia, and it occurs when deep layers of the brain white matter are damaged by intracerebral atherosclerosis.

I67.5 Moyamoya disease

Moyamoya disease is characterized by the progressive occlusion of the arteries around the circle of Willis area of the brain, which if untreated can eventually cause strokes or hemorrhage. The cause is unknown but thought to be hereditary.

I67.7 Cerebral arteritis, not elsewhere classified

Cerebral arteritis is inflammation of the small and medium-sized arteries in the brain, also known as cerebral vasculitis or central nervous system vasculitis.

I67.83 Posterior reversible encephalopathy syndrome

Also referred to as PRES, posterior reversible encephalopathy syndrome is a condition of cortical and subcortical edema that can cause headaches, seizures, confusion, and loss of vision. This condition is prevalent in chronic kidney disease patients because of their susceptibility to hypertension and uremia.

I69.- Sequelae of cerebrovascular disease

This category classifies conditions that are sequela or late effects of conditions classified to categories I60-I67. Late effects of cerebrovascular disease are classified according to the neurological deficit; the causal condition of the sequela, such as nontraumatic subarachnoid, intracerebral, intracranial hemorrhages, cerebral infarctions, or other and unspecified cerebrovascular diseases; and the specific deficit or sequela, such as cognitive deficits, speech deficits, mono and hemiplegias, dysphagia, ataxia, and other deficits.

Focus Point

Disturbance of vision is located in the "other" sequela subcategory.

I69.0- Sequelae of nontraumatic subarachnoid hemorrhage

This subcategory classifies conditions that are sequelae or late effects of nontraumatic subarachnoid hemorrhage. A subarachnoid hemorrhage is an extravasation of blood into the subarachnoid space. Nontraumatic subarachnoid hemorrhage is due to primary disease such as arteriosclerotic aneurysm, arteriovenous malformation, or hemorrhagic diathesis. The episodes are usually sudden in nature and account for 5 percent to 10 percent of all cerebrovascular accidents. These sequelae codes are reported for conditions specified as residuals, which may occur at any time after the onset of the causal condition. The specific deficits are further subdivided by defined conditions within the subcategory.

I69.01- Cognitive deficits following nontraumatic subarachnoid hemorrhage

Cognitive deficits include impairment conditions related to mental functions regarding information exchange and comprehension as well as how these functions are applied to the patient's actions. These deficits are categorized into domains as follows:

I69.010 Attention and concentration deficit following nontraumatic subarachnoid hemorrhage

These types of disorders indicate inability to focus and pay attention to the task at hand, with problems concentrating, often manifested by what appears to be daydreaming.

I69.011 Memory deficit following nontraumatic subarachnoid hemorrhage

Difficulty with short-term or long-term recall of events.

I69.012 Visuospatial deficit and spatial neglect following nontraumatic subarachnoid hemorrhage

These deficits affect a person's ability to recognize objects and their relationships to one another, differentiating between light and dark, and/or recognizing places or faces. Spatial neglect often causes the patient to be unable to respond or react to stimuli.

I69.013 Psychomotor deficit following nontraumatic subarachnoid hemorrhage

These affect hand-eye coordination tasks that require thought and motion in combination.

I69.014 Frontal lobe and executive function deficit following nontraumatic subarachnoid hemorrhage

The executive function includes time management skills, which allow the patient to plan, recognize details, pay attention, and focus, as well as adjust behavior based on past experiences.

I69.015 Cognitive social or emotional deficit following nontraumatic subarachnoid hemorrhage

This kind of deficit affects how a patient controls behavior and emotions, empathy, and skills that help solve problems.

I69.02- Speech and language deficits following nontraumatic subarachnoid hemorrhage

These deficits are classified as communication difficulties that affect articulation, language use, and/or voice imperfections. Speech and language deficits are categorized into domains as follows:

I69.020 Aphasia following nontraumatic subarachnoid hemorrhage

The partial or total loss of ability to comprehend language or communicate through speaking, the written word, or sign language.

I69.021 Dysphasia following nontraumatic subarachnoid hemorrhage

A speech impairment manifested by incoordination and inability to arrange words in their proper order.

I69.022 Dysarthria following nontraumatic subarachnoid hemorrhage

Dysarthria is difficulty pronouncing words.

I69.023 Fluency disorder following nontraumatic subarachnoid hemorrhage

Fluency disorders often fit into a stuttering diagnosis group, meaning actions relate to repetition or hesitations in speech patterns.

I69.03- Monoplegia of upper limb following nontraumatic subarachnoid hemorrhage

I69.04- Monoplegia of lower limb following nontraumatic subarachnoid hemorrhage

Monoplegia is the loss or impairment of motor function in one arm or one leg.

I69.05- Hemiplegia and hemiparesis following nontraumatic subarachnoid hemorrhage

Hemiplegia is the paralysis of one side of the body. Hemiparesis is weakness of one side of the body.

I69.06- Other paralytic syndrome following nontraumatic subarachnoid hemorrhage

Sequelae conditions such as paraplegia, paraparesis, quadriplegia, quadriparesis, or locked-in state are classified here. Paraplegia is the loss or impairment of motor function in both of the legs and can involve the trunk from the waist down. Quadriplegia, also referred to as tetraplegia, involves some degree of loss or impairment of all four arms and legs and can involve the trunk. Locked-in state or syndrome is a paralytic loss of movement in all voluntary muscles except those controlling the eyes. Although the patient is cognitively aware, he or she is often thought to be unconscious because of the inability to communicate except with eye movements. These conditions when due to transient ischemic attack (TIA) or small stroke may resolve completely, but the amount of recovery depends on the extent of damage, diagnosis time, and level of treatment provided.

I69.09- Other sequelae of nontraumatic subarachnoid hemorrhage

This subcategory includes various conditions that can be residual effects of CVA that are not included in the other subcategories.

I69.090 Apraxia following nontraumatic subarachnoid hemorrhage

This is a neurologic disorder that inhibits the patient's ability to perform motor skill movements even though the muscles are intact. The disorder can be manifested in a few ways: Orofacial apraxia affects the voluntary movement of the facial muscles, speech apraxia inhibits the movement of the tongue or mouth in order to speak, and other forms may affect a patient's ability to move the extremities.

I69.091 Dysphagia following nontraumatic subarachnoid hemorrhage

This disorder is defined as swallowing difficulty wherein getting the food or beverage from the mouth into the stomach is difficult and, in some cases, impossible. Infrequent bouts of dysphagia may occur when food is eaten too quickly or not chewed well and is not cause for concern; however, recurrent and continuous episodes of dysphagia may be a sign of an underlying condition requiring medical intervention.

I69.092 Facial weakness following nontraumatic subarachnoid hemorrhage

Facial weakness or droop is the reduction or complete loss of movement within the facial muscles, often due to nerve damage from a stroke. It can occur on either or both sides of the face.

I69.093 Ataxia following nontraumatic subarachnoid hemorrhage

Ataxia describes the decreased ability to perform voluntary muscle functions that affect balance and coordination and may manifest in speech problems and difficulty swallowing and making eye and other movements, often due to cerebellum damage or trauma. Medical treatment and additional therapies such as physical, occupational, and speech therapies may be necessary as well as the use of walkers for more stable ambulation.

I69.1- Sequelae of nontraumatic intracerebral hemorrhage

This subcategory classifies conditions that are sequelae, or late effects, of nontraumatic intracerebral hemorrhage. A nontraumatic intracerebral hemorrhage, also referred to as intraparenchymal hemorrhage, is a spontaneous extravasation of blood within the brain and includes sites documented as cerebrum (hemisphere), intraventricular, brainstem, and cerebellum. Etiologies include hypertension with microaneurysmal formation, bleeding diathesis (leukemia, thrombocytopenia, and hemophilia), disseminated intravascular coagulation, anticoagulant therapy, liver disease, cerebral amyloid angiopathy, AV malformation, and brain neoplasms. These sequelae codes are reported for conditions specified as residuals, which may occur at any time after the onset of the causal condition. The specific deficits are further subdivided by defined conditions within the subcategory.

I69.11- Cognitive deficits following nontraumatic intracerebral hemorrhage

Cognitive deficits group impairment conditions related to mental functions regarding information exchange and comprehension as well as how these functions are applied to the patient's actions. These deficits are categorized into domains as follows:

I69.110 Attention and concentration deficit following nontraumatic intracerebral hemorrhage

These types of disorders indicate inability to focus and pay attention to the task at hand, with problems concentrating, often manifested by what appears to be daydreaming.

I69.111 Memory deficit following nontraumatic intracerebral hemorrhage

Memory deficit is characterized by difficulty with short-term or long-term recall of events.

I69.112 Visuospatial deficit and spatial neglect following nontraumatic intracerebral hemorrhage

These deficits affect a person's ability to recognize objects and their relationships to one another, differentiating between light and dark, and/or recognizing places or faces. Spatial neglect often causes the patient to be unable to respond or react to stimuli.

I69.113 Psychomotor deficit following nontraumatic intracerebral hemorrhage

These deficits affect hand-eye coordination tasks that require thought and motion in combination.

I69.114 Frontal lobe and executive function deficit following nontraumatic intracerebral hemorrhage

The executive function includes time management skills that allow the patient to plan, recognize details, pay attention, and focus, as well as adjusting behavior based on past experiences.

I69.115 Cognitive social or emotional deficit following nontraumatic intracerebral hemorrhage

These deficits affect how a patient controls behavior and emotions, empathy, and skills that assist in solving problems.

I69.12- Speech and language deficits following nontraumatic intracerebral hemorrhage

These deficits are classified as communication difficulties that affect articulation, language use, and/or voice imperfections. Speech and language deficits are categorized into domains as follows:

I69.120 Aphasia following nontraumatic intracerebral hemorrhage

The partial or total loss of the ability to comprehend language or communicate through speaking, the written word, or sign language.

I69.121 Dysphasia following nontraumatic intracerebral hemorrhage

A speech impairment manifested by incoordination and inability to arrange words in their proper order.

I69.122 Dysarthria following nontraumatic intracerebral hemorrhage

Dysarthria is difficulty pronouncing words.

I69.123 Fluency disorder following nontraumatic intracerebral hemorrhage

Fluency deficits often fit into a stuttering diagnosis group, meaning actions relate to repetition or hesitations in speech patterns.

I69.13- Monoplegia of upper limb following nontraumatic intracerebral hemorrhage

I69.14- Monoplegia of lower limb following nontraumatic intracerebral hemorrhage

Monoplegia is the loss or impairment of motor function in one arm or one leg.

I69.15- Hemiplegia and hemiparesis following nontraumatic intracerebral hemorrhage

Hemiplegia is the paralysis of one side of the body. Hemiparesis is weakness of one side of the body.

I69.16- Other paralytic syndrome following nontraumatic intracerebral hemorrhage

Sequelae conditions such as paraplegia, paraparesis, quadriplegia, quadriparesis, or locked-in state are classified here. Paraplegia is the loss or impairment of motor function in both of the legs and can involve the trunk from the waist down. Quadriplegia, also referred to as tetraplegia, involves some degree of loss or impairment of all four arms and legs and can involve the trunk. Locked-in state or syndrome is a paralytic loss of movement in all voluntary muscles except those controlling the eyes. Although the patient is cognitively aware, he or she is often thought to be unconscious because of the inability to communicate except with eye movements. These conditions when due to transient ischemic attack (TIA) or small stroke may resolve completely, but the amount of recovery depends on the extent of damage, diagnosis time, and level of treatment provided.

I69.19- Other sequelae of nontraumatic intracerebral hemorrhage

This subcategory includes various conditions that can be residual effects of cardiovascular accident (CVA) that are not included in the other subcategories.

I69.190 Apraxia following nontraumatic intracerebral hemorrhage

Apraxia is a neurologic disorder that inhibits the ability of the patient to perform motor skill movements even though the muscles are intact. It can manifest in a few ways: Orofacial apraxia affects the voluntary movement of the facial muscles, speech apraxia inhibits the movement of the tongue or mouth in order to speak, and other forms may affect a patient's ability to move the extremities.

I69.191 Dysphagia following nontraumatic intracerebral hemorrhage

Dysphagia is simply defined as swallowing difficulty wherein getting the food or beverage from the mouth into the stomach is difficult and, in some cases, impossible. Infrequent bouts of dysphagia may occur when food is eaten too quickly or not chewed well and is not cause for concern; however, recurrent and continuous episodes of dysphagia may be a sign of an underlying condition requiring medical intervention.

I69.192 Facial weakness following nontraumatic intracerebral hemorrhage

Facial weakness or droop is the reduction or complete loss of movement within the facial muscles, often due to nerve damage from a stroke. It can occur on either or both sides of the face.

I69.193 Ataxia following nontraumatic intracerebral hemorrhage

Ataxia describes the decreased ability to perform voluntary muscle functions that affect balance and coordination and may manifest in speech problems and difficulty swallowing and making eye and other movements, often due to cerebellum damage or trauma. Medical treatment and additional therapies such as physical, occupational, and speech therapies may be necessary as well as the use of walkers for more stable ambulation.

I69.2- Sequelae of other nontraumatic intracranial hemorrhage

This subcategory classifies conditions that are sequelae, or late effects, of nontraumatic intracranial hemorrhage. The intracranial hemorrhage is bleeding within the skull in the subdural, extradural, or epidural space. The subdural space is the potential space that results from the separation of the arachnoid mater from the dura mater as a result of trauma, pathologic process, or the absence of cerebrospinal fluid. The epidural space is the potential space between the endosteum of the cranium (skull) and the dura mater, the outermost layer of a three-layer membrane that covers the brain. Another term used to refer to the epidural space is extradural space, which is nearly synonymous except that the term epidural implies bleeding in immediate proximity to the dura mater while extradural implies bleeding that may be unconnected to the membrane itself, such as hemorrhage from the skull vessels. These sequelae codes are reported for conditions specified as residuals, which may occur any time after the onset of the causal condition. The specific deficits are further subdivided by defined conditions within the subcategory.

I69.21- Cognitive deficits following other nontraumatic intracranial hemorrhage

Cognitive deficits group impairment conditions related to mental functions regarding information exchange and comprehension as well as how these functions are applied to the patient's actions. These deficits are categorized into domains as follows:

I69.210 Attention and concentration deficit following other nontraumatic intracranial hemorrhage

These types of disorders indicate inability to focus and pay attention to the task at hand, with problems concentrating, often manifested by what appears to be daydreaming.

I69.211 Memory deficit following other nontraumatic intracranial hemorrhage

This deficit leads to difficulty with short-term or long-term recall of events.

I69.212 Visuospatial deficit and spatial neglect following other nontraumatic intracranial hemorrhage

These deficits affect a person's ability to recognize objects and their relationships to one another, differentiating between light and dark, and/or recognition of places or faces. Spatial neglect often causes the patient to be unable to respond or react to stimuli.

I69.213 Psychomotor deficit following other nontraumatic intracranial hemorrhage

Psychomotor problems affect hand-eye coordination tasks that require thought and motion in combination.

I69.214 Frontal lobe and executive function deficit following other nontraumatic intracranial hemorrhage

The executive function includes time management skills that allow the patient to plan, recognize details, pay attention, and focus, as well as adjust behavior based on past experiences.

I69.215 Cognitive social or emotional deficit following other nontraumatic intracranial hemorrhage

These deficits affect how a patient controls behavior and emotions, empathy, and skills that assist in solving problems.

I69.22- Speech and language deficits following other nontraumatic intracranial hemorrhage

These deficits are classified as communication difficulties that affect articulation, language use, and/or voice imperfections. Speech and language deficits are categorized into domains as follows:

I69.220 Aphasia following other nontraumatic intracranial hemorrhage

The partial or total loss of the ability to comprehend language or communicate through speaking, the written word, or sign language.

I69.221 Dysphasia following other nontraumatic intracranial hemorrhage

A speech impairment manifested by incoordination and inability to arrange words in their proper order.

I69.222 Dysarthria following other nontraumatic intracranial hemorrhage

Dysarthria is difficulty pronouncing words.

I69.223 Fluency disorder following other nontraumatic intracranial hemorrhage

These are deficits that often fit into a stuttering diagnosis group, meaning actions relate to repetition or hesitations in speech patterns.

I69.23- Monoplegia of upper limb following nontraumatic intracranial hemorrhage

I69.24- Monoplegia of lower limb following nontraumatic intracranial hemorrhage

Monoplegia is the loss or impairment of motor function in one arm or one leg.

I69.25- Hemiplegia and hemiparesis following other nontraumatic intracranial hemorrhage

Hemiplegia is the paralysis of one side of the body. Hemiparesis is weakness of one side of the body.

I69.26- Other paralytic syndrome following other nontraumatic intracranial hemorrhage

Sequelae conditions such as paraplegia, paraparesis, quadriplegia, quadriparesis, or locked-in state are classified here. Paraplegia is the loss or impairment of motor function in both of the legs and can involve the trunk from the waist down. Quadriplegia, also referred to as tetraplegia, involves some degree of loss or impairment of all four arms and legs and can involve the trunk. Locked-in state or syndrome is a paralytic loss of movement in all voluntary muscles except those controlling the eyes. Although the patient is cognitively aware, he or she is often thought to be unconscious because of the inability to communicate except with eye movements. These conditions when due to transient ischemic attack (TIA) or small stroke may resolve completely, but the amount of recovery depends on the extent of damage, diagnosis time, and level of treatment provided.

I69.29- Other sequelae of other nontraumatic intracranial hemorrhage

This subcategory includes various conditions that can be residual effects of cardiovascular accident (CVA) that are not included in the other subcategories.

I69.290 Apraxia following other nontraumatic intracranial hemorrhage

Apraxia is a neurologic disorder that inhibits the patient's ability to perform motor skill movements even though the muscles are intact. The disorder and can be manifested in a few ways: Orofacial apraxia affects the voluntary movement of the facial muscles, speech apraxia inhibits the movement of the tongue or mouth in order to speak, and other forms may affect a patient's ability to move the extremities.

I69.291 Dysphagia following other nontraumatic intracranial hemorrhage

Dysphagia is simply defined as swallowing difficulty wherein getting the food or beverage from the mouth into the stomach is difficult and, in some cases, impossible. Infrequent bouts of dysphagia may occur when food is eaten too quickly or not chewed well and is not cause for concern; however, recurrent and continuous episodes of dysphagia may be a sign of an underlying condition requiring medical intervention.

I69.292 Facial weakness following other nontraumatic intracranial hemorrhage

Facial weakness or droop is the reduction or complete loss of movement within the facial muscles, often due to nerve damage from a stroke. It can occur on either or both sides of the face.

I69.293 Ataxia following other nontraumatic intracranial hemorrhage

Ataxia describes the decreased ability to perform voluntary muscle functions that affect balance and coordination and may manifest in speech problems and difficulty swallowing and making eye and other movements, often due to cerebellum damage or trauma. Medical treatment and additional therapies such as physical, occupational, and speech therapies may be necessary as well as the use of walkers for more stable ambulation.

I69.3- Sequelae of cerebral infarction

This subcategory classifies conditions that are sequelae, or late effects, of ischemic, nonhemorrhagic cerebral infarction. Cerebral infarction can result from a blocked blood vessel due to a thrombus, embolus, or a constriction or narrowing of an artery in the head or neck (stenosis). A thrombus is a mass of platelets, fibrin, and other blood components that form within the precerebral or cerebral vessels that supply blood to the brain. Precerebral artery occlusions include the carotid, basilar, and vertebral arteries while cerebral arteries involve the middle, anterior, posterior, or cerebellar artery. Conditions documented as late effects from stroke with no further specification as to the type of stroke are also classified here. These sequelae codes are reported for conditions specified as residuals, which may occur at any time after the onset of the causal condition. The specific deficits are further subdivided by defined conditions within the subcategory.

I69.31- Cognitive deficits following cerebral infarction

Cognitive deficits group impairment conditions related to mental functions regarding information exchange and comprehension as well as how these functions are applied to the patient's actions. These deficits are categorized into domains as follows:

I69.310 Attention and concentration deficit following cerebral infarction

These types of disorders involve the inability to focus and pay attention to the task at hand, with problems concentrating, often manifested by what appears to be daydreaming.

I69.311 Memory deficit following cerebral infarction

This deficit leads to difficulty with short-term or long-term recall of events.

I69.312 Visuospatial deficit and spatial neglect following cerebral infarction

These deficits affect a person's ability to recognize objects and their relationships to one another, differentiating between light and dark, and/or recognition of places or faces. Spatial neglect often causes the patient to be unable to respond or react to stimuli.

I69.313 Psychomotor deficit following cerebral infarction

Psychomotor deficits affect hand-eye coordination tasks that require thought and motion in combination.

I69.314 Frontal lobe and executive function deficit following cerebral infarction

The executive function includes time management skills which allow the patient to plan, recognize details, pay attention, and focus, as well as adjust behavior based on past experiences.

I69.315 Cognitive social or emotional deficit following cerebral infarction

These kinds of deficits affect how a patient controls behavior and emotions, empathy, and skills that assist in solving problems.

I69.32- Speech and language deficits following cerebral infarction

These deficits are classified as communication difficulties that affect articulation, language use, and/or voice imperfections. Speech and language deficits are categorized into domains as follows:

I69.320 Aphasia following cerebral infarction

The partial or total loss of the ability to comprehend language or communicate through speaking, the written word, or sign language.

I69.321 Dysphasia following cerebral infarction

Dysphasia is a speech impairment manifested by incoordination and inability to arrange words in their proper order.

I69.322 Dysarthria following cerebral infarction

Dysarthria is difficulty pronouncing words.

I69.323 Fluency disorder following cerebral infarction

Fluency disorders often fit into a stuttering diagnosis group, meaning actions relate to repetition or hesitations in speech patterns.

I69.33- Monoplegia of upper limb following cerebral infarction

I69.34- Monoplegia of lower limb following cerebral infarction

Monoplegia is the loss or impairment of motor function in one arm or one leg.

I69.35- Hemiplegia and hemiparesis following cerebral infarction

Hemiplegia is the paralysis of one side of the body. Hemiparesis is weakness of one side of the body.

I69.36- Other paralytic syndrome following cerebral infarction

Sequelae conditions such as paraplegia, paraparesis, quadriplegia, quadriparesis or locked in state are classified here. Paraplegia is the loss or impairment of motor function in both of the legs and can involve the trunk from the waist down. Quadriplegia also referred to as tetraplegia, involves some degree of loss or impairment of all four arms and legs, and can involve the trunk. Locked-in state or syndrome is a paralytic loss of movement in all voluntary muscles except those controlling the eyes. Although the patient is cognitively aware, he or she is often thought to be unconscious because of the inability to communicate except with eye movements. These conditions when due to transient ischemic attack (TIA) or small stroke may resolve completely, but the amount of recovery depends on the extent of damage, diagnosis time, and level of treatment provided.

I69.39- Other sequelae of cerebral infarction

This subcategory includes various conditions that can be residual effects of cardiovascular accident (CVA) that are not included in the other subcategories.

I69.390 Apraxia following cerebral infarction

This is a neurologic disorder that inhibits the ability of the patient to perform motor skill movements even though the muscles are intact. The condition can be manifested in a few ways: Orofacial apraxia affects the voluntary movement of the facial muscles, speech apraxia inhibits the movement of the tongue or mouth in order to speak, and other forms may affect a patient's ability to move the extremities.

I69.391 Dysphagia following cerebral infarction

Dysphagia is simply defined as swallowing difficulty wherein getting the food or beverage from the mouth into the stomach is difficult and, in some cases, impossible. Infrequent bouts of dysphagia may occur when food is eaten too quickly or not chewed well and is not cause for concern; however, recurrent and continuous episodes of dysphagia may be a sign of an underlying condition requiring medical intervention.

I69.392   Facial weakness following cerebral infarction

Facial weakness or droop is the reduction or complete loss of movement within the facial muscles, often due to nerve damage from a stroke. It can occur on either or both sides of the face.

I69.393   Ataxia following cerebral infarction

Ataxia describes the decreased ability to perform voluntary muscle functions that affect balance and coordination and may manifest in speech problems and difficulty swallowing and making eye and other movements, often due to cerebellum damage or trauma. Medical treatment and additional therapies such as physical, occupational, and speech therapies may be necessary as well as the use of walkers for more stable ambulation.

I69.8-   Sequelae of other cerebrovascular diseases

This subcategory classifies conditions that are sequelae or late effects of varied diseases and disorders of the cerebral vasculature, including nonruptured dissection or aneurysm of the cerebral arteries, atherosclerosis, hypertensive encephalopathy, arteritis, vasospasm, and other nontraumatic specified conditions. These sequelae codes are reported for conditions specified as residuals, which may occur at any time after the onset of the causal condition. The specific deficits are further subdivided by defined conditions within the subcategory.

I69.81-   Cognitive deficits following other cerebrovascular disease

Cognitive deficits group impairment conditions related to mental functions regarding information exchange and comprehension as well as how these functions are applied to the patient's actions. These deficits are categorized into domains as follows:

I69.810   Attention and concentration deficit following other cerebrovascular disease

These types of disorders indicate the inability to focus and pay attention to the task at hand, with problems concentrating, often manifested by what appears to be daydreaming.

I69.811   Memory deficit following other cerebrovascular disease

This deficit is characterized by difficulty with short-term or long-term recall of events.

I69.812   Visuospatial deficit and spatial neglect following other cerebrovascular disease

These deficits affect a person's ability to recognize objects and their relationships to one another, differentiating between light and dark, and/or recognizing places or faces. Spatial neglect often causes the patient to be unable to respond or react to stimuli.

I69.813   Psychomotor deficit following other cerebrovascular disease

Psychomotor deficits affect hand-eye coordination tasks that require thought and motion in combination.

I69.814   Frontal lobe and executive function deficit following other cerebrovascular disease

The executive function determines time management skills that allow the patient to plan, recognize details, pay attention, and focus, as well as adjust behavior based on past experiences.

I69.815   Cognitive social or emotional deficit following other cerebrovascular disease

These deficits affect how a patient controls behavior and emotions, empathy, and skills that assist in solving problems.

I69.82-   Speech and language deficits following other cerebrovascular disease

These deficits are classified as communication difficulties that affect articulation, language use, and/or voice imperfections. Speech and language deficits are categorized into domains as follows:

I69.820   Aphasia following other cerebrovascular disease

The partial or total loss of ability to comprehend language or communicate through speaking, the written word, or sign language.

I69.821   Dysphasia following other cerebrovascular disease

A speech impairment manifested by incoordination and inability to arrange words in their proper order.

I69.822   Dysarthria following other cerebrovascular disease

Dysarthria is difficulty pronouncing words.

I69.823   Fluency disorder following other cerebrovascular disease

Fluency disorders often fit into a stuttering diagnosis group, meaning actions relate to repetition or hesitations in speech patterns.

I69.83- Monoplegia of upper limb following other cerebrovascular diseases

I69.84- Monoplegia of lower limb following other cerebrovascular diseases

Monoplegia is the loss or impairment of motor function in one arm or one leg.

I69.85- Hemiplegia and hemiparesis following other cerebrovascular disease

Hemiplegia is the paralysis of one side of the body. Hemiparesis is weakness of one side of the body.

I69.86- Other paralytic syndrome following other cerebrovascular disease

Sequelae conditions such as paraplegia, paraparesis, quadriplegia, quadriparesis, or locked-in state are classified here. Paraplegia is the loss or impairment of motor function in both of the legs and can involve the trunk from the waist down. Quadriplegia, also referred to as tetraplegia, involves some degree of loss or impairment of all four arms and legs and can involve the trunk. Locked-in state or syndrome is a paralytic loss of movement in all voluntary muscles except those controlling the eyes. Although the patient is cognitively aware, he or she is often thought to be unconscious because of the inability to communicate except with eye movements. These conditions when due to transient ischemic attack (TIA) or small stroke may resolve completely, but the amount of recovery depends on the extent of damage, diagnosis time, and level of treatment provided.

I69.89- Other sequelae of other cerebrovascular disease

This subcategory includes various conditions that can be residual effects of cardiovascular accident (CVA) that are not included in the other subcategories.

I69.890 Apraxia following other cerebrovascular disease

Apraxia is a neurologic disorder that inhibits the ability of the patient to perform motor skill movements even though the muscles are intact. It can be manifested in a few ways: Orofacial apraxia affects the voluntary movement of the facial muscles, speech apraxia inhibits the movement of the tongue or mouth in order to speak, and other forms may affect a patient's ability to move the extremities.

I69.891 Dysphagia following other cerebrovascular disease

Dysphagia is simply defined as swallowing difficulty wherein getting the food or beverage from the mouth into the stomach is difficult and, in some cases, impossible. Infrequent bouts of dysphagia may occur when food is eaten too quickly or not chewed well and is not cause for concern; however, recurrent and continuous episodes of dysphagia may be a sign of an underlying condition requiring medical intervention.

I69.892 Facial weakness following other cerebrovascular disease

Facial weakness or droop is the reduction or complete loss of movement within the facial muscles, often due to nerve damage from a stroke. It can occur on either or both sides of the face.

I69.893 Ataxia following other cerebrovascular disease

Ataxia describes the decreased ability to perform voluntary muscle functions that affect balance and coordination and may manifest in speech problems and difficulty swallowing and making eye and other movements, often due to cerebellum damage or trauma. Medical treatment and additional therapies such as physical, occupational, and speech therapies may be necessary as well as the use of walkers for more stable ambulation.

> **Focus Point**
>
> If documentation lacks the specific information on the causal condition needed to use one of the preceding subcategories I69.1-, I69.2-, and I69.3-, or I69.8-, report codes from subcategory I69.9.- Sequelae of unspecified cerebrovascular diseases.

Diseases of Arteries, Arterioles and Capillaries (I70-I79)

This code block includes conditions affecting the arteries, arterioles, and capillaries, including atherosclerosis, aneurysm, peripheral vascular disease, embolism and thrombosis, arteritis, and stricture.

The categories in this code block are as follows:

I70	Atherosclerosis
I71	Aortic aneurysm and dissection
I72	Other aneurysm
I73	Other peripheral vascular diseases
I74	Arterial embolism and thrombosis
I75	Atheroembolism
I76	Septic arterial embolism
I77	Other disorders of arteries and arterioles
I78	Diseases of capillaries
I79	Disorders of arteries, arterioles and capillaries in diseases classified elsewhere

I70.-   Atherosclerosis

Atherosclerosis is a form of arteriosclerosis characterized by irregularly distributed atheromas accumulating within the tunica intima of arteries. The deposits are associated with calcification and fibrosis, reducing the size of the arterial lumen and resulting in obstructive ischemia.

I70.92   Chronic total occlusion of artery of the extremities

Chronic total occlusion of an extremity artery usually develops over a long period of time, although partial occlusion is initially present. The presence of a collateral blood supply can cause a wide variation in symptoms and may actually allow worsening of an occlusion even though symptoms may be relatively mild. Since a total occlusion is more difficult to cross than a partial occlusion, treatment with angioplasty and/or stenting is significantly more complex.

I71.-   Aortic aneurysm and dissection

Aortic aneurysms are circumscribed dilations of the aorta. Generally, an aneurysm is considered clinically significant if its diameter is twice that of the normal artery. A dissecting aneurysm is characterized by blood entering through a split or tear in the intima of the artery wall or by interstitial hemorrhage.

Focus Point

When an aneurysm develops at an adjoining site such as aortoiliac, code each site separately, unless a code is provided that identifies the adjoining site, such as thoracoabdominal aorta.

I71.00   Dissection of unspecified site of aorta

I71.01   Dissection of thoracic aorta

I71.02   Dissection of abdominal aorta

I71.03   Dissection of thoracoabdominal aorta

Aortic dissection is a tear in the aorta that causes bleeding into the aorta wall. This can occur in the thoracic portion, abdominal portion, or thoracoabdominal portion. The tear initially creates two passages for blood: one passage continues to promote normal blood flow and the other allows accumulation of blood. As this disease progresses, the tear increases in size and the accumulation of blood grows, causing pressure on other branches of the aorta. While the specific cause of this disorder is still unknown, it is thought to be brought on by atherosclerosis and hypertension, as well as injury to the chest or abdomen. A large dissection can be fatal.

I71.1   Thoracic aortic aneurysm, ruptured

I71.2   Thoracic aortic aneurysm, without rupture

A thoracic aortic aneurysm (TAA) is a circumscribed dilation in a weakened portion of the aorta in the chest. An aneurysm is considered clinically significant if its diameter is twice the size of the normal artery. Aortic aneurysms are often asymptomatic but large thoracic aneurysms may cause pain in the jaw, neck, chest, or upper back. Other symptoms include coughing, hoarseness, or difficulty breathing. Large TAAs are at risk for rupture. If rupture occurs, internal bleeding occurs and without emergent treatment can rapidly lead to shock and death.

I71.3   Abdominal aortic aneurysm, rupture

I71.4   Abdominal aortic aneurysm without rupture

An abdominal aortic aneurysm is defined as an enlargement of the aorta, the primary blood vessel feeding the abdomen, pelvis, and legs. This enlargement may become so severe that it causes a rupture of the vessel itself. This condition may take time to develop, often with no symptoms at all, and may be an incidental finding. If the aneurysm grows quickly, symptoms may include abdominal pain, fainting, nausea and vomiting, increased heart rate, and clammy skin. Radiological tests are performed to locate and measure the aneurysm to determine size and severity. If the patient is asymptomatic and the aneurysm size is less than 2 inches, typically the approach is wait-and-see monitoring, with ultrasounds performed perhaps twice a year to evaluate for growth. For symptomatic patients and large aneurysms, surgery is required to repair the defect either by graft or stent placement. Ruptured aneurysms require immediate intervention and have a mortality rate of one in five.

I72.- Other aneurysm

An aneurysm occurs when an artery bulges in a weak area of the arterial wall due to blood flow pressure. Aneurysms occurring outside the aorta in peripheral vessels are classified here. The most common location for a peripheral aneurysm is in the popliteal artery that runs down the back of the leg. Aneurysms also occur in the femoral artery, carotid artery, renal artery, and iliac artery and other sites in the upper and lower extremities. If a patient is diagnosed with a peripheral aneurysm in one leg, it is not uncommon to find an aneurysm in the other leg as well. Symptoms vary based on the location, size, and amount of blockage caused by an aneurysm.

I72.0   Aneurysm of carotid artery

The carotid artery subcategory includes the primary arteries that deliver blood to the brain, neck, and face on either side of the neck. The common carotid artery divides into the internal carotid artery, which delivers blood to the brain, and the external carotid artery, which delivers blood to the face and neck. Carotid artery aneurysms and pseudoaneurysms pose a risk for transient ischemic attacks (TIA) or stroke but are not common, generally occurring from trauma or previous surgical procedures. Such aneurysms can be treated successfully with endovascular stents or bypass.

Focus Point

Only aneurysms of the internal carotid artery involving the extracranial portion (neck) is reported here. Any internal carotid aneurysm of the intracranial portion or one documented as unspecified is reported with I67.1.

I72.1   Aneurysm of artery of upper extremity

Upper extremity vessels supply blood to the upper extremities and begin at the subclavian artery as it enters the axillary artery at the area of the first rib. The axillary artery then forms the brachial artery within the upper arm. At the level of the elbow, the brachial artery branches off to form the radial and ulnar arteries, which in turn further branch off to supply blood to the fingers. Aneurysms in these arteries are most often caused by a previous trauma. Surgical treatment is recommended for upper artery extremity aneurysms because of the risk of complications from embolism, thrombus, or clots.

I72.2   Aneurysm of renal artery

Aneurysm affecting the renal artery, which extends from the abdominal aorta into the kidneys, is rare. The average age of presentation is between 40 and 60 years, and more women than men have the aneurysms because of the increased incidence of fibromuscular dysplasia among females. Patients are typically asymptomatic with discovery incidental during other imaging; if symptoms are experienced, they are those related to hypertension or hematuria. Rupture of a renal artery aneurysm carries a high mortality risk in pregnant woman and fetuses.

I72.3   Aneurysm of iliac artery

The common iliac artery begins at the abdominal aorta, where it meets the lumbar spine around the fourth vertebra, splitting off into the right and left iliac arteries, which continue down the body to the point of the pelvis. At this junction, the arteries divide into the internal iliac and external iliac arteries. The internal iliac delivers blood to the pelvic organs, while the external iliac directs blood to the lower extremities. Aneurysms in the iliac arteries are uncommon but can be life-threatening if rupture occurs. Causes are typically atherosclerosis or prior surgical trauma, but infections can also be a factor. If surgery is indicated, endovascular stent grafts can be deployed.

I72.4   Aneurysm of artery of lower extremity

This artery begins at the external iliac artery and becomes the femoral artery within the thigh, which divides to form the popliteal, anterior, and posterior tibial arteries, located at the area of the knee and continuing to the lower leg to deliver blood to the feet and toes. Femoral and popliteal aneurysms can lead to dangerous blood loss if ruptured or create blood clots with resultant amputation of a limb. The major cause is thought to be atherosclerosis, although trauma to the artery can also be a factor.

I72.5   Aneurysm of other precerebral arteries

Precerebral arteries include the basilar artery, which begins at the base of the skull off of the vertebral arteries and supplies blood to the cerebellum, brainstem, and occipital regions. Basilar artery aneurysms are a common site as posterior circulation has been known to cause ischemic strokes. They are more difficult to treat because of their proximity to the brainstem and because they often have already caused bleeding and thrombosis to occur by the time they are discovered.

I72.6   Aneurysm of vertebral artery

This artery begins at the subclavian, moving up the neck and delivering blood to the occipital region and spinal column. Extracranial, cervical vertebral aneurysms are rare but can lead to dissection.

I73.-   Other peripheral vascular diseases

Peripheral vascular disease encompasses conditions that affect the blood vessels outside of the heart and brain. These conditions result from inadequate blood flow within the vessels and result in circulation disorders and symptoms. Peripheral vascular disease may be functional, meaning there is no structural defect, or organic, meaning that structural defects within the vessels, such as inflammation or plaque buildup, are present, which may lead to circulation symptoms.

I73.0-   Raynaud's syndrome

Raynaud's syndrome is a rare blood vessel disorder that primarily affects the arteries of the fingers and toes causing the blood vessels to constrict due to cold or emotional distress. When this happens blood cannot reach the skin and soft tissues and the skin turns white with blue mottling. When the blood vessels open again the skin turns red and the digits may throb or tingle. Severe cases of Raynaud's syndrome can result in gangrene (tissue death) caused by the loss of blood supply.

I73.81   Erythromelalgia

Erythromelalgia is a rare condition in which maldistribution of blood flow causes redness, pain, increased skin temperature, and burning sensations in various parts of the body, most frequently occurring in the extremities but also the torso, ears, and face. This condition may manifest on one or both sides of the body and may affect external tissues and internal organs. Heat exposure may trigger a flare. Patients generally have heat intolerance and sensitivity to alcohol and spicy foods. Body position may also contribute to symptoms. Onset and progression vary from gradual to rapid and severity may be mild to debilitating episodes. The cause of primary erythromelalgia is unknown.

I73.89   Other specified peripheral vascular diseases

Other peripheral vascular diseases includes acrocyanosis (longstanding cyanosis of the hands and sometimes the feet or face), simple and vasomotor acroparesthesia ("pins and needles" sensations), erythrocyanosis (swelling and dusky red discoloration of limbs due to cold exposure), and other conditions for which a more specific code is not available.

I74.-   Arterial embolism and thrombosis

An arterial embolism is a partial or complete obstruction of an artery due to the migration of a blood clot or other foreign material. An arterial thrombosis is the formation of a blood clot within the lumen of an artery. In each case, infarction of the tissues perfused by the artery is a potential complication. Arterial embolism and thrombosis is classified by site. Specific codes are available for the abdominal aorta, thoracic aorta, and iliac arteries. Other codes identify only the general region and include codes for the upper extremities, lower extremities, and other arteries.

I74.01   Saddle embolus of abdominal aorta

A saddle embolus is one of the most severe forms of embolism and is associated with sudden, high mortality rates. A saddle embolus is so named because it straddles the bifurcation of a blood vessel. This type of embolus is often large in diameter and can cause catastrophic circulatory obstructions. The embolus typically originates in the lower extremity veins, migrates to the vena cava, and flows through the heart into the aorta. The most common site for a saddle embolus is the aorta. Aortic saddle embolus (ASE) is a lodging of the embolus at the aortic bifurcation. Symptoms associated with ASE include bilateral lower extremity ischemia and rest pain. Some ASE include extension of the clot to the iliac bifurcation.

I75.-   Atheroembolism

Atheroembolism occurs when fragments of plaque break off from the original location and travel elsewhere in the body developing an embolism in another artery. This category reports atheroembolisms that become lodged within arteries of the extremities, kidneys, or other peripheral artery sites. Codes for the extremities identify the site as upper or lower extremity and then specify laterality as right, left, or bilateral.

I75.81   Atheroembolism of kidney

Atheroembolism of the kidney occurs when plaque breaks off, moves through the vascular system, and deposits within the small arteries of the kidneys causing an inflammatory response, narrowing, and obstruction of these vessels. Narrowing and obstruction of the kidney vasculature by atheroembolism results in inadequate blood supply that can lead to renal failure. Due to the progressive nature of this condition, the ultimate goal of treatment is to slow progression and reduce risk factors.

I76   Septic arterial embolism

A septic arterial embolism may originate from an infective process of the heart or lungs, such as endocarditis or a lung abscess. The embolic material passes through the systemic arterial system and becomes lodged in a blood vessel. Septic arterial emboli can affect small vessels practically anywhere in the body, including the brain, retina, or digits.

I77.-   Other disorders of arteries and arterioles

Arteries transport oxygen-rich blood away from the heart to all organs and cells of the body. Elastic or conducting arteries have the largest diameter of all arteries in the body and muscular (distributing) arteries are midsize arteries that are branches off of the elastic arteries. Branching into increasingly smaller arteries, the muscular arteries eventually branch out into the microscopic arterioles that control blood flow into the capillary networks. This category captures codes for conditions affecting the arteries and arterioles, such as fistulas, strictures, ruptures, and necrosis.

I77.0   Arteriovenous fistula, acquired

Acquired arteriovenous fistula is an abnormal connection between an artery and a vein. Normally blood flows from arteries to arterioles to capillaries and then back to the heart through the venous system. When an abnormal connection forms between an artery and vein, the blood supply bypasses the capillaries, impeding blood and nutrients from reaching the tissue and cells, which are normally perfused by the bypassed capillaries. Symptoms include discoloration of the overlying skin, purplish bulging veins, and edema of the affected tissues. Treatment depends on the site and size of the arteriovenous fistula. Small asymptomatic arteriovenous fistulas may be monitored. However, large fistulas may require repair using an interventional radiology or surgical procedure.

I77.1   Stricture of artery

A stricture of an artery is narrowing of the lumen and in this instance the narrowing is located in an artery for which there is not a more specific code.

I77.2   Rupture of artery

Rupture of artery indicates an artery that tears or breaks apart and in this instance the rupture occurs in an artery for which there is not a more specific code.

I77.3   Arterial fibromuscular dysplasia

This condition may also be referred to as arterial fibromuscular hyperplasia. Dysplasia, or hyperplasia, of the arteries refers to an increase in the number of cells in the artery wall. The overgrowth of cells may occur in the fibrous tissue or the muscular tissue of the artery. The overgrowth may affect any of the three layers (tunica intima, tunica media, or adventitia), but the most common type and site is fibrous dysplasia of the tunica media (middle layer). Fibrous dysplasia causes thickening of the artery. This condition usually affects the small and medium arteries.

I77.4   Celiac artery compression syndrome

The celiac artery is the first major branch off the abdominal aorta. It supplies blood to the stomach, liver, spleen, and distal portion of the esophagus, a region also referred to as the foregut. Celiac artery compression syndrome, also called median arcuate ligament syndrome, occurs when the celiac artery becomes restricted due to compression by the median arcuate ligament in the diaphragm. The main symptom is pain, which may be chronic or may occur only after eating. Pain is often severe enough that it is debilitating. Treatment involves surgical release of the median arcuate ligament.

I77.5   Necrosis of artery

Necrosis refers to tissue death, in this case affecting an artery. Tissue death typically occurs when blood supply to the tissues is interrupted.

I77.6   Arteritis, unspecified

Arteritis is an inflammation of an artery. This code is used when the cause of the inflammation is not specified and/or when there is not a more specific code for a particular site when the site is documented.

I77.7-   Other arterial dissection

Arterial dissections occur when an area in the inner lining of the artery tears and blood enters the wall of the vessel and widens the space between the wall layers. The pathology of a dissection has two primary outcomes: the tear can activate the clotting mechanism in the blood, forming a clot (thrombus) that can obstruct the lumen of the artery or break off and migrate to other parts of the body; or the pooling of blood in the arterial wall can expand the wall into the arterial lumen, obstructing the vessel itself. Either event increases the risk of secondary consequences, such as rupture of the artery, acute myocardial infarction, cerebrovascular hemorrhages, renal failure, or paralysis. Arterial dissection is particularly high risk when it involves the aorta, or a coronary, cerebral, or precerebral artery. Dissections occur both as a result of trauma and spontaneously.

I77.81-   Aortic ectasia

Aortic ectasia is a diffuse and irregular dilation of the aorta that is less than 3 cm in diameter. This diagnosis describes aortic vessel dilation in the absence of aneurysm formation.

Diseases of Veins, Lymphatic Vessels and Lymph Nodes, Not Elsewhere Classified (I80-I89)

Lymphatic vessels originate in spaces between cells called lymph capillaries, which are distributed throughout the body (excluding avascular tissue, the central nervous system, splenic pulp, and bone marrow). The vessels contain lymph nodes at various intervals. The lymphatics of the skin converge with the lymphatics of the viscera to form the lymphatic channels (the thoracic duct and the right lymphatic duct). The thoracic duct receives lymph from the left side of the head, neck, and chest; the left upper extremity; and the entire body below the ribs. The right lymphatic duct collects lymph from the right jugular trunk, which drains the right side of the head and neck; from the right subclavian trunk, which drains the right upper extremity; and from the right bronchomediastinal trunk, which drains the right side of the thorax, right lung, right side of the heart, and part of the convex surface of the liver. Skeletal muscle contractions and respiratory movements are factors maintaining lymph flow.

The categories in this code block are as follows:

I80	Phlebitis and thrombophlebitis
I81	Portal vein thrombosis
I82	Other venous embolism and thrombosis
I83	Varicose veins of lower extremities
I85	Esophageal varices
I86	Varicose veins of other sites
I87	Other disorders of veins
I88	Nonspecific lymphadenitis
I89	Other noninfective disorders of lymphatic vessels and lymph nodes

I80.- Phlebitis and thrombophlebitis

Phlebitis is inflammation of a vein. Thrombophlebitis is a partial or complete obstruction of a vein with secondary inflammatory reaction in the wall of the vein. Thrombophlebitis can develop from prolonged sitting, immobility, or bedrest that may be occasioned by long distance traveling, major injuries, paralysis, surgery, or pregnancy. Surgery that involves the legs or pelvis, existing heart or circulation problems, hormone replacement therapy, obesity, age, and certain genetic conditions that make blood clotting more likely than usual increase the risk. Phlebitis and thrombophlebitis of the lower extremities are classified by depth of the vein, which includes superficial and deep veins. Superficial veins include the femoropopliteal and greater and lesser saphenous veins. Deep veins of the lower extremities include the iliac, femoral, popliteal, and tibial veins. Superficial phlebitis and thrombophlebitis codes of the lower extremity identify laterality but do not identify the vein. Deep vein phlebitis and thrombophlebitis codes identify the specific vein and laterality in the lower extremity. A single nonspecific code is available for reporting phlebitis and thrombophlebitis of the upper extremities and other sites.

I80.1- Phlebitis and thrombophlebitis of femoral vein

I80.2- Phlebitis and thrombophlebitis of other and unspecified deep vessels of lower extremities

The formation of a blood clot, or thrombus, in the deep veins of the leg not only impedes blood circulation, but also may become life-threatening if the clot or pieces of the blood clot break loose and travel to the lungs where they lodge in an artery, causing pulmonary embolism. People develop deep vein thrombosis from prolonged sitting, immobility, or bedrest that may be

occasioned by long distance traveling, major injuries, paralysis, surgery, or pregnancy. Surgery that involves the legs or pelvis, existing heart or circulation problems, hormone replacement therapy, obesity, age, and certain genetic conditions that make blood clotting more likely than usual increase the risk. When a thrombus forms, blood flow back to the heart is impeded, causing redness, swelling, and pain in the leg below the clot that may be perceived as aching or tightness.

I81 Portal vein thrombosis

Portal vein thrombosis is inflammation and blood clot in the main vein of the liver, which increases the pressure in the portal vein and causes portal hypertension. It can also cause splenomegaly and esophageal or gastric varices. Portal vein thrombosis is most commonly caused by liver cirrhosis, which slows the flow of blood through the liver making it more likely to clot. It can eventually progress to Budd-Chiari syndrome.

Schematic Showing the Portal Vein

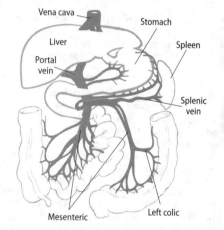

I82.- Other venous embolism and thrombosis

This category identifies Budd-Chiari syndrome, which is a hepatic vein clot, and thrombophlebitis migrans, which is characterized by clots that recur in different locations.

Focus Point

Even though embolisms of veins such as portal, pulmonary, and vena cava are located in the circulatory chapter, some are in other chapters, including mesenteric, which can be found in subcategory K55.0- Acute vascular disorder of the intestine, in Chapter 11 Diseases of the Digestive System.

I82.0   Budd-Chiari syndrome

Budd-Chiari syndrome is caused by a thrombus in the main vein that leaves the liver. It is characterized by hepatomegaly, ascites, jaundice, and abnormal liver function tests. Without treatment, progression to liver failure and death are likely.

I82.4-   Acute embolism and thrombosis of deep veins of lower extremity

This subcategory describes a new current condition in which a blood clot forms in (thrombus) or is transported to (embolus) the deep veins of the legs. A thrombus forms in the deep veins of the legs causing narrowing and blockage of blood flow. An embolism occurs when a thrombus or piece of thrombus breaks away and moves to a vein in another part of the body, becoming lodged within that vessel, and can obstruct blood flow. Acute embolism and thrombosis codes for the deep veins of the lower extremities are specific to site (femoral, iliac, popliteal, tibial, and other specified deep vein of the lower extremity) and laterality (right, left, bilateral).

> **Focus Point**
>
> *A thrombus or embolus within the femoral veins puts the patient at risk for a pulmonary embolism and typically requires hospitalization for monitoring and treatment to prevent the clot from traveling to the lungs.*

I82.5-   Chronic embolism and thrombosis of deep veins of lower extremity

This subcategory describes a long-term condition in which one or more blood clots (thrombus) form in or are transported to (embolus) the deep veins of the legs. A thrombus that forms in the deep veins of the legs causes narrowing and blockage of blood flow. An embolism occurs when a thrombus or piece of thrombus breaks away and moves to a vein in another part of the body, becoming lodged within that vessel, which can obstruct blood flow. Chronic embolism and thrombosis codes for the deep veins of the lower extremities are specific to site (femoral, iliac, popliteal, tibial, and other specified deep vein of the lower extremity) and laterality (right, left, bilateral).

I82.6-   Acute embolism and thrombosis of veins of upper extremity

This subcategory describes a new current condition in which a blood clot forms in (thrombus) or is transported to (embolus) the veins of the arms. A thrombus forms in the superficial or deep veins of the arms causing narrowing and blockage of blood flow. An embolism occurs when a thrombus or piece of thrombus breaks away and moves to a vein in another part of the body, becoming lodged within that vessel, which can obstruct blood flow. Acute embolism and

thrombosis codes for superficial and deep veins of the arms are specific to the depth of the vessel (superficial, deep), but are not specific to site. Laterality (right, left, bilateral) is a component of the code.

I82.7-   Chronic embolism and thrombosis of veins of upper extremity

This subcategory describes a long-term condition in which one or more blood clots (thrombus) form in or are transported to (embolus) the veins of the arms and shoulder regions. A thrombus forms in the veins of the upper extremity causing narrowing and blockage of blood flow. An embolism occurs when a thrombus or piece of thrombus breaks away and moves to a vein in another part of the body, becoming lodged within that vessel, which can obstruct blood flow. Chronic embolism and thrombosis codes for the deep veins of the upper extremities are specific to site (axillary, subclavian, internal jugular, and other specified deep vein of the upper extremity) and laterality (right, left, bilateral). There is also a separate designation for superficial veins of the upper extremity that is not specific to site but does specify laterality.

I83.-   Varicose veins of lower extremities

Varicose veins are dilated, elongated, and tortuous networks in the subcutaneous venous system resulting from valvular incompetence. The condition develops predominantly in the lower extremities. Most commonly, the long saphenous vein and its tributaries are involved, but the short saphenous vein also may be affected. Symptoms include night cramps, localized pain, edema, inflammation, or hemorrhage and a dull aching or fatigue exacerbated by standing in place.

I83.0-   Varicose veins of lower extremities with ulcer

Varicose veins of lower extremities with ulcer result when the long-standing pooling of blood and subsequent tissue pressure due to the varicose veins cause a drop in oxygenation of the surrounding skin and an ulcer develops. Slow to heal, these ulcers are often chronic.

I83.1-   Varicose veins of lower extremities with inflammation

Varicose veins of lower extremities with inflammation is phlebitis that may occur as the result of an injury or spontaneously. It is manifested by redness and tenderness along the path of a superficial vein. The area may be hard, warm, and swollen, with itching and burning pain. The patient may have a low-grade fever as well.

I83.2-   Varicose veins of lower extremities with both ulcer and inflammation

Varicose veins of lower extremities with ulcer and inflammation result when the long-standing pooling of blood and subsequent tissue pressure due to the varicose veins cause a drop in oxygenation of the surrounding skin and an ulcer develops. Slow to heal, these ulcers are often chronic. The ulcer is complicated by inflammation, which is manifested by redness and tenderness along the path of a superficial vein. The area may be hard, warm, and swollen, with itching and burning pain. The patient may have a low-grade fever as well.

I85.-   Esophageal varices

Esophageal varices are distended, enlarged veins that are in the walls of the lower esophagus. This condition can be considered idiopathic or primary or can be considered secondary, if caused by cirrhosis, alcoholic, or other liver disease. A common cause is cirrhosis, where scarring slows the extra blood flow through the liver and redirects the extra blood through the esophageal veins. Combination codes indicate whether bleeding is present.

I86.-   Varicose veins of other sites

Varicose veins are dilated, elongated, and tortuous networks in the venous system resulting from valvular incompetence. This subcategory includes varicose veins of sublingual, scrotal, pelvic, vulval, gastric, and other specified sites.

Focus Point

Hemorrhoids and perianal venous thrombosis are not located in this chapter but can be found in category K64 of Chapter 11 Diseases of the Digestive System.

I87.-   Other disorders of veins

After the capillary exchange of oxygen, nutrients, hormones, and other byproducts takes place, the blood flows through the venules, which become larger veins, and is returned back to the right atrium of the heart via the inferior and superior vena cava. This category identifies disorders of the vessels or valves within the vessels that can disrupt this venous process, such as postthrombotic syndrome, compression of vein, insufficiency, or chronic venous hypertension.

I87.0-   Postthrombotic syndrome

Postthrombotic syndrome occurs as a complication of deep vein thrombosis and is symptomatic of chronic venous deficiency. It is typically caused by venous hypertension due to vein damage or incomplete closure of the venous valves. When blood clots form and grow they attach to venous walls leading to decreased blood flow and permanent damage to the vein itself. Normally valves within the leg veins prevent the reverse flow of blood. However, damage to these valves renders them incompetent and results in the vein not being able to push the blood back to the heart, which causes blood pooling within the legs.

I87.01-   Postthrombotic syndrome with ulcer

One of the complications of postthrombotic syndrome is skin ulcers. Ulcers form when the increased pressure of blood in the affected veins puts pressure directly on the surrounding tissues. This pressure, along with a drop in oxygenation of the surrounding skin, causes an ulcer to develop. Slow to heal, these ulcers are often chronic.

Focus Point

Postthrombotic syndrome with ulcer is not a common complication except in the popliteal vein when there is also valve incompetence.

I87.02-   Postthrombotic syndrome with inflammation

Phlebitis, or inflammation of the vein, is another complication of postthrombotic syndrome.

I87.03-   Postthrombotic syndrome with ulcer and inflammation

Inflammation and ulcer may occur together in postthrombotic syndrome.

I87.1   Compression of vein

Compression of a vein describes conditions where any vein is squeezed together between other structures or tissues causing narrowing or stricture that reduces blood flow. Included in this subcategory is vena cava syndrome, a slow growing condition for which the diagnosis is often not made until significant symptoms exist, which can become life-threatening. It occurs due to compression of the superior or inferior vena cava, the large veins flowing into the heart.

I87.2   Venous insufficiency (chronic) (peripheral)

Venous insufficiency describes conditions where the blood flow back to the heart is deficient in some way, thereby reducing adequate supply and circulation. This condition may appear in superficial veins, deep veins, or perforating veins. Within the veins are valves that direct the blood flow toward the heart. These valves close when muscles relax, as when sitting or lying down, preventing the blood from collecting in the extremities, particularly the legs. This collection of blood causes the venous pressure to rise in these areas. The deep and perforating veins can handle short durations of increased pressure. However, in some people extensive sitting or standing leads to stretching of the vein walls and damage to the valves leading to venous insufficiency.

Without adequate treatment, chronic venous insufficiency can lead to dermal changes in the lower extremities, known as stasis dermatitis. Initially the skin may look scaly and erythematous, and become weepy and/or hyperpigmented. These skin changes can leave the patient vulnerable to bacterial invasion, leading to infection. In severe cases, skin ulcers or a painful condition called lipodermatosclerosis can also develop.

I87.3- Chronic venous hypertension (idiopathic)

Chronic venous hypertension is a condition where high blood pressure is noted within any vein and the underlying cause is unknown. The increase in pressure within the veins suggests an insufficiency in the blood flowing back toward the heart. It may occur due to conditions such as obesity and pregnancy, or as the result of surgery that puts pressure on the venous system (e.g., hip surgery). Chronic venous hypertension can result in the same type of complications seen in postthrombotic syndrome: ulceration and inflammation.

I87.30- Chronic venous hypertension (idiopathic) without complications

Chronic venous hypertension without complications may still be treated with compression stockings, elevating the legs, and paying close attention to skin care of the legs.

I87.31- Chronic venous hypertension (idiopathic) with ulcer

Chronic venous hypertension with ulcer occurs when the tissues fail to receive an adequate amount of oxygen and nutrients. The ulcers may be very slow to heal and may be chronic.

I87.32- Chronic venous hypertension (idiopathic) with inflammation

Chronic venous hypertension with redness and tenderness along the path of a superficial vein is an indication of inflammation of the vein.

I87.33- Chronic venous hypertension (idiopathic) with ulcer and inflammation

Ulcer and inflammation can complicate chronic venous hypertension.

I87.8 Other specified disorders of veins

Other forms of circulation disorders may include hardening of the vein walls or collateral circulation where the communication between affected blood vessels develops a new path due to obstruction of the intended path of blood flow.

I88.- Nonspecific lymphadenitis

Lymphadenitis refers to an enlargement or inflammation of lymph nodes whose primary function is to act as a filter for abnormal cells that are in the lymph fluid. It is often a benign response that serves as a sign of a localized or systematic infection.

I88.0 Nonspecific mesenteric lymphadenitis

Mesenteric lymphadenitis is persistent inflammation of one or more lymph nodes in the peritoneal fold that encases the abdominal organs, also referred to as Brennemann's syndrome.

I88.1 Chronic lymphadenitis, except mesenteric

Chronic lymphadenitis is characterized by prolonged inflammation of the lymph nodes. Lymphadenitis may be generalized or restricted to regional lymph nodes.

I89.- Other noninfective disorders of lymphatic vessels and lymph nodes

This category represents other disorders of a noninfective nature that are identified by inflammation or enlargement of lymph nodes, such as lymphedema and lymphangitis.

I89.0 Lymphedema, not elsewhere classified

This code includes some forms of elephantiasis, which is a condition caused by obstruction of the lymphatic system that in turn creates a buildup of lymph fluid resulting in abnormal enlargement of the affected body area. Some of the types of elephantiasis included here are telangiectodes, streptococcal, glandular, and scrotal.

> **Focus Point**
>
> *Some forms of elephantiasis are caused by parasitic, thread-like roundworms that occupy the lymphatic system. These codes are located in category B74 in Chapter 1 Certain Infectious and Parasitic Diseases.*

Other and Unspecified Disorders of the Circulatory System (I95-I99)

This block of codes represents conditions such as various types of hypotension and gangrene. Additionally, intraoperative and postprocedural complications are located in this block.

The categories in this code block are as follows:

I95	Hypotension
I96	Gangrene, not elsewhere classified
I97	Intraoperative and postprocedural complications and disorders of circulatory system, not elsewhere classified
I99	Other and unspecified disorders of circulatory system

I95.-   Hypotension

Hypotension is low blood pressure, which is essentially the pressure within the arteries as the heart pumps blood. This measurement is recorded when the heart beats to pump the blood (systolic) and when the heart is resting between beats (diastolic). Adults typically have a normal blood pressure reading of less than 120/ 80 mm Hg (systolic/diastolic millimeters of mercury). A patient diagnosed with hypotension has a blood pressure reading of 90/60 or lower. The body has a natural balance with blood pressure in that when a rise or drop in pressure occurs it signals cells within the arteries to assist in stabilizing the blood pressure. In these conditions, the body cannot adequately keep up with the regulation or cannot find the balance fast enough. Some people may have a blood pressure that is below normal on a regular basis without displaying any symptoms of this condition. Medical treatment is sought when dizziness or fainting occurs.

I95.1   Orthostatic hypotension

Orthostatic hypotension is low blood pressure due to positional changes, as when sitting or lying down and then standing up. Oftentimes, this may make a patient light-headed. This type of hypotension, also called "postural hypotension," is a common type of low blood pressure.

I95.2   Hypotension due to drugs

Also referred to as iatrogenic hypotension, hypotension due to drugs is abnormally low blood pressure due to an adverse effect of medication.

I95.3   Hypotension of hemodialysis

Hypotension of hemodialysis is a fairly common complication for patients undergoing hemodialysis. It may be due to underlying conditions and fluid shifts that occur during the procedure.

I97.-   Intraoperative and postprocedural complications and disorders of circulatory system, not elsewhere classified

This category includes complications of procedures of the circulatory system such as hemorrhage and hematomas, accidental puncture or lacerations, and postprocedural cardiac dysfunctions such as heart failure, cardiac arrest, or insufficiency. Codes for intraoperative and postprocedural cerebrovascular infarction (stroke/CVA) are also located in this category.

I97.2   Postmastectomy lymphedema syndrome

Postmastectomy syndrome is a form of lymphedema due to excision of the axillary lymphatic structures during mastectomy. Edema in arms and hands develops from pooling of interstitial fluids, due to reduced lymphatic circulation.

Chapter 10: Diseases of the Respiratory System (JØØ-J99)

This chapter classifies diseases and disorders of the two main parts of the respiratory system: the upper respiratory tract and the lower respiratory tract. The upper respiratory tract contains the nose (external, nasal cavity), sinuses (frontal, ethmoid, sphenoid, maxillary), pharynx (nasopharynx, oropharynx), larynx (true and false vocal cords, glottis), and trachea. The lower respiratory tract contains the bronchi (left, right, main, carina), and lungs (intrapulmonary bronchi, bronchioli, lobes, alveoli, pleura).

This complex of organs is responsible for pulmonary ventilation and the exchange of oxygen and carbon dioxide between the lungs and ambient air. The organs of the respiratory system also perform nonrespiratory functions such as warming and moisturizing the air passing into the lungs, providing airflow for the larynx and vocal cords for speech, and releasing excess body heat in the process of thermoregulation for homeostasis. The lungs also perform important metabolic and embolic filtering functions by excreting gaseous wastes. Air moves into the lungs and bronchial tubes, reaching the alveoli. Running by these alveoli are capillaries carrying blood that has traveled through the body and been pumped from the right side of the heart through the pulmonary artery and then into capillaries. The alveoli transport the oxygen to the capillaries where hemoglobin helps the oxygen flow into the bloodstream. As the oxygen is absorbed, the carbon dioxide is extracted from the capillaries into the alveoli and is exhaled as a waste gas. The oxygenated blood then travels through the pulmonary vein to the left side of the heart, which pumps it to the rest of the body. Any malfunction in this process leads to cell death within the tissues of the various organs of the body due to the reduced amount of oxygen distributed to these organs and it may cause excess waste to accumulate within the body's tissues.

An instructional note at the beginning of this chapter directs that if a respiratory condition exists in more than one site and does not have its own specific, separate entry in the Alphabetic Index it should be classified to the lower anatomical site.

Since inhaled tobacco smoke travels from the mouth through the upper airway, reaching the alveoli, tobacco use has proven implications on the entire respiratory system, prompting directions indicating that a code for tobacco exposure, use, or dependence be added if applicable.

The chapter is broken down into the following code blocks:

JØØ-JØ6   Acute upper respiratory infections

JØ9-J18   Influenza and pneumonia

J2Ø-J22   Other acute lower respiratory infections

J3Ø-J39   Other diseases of upper respiratory tract

J4Ø-J47   Chronic lower respiratory diseases

J6Ø-J7Ø   Lung diseases due to external agents

J8Ø-J84   Other respiratory diseases principally affecting the interstitium

J85-J86   Suppurative and necrotic conditions of the lower respiratory tract

J9Ø-J94   Other diseases of the pleura

J95   Intraoperative and postprocedural complications and disorders of respiratory system, not elsewhere classified

J96-J99   Other diseases of the respiratory system

Acute Upper Respiratory Infections (JØØ-JØ6)

Infections of the upper respiratory system are those that affect the nose or nares, nasal cavity, nasopharynx, sinuses, oropharynx, hypopharynx, larynx, trachea, and epiglottis. Acute infections are generally sudden in onset with immediately recognizable signs and symptoms, such as fever, chills, and body aches.

The categories in this code block are as follows:

JØØ   Acute nasopharyngitis (common cold)

JØ1   Acute sinusitis

JØ2   Acute pharyngitis

JØ3   Acute tonsillitis

JØ4   Acute laryngitis and tracheitis

JØ5   Acute obstructive laryngitis [croup] and epiglottitis

JØ6   Acute upper respiratory infections of multiple and unspecified sites

Focus Point

Pneumonia and influenza are excluded from this code block and can be found in the next block JØ9-J18.

J00   Acute nasopharyngitis [common cold]

This code classifies nasopharyngitis, rhinitis, coryza, or nasal catarrh of an acute nature. Acute nasopharyngitis is the most common of the upper respiratory infections and is characterized by edema of the nasal mucous membrane, discharge, and obstruction.

J01.-   Acute sinusitis

Acute sinusitis is a sudden and severe inflammation or infection of the paranasal sinuses. The paranasal sinuses are air spaces adjacent to the nose that open into the nasal passages for the exchange of air and mucus. Anything that triggers a swelling in the nose, such as an infection or an allergic reaction, can affect the sinuses. When a virus causes inflammation in the mucous membranes of the nose and sinuses, bacteria and secretions including pus can get trapped in the sinuses. The bacteria then multiply causing acute sinusitis. Most sinus infections are caused by *Streptococcus*, *Pneumococcus*, *Haemophilus influenza*, and *Staphylococcus*. In the case of immuno-compromised patients, the infectious agents are more likely to be due to aspergillosis, candidiasis, or fungal infections of the order Mucorales. Sinusitis is classified according to the site of infection. The maxillary sinuses are located behind each cheekbone. The frontal sinuses are located above the eyes. The ethmoidal sinuses are located between the eyes on either side of the nose, behind the bridge of the nose. The sphenoidal sinuses are located behind the eyes, on either side of the upper nose. Pansinusitis is an infection involving all the paranasal sinuses on one or both sides. The code for other site is used for a sinus infection involving more than one sinus, but is not pansinusitis. Acute sinusitis is also classified by whether or not the acute condition is recurrent. If the condition is not recurrent it is reported with the unspecified code. Included in the definition of acute sinusitis are abscess, empyema, and suppuration. Acute sinusitis is usually preceded by an acute respiratory infection.

Focus Point

A second code from Chapter 1 Certain Infectious and Parasitic Diseases (B95-B97) can be reported to identify the infectious agent.

J02.-   Acute pharyngitis

Pharyngitis is the medical term for sore throat. Acute pharyngitis is an acute inflammatory disorder of the posterior pharynx, which may be caused by a virus or bacteria. Frequently, coryza or other communicable disease precedes acute pharyngitis. The majority of sore throats are caused by viruses, however they are occasionally caused by bacterial infections including *Streptococcus*, *Mycoplasma pneumoniae*, and *Chlamydia pneumoniae*.

J02.0   Streptococcal pharyngitis

Streptococcal pharyngitis, more commonly referred to as strep throat, is a contagious, bacterial infection caused by Group A *Streptococcus*, also called *Streptococcus pyogenes*. It is most common in ages 5 through 15, although it can affect individuals of any age and occurs most often from late fall through early spring. Strep throat is a common bacterial infection. It presents with a red sore throat that may have white or yellow spots, fever, and swollen lymph glands in the neck. The infection responds readily to antibiotics, although it usually goes away in three to seven days with or without treatment. Antibiotics may only shorten the infection by one day, but physicians usually choose to treat patients because the contagious period is shortened. Antibiotic treatment also lowers the risk of developing other complications. Strep throat can be transmitted when the infected person breathes, sneezes, or coughs, since strep bacteria is an airborne illness. After being exposed to strep, it may take two to five days to develop symptoms.

Focus Point

Untreated streptococcal pharyngitis can cause complications such as rheumatic fever and kidney inflammation.

J03.-   Acute tonsillitis

The palatine tonsils are masses of lymphatic tissue found on both sides of the back of the throat, above and behind the tongue. They are responsible for protecting the body against infection. When bacteria and viruses attempt to infect the body through the nose or mouth, the tonsils serve as a filter and surround the organisms in white blood cells. This can cause a low-grade infection in the tonsils. Occasionally, infections are too much for the tonsils to control and the tonsils become infected themselves, a condition called tonsillitis. The infection may also be present in surrounding areas, causing inflammation of the throat and pharynx as well. Acute tonsillitis is a sudden, severe inflammation of the palatine tonsils with the infective agent most commonly streptococcal or viral. Tonsillitis may be accompanied by throat pain, high fever, and, in some cases, vomiting. The codes in this section are classified by whether the acute tonsillitis is recurrent and by whether the infectious organism is *Streptococcus*, another specified organism, or whether the organism is unspecified. Acute streptococcal tonsillitis occurs as a sudden onset infection and inflammation. It is caused by Group A *Streptococcus*, also called *Streptococcus pyogenes*, and can occur as a single isolated episode or repeatedly as a recurrent infection. It is treated with and usually responds readily to antibiotics. For recurrent infections, surgical removal is indicated if the patient has had three or more tonsil or adenoid infections per year for three years in a row, or if the infection does not respond to beta-lactamase-resistant antibiotics.

J04.- Acute laryngitis and tracheitis

Sudden and severe inflammation of the larynx (voice box) or trachea associated with infection is classified to this category. Laryngitis and tracheitis usually follow an upper respiratory infection, but may occur during the course of pneumonia, bronchitis, flu, or measles. The condition is classified by site.

J04.0 Acute laryngitis

This site involves the vocal cords and voice box.

J04.1- Acute tracheitis

This site involves the trachea and is further differentiated by whether or not the inflammation of the trachea is complicated by obstruction. Obstruction occurs when the inflammation becomes so severe that it impedes breathing. Symptoms of obstruction include difficulty breathing, swallowing, or talking.

J04.2 Acute laryngotracheitis

This site involves the vocal cords, voice box, and trachea.

J04.3- Supraglottitis, unspecified

This is a nonspecific code for inflammation involving the region above the epiglottis. The epiglottis is the flap of tissue in the upper aspect of the trachea. Supraglottitis can occur with or without obstruction. Obstruction occurs when the inflammation becomes so severe that it impedes breathing. Symptoms of obstruction include difficulty breathing, swallowing, or talking.

J05.- Acute obstructive laryngitis [croup] and epiglottitis

Acute obstructive laryngitis, also called croup, is an infection of the upper airways that is typically seen in early childhood and involves the larynx (vocal cords), trachea (windpipe), and bronchial tubes. Acute epiglottitis is an inflammation of the epiglottis, a flap of tissue in the upper aspect of the trachea that is covered by a mucous membrane.

J05.0 Acute obstructive laryngitis [croup]

Croup is an infection of the upper airways that is typically seen in early childhood and involves the larynx (vocal cords), trachea (windpipe), and bronchial tubes. It is characterized by inflammation that obstructs breathing causing a high-pitched wheezing

sound (stridor) on respiration and barking cough. Parainfluenza virus is usually the infective agent, although respiratory syncytial virus can also cause croup.

J05.1- Acute epiglottitis

Acute epiglottitis is an inflammation of the epiglottis and surrounding soft tissues usually due to an infection by *Hemophilus influenzae, Pneumococcus,* or Group A *Streptococcus.* The inflammation can occur with or without obstruction of the larynx. Acute epiglottitis with obstruction is a rare but potentially life-threatening condition. Signs and symptoms of acute epiglottitis include high fever, sore throat, dysphagia, stridor, and respiratory distress.

Influenza and Pneumonia (J09-J18)

Pneumonia and influenza are inflammations in the alveolar parenchyma of the lung caused by microbial infection. Pneumonia is a serious infection/inflammation of one or both of the lungs in which the alveoli (air sacs) fill with pus or liquid rather than oxygen making it difficult to breath and difficult for oxygen to pass into the bloodstream. Pneumonia is caused by a wide variety of pathogens including viral, bacterial, fungal, protozoal, mycobacterial, mycoplasmal, or rickettsial microorganisms. Influenza is an acute respiratory infection caused by orthomyxoviruses and is characterized by the abrupt onset, chills, fever, dry cough, muscle aches, and headache. Influenza may be complicated by secondary bacterial infection. Influenza is generally transmitted person-to-person by direct contact and airborne droplets. It commonly occurs in epidemics, which develop and spread rapidly. Human influenza is categorized into three main types: A, B, and C. Influenza A viruses are further classified by subtype, according to the presence of glycoproteins hemagglutinin (HA) or neuraminidase (NA). Influenza virus type A is the most common and causes epidemics of varying severity. Influenza virus type B is associated with more limited epidemics and has been linked to Reye's syndrome. Influenza virus type C is an uncommon strain that causes very mild upper respiratory symptoms.

The categories in this code block are as follows:

J09	Influenza due to certain identified influenza viruses
J10	Influenza due to other identified influenza virus
J11	Influenza due to unidentified influenza virus
J12	Viral pneumonia, not elsewhere classified

J13	Pneumonia due to Streptococcus pneumoniae
J14	Pneumonia due to hemophilus influenzae
J15	Bacterial pneumonia, not elsewhere classified
J16	Pneumonia due to other infectious organisms, not elsewhere classified
J17	Pneumonia in diseases classified elsewhere
J18	Pneumonia, unspecified organism

Focus Point

One difference between pneumonia and influenza can be identified through the cough. A cough associated with pneumonia is productive and produces yellow, green, or brown sputum while a cough due to influenza is generally dry or is accompanied by thin, clear, or white sputum.

J09.- Influenza due to certain identified influenza viruses

Codes in this category describe only novel influenza A viruses. Novel influenza A viruses are those described as avian or bird influenza, swine influenza, or influenza of other animal origin. This type of influenza is also sometimes described using a designation such as H5N1. All flu viruses are named and identified using two surface proteins: hemagglutinin (H) and neuraminidase (N). Each time a new virus is identified it is given a new designation using the letter H followed by a number and the letter N followed by a number. Flu viruses that begin with H5 or H7 are avian (bird) flu viruses and are included in this category.

Focus Point

Codes in this category represent specific forms of influenza and should only be assigned if the specific infectious agent (e.g., Novel influenza A virus) is documented as confirmed. The specific codes in category J09 should not be assigned if the corresponding documentation contains terminology such as "possible," "suspected," or "probable." In these instances, assign the appropriate code for the presenting symptoms.

J09.X- Influenza due to identified novel influenza A virus

Influenza A causes significant morbidity and mortality worldwide. Novel influenza A includes all human infections with influenza A viruses that are different from currently circulating human influenza viruses. These include viruses subtyped as nonhuman in origin and those that are unsubtypable with standard laboratory methods. New forms can spread widely due to the lack of existing immunity in exposed populations. The novel H1N1, also known as swine flu, is notable for a 2009 pandemic and has since been a

seasonal human flu with an uptick of occurrence again in 2014. The novel H1N1 or swine flu virus is known to circulate in pigs, but it is not caused by ingesting improperly cooked pork and products. Novel influenza A is transmitted similarly to seasonal influenza by contact with airborne or surface respiratory secretions of infected persons. General symptoms mimic those of other influenza infection, including fever, body aches, chills, and fatigue. Respiratory symptoms include cough and sore throat. Respiratory novel influenza A infection may manifest as pneumonia (including bronchopneumonia), laryngitis, pharyngitis, or acute upper respiratory infection. Gastrointestinal symptoms may include diarrhea and nausea and vomiting. Avian influenza, (H5N1) an infection caused by bird influenza viruses, can occur in humans even though the virus is predominantly found in birds. These viruses do not typically infect humans and there is no evidence that it can be spread by person-to-person contact. The approximately 650 cases reported worldwide from 2003 to 2014 mostly resulted from contact with infected domesticated chickens, ducks, or turkeys, or from surfaces contaminated with secretions or excretions from these infected birds. Codes in this category are further broken down into subcategories that contain combination codes describing manifestations and complications of the novel influenza A virus infection.

J09.X1 Influenza due to identified novel influenza A virus with pneumonia

This code is used only for identified novel influenza A virus in combination with any type of pneumonia.

J09.X2 Influenza due to identified novel influenza A virus with other respiratory manifestations

This code is used to specify respiratory conditions such as laryngitis, pharyngitis, sinusitis, pleural effusion, or other respiratory manifestations.

J09.X3 Influenza due to identified novel influenza A virus with gastrointestinal manifestations

This code is only for gastroenteritis that is specified as "due to" novel influenza A virus. Other viral gastroenteritis is located in Chapter 1 Certain Infectious and Parasitic Diseases.

J09.X9 Influenza due to identified novel influenza A virus with other manifestations

This subcategory includes manifestations that may occur due to identified novel influenza A virus such as encephalopathy, myocarditis, otitis media, or other manifestations. An additional code is needed to identify the specific manifestation.

J10.- Influenza due to other identified influenza virus

Influenza is an acute respiratory infection due to orthomyxoviruses characterized by abrupt onset, chills, fever, dry cough, muscle aches, and headache and may be followed by a secondary bacterial infection. This category represents other identified influenza viruses such as Influenza B or C. Influenza B is less common than A but can cause seasonal flu outbreaks and generally only in humans. Influenza B spreads slower than influenza A but faster than influenza C. Influenza C is different from A and B as it presents with mild or no respiratory symptoms and rarely causes epidemics.

J10.0- Influenza due to other identified influenza virus with pneumonia

This subcategory is used only for other identified influenza viruses such as B and C, in combination with any type of pneumonia. The fifth character represents whether the type of pneumonia is unspecified type, the same as the identified influenza virus, or another type of pneumonia.

J10.1 Influenza due to other identified influenza virus with other respiratory manifestations

This code is used to specify respiratory conditions such as laryngitis, pharyngitis, sinusitis, pleural effusion, or other respiratory manifestations that occur due to the other identified influenza such as B or C.

J10.2 Influenza due to other identified influenza virus with gastrointestinal manifestations

This code is only for gastroenteritis or stomach flu that is specified as "due to" an identified influenza virus such as B or C influenza virus.

J10.8- Influenza due to other identified influenza virus with other manifestations

This subcategory includes combination codes with the fifth character representing manifestations that may occur due to identified influenza viruses such as B or C, and includes encephalopathy, myocarditis, otitis media, or other manifestations such as Reye's syndrome.

J12.- Viral pneumonia, not elsewhere classified

Pneumonia is a serious infection/inflammation of one or both of the lungs in which the alveoli (air sacs) fill with pus or liquid rather than oxygen making it difficult to breath and difficult for oxygen to pass into the bloodstream. In pneumonia, chest x-rays show infiltration or consolidation. Viral pneumonias tend to develop more gradually and with initially milder symptoms than bacterial pneumonia, but both can vary in severity. Viral pneumonias occur most commonly in younger children, older adults, or those with a weakened immune system. If treated, antivirals are used for viral pneumonias as antibiotics are not effective against viral infections. Depending on which virus is involved, the symptoms, severity, and treatment can vary.

Focus Point

Check the Alphabetic Index closely to determine the appropriate code assignment for pneumonia. Codes for pneumonia are found in various chapters and categories depending on etiology. For example, Candida pneumonia is found in Chapter 1 Infectious and Parasitic Diseases, pneumonia occurring in newborns is found in Chapter 16 Certain Conditions Originating in the Perinatal Period, and interstitial and aspiration pneumonia not due to virus, are both located later in this chapter.

J12.0 Adenoviral pneumonia

Adenovirus is classified as medium sized adenoidal-pharyngeal-conjunctival virus, causing upper respiratory infections and viral pneumonia. Of the 50 or more identified serotypes causing respiratory infections in humans, only six are commonly associated with pneumonia. While adenoviruses are a rare cause of pneumonia in adults, they are responsible for approximately 20 percent of all childhood pneumonias and occur most often in children younger than 5 years of age.

J12.1 Respiratory syncytial virus pneumonia

Respiratory syncytial virus (RSV) is a common cause of mild respiratory disease in adults but can be a serious source of pneumonia in young children. RSV most often occurs seasonally, usually from late fall to early spring. Infants are most vulnerable to the disease.

J12.2 Parainfluenza virus pneumonia

There are several types of human parainfluenza virus (HPIV) that cause pneumonia, although generally it is HPIV1, which occurs during the fall, and HPIV3, which occurs year round but peaks in spring.

J12.3 Human metapneumovirus pneumonia

Although it has likely been around much longer, human metapneumovirus (hMPV) was first recognized in 2001 and most often affects young children or older adults. It is spread easily and occurs most commonly in the U.S. in late winter and early spring. It ranks second, behind RSV, as the most common cause of lower respiratory infections in children. Symptoms of pneumonia include severe cough, difficulty breathing, rapid respiratory rate, and wheezing.

J12.8- Other viral pneumonia

This category contains a specific code for SARS-associated corona virus and a second code for other viral pneumonia not classified elsewhere.

J12.81 Pneumonia due to SARS-associated coronavirus

Severe acute respiratory syndrome (SARS) is a severe form of viral pneumonia associated with the coronavirus first identified in a 2003 outbreak. Symptoms include fever, dry cough, dyspnea, headache, hypoxemia, lymphopenia, with possible respiratory failure and alveolar damage.

Focus Point

A notice on the CDC Website states that no known cases of SARS have been reported anywhere in the world since 2004.

J13 Pneumonia due to Streptococcus pneumoniae

Streptococcus pneumoniae, also called pneumococcal pneumonia, is a bacterial pneumonia caused by a gram positive coccus and is the leading cause of pneumonia in all ages. It is commonly found in the nose and throat and can be carried by people who do not exhibit symptoms of illness. Those who do become ill are mostly young children or older adults. *S. pneumoniae* goes through four stages of progression as a result of the body's inflammatory response. First, a serous fluid builds up in the alveoli and then spreads the organism throughout the lungs. The neutrophils and red blood cells invade the alveoli crowding out the bacteria. Finally, macrophages destroy the residue. This response causes fluid build-up in the lungs and if untreated may cause bacteremia of the blood.

J14 Pneumonia due to Hemophilus influenzae

Hemophilus influenzae is a small (1 μm X 0.3 μm), pleomorphic, gram-negative coccobacillus that can lead to infections within the respiratory tract including pneumonia. There are six identified types of *Hemophilus influenzae*, which are designated with the letters a through f. The one that is most often discussed is *Hemophilus influenzae* Type b (Hib). These bacteria are spread through sneezing, coughing, and touching.

Focus Point

It is important to note that children are immunized against type B (Hib) to prevent serious and even deadly infections, such as pneumonia. There are no vaccines for other types.

J15.- Bacterial pneumonia, not elsewhere classified

Bacterial pneumonia is an infection in one or both lungs causing the alveoli to fill with pus, fluid, and cell debris. It interferes with the gas exchange of oxygen and carbon dioxide in the lungs and causes dyspnea. The infection can be community or health care acquired with infection spread through airborne droplets or skin-to-skin contact. This category includes types of bacterial bronchopneumonia other than *S. pneumoniae* or *H. influenzae*.

Focus Point

Symptoms for bacterial and viral pneumonia are similar although symptoms for bacterial tend to occur more quickly while viral are often not as obvious and slower to progress.

J15.0 Pneumonia due to Klebsiella pneumoniae

Klebsiella pneumoniae is not a common cause of pneumonia in the healthy individual. Lung infections due to *K. pneumoniae* typically occur only in individuals with other debilitating disease processes and in older alcoholics. The bacterium is spread by person-to-person contact or direct contact with contaminated surfaces. It is not spread through the air. In the hospital setting, the presence of invasive devices increases risk of development. Presenting symptoms include acute fever, chills, and hemoptysis that can lead to cavitating lesions, lung abscess, and empyema.

Focus Point

K. pneumoniae is showing increasing resistance to antibiotics, particularly the carbapenem class. Use an additional code from category Z16 to identify any documented resistance to antibiotics.

J15.1 Pneumonia due to Pseudomonas

Pseudomonas pneumonia is caused by a common gram-negative bacterium called *Pseudomonas aeruginosa*, which is a common cause of hospital acquired pneumonia often through ventilator tubing or bronchoscopes. The incidence of infection is higher in immunocompromised individuals and those with chronic disease in hospital and community settings. Those at higher risk for bacterial pneumonia are infants, children or adults older than 65, those with impaired immunity, chronic diseases, smokers, or those taking immunosuppressant drugs.

J15.21- Pneumonia due to staphylococcus aureus

Staphylococcus aureus is a bacterium that causes a wide spectrum of infectious diseases including pneumonia. In recent years, some *S. aureus* strains have become resistant to a number of antibiotics. Pneumonia due to *S. aureus* typically occurs in the hospital setting, but is also a rare cause of community acquired pneumonia. *S. aureus* pneumonia is classified based on susceptibility or resistance to beta lactam antibiotics.

J15.211 Pneumonia due to Methicillin susceptible Staphylococcus aureus

The term methicillin-susceptible *Staphylococcus aureus* (MSSA) identifies strains of *S. aureus* that are susceptible or treatable with the traditional beta lactam class of antibiotics such as penicillin, methicillin, and cephalosporins. MSSA causes a number of infectious conditions including pneumonia.

J15.212 Pneumonia due to Methicillin resistant Staphylococcus aureus

Methicillin-resistant *S. aureus* (MRSA) is a variant form of the bacterium that is resistant to the traditional beta lactam class of antibiotics such as penicillin, methicillin, and cephalosporins. Sometimes referred to as a "superbug," MRSA is a major cause of hospital-acquired infections, as well as community-acquired infections. Community acquired MRSA infections (CA-MRSA) are generally not life-threatening. Due to clinical challenges, MRSA is more difficult and costly to combat than MSSA, and generally poses a greater public health threat due to its multidrug resistance.

J15.5 Pneumonia due to Escherichia coli

Escherichia coli (E. coli) are a large and diverse group of bacteria that range from relatively harmless to those that cause serious, life-threatening infections. *E. coli* is a rare cause of pneumonia in otherwise healthy individuals. It can be found as a hospital acquired condition but when it is community acquired, it mainly affects the immunocompromised or those with chronic diseases. This type of pneumonia usually presents as a lower lobe pneumonia and can be complicated by empyema.

Focus Point

E. coli pneumonia is commonly associated with an E. coli urinary tract infection that has spread to the bloodstream and then to the lungs.

J15.7 Pneumonia due to Mycoplasma pneumoniae

Mycoplasma bacteria are the smallest free-living (nonparasitic) organisms. This genus of bacteria is also unique in that it lacks a cell wall, a characteristic that makes it resistant to many antimicrobial medications. *Mycoplasma pneumoniae* infects mucosal surfaces of the bronchi and lungs. It is a common cause of community acquired pneumonia as it is easily spread from person-to-person. It typically is a mild form of pneumonia and is often referred to as atypical or walking pneumonia. The condition is characterized by a nine- to 12-day incubation period in most instances, and typically results in symptoms of an upper respiratory infection, dry cough, and fever.

J18.- Pneumonia, unspecified organism

In some instances it is not possible to identify the pathogenic organism that has caused the pneumonia. Even when the casual organism is not known, the site of the infection may be more specifically identified as occurring in the bronchus and lungs or in the lobes.

J18.Ø Bronchopneumonia, unspecified organism

This code identifies bronchopneumonia that affects both lungs and bronchi without specification of the causal organism.

J18.1 Lobar pneumonia, unspecified organism

This code specifies lobar pneumonia that affects one or more sections or lobes of the lungs without specification of causal organism.

J18.2 Hypostatic pneumonia, unspecified organism

Hypostatic pneumonia, unspecified organism, is specifically associated with a lack of movement over a long period of time. Fluids settle in the patient's lungs, causing the pneumonia. This condition often affects elderly, debilitated, or bedridden people. There may be an organism that is causing the pneumonia, but this particular code does not require that the organism be specifically identified.

Other Acute Lower Respiratory Infections (J2Ø-J22)

This category includes inflammations and infections of the bronchi and bronchioli that have a sudden onset.

The categories in this code block are as follows:

J2Ø	Acute bronchitis
J21	Acute bronchiolitis
J22	Unspecified acute lower respiratory infection

J2Ø.- Acute bronchitis

Acute bronchitis is a sudden and severe inflammation of the main air passageways in the lungs (bronchi), causing production of large quantities of mucus that obstruct the airways and make it hard to breathe. Even bronchitis that lasts up to 9Ø days is normally still considered acute. Bronchitis occurs most often during the winter and is caused more frequently by viruses than bacteria. Acute bronchitis may have an infectious or irritative etiology; however, only bronchitis due to infectious organisms is classified here.

J20.0 Acute bronchitis due to Mycoplasma pneumoniae

Mycoplasma bacteria are the smallest free-living (nonparasitic) organisms. This genus of bacteria is also unique in that it lacks a cell wall, a characteristic that makes it resistant to many antimicrobial medications. *Mycoplasma pneumoniae* infects mucosal surfaces of the bronchi and lungs. It is a common cause of community acquired infections as it is easily spread from person-to-person. In this case, the infection is limited to the bronchi.

J20.1 Acute bronchitis due to Hemophilus influenzae

Hemophilus influenzae is a small (1 μm X 0.3 μm), pleomorphic, gram-negative coccobacillus that can lead to infections within the respiratory tract. The bacteria are spread through sneezing, coughing, and touching. There are six identified types of *H. influenzae*, which are designated with the letters a through f. The one that is most often discussed is *H. influenzae* Type b (Hib).

J20.2 Acute bronchitis due to streptococcus

Streptococcus, the gram negative bacteria commonly linked with strep throat, can also cause acute bronchitis, which is usually in the form of an exacerbation of a chronic bronchitis.

J20.3 Acute bronchitis due to coxsackievirus

Coxsackievirus is an enterovirus that appears in the human digestive tract and is spread by unwashed hands and contaminated surfaces. It is characterized by cough, fever, and tachypnea. Due to the fecal-oral route of transmission, this virus tends to spread amongst children quickly, especially during warm weather months.

J20.4 Acute bronchitis due to parainfluenza virus

Parainfluenza virus is one of many viruses leading to respiratory infections, most often mild in older children and adults since they have been exposed and the body has built up immunity to the virus. However, infants and people with weakened immune systems experience more severe symptoms.

J20.5 Acute bronchitis due to respiratory syncytial virus

Respiratory syncytial virus, commonly known as RSV, is a large contributor to respiratory infections among children. RSV is highly contagious and is spread through contaminated surfaces and coughing, sneezing, and touching.

Focus Point

RSV causes bronchiolitis more often than bronchitis. To report RSV bronchiolitis, use code J21.0.

J20.6 Acute bronchitis due to rhinovirus

Rhinovirus is one of 200 viruses that contribute to the common cold, but it can also cause inflammation of the bronchi. It can survive about three hours on the skin and other surfaces. There is no treatment for the virus, only management of the symptoms until the virus has run its course.

J20.7 Acute bronchitis due to echovirus

One of the viruses that can cause bronchitis, echovirus, or enteric cytopathic human orphan virus, can cause gastrointestinal, skin, and respiratory infections spread by contaminated feces or particles in the air from infected people. This type of infection is common and is often mild, although in one of five cases the infection leads to viral meningitis. This type of infection often resolves itself; however, in more severe cases, immune system therapy may help people with weak immune systems.

J21.- Acute bronchiolitis

Bronchiolitis is a similar condition to bronchitis, a sudden and severe inflammation and infection, but affecting the small airways called bronchioles within the lung. As a result of the infection and inflammation, mucus accumulates in these airways and makes it difficult for air to flow freely through the lungs. Bronchiolitis is usually preceded by an upper respiratory infection. Symptoms of bronchiolitis include coughing and wheezing, which may progress to difficulty breathing. Bronchiolitis is a common manifestation of lower respiratory viral infection in young children and infants.

J21.0 Acute bronchiolitis due to respiratory syncytial virus

Respiratory syncytial virus, commonly known as RSV, is a common cause of bronchiolitis in children. Bronchiolitis affects the small airways that lead to the lungs causing inflammation, congestion, and difficulty breathing. RSV is highly contagious and is spread through contaminated surfaces and coughing, sneezing, and touching.

J21.1 Acute bronchiolitis due to human metapneumovirus

Human metapneumovirus (hMPV) was discovered in 2001 but has no doubt been contributing to respiratory infections for more than 50 years. While most people experience mild symptoms, hMPV is a common cause of bronchiolitis in infants. Bronchiolitis and other more severe respiratory manifestations have been reported in people younger than age 1 and within the elderly population and those with weak immune systems. Infection often occurs three to five days after exposure by close contact with an infected person or surface containing the virus. Transplant patients are among those at highest risk for hMPV infection.

Other Diseases of Upper Respiratory Tract (J30-J39)

Other diseases of the upper respiratory tract include conditions other than those described as acute that affect the nose, sinuses, tonsils, adenoids, larynx, vocal cords, or the surrounding soft tissues.

The categories in this code block are as follows:

J30	Vasomotor and allergic rhinitis
J31	Chronic rhinitis, nasopharyngitis and pharyngitis
J32	Chronic sinusitis
J33	Nasal polyp
J34	Other and unspecified disorders of nose and nasal sinuses
J35	Chronic diseases of the tonsils and adenoids
J36	Peritonsillar abscess
J37	Chronic laryngitis and laryngotracheitis
J38	Diseases of the vocal cords and larynx, not elsewhere classified
J39	Other diseases of upper respiratory tract

J30.- Vasomotor and allergic rhinitis

Rhinitis is an inflammation of the mucous membranes of the nasal passages. Allergic rhinitis is caused by an allergic reaction to airborne substances such as pollen or less commonly due to an allergic reaction to food. There are two types of allergic rhinitis: seasonal and perennial. Allergic rhinitis due to pollen is a type of seasonal rhinitis while that due to dust mites or animal hair or dander are perennial types. Both types of allergies can develop at any age, although childhood through early adulthood onset is most common. Vasomotor rhinitis is a noninfectious and nonallergic type of rhinitis for which the cause is often unknown.

J30.0 Vasomotor rhinitis

Vasomotor rhinitis is a noninfectious and nonallergic type of rhinitis for which the cause is often unknown. Suspected causes include dry air, air pollution, and certain medications. Symptoms often mimic those of allergic rhinitis and include congestion, runny nose, and sneezing. A diagnosis of vasomotor rhinitis is typically made after ruling out allergens as the cause.

J30.1 Allergic rhinitis due to pollen

Allergic rhinitis due to pollen is a seasonal type of allergy that occurs when airborne plant pollens are at their highest levels, generally in spring and summer. It is often referred to as hay fever. The triggers may include trees, grass, and ragweed pollens.

J30.5 Allergic rhinitis due to food

Some people are sensitive to food and will experience nasal congestion and runny nose when eating these foods. Hot spicy foods and alcohol are commonly associated with allergic rhinitis.

J30.8- Other allergic rhinitis

Home or workplace airborne pollutants are usually the cause of the perennial type. Common perennial allergens include mold, dust mites, and animal hair and dander. Oftentimes, the animal need not be present to cause the reaction to animal dander; it can occur upon exposure to the allergens left in a room where the animal has previously been.

J31.- Chronic rhinitis, nasopharyngitis and pharyngitis

Chronic rhinitis is persistent inflammation and swelling of the mucous membrane of the nose. Structural problems or chronic infections are the most common causes of chronic rhinitis. Symptoms of rhinitis include rhinorrhea (runny nose), congestion, sneezing, pus-filled discharge from the nose, and frequent bleeding. Chronic pharyngitis is a persistent, long-standing sore throat and nasopharyngitis is persistent inflammation of the nose and throat. Chronic inflammation of the nose and/or throat can be the result of an infective agent or due to an allergy or exposure to an irritant.

> **Focus Point**
>
> *Chronic rhinitis due to an allergen is located in category J30 Vasomotor and allergic rhinitis.*

J32.- Chronic sinusitis

Chronic sinusitis is persistent inflammation of the sinuses and includes any persistent abscess, empyema, or infection of the nasal sinuses. It can be caused by an infective agent or by exposure to an allergic agent or irritant. Code selection is based on site: maxillary, frontal, ethmoidal, sphenoidal, pansinusitis, or other sites. The maxillary sinus cavities are located behind the cheekbone. The frontal sinus cavities are located above the eyes. The ethmoid sinus cavities are located between the eyes on either side of the nose. The sphenoid sinus cavities are located behind the eyes on either side of the nose. Pansinusitis involves all of the paranasal sinuses on one or both sides. Other sites are used for sinusitis of more than one sinus but not all of the sinuses.

J33.- Nasal polyp

A nasal polyp is a soft, painless, benign growth arising from the mucosa of the nasal cavity or sinuses. Nasal polyps are a natural reaction to chronic sinusitis due to infection or allergy. Polyps most commonly form around the ostia of the maxillary sinus, and are classified according to whether they are located in the nose or sinuses with a separate category for polypoid sinus degeneration. Polypoid sinus degeneration includes Woakes' syndrome, also called Woakes' ethmoiditis, which is characterized by recurrent nasal polyps arising from the ethmoid sinuses resulting in broadening of the nose; the condition is thought to be hereditary. Polyps may be asymptomatic or they may block the nasal airways or promote chronic sinus infection.

J34.- Other and unspecified disorders of nose and nasal sinuses

This category includes conditions such as cellulitis, furuncles, carbuncles, and cysts of the nose and nasal sinuses, along with the other conditions that follow.

J34.2 Deviated nasal septum

The nasal septum is a thin wall composed of cartilage and bone that separates the two nostrils. A deviated nasal septum is one that is crooked or displaced from the midline. It is a common disorder that often requires no treatment. However, in some cases, the deviation in the septum causes obstructions in the nasal passages that lead to chronic conditions like sinusitis or epistaxis. If the deviation predisposes the patient to chronic problems, the condition may be treated surgically.

J34.3 Hypertrophy of nasal turbinates

The nasal turbinates are ridges of bone and soft tissue that project from the sidewalls of the nasal passages. There are three turbinates in each nasal passage: inferior, middle, and superior. The turbinates help to cleanse and humidify the air. An overgrowth of the bone or soft tissue that comprises the nasal turbinates is referred to as hypertrophy. Hypertrophy of the nasal turbinates can cause obstruction of the nasal passages.

J34.81 Nasal mucositis (ulcerative)

Nasal mucositis is a painful inflammation of the mucous membranes of the nose that may be complicated by ulceration of the mucosal tissue. Mucositis is often a complication of antineoplastic, immunosuppressive, or radiation therapy as mucosal tissues are especially vulnerable to damage by chemotherapy, radiation therapy, and immune system diseases.

Focus Point

Nasal mucositis is coded in the respiratory chapter, but mucositis can also occur throughout the body at any site where there are mucous membranes, through the entire digestive tract—anywhere from the mouth and esophagus to the rectum, and also in genital areas.

J36 Peritonsillar abscess

A peritonsillar abscess is a collection of pus in the soft tissue of the peritonsillar space. The peritonsillar space is located between the capsule of the palatine tonsils and the pharyngeal constrictor muscles, and extends

from the anterior to posterior tonsillar pillars and from the torus tubarius superiorly to the pyriform sinus inferiorly. Use this code to report an abscess of the tonsil or peritonsillar cellulitis.

J37.- Chronic laryngitis and laryngotracheitis

Chronic laryngitis, a persistent inflammation of the larynx, and laryngotracheitis, a persistent inflammation of the larynx and trachea, are related to allergic reactions, inhalation of irritants, gastroesophageal reflux, or voice overuse. Inflammation affects the quality of the voice, which may be compromised, hoarse, or absent.

J38.- Diseases of vocal cords and larynx, not elsewhere classified

A wide variety of conditions that affect the vocal cords and larynx are classified here. Conditions classified here that may affect both sites include paralysis, polyps, abscess, and cellulitis. Conditions that affect the vocal cords that are classified here include nodules, granuloma, leukokeratosis, and leukoplakia. Conditions that affect the larynx include edema, laryngeal spasm, stenosis, necrosis, pachyderma, perichondritis, and ulcer.

J38.0- Paralysis of vocal cords and larynx

The vocal cords, also called vocal folds, are comprised of two bands of muscle tissue located in the larynx that open during respiration, close during swallowing, and vibrate during speech. Vocal cord paralysis and paralysis of the larynx are characterized by failure of the vocal folds to open and close properly. This affects speech and because the vocal cord paralysis causes the vocal cords to remain open, it is possible to aspirate foreign substances into the bronchi and lungs. Paralysis can occur on one or both sides and laterality is a component of these codes.

Focus Point

This category includes Gerhardt's syndrome, which is paralysis of the vocal cords causing inspiratory dyspnea.

J38.5 Laryngeal spasm

Laryngeal spasm is caused by an involuntary muscle contraction of the vocal cords that occurs during inspiration momentarily blocking air from entering the trachea and lower respiratory tract. Laryngeal spasm often occurs during sleep causing the person to wake due to the inability to inhale. Laryngeal spasm occurring at night may also be referred to as Millar's or Wichmann's asthma, laryngismus stridulus, or spasmodic false croup. These nighttime spasms occur in the glottis and windpipe and are accompanied by a spasmodic inspiration and a crowing noise. Laryngeal spasms typically last only a minute or two from the time the vocal cords close to the time they relax and slowly reopen. However, if the attack persists, the face and extremities may become purple, and the episode may include muscle spasms of the extremities. As the vocal cords reopen, inhalation causes high-pitched breath sounds that resolve as the vocal cords relax.

J39.- Other diseases of upper respiratory tract

Diseases classified here include abscess of the pharynx. There are two specific codes: one for retropharyngeal and parapharyngeal abscess and the other for abscess of the pharynx. Other conditions classified here include cyst or edema of the pharynx and hypersensitivity reaction of an unspecified site.

J39.2 Other diseases of pharynx

This code includes Tornwaldt's cyst, which is a fairly common superficial nasopharyngeal mucosal cyst that is usually asymptomatic unless it becomes infected; infection can cause purulent exudate and drainage, sore throat, and eustachian tube complications.

Chronic Lower Respiratory Diseases (J40-J47)

Chronic bronchitis, chronic obstructive pulmonary disease (COPD), emphysema, and asthma are grouped into the chronic lower respiratory disease group, which affects the bronchus and lungs. These conditions comprise some of the leading causes of death in the U.S. A vast majority of these illnesses are attributable to cigarette smoking, although other risk factors include environmental exposures and genetic predisposition.

The categories in this code block are as follows:

J40	Bronchitis, not specified as acute or chronic
J41	Simple and mucopurulent chronic bronchitis
J42	Unspecified chronic bronchitis
J43	Emphysema
J44	Other chronic obstructive pulmonary disease
J45	Asthma
J47	Bronchiectasis

J41.- Simple and mucopurulent chronic bronchitis

Chronic bronchitis is defined as a persistent cough with sputum production occurring on most days for at least three months of the year for at least two years. Simple chronic bronchitis includes smoker's cough as the most common etiology is cigarette smoking, but it also may be caused by environmental pollution or inhalation of irritant chemicals. Mucopurulent

bronchitis is persistent, purulent, and recurrent. Simple and mucopurulent types of bronchitis can occur together and this condition is classified as "mixed" chronic bronchitis.

J43.- Emphysema

Emphysema is a condition of the respiratory system that restricts the airflow during exhalation because the bronchioles and alveoli deteriorate gradually. This causes a loss of lung elasticity, which can result in significant breathing difficulty. As this condition progresses, the spherical air sacs within the lungs become irregular and contain holes, reducing not only the number of air sacs but also the amount of oxygen that can circulate into the blood from the lungs (a decrease in the gas exchange). As the air sacs deteriorate, the openings collapse, trapping air within the lungs. Treatment for this condition can slow down the deterioration; however, once the damage is done, it cannot be reversed or cured. Smoking and air pollution are main contributors to emphysema.

J43.0 Unilateral pulmonary emphysema [MacLeod's syndrome]

MacLeod's syndrome is a form of emphysema in which one lung becomes somewhat transparent in conjunction with the reduced oxygen and carbon dioxide exchange within the blood. MacLeod's syndrome is also known as Swyer James syndrome or SJS.

J43.1 Panlobular emphysema

Panlobular emphysema affects all parts of the lobes within the lungs. The right lung has three lobes and the left lung has two lobes, and each lobe further divides into hundreds of smaller lobules each containing a bronchiole and its own group of alveoli. A person with panlobular emphysema has a condition directly affecting all of these areas.

J43.2 Centrilobular emphysema

Centrilobular emphysema occurs mainly in the central part of the lobule and is the most common form of emphysema. This form occurs most often in the central portion of the upper lobes and is more frequently seen in men than women. Smoking and dust inhalation are the primary risk factors associated with this type of emphysema.

J43.9 Emphysema, unspecified

This code includes emphysematous blebs, which are blisters larger than 1 mm within an emphysematous lung that contain blood or serum. It is a fairly generic term, referring more to a symptom that occurs during emphysema than to a disease process itself.

J44.- Other chronic obstructive pulmonary disease

Chronic airway obstruction is a nonspecific condition characterized by a chronic or recurrent reduction in expiratory airflow within the lung. Chronic obstructive pulmonary disease (COPD) and chronic obstructive lung disease (COLD) are the two most common descriptive diagnostic terms for conditions assigned to this code category. Signs and symptoms of chronic airway obstruction include dyspnea on exertion with reduced exercise tolerance, sputum-productive cough, ronchi, decreased intensity of breath sounds, and prolonged expiration. Obstructive chronic bronchitis is chronic bronchitis combined with obstructive lung disease. Chronic bronchitis is defined as a persistent cough with sputum production occurring on most days for at least three months of the year for at least two years. Obstructive chronic bronchitis is characterized by an increased mass of mucous glands in the lungs, resulting in an increase in the thickness of the bronchial mucosa. Its most common etiology is cigarette smoking, but it also may be caused by environmental pollution or inhalation of irritant chemicals. Chronic obstructive asthma is used to identify obstructive forms of asthma in obstructive lung disease. Patients with chronic obstructive pulmonary disease with asthma have a continuous obstruction to airflow on expiration, which is different than patients with nonobstructive asthma, who wheeze during an asthma attack, but return to normal breathing once the attack subsides. The fourth character identifies whether the chronic obstructive pulmonary disease is complicated by an acute lower respiratory infection or whether the condition is exacerbated or decompensated. The unspecified option is the appropriate choice when neither of those conditions applies.

Focus Point

This category now includes chronic obstructive bronchitis and chronic obstructive asthma as inclusion terms in the J44 code set. If asthma is documented, the type of asthma (identified in category J45) must be coded separately.

J45.- Asthma

Asthma is the narrowing of the airways due to increased responsiveness of the trachea and bronchi to various stimuli. Asthma is reversible, changing in severity spontaneously or as a result of treatment. Asthma is associated with bronchospasm and pathologic features such as increased mucous secretion, mucosal edema and hyperemia, hypertrophy of bronchial smooth muscle, and acute inflammation. Extrinsic asthma is asthma due to allergenic exposure to substances such as pollen, house dust, animal dander, molds, food or beverages, vapors, or drugs. Most prevalent in children, this condition is associated with abnormally high levels of

IgE immunoglobulins, indicating an allergic reaction. Intrinsic asthma is asthma due to nonallergenic factors such as emotional stresses, fatigue, endocrine changes, irritants (nonallergenic) such as dust and chemicals, and acute respiratory infection. More prevalent in adults, intrinsic asthma is associated with normal IgE immunoglobulin levels, indicating a nonallergic reaction. Asthma codes are assigned based on severity, which may be mild intermittent, mild persistent, moderate persistent, or severe. Asthma is further classified as uncomplicated, with acute exacerbation, or with status asthmaticus. An exacerbation of a patient's condition is simply an increase in the seriousness of his or her disease, typically marked by a greater intensity of signs and symptoms. Status asthmaticus refers to a prolonged, severe asthmatic attack or airway obstruction (mucous plug) not relieved by bronchodilators.

Focus Point

Because manifestations of extrinsic and intrinsic diseases commonly occur in the same patient, both are now inclusions in all of the asthma codes. If documentation identifies exacerbation and status asthmaticus, only the status asthmaticus is coded since it is the more life-threatening condition.

J45.2- Mild intermittent asthma

Mild intermittent asthma is classified based on the following indications:

- Symptom frequency twice a week or less
- Waking at night due to symptoms twice a month or less
- Necessary use of immediate relief inhaler twice a week
- Little or no interference with daily activities
- Normal peak flow readings between symptoms
- Not requiring the use of oral steroids to control or requiring them only once per year

J45.3- Mild persistent asthma

Mild persistent asthma is classified based on the following indications:

- Symptom frequency more than two days a week, but not every day
- Waking at night due to symptoms three to four times a month
- Necessary use of immediate relief inhaler more than two times a week
- Minor interference with daily activities
- Peak flow readings equal to 80 percent of personal norm
- Requiring the use of oral steroids twice a year

J45.4-   Moderate persistent asthma

Moderate persistent asthma is classified based on the following indications:

- Daily symptoms

- Waking at night due to symptoms more than one time a week

- Necessary use of immediate relief inhaler daily

- Some interference with daily activities

- Peak flow reading from 60 to 80 percent of personal norm

- Requiring the use of oral steroids twice a year

J45.5-   Severe persistent asthma

Severe persistent asthma is classified based on the following indications:

- Frequent symptoms throughout the day

- Waking at night due to symptoms often every night

- Necessary use of immediate relief inhaler several times daily

- Symptoms that severely limit daily activities

- Peak flow readings less than 60 percent of personal norm

- Requiring the use of oral steroids two or more times a year

J47.-   Bronchiectasis

Bronchiectasis is dilation of the bronchi with mucous production and persistent cough. Mounier-Kuhn syndrome is a form of bronchiectasis. The fourth character identifies whether an acute lower respiratory infection is present or whether the condition is exacerbated or decompensated. The uncomplicated option is the appropriate choice when neither of those conditions applies.

Lung Diseases Due to External Agents (J60-J70)

Conditions classified here include pneumoconiosis due to inorganic dusts; pneumoconiosis associated with tuberculosis; airway disease or hypersensitivity due to organic dusts; respiratory conditions due to inhalation of chemicals, gases, fumes, or vapors; pneumonitis due to solids or liquids; and respiratory conditions due to other external agents.

Pneumoconiosis is a condition caused by inhaling inorganic dust particles, typically associated with occupations that require regular exposure to mineral dusts. This condition is a form of interstitial lung

disease that contributes to the inflammation of the air sacs, causing the lung tissue to harden. There is no cure for this disease, and treatment is focused on managing the patient's symptoms.

Lung diseases due to organic dusts fall into two categories: airway disease and hypersensitivity. In airway disease it is the organic dust that causes the lung condition, while in hypersensitivity it is an allergic reaction to the dust that causes the lung disease.

Respiratory conditions due to inhalation of chemicals, gases, fumes, and vapors may be acute (subacute) or chronic. Acute conditions classified in this code block include bronchitis, pneumonitis, pulmonary edema, upper respiratory inflammation, and reactive airway dysfunction syndrome when the cause is specified as due to inhalation of a chemical, gas, fume, or vapor. Chronic conditions include bronchitis, pulmonary edema, emphysema, obliterative bronchiolitis, and pulmonary fibrosis specified as due to the same causes.

Pneumonitis is an inflammation of the lung tissue and pneumonitis due to inhalation of food, vomit, oils, essences, or other solids or liquids is classified in category J69.

Other respiratory conditions caused by radiation, drugs, smoke inhalation, and other external agents are classified in category J70. Codes identify the general type of external agent and whether the respiratory condition is acute or chronic.

The categories in this code block are as follows:

J60	Coalworker's pneumoconiosis
J61	Pneumoconiosis due to asbestos and other mineral fibers
J62	Pneumoconiosis due to dust containing silica
J63	Pneumoconiosis due to other inorganic dusts
J64	Unspecified pneumoconiosis
J65	Pneumoconiosis associated with tuberculosis
J66	Airway disease due to specific organic dust
J67	Hypersensitivity pneumonitis due to organic dust
J68	Respiratory conditions due to inhalation of chemicals, gases, fumes and vapors
J69	Pneumonitis due to solids and liquids
J70	Respiratory condition's due to other external agents

J60 Coalworker's pneumoconiosis

Coalworker's pneumoconiosis affects people who work in mines, manufacturing, or shipping of coal and graphite products with regular inhalation of these particles. It is characterized by the deposit of coal dust in the lungs and the formation of black nodules on the bronchioles, which results in focal emphysema. This condition is often referred to as black lung disease or anthracosis, and the progress can often be halted if further exposure to coal dust is prevented.

J61 Pneumoconiosis due to asbestos and other mineral fibers

Asbestosis is a generic term for a group of minerals that cause this form of lung disease. These minerals are taken from underground deposits and have been historically used in insulation, tiles, and automobile parts. People who work in these industries are not the only groups that develop this condition. Those who live or work in structures that contain asbestos products that have begun to break down have also been known to acquire this condition; however, symptoms do not often occur until 20 years or more after exposure. In these patients, chest films often show small linear opacities distributed throughout the lung. In addition, asbestosis can lead to mesothelioma, a rare form of cancer in which malignant cells are found in the sac lining of the chest or abdomen. This disease tends to be progressive, beginning with shortness of breath, progressing eventually to respiratory failure.

J62.- Pneumoconiosis due to dust containing silica

Inhalation of silica dust is the most common cause of pneumonoconiosis. Silicosis is a pneumoconiosis that usually follows long-term inhalation of small particles of crystalline free silica in industries such as metal mining (lead, hard coal, copper, silver, gold), metal casting, pottery making, and sandstone and granite cutting. The etiology involves alveolar macrophages that engulf particles of free silica and enter the lymphatics and interstitial tissue. The macrophages cause the release of toxic enzymes, and fibrosis of the lung parenchyma occurs. When a macrophage dies, the silica particles are released and engulfed by other macrophages, and the process is repeated. Patients with simple nodular silicosis have no respiratory symptoms and usually no respiratory impairment. They may cough and raise sputum, but these symptoms are due to industrial bronchitis and occur as often in persons with normal x-rays. Conglomerate silicosis may lead to severe shortness of breath, cough, and sputum, with severity related to the size of the conglomerate in the lungs. Extensive masses can cause severe disability. Exposure of 20 to 30 years is usually necessary before the disease becomes apparent, although it can develop in less than 10 years when the exposure to dust is extremely high (i.e., in industries such as tunneling, abrasive soap making, and sandblasting). No effective treatment is known other than lung transplantation.

J62.0 Pneumoconiosis due to talc dust

Talc is a type of silica and pneumoconiosis is caused by regular exposure to talc dust often present in industries such as cosmetics, pharmaceutical, paper, ceramics, and electronics manufacturing. This stage of the disease is considered "simple pneumoconiosis"; continued overexposure leads to fibrosis.

J62.8 Pneumoconiosis due to other dust containing silica

Pneumoconiosis due to all other dusts containing silica excluding talc dust are included here.

J63.- Pneumoconiosis due to other inorganic dusts

Parenchymal lung diseases due to chronic inhalation of inorganic (mineral) dusts are called pneumoconiosis. Diagnosis depends on a history of exposure to the inorganic dust and clinical manifestations.

J63.0 Aluminosis (of lung)

Aluminosis may also be referred to as aluminum lung. Typically, this condition afflicts those working in explosive or abrasive aluminum manufacturing, particularly aluminum welders or polishers. Recent studies show a small portion of these workers develop this condition over the course of 25 years or more of exposure.

J63.1 Bauxite fibrosis (of lung)

Bauxite fibrosis of the lung is due to inhalation of bauxite dust, which can be found in combinations of hydrated aluminum oxides that include iron and silicon. Those who work with abrasive materials in spark plugs and furnaces are exposed to this type of dust.

J63.2 Berylliosis

Berylliosis is caused by the light-weight metallic element beryllium, which is used in aerospace, semiconductor, electrical industries, and also found in copper alloy in springs. The most common use of this element is in electric light bulbs and fluorescent tubes. Pneumoconiosis due to beryllium may also be called beryllium disease, beryllium poisoning, or beryllium granulomatosis. The condition is characterized by generalized granulomatous disease caused by inhalation of dust or fumes containing beryllium compounds and products. This condition was first recognized in the 1940s as an occupational lung disease. It remains very rare. Symptoms of chronic berylliosis include cough, chest pain, weight loss, and fatigue, although the patient may not develop any of these until 20 years after exposure has ceased.

Focus Point

Acute berylliosis is classified as a chemical pneumonitis and is reported with code J68.0.

J63.3   Graphite fibrosis (of lung)

Graphite fibrosis of the lung is caused by the dust from graphite, which is one of many mineral forms of carbon with a wide variety of uses. Graphite can be mixed with clay as is done for making pencils and has uses in lubricants, polish, batteries, and nuclear reactor cores.

J63.4   Siderosis

Siderosis, also called welder's or silver polisher's lung, arises from exposure to iron particles or dust. A person with this condition may not display any symptoms, but a chest x-ray will show an abnormality in one or both of the lungs.

J63.5   Stannosis

Stannosis results from overexposure to tin dust (stannic or tin oxide) and can be seen on a chest x-ray presenting as dense masses. These oxides are often used in the production of glass, enamels, and ceramic glazes.

J66.-   Airway disease due to specific organic dust

Lung diseases due to organic dusts fall into two categories: airway disease and hypersensitivity. In airway disease it is the organic dust that causes the lung condition, while in hypersensitivity it is an allergic reaction to the dust that causes the lung disease. This category classifies airway disease due to cotton, flax, hemp, and other unprocessed fibers.

J66.0   Byssinosis

Byssinosis, also referred to as brown lung disease, causes narrowing of air passages, like asthma. The primary cause of this condition is inhalation of cotton, which is frequently used in the textile industry.

J66.1   Flax-dressers' disease

Flax-dresser's disease is a form of byssinosis that is caused by inhaling remnants of flax, which is grown for the seed it produces and the oil component of that seed. The oil produced has many industrial, household, and animal uses, such as paint, varnish, ink, and protein meal for livestock. Recently flax seed has been recognized as a beneficial additive to human food due to the fatty acids in the oil.

J66.2   Cannabinosis

Cannabinosis is another form of byssinosis specific to the inhalation of hemp and other unprocessed fibers within the textile manufacturing industry. People working in factories that produce yarn, thread, and fabric containing hemp are at increased risk of developing this condition.

J67.-   Hypersensitivity pneumonitis due to organic dust

Hypersensitivity pneumonitis occurs when fine dust of natural materials is inhaled and causes an allergic reaction and inflammation of the lungs. Allergy to the substance can take months or years to develop but damage can be reversed if the allergen is avoided in the early stages of the disease. Once lung scarring and pulmonary fibrosis sets in, the damage is permanent. The most common type of hypersensitivity pneumonitis is farmer's lung, which is caused by exposure to moldy hay, grain, and straw. Other causes include organisms growing in air conditioner ventilation systems, fungus in humidifiers and heating systems, coffee beans, bird droppings, cork, and many other substances.

J67.0   Farmer's lung

Farmer's lung is caused by the antigen *Micropolyspora faeni* or *Thermoactinomyces vulgaris* in moldy hay.

J67.1   Bagassosis

Bagassosis is caused by the antigen *Micropolyspora faeni* or *Thermoactinomyces vulgaris* in sugarcane waste.

J67.2   Bird fancier's lung

Bird fancier's lung is caused by an antigen found in bird droppings from parakeets, pigeons, and chickens.

J67.3   Suberosis

Suberosis is caused by antigens found in moldy cork dust which is why the condition is also called cork-handler's lung.

J67.4   Maltworker's lung

Malt worker's lung is caused by *Aspergillus clavatus* or *Aspergillus* fumigatus, antigens that are found in moldy barley or malt.

J67.5   Mushroom-worker's lung

Mushroom-workers lung is caused by *Micropolyspora faeni* or *Thermoactinomyces vulgaris*, antigens in mushroom compost.

J67.6   Maple-bark-stripper's lung

Maple bark-stripper's lung is caused by the antigen *Cryptostroma corticale*, found in infected maple bark.

J68.- Respiratory conditions due to inhalation of chemicals, gases, fumes and vapors

This category includes several respiratory conditions that may occur due to the inhalation of chemical or gas fumes and vapors. Some of the codes in these subcategories represent conditions that can be caused by these substances such as bronchitis, pneumonitis, pulmonary edema, emphysema, bronchiolitis, and pulmonary fibrosis. Many of these exposures are occupationally related although some can be caused by common household substances such as chlorine bleach and ammonia.

J68.0 Bronchitis and pneumonitis due to chemicals, gases, fumes and vapors

Chemical pneumonitis is inflammation of the lungs induced by the inhalation of, or choking on, chemicals, gases, fumes, and vapors including common substances such as chlorine gas (from chlorine bleach), ammonia, pesticide noxious fumes, and fertilizer dust. It occurs acutely or chronically over prolonged exposure to the chemical. Some conditions classified here include silo-filler's bronchitis or pneumonitis and acute bronchitis due to beryllium, cadmium, crack cocaine, fluorocarbon-polymer, manganese, nitrogen dioxide, and vanadium.

J69.- Pneumonitis due to solids and liquids

Pneumonitis due to solids and liquids is an inflammation of the lung tissue caused by aspiration of foreign material into the tracheobronchial tree. Aspiration of gastric contents or toxic materials such as petroleum distillates often causes pneumonia or pneumonitis due to an inflammatory response in the lungs and lung parenchyma.

J69.0 Pneumonitis due to inhalation of food and vomit

Aspiration of gastric contents often causes pneumonia or pneumonitis due to an inflammatory response in the lungs and lung parenchyma. Signs and symptoms of pneumonitis due to inhalation of food or vomitus include a history of feeding disorder, convulsive disorder, marked debility or disturbance of consciousness, drug or alcohol intoxication, rales, dyspnea, cyanosis, hypotension, and tachycardia.

Focus Point
Neonatal aspiration pneumonitis is not coded to this category and should be assigned to a code in category P24.

J69.1 Pneumonitis due to inhalation of oils and essences

Lipid pneumonia is a chronic syndrome due to the repeated aspiration of oil-containing substances such as mineral oil, cod liver oil, and oily nose drops. It is characterized by chronic granulomatous inflammation with fibrosis. It progresses slowly and is often asymptomatic with detection noted incidentally on a chest x-ray.

Focus Point
This code excludes endogenous lipid pneumonia, which is caused by retention of lipids in the lung parenchyma released during the breakdown of tissue. Endogenous lipid pneumonia is reported with code J84.89.

J70.- Respiratory conditions due to other external agents

Other external agents can cause acute or chronic respiratory conditions that can affect the entire lung or the interstitium. The interstitium is the network of tissue (walls) that contains thin layers of cells and blood vessels that surround and support the air sacs (alveoli).

J70.0 Acute pulmonary manifestations due to radiation

Radiation pneumonitis most commonly occurs in those who undergo radiation therapy for lung and other cancers in the thoracic cavity. Radiation causes inflammation and decreases the production of surfactant, which keeps lungs expanded. Symptoms usually occur one to six months after completing therapy. Pneumonitis usually resolves with treatment.

J70.1 Chronic and other pulmonary manifestations due to radiation

This code includes pulmonary fibrosis (scarring of lung), which can occur if radiation pneumonitis is untreated or persists. This condition is often permanent.

J70.5 Respiratory conditions due to smoke inhalation

The injury referred to as "smoke inhalation" occurs when the products of combustion during a fire are inhaled into the respiratory tract. The materials being burned, the degree of heat generated by the combustion, and the amount of oxygen available determine the type of smoke produced and thus, the complexities of the inhalation injury. Three primary mechanisms combine to create inhalation injury: asphyxiation, pulmonary irritation, and thermal damage of the airways. Combustion utilizes oxygen, consuming the amount available. The subsequent rise in carbon monoxide causes tissue hypoxia by further decreasing the capacity for circulating oxygen leading to metabolic acidosis and depressed myocardial contractility. Additionally, the combustion of certain products can produce noxious gasses that result in immediate respiratory arrest. Airborne irritants released during combustion cause an inflammatory response of the tissues, the degree of which is determined by their solubility in water. Highly soluble substances cause injury to the upper airway, intermediate soluble substances cause both upper and lower tract injuries, and those with low water solubility have a particularly adverse effect on the lungs.

Focus Point

Use additional codes to identify any associated secondary respiratory conditions (e.g., respiratory failure).

Other Respiratory Diseases Principally Affecting the Interstitium (J80-J84)

This block of codes is comprised of diseases that are considered interstitial lung diseases and disorders. The American Thoracic Society (ATS) and the American College of Chest Physicians (ACCP) requested specific classification codes to differentiate between interstitial lung diseases. Each type of interstitial lung disease is distinctive in presentation, pathophysiology, and clinical course.

The interstitium is the network of tissue (walls) that contains thin layers of cells and blood vessels that surround and support the air sacs (alveoli). A condition located in this block is acute respiratory distress syndrome (ARDS), which occurs when fluid causes the collapse of the alveolar space resulting in hypoxia. Some of the other interstitial lung diseases, which are also considered "lung scarring" conditions, included here are pulmonary edema, pulmonary eosinophilia, allergic pneumonia, fibrosis and cirrhosis of the lung, and idiopathic interstitial lung disease.

The categories in this code block are as follows:

J80	Acute respiratory distress syndrome
J81	Pulmonary edema
J82	Pulmonary eosinophilia, not elsewhere classified
J84	Other interstitial pulmonary disease

J80   Acute respiratory distress syndrome

Acute respiratory distress syndrome (ARDS) is a sudden failure of the respiratory system. In ARDS, the alveoli become inflamed and engorged with fluid, resulting in flooding and collapse of the alveolar space. As a result, pulmonary gas exchange is compromised and the patient becomes hypoxic. ARDS usually occurs only in critically ill patients. It is often associated with sepsis and shock. Symptoms of ARDS include dyspnea, tachypnea, hypoxemia, left atrial hypertension,

pulmonary hypertension, and cyanosis. Diagnosis can be confirmed by the identification of abnormalities on chest x-ray. Prognosis is variable, dependent upon the underlying etiologies and health status of the patient at the time of the critical illness. Treatment requires intensive care management with ventilatory and hemodynamic support and adjuvant drug therapies. ARDS is also called shock lung.

J81.-   Pulmonary edema

Pulmonary edema is caused by excessive fluid within the lungs. This excess fluid accumulates in the air sacs making it difficult to breath. The condition may be acute or chronic.

Focus Point

Chronic pulmonary edema may be a symptom of left ventricular heart failure. When left ventricular heart failure is the cause of the pulmonary edema, only the left ventricular heart failure is reported.

J82   Pulmonary eosinophilia, not elsewhere classified

An eosinophil is a leukocyte in the blood that normally constitutes 1 to 3 percent of the white blood cells. Eosinophilia is an increase in the number of eosinophils that accompanies an inflammatory or allergic response. This increase can be caused by extrinsic or intrinsic factors. Loeffler's syndrome or PIE syndrome is one type of pulmonary eosinophilia classified here that is a mild form due to an extrinsic response from inhalation or ingestion of substances such as infectious agents including fungi, mycobacteria, or medications. Tropical eosinophilia, also referred to as Weingarten's syndrome, is classified here.

J84.-   Other interstitial pulmonary diseases

The interstitium is the network of tissue (walls) that contains thin layers of cells and blood vessels that surround and support the air sacs (alveoli). Other interstitial pulmonary diseases classified here include some types of fibrosis, idiopathic interstitial pneumonia, and lymphoid interstitial pneumonia. The manifestation code for interstitial pulmonary diseases with fibrosis in diseases classified elsewhere is also included in this category.

J84.01   Alveolar proteinosis

Alveolar proteinosis is a rare condition of reduced ventilation due to proteinaceous deposits on alveoli. The build-up of deposits is thought to be due to a defect in the ability of alveolar macrophages to break-down and remove excess surfactant and other inhaled particles. Symptoms include dyspnea, cough, chest pain, and hemoptysis. It affects more men than women with average age between 30 and 50.

J84.02   Pulmonary alveolar microlithiasis

Pulmonary alveolar microlithiasis (PAM) is a rare chronic disease of unknown cause in which small calcium deposits (calculi) form in the alveoli resembling sand-like particles on x-ray. The disease is usually discovered incidentally from birth to 40 years of age. Patients can be asymptomatic with normal or mild restrictive pulmonary function although in some cases it can progress to pulmonary fibrosis or respiratory failure. Lung transplantation is the only known effective treatment.

J84.112   Idiopathic pulmonary fibrosis

Idiopathic pulmonary fibrosis (IPF) is a chronic disease of unknown cause characterized by scarring and thickening of the lungs. IPF most commonly affects males older than age 50. The chief symptom is progressive dyspnea. Additional symptoms include pleuritic chest pain, dry paroxysmal cough, and shortness of breath. Clinical signs include decreased vital capacity and impaired gas exchange, abnormal breath sounds (crackles), cyanosis, and clubbing of the distal phalanges. Disease progression varies from gradual to rapid, with complications that include chronic hypoxemia, polycythemia, pulmonary hypertension, and respiratory failure. IPF may be associated with certain connective tissue diseases (e.g., rheumatoid arthritis, SLE, scleroderma).

J84.113   Idiopathic non-specific interstitial pneumonitis

Nonspecific interstitial pneumonitis (NSIP) is a specific type of fibrosing interstitial pneumonia, a group of lung diseases that cause scarring of the lung. NSIP commonly occurs in female nonsmokers between 40 to 50 years of age, with unknown causation. Initial onset of symptoms may be subacute or gradual in nature, with a duration prior to diagnosis that may range from six months to a few years. Symptoms include weight loss, breathlessness, cough, and fatigue. Pulmonary function studies indicate a restrictive pattern with exercise-induced hypoxemia. The histology of NSIP varies widely in regard to presenting features and severity, marked by the degrees of fibrosis. However, NSIP findings are distinct histologically from the usual interstitial pneumonia pattern, having a characteristic homogenous inflammation and fibrosis. NSIP may mimic other clinical causes, including collagen vascular disease, hypersensitivity pneumonitis, drug-induced pneumonitis, infection, and immunodeficiency. NSIP has been found to occur in patients with HIV, sometimes mimicking pneumocystis pneumonia.

J84.114   Acute interstitial pneumonitis

Acute interstitial pneumonitis (AIP) is a rapidly progressive, histologically distinct, and potentially fatal form of interstitial pneumonia of unknown cause. AIP is characterized by rapid disease progression and high mortality rate. Onset occurs at approximately 50 years of age, and affects both sexes equally. Medical history is often remarkable for prior illness suggestive of a viral upper respiratory infection. Symptoms mimic that of viral syndrome with myalgias, arthralgias, fever, chills, and malaise. Disease progression occurs rapidly within seven to 14 days from onset, resulting in respiratory failure.

J84.115   Respiratory bronchiolitis interstitial lung disease

Respiratory bronchiolitis interstitial lung disease (RB-ILD) is a condition affecting smokers, which is characterized by small airway (bronchiole) inflammation and interstitial lung disease. Histopathology is remarkable for pigmented intraluminal macrophages, alveolar septal scarring, and mucus stasis within the bronchioles. The condition is largely asymptomatic at the bronchiolitis stage; however, when the patient develops interstitial disease, pulmonary symptoms (cough, dyspnea on exertion) and abnormal clinical signs (crackles on examination) occur.

J84.116   Cryptogenic organizing pneumonia

Cryptogenic organizing pneumonia (COP) is an idiopathic condition characterized by granular obstructions of the alveolar ducts and spaces with secondary inflammation. Most patients present with a persistent flu-like syndrome, which includes progressive dyspnea on exertion, cough, fever, fatigue, and weight loss. Clinical signs include crackles on pulmonary exam. Histologically, COP is an organizing pneumonia characterized by scarification as opposed to resolution and resorption of exudates. This scarification process is caused by the pathological plugging or filling of the alveoli and bronchioles by loose plugs of connective tissue. The tissue changes inherent in COP occur in the alveolar ducts and alveoli, occasionally exhibiting a "honeycomb" appearance or polyposis.

J84.117   Desquamative interstitial pneumonia

Desquamative interstitial pneumonia (DIP) is a chronic lung inflammation characterized by the accumulation of numerous pigmented macrophages within the alveoli. DIP is distinguished from other interstitial pulmonary fibrosis in its diffuse, uniform distribution of histopathological features. It is primarily associated with the effects of cigarette smoking, occurring almost exclusively in current or former smokers, and often associated with emphysema. Onset occurs typically in midlife, although some patients present between the ages of 30 and 40. It affects a greater proportion of men than women.

J84.2   Lymphoid interstitial pneumonia

Lymphoid interstitial pneumonia (LIP) presents as a syndrome of fever, dyspnea, and cough with pulmonary infiltrates on diagnostic imaging. LIP may be considered a histological variant of diffuse pulmonary lymphoid hyperplasia, which is predominately characterized by interstitial changes due to infiltration of lymphocytes and plasma cells. As the condition progresses, lung nodules may occur, and fibrosis becomes more diffusely distributed throughout the pulmonary interstitium with extensive infiltration of the alveolar septa. Causation remains uncertain, although it is commonly associated with autoimmune lymphoproliferative disorders (e.g., rheumatoid arthritis, myasthenia gravis, Sjögren syndrome, lupus) and certain retrovirus infections (e.g., HIV, Epstein-Barr, HTLV1). Onset is often gradual, with initial symptoms presenting as cough and breathlessness.

J84.81   Lymphangioleiomyomatosis

Lymphangioleiomyomatosis (a.k.a., lymphangiomyomatosis, LAM) is a rare, progressive lung disease that almost exclusively affects women of childbearing age. Pathophysiology is the result of an abnormal proliferation of smooth muscle growth resulting in cystic leiomyoma formation throughout the lungs and pulmonary structures, causing obstruction. LAM may initially be misdiagnosed as asthma or COPD. Onset of disease can occur prior to the presence of detectable anomalies on diagnostic imaging or pulmonary function tests. Once symptomatic, spirometry demonstrates chronic airway obstruction. High resolution CT (HRCT) is essential to diagnosis and elimination of other causal disease. Characteristic thoracic findings include diffuse, thin walled cysts, thoracic adenopathy, pleural effusion, and ground-glass opacities (GGO). Abdominal HRCT findings may be consistent with retroperitoneal adenopathy and angiomyolipoma of the kidney, liver, and spleen with thickened vasculature and adipose tissue. Symptoms include nonproductive cough, hemoptysis, and pulmonary vascular congestion. LAM is associated with tuberous sclerosis complex, in which patients also suffer renal angiomyolipomas. LAM is characterized by the infiltration of the lung with neoplastic smooth muscle cells of unknown origin and cystic destruction of lung tissue. Exacerbation correlates with fluctuations in hormone levels associated with pregnancy, menstruation, and synthetic estrogen use. Treatment may include antiestrogen hormonal therapies, such as progesterone or gonadotropin-releasing hormone antagonists. Procedural intervention may be necessary to manage pleural effusions. Eventually, bilateral lung transplant is indicated. However, the disease has been known to recur postoperatively, with abnormal smooth muscle proliferation in the transplanted lung.

J84.82   Adult pulmonary Langerhans cell histiocytosis

Adult pulmonary Langerhans cell histiocytosis (PLCH) is a rare interstitial lung disorder of unknown etiology characterized by the destructive granulomatization of accumulated Langerhans' cells in the distal bronchioles. Presenting symptoms include dyspnea and cough, although some patients may experience chest pain due to associated pneumothorax or bone lesions. In adults, PLCH usually occurs as a single-system disease, characterized by focal Langerhans' cell granulomas infiltrating and destroying distal bronchioles. The typical high resolution CT (HRCT) pattern combines small nodules with or without cavitation and cysts predominantly involving upper lungs with relative sparing of the lung bases. Diagnosis may be confirmed by biopsy for identification of Langerhans' cell granulomas in tissue samples.

J84.84-   Other interstitial lung diseases of childhood

Pediatric interstitial lung disease (ILD) includes a spectrum of relatively rare chronic respiratory disorders in infants and children characterized by lung damage due to fibrotic and inflammatory changes of the alveolar walls. Common symptoms include dyspnea, diffuse infiltrates, and abnormal pulmonary function tests with impaired gas exchange and associated ventilatory defect. Although high resolution CT (HRCT) scan assists in the diagnostic process, lung biopsy is often essential for definitive diagnosis, since ILD classification is largely based on distinguishing characteristic histopathological features. Prognosis varies according to clinical presentation and comorbid conditions. In general, treatment consists of corticosteroid and oxygen therapy.

J84.841   Neuroendocrine cell hyperplasia of infancy

Neuroendocrine cell hyperplasia of infancy (NEHI) is an interstitial lung disease (ILD) of childhood of uncertain etiology that adversely affects pulmonary function. Signs and symptoms include respiratory distress with tachypnea, hypoxemia, and audible crackles on exam. High resolution CT (HRCT) findings that distinguish NEHI from other forms of childhood ILD include pulmonary hyperexpansion and prominent ground-glass opacifications (GGO). Laboratory findings include normal serum KL-6 levels, in contrast to the abnormal findings associated with other diseases.

J84.842   Pulmonary interstitial glycogenosis

Pulmonary interstitial glycogenosis (PIG) is a disorder of the newborn or infant that is characterized by tachypnea, hypoxemia, and diffuse pulmonary infiltrates. Histopathological features are remarkable for proliferation of histocytic cell types with abundant cytoplasmic glycogen within the alveolar interstitium, with minimal infiltration. These abnormal findings result in significant thickening of the alveolar space, with impaired oxygen exchange. Surfactant mutations of the lung make up a group of genetic disorders resulting in potentially fatal pediatric lung disease. Onset of disease occurs typically within the perinatal period, although lung disease has been diagnosed later in childhood and onset of symptoms seems to depend on the specific surfactant mutation. Surfactant mutations are a leading indication for pediatric lung transplantation.

J84.843 Alveolar capillary dysplasia with vein misalignment

Congenital alveolar capillary dysplasia with misalignment of pulmonary veins (ACDMPV) is a disorder of the lungs characterized by anomalous development of the pulmonary vasculature, with rapidly progressive respiratory failure and severe pulmonary hypertension. The existing capillaries become malpositioned within the walls of the alveoli, resulting in progressive thickening of the pulmonary arterioles with pulmonary arteriovenous malformations. These changes impair the exchange of pulmonary gases (oxygen and carbon dioxide) and restrict blood flow ultimately resulting in pulmonary hypertension. Onset of ACDMPV occurs in the immediate neonatal period. The condition is often fatal, despite therapeutic interventions for pulmonary hypertension, advanced ventilation strategies, and extracorporeal membrane oxygenation (ECMO). ACDMPV may be associated with other or multiple congenital anomalies, including disruption of the normal right-left asymmetry of thoracic and abdominal internal organs.

Suppurative and Necrotic Conditions of the Lower Respiratory Tract (J85-J86)

Conditions classified here include pus producing conditions that may lead to tissue death in the lower respiratory tract. The term pyothorax refers to conditions such as empyema and purulent, suppurative, or septic pleurisy, which are located in this block of codes, along with necrosis of lungs and abscesses of lungs, pleura, or mediastinum. Pleurisy, also called pleuritic chest pain, is the inflammation of the pleural membrane that lines the chest cavity and contains the lung. This category includes pleurisy that is suppurative or purulent, which are both defined as an accumulation or discharge of pus. Sharp pain brought on by breathing and coughing is the most common symptom. When this fluid becomes infected, additional symptoms occur and this condition is then known as empyema. A fistula, or communication between the pleural cavity to another structure, may be present in empyema or suppurative pleurisy.

> **Focus Point**
>
> *Pleurisy with exudate or effusion that is not specified as purulent, suppurative, septic, or staphylococcal is coded in the next block of codes in category J90 Pleural effusion, not elsewhere classified. Tuberculosis with pleurisy is located in Chapter 1 Certain Infectious and Parasitic Diseases. Pleurisy, not specified with any of the previous descriptors (unspecified or acute) is considered a symptom and is coded in Chapter 18 Symptoms, Signs and Abnormal Clinical and Laboratory Findings.*

The categories in this code block are as follows:

J85	Abscess of lung and mediastinum
J86	Pyothorax

J85.- Abscess of lung and mediastinum

An abscess is an enclosed collection of purulent material caused by the liquefaction of infected tissue. Abscess of the lung can occur with or without pneumonia. Gangrene may result from death of lung tissue as a complication of a severe lung infection.

J85.0 Gangrene and necrosis of lung

Necrosis is defined as the death of cell tissue and gangrene is the potentially life-threatening condition that is caused by considerable necrosis. Lung gangrene is a rare complication of a severe lung infection and can lead to sepsis, multiple-organ failure, and death.

J85.1 Abscess of lung with pneumonia

J85.2 Abscess of lung without pneumonia

Lung abscess occurs when there is death of the pulmonary tissues that form cavities of necrotic debris or fluid. Primary abscesses are caused by infections such as *Staphylococcus,* anaerobic bacteria, or aspergillus. Secondary abscesses are due to a preexisting condition, such as an obstruction, an immunocompromised state, or an infection that has spread from another location in the body. A frequent cause of lung abscess is aspiration pneumonia with periodontal disease in which the gingival bacteria is aspirated. In most cases, symptoms are slow to develop except when the infection is caused by *Staphylococcus aureus,* in which case they appear suddenly and can be fatal if not treated immediately. Most abscesses of the lung are treated with antibiotics. In some rare cases, a bronchoscopy is performed and a tube is inserted to drain the abscess.

J86.- Pyothorax

Pyothorax is a collection of pus in the pleural space. It is commonly caused by an infection that spreads from the lung, such as bacterial pneumonia or a lung abscess. As the pus builds up it puts pressure on the lungs making it difficult to breathe. The most common organisms that cause this condition are *S. pneumoniae, S. aureus,* and Group A *Streptococcus.* Signs and symptoms include chest pain, shortness of breath, weakness, fever, and hemoptysis. Treatment includes antibiotics and surgical intervention for infection that is persistent or resistant to antibiotic therapy.

J86.0   Pyothorax with fistula

A pyothorax may be associated with a fistula, which in this case is an abnormal connection between respiratory structures or respiratory structures and another site, such as the skin or liver. Fistulas can result from infection, inflammation, injury, or surgery.

Other Diseases of the Pleura (J90-J94)

The pleura are thin membranes covering the lungs and lining the inside of the chest wall. The pleura surround the lungs and are divided into the visceral and parietal layers. The visceral layer encapsulates the lung surface and the area between the lobes, while the parietal layer covers the inside surface of the chest wall. The area between these layers is the pleural cavity, which contains pleural fluid produced by the membranes. That fluid functions as a lubricant to decrease friction during respiration. The categories in this block represent various conditions that affect the pleura, such as effusions, plaques, and air leaks.

The categories in this code block are as follows:

J90	Pleural effusion, not elsewhere classified
J91	Pleural effusion in conditions classified elsewhere
J92	Pleural plaque
J93	Pneumothorax and air leak
J94	Other pleural conditions

J90   Pleural effusion, not elsewhere classified

Pleural effusion is the accumulation of fluid in the pleural space. Transudative and exudative pleurisy and pleural effusions without further specification are included in this code. Pleural effusion may be preceded by pleuritic chest pain caused by inflammation of pleural membranes, but the pain often subsides as fluid accumulates. As fluid accumulates, the fluid compresses the lung causing shortness of breath. Other signs and symptoms of pleural effusion include decreased tactile fremitus, pleural friction rub, dullness to percussion, egophony, and distant breath sounds. Pleural effusion is a common manifestation of systemic and intrathoracic diseases and treatment requires identifying and treating the underlying disease.

> **Focus Point**
>
> *Pleural adhesions without a diagnosis of pleural effusion are reported with code J94.8.*

J91.-   Pleural effusion in conditions classified elsewhere

Conditions classified here report pleural effusions that are manifestations of other diseases, such as malignant neoplasms or other diseases processes that cause fluid to accumulate in the pleural cavity.

J91.0   Malignant pleural effusion

Malignant pleural effusion is a common complication of advanced or disseminated malignant neoplasm resulting in the accumulation of fluid in the pleural space. Malignant pleural effusion commonly occurs as a result of a primary cancerous neoplastic process in the lung or breast or other malignancies within the chest cavity. Malignant pleural effusions may also be attributed to the presence of a metastatic secondary neoplasm of the pleura from primary tumors elsewhere in the body, or they may arise as a primary neoplasm of the pleura, as a thoracic lymphoma, or as an integral part of progressive primary lung cancer. As the malignant fluid accumulates in the pleural space, the lung collapses, resulting in chest pain, cough, hypoxia, and shortness of breath.

J92.-   Pleural plaque

Pleural plaques are areas of fibrous thickening that form on the parietal or visceral pleura, the membranes that line the ribs and lungs respectively. Studies indicate that 80 percent of patients with pleural plaque have been exposed to some form of asbestos This plaque is typically benign in nature, and treatment focuses on symptoms, if any are present. Patients with pleural plaque have an elevated risk of diffuse pleural fibrosis.

J93.-   Pneumothorax and air leak

A pneumothorax is an abnormal leakage of air into the pleural space, which displaces lung capacity. There are several clinical subtypes of pneumothorax attributed to separate causal factors or clinical presentations. Spontaneous pneumothorax may be primary or secondary and thus related to various other conditions.

J93.0   Spontaneous tension pneumothorax

Spontaneous tension pneumothorax is a life-threatening condition resulting in severe hypoxia recalcitrant to oxygen therapy, hypotension, and mental status change. The mediastinal structures become displaced, compromising cardiopulmonary function. Immediate intervention by emergency thoracic decompression is required.

J93.11   Primary spontaneous pneumothorax

A primary spontaneous pneumothorax (PSP) can occur in otherwise healthy people in the absence of comorbid (primary) lung disease or injury. The symptoms are usually mild, consisting of mild pleuritic chest pain and breathlessness, and rarely progresses to tension pneumothorax. As a result, treatment may be delayed or absent altogether if the condition resolves spontaneously.

J93.12   Secondary spontaneous pneumothorax

Secondary spontaneous pneumothorax (SSP) occurs secondary to an underlying disease. As a result, symptoms may be more severe if the health status of the patient has been compromised. Conditions that can cause a secondary pneumothorax include cystic fibrosis, spontaneous rupture of the esophagus, Marfan's syndrome, lymphangioleiomyomatosis, metastatic cancer, primary lung cancer, catamenial, pneumocystis carinii pneumonia, and eosinophilic pneumonia.

J94.-   Other pleural conditions

Other conditions that affect the thin membranes covering the lungs and lining the inside of the chest wall and the cavity formed by these membranes are reported here.

J94.0   Chylous effusion

Chylous pleural effusion is fluid within the pleural space that appears opaque and white, but the fluid is no longer opaque when combined with ether. This condition is due to the leaking of lymph contents into the space, usually as a result of thoracic duct damage or injury or mediastinal lymphoma.

J94.1   Fibrothorax

Fibrothorax is simply fibrosis within the pleural lining of the lungs. It is commonly seen as a stiff layer surrounding the lung and is attributed to traumatic hemothorax or pleural effusion.

J94.2   Hemothorax

Hemothorax occurs when blood accumulates within the pleural cavity. While the most common contributor to this condition is trauma to the chest, only nontraumatic causes are included here. Some underlying conditions that may lead to hemothorax include clotting defects, necrosis of lung tissue, cancer of the lung or within the pleura, central venous catheter placement, tuberculosis (TB), or surgery.

J94.8   Other specified pleural conditions

Hydropneumothorax is included in this code and is defined as the presence of both air (pneumothorax) and fluid other than blood (hydrothorax) in the pleural space. Hydrothorax without pneumothorax is also included here.

Intraoperative and Postprocedural Complications and Disorders of Respiratory System, Not Elsewhere Classified (J95)

ICD-10-CM groups all of the intraoperative and post-procedural complications into one block of codes that is located in each of the body system chapters. Located here are any complications of medical or surgical procedures performed on the respiratory system.

The categories in this code block are as follows:

J95		Intraoperative and postprocedural complications and disorders of respiratory system, not elsewhere classified
J95.-		Intraoperative and postprocedural complications and disorders of respiratory system, not elsewhere classified

Among the respiratory complications classified here are hemorrhage, hematoma, punctures, lacerations, and those related to tracheostomies. Postprocedure pneumothorax, pulmonary insufficiency and respiratory failure, ventilator associated pneumonia, and mechanical complications related to ventilation are also found in this category.

J95.0-   Tracheostomy complications

A tracheostomy is a surgically created artificial opening into the windpipe (trachea) with insertion of a tube to facilitate breathing. It can be a temporary stoma or permanent. Some of the complications that can occur are hemorrhage or infection of the site, tracheal stenosis, tracheo-esophageal fistula, and malfunction (mechanical) of the tubing, such as obstruction or displacement of tubing.

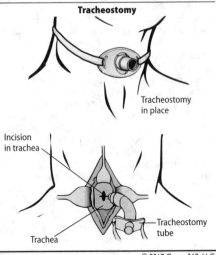

Tracheostomy

Tracheostomy in place

Incision in trachea

Trachea

Tracheostomy tube

J95.4 Chemical pneumonitis due to anesthesia

Also called Mendelson's syndrome, this condition is caused by the aspiration of gastric acids, blood, or bile during anesthesia and is thought to be precipitated by the absence of laryngeal reflexes. Symptoms include dyspnea, wheezing, tachycardia, tachypnea, and cyanosis.

Focus Point

Note that chemical pneumonitis due to anesthesia during obstetrical procedures is not coded in this chapter. It is located in Chapter 15 Pregnancy, Childbirth and the Puerperium.

J95.5 Postprocedural subglottic stenosis

Subglottic stenosis is defined as a narrowing of the trachea (windpipe), which causes shortness of breath, wheezing, and hoarseness. It occurs most often in patients who have been intubated or on a ventilator.

J95.811 Postprocedural pneumothorax

An iatrogenic pneumothorax occurs as the result of air being introduced into the pleural space or by incidental lung puncture during or following a medical or surgical procedure. Tension pneumothorax may also occur in patients receiving mechanical ventilation. In these cases, sedation may obscure the diagnosis that otherwise results in sudden deterioration of the patient's cardiorespiratory status.

J95.812 Postprocedural air leak

Occasionally, an air leak may persist following a chest tube insertion for the treatment of spontaneous pneumothorax. It is a minor condition that often resolves spontaneously and requires little or no intervention. In the event that intervention is required, the air leak may be repaired thoracoscopically, with pleurodesis, or in cases of persistent air leak, by insertion of endobronchial valves.

J95.82- Postprocedural respiratory failure

Postprocedural respiratory failure (PRF) is a complication that is associated with increased use of resources (e.g., mechanical ventilation, prolonged hospitalization) and mortality risk. The risk of PRF can be reduced, but not eliminated, through evidence-based interventions, such as preoperative smoking cessation and perioperative lung expansion exercises and increased postoperative monitoring. Patients at increased risk for serious pulmonary complications include those who undergo thoracic surgery, react adversely to anesthetics, suffer spinal cord or head trauma injuries, have chronic lung disease, are smokers, or are obese. In the immediate postoperative period, patients should be monitored for changes in respiratory status including cyanosis, shortness of breath, low oxygen saturation levels, and increased CO2 levels in the blood. Treatment includes increased supplemental oxygen and identification and management of underlying causal factors (i.e., infection, heart failure, chronic lung disease). Mechanical ventilation and respiratory support techniques assist in maintaining oxygenation and facilitate optimal lung function. Once stabilized, suctioning of the lungs and breathing exercises keep the airways cleared of obstruction throughout the patient's recovery.

J95.84 Transfusion-related acute lung injury (TRALI)

Transfusion related acute lung injury (TRALI) is a relatively rare, but serious, pulmonary complication of blood transfusion. The signs and symptoms that occur posttransfusion include acute respiratory distress, noncardiogenic pulmonary edema, cyanosis, hypoxemia, hypotension, fever, and chills. Onset usually occurs within one to two hours of transfusion, with rapid progression during four to six hours posttransfusion. White blood cell response to antigens leads to increased vascular permeability of the pulmonary microvasculature. This capillary injury results in pulmonary edema. Treatment involves stopping the transfusion followed by supportive measures. Most often, face-mask continuous positive airway pressure and added oxygen or ventilation with hemodynamic support are required. The vast majority of cases resolve within 96 hours if properly treated, often with complete resolution and little sequelae. Renal failure or other antibody-related organ damage has occurred in some cases.

Other Diseases of the Respiratory System (J96-J99)

This final block of codes for the respiratory system includes various conditions of different sites that do not fit into other classifications. Conditions of the lungs, bronchus, mediastinum, and diaphragm are included. Some of the diseases and disorders located in this code block are acute and chronic respiratory failure, acute bronchospasm, stenosis, ulcer or calcifications of the bronchus, pulmonary collapse, and emphysema not classified in other categories. Diseases of the mediastinum, such as fibrosis, hernia or mediastinitis, and diaphragm disorders, such as paralysis of diaphragm or diaphragmatitis, are also contained in this section.

The categories in this code block are as follows:

J96	Respiratory failure, not elsewhere classified
J98	Other respiratory disorders
J99	Respiratory disorders in diseases classified elsewhere

J96.- Respiratory failure, not elsewhere classified

Failure of the gas exchange function of oxygenation, carbon dioxide elimination, and/or ventilation that is severe enough to impair or threaten the functioning of vital organs constitutes respiratory failure. With failure of oxygenation, the tissues of the lung are not functioning properly. An example of failure of oxygenation would be an acute exacerbation of bronchial asthma in a patient with emphysema. With failure of ventilation, airflow in and out of the lungs is impaired, for example, by compression of the trachea caused by metastatic carcinoma of the thoracic lymph nodes. Respiratory failure is classified as hypoxemic or hypercapnic. Hypoxia is a reduction of adequate oxygen level in the blood typically characterized by oxygen lower than 60 mm Hg with normal or low arterial carbon dioxide. Hypercapnia is an abnormally high carbon dioxide level in the blood of over 50 mm Hg. It is common for people with hypercapnic respiratory failure to also be hypoxemic. Signs and symptoms of respiratory failure include headache, cyanosis, dyspnea, impaired motor function, restlessness, confusion, anxiety, delirium, and occasionally symptoms of depressed consciousness, tachypnea, tachycardia, and tremor. The subcategories in this category include a fourth character to indicate whether the respiratory failure is acute, chronic, or acute on chronic. The code is further defined by a fifth character that represents whether hypoxia or hypercapnia was present or unspecified.

Focus Point

If respiratory failure is documented with hypoxia and hypercapnia, separate codes are necessary to indicate that both are present.

J98.- Other respiratory disorders

Some diseases that do not fit well into other code categories, such as bronchospasm, pulmonary atelectasis and collapse, interstitial and compensatory emphysema, and other disorders of the lung and diaphragm are included here.

J98.01 Acute bronchospasm

Acute bronchospasm is an abnormal contraction of the smooth muscle of the bronchi, causing narrowing and obstruction of the airway. The physiology of a bronchospasm consists of an autonomic contraction of the pulmonary muscles, often coupled with inflammation of the pleura. The bronchus becomes constricted and the mucosa inflamed, which reduces the airway's diameter and restricts breathing. When the bronchial mucosa is irritated or inflamed, it produces sticky mucus that can also plug the bronchus and further restrict airflow.

J98.1- Pulmonary collapse

Pulmonary collapse is incomplete expansion of lobules (clusters of alveoli) or lung segments.

J98.11 Atelectasis

Atelectasis is partial or complete lung collapse, which impairs gas exchange, resulting in hypoxia. Atelectasis may be due to obstructions, such as mucous plugs, neoplasms and foreign bodies, or to external compression of the lungs from conditions such as pleural effusion, enlarged thoracic lymph nodes, or pneumothorax. Slowly developing or minor atelectasis may be asymptomatic. Signs and symptoms of more rapidly developing or massive atelectasis include decreased breath sounds, dull chest percussions, sudden dyspnea, cyanosis, hypotension, tachycardia, elevated temperature, peripheral circulatory collapse or shock, diaphoresis, and substernal or intercostal retraction.

J98.19 Other pulmonary collapse

Included in this subcategory is Brock's syndrome or right middle lobe syndrome (RMLS), a type of persistent atelectasis or collapse that occurs in the right middle lobe. One cause of RMLS is enlarged hilar lymph nodes or tumor compressing on the bronchus of the right middle lobe. Other cases most commonly seen in children have been associated with asthma, although the mechanism is unknown; likely contributors are mucus plugging, inflammation, and bronchospasm. Anatomical characteristics make this area of the lung more susceptible because of its narrow lobar bronchus diameter and acute drainage angles.

J98.2 Interstitial emphysema

Interstitial emphysema, also called mediastinal emphysema or Hamman's syndrome, is described as a condition of spontaneous, idiopathic pneumomediastinum with subcutaneous emphysema. It is usually mild and self-limiting with symptoms such as chest pain, dyspnea, and dysphonia and can often be detected by a phenomenon called Hamman's sign. Hamman's is an unusual rasping sound in the chest that is concurrent with the heartbeat. It is most often seen in young adults and peri- or postpartum women.

J98.3 Compensatory emphysema

Compensatory emphysema is a condition of overdistension of lung tissue into a void created when adjacent tissue was excised or damaged.

J98.51 Mediastinitis

Mediastinitis is an inflammation of the mediastinum, or chest cavity, which may be acute, occurring suddenly, or chronic, occurring after a long-term infection. Underlying causes are usually related to either a procedure requiring a median sternotomy (such as coronary artery bypass grafting) or a tear in the esophagus. The disorder is a life-threatening condition that carries an extremely high mortality if not recognized early and properly treated. Antibiotics are the first line of treatment, but surgical measures, such as withdrawing fluid from infected tissues, may be necessary in certain situations.

J98.59 Other diseases of mediastinum, not elsewhere classified

One of the conditions included here is fibrosis of the mediastinum, also called sclerosing mediastinitis, a rare condition caused by growth of collagen, fibrosis tissue, and inflammatory cells within the mediastinum. It can be idiopathic or a late effect of histoplasmosis. It is thought that the condition occurs when fungal antigens from lymph nodes in the mediastinum leak and cause a hypersensitive reaction, leading to a fibrotic response. Other potential precipitants include tuberculosis, radiation therapy to the area, or other infections.

J98.6 Disorders of diaphragm

Paralysis of the diaphragm is included in the code and can be unilateral or bilateral. Unilateral is usually asymptomatic and found incidentally on an x-ray and usually affects the left hemidiaphragm. Bilateral paralysis is symptomatic with dyspnea, rapid shallow breathing, and respiratory failure. Unilateral paralysis is most commonly caused by lung cancer with nerve compression while bilateral paralysis is usually caused by a motor neuron disease, such as muscular dystrophy or Guillain-Barre syndrome. Both are more common in men than women.

Chapter 11: Diseases of the Digestive System (K00-K95)

This chapter classifies diseases and disorders of the organs comprising the alimentary (digestive) tract, the long, muscular tube that begins at the mouth and ends at the anus. The major digestive organs include the pharynx, esophagus, stomach, and intestines. Supporting structures include the salivary and parotid glands, jaw, teeth, tongue, biliary tract, and peritoneum.

Accessory organs or structures that support the digestive process from outside this continuous tube are also included in this chapter: gallbladder, pancreas, and liver. These organs provide secretions that are critical to food absorption and use of nutrients by the body.

The digestive system is a group of organs that breaks down and changes food chemically for absorption as simple, soluble substances by blood, lymph systems, and body tissues. Digestion involves mechanical and chemical processes. Mechanical actions include chewing in the mouth, churning action in the stomach, and intestinal peristaltic action. These mechanical forces move the food through the digestive tract and mix it with secretions containing enzymes, which accomplish three chemical reactions: the conversion of carbohydrates to simple sugars, the breakdown of proteins into amino acids, and the conversion of fats into fatty acids and glycerol.

The stomach churns and mixes the food with hydrochloric acid and enzymes and gradually releases materials into the upper small intestine (the duodenum) through the pyloric sphincter. The majority of the digestive process occurs in the small intestine where most foods are hydrolyzed and absorbed. The products of digestion are actively or passively transported through the wall of the small intestine and assimilated into the body. The stomach and the large intestine (colon) can also absorb water, alcohol, certain salts and crystalloids, and some drugs. Water-soluble digestive products (minerals, amino acids, and carbohydrates) are transferred into the blood system and transported to the liver. Many fats, resynthesized in the intestinal wall, are picked up by the lymphatic system and enter the blood stream through the vena caval system, bypassing the liver. Remaining undigested matter is passed into the large intestine (the colon) where water is extracted. This solid mass (the stool) is propelled into the rectum, where it is held until excreted through the anus.

Diseases and disorders that interfere with this function, called functional disorders, are classified here, along with diseases and disorders that affect the organs of the digestive tract even when the condition has no direct effect on digestion. For example, dental caries have a direct effect on digestion because they interfere with mastication, the mechanical breakdown of food by chewing. Portal hypertension does not directly affect digestion, but is included in this chapter because it represents a disease of a digestive system organ. Portal hypertension would have no discernible effect on the digestive process until the disease has progressed to the point that the liver can no longer perform its function as a digestive organ.

In ICD-10-CM, conditions are organized into code blocks of related conditions or diseases.

The chapter is broken down into the following code blocks:

K00-K14	Diseases of oral cavity and salivary glands
K20-K31	Diseases of esophagus, stomach and duodenum
K35-K38	Diseases of appendix
K40-K46	Hernia
K50-K52	Noninfective enteritis and colitis
K55-K64	Other diseases of intestines
K65-K68	Diseases of peritoneum and retroperitoneum
K70-K77	Diseases of liver
K80-K87	Disorders of gallbladder, biliary tract and pancreas
K90-K95	Other diseases of the digestive system

Excluded from this chapter are codes pertaining to disorders and diseases of the jaw, such as temporomandibular joint disorders (TMJ), hyperplasia, and malocclusions of the maxillary and mandible. These conditions are classified in Chapter 13 Diseases of the Musculoskeletal System and Connective Tissue.

Diseases of the Oral Cavity and Salivary Glands (K00-K14)

This code block includes diseases and disorders of the jaw, salivary and parotid glands, teeth, gingiva and periodontium, lips, oral mucosa, and tongue.

The categories in this code block are as follows:

K00	Disorders of tooth development and eruption
K01	Embedded and impacted teeth
K02	Dental caries

K03	Other diseases of hard tissues of teeth
K04	Diseases of pulp and periapical tissues
K05	Gingivitis and periodontal diseases
K06	Other disorders of gingiva and edentulous alveolar ridge
K08	Other disorders of teeth and supporting structures
K09	Cysts of oral region, not elsewhere classified
K11	Diseases of salivary glands
K12	Stomatitis and related lesions
K13	Other diseases of lip and oral mucosa
K14	Diseases of tongue

K00.- Disorders of tooth development and eruption

This category includes disorders of tooth development and eruption in all patients regardless of age. It is one of the few categories in ICD-10-CM that classifies congenital anomalies and hereditary disturbances outside of Chapter 17 Congenital Malformations, Deformations, and Chromosomal Abnormalities.

Focus Point

Most conditions classified here relate to disorders of the development of teeth rather than trauma. Traumatic injuries to teeth and supporting structures may be more appropriately classified to the injury codes in Chapter 19.

K00.3 Mottled teeth

Mottled teeth refers to abnormalities in the color of the tooth enamel, such as white spots, dark lines, and frosted edges. One cause of mottled teeth is dental fluorosis, which is abnormalities in tooth enamel due to excessive amounts of fluoride in supplements, in drinking water, or in combination. Dental fluorosis can be particularly evident in communities with drinking water containing fluoride in amounts greater than two parts per million. The signs are whitish flecks or spots, particularly on the front teeth, or dark spots or stripes, and in more severe cases the enamel may become rough or pitted. Discoloration of enamel can also be due to other causes and diagnostic workup is required to determine the cause and proper treatment.

K02.- Dental caries

Dental caries are a demineralization of the tooth enamel caused by acids produced by bacteria, particularly *Streptococcus mutans*. The bacteria that cause caries are microflora and are present not only in the oral cavity but also in the gastrointestinal tract and other parts of the body. Variations in intraoral mechanical forces, such as chewing or grinding of the teeth, affect formation of bacteria and plaque on the teeth that can lead to dental caries. Other causes are

related to feeding behaviors, such as baby bottle tooth decay in infants. Craniofacial problems, neurologic abnormalities, or impaired cognitive abilities can interfere with proper dental care and also result in dental caries. Primary prevention measures include fluoride therapy, fissure-sealant therapy, dietary counseling, and oral-hygiene measures. Dental caries are classified by the surface type or by site and by the depth of the decay.

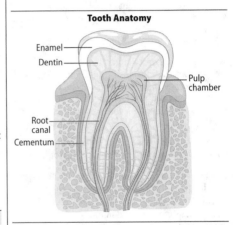

Tooth Anatomy

K02.5- Dental caries on pit and fissure surface

Pit and fissure decay begins in the narrow grooves on the top of the crown and the cheek side of the back teeth and progresses rapidly. Enamel and dentin comprise the hard tissues of the exposed portions of the teeth (above the root). Enamel is the hardest and outermost surface. The second layer and largest portion of the teeth is the dentin; although softer than enamel, it is still harder than bone. Pulp is a soft tissue lying below the dentin. Caries may be limited to the enamel or penetrate into the dentin or pulp.

K02.6- Dental caries on smooth surface

Smooth surface decay grows the slowest and begins as a white spot where bacteria are dissolving the calcium of the enamel. Enamel and dentin comprise the hard tissues of the exposed portions of the teeth (above the root). Enamel is the hardest and outermost surface. The second layer and largest portion of the teeth is the dentin; although softer than enamel, it is still harder than bone. Pulp is a soft tissue lying below the dentin. Caries may be limited to the enamel or penetrate into the dentin or pulp.

K02.7 Dental root caries

Root decay occurs in the cementum covering the root surface when gums have receded. Cementum is a hard tissue that covers the root of the tooth; it is harder than bone but not as hard as enamel or dentin.

K03.- Other diseases of hard tissues of teeth

Enamel, dentin, and cementum comprise the three hard tissues of the teeth. Enamel is the hardest and outermost surface and is formed by ameloblasts. It allows the tooth to withstand chewing pressure and temperature changes. Once formed, enamel cannot regrow or repair; however, it can regain minerals and halt decay or dental caries. The second layer and largest portion is the dentin, which is made from odontoblasts; although softer than enamel, it is still harder than bone. It contains tubules of dentinal fibers that can transfer not only pain, but nutrition throughout the tooth. Finally, the last hard tissue is the cementum, which covers the root of the tooth and is also harder than bone but not as hard as enamel or dentin. The codes in this category affect these hard surfaces.

K03.0 Excessive attrition of teeth

Attrition is the normal wearing away of the substance or structure of the teeth through regular use. Excessive attrition indicates that the substance or structure of the teeth is wearing away faster than would be expected based on the patient's age and general health status.

K03.1 Abrasion of teeth

Abrasion is wearing away of a tooth through an unnatural mechanical process such as brushing too hard or improperly or using the teeth for purposes other than chewing (e.g., holding or biting hard objects, and tongue jewelry that hits the teeth).

K03.2 Erosion of teeth

Erosion is a progressive eating away or destruction of the hard substance of a tooth by a chemical, not bacterial, process. Some examples include drinking too many carbonated beverages or high acid fruit juices. Erosion can also be caused by gastroesophageal reflux disease (GERD) or the eating disorders anorexia and bulimia.

K03.3 Pathological resorption of teeth

Pathological resorption occurs when calcified tissue of the root is lost from the tooth through an absorption and removal process happening within the cementum and dentin, into the root canal. This condition may be triggered by occlusive trauma and disease, such as neoplastic activity. Internal resorption is an unusual form of pathological resorption that begins in the center of the tooth, with inflamed and hyperplastic pulp tissue filling the resorbed central area and showing pink through the crown of the tooth.

K03.81 Cracked tooth

A cracked tooth is characterized by a break or opening that extends from the chewing surface of the tooth vertically toward the root but does not completely divide the tooth into two segments. There are multiple types of cracked teeth. Treatment and outcome depend largely on the type, location, and extent of the crack. Root canal therapy is often required to treat the injured pulp, and a crown is placed to hold and protect the cracked tooth. If the crack extends below the gingival tissue line, extraction is required.

K04.- Diseases of pulp and periapical tissues

The center of the tooth and its soft tissues are known as the pulp. The pulp extends from the bottom of the crown to the bottom of the root and is made up of blood vessels that carry oxygen and nutrients back and forth from the heart. Nerves lining the pulp respond to heat, cold, and pressure.

K04.0- Pulpitis

Comprising living cells and connective tissue, the pulp is situated in the center of the tooth below the dentin. Inflammation of the dental pulp, pulpitis, is a consequence of damage to the dentin. Trauma, cavities, and repetitive dental repair are the primary etiologies, with tooth pain the most prominent symptom. Reversibility of the condition largely depends on whether necrosis and/or infection are present.

K04.01 Reversible pulpitis

Pain is minor with reversible pulpitis typically experienced only when some sort of stimulus, such as something sweet or cold, is applied. The pain is precise and the affected tooth easily identified. The tooth can be saved often simply by filling a cavity or through other minor restoration procedures.

K04.02 Irreversible pulpitis

Irreversible pulpitis occurs when there is inadequate circulation to the pulp and the pulp begins to necrose. Pain experienced is excruciating, often radiating beyond the affected tooth, so much so that it is hard for the patient to precisely identify the culprit tooth. In addition to necrosing, the tooth may be more easily susceptible to infection, which can further tooth damage as well as lead to abscess formation. Treatment options for irreversible pulpitis include root canal or extraction.

K04.1 Necrosis of pulp

Necrosis of dental pulp is a condition in which the pulp has been killed by acute or chronic inflammation; because the pulp is dead, pulp extirpation or tooth extraction is necessary.

K04.4 Acute apical periodontitis of pulpal origin

Acute apical periodontitis is severe inflammation of the periodontal ligament, resulting from inflammation or necrosis of the pulp. Signs and symptoms include swollen and red gums that may drain thick purulent material. There is sensitivity of the teeth to hot or cold, possible fever, and swollen glands of the neck.

Throbbing pain that radiates along the jaw may also be present. In severe cases, a swollen area of the jaw may also be present. Biting or closing the mouth tightly also increases pain.

K04.6   Periapical abscess with sinus

K04.7   Periapical abscess without sinus

Periapical tissue surrounds the base of the tooth. A periapical abscess is an infection of the pulp and periapical tissue. The presence of an abscess, which is a collection of pus, requires immediate dental attention and antibiotics to control the infection. Treatment may include a root canal or, in extreme cases, an apicoectomy to drain the abscess prior to a root canal. This condition may occur with or without a sinus. A sinus, also called a fistula, is an abnormal opening connecting one structure with another. In this case, the sinus connects underlying dental structures or the alveolar process to the oral mucosa, which allows the abscess to drain.

K05.-   Gingivitis and periodontal diseases

Gingival and periodontal diseases include acute and chronic gingivitis and acute and chronic periodontitis. There may be no symptoms in the early stages of gingivitis. Signs and symptoms of advanced gingivitis and periodontitis include blood on the tooth brush when brushing the teeth, swollen and red gums, tenderness when the gums are touched, pus around the teeth, bad taste in the mouth, and visible deposits of tartar or calculus on the teeth.

K05.0-   Acute gingivitis

Acute gingivitis, an inflammation of the gums, has a sudden onset, is of short duration, and is painful.

K05.00   Acute gingivitis, plaque induced

Acute gingivitis, characterized by inflammation and pain, is often attributed to plaque. Plaque is a soft, sticky substance containing millions of microorganisms that adheres to the teeth. If gingivitis remains untreated, progression to periodontitis is possible.

> **Focus Point**
>
> *Diabetes, leukemia, or other systemic diseases can aggravate plaque-associated gingivitis. Endocrine changes such as puberty or pregnancy; medications such as nifedipine, cyclosporin, and phenytoin; and malnutrition or vitamin C deficiency may also exacerbate gingivitis.*

K05.01   Acute gingivitis, non-plaque induced

Non-plaque-induced acute gingivitis can be the result of bacterial pathogens such as *Neisseria gonorrhoeae* or viral or fungal infections; mucocutaneous disorders such as lichen planus or pemphigoid; allergic reactions to restorative substances, toothpaste, or chewing gum; or physical, chemical, or thermal trauma. Underlying factors also include genetic disorders, such as hereditary gingival fibromatosis.

K05.1-   Chronic gingivitis

Chronic gingivitis has a slower onset than the acute condition, a longer duration, and is often painless.

K05.10   Chronic gingivitis, plaque induced

Chronic gingivitis, characterized by prolonged inflammation of the gums, is often attributed to plaque. Plaque is a soft, sticky substance containing millions of bacteria that adheres to the teeth.

K05.11   Chronic gingivitis, non-plaque induced

Causes of non-plaque induced chronic gingivitis include underlying illnesses and certain medications that make a person more susceptible to the development of gingivitis. Chronic conditions that predispose a person to chronic gingivitis include diabetes, Addison's disease, HIV, other conditions affecting the immune system, and Sjogren's syndrome. Long-term use of steroids also predisposes a person to chronic gingivitis as do antiepileptic drugs, high blood pressure medications, and drugs that suppress the immune system such as those used to prevent organ rejection in organ transplant recipients.

K05.2-   Aggressive periodontitis

The soft tissue lining the mouth and surrounding the teeth is known as the gingiva or gums. Healthy gums protect the portion of the tooth that lies below the gum line. When proper oral hygiene is not practiced, plaque and bacteria can accumulate below the gums, leading to gingival and/or periodontal disease. Periodontitis is an advanced stage of gingival inflammation that can lead to bone loss, periodontal pockets, tooth migration, and eventually tooth loss.

The aggressive form of periodontitis is characterized by an early age at onset, often at or before puberty, although it has been seen in older adults. The disease progresses rapidly, involving multiple teeth, and periodontal tissue loss out of proportion to the amount of plaque observed. There are two forms of the disease: localized and generalized. Localized is defined as less than 30 percent tooth involvement and generalized as greater than or equal to 30 percent tooth involvement. Both are frequently associated with the periodontal pathogen *Actinobacillus actinomycetemcomitans*. Severity is also a part of the classification and is determined by the amount of clinical attachment loss (CAL), which is designated as slight (1 to 2 mm CAL), moderate (3 to 4 CAL), or severe (>5 mm CAL).

K05.3-   Chronic periodontitis

The term chronic periodontitis signifies the progression of the inflammatory disease of the body and ligamentous supporting tissues of the teeth over time as a result of failure to treat the disease in the acute stage. This does not mean that the disease is untreatable, but patients with severe and widespread chronic periodontitis have a high risk for tooth loss. The chronic condition typically progresses slowly, although there may be spurts of destruction. The disease progression rate is also influenced by local factors, systemic diseases, and extrinsic factors such as smoking. Chronic periodontitis is further classified as localized or generalized depending on the extent of the disease, which is based on the percentage of sites involved, with localized defined as less than 30 percent involvement and generalized as greater than or equal to 30 percent. Severity is determined by the amount of clinical attachment loss (CAL) and is designated as slight (1 to 2 mm CAL), moderate (3 to 4 mm CAL), or severe (>5 mm CAL).

K06.-   Other disorders of gingiva and edentulous alveolar ridge

This category includes diseases of the soft tissue lining of the mouth (gingiva), to which the teeth are attached. The alveolar ridge is a column of bone in the mouth that surrounds and anchors the teeth; when described as edentulous, the teeth are absent.

K06.0-   Gingival recession

Gingival recession involves the progressive loss of gum tissue with the gums receding back, potentially exposing the roots of the teeth. For a diagnosis of gingival recession, there are two elements required. The first is whether recession is generalized (multiple teeth in an area that require treatment), or localized (limited to individual teeth in an area of the mouth). The second element is the degree of recession, which is indicated by minimal, moderate, or severe. The most common causes of gingival recession are overaggressive brushing, whitening toothpastes that contain abrasives, orthodontics and tooth position, poor oral hygiene, and chewing tobacco.

K06.01-   Gingival recession, localized

This subcategory includes localized (<30%) gingival recession limited to individual teeth in an area of the mouth often related to plaque or even trauma. Unique codes in this subcategory specify the degree of recession, which is indicated by minimal, moderate, or severe.

K06.02-   Gingival recession, generalized

This subcategory includes generalized (>30%) gingival recession affecting multiple teeth in an area that require treatment, and is often due to poor oral hygiene and/or untreated periodontal disease. Unique codes in this subcategory specify the degree of recession, which is indicated by minimal, moderate, or severe.

K06.3   Horizontal alveolar bone loss

Between vertical and horizontal bone loss, horizontal is the most common type encountered in periodontal disease. In horizontal alveolar bone loss, the bone loss is perpendicular to the vertical axis of the tooth with the height of the bone in relation to the tooth uniformly decreased, due to a somewhat even degree of bone resorption. This condition typically occurs with chronic generalized periodontitis.

K08.-   Other disorders of teeth and supporting structures

This category covers an assortment of disorders including exfoliation or premature loss of teeth. These conditions may result from a systemic disease that affects the immune system or connective tissue such as neutropenia, HIV, or diabetes among many others. This category also contains codes for loss of teeth, jaw atrophy, complications of tooth restoration, and retained dental root.

K08.1-   Complete loss of teeth

Complete loss of teeth, also called complete edentulism, is divided into four classes, defined by the level of difficulty or complexity in treatment. Class IV is the most debilitating, requiring reconstructive surgery when all teeth are missing. Treatment is primarily prosthodontic in nature with missing teeth or adjacent structures being restored or replaced with artificial, biocompatible substitutes. Tooth loss can be due to a variety of causes. Congenital conditions such as Papillon Lefèvre syndrome, systemic conditions such as Langerhans cell histiocytosis, loss of supporting structures, trauma, periodontal disease, and dental caries are some conditions that may be responsible for loss of teeth. Tooth loss is classified by etiology (cause), which includes trauma, periodontal disease, caries, or other cause, and by severity, which ranges from Class I to Class IV.

Focus Point

Papillion-Lefèvre syndrome is a genetic disorder caused by a deficiency in the cathepsin C enzyme and is characterized by the severe destruction of periodontium, resulting in the loss of all primary and permanent teeth by age 14.

Langerhans cell histiocytosis, also known as Hand-Schüller-Christian disease or histiocytosis X, is a set of closely related disorders characterized by proliferation of Langerhans cells (epidermal dendritic cells).

K08.2- Atrophy of edentulous alveolar ridge

The alveolar ridge, also called the alveolar process, is a ridge of bone just behind the teeth on the upper (maxilla) and lower (mandible) jawbones that forms the root cavities or sockets for the teeth. Edentulous ridges have lost the teeth that were once held in those sockets. Atrophy presents as a wasting and shrinking of the size of the alveolar ridge that previously held the teeth. Severe atrophy may present as small, knife-like edges along the alveolar ridge with a sunken appearance to the mouth and lips, leaving a protruding chin, especially with anterior atrophy of the maxilla and mandible. Severe forms require oral maxillofacial surgery to reconstruct the maxilla and/or mandible. Bone grafts may be used for ridge augmentation, along with placement orthopedic bone plates, reconstruction of the vestibule of the mouth, and complete dentures. This condition is classified by site and severity of the atrophy.

K08.4- Partial loss of teeth

Partial loss of teeth, also called partial edentulism, is the loss of one or several teeth. Edentulism is divided into four classes, defined by how compromised the presenting diagnostic criteria are in partial edentulism. Class IV is the most debilitating and in partial tooth loss refers to the most severely compromised oral manifestations with poor outcome prognosis. Treatment is primarily prosthodontic in nature with missing teeth or adjacent structures being restored or replaced with artificial, biocompatible substitutes. Tooth loss is classified by etiology (cause), which includes trauma, periodontal disease, caries, or other cause, and by severity, which ranges from Class I to Class IV.

K08.5- Unsatisfactory restoration of tooth

Restorations are defined as materials or methods used to replace lost teeth or tooth structure, such as fillings, inlays, onlays, crowns, bridges, or complete or partial dentures. Dental restorative materials used include amalgam, composite resin, silicate, acrylic, synthetic, and plastic. These methods are not permanent and may suffer failure over time. The restoration may develop recurrent cavities, become defective due to marginal breakdown, undergo corrosion or discoloration, fracture, and partially or completely fall out. Unsatisfactory restoration may also damage the remaining tooth structure surrounding the restoration, which may fracture or cause other injury to the tooth.

K08.51 Open restoration margins of tooth

Restoration problems may appear as open margins surrounding restoration sites, causing an increased potential for plaque retention and gingival inflammation.

K08.52 Unrepairable overhanging of dental restorative materials

Overhanging restorative materials extend beyond the region of the tooth or cavity preparation site. An unrepairable overhanging of dental restorative materials promotes plaque accumulation and causes nondestructive subgingival flora to become destructive. When the overhanging material cannot be reconfigured, the entire restoration must be removed to prevent complications such as bleeding, gingivitis, and loss of bone density in the region around the overhanging dental restorative materials. Any conditions resulting from the overhanging materials, such as periodontitis, must be treated in addition to correcting the restoration.

K08.53- Fractured dental restorative material

Fracturing of dental restorative materials occurs when the restoration fissures, cracks, or breaks. Fractured dental restorative material allows bacterial entry, resulting in pulp and periapical disease. Fracturing is classified based on whether there is loss of the restorative material along with the fracture.

K08.54 Contour of existing restoration of tooth biologically incompatible with oral health

Tooth restoration requires matching of the diseased tooth contour with that of the restored tooth contour. This includes matching size, shape, and height, as well as ridges and depressions in the native tooth. When the restoration does not match the contour of the native tooth it can affect the alignment and health of the remaining teeth, as well as the underlying structures. Restoration resulting in biologically incompatible contours, known as unacceptable morphology, can lead to development of chronic dental lesions and bone loss.

K08.56 Poor aesthetic of existing restoration of tooth

Restoration of the teeth also requires matching of the color and other features of the native teeth. Poor aesthetics refers to restoration resulting in an undesirable appearance of the restored tooth.

K08.8- Other specified disorders of teeth and supporting structures

This residual subcategory contains disorders not found elsewhere but that still relate to teeth and their supporting structures. Specific conditions captured in this subcategory include unspecified enlargement of alveolar ridge, irregular alveolar process, and toothache NOS.

K08.81 Primary occlusal trauma

Excessive forces on the teeth may cause chips, stress cracks, and significant signs of wear that alter the patient's bite (occlusion). In primary occlusal trauma, this is caused by excessively heavy biting forces exerted by the patient and causing damage to otherwise normal tooth structures. There is no secondary disease-related cause. Culprit biting habits can include excessive chewing on inanimate objects such as ice, fingernails, or pens or bruxism (teeth grinding or jaw clenching).

K08.82 Secondary occlusal trauma

When there is some periodontal attachment loss and when once-tolerated biting forces are now too excessive for the damaged tooth structures to withstand, secondary occlusal trauma can occur. The weakened condition of the periodontal attachments put the teeth at risk for trauma from forces that would typically not be problematic.

K11.- Diseases of salivary glands

The major salivary glands are paired glands that secrete a predominantly alkaline fluid that moistens the mouth, softens food, and aids in digestion. The three major salivary glands include the submandibular glands located under the lower jaw, the sublingual glands beneath the tongue, and the parotid glands in front of each ear. Saliva is antimicrobial and works against a host of bacteria associated with oral and systemic diseases. Large salivary mucins are antiviral as are cystatin that are active against herpes viruses. Saliva also contains histatin, anti-fungal proteins that are potent inhibitors of candida, which is normally kept in check at extremely low levels in the mouth. The sublingual glands secrete the enzyme lysozyme, which destroys bacterial invasion by degrading bacterial membranes, inhibiting the growth and metabolism of certain bacteria, and disrupting bacterial enzyme systems. The saliva of the parotid gland contains the enzyme amylase that aids in the digestion of carbohydrates. In addition to these glands, there are hundreds of minor saliva glands in the lips, inner cheek area (buccal mucosa), and in other linings of the mouth and throat.

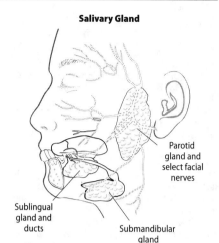

Salivary Gland

Parotid gland and select facial nerves

Sublingual gland and ducts

Submandibular gland

K11.0 Atrophy of salivary gland

Atrophy is a wasting away or death of salivary gland tissue.

K11.1 Hypertrophy of salivary gland

Hypertrophy is overgrowth or overdevelopment of tissue of the salivary glands.

K11.2- Sialoadenitis

If the flow of saliva from a salivary gland is reduced or obstructed bacteria starts to grow. The bacteria cause an infection that results in inflammation of the salivary gland known as sialoadenitis. The infection is often the result of dehydration with overgrowth of the oral flora. Sialoadenitis occurs most often in the parotid and submandibular glands. It may be caused by *Staphylococcus aureus*, *Streptococcus viridans*, *Haemophilus influenzae*, *Streptococcus pyogenes*, or *Escherichia coli*. Signs and symptoms include difficulty opening the mouth or swallowing, erythema, fever, malaise, and pain. Treatment includes antibiotics and increased fluids that in turn increase saliva production and decrease swelling. Sialoadenitis is classified as acute, acute recurrent, chronic, or unspecified.

K11.3 Abscess of salivary gland

Abscess of a salivary gland, characterized by a collection of pus in the salivary gland and surrounding tissues, is a complication of a salivary gland infection. The abscess is caused by a bacterial infection such as *Staphylococcus aureus*, *Streptococcus viridans*, *Haemophilus influenzae*, *Streptococcus pyogenes*, or *Escherichia coli*. Treatment requires incision and drainage of the abscess and administration of antibiotics.

Chapter 11: Diseases of the Digestive System (K00-K95)

Focus Point

Any infection of the submandibular gland can cause a submandibular abscess, a serious condition with the potential to expand to the deep spaces of the neck. In rare cases, continued progression of infection can lead to a life-threatening infection of the submental and sublingual spaces.

K11.5   Sialolithiasis

Sialolithiasis is the formation or presence of a salivary calculus, which occurs when the chemicals in saliva crystallize into a solid concretion that blocks the salivary ducts. This results in pain and swelling of the gland. Salivary calculi account for more than 50 percent of major salivary gland diseases and are the most common cause of acute and chronic salivary gland infections. Signs and symptoms include difficulty opening the mouth or swallowing, erythema, fever, malaise, and pain. Treatment involves removing the calculus and administration of antibiotics for the infection.

K12.-   Stomatitis and related lesions

Stomatitis is any inflammatory condition of the oral mucosa and may include oral tissue infections or inflammatory conditions of the periodontium, dentition, or periapicals. Oral mucositis is a form of stomatitis and typically presents as redness or ulcerations. Treatment of stomatitis varies, depending on the underlying cause. An infectious or systemic cause can often be treated with medication. Correction of underlying vitamin B12, iron, or folate deficiencies is indicated for chronic problems with aphthous stomatitis. Medication can also be applied to oral canker sores.

K12.3-   Oral mucositis (ulcerative)

Oral mucosal inflammation, or mucositis, affects the tissues that line the mouth. Mild cases of mucositis may respond to topical pain relief medication such as gels or creams. Analgesics such as acetaminophen may be helpful for relieving moderate pain, and severe pain may require stronger oral or injectable pain medications. Symptom improvement may also be obtained with allopurinol or vitamin E.

K12.31   Oral mucositis (ulcerative) due to antineoplastic therapy

Oral mucositis is a frequent, debilitating complication of antineoplastic therapy, caused by chemotherapy. It occurs when the epithelial cells lining the mouth, throat, esophagus, stomach, and small and large intestines break down, leaving the mucosal tissue susceptible to infection and ulceration. Manifestations can include ulcers in the soft tissues of mucosal surfaces throughout the body, particularly the mouth. Oral mucositis occurs in 20 percent to 40 percent of patients treated solely with chemotherapy. In patients receiving combination chemotherapy and radiation therapy, particularly those with head and neck cancer, the occurrence rate increases to up to 50 percent.

Focus Point

Since the ability of cells to reproduce is affected by antineoplastic therapy, healing of the oral mucosa is slowed, leaving the patient more susceptible to opportunistic mouth infections. Damaged mucosa is a point of entry for bacteria and fungi, and mucositis is also associated with febrile neutropenia.

K12.33   Oral mucositis (ulcerative) due to radiation

A frequent, debilitating complication of radiation treatment, oral mucositis occurs when the epithelial cells lining the mouth break down, leaving the mucosal tissue susceptible to infection. Manifestations include inflammation and ulcers in the soft tissues of mucosal surfaces.

K13.-   Other diseases of lip and oral mucosa

This category includes lip diseases, cheek and lip biting, leukoplakia, granuloma lesions of oral mucosa, fibrosis of oral submucosa, and hyperplasia of oral mucosa.

Focus Point

Cancrum oris, a gangrenous, ulcerative inflammatory lesion of mouth, is caused by an infection and is classified in Chapter 1 Certain Infectious and Parasitic Diseases.

K13.0   Diseases of lips

A number of conditions affecting the lips are classified here, including cheilitis. Cheilitis is an inflammation of the lips, most commonly of the lower lip, that typically affects young children and babies but can occur in all ages. Causes are infections, allergic reaction, or photosensitivity. Inflammation may involve the sides of the lips where the upper and lower lips join and is called angular cheilitis. Angular cheilitis is characterized by fissures that can cause pain and bleeding. Cheilitis glandularis (glandular cheilitis) is characterized by enlargement and eversion of the lower lip that exposes the underlying mucosa. When this occurs, the delicate mucosal tissue dries out leading to erosion, crusting, ulceration, and, in some cases, infection. Cellulitis of lips is also captured with this code.

K13.21 Leukoplakia of oral mucosa, including tongue

Leukoplakia is one or more benign, firm, white patches that form in the inside of the mouth, including cheeks and tongue. Although usually not dangerous, some cancers have been seen occurring next to these patches. The cause of them is unknown, although the condition appears more often with smokers.

K13.22 Minimal keratinized residual ridge mucosa

K13.23 Excessive keratinized residual ridge mucosa

Keratinized tissue is made up of keratin, the main protein constituent in the epidermis, hair, and nails. Soft keratin is found in epithelial tissue. Healthy attached keratinized mucosa that presents in an even thickness on residual ridge gingiva in the edentulous patient is ideal for denture stability, because dentures rely on the residual alveolar ridge and oral mucosa for support and retention. However, sometimes the keratinized epithelium present on a residual ridge is in excess. In these cases, the amount of tissue must be decreased before restorative measures can be carried out. This condition is classified based on the amount of keratinized residual ridge mucosa, which is differentiated as minimal or excessive.

K14.- Diseases of tongue

This category contains codes defining an assortment of maladies affecting the tongue, including abscesses, ulcerations, black hairy tongue, fissured tongue, tongue pain, and other ailments.

K14.1 Geographic tongue

Geographic tongue is a common and harmless condition in which one or more irregularly shaped patches appear on the tongue in a design that may resemble a map of a country. The center area is redder than the rest of the tongue and the edges of the patch are whitish in color. The etiology is unknown, although a viral infection is assumed, and it may be associated with a variety of inflammatory or allergic conditions as well. Geographic tongue often goes away without treatment, but can be treated with topical steroids.

K14.3 Hypertrophy of tongue papillae

Black hairy tongue is classified here. It is characterized by dark discolored areas on the surface of the tongue. The discoloration is caused by trapping of pigment and bacteria by the filiform papillae that cover the top surface of the tongue.

Diseases of the Esophagus, Stomach, and Duodenum (K20-K31)

This category includes diseases and disorders of the esophagus, a muscular, tubular structure that serves as a conduit for the passage of food and water from the pharynx to the stomach. Transportation of food and fluids from the mouth to the stomach is accomplished by a combination of gravity and peristaltic waves in the esophagus. The esophagus is equipped with two sphincters. The first is the pharyngeal-esophageal sphincter located at the level of the cricoid cartilage; the second is the gastroesophageal sphincter (also known as the lower esophageal sphincter) located at the level of the esophageal hiatus of the diaphragm.

As food is eaten, it passes from the mouth through the esophagus and to the stomach. Acids in the stomach break down the food. These acids are prevented from entering the esophagus by the lower esophageal sphincter. The contractile activity of the stomach helps to mix, grind, and evacuate small portions of chyme into the small bowel, while the rest of the chyme is mixed and ground. Anatomically, the stomach can be divided into three major regions: fundus (the most proximal), corpus, and antrum. One of the primary critical functions of the stomach is to store partially digested food that is then churned, mixed, and moved into the duodenum. In addition, the stomach is a secretory organ that secretes gastric juices and an intrinsic factor necessary for the absorption of vitamin B12. The stomach also absorbs some drugs, water, alcohol, and lactic fatty acids; produces gastrin hormone for digestive regulation; and helps destroy swallowed pathogenic bacteria.

The categories in this code block are as follows:

K20	Esophagitis
K21	Gastro-esophageal reflux disease
K22	Other diseases of esophagus
K23	Disorders of esophagus in diseases classified elsewhere
K25	Gastric ulcer
K26	Duodenal ulcer
K27	Peptic ulcer, site unspecified
K28	Gastrojejunal ulcer
K29	Gastritis and duodenitis
K30	Functional dyspepsia
K31	Other diseases of stomach and duodenum

K20.- Esophagitis

Esophagitis is an inflammation and swelling of the esophagus that is often very painful. Symptoms usually resolve quickly once the cause has been eliminated.

K20.0 Eosinophilic esophagitis

Eosinophilic esophagitis is an inflammation (often severe) of the esophagus that affects the ability to swallow. In children, this often results in malnutrition and failure to thrive. Eosinophilic esophagitis selectively affects the lining of the esophagus. It is characterized by the accumulation of eosinophil cells in the esophageal tissue, causing inflammation. In eosinophilic esophagitis, eosinophil accumulation occurs in the absence of known causes for eosinophilia (e.g., allergies, drug reactions, parasitic infection, connective tissue disease, or malignancy).

Focus Point

Eosinophilic gastrointestinal disorders (EGID) can selectively affect any region of the gastrointestinal tract resulting in the accumulation of eosinophil cells in the lining of the affected region, which causes inflammation.

K20.8 Other esophagitis

Other esophagitis includes inflammation and swelling of the esophagus due to an infection that has resulted in abscess formation.

K20.9 Esophagitis, unspecified

This code includes infectional, chemical, peptic, necrotic, alkaline, chronic, and postoperative esophagitis. Esophagitis due to infection is relatively rare.

Focus Point

Chemical esophagitis should not be confused with a chemical corrosive burn of the esophagus. A chemical burn, classified as corrosion, is caused by ingestion and regurgitation of caustic liquids or solids and is reported with code T28.6- Corrosion of esophagus. Corrosive burns of the esophagus vary in severity and may manifest with sloughing of the mucous membrane, edema, and inflammation of the submucosa, thrombosis of the esophageal vessels, perforation, and mediastinitis. Caustic agents that result in corrosive burns can cause severe tissue damage and may constitute a medical emergency depending on the strength of the chemical and the length of time the chemical remains in the esophagus.

K21.- Gastro-esophageal reflux disease

Normally, the gastroesophageal sphincter prevents the reflux of gastric juice into the esophagus, but a variety of conditions can compromise sphincter function leading to gastroesophageal reflux disease, also called GERD. GERD may occur with or without esophagitis.

Esophagitis due to GERD may be called reflux or regurgitant esophagitis, and is the most common form of esophagitis. It is caused by reflux of acid and pepsin from the stomach into the esophagus. Signs and symptoms of GERD with esophagitis include heartburn after eating or while resting in a recumbent position, chest pain sometimes masquerading as angina pectoris, regurgitation (water brash), and dysphagia due to inflammatory edema or stricture in the distal esophagus. GERD without esophagitis sometimes occurs, most often at night and may be asymptomatic.

Focus Point

Hiatal hernia is an underlying cause of sphincter incompetence and gastroesophageal reflux disease. Other causes are pregnancy, certain drugs (e.g., anticholinergic agents, calcium channel blockers, beta-adrenergic agonists), scleroderma, obesity, placement of nasogastric tubes, and surgical vagotomy.

K22.- Other diseases of esophagus

A variety of other diseases of the esophagus are classified here, including ulcer, obstruction, perforation, esophageal spasm, as well as others.

K22.0 Achalasia of cardia

Achalasia is a neuromuscular disorder characterized by an absence of peristalsis, dilation of the body of the esophagus, and a conically narrowed cardioesophageal junction. The dominant symptom is difficulty swallowing (dysphagia).

Focus Point

Achalasia of cardia, also referred to as cardiospasm, should not be confused with diffuse esophageal spasm. Cardiospasm refers to a reflex spasm in the cardia of the stomach that is the result of the narrowing of the cardioesophageal junction. Diffuse esophageal spasm, classified as dyskinesia of the esophagus and reported with code K22.4, is a generalized spasm of the entire esophagus.

K22.4 Dyskinesia of esophagus

Dyskinesia of the esophagus is a generalized spasm of the esophagus caused by contractions throughout the length of the esophagus that are uncoordinated, simultaneous, and/or extremely rapid rather than the coordinated, sequential contractions seen in normal esophageal peristalsis.

K22.5 Diverticulum of esophagus, acquired

A diverticulum is a pouch that protrudes outward, in this case from the esophageal lining. The most common type is Zenker's diverticula, which is located at the back of the throat (pharyngoesophageal). This type occurs most often in the elderly, growing slowly and eventually causing dysphagia, regurgitation, and aspiration pneumonia. Other sites where esophageal diverticula occur include midthoracic (mid-chest) and epiphrenic (above the diagram) regions.

K22.6   Gastro-esophageal laceration-hemorrhage syndrome

Gastroesophageal laceration-hemorrhage syndrome refers to a vertical tear of the esophagus or cardioesophageal junction. More commonly known as Mallory-Weiss syndrome, this condition follows prolonged or forceful vomiting.

K22.7-   Barrett's esophagus

Barrett's esophagus is a condition that develops in some people who have chronic gastroesophageal reflux disease (GERD) and inflammation of the esophagus (esophagitis). The chronic exposure of the cells in the lower esophagus to gastric acid damages the normal squamous cells that line the esophagus. The damaged squamous cells are then replaced by columnar cells, which is a process known as metaplasia. Barrett's esophagus is a kind of metaplasia. The metaplastic columnar lining comes in three types: two types are comparable to groups of cells found in regions of the stomach lining and the third type is comparable to groups of cells found in the small intestine. This intestinal type of metaplasia is important because it can potentially lead to the development of cancer. The cells of Barrett's esophagus are classified into four general categories: nondysplastic, low-grade dysplasia, high-grade dysplasia, and frank carcinoma.

K22.70   Barrett's esophagus without dysplasia

In nondysplastic Barrett's esophagus, the tissue does not exhibit features indicative of precancerous changes. The nondysplastic type still requires annual observation with endoscopy.

K22.71-   Barrett's esophagus with dysplasia

Dysplasia is defined as abnormal tissue development and is the earliest form of precancerous lesion recognizable in a biopsy. Low-grade patients are generally advised to undergo annual observation with endoscopy. In high-grade dysplasia, the risk of developing cancer might be at 10 percent or greater per patient-year. High-grade dysplasia patients are generally advised to undergo surgical treatment. Barrett's dysplasia is classified based on the severity or grade of the dysplasia.

K25.-   Gastric ulcer

Gastric ulcers result from discreet tissue destruction within the lumen of the stomach. The destruction is due to the action of hydrochloric (gastric) acid and pepsin on areas of gastric mucosa having a decreased resistance to ulceration. Gastric ulcers often result from an infection with *Helicobacter pylori* or the use of nonsteroidal antiinflammatory drugs (NSAID). Signs and symptoms of gastric ulcer include pain exacerbated by eating, weight loss, repeated vomiting (which is a sign of possible gastric outlet obstruction), vomiting of frank red blood or "coffee ground" material, and black, tarry, or heme positive stools if the ulcer is bleeding. A breath test is often performed to detect the presence of *Helicobacter pylori*. The combination codes contained in this category indicate whether the ulcer is acute or chronic and identify the presence or absence of hemorrhage and/or perforation. The most common ulcer complication is gastrointestinal bleeding or hemorrhage, which occurs when the ulcerated tissue of the organ grows so thin that the gastric acids begin to erode the GI blood vessels. Perforation occurs when the ulcer erodes the wall of the gastrointestinal organ, potentially spilling the stomach or intestinal contents into the abdominal cavity. Further complications from the spillage can lead to more serious conditions, such as peritonitis and pancreatitis.

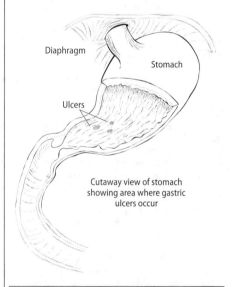

Diaphragm

Stomach

Ulcers

Cutaway view of stomach showing area where gastric ulcers occur

---

Focus Point

Associated conditions include acute and/or chronic blood loss anemia and gastric outlet obstruction. Gastric outlet obstruction is no longer included as a complication within the ulcer code sets. According to the Alphabetic Index, K31.1 Adult hypertrophic pyloric stenosis, is the appropriate code for this condition and would be coded separately.

K26.- Duodenal ulcer

Duodenal ulcers are formed in the first segment of the small intestine (duodenum) by discreet tissue destruction due to the actions of hydrochloric (gastric) acid and pepsin on areas of the mucosa having a decreased resistance to ulceration. Duodenal ulcers occur about five times more frequently than gastric ulcers and most often result from an infection with *Helicobacter pylori* or the use of nonsteroidal antiinflammatory drugs (NSAID). About 95 percent occur in the area of the duodenal bulb or cap. Signs and symptoms of a duodenal ulcer include pain with cramps, burning, gnawing, heartburn, vomiting of highly acidic fluid with no retained food, deep epigastric tenderness, voluntary muscle guarding, unilateral rectus spasm over duodenal bulb, and melena and occult blood in stools when bleeding is present. Pain diminishes by eating, but recurs two to three hours later. The combination codes contained in this category indicate whether the ulcer is acute or chronic and the presence or absence of hemorrhage and/or perforation. The most common ulcer complication is gastrointestinal bleeding or hemorrhage, which occurs when the ulcerated tissue of the duodenum grows so thin that the gastric acids begin to erode the blood vessels. Perforation occurs when the ulcer erodes the wall of the duodenum, potentially spilling the stomach or intestinal contents into the abdominal cavity.

K27.- Peptic ulcer, site unspecified

This category classifies acute or chronic benign ulcer occurring in a portion of the digestive tract accessible to gastric secretions. Peptic ulcers result from the corrosive action of acid gastric juice on vulnerable epithelium. A code from this category should only be assigned when the site of gastrointestinal tract ulcer has not been documented. The combination codes contained in this category indicate whether the ulcer is acute or chronic and the presence or absence of hemorrhage and/or perforation.

K28.- Gastrojejunal ulcer

This category classifies ulcer formation at or proximal to the junction of a previous gastrojejunal anastomosis. The signs and symptoms, diagnostics, therapies, and associated conditions are virtually the same as for gastric or duodenal ulcers. The combination codes contained in this category indicate whether the ulcer is acute or chronic and the presence or absence of hemorrhage and/or perforation.

K29.- Gastritis and duodenitis

Gastritis is an inflammation of the lining of the stomach and duodenitis is inflammation of the duodenum. Causes, which are the same for both disorders, include alcohol, prolonged irritation from the use of nonsteroidal antiinflammatory drugs (NSAIDs), infection with the bacteria *Helicobacter pylori*, pernicious anemia, degeneration related to age,

or chronic bile reflux. Symptoms include upper abdominal pain aggravated by eating, indigestion, anorexia, nausea, vomiting, and dark stools. Diagnosis may be made based on symptoms or by endoscopic examination. Treatment of gastritis or duodenitis depends on the cause but may include H2 blockers and antacids to reduce acid production or antibiotic therapy when the inflammation is caused by bacterial infection.

> **Focus Point**
>
> *Untreated gastritis or duodenitis can progress to erosion, ulceration, and bleeding. Complications include severe loss of blood and an increased risk of gastric or duodenal cancer.*

K29.0- Acute gastritis

Gastritis that occurs suddenly is called acute gastritis. A mucosal lining protects the walls of the stomach from stomach acids that are needed to digest food. Occasionally this mucosal barrier becomes weak and allows the digestive acids to damage and inflame the stomach lining. In acute gastritis, the stomach lining appears red, irritated, and swollen on gastroscopy, and it may have areas of bleeding. Common causes of acute gastritis include bacteria, viruses, stress, ingestion of corrosive substances, and certain medications. Mild, uncomplicated gastritis typically resolves within a few days and may not require treatment. Acute gastritis is classified as with or without bleeding.

K29.6- Other gastritis

A condition called Ménétrier's disease is included in this subcategory. In Ménétrier's disease an overgrowth of mucous cells forms ridges in the stomach wall. These cells release too much mucus and allow proteins to leak into the stomach from the blood, causing low protein in the blood. It also decreases stomach acid by reducing the acid producing cells. It may also be referred to as hypoproteinemic hypertrophic gastropathy. Conditions included here are classified as with or without bleeding.

K31.- Other diseases of stomach and duodenum

Included in this category are conditions sometimes referred to as functional disorders. The term functional generally applies to disorders described by symptoms when no organic explanation is identified. An assortment of ailments are included in this category such as volvulus or twisting of duodenum, fistulas, polyps and Dieulafoy lesion, which is a rare condition but one that can be life-threatening.

K31.1 Adult hypertrophic pyloric stenosis

Adult hypertrophic pyloric stenosis is an acquired condition that occurs when the opening between the stomach and the duodenum becomes narrowed. The narrowing may be due to overgrowth (hypertrophy) of the pyloric muscle or overgrowth of the pyloric muscle cells (hyperplasia). Narrowing of the pylorus may be primary or of undetermined cause or secondary meaning that another condition such as pyloric ulcer, gastritis, pylorospasm, or gallbladder disease is responsible for the narrowing. Gastric outlet obstruction is included here and occurs when an ulcer causes scarring or swelling and this swelling prevents the contents of the stomach from properly emptying into the duodenum.

K31.6   Fistula of stomach and duodenum

A fistula is an abnormal connection between two structures. A fistula of the stomach or duodenum allows the contents from the structures to leak to and from the structure where the fistula terminates. The connection may occur between the stomach or duodenum and another portion of the digestive tract such as the esophagus, jejunum, or colon.

Focus Point

Report K31.6 when the G-tube site fails to spontaneously close following removal of the G-tube. This condition, which requires surgical closure, is not considered a complication of the G-tube. This code reports only fistulas between the stomach or duodenum and other structures of the gastrointestinal tract. Enterocutaneous fistulas are reported with K63.2. Fistulas between the gastrointestinal tract and the uterus, vagina, or bladder are reported with codes from Chapter 14 Diseases of the Genitourinary System.

K31.81-   Angiodysplasia of stomach and duodenum

Angiodysplasia is an abnormality of the blood vessels in the lining of the stomach or duodenum that occurs primarily in the elderly. These abnormal blood vessels are subject to bleeding that can cause anemia. Watermelon stomach, which is included in this code, is a hemorrhagic condition that is characterized by a watermelon stripe-like appearance in the lining of the stomach. This code is classified based on the presence or absence of bleeding.

K31.83   Achlorhydria

Achlorhydria is the absence of hydrochloric acid in the stomach. There are varying degrees of achlorhydria, although, the older the patient, the greater the deficiency, which may include complete absence of hydrochloric acid. Symptoms frequently occur several hours after eating and include flatulence and often alternating constipation and diarrhea.

K31.84   Gastroparesis

Gastroparesis is a disorder in which the stomach takes too long to empty its contents. Cause is unknown, although disruption of nerve stimulation to the intestine is a possible cause. Symptoms of gastroparesis are nausea, vomiting, an early feeling of fullness when eating, weight loss, abdominal bloating,

and abdominal discomfort. In most cases, gastroparesis is usually a chronic condition, although treatment does help manage the condition. Risk factors include diabetes, systemic sclerosis, anorexia nervosa, previous vagotomy, previous gastrectomy, visceral neuropathy, and use of anticholinergic medication.

Focus Point

Gastroparesis is often a complication of Type I diabetes; it occurs less often in people with Type II diabetes. A diabetic code from Chapter 4 Endocrine, Nutritional and Metabolic Diseases, must be coded first.

Diseases of Appendix (K35-K38)

The vermiform appendix is a short tube that is closed at one end and attached to the cecum at the other. The appendix, like the rest of the intestine, is formed by a muscular wall that is lined with mucosal tissue. The muscular wall contracts to expel the mucus and other debris that collects in the appendix into the cecum. Blockage of the opening to the cecum can cause inflammation of the appendix and other complications.

The categories in this code block are as follows:

K35	Acute appendicitis
K36	Other appendicitis
K37	Unspecified appendicitis
K38	Other diseases of appendix

K35.-   Acute appendicitis

Appendicitis is inflammation of the vermiform appendix. Acute appendicitis is usually initiated by obstruction of the appendiceal lumen by a fecalith, inflammation, neoplasm, or foreign body. The obstruction is followed by infection, edema, and frequently infarction of the appendiceal wall. Intraluminal tension develops rapidly and tends to cause mural necrosis and perforation. Signs and symptoms of acute appendicitis include abdominal pain, usually beginning with epigastric or periumbilical pain associated with one or two episodes of vomiting. The abdominal pain may shift during the next 12 hours to the right lower quadrant (McBurney's point) where it persists as steady soreness aggravated by walking or coughing. Other symptoms include anorexia, moderate malaise, slight to moderate fever, constipation (or occasionally diarrhea), rebound tenderness, and spasm.

Focus Point

Appendicitis is the most common nonobstetrical complication of pregnancy.

K35.2 Acute appendicitis with generalized peritonitis

K35.3 Acute appendicitis with localized peritonitis

Acute appendicitis with generalized peritonitis is a condition where the appendix perforates, releasing infectious contents into the abdominal cavity. This fluid can develop into an infection of the peritoneum, which is referred to as generalized peritonitis. A perforated appendix is generally treated with intravenous antibiotics. Acute appendicitis with localized peritonitis occurs when the inflammation and infection of the peritoneum is limited to the region of the appendix. Appendicitis with localized peritonitis may present with a peritoneal abscess, which occurs when infection from a perforated appendix is walled off from the rest of the body and develops into a pus-filled sac. Scar tissue then surrounds the appendix and separates it from the rest of the abdomen, preventing spread of infection.

K35.8- Other and unspecified acute appendicitis

Acute appendicitis without mention of peritonitis is the phase of appendicitis referred to as early appendicitis. No gangrene, perforation, or abscess is present. Acute appendicitis without localized or generalized peritonitis is reported with the code for unspecified acute appendicitis. Other appendicitis is reported for inflammation of the appendix that is chronic or intermittent (recurrent).

Hernia (K40-K46)

A hernia of the abdominal cavity is the protrusion of tissue, an organ, or part of an organ through an abnormal opening in the wall of the body cavity in which it is normally confined. The majority of hernias are abdominal resulting from herniation of abdominal contents through the internal or external inguinal rings, femoral rings, or defects in the abdominal wall resulting from trauma or improper healing after a surgical procedure. A hernia that can be pushed back into the abdominal cavity (called a reducible hernia) is not considered an immediate health threat, though it does require surgery to repair the hernia. A hernia that cannot be pushed back in (called a nonreducible hernia) may lead to dangerous complications such as the obstruction of the flow of the intestinal contents or intestinal blood supply (strangulation), leading to tissue death, and requires immediate surgery.

The categories in this code block are as follows:

K40	Inguinal hernia
K41	Femoral hernia
K42	Umbilical hernia
K43	Ventral hernia
K44	Diaphragmatic hernia
K45	Other abdominal hernia
K46	Unspecified abdominal hernia

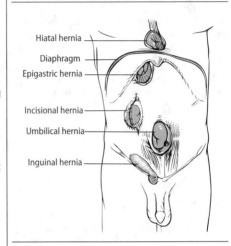

Hiatal hernia
Diaphragm
Epigastric hernia
Incisional hernia
Umbilical hernia
Inguinal hernia

Focus Point

A hernia that is both obstructed and with gangrene is coded to "with gangrene."

K40.- Inguinal hernia

An inguinal hernia occurs when a loop of intestine enters the inguinal canal, a tubular passage through the lower layers of the abdominal wall. A direct inguinal hernia creates a bulge in the groin area, and an indirect hernia descends into the scrotum. Inguinal hernias occur less often in women than men. Hernias are caused by congenital (defects at birth) or age-related weaknesses in the abdominal walls. In males, they are often congenital and caused by an improper closure of the abdominal cavity. They can also be caused by an increase in pressure within the abdominal cavity due to heavy lifting, straining, violent coughing, obesity, or pregnancy. The primary sign is a protrusion in the groin area between the pubis and the top of the leg in the area known as the inguinal region of the abdomen. Symptoms include pain during urination or a bowel movement or when lifting a heavy object that may be sharp and immediate, a dull aching sensation, nausea, and constipation. Symptoms typically get worse toward the end of the day or after standing for long periods of time and may disappear when lying down. Inguinal hernias are classified based on laterality, the presence or absence of complications, and whether or not the condition is recurrent.

K41.- Femoral hernia

A femoral hernia, also called a femorocele, occurs when a small part of the intestine protrudes through the femoral canal wall, which is located just below the inguinal ligament in the groin. It is often misdiagnosed as an inguinal hernia and often is too small for a doctor to feel during an exam. Although femoral hernias are relatively uncommon, they are three times more likely to occur in women than in men due to straining in childbirth. Femoral hernias are classified based on laterality, the presence or absence of complications, and whether or not the condition is recurrent.

K42.- Umbilical hernia

An umbilical hernia occurs around the umbilicus (navel). Umbilical hernias are commonly present at birth. Premature babies and those with low birth weight are at increased risk. Umbilical hernias can also be caused by an increase in pressure within the abdominal cavity due to heavy lifting, straining, violent coughing, obesity, or pregnancy. The primary sign of an umbilical hernia is a protrusion by the navel area that may manifest in infants while crying, coughing, or during a bowel movement. Umbilical hernias are usually not painful in infants and young children but may cause pain in older children and adults. Most congenital umbilical hernias resolve spontaneously by age 1. Surgical repair is recommended for hernias that do not resolve by age 4. Umbilical hernias are classified based on the presence or absence of obstruction and/or gangrene.

K43.- Ventral hernia

Ventral hernias are sometimes called abdominal hernias because the loop of bowel protrudes through the abdominal wall muscles. The condition may occur at the incision site of a previous surgery where tissue has stretched and weakened. It may also be a birth defect due to incomplete closure of the abdominal wall. Ventral hernias are classified based on the specific type and the presence or absence of complications. The fourth character identifies whether the ventral hernia is incisional, parastomal, or other type. The fifth character identifies the presence or absence of an obstruction and/or gangrene.

> **Focus Point**
>
> *Two codes are required to report the diagnosis of incarcerated incisional hernia with small bowel obstruction due to adhesions. Sequence the code for the incisional hernia with obstruction first, followed by the code for peritoneal adhesions.*

K44.- Diaphragmatic hernia

A diaphragmatic hernia is a protrusion of part of the stomach through the esophageal hiatus of the diaphragm. The esophageal hiatus is the opening in the diaphragm between the central tendon and the hiatus aorticus where the esophagus and the two

vagus nerves pass. Clinicians recognize two different types of esophageal hiatal hernias: paraesophageal and sliding. Sliding is the more common type of diaphragmatic hernia. With a sliding hiatal hernia, the upper stomach, along with the cardioesophageal junction, herniates upward into the posterior mediastinum. The stomach displacement may be stationary, or it may actually slide in and out of the thorax with movement, after a large meal, or with alterations of pressure in the abdominal and thoracic cavities. Paraesophageal hiatal hernia is characterized by all or part of the stomach herniating into the thorax immediately adjacent and to the left of a nondisplaced gastroesophageal junction. Both types are reported with the same codes based on whether the diaphragmatic hernia is uncomplicated or complicated by obstruction or gangrene.

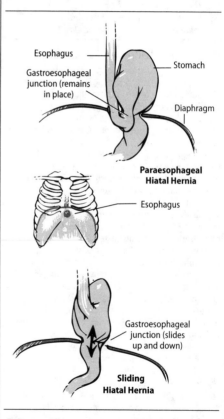

Esophagus

Gastroesophageal junction (remains in place)

Stomach

Diaphragm

Paraesophageal Hiatal Hernia

Esophagus

Gastroesophageal junction (slides up and down)

Sliding Hiatal Hernia

> **Focus Point**
>
> *Conditions associated with diaphragmatic hernia include reflux esophagitis, esophageal stricture, polyps, ulcer formation with or without bleeding, carcinoma, and Saint's triad (hiatal hernia, gallbladder disease, and colon diverticulosis). Associated conditions are reported additionally.*

Noninfective Enteritis and Colitis (K50-K52)

Inflammatory bowel disease that is not due to an infection is classified here.

The categories in this code block are as follows:

K50   Crohn's disease [regional enteritis]

K51   Ulcerative colitis

K52   Other and unspecified noninfective gastroenteritis and colitis

Focus Point

Infectious forms of gastroenteritis or colitis codes are located in Chapter 1 Certain Infectious and Parasitic Diseases. Diarrhea not caused by another condition and not otherwise specified is found in Chapter 18 Symptoms, Signs, and Abnormal Clinical and Laboratory Findings, Not Elsewhere Classified

K50.-   Crohn's disease [regional enteritis]

Crohn's disease is a form of inflammatory bowel disease characterized by chronic granulomatous disease. Granulomas are nodular inflammatory lesions, usually small or granular, firm, persistent, and containing compactly grouped modified phagocytes. Also known as regional enteritis, Crohn's disease is identified by its characteristic cobblestone appearance where segments of diseased bowel are located between regions of healthy bowel tissue, hence the name regional enteritis. It most often affects the large intestines but may occur anywhere in the gastrointestinal tract (e.g., mouth, esophagus, stomach, duodenum, large intestine, appendix, rectum, and anus). Crohn's disease can lead to several complications, including obstruction, abscess, fistula, and hemorrhage. The formation of strictures and adhesions that narrow the lumen can block the passageway of intestinal contents and cause an intestinal obstruction. In Crohn's disease, fistulae, abnormal passages from one epithelial surface to another, can develop between two loops of bowel, between the bowel and bladder, between the bowel and vagina, and between the bowel and skin. Abscesses are another complication and occur most often in the abdominal and perianal regions.

Focus Point

Combination codes capture Crohn's disease, site, and associated complications of rectal bleeding, intestinal obstruction, fistula, and abscess. Manifestations and conditions associated with Crohn's disease, such as pyoderma gangrenosum and malabsorption, are reported additionally.

K50.00   Crohn's disease of small intestine without complications

This code captures regional duodenitis, regional ileitis, terminal ileitis, jejunoileitis, and jejunitis. Crohn's disease without current complications is classified here.

K50.01-   Crohn's disease of small intestine with complications

This subcategory includes conditions such as ileitis, terminal ileitis, and jejunoileitis. In some rare cases, Crohn's disease can also cause inflammation in the stomach and the duodenum. For Crohn's disease of the small intestine with complications, combination codes provide a sixth character that describes the specific complications of rectal bleeding, intestinal obstruction, fistula, and abscess. There are also codes for other and unspecified complications.

Focus Point

If Crohn's disease of the small intestine is present with a rectal abscess, it would still be appropriate to use the combination code with a fifth character indicating with abscess, even though it is located in another part of the intestinal tract. A code for the rectal abscess would be added in order to specify the site of the abscess.

K50.10   Crohn's disease of large intestine without complications

This code captures Crohn's disease without current complications for sites in the large intestine, including the cecum, ascending colon, hepatic flexure, transverse colon, splenic flexure, descending colon, sigmoid colon, and rectum.

K50.11-   Crohn's disease of large intestine with complications

These subcategories include sites in the large intestine including the cecum, ascending colon, hepatic flexure, transverse colon, splenic flexure, descending colon, sigmoid colon, and rectum. For Crohn's disease of the large intestine with complications, combination codes provide a sixth character that describes the specific complications of rectal bleeding, intestinal obstruction, fistula, and abscess. There are also codes for other and unspecified complications.

K51.-   Ulcerative colitis

Ulcerative colitis is a disease that causes inflammation and ulcers in the top layers of the lining of the large intestine. The inflammation usually occurs in the rectum and lower part of the colon, but it may affect the entire colon and makes the colon empty frequently, causing diarrhea. Ulcers form in places where the inflammation has killed colon cells; the ulcers bleed and produce pus and mucous. Ulcerative colitis rarely affects the small intestine except for the lower section, called the ileum. The disease can be difficult to diagnose because its symptoms are similar to other intestinal disorders such as irritable bowel syndrome and Crohn's disease. The most common symptoms of ulcerative colitis are abdominal pain and bloody diarrhea. Patients also may experience fatigue, weight loss, and rectal bleeding. Symptoms can go into remission for months or years and then suddenly flare up. Treatment for ulcerative colitis depends on the seriousness of the disease. Most people are treated with medication, although in severe cases, a patient may need surgery to remove the diseased colon.

Focus Point

Combination codes capture the site of the ulcerative colitis and associated complications of rectal bleeding, intestinal obstruction, fistula, and abscess.

K51.0- Ulcerative (chronic) pancolitis

Pancolitis is a severe ulcerative colitis that involves the entire large intestine in varying degrees from the cecum to the rectum. This may also be referred to as universal colitis. Patients that experience this condition, especially for long periods of time, are predisposed to developing colon cancer.

K51.00 Ulcerative (chronic) pancolitis without complications

This code describes pancolitis without current complications.

K51.01- Ulcerative (chronic) pancolitis with complications

For ulcerative pancolitis with complications, combination codes provide a sixth character that describes the specific complications of rectal bleeding, intestinal obstruction, fistula, and abscess. There are also codes for other and unspecified complications.

K51.4- Inflammatory polyps of colon

Inflammatory polyps of colon have previously been referred to as pseudopolyposis, but that term is no longer commonly used. It is a condition of numerous pseudopolyps in the colon and rectum, due to longstanding alternation of ulceration and granulation tissue formation during the healing phase. This process leaves polyps that are inflammatory, not neoplastic.

K51.40 Inflammatory polyps of colon without complications

This code describes inflammatory polyps without current complications.

K51.41- Inflammatory polyps of colon with complications

For this condition with complications, combination codes provide a sixth character that describes the specific complications of rectal bleeding, intestinal obstruction, fistula, and abscess. There is also a code for other or unspecified complication.

K52.- Other and unspecified noninfective gastroenteritis and colitis

Inflammatory conditions of the stomach and intestines due to radiation, drugs or toxins, and food allergies are a few types of noninfective gastroenteritis and colitis classified here.

K52.2- Allergic and dietetic gastroenteritis and colitis

The disorders in this subcategory include hypersensitivities to food, as well as other allergic conditions that result in inflammation of the GI tract, particularly the stomach and colon. The conditions found in this subcategory do not involve any infectious processes, unlike other categories in this chapter.

K52.21 Food protein-induced enterocolitis syndrome

K52.22 Food protein-induced enteropathy

The underlying pathology for these two conditions is a prompting of the immune system in response to certain food proteins. Unlike the more "classic" food allergies, food protein-induced allergy symptoms are typically limited to the gastrointestinal system only. Cow's milk is the most common inciting agent, but other foods can also trigger a reaction, including gluten-containing foods and soy. The underlying variance between these two conditions primarily relates to symptom severity.

Food protein-induced enterocolitis syndrome (FPIES) typically affects infants and children under the age of 3. It commonly manifests itself with chronic vomiting and diarrhea, leading to dehydration and failure to thrive. FPIES may be difficult to diagnose because the allergic response may be delayed by several hours after someone comes in contact with the trigger food. Patients with food protein-induced enteropathy experience vomiting and diarrhea but not to the extent that is seen in FPIES. Treatment of both conditions primarily involves symptom management during acute episodes and avoidance of the trigger foods.

K52.3 Indeterminate colitis

A patient with indeterminate colitis cannot be diagnosed with either ulcerative colitis or Crohn's disease, although they may have symptoms of either or both. None of the standard diagnostic testing for these conditions, such as colonoscopy, imaging, laboratory tests, or biopsy can unequivocally provide a clear diagnosis. Some patients may go on to develop ulcerative colitis or Crohn's disease, but others may have long-standing durable indeterminate colitis.

K52.81 Eosinophilic gastritis or gastroenteritis

K52.82 Eosinophilic colitis

Eosinophilic gastroenteritis is an inflammation at multiple levels of the gastrointestinal tract and eosinophilic colitis is an inflammation of only the colon. Eosinophilic gastrointestinal disorders (EGID) selectively affect the lining of the gastrointestinal tract through the accumulation of eosinophil cells in the intestinal tissue, causing inflammation. In this disease, eosinophil accumulation occurs in the absence of known causes for eosinophilia (e.g., drug reactions, parasitic infection, connective tissue disease, or malignancy). Treatment for EGIDs can include limiting the diet to avoid antigens that trigger disease symptoms, use of a feeding tube, treatment with steroids, and other specific therapy (such as treatment with anti-interleukin-5 antibody). Eosinophilic gastritis is inflammation of the stomach, usually the entire stomach wall, although involvement may be limited to the serosal or muscle layers. Complications include ascites and peritonitis. Eosinophilic gastroenteritis is inflammation at multiple levels of the gastrointestinal tract. Symptoms include severe abdominal pain and vomiting. Eosinophilic colitis is inflammation of the colon that causes severe abdominal pain, diarrhea, and blood in the stool.

K52.83- Microscopic colitis

Colitis is an inflammation of the large intestine. Typically colonic tissue that is inflamed will appear as such when observed via an endoscopic procedure. Beyond the symptom of watery diarrhea, a patient with microscopic colitis does not have evidence of colonic abnormalities except under microscopic examination.

K52.831 Collagenous colitis

K52.832 Lymphocytic colitis

Collagenous and lymphocytic colitis are both classified as microscopic colitis conditions. A patient may have chronic watery, nonbloody diarrhea while radiographic and endoscopic studies of their GI system are normal. Only a mucosal biopsy procedure can show specific inflammatory changes related to each of these conditions. In collagenous colitis, a thickened, nonelastic band of tissue made of a protein (collagen), is found just beneath the lining of the colon. When biopsy samples indicate an increased number of lymphocytes within the lining of the colon, lymphocytic colitis is diagnosed. Additional distinguishing factors include age and sex. Collagenous colitis is more frequently diagnosed in women, most often in their 50s. Lymphocytic colitis is more evenly distributed between the sexes, and the age at onset is usually a bit later, in the 60s. These forms of colitis are not considered as severe as inflammatory bowel disease (Crohn's disease or

ulcerative colitis), and treatment is directed primarily at the watery, nonbloody diarrhea, with bulk-forming agents or other various antidiarrheals that slow the contractions that move bowel contents forward. Additional therapies may include antibiotics or anti-inflammatory medications.

Other Diseases of Intestines (K55-K64)

Conditions classified here are other diseases and disorders that involve the small and large intestines, such as disorders of blood vessels that supply the intestine, some types of intestinal obstructions, diverticulosis and diverticulitis, functional disorders such as irritable bowel syndrome, and certain conditions affecting the rectum and anus.

The categories in this code block are as follows:

K55	Vascular disorders of intestine
K56	Paralytic ileus and intestinal obstruction without hernia
K57	Diverticular disease of intestine
K58	Irritable bowel syndrome
K59	Other functional intestinal disorders
K60	Fissure and fistula of anal and rectal regions
K61	Abscess of anal and rectal regions
K62	Other diseases of anus and rectum
K63	Other diseases of intestine
K64	Hemorrhoids and perianal venous thrombosis

K55.- Vascular disorders of intestine

There are three arteries that supply blood to the intestines: the celiac artery, superior mesenteric artery, and inferior mesenteric artery. When one or more of these arteries become partially or completely blocked by atherosclerotic plaque, an embolus, or a thrombus, intestinal tissue injury or death (necrosis) may occur. Vascular disorders classified here are differentiated only as acute or chronic, not by the specific condition, which may be documented as acute or chronic ischemia, intestinal infarction, or ischemic inflammation (enteritis, colitis). Conditions may also be designated based on the blood vessel that is affected, such as mesenteric embolism or thrombus.

K55.0- Acute vascular disorders of intestine

Codes in this subcategory are classified based on the type of vascular disorder, in particular ischemia or infarction, and the part of the intestine affected and the extent of the effect. In early stages, the patient may appear in more pain and sicker than the physical exam suggests; however, in a short time span, complications such as metabolic acidosis, hypovolemia, septic shock, and multi-organ failure can occur.

K55.01- Acute (reversible) ischemia of small intestine

K55.02- Acute infarction of small intestine

K55.03- Acute (reversible) ischemia of large intestine

K55.04- Acute infarction of large intestine

Infarction and ischemia are direct consequences of a decreased blood supply to the intestine. Low blood pressure, atrial or venous blood clots, adhesions, or intestinal herniation are just a few underlying etiologies that can lead to intestinal ischemia or infarction. With continued vascular compromise, the bowel can become necrotic and/or gangrenous.

K55.1 Chronic vascular disorders of intestine

Chronic visceral ischemic syndromes are associated with atherosclerotic lesions obstructing the celiac trunk, superior mesenteric artery, and inferior mesenteric artery due to embolism, mesenteric venous thrombosis, and aneurysms. Narrowing of the superior mesenteric artery often presents with intense abdominal pain with vomiting or loose bowel movements. Gradual occlusion of this artery causes severe pain around the navel within one hour of eating because of the increased demand for blood to the intestines for digestion. The abdomen becomes distended and the stool becomes bloody. The intestine becomes gangrenous because of the lack of blood being supplied to the area. Surgical intervention for embolectomy or bypass reconstruction of the obstructing lesions is usually necessary to avoid extensive intestinal necrosis or death. Wilkie's syndrome, an obstruction of the duodenum, is included here.

K55.3- Necrotizing enterocolitis

Necrotizing enterocolitis (NEC) is a serious GI condition that primarily affects preterm and otherwise unhealthy neonates. It involves intestinal necrosis and most commonly occurs after enteral feedings. Initial symptoms usually include feeding difficulties and bloody or bilious gastric residuals (after feedings), followed by abdominal distension, bilious emesis, and gross blood in stool. The diagnosis is made based on blood in the stool and the presence of pain. Treatment involves stopping feedings, NG suction, broad-spectrum antibiotics, fluid resuscitation, TPN, and in some severe cases, surgery.

K55.31 Stage 1 necrotizing enterocolitis

K55.32 Stage 2 necrotizing enterocolitis

K55.33 Stage 3 necrotizing enterocolitis

The original staging of necrotizing enterocolitis (NEC) was developed in 1978 by Dr. Martin Bell. Stage 1 represents the mildest form of the condition, and because the diagnosis of NEC is often questionable, some patients are categorized as in this stage until a firm diagnosis is made. Stage 2 is for those patients who have the classic radiological sign of pneumatosis intestinalis, characterized by gas in the bowel wall. Frank blood may be seen in the stool, abdominal distension may be marked, and radiology may show persistent or unchanging bowel loops and the development of portal vein gas. The most severe cases of NEC are classified as stage 3. Patients have all of the symptoms of the other stages of the disease, along with a deterioration of vital signs, evidence of septic shock, or marked gastrointestinal bleeding. The patient may also have pneumoperitoneum on abdominal films and bowel necrosis, requiring surgical intervention.

K56.- Paralytic ileus and intestinal obstruction without hernia

Intestinal (bowel) obstruction occurs when the internal lumen of the intestine becomes partially or completely blocked, and bowel contents cannot move through the bowel and be excreted through the anus. There are a number of conditions other than hernia that can result in bowel obstruction.

K56.0 Paralytic ileus

Paralytic ileus, also known as adynamic ileus, is a neurogenic impairment of peristalsis that can lead to complete intestinal obstruction. The intraabdominal etiologies for paralytic ileus include gastrointestinal surgery, peritoneal irritations (e.g., intraabdominal hemorrhage, ruptured viscus, pancreatitis, or peritonitis), or anoxic organic obstruction. Other etiologies include drugs with anticholinergic properties, renal colic, vertebral fractures, spinal cord injuries, uremia, severe infection, diabetic coma, and electrolyte imbalances.

K56.1 Intussusception

Intussusception occurs when one part of the intestine prolapses over an adjoining area of intestine, a finding sometimes referred to as telescoping. This cuts off blood supply to the affected area and blocks food and liquids from passing through the intestine. It occurs most often in young children, boys four times more than girls, but can occur rarely in adults. This serious condition can lead to dehydration, infection, shock, rupture, or necrosis of the bowel and is considered a medical emergency.

K56.2   Volvulus

Volvulus is an abnormal twisting of a loop of intestine also more likely to affect children than adults. It produces the same results as intussusception of blockage, ischemia, and necrosis.

K56.41   Fecal impaction

A fecal impaction is an obstructive, immobile mass of hardened stool in the rectum as a result of chronic constipation. Immobile patients, those with neurological diseases, and patients on certain chronic medications are at risk for chronic constipation with subsequent fecal impaction. Symptoms include cramping, abdominal pain, rectal pain, diarrhea, straining, and rectal bleeding. Complications include rectal tear, rectal fissure, hemorrhoids, rectal ulcer, and necrosis of rectal tissues. Prevention measures include a high fiber diet, stool softeners, physical exercise, and increased fluid intake. Laxative use is contraindicated for fecal impaction, as it may result in bowel damage due to traumatic expulsion of the mass. Disimpaction procedures include enemas to soften the mass with digital manipulation by the physician. In severe obstructed cases, surgical intervention may be necessary.

K56.5-   Intestinal adhesions [bands] with obstruction (postinfection)

Intestinal adhesions with bowel obstruction are fibrous bands of scar tissue that can block the intestines either completely or partially. Intestinal adhesions can be attributed to previous infection, abscess, trauma, and unknown causes. Adhesions from previous surgery are the most common cause of intestinal obstruction in the United States and do not generally require a surgical complication code. Although adhesions or solitary adhesion bands are a common cause of intestinal obstruction, adhesions following surgery are not necessarily due to the surgery. In many cases, intestinal adhesions are due to an infectious or inflammatory cause, such as acute appendicitis, diverticulitis, cholecystitis, pelvic infections, Crohn's disease, or chronic peritonitis. Intestinal obstruction varies in severity, from partial or intermittent obstruction that usually resolves without intervention (especially of the small intestine) to complete obstruction requiring surgery as it may lead to intestinal gangrene and perforation. When significant obstruction is present, lysis of adhesions is usually performed. Physicians often document intestinal obstruction as partial versus complete, but intestinal obstruction can be coded as unspecified whether partial or complete.

Focus Point

Intestinal adhesions or bands causing obstruction that are due to a surgery (postprocedural) are not coded in this subcategory but are reported with a code from subcategory K91.3-.

K56.6-   Other and unspecified intestinal obstruction

This subcategory classifies intestinal obstruction due to other specified and unspecified causes. If specified causes of intestinal obstruction such as tumors or inflammatory bowel diseases such as Crohn's disease, diverticulitis, or ulcers are documented, the code for the specific condition would be used. This subcategory would only be used if a more specific condition is not documented or represented elsewhere by another code. Examples of obstructions that may be coded here are stenosis, stricture unspecified, obstruction of unknown cause, or not elsewhere coded. Intestinal obstruction varies in severity, from partial or intermittent obstruction that usually resolves without intervention (especially of the small intestine) to complete obstruction that requires surgery as it may lead to intestinal gangrene and perforation. Physicians often document intestinal obstruction as partial versus complete, but intestinal obstruction can be coded as unspecified as to partial versus complete.

K57.-   Diverticular disease of intestine

Diverticula are sac-like herniations of the mucosal lining that can occur at any site in the small or large intestine, although they tend to occur in higher-pressure areas, such as the sigmoid colon. Diverticula consist of a mucosal coat and serosa and usually herniate through the muscularis of the colon with the herniation or dissection occurring along the course of nutrient vessels. Diverticula may be described as true or false. True diverticula contain all layers of the bowel and are rare in the colon. False diverticula consist of mucosa and submucosa that have herniated through the muscularis. Diverticulosis refers to the presence of sac-like herniations in the mucosal lining. Diverticulitis refers to inflammation of the diverticula. Diverticular disease may be complicated by bleeding, abscess, and/or perforation. Diverticular disease is classified by site, whether or not inflammation (diverticulitis) is present, and by the presence of absence of other complications.

Focus Point

For coding purposes, the terms "true" and "false" have no significance and should be treated as nonessential modifiers. Both true and false diverticula are reported with codes from category K57.

K58.-   Irritable bowel syndrome

Irritable bowel syndrome (IBS) is not typically diagnosed with a specific test or diagnostic study. Rather, a physician reviews a constellation of symptoms and takes a detailed history, conducts a physical examination, and may use some limited testing to help make a diagnosis.

K58.0 Irritable bowel syndrome with diarrhea

K58.1 Irritable bowel syndrome with constipation

K58.2 Mixed irritable bowel syndrome

The most common symptoms of irritable bowel syndrome (IBS) include intermittent upper abdominal discomfort or pain (dyspepsia), feelings of bowel urgency, early feeling of fullness (satiety), bloating, feeling of "incomplete" bowel emptying, heartburn, and/or nausea. IBS with diarrhea is sometimes referred to as IBS-D. Most people define diarrhea as loose or watery stools. Others think of diarrhea as frequent bowel movements. IBS with constipation is sometimes referred to as IBS-C or constipation-predominant IBS. This can take the form of infrequent stools, difficulty or straining at stools, the sensation of wanting to go but not being able to, or feeling of being unable to completely empty during a bowel movement. Some patients have both constipation and diarrhea, just at different times, which is categorized as mixed irritable bowel syndrome.

K59.- Other functional intestinal disorders

Diarrhea and various forms of constipation are just a few of the conditions captured in this category.

K59.0- Constipation

Constipation is defined by less frequent than normal or difficult bowel movements; while the frequency differs for each person, any length of time beyond three days is not typical and leads to even more difficult bowel movements. Symptoms include reduction in frequency specific to the person's normal schedule, feeling incompletely evacuated, abdominal pain, decreased amount of feces, and having to strain to produce a bowel movement. Many underlying reasons can lead to constipation as well as several home remedies and over-the-counter aids to help relieve constipation. However, medical intervention may be necessary if other symptoms include abdominal pain and/or cramps in addition to having no gas or bowel movements.

K59.01 Slow transit constipation

Slow transit constipation (STC), also referred to as neuronal intestinal dysplasia (NID), occurs when peristalsis within the large intestine decreases due to irregularities with the enteric nerves. This unusually slow disposal of feces may lead to lifelong problems, including constipation and uncontrolled bowel movements for which there is no remedy. The symptoms are similar to typical constipation with the addition of uncontrolled defecation and decreased appetite and, less commonly, blood in stool, hemorrhoids, and diarrhea. Diagnosis is difficult when standard constipation radiological studies are performed; therefore it is recommended that a continence specialist perform an evaluation with colonic nuclear transit study and/or full-thickness laparoscopic biopsy. While there is no cure, the condition can be managed by medication aimed at increasing bowel motility, enemas to help flush out the rectum, and interferential electrical stimulation therapy. In extreme cases, surgery may be an option, but this course of action depends on the area of bowel affected and the severity of the condition.

> **Focus Point**
>
> *Although the symptoms of slow transit constipation (STC) may be similar to those of a congenital condition known as Hirschsprung's disease, Hirschsprung's is due to lack of peristalsis caused by the absence of nerve cells in the rectum and/or intestine. This congenital anomaly is reported with Q43.1.*

K59.02 Outlet dysfunction constipation

Outlet constipation may also be referred to as pelvic floor dysfunction. It indicates a problem with the muscles of the pelvic floor during attempted bowel movements. Because the majority of patients with this condition have a normal colon transit time, the cause is typically not due to any muscle or neurologic disorder. The feces reach the rectum, but evacuation does not occur, which leads to lengthy straining, softer than normal feces, and discomfort during bowel movements. The final determination of this condition is still uncertain and while typical medical treatment does not provide much relief, some patients do well with biofeedback and/or relaxation treatments.

K59.03 Drug induced constipation

Many medications can lead to drug-induced constipation, including many narcotics. These medications tend to slow down the digestive tract, thereby causing a decrease in the frequency of bowel movements and creating harder, more difficult to pass feces. Several natural remedies can be helpful such as prunes and fiber in the form of psyllium. A couple of prescription drugs also can help, such as methylnaltrexone or naloxegol.

K59.04 Chronic idiopathic constipation

Chronic idiopathic constipation (CIC) also includes functional constipation and follows the typical constipation symptoms. In more severe cases, it may require manual removal of the feces, which can also contribute to injury or bleeding around the anus. The cause of this type of constipation is not known and does not appear to be any underlying condition or medication. Additional symptoms to watch for that would lead to a more serious diagnosis/condition include blood in the stool, symptoms occurring after the age of 50, family history of intestinal cancer or other inflammatory bowel conditions, fever with decreased blood count, and weight loss. Treatment may be as simple as lifestyle and diet changes with increased fiber and water intake and/or medications such as laxatives and stool softeners.

K59.3- Megacolon, not elsewhere classified

Megacolon is generally described as a dilatation of the colon not caused by mechanical obstruction. Most physicians agree with the following measurements as guidelines: greater than 12 cm in diameter for the cecum, greater than 6.5 cm in the rectosigmoid region, and greater than 8 cm for the ascending colon.

K59.31 Toxic megacolon

Toxic megacolon is a potentially lethal condition and features signs of systemic toxicity, such as dehydration, altered mental status, electrolyte abnormality, or hypotension. It can be a complication of inflammatory bowel disease (such as Crohn's disease). The condition is diagnosed based on a history and physical, diagnostic radiological studies, and lab tests such as complete blood count (CBC) and electrolyte studies. A patient with toxic megacolon is typically treated with surgery, particularly if bowel perforation is present. If not treated quickly, toxic megacolon can progress to sepsis, shock, and coma.

K60.- Fissure and fistula of anal and rectal regions

The last part of the rectum (anal canal) is a section about 1.5 inches long, which ends with the anus. Common conditions affecting the anus and rectal regions are anal fissures and anal, rectal, or anorectal fistula. An anal fissure is a tear in the lining of the anus. A fistula is a channel or tract that develops in the presence of inflammation and infection.

K60.0 Acute anal fissure

K60.1 Chronic anal fissure

K60.2 Anal fissure, unspecified

Anal fissures are frequently caused by constipation when a dry bowel movement results in a break in the tissue. However, fissures can also occur with severe bouts of diarrhea, inflammation, injury to the anal canal during childbirth, and laxative abuse. A fissure can be painful during and following bowel movements because of the muscles that control the passage of stool and keep the anus tightly closed at other times. When those muscles expand, it stretches the fissure open causing pain. A fistula is a channel or tract that develops in the presence of inflammation and infection. The channel usually runs from the rectum to an opening in the skin around the anus. Since fistulas are infected channels, there is usually some drainage.

K62.- Other diseases of anus and rectum

Conditions affecting the anus and rectum that do not fit well into more specific categories are classified here. These include polyps, prolapse, narrowing (stenosis, stricture) of the lumen, bleeding, ulcers, inflammation of the rectum due to radiation treatment, and other conditions.

K62.81 Anal sphincter tear (healed) (nontraumatic) (old)

There are two muscles, the internal anal sphincter and the external anal sphincter, that surround the anus and keep the anal openings closed. The internal anal sphincter holds stool in the rectum. When the rectum is full a reflex causes the rectum to open allowing stool to pass into the anus for defecation. The external anal sphincter holds stool in the anus until it is voluntarily relaxed during a bowel movement. Either of these two muscles can tear, resulting in an inability to hold stool in the anus, which may lead to fecal incontinence.

K62.82 Dysplasia of anus

Anal dysplasia, also called anal intraepithelial neoplasia or AIN, refers to the presence of abnormal cells in the lining of the anal canal. AIN is caused by human papillomavirus (HPV). To diagnosis AIN, a cytologic smear from the anal canal must be obtained and a histological evaluation of the cells performed. This may be referred to as an anal PAP smear. Following an anal PAP smear, the cells are classified based on their appearance. A result showing low-grade squamous intraepithelial lesion (LSIL) is classified as mild dysplasia, while high-grade squamous intraepithelial lesion (HSIL) represents moderate to severe dysplasia.

Focus Point

Only mild to moderate dysplasia, also referred to as anal intraepithelial neoplasia I or II (AIN I, AIN II), is classified here. Severe anal dysplasia, also referred to as anal intraepithelial neoplasia III (AIN III), is classified as carcinoma in situ of the anus and is reported with a code from the neoplasm chapter.

K63.- Other diseases of intestine

Conditions affecting the intestine that do not fit well into more specific categories are classified here, along with conditions that are not documented with sufficient detail to allow assignment of a more specific code.

K63.4 Enteroptosis

This condition is characterized by an abnormal prolapse of part of the intestine below its normal position. Enteroptosis, also referred to as Glenard's disease, can be caused by obesity or muscle weakness.

K63.81   Dieulafoy lesion of intestine

This obscure, potentially life-threatening condition can cause acute, massive GI hemorrhage. It manifests as an abnormally dilated submucosal artery, which is often hard to diagnose. It occurs most frequently in the stomach, followed by the duodenum and the colon. It can affect any age group and affects men twice as often as women.

K64.-   Hemorrhoids and perianal venous thrombosis

Hemorrhoids are dilated veins of the hemorrhoidal plexus in the lower rectum. Generally caused by too much straining or pressure on the veins, they can be painful, but are not usually a serious medical condition. External hemorrhoids occur in the region of the external anal sphincter and are covered by the skin of the anal canal. Internal hemorrhoids occur in the rectum and are covered with rectal mucosa. Internal hemorrhoids typically cannot be seen or felt unless they prolapse through the anal canal. Internal hemorrhoids are classified by severity based on whether or not they prolapse through the anal canal during straining with a bowel movement and whether or not the prolapsed hemorrhoid spontaneously retracts into the rectum, can be manually manipulated into the rectum, or cannot be returned to rectum.

K64.0   First degree hemorrhoids

These internal hemorrhoids may be with or without hemorrhage and they do not prolapse outside of the anal canal.

K64.1   Second degree hemorrhoids

These internal hemorrhoids may be with or without hemorrhage and they prolapse with straining outside the anal canal, but spontaneously retract.

K64.2   Third degree hemorrhoids

These internal hemorrhoids may be with or without hemorrhage and they prolapse with straining, requiring manual replacement back inside the anal canal.

K64.3   Fourth degree hemorrhoids

These internal hemorrhoids may be with or without hemorrhage, prolapse with straining outside the anal canal, and cannot be manually replaced. Internal fourth degree hemorrhoids may become severe enough to need tying off to reduce the blood flow to the hemorrhoids, allowing them to dissipate.

K64.4   Residual hemorrhoidal skin tags

K64.5   Perianal venous thrombosis

External hemorrhoids develop under the sensitive perianal skin and can itch and bleed when irritated. Usually painless, they may become a hard, painful lump if a blood clot or venous thrombosis develops. When a venous thrombosis is contained within the perianal blood vessel, the external hemorrhoid is classified as a perianal venous thrombosis. When no thrombosis is present in the external hemorrhoid, the condition is classified as a residual hemorrhoid or skin tag.

Diseases of the Peritoneum and Retroperitoneum (K65-K68)

The peritoneum is a membrane that lines the abdominal wall (parietal peritoneum) and covers most of the organs in the abdomen (visceral peritoneum). The space between the parietal peritoneum and the visceral peritoneum is called the peritoneal cavity. The retroperitoneum is part of the abdominal cavity. It is the space behind the posterior parietal peritoneum and in front of the posterior aspect of the abdominal wall. It contains the adrenal glands, kidneys, ureters, aorta and inferior vena cava, esophagus, rectum, parts of the duodenum and colon, and parts of the pancreas.

The categories in this code block are as follows:

K65	Peritonitis
K66	Other disorders of peritoneum
K67	Disorders of peritoneum in infectious diseases classified elsewhere
K68	Disorders of retroperitoneum

K65.-   Peritonitis

The term peritonitis encompasses a number of inflammatory conditions affecting the peritoneum. Peritonitis is an inflammation of the peritoneum; peritoneal abscess is a collection of pus in the peritoneum; choleperitonitis is an inflammation of the peritoneum due to bile; and sclerosing mesenteritis is a rare disorder characterized by inflammation and scar tissue formation of the tissue that surrounds and supports the intestines. These inflammatory conditions may arise in response to agents such as bacteria, viruses, bile, hydrochloric acid, and chemicals such as continuous ambulatory peritoneal dialysis (CAPD) fluid. Other causative agents include parasites, fungi, and foreign bodies. Ruptured viscus and surgical procedures are two common underlying factors in secondary peritonitis. Chronic peritonitis can lead to dense, widespread abdominal adhesions.

K65.3   Choleperitonitis

Choleperitonitis is an infection and inflammation of the peritoneum caused by the escape of bile from the gallbladder or bile ducts into the peritoneal cavity. This may occur due to nontraumatic rupture of the gallbladder or bile duct or intraabdominal trauma with injury to these structures.

K65.4   Sclerosing mesenteritis

Sclerosing mesenteritis is a rare disease process that forms mesenteric masses or areas of thickening, more commonly of the small bowel but also the mesocolon. The disease usually presents around age 60, with a higher predominance in men. Signs and symptoms include abdominal pain, masses, diarrhea, nausea, vomiting, and weight loss. Sclerosing mesenteritis is a combination of fat necrosis, chronic inflammation, and fibrosis occurring in the mesentery, commonly manifesting as a single mass of diffuse thickening, although additional lesions are sometimes reported. Masses are hard and gritty and may be from 1 to 40 cm in size. Patients may require surgical resection when bowel obstruction occurs. The numerous other terms applied to this disease process, such as mesenteric panniculitis, retractile mesenteritis, and mesenteric lipodystrophy share the same common clinical and histological features and are generally considered to be different spectrums of the single disease.

K68.-   Disorders of retroperitoneum

Retroperitoneal abscesses and other disorders of the retroperitoneum are classified here.

K68.12   Psoas muscle abscess

The psoas muscle is located in the iliopsoas compartment behind the transversalis fascia and connects the lumbar vertebrae to the femur and flexes the trunk or thigh. Psoas muscle abscess may also be documented as retrofascial in location because the psoas muscle is located in the retrofascial space, which is the posterior aspect of the peritoneum. Psoas muscle abscess is a rare condition. The abscess site may be externally visible on the flank or down the anterior thigh. Symptoms include fever, flank pain, and inability to fully move the hip. Historically, the most common cause of psoas abscess was tuberculosis. Today psoas abscess is more commonly associated with severe kidney or other infections caused by a number of organisms including staphylococcus.

Diseases of the Liver (K70-K77)

The liver is the largest gland in the body and serves many metabolic purposes including glycogen storage, digestion of fats and proteins, bile production, synthesizing blood clotting factors, processing medications, and removing toxins from the body.

The categories in this code block are as follows:

K70	Alcoholic liver disease
K71	Toxic liver disease
K72	Hepatic failure, not elsewhere classified
K73	Chronic hepatitis, not elsewhere classified
K74	Fibrosis and cirrhosis of liver
K75	Other inflammatory liver diseases
K76	Other diseases of liver
K77	Liver disorders in diseases classified elsewhere

K70.-   Alcoholic liver disease

Chronic alcohol use leads to three forms of liver disease: steatosis (fatty liver), hepatitis, and cirrhosis. The conditions have many overlapping features.

K70.0   Alcoholic fatty liver

Alcoholic fatty liver disease is an accumulation of an excessive amount of fat cells in the liver tissue due to the consumption of alcohol. Fatty liver occurs when more than 5 percent to 10 percent of the total weight of the liver is composed of fat cells. Fatty liver typically develops following prolonged periods of moderate to heavy alcohol consumption but can also occur after a short period of excessive alcohol intake. Fatty liver disease is reversible but requires abstinence from alcohol for a period of time and then continuing to abstain from alcohol or limiting alcohol intake after the condition has resolved.

K70.10   Alcoholic hepatitis without ascites

K70.11   Alcoholic hepatitis with ascites

Hepatitis is an inflammation of the liver, in this case due to alcohol. Mild alcoholic hepatitis may cause few symptoms. However, as the severity and duration of the liver inflammation increases, symptoms may include feeling generally unwell, the skin may become jaundiced due to elevated bilirubin levels, and there may be pain over the liver. Hepatitis may be complicated by ascites, which is an accumulation of fluid in the abdominal cavity. Ascites is characterized by abdominal distension and weight gain due to the accumulation of fluid. Other symptoms include swelling (edema) of the legs, particularly around the ankles, and shortness of breath from accumulation of fluid in the abdomen, which puts pressure on the thoracic cavity and lungs. Alcoholic hepatitis is classified as with or without ascites.

K70.2   Alcoholic fibrosis and sclerosis of liver

Hepatic fibrosis is the formation of scar tissue in the liver due to tissue injury and, in this case, the injury is caused by excessive consumption of alcohol. Hepatic sclerosis is a disruption of the liver vasculature, particularly the microcirculation in the liver, caused by the formation of scar tissue in the liver.

K70.30   Alcoholic cirrhosis of liver without ascites

K70.31   Alcoholic cirrhosis of liver with ascites

Cirrhosis of the liver is a chronic, progressive disease characterized by damage to the hepatic parenchymal cells and nodular regeneration, fibrosis formation, and disturbance of the normal architecture. Two different types of cirrhosis have been described based on the amount of regenerative activity in the liver: chronic sclerosing cirrhosis in which the liver is small and hard and nodular cirrhosis in which the liver may be initially quite enlarged. In alcoholic cirrhosis, the liver tends to shrink and become fibrotic. Alcoholic cirrhosis accounts for about 60 percent of all cirrhosis cases and the risk appears to rise with the amount of alcohol consumed daily. Cirrhosis may be complicated by ascites, which is an accumulation of fluid in the abdominal cavity. Ascites is characterized by abdominal distension and weight gain due to the accumulation of fluid. Other symptoms include swelling (edema) of the legs, particularly around the ankles, and shortness of breath from accumulation of fluid in the abdomen, which puts pressure on the thoracic cavity and lungs. Alcoholic cirrhosis is classified as with or without ascites.

K70.40   Alcoholic hepatic failure without coma

K70.41   Alcoholic hepatic failure with coma

Alcoholic hepatitis or cirrhosis can lead to hepatic failure, also called liver failure or end-stage liver disease. Liver failure occurs when normal liver tissue is replaced by scar tissue. The scar tissue affects the structure of the liver, damaging liver cells and causing them to die. As more normal liver tissue is replaced with scar tissue, the liver loses its ability to function. The scar tissue also affects the blood vessels in the liver, which may eventually cause portal hypertension. Alcoholic liver failure is classified as with or without coma. Coma is caused by hepatic encephalopathy, which is a deterioration of brain function due to the inability of the damaged liver to remove toxins from the blood. Intoxication with ammonia is also implicated in hepatic encephalopathy. Ammonia is a byproduct of protein digestion that the diseased liver fails to convert into urea. Hepatic encephalopathy is characterized by slow or rapid onset of bizarre behavior, disorientation, flapping tremors in extended arms, hyperactive reflexes, and later lethargy and coma.

K71.-   Toxic liver disease

Toxic liver disease, also called toxic hepatitis or hepatotoxicity, refers to liver damage that is chemical or drug-induced. Some causes include exposure to industrial chemicals such as dry cleaning solvents, herbicides, and vinyl chloride; over use of over-the-counter pain relievers such as acetaminophen, aspirin, ibuprofen, and naproxen; several prescription medications including Augmentin, Lipitor, Crestor, and others; and even some herbs and supplements. Some drugs directly harm the liver but others are transformed into injurious chemicals by the liver itself. Overdoses or long-term exposure can sometimes cause irreversible harm.

Focus Point

Because this type of hepatitis is caused by a drug or chemical, it is necessary to first code for poisoning due to a drug or toxin, if applicable. If toxic liver disease is not considered a poisoning, but an adverse effect, use an additional secondary code for the adverse effect to identify the drug.

K71.0   Toxic liver disease with cholestasis

This combination code identifies chemical or drug induced hepatitis with cholestasis. Cholestasis is an impairment of bile flow, which allows bilirubin to escape and accumulate in the bloodstream rather than bind with bile and move along its normal course through the digestive tract where it would be eliminated in the stool.

K71.10   Toxic liver disease with hepatic necrosis, without coma

K71.11   Toxic liver disease with hepatic necrosis, with coma

Hepatic necrosis that occurs due to toxic liver disease is an acute injury to the liver tissues resulting in pathologic death of liver cells, usually parenchymal cells, affecting all or part of the liver. This can result in liver dysfunction or failure. Symptoms are typically systemic and include nausea, weakness, fatigue, and abdominal pain. If the toxic substance is identified and removed, liver dysfunction can sometimes be reversed. In toxic liver disease, necrosis is classified with or without coma.

K71.2   Toxic liver disease with acute hepatitis

Acute hepatitis is inflammation of hepatocytes (liver cells) that lasts less than six months. In acute hepatitis due to a drug, chemical, or toxin, the inflammation typically occurs abruptly and may be accompanied by fever, chills, rash, itching, joint pain, headache, abdominal pain, nausea, and vomiting. Treatment involves discontinuing the drug or eliminating exposure to the chemical or toxin and supportive care until the inflammation resolves.

K71.3   Toxic liver disease with chronic persistent hepatitis

K71.4   Toxic liver disease with chronic lobular hepatitis

When inflammation of hepatocytes (liver cells) continues for more than six months, hepatitis is classified as chronic. In chronic persistent hepatitis, inflammation is limited to the portal tracts and death of hepatocytes (liver cells) is not seen. In chronic lobular hepatitis, there is inflammation of the portal tracts accompanied with inflammation of the liver parenchyma adjacent to the portal tracts that is usually localized to a single lobe. In chronic lobular hepatitis there is some necrosis (death) of hepatocytes but the necrosis is typically limited to the connective tissues around the portal tract. Even though the inflammation may last for years, these two types of hepatitis generally do not progress to more serious liver disease so extensive liver damage resulting in cirrhosis does not occur and the prognosis for recovery is good.

K71.50   Toxic liver disease with chronic active hepatitis without ascites

K71.51   Toxic liver disease with chronic active hepatitis with ascites

Chronic active hepatitis refers to inflammation and necrosis of hepatocytes (liver cells) for a period lasting longer than six months. Chronic active hepatitis is a serious condition that can result in permanent liver damage, including cirrhosis and liver failure, and can also lead to liver cancer. Toxic liver disease with lupoid hepatitis is included here. Lupoid hepatitis is an autoimmune hepatitis that occurs when the body launches a cell-mediated attack on its own tissues, and in this case the autoimmune response is triggered by a drug, chemical, or other toxin. Toxic liver disease with chronic active hepatitis is classified based on the presence or absence of ascites, which is an accumulation of fluid in the peritoneal cavity.

K71.7   Toxic liver disease with fibrosis and cirrhosis of liver

Liver fibrosis is caused by chronic liver disease, in this case due to a drug or toxin, that results in damage to liver tissues with replacement of healthy tissue by scar tissue. Cirrhosis of the liver is a chronic, progressive disease characterized by damage to the hepatic parenchymal cells and nodular regeneration, fibrosis formation, and disturbance of the normal architecture.

K73.-   Chronic hepatitis, not elsewhere classified

Chronic hepatitis refers to inflammation of hepatocytes (liver cells) lasting longer than six months. Depending on the specific type, the prolonged inflammation may have a relatively benign outcome resolving on its own over the course of several years or may progress to more serious liver disease including liver failure or liver cancer. Chronic hepatitis for which the etiology is not known or for which there is not a more specific code is classified here.

K73.0   Chronic persistent hepatitis, not elsewhere classified

K73.1   Chronic lobular hepatitis, not elsewhere classified

When inflammation of hepatocytes (liver cells) continues for more than six months, hepatitis is classified as chronic. In chronic persistent hepatitis, inflammation is limited to the portal tracts and death of hepatocytes (liver cells) is not seen. In chronic lobular hepatitis, there is inflammation of the portal tracts accompanied with inflammation of the liver parenchyma adjacent to the portal tracts that is usually localized to a single lobe. In chronic lobular hepatitis there is some necrosis (death) of hepatocytes but the necrosis is typically limited to the connective tissues around the portal tract. Even though the inflammation may last for years, these two types of hepatitis generally do not progress to more serious liver disease so extensive liver damage resulting in cirrhosis does not occur and the prognosis for recovery is good.

K73.2   Chronic active hepatitis, not elsewhere classified

Chronic active hepatitis refers to inflammation and necrosis of hepatocytes (liver cells) for a period lasting longer than six months. Chronic active hepatitis is a serious condition that can result in permanent liver damage including cirrhosis and liver failure and can also lead to liver cancer.

K74.-   Fibrosis and cirrhosis of liver

This category represents liver fibrosis and cirrhosis that is not caused by alcohol use or toxic liver disease. Liver fibrosis is caused by chronic liver disease that results in damage to liver tissues with replacement of healthy tissue by scar tissue. Cirrhosis of the liver is a chronic, progressive disease characterized by damage to the hepatic parenchymal cells and nodular regeneration, fibrosis formation, and disturbance of the normal architecture. Hepatitis due to viral infections, or viral hepatitis, is most commonly caused by one of the five unrelated hepatotropic viruses.

K74.0   Hepatic fibrosis

Hepatic fibrosis is the formation of scar tissue in the liver due to tissue injury. Hepatic fibrosis results from an over accumulation of proteins including collagen and is caused by chronic liver disease. The main causes other than alcohol abuse are Hepatitis C (HCV) infection and nonalcoholic steatohepatitis (NASH).

K74.1   Hepatic sclerosis

Hepatic sclerosis is a chronic liver disease characterized by the deterioration of liver tissues and replacement by fibrous scar tissue. In hepatic sclerosis there is a disruption of the liver vasculature, particularly the microcirculation in the liver, caused by the formation of scar tissue in the liver.

K75.- Other inflammatory liver diseases

This category includes inflammatory conditions that are caused by infection, such as a liver abscess; vascular disease, such as inflammation of the portal vein; hepatitis caused by autoimmune disease; and nonalcoholic steatohepatitis (fatty liver), as well as others.

K75.4 Autoimmune hepatitis

Autoimmune hepatitis may be described as the body's immune system attacking the liver. The body's immune cells mistake the liver's normal cells as harmful invaders. Although the causal mechanism is largely unknown, precipitating factors may include genetic predisposition, preexisting immune or other diseases, or exposures to certain drugs or toxins. In general, autoimmune hepatitis primarily affects women between the ages of 15 and 40. It is characterized by continuing hepatocellular inflammation and necrosis, which tends to progress to cirrhosis. Immune serum markers frequently are present, and the disease may be associated with other autoimmune diseases. However, two clinical categories exist: Type I or Type II. Type I is more common in North America and affects patients at any age, although it is more prevalent among women. About half of patients with type I autoimmune hepatitis suffer from other autoimmune disorders, such as Type 1 diabetes, proliferative glomerulonephritis, thyroiditis, Graves' disease, Sjögren's syndrome, autoimmune anemia, and ulcerative colitis. Type II autoimmune hepatitis is less common, typically affecting girls ages 2 to 14, although it has been known to affect adults as well. Symptoms of autoimmune hepatitis range from mild to severe, and may include hepatomegaly, jaundice, ascites, joint pain, and pruritus. Diagnosis may be confirmed by biopsy. Treatment is often focused on the underlying condition.

Focus Point

Lupoid hepatitis, a type of autoimmune hepatitis, is reported with a code from subcategory K71.5- when the cause is due to drugs or toxins.

K75.81 Nonalcoholic steatohepatitis (NASH)

Nonalcoholic steatohepatitis, or NASH, is a common, often silent, liver disease. It resembles alcoholic liver disease but occurs in people who drink little or no alcohol. The major feature in NASH is fat in the liver, along with inflammation and damage. NASH can be severe and can lead to cirrhosis, a condition in which the liver is permanently damaged and scarred and is no longer able to work properly.

K76.- Other diseases of liver

This category classifies diseases of the liver that do not fit well into a more specific category. A number of liver diseases caused by circulatory disorders are included here.

K76.4 Peliosis hepatis

Peliosis hepatis is an uncommon condition characterized by randomly distributed, multiple blood-filled cystic cavities throughout the liver. It is usually asymptomatic but has been known to develop into overt liver disease and can even cause rupture with hemorrhage. Mild cases are generally detected incidentally when liver function tests show abnormal results or when the cysts are seen on ultrasound.

K76.6 Portal hypertension

Portal hypertension occurs when there is an increase in blood pressure of the portal venous system (portal vein and its branches) due to blockages in the liver vessels from liver damage. Esophageal or gastric varices can develop as a result of the pressure and can rupture and bleed. Another potential complication is an enlarged spleen, which can result in decreased numbers of white blood cells and increased circulating platelets that in turn increase risk of infection and bleeding.

K76.7 Hepatorenal syndrome

Hepatorenal syndrome is combined liver and kidney failure that is usually caused by serious injury to the liver associated with hemorrhage, shock, and acute renal insufficiency.

K76.81 Hepatopulmonary syndrome

Hepatopulmonary syndrome (HPS) is a complication of advanced acute or chronic liver disease, which has progressed to the point where the lungs are affected, resulting in dyspnea and hypoxia. Although it is most prevalent among adults, a pediatric patient with liver disease may also develop HPS. It is commonly associated with cirrhosis of the liver, acute ischemic hepatitis, and noncirrhotic portal hypertension. The liver plays an important role in regulating blood vessel tone in the lungs. As such, when the liver is damaged, it can cause microvascular dilation of the pulmonary vasculature, which causes intrapulmonary shunting of blood from the lungs to the heart.

Disorders of Gallbladder, Biliary Tract, and Pancreas (K80-K87)

The gallbladder, biliary tract, and pancreas are accessory organs or structures that support the digestive process. These organs provide secretions that are critical to food absorption and use of nutrients by the body.

The categories in this code block are as follows:

K80	Cholelithiasis
K81	Cholecystitis
K82	Other diseases of gallbladder
K83	Other diseases of biliary tract

K85   Acute pancreatitis

K86   Other diseases of pancreas

K87   Disorders of gallbladder, biliary tract and pancreas in diseases classified elsewhere

K80.-   Cholelithiasis

Cholelithiasis refers to the presence or formation of concretions (calculi or "gallstones") in the gallbladder. The concretions contain cholesterol, calcium carbonate, or calcium bilirubinate in pure forms or in various combinations. Many factors contribute to concretion formation, but they generally can be grouped into three categories: abnormal composition of bile, abnormal contractility of the gallbladder, and abnormal epithelial secretions. Signs and symptoms of cholelithiasis include cramps or severe epigastric pain, nausea and vomiting, heartburn, eructation, flatulence, sensation of dullness in stomach, jaundice, distention of gallbladder, and pain on palpation of gallbladder. However, cholelithiasis is asymptomatic in many patients.

Cholelithiasis

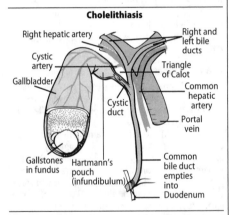

K80.00   Calculus of gallbladder with acute cholecystitis without obstruction

K80.01   Calculus of gallbladder with acute cholecystitis with obstruction

Acute cholecystitis is sudden onset inflammation of the gallbladder, which in this case is associated with the presence of gallstones or calculi in the gallbladder or cystic duct. The acute inflammation is most often caused by an obstruction of the cystic duct by gallstones or biliary sludge that has obstructed the gallbladder neck. This creates pressure within the gallbladder, which along with cholesterol supersaturated bile, elicits an acute inflammatory response. This condition is classified based on the presence or absence of obstruction of the cystic duct or gallbladder.

K80.3-   Calculus of bile duct with cholangitis

When there are concretions, called calculi or gallstones, in the system of bile ducts called the biliary tree, the condition is referred to as choledocholithiasis. Common duct stones usually originate in the gallbladder, but may form spontaneously in the common duct following cholecystectomy. Cholangitis, an inflammation or infection of the cystic or common bile duct, is also referred to as ascending cholangitis because it most often occurs when obstructive gallstones allow bacteria to ascend from the duodenum causing a common bile duct infection. Cholangitis may become life-threatening if it progresses to bacteremia and sepsis. Symptoms that suggest choledocholithiasis with cholangitis include Charcot's triad. Charcot's triad is a symptom complex consisting of frequently recurring attacks of severe, persistent, right upper quadrant pain lasting for hours; chills and fever associated with severe colic; and a history of jaundice chronologically associated with abdominal pain.

> **Focus Point**
>
> *Cholangitis and cholecystitis may occur together when there is a calculus in a bile duct. Codes from subcategory K80.3- should not be reported when both conditions are present. Use codes in subcategory K80.4- when documentation indicates that both conditions are present.*

K80.4-   Calculus of bile duct with cholecystitis

When there are concretions, called calculi or gallstones, in the system of bile ducts called the biliary tree, the condition is referred to as choledocholithiasis. Common duct stones usually originate in the gallbladder, but may form spontaneously in the common duct following cholecystectomy. Cholecystitis is an inflammation of the gallbladder that may manifest as an acute or chronic condition and can be present with choledocholithiasis either alone or along with cholangitis. An acute inflammation of the gallbladder occurs suddenly and is usually caused by an obstruction at the outlet of the gallbladder, with consequent edema and congestion that can result in serious complications such as gangrene and perforation. Chronic cholecystitis is a mild symptomatic inflammation of the gallbladder that continues over a long period of time. In addition, an acute episode of cholecystitis can be superimposed on chronic cholecystitis. Codes in this subcategory are assigned based on whether cholecystitis is acute, chronic, or acute on chronic, and whether or not the choledocholithiasis with cholecystitis is complicated by obstruction of the bile duct or gallbladder.

K80.5- Calculus of bile duct without cholangitis or cholecystitis

Choledocholithiasis, the presence of calculi or gallstones in the biliary ducts, without inflammation of the ducts and without inflammation of the gallbladder is classified here. The presence of calculi in the biliary ducts may be complicated by obstruction of the biliary ducts or the gallbladder.

> **Focus Point**
>
> *Secondary pancreatitis, biliary cirrhosis, and hypoprothrombinemia may complicate choledocholithiasis and are reported additionally.*

K81.- Cholecystitis

Cholecystitis is an inflammation of the gallbladder. Only inflammation of the gallbladder that is not due to the presence of gallstones or calculi in the gallbladder or bile ducts is classified here.

K81.0 Acute cholecystitis

K81.1 Chronic cholecystitis

K81.2 Acute cholecystitis with chronic cholecystitis

An acute inflammation of the gallbladder occurs suddenly and is usually caused by an obstruction at the outlet of the gallbladder, with consequent edema and congestion that can result in serious complications such as gangrene and perforation. Other causes of acute cholecystitis include obstruction of the cystic duct by another process (such as a malignant tumor), bile stasis ("sludge" formation, which is a precipitant of calcium bilirubinate calculi formation), or infection due to organisms such as *Escherichia coli*, *E. clostridia*, or *Salmonella typhi*. Chronic cholecystitis is a mild symptomatic inflammation of the gallbladder that continues over a long period of time. Chronic cholecystitis rarely occurs in the absence of cholelithiasis, but can occur in conditions such as cholesterolosis and adenomatous hyperplasia. Acute and chronic forms may occur together.

K82.- Other diseases of gallbladder

This category identifies conditions such as obstructions of the cystic duct or gallbladder that are not due to cholelithiasis, perforations, adhesions, mucocele, strawberry gallbladder, and other disorders of the gallbladder or cystic duct.

K82.1 Hydrops of gallbladder

Hydrops (mucocele) of the gallbladder is a noninflammatory condition that occurs when the gallbladder fills with mucoid or clear, watery fluid and becomes distended. It is generally caused by an impacted calculus in the gallbladder neck or cystic duct.

> **Focus Point**
>
> *Hydrops of gallbladder should not be confused with gallbladder empyema, a condition where the gallbladder is filled with pus. The appropriate code for gallbladder empyema is K81.0 Acute cholecystitis.*

K82.4 Cholesterolosis of gallbladder

Cholesterolosis is also referred to as strawberry gallbladder because of its appearance of yellow deposits on the mucosal surface of the gallbladder resembling a strawberry. These accretions form from abnormal deposits of cholesterol esters, precursors, and triglycerides. The stippled accumulation of lipids is a benign condition, but can lead to similar complications as those caused by gallstones.

K83.- Other diseases of biliary tract

This category includes conditions of the bile duct such as occlusions that are not due to cholelithiasis, perforations, fistulas, cysts, cholangitis, and other diseases.

K83.0 Cholangitis

Cholangitis classified here refers to an infection or inflammation of the common bile duct not due to calculus. Sclerosing cholangitis, an inflammation that causes scars within the bile ducts, is one of the conditions included in this code. This chronic scarring leads to narrowing of the ducts, repeated infections, and eventual liver failure. The only cure for this condition is a liver transplant.

K83.1 Obstruction of bile duct

Obstruction of the bile duct may occur due to an occlusion, stenosis, or stricture of the bile duct. Obstruction results in a condition called cholestasis or bile stasis, which refers to the inability of bile to flow from the liver to the duodenum. When the flow of bile is obstructed, the two major components of bile, bilirubin and bile acids, accumulate in the blood causing jaundice (yellowing of the skin) and pruritus (itching). Mirizzi's syndrome, an extrinsic extrahepatic bile duct obstruction that is caused by compression from an impacted calculus in the Hartmann's pouch of the gallbladder or the cystic duct, is classified here.

K85.- Acute pancreatitis

Acute pancreatitis is a sudden inflammation of the pancreas that resolves within a short period of time with proper treatment. The primary symptom of acute pancreatitis is pain that may range from mild abdominal discomfort to severe and debilitating pain. Pain tends to be centered in the upper abdomen and may radiate into the back. Other symptoms include swollen and tender abdomen, nausea and vomiting, fever, and elevated heart rate. Pancreatitis can be caused by gallstones (biliary), alcohol, drugs, or may be idiopathic. Acute pancreatitis is classified based on type or cause and on whether necrosis, with or without infection, is present.

K85.0- Idiopathic acute pancreatitis

Acute pancreatitis develops due to inflammation of the exocrine pancreas and, while routine examinations typically determine the cause in 75 percent to 90 percent of instances, 10 percent to 25 percent of the cases remain idiopathic. Assessment and treatment are necessary to prevent recurrence the condition evolving into chronic pancreatitis, leading to functional complications. Acute pancreatitis can become serious when organ failure or pancreatic necrosis is involved with a mortality rate of 2 percent to 7 percent in spite of aggressive treatment.

K85.1- Biliary acute pancreatitis

Biliary acute pancreatitis caused by gallstones is the primary cause of pancreatitis, which can lead to serious complications. When gallstones obstruct the pancreatic duct, the pancreatic enzymes are trapped inside the pancreas, causing inflammation. While most cases achieve full recovery, almost a third of cases require physicians from multiple specialties to manage and treat the condition, often requiring a cholecystectomy. Complications such as necrosis and respiratory system disorders may require hospitalization. This diagnosis should be considered for patients with a history of biliary colic; however, other causes may contribute, such as overuse of alcohol, medications, genetics, infections, and complications of surgery.

K85.2- Alcohol induced acute pancreatitis

K85.3- Drug induced acute pancreatitis

The top three causes of acute pancreatitis are gallstones, alcohol, and drugs, in that order. Acute pancreatitis can present after an episode of heavy alcohol binge drinking. Reports of acute pancreatitis based on drug complications are limited in terms of identifying the specific drug that may lead to this complication since over 500 medications have been suggested. The best way to determine the cause is to eliminate the specific drug or alcohol while investigating other potential triggers of the pancreatitis in order to evaluate the optimal course of action for treatment.

Focus Point

Episodic binge drinking can cause acute pancreatitis, which is reported with K85.2- Alcohol induced acute pancreatitis. Prolonged alcohol abuse is a leading cause of chronic pancreatitis, which is reported with code K86.0 Alcohol-induced chronic pancreatitis, along with a code to identify the alcohol abuse or dependence from chapter 5.

K86.- Other diseases of pancreas

The pancreas is a glandular organ that has both an endocrine and exocrine function. It is more commonly known for its role in glucose maintenance and the production of insulin, yet it also plays an important role in digestion by secreting a fluid called pancreatic juice. This juice contains enzymes that digest carbohydrates, fats, proteins, and nucleic acids. The pancreas also helps neutralize the acidic chyme that leaves the stomach and enters the intestine. Conditions other than acute pancreatitis can be found in this category.

Focus Point

Pancreatitis can arise from cytomegalovirus, which is spread from direct person-to-person contact and is usually harmless but can cause severe disease in people with compromised immune systems. The appropriate code for cytomegaloviral pancreatitis can be found in Chapter 1 Certain Infectious and Parasitic Diseases.

K86.0 Alcohol-induced chronic pancreatitis

Alcohol-induced chronic pancreatitis is a prolonged inflammation of the pancreas caused by long-term, heavy alcohol use. Long-term, heavy alcohol use is responsible for 45 percent of all cases of chronic pancreatitis. Alcohol induced chronic pancreatitis is often initially asymptomatic. When chronic pancreatitis becomes symptomatic it is characterized by pain in the upper abdomen that radiates to the back, swollen and tender abdomen, nausea and vomiting, fever, and elevated heart rate. Other symptoms include weight loss due to poor absorption of nutrients from food and diabetes caused by damage to the insulin producing cells of the pancreas.

K86.1 Other chronic pancreatitis

Chronic pancreatitis is characterized by prolonged inflammation of the pancreas. Chronic pancreatitis not due to alcohol is classified here. Causes of chronic pancreatitis include gallstones, hereditary conditions, cystic fibrosis, high triglycerides, and some medications. However, in up to 25 percent of cases, the cause of chronic pancreatitis cannot be determined. Chronic pancreatitis is often initially asymptomatic. When chronic pancreatitis becomes symptomatic it is characterized by the same symptoms as acute pancreatitis, including pain in the upper abdomen that radiates to the back, swollen and tender abdomen, nausea and vomiting, fever, and elevated heart rate.

Other symptoms include weight loss due to poor absorption of nutrients from food and diabetes caused by damage to the insulin producing cells of the pancreas.

K86.81   Exocrine pancreatic insufficiency

Exocrine pancreatic insufficiency (EPI) occurs when decreased enzymes contribute to difficulty with digestion, which may be caused by an underlying medical condition also affecting the pancreas. The primary cause of EPI for adults is chronic pancreatitis due to the passage of time and inflammatory process that damages the pancreas, including enzyme and insulin production. A person with this condition cannot digest fats, proteins, or carbohydrates effectively, which inhibits the body's ability to absorb essential nutrients and contributes to various gastrointestinal complaints. Treatment plans often include a healthy diet in addition to enzyme replacements and additional vitamins and/or supplements.

K86.89   Other specified diseases of pancreas

Several conditions may be assigned this code based on the following inclusion terms provided:

- Aseptic pancreatic necrosis, unrelated to acute pancreatitis: A condition leading to tissue death within the pancreas due to enzyme activation before leaving the pancreas and entering the duodenum, leading to cell death, atrophy, and eventually septic complications.

- Atrophy of pancreas: A deterioration of the pancreas that is typically a complication of chronic pancreatitis and most often caused by alcoholism. However, other contributing conditions include autoimmune disease, cystic fibrosis, and familial pancreatitis.

- Calculus of pancreas: Stone(s) in the pancreas consisting of calcium carbonate along with salt and other inorganic matter.

- Cirrhosis of pancreas: Deterioration of pancreatic cells leading to inflammation, destruction, and formation of scar tissue.

- Fibrosis of pancreas: Typically brought on due to necrosis, inflammation or obstruction; however, initially an injury to the pancreas affecting the cells precipitates all of these.

- Pancreatic fat necrosis, unrelated to acute pancreatitis: Enzymes in the pancreas activate before leaving the organ, causing inflammation and necrosis of the fat and vessels.

- Pancreatic infantilism: Decreased development of the organ due to deficient production of islet hormones, specifically insulin.

Other Diseases of the Digestive System (K90-K95)

Conditions classified here relate to disorders that prevent the intestinal tract from absorbing nutrients, some symptoms associated with digestive system disorders, and complications related to procedures and artificial openings of the digestive system.

The categories in this code block are as follows:

K90	Intestinal malabsorption
K91	Intraoperative and postprocedural complications and disorders of digestive system, not elsewhere classified
K94	Complications of artificial openings of the digestive system
K95	Complications of bariatric procedures

K90.-   Intestinal malabsorption

The mucosal layer of the intestine is a crucial barrier that prevents bacteria, antigens, and undigested food from seeping through the gastrointestinal wall and into the systemic circulation. However, nutrients and fluids must be able to pass through the mucosal layer. When a condition such as inflammation, disease, or injury of the mucosal layer occurs, absorption of nutrients may be adversely affected and this is called intestinal malabsorption. This condition can result in nutrient deficiencies and weight loss. A common symptom is abnormal appearing stools.

K90.0   Celiac disease

Celiac disease, also called nontropical sprue, celiac sprue, gluten intolerant enteropathy, Gee-Herter syndrome, or gluten sensitive enteropathy, is a condition in which there is a chronic inflammatory reaction to certain proteins, commonly referred to as glutens, found in some cereal grains. This reaction destroys the villi in the small intestine, with resulting malabsorption of nutrients. The disease affects both sexes and it can begin at any age, from infancy (as soon as cereal grains are introduced) to later life (even though the individual has consumed cereal grains all along). The onset of the disease seems to require genetic predisposition and some kind of trigger, such as overexposure to wheat, a pregnancy, an operation, or a viral infection.

K90.1   Tropical sprue

Tropical sprue, also known as tropical steatorrhea, is a disease causing absorption problems within the small bowel. Symptoms may appear as celiac disease; however, this is not an autoimmune condition but more of an infection by unknown bacteria. The condition most often affects people living or visiting a tropical climate who present with diarrhea, fever, and discomfort, which then evolve into more serious deficiencies. Medical treatment includes fluids, antibiotics, and vitamins or supplements. Without treatment the condition may become chronic.

K90.2   Blind loop syndrome, not elsewhere classified

This condition is caused by the formation of an abnormal bypass of the small intestine. This bypassed area is called a "blind loop" and prevents food from moving normally through the gastrointestinal tract. The small intestine normally contains few bacteria, but when a blind loop is present, stagnant food in the blind loop causes overgrowth of bacteria leading to bacterial derangement that disrupts the digestive process and inhibits the absorption of nutrients. Also called stasis syndrome or stagnant loop syndrome, some causes of this condition are inflammatory bowel disease, diabetes, and scleroderma.

K90.3   Pancreatic steatorrhea

Pancreatic steatorrhea is characterized by excess fat found in feces due to lack of pancreatic enzymes within the intestine. Treatment in the form of enzyme supplements typically restores the normal processing within the pancreas, and the digestive tract functions normally. In some cases additional steps, including diet restrictions and/or abstinence from alcohol, are needed to restore normal.

K90.41   Non-celiac gluten sensitivity

Gluten sensitivity often appears as celiac disease in that the patients cannot handle gluten but do not exhibit the same damage or produce the same antibodies as those with celiac disease. Furthermore, symptoms extend beyond the typical gastrointestinal issues and may manifest in headaches, joint pain, and extremity numbness. There are currently no methods of testing for this condition and the condition is instead diagnosed by process of elimination, starting with allergy tests and celiac testing and then diet modification to eliminate gluten.

K90.81   Whipple's disease

Whipple's disease is an infection primarily occurring in the small intestine, caused by a rare bacteria called *Tropheryma whipplei* (*T. whipplei*). Lesions and thickening of intestinal tissues damages the villi and impairs the breakdown of foods and proper absorption of nutrients, leading to diarrhea and malnutrition. The bacteria can also infect other parts of the body such as the joints, brain, and heart.

K91.-   Intraoperative and postprocedural complications and disorders of digestive system, not elsewhere classified

A variety of complications can occur during or following procedures on the digestive system. Some complications such as dumping syndrome and malabsorption relate directly to digestive system procedures, while other complications such as hemorrhage, accidental puncture, and laceration can occur due to a digestive system procedure or a procedure on organs that are in close proximity to digestive system organs.

K91.1   Postgastric surgery syndromes

Dumping syndrome is classified to this category and represents a constellation of symptoms that include reflux, vomiting, nausea, diaphoresis, and diarrhea. These symptoms are related to increased transit of undigested food directly into the small bowel that may occur after complete or partial gastrectomy and gastric bypass surgery. Treatment involves adjusting the diet, although in severe cases medication or additional surgery is needed.

K91.2   Postsurgical malabsorption, not elsewhere classified

Blind loop syndrome as a complication of surgery is included in this code. Postsurgical blind loop syndrome is most often associated with partial or complete gastrectomy for ulcers or malignant neoplasms of the stomach and gastric bypass procedures performed to treat obesity. This condition is caused by the formation of an abnormal bypass of the small intestine. This bypassed area is called a blind loop and prevents food from moving normally through the gastrointestinal tract. The small intestine normally contains few bacteria, but when a blind loop is present, stagnant food in the blind loop causes overgrowth of bacteria leading to bacterial derangement that disrupts the digestive process and inhibits the absorption of nutrients.

K91.3-   Postprocedural intestinal obstruction

This subcategory classifies intestinal obstruction documented as a postoperative complication. The most common postprocedural intestinal obstruction is paralytic ileus. Generally, a postoperative obstructive ileus that is present for up to three days after a surgical procedure is considered an expected outcome of the procedure and not reported as a complication. However, a failure to return to normal bowel function after three days, which requires treatment such as nasogastric tube, rectal tube, NPO status is most likely a postprocedural intestinal obstruction. Physicians often document postprocedural intestinal obstruction as partial versus complete, but the intestinal obstruction can be coded as unspecified as to partial versus complete.

K91.850 Pouchitis

Pouchitis is inflammation of an internal ileoanal pouch, surgically created following resection of the colon or rectum. The ileoanal pouch (pull-through) and the continent ileostomy (Kock pouch) are surgical alternatives to a standard ileostomy, which uses an external appliance for stool collection. The internal pouch eliminates the need to wear an external ostomy device. In pouch creation, the small intestine (ileum) is used to create an internal pouch for collection of stool. The surgery may be performed for treatment of ulcerative colitis or familial adenomatous polyposis. Inflammation of the pouch (pouchitis) is one of the most common postsurgical complications. Symptoms may mimic those of ulcerative colitis, with diarrhea, rectal bleeding, crampy abdominal pain, fecal urgency, or incontinence. Additional symptoms may include fever, loss of appetite, dehydration, joint pain, and malaise. Approximately one third of patients with an ileoanal pouch experience at least one episode of pouchitis. Patients with concomitant autoimmune or inflammatory disease have a higher incidence of occurrence. Pouchitis is typically treated with a short course of antibiotics, suggesting an infectious etiology. Chronic pouchitis is relatively rare, but when it does occur, surgical conversion to a standard ileostomy may be necessary.

K91.86 Retained cholelithiasis following cholecystectomy

Retained gallstones are a relatively common occurrence following cholecystectomy, especially following laparoscopic cholecystectomy. During surgery, gallstones may dislodge into the bile duct, be pushed into the gastrointestinal tract, or be displaced into the abdominopelvic cavity. Retained stones can cause obstruction or infection, although in some cases displaced or retained stones remain asymptomatic. Symptoms indicative of retained stones in the bile ducts include biliary colic symptoms, right upper quadrant and postprandial pain, and digestive problems. Stones that are incidentally displaced or spilled into the pelvic cavity can cause symptoms that mimic gynecological disease and can cause pain, dysmenorrhea, and pelvic adhesive disease that may impair fertility.

K92.- Other diseases of digestive system

This category contains codes for symptoms and other conditions that do not fit well into a more specific category.

K92.0 Hematemesis

Gastrointestinal bleeding as evidenced by vomiting of blood is referred to as hematemesis. Hematemesis may present as frank red blood or partially digested dark or black blood flecks in vomitus. Hematemesis usually is indicative of bleeding of the upper gastrointestinal tract.

K92.1 Melena

Melena is the presence of partially digested blood, which presents as dark tarry stools. Also classified here is hematochezia, which is the passage of frank red blood in stools. Passage of frank red or partially digested blood in the stools may be due to a condition in the upper or lower GI tract.

K92.81 Gastrointestinal mucositis (ulcerative)

Mucosal inflammation, or mucositis, affects the tissues that line the gastrointestinal tract. A frequent, debilitating complication of chemotherapy or radiation treatment, mucositis occurs when the epithelial cells lining the GI tract break down, leaving the mucosal tissue susceptible to infection and ulceration. Some non-chemotherapeutic drugs may also cause adverse reactions that manifest as mucositis. Complications of mucositis range from mild symptoms that require little intervention to severe, sometimes fatal problems such as malnutrition, hypovolemia, or electrolyte abnormalities. Nausea and vomiting are frequent side-effects of antineoplastic therapy and may further complicate the mucositis.

Focus Point

Gastrointestinal mucositis is classified as an adverse effect when it is associated with antineoplastic drugs, other medications, or radiotherapy. The appropriate code for the causative agent is reported additionally.

Gastrointestinal mucositis does not include mucositis of the mouth and oral soft tissue, which is reported with a code from subcategory K12.3-.

K94.- Complications of artificial openings of the digestive system

This category includes complications of surgically created artificial openings such as colostomies, enterostomies, gastrostomies, and esophagostomies.

K94.0- Colostomy complications

A colostomy creates an opening through the abdomen into the colon when the colon, rectum, or anus does not function properly due to disease or injury; this allows the body to eliminate the waste that would normally progress through the large intestine.

As with any surgery, there are potential complications to the colostomy procedure such as hemorrhage, infection, malfunction, leaking, or injury to adjacent organs. When leaking, hemorrhage, swelling, pain, fever, and/or rectal bleeding occur without resolution from medication or postoperative instructions, the surgeon should be contacted as these symptoms may indicate an infection or more serious complications.

The surgical team typically provides information on all possible complications to the procedure as well as ways to prevent or minimize these complications:

- Discharge from the rectum: Mucus production within the bowel lining does not cease once a colostomy is created.
- Parastomal hernia: This may occur when a portion of the intestines migrates through the muscles around the stoma, producing a mass under the skin surface.
- Stoma blockage: Obstruction due to food accumulation. Often decreasing intake of solid food while increasing fluid helps relieve this, but if symptoms progress or worsen, the stoma nurse should be contacted in case immediate medical attention is required.
- Skin problems: Skin surrounding the stoma that has become irritated.
- Stomal fistula: A tunnel under the skin adjacent to the stoma.
- Stoma retraction: When the stoma falls under the level of the skin after initial healing, often causing leaking problems.
- Stoma prolapse: Advancement of the stoma further above skin level.
- Stomal stricture: Development of scarring, causing restriction.
- Stomal ischemia: Decrease in blood flow to the area.

K94.1- Enterostomy complications

An enterostomy creates an opening into the abdomen to access the small intestine to insert a drainage or feeding tube and includes ileostomies and jejunostomies. Complications for this procedure may include:

- Infection
- Migration of tube
- Obstruction
- Leaking
- Incision separation

Although this procedure is not considered a high-risk operation, about 40 percent of ileostomy procedures result in some complication while 15 percent may require further surgical intervention to correct the problem.

K94.2- Gastrostomy complications

A gastrostomy is performed to insert a feeding tube through the skin directly into the stomach. Minor complications include tube malfunction, bleeding, or infection. The following major complications are not common, but can lead to necrotizing fasciitis or colocutaneous fistula:

- Necrotizing fasciitis: Necrosis of tissues requiring prompt medical treatment with debridement.
- Hemorrhage: Bleeding may occur around the stoma or from within the tract and is most often controlled by applying pressure to the wound or adjustment of the bumper; only in rare instances is surgery needed to control the bleeding.
- Leaking: Leaking is often seen initially after placement, although it may occur later for patients with other conditions such as malnutrition or hyperglycemia. In some cases removal and reinsertion at a later time may be required.
- Ulcers: These can develop when an internal mechanism is too tight against the gastric wall and, while loosening of components often corrects the problem, sometimes the mechanism is removed and replaced with a more flexible variety.
- Gastric outlet obstruction: Obstruction may occur if the tube moves into the duodenum away from

the wall of the abdomen. Proper positioning should be able to prevent this complication.

- Tube dislocation: Dislocation is often a result of pressure or pulling on the tube, which may require removal and reinsertion in conjunction with antibiotics to avoid peritonitis.

Focus Point

Report K31.6 when the G-tube site fails to spontaneously close following removal of the G-tube. This condition, which requires surgical closure, is not considered a complication of the G-tube. This code reports only fistulas between the stomach or duodenum and other structures of the gastrointestinal tract. Enterocutaneous fistulas are reported with K63.2. Fistulas between the gastrointestinal tract and the uterus, vagina, or bladder are reported with codes from Chapter 14 Diseases of the Genitourinary System.

K94.3- Esophagostomy complications

An esophagostomy is created to form an opening into the esophagus for tube feeding. Minor complications associated with this procedure could range from obstruction, head/neck swelling, dermatitis/cellulitis, or inflammation due to infections and abscess.

Tube obstructions can be more common, usually resolved by flushing water through the tube, but in some instances clearing the obstruction with a guidewire may be necessary. Cellulitis and inflammation may increase depending on the type of sutures used and can be corrected with tube removal and wound care.

K95.- Complications of bariatric procedures

Bariatric surgery, also called weight reduction surgery, is performed to treat morbid obesity in patients, particularly those who have a significant medical condition, such as diabetes mellitus or hypertension, and are unable to lose weight using traditional methods of weight loss. Many different types of bariatric surgery are available, including Roux-En-Y gastric bypass, gastric "sleeve" (stomach stapling), combination bypass and banding (vertical bypass), duodenal switch bypass, and laparoscopic adjustable gastric banding. Bariatric procedures carry certain complication risks, including infections, hemorrhage, obstructions, and device malfunctions. Some complications that occur during the immediate postoperative period, such as regurgitation, nausea, acid reflux, constipation, and diarrhea, are typically self-limited, and can often be treated medically. However, the presence of persistent abdominal pain, hemorrhage, and fever may indicate a serious complication requiring urgent intervention. The risks associated with bariatric procedure complications are dependent upon multiple risk factors, including the type of bariatric surgery performed, the patient's medical history, and the patient's compliance with

lifestyle adjustments and self-care measures required to ensure the success of the surgery. The fact that devices (e.g., bands, ports, tubing) are often left in situ in bariatric procedures carries additional risks. Bariatric procedures that include a port and/or a tube connecting port and/or banding can malfunction and or become displaced, requiring repair or repositioning procedures.

K95.0- Complications of gastric band procedure

Gastric banding procedures are commonly performed via a laparoscopic approach, reducing the risk for certain complications associated with open abdominal surgery. However, gastric banding is not without procedural risk. Gastric band associated complications are divided into infection due to gastric band procedure and other complications.

K95.01 Infection due to gastric band procedure

Infection due to gastric band procedure may manifest as an intraabdominal infection or abscess or a port site infection. The gastric band is a foreign body that is introduced into the abdominal cavity and may predispose the patient to intraabdominal infection or abscess. Port-site infections are classified as early or late. Early port-site infection causes redness, swelling, and pain and typically manifests as cellulitis. Late port-site infections usually result from gastric band erosion that initially causes intraabdominal infection that migrates up the tubing to the port site. Late port-site infections can lead to sepsis if not recognized and promptly treated.

K95.09 Other complications of gastric band procedure

Pouch enlargement is one of the more common complications of gastric band procedure. Pouch enlargement refers to distension of the proximal portion of the stomach above the gastric band and it may be accompanied by dilation of the distal aspect of the esophagus. Pouch enlargement is a pressure related complication that may be caused by overinflation of the gastric band or by overeating, both of which can cause elevated pressure in the pouch. The condition is treated by deflating the band and/or dietary changes, which include maintaining a low calorie diet and limiting portion size.

Focus Point

Mechanical complications of the gastric band device, such as breakdown, displacement, malfunction, and malposition, are located in Chapter 19 Injury, Poisoning and Certain Other Consequences of External Causes.

Focus Point

Report K31.6 when the G-tube site fails to spontaneously close following removal of the G-tube. This condition, which requires surgical closure, is not considered a complication of the G-tube. This code reports only fistulas between the stomach or duodenum and other structures of the gastrointestinal tract. Enterocutaneous fistulas are reported with K63.2. Fistulas between the gastrointestinal tract and the uterus, vagina, or bladder are reported with codes from Chapter 14 Diseases of the Genitourinary System.

This chapter classifies diseases and disorders of the epidermis, dermis, subcutaneous tissue, nails, sebaceous glands, sweat glands, and hair and hair follicles. The skin is the largest organ system, covering the entire external surface of the body. Known as the integumentary system, the skin serves many purposes. It protects tissue layers from damage and provides waterproofing and cushioning. It also helps the body excrete wastes properly and regulate temperature, and provides the nerves with a surface for originating sensory receptors.

The top layer of the skin is known as the epidermis. This thinner portion of the skin mainly exists to absorb nutrients and to protect deeper tissue layers. The deeper and thicker layer of the skin is the dermis. The dermis is the connective tissue layer and contains the sweat glands, sebaceous glands, hair roots and follicles, blood vessels, sensory receptors, and other important structures of the integumentary system. Beneath the dermis is the hypodermis, or subcutaneous layer. This layer is not part of the skin itself, but the tie between the integumentary system and the fascia below.

The sweat glands, also known as sudoriferous glands, are found throughout the body. There are three to four million of these glands, which release perspiration onto the surface of the skin through small holes called pores. This process helps regulate body temperature by releasing perspiration and allowing it to evaporate.

The sebaceous glands secrete sebum, an oily substance that keeps the skin and hair from drying out. The sebaceous glands are attached to a portion of the hair follicles. The hair and follicles are quite a complex system, allowing for continuous growth and regeneration. Hair, itself, can be thought of as a recycling system, using dead, keratinized epidermal cells to bond with proteins to create the hair within the follicle. The hair shaft grows out from the follicle, through the epidermis, and out of the skin entirely. The function of hair depends on its location—in some locations it helps avoid heat loss, while in other locations it protects from foreign bodies.

The chapter is broken down into the following code blocks:

LØØ-LØ8	Infections of the skin and subcutaneous tissue
L1Ø-L14	Bullous disorders
L2Ø-L3Ø	Dermatitis and eczema
L4Ø-L45	Papulosquamous disorders
L49-L54	Urticaria and erythema
L55-L59	Radiation-related disorders of the skin and subcutaneous tissue
L6Ø-L75	Disorders of skin appendages
L76	Intraoperative and postprocedural complications of skin and subcutaneous tissue
L8Ø-L99	Other disorders of the skin and subcutaneous tissue

Infections of the Skin and Subcutaneous Tissue (LØØ-LØ8)

Infections of the skin and subcutaneous tissue range from staphylococcal scalded skin syndrome and impetigo to cutaneous abscess, furuncle, and carbuncle. Cellulitis, lymphangitis, acute lymphadenitis, pyoderma, and pilonidal cyst and sinus are also classified here.

The categories in this code block are as follows:

LØØ	Staphylococcal scalded skin syndrome
LØ1	Impetigo
LØ2	Cutaneous abscess, furuncle and carbuncle
LØ3	Cellulitis and acute lymphangitis
LØ4	Acute lymphadenitis
LØ5	Pilonidal cyst and sinus
LØ8	Other local infections of skin and subcutaneous tissue

Focus Point

When assigning a code from categories LØØ-LØ8, also assign a secondary code from categories B95-B97 to identify the infective organism, when the infective organism is documented.

LØØ   Staphylococcal scalded skin syndrome

Staphylococcal skin infection primarily affects children younger than 5 years of age, and is characterized by eruptions ranging from a localized bullous to widespread, easily ruptured fine vesicles and bullae. This results in marked exfoliation (shedding) of large planes of skin leaving raw edges and giving the skin its characteristic "scalded" appearance.

L01.-   Impetigo

Impetigo is an acute, superficial, highly contagious skin infection commonly occurring in children. Skin lesions usually appear on the face and consist of subcorneal vesicles and bullae that burst and form yellow crusts. Usually caused by streptococci, staphylococci, or both, impetigo occurs most frequently after a minor skin injury such as a cut, scrape, or insect bite but infrequently may also develop on healthy skin. Signs and symptoms of impetigo include skin lesions, itching, and mild pain. A gram stain and culture of the lesion identify the infective organism, and antistreptolysin-O (ASO) titers detect streptococcal infection. Therapies include triple antibiotic ointment (bacitracin, Polysporin, and neomycin).

L01.01   Non-bullous impetigo

Non-bullous impetigo originates as small vesicles or pustules that break, exposing a red, moist base, with secretion that form a honey-yellow to white-brown crust. Mild lymphadenopathy is also often present. Non-bullous impetigo usually resolves on its own within two weeks.

L01.02   Bockhart's impetigo

Also called follicular pyoderma, Bockhart's impetigo is an infection of the hair follicles with *Staphylococcus aureus*. Yellow pustules form in the follicles in the face, scalp, and limbs and can be caused by shaving, insect bites, or scratches.

L01.03   Bullous impetigo

Bullous impetigo is considered to be less contagious than non-bullous, and also differs in that it can affect the buccal membranes. The fragile bullae form rapidly, break early, and heal centrally, leaving crusted erosions.

L02.-   Cutaneous abscess, furuncle and carbuncle

An abscess is a collection of pus under the skin resulting from an acute or chronic localized infection associated with tissue destruction. An abscess is an infection caused by streptococci, staphylococci, or other organisms. Those occurring in the integumentary system are called cutaneous abscesses. Signs and symptoms of other cellulitis and abscess include edema, warmth, redness, pain, and interference with function. Often a cutaneous abscess requires incision and drainage to heal appropriately. Carbuncles and furuncles are infections caused by aerobic or anaerobic bacterial organisms. A furuncle, more commonly known as a boil, is a localized skin infection typically caused by the *Staphylococcus aureus* bacterium. A furuncle is a specific type of abscess that usually begins in a gland or hair follicle, where a core of dead tissue is formed, causing pain, redness, and swelling. The dead tissue may simply reabsorb into the system, which resolves the problem, or it may

spontaneously extrude itself. In some instances, surgical removal of the necrotic tissue may be required. A carbuncle is larger than a furuncle and typically consists of several interconnected sites of infection that eventually discharge pus to the skin's surface. Carbuncles are also often caused by the *Staphylococcus aureus* bacterium and can vary greatly in size. Some carbuncles can be small, similar to the size of a pea, but others can grow to be quite large, greater than the size of a golf ball. Much like furuncles, some carbuncles heal on their own by reabsorption into the system or spontaneous extrusion. However, sometimes surgical treatment and antibiotics are required.

Signs and symptoms of carbuncles and furuncles include pain, fluctuating or fixed mass, and fever, chills, and malaise with furuncle in active stage. A gram stain and culture (if open wound or pus is present) may be performed to identify the infective organism.

> **Focus Point**
>
> *In ICD-10-CM, individual codes are available for cutaneous abscess, furuncle, and carbuncle each with specific sites, in addition to laterality. The organism should be also coded separately if known.*

L03.-   Cellulitis and acute lymphangitis

Cellulitis is an infection of the dermis and subcutaneous tissues, more severe in patients with lower resistance to infection (e.g., diabetics). Signs and symptoms of cellulitis include edema, warmth, redness, and pain. Therapies include antimicrobials. The lymph system is a network of lymph nodes, ducts and vessels (channels), and organs that provide lymph fluid from tissues into the bloodstream. Not to be confused with lymphadenitis, which is an inflammation of the lymph node(s), lymphangitis is an inflammation of one or more lymphatic channels or vessels, usually resulting from an acute streptococcal infection of one of the extremities. It is characterized by fine red streaks extending from the infected area to the axilla or groin and by fever, chills, headache, and myalgia. The infection may spread to the bloodstream.

> **Focus Point**
>
> *Many anatomical sites of cellulitis are not included in this chapter. Cellulitis of the eyelid and orbit are located in Chapter 7 Diseases of the Eye and Adnexa; cellulitis of the ear is found in Chapter 8 Diseases of Ear and Mastoid Process; cellulitis of the mouth, lip, anus, and rectum are all located in Chapter 11 Diseases of the Digestive System; and cellulitis of the breast, male and female genitals, is found in Chapter 14 Diseases of the Genitourinary System.*

L03.011   Cellulitis of right finger

Cellulitis of the finger includes a condition called felon, also referred to as whitlow, which is an infection in the fleshy tip of the finger that develops an abscess. Complications may occur if not treated. A felon can constrict the blood flow to the finger and also cause infection in the bone. *Staphylococcus aureus*, a bacterium, is the most common cause of this condition, but it may also be caused by fungus and the herpes virus. Common symptoms include throbbing pain, warmth, inflammation, and tenderness.

L04.-   Acute lymphadenitis

Acute lymphadenitis is sudden, severe inflammation and/or enlargement of the lymph nodes. The lymphatic system is a network of nodes, vessels, and organs. It is part of the immune system, which protects the body against infection, inflammation, and cancer. This condition arises when the lymph nodes are infected by bacteria, fungi, virus, cancer cells, or inflammation. Lymphadenitis may affect a central cluster of nodes in the area of a localized infection or may be generalized, involving a number of lymph nodes. The condition may be unilateral or bilateral. Lymphadenitis is a common complication of cellulitis or other bacterial infections caused by *Streptococcus*, *Staphylococcus*, or other organisms. Signs and symptoms may include local pain, tenderness, and erythema. Therapies include antimicrobials (penicillin).

L05.-   Pilonidal cyst and sinus

A pilonidal cyst is a skin pocket containing hair and skin debris that is almost always located in the back over the coccyx, just above the cleft of the buttocks. The condition occurs when hair becomes embedded or ingrown. Infected pilonidal cysts are quite painful and may result in sinus formation with an opening in the skin at a postanal dimple and drainage of purulent material. Signs and symptoms of pilonidal cyst include edema, warmth, redness, pain, and interference with function. A gram stain and culture of the lesion identify the infective organism. Therapies include incision and drainage or circumferential excision. The subcategory codes also indicate whether an abscess was present or not.

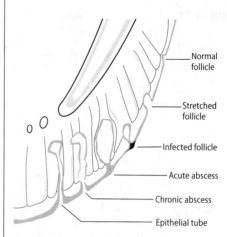

L08.-   Other local infections of skin and subcutaneous tissue

This category classifies other local infections of the skin and subcutaneous tissue including pyoderma, erythrasma, pyoderma vegetans, and omphalitis not occurring in a newborn.

L08.0   Pyoderma

Pyoderma refers to any pyogenic or pus producing superficial skin infection that is not documented as a specified condition classified to another category such as impetigo, furuncle, carbuncle, folliculitis, etc. Also included in this code is dermatitis gangrenosa, which is a cutaneous *Clostridium* infection causing necrosis and skin sloughing. Ecthyma is also represented by this code and is an ulcerative pyoderma caused by group A beta-hemolytic streptococci that extends into the dermis similar to a deeper impetigo.

L08.1   Erythrasma

Erythrasma is a chronic, superficial skin infection of brown scaly patches, commonly found in skin folds, caused by the gram-positive bacterium *Corynebacterium minutissimum*. It is most prevalent in the overweight or diabetic population.

L08.81   Pyoderma vegetans

Pyoderma vegetans is characterized by the formation of large, elevated plaques with multiple pustular eruptions and ulcerations. It is believed to be a bacterial disease affecting the immunosuppressed and it is thought that the immunological dysfunction may induce the development of the vegetations. Some of the conditions that have been associated with this are HIV, ulcerative colitis, diffuse T-cell lymphoma, and chronic myeloid leukemia (CML).

L08.82   Omphalitis not of newborn

Normally presenting as superficial cellulitis with discharge, omphalitis is an infection of the umbilical stump that can spread through the abdominal wall and progress to necrotizing fasciitis, myonecrosis, or systemic disease. Although more prevalent in newborns and children, it is occasionally found in adults, associated with inadequate hygiene or a deeper than normal umbilical cord opening possibly caused by obesity.

L08.89   Other specified local infections of the skin and subcutaneous tissue

Spiegler-Fendt sarcoid and Andrew's disease are included in this code. Spiegler-Fendt sarcoid is a rare form of a recurrent benign lymphoreticular tissue consisting of yellow to purple, rubbery lesions that have a tendency to spread. It is more common in women than men and can also be referred to as Kaposi-Spiegler sarcomatosis or Bäfverstedt syndrome. Andrew's disease is a condition of pustulosis palmoplantaris where an infection, usually positive for staphylococci or streptococci, is involved. It typically originates in the midpalm or soles as pustules that spread outward and eventually dry out to form a honeycomb structure covered by dry scales. Most often it follows an infection of teeth, sinus, or tonsils affecting the middle aged.

Bullous Disorders (L10-L14)

Bullae are fluid filled lesions that form at some level of the skin that are usually considered larger than vesicles (top of pin size) or blisters (under 1 centimeter). The skin covering the bullae acts as a protective barrier against infection.

The categories in this code block are as follows:

L10	Pemphigus
L11	Other acantholytic disorders
L12	Pemphigoid
L13	Other bullous disorders
L14	Bullous disorders in diseases classified elsewhere

L10.-   Pemphigus

These are chronic, relapsing, sometimes fatal autoimmune skin diseases that result in vesicles, bullae, and autoantibodies against intracellular connections and cause acantholysis.

L10.0   Pemphigus vulgaris

Pemphigus vulgaris is the most common of pemphigus cases and is an autoimmune disease of the intraepithelial region causing blistering of skin and mucous membranes. It can lead to painful erosions of the skin and become life-threatening.

L10.1   Pemphigus vegetans

Pemphigus vegetans is a variation of pemphigus vulgaris in which the bullae erosions form excessive crusting and vegetating lesions of granulation tissue.

L10.2   Pemphigus foliaceous

Pemphigus foliaceous, a chronic autoimmune disease, is typically a benign type of pemphigus that causes superficial blisters and rarely extends to involve the mucous membranes.

L10.4   Pemphigus erythematosus

Also referred to as Senear-Usher syndrome, this is suggested to be a multiple autoimmune disorder with features of lupus erythematosus and pemphigus foliaceus. It may occur especially in sun exposed parts of the body, and presents as small bullae or superficially eroded lesions that ooze and crust.

L10.81   Paraneoplastic pemphigus

This autoimmune condition is precipitated by an underlying neoplasm in which blistering of the epithelia is induced by tumor antigens that evoke a cellular immune response.

L11.-   Other acantholytic disorders

The term acantholytic is defined as a breakdown of intercellular connections of the epidermis resulting in loss of cohesion between the epidermal cells and causing multiple skin disorders.

L11.1   Transient acantholytic dermatosis [Grover]

Commonly called Grover's disease, the term "transient" is misleading since this condition can persist for 10 to 12 months or more. It manifests as intense itching red pustules in the chest area that can eventually spread to neck and limbs, but sparing the scalp, palms, and soles. Etiology is unknown, although it appears to be frequently associated with sweating or heat. It most commonly affects middle aged men and some women.

L12.-   Pemphigoid

The definition of pemphigoid is chronic, benign eruption of blisters on the skin. Pemphigoid is seen chiefly in the elderly and in individuals with autoimmune disease. Signs and symptoms of pemphigoid include tense bullae on normal or reddened skin.

L12.0   Bullous pemphigoid

Bullous pemphigoid presents with large, fluid-filled blistering at the site of the attack and is accompanied by itching and pain. It is a rare autoimmune condition that is more common in people older than age 60. Etiology is unknown but may sometimes be triggered by certain medications.

L12.1   Cicatricial pemphigoid

Cicatricial pemphigoid presents with blistering, eventually causing scarring, in the mucous membranes, conjunctiva, and in about a third of the cases the skin. The skin lesions can manifest as bullae that may be hemorrhagic. When the scalp is affected, it can cause alopecia (hair loss). It is a rare, chronic autoimmune disease occurring most often in people older than age 60. The scarring can cause decreased vision, blindness, or supraglottic stenosis. It is also referred to as mucous membrane pemphigoid.

L13.-   Other bullous disorders

This category of codes includes conditions such as Duhring's disease, Sneddon-Wilkinson disease, and other bullous disorders.

L13.0   Dermatitis herpetiformis

Dermatitis herpetiformis is a chronic, multisystem disease that manifests in the cutaneous system. It is seen as an extremely pruritic eruption of various lesions on the extensor surfaces, such as elbows and knees. When healing, it frequently leaves hyperpigmentation or hypopigmentation and occasional scarring. It is caused by IgA deposits in the papillary dermis triggering an immunologic response usually associated with an asymptomatic gluten-sensitive enteropathy or celiac disease. Although it is a lifelong disease, it is common to experience exacerbations and remissions. Also referred to as Duhring's disease, it can affect any age but is rare in children.

L13.1   Subcorneal pustular dermatitis

This relapsing condition, also referred to as Sneddon-Wilkinson disease, is relatively rare, most often affecting women older than age 40. It presents as pustular eruptions in the flexor surfaces of the limbs and trunk. Multiple subtypes have been found but the etiology is unknown.

Dermatitis and Eczema (L20-L30)

Dermatitis is inflammation of the skin and eczema is one form of dermatitis. Contact dermatitis, a fairly common form of the condition, is inflammation that results from an allergic reaction (allergic contact dermatitis) or exposure to some type of skin irritant (irritant contact dermatitis).

Dermatitis and eczema can be something as simple as redness of the skin or a bumpy rash to something more serious such as blisters.

Focus Point

ICD-10-CM uses the terms *dermatitis* and *eczema* interchangeably.

The categories in this code block are as follows:

L20	Atopic dermatitis
L21	Seborrheic dermatitis
L22	Diaper dermatitis
L23	Allergic contact dermatitis
L24	Irritant contact dermatitis
L25	Unspecified contact dermatitis
L26	Exfoliative dermatitis
L27	Dermatitis due to substances taken internally
L28	Lichen simplex chronicus and prurigo
L29	Pruritus
L30	Other and unspecified dermatitis

L20.-   Atopic dermatitis

Atopic dermatitis is a chronic skin condition. It is characterized by skin that is erythematous and irritated. It commonly develops a fluid-filled rash that may drain clear fluid. In time, the rash crusts over and begins to peel. There are many conditions that contribute to atopic dermatitis such as allergies, asthma, and a family history of dry skin. Signs and symptoms of atopic dermatitis include severe pruritus, erythema, inflammation, crusting, scaling, and exudation.

L20.0   Besnier's prurigo

Besnier's prurigo is a form of atopic dermatitis associated with pregnancy. Also known as prurigo gestationis, it is a dermatological condition of pregnancy typically affecting women between the 20th and 34th week of gestation. It normally consists of an eruption of itchy, red papules that can be excoriated as well. There are several treatments that can make the patient more comfortable, although given the pregnancy, not all prescription treatments are an option.

L20.81   Atopic neurodermatitis

Neurodermatitis is characterized by a cycle of recurring intensely itchy eczema following by scratching, which can cause it to worsen and become infected. The more it is scratched, the worse the itching can become with sleep disruption and thickening and darkening of the skin. It affects more women than men usually occurring between 30 and 40 years of age. Effective treatment requires cessation of scratching, which makes the condition more difficult to treat.

L20.82   Flexural eczema

Flexural eczema is a form of atopic dermatitis found in the flexures of the body, such as the inside of the elbows, wrists, and knees. This type of dermatitis often affects children, although it isn't exclusive to youth. It typically results in lichenification, which is a thickening and hardening of the epidermis that often results in an exaggeration of its normal markings. It also causes cracking and weeping of the area.

L21.-   Seborrheic dermatitis

Seborrheic dermatitis is an inflammatory, scaly condition of the skin predominantly affecting the scalp and face. Signs and symptoms include dandruff, itching, dry skin, and crusted scalp lesion ("cradle cap") in infants.

L21.0   Seborrhea capitis

Seborrhea capitis is often called cradle cap in infants. It is characterized by erythematous, swollen, and greasy yellowish scales on the scalp, particularly the crown. The margins of the lesions are well defined and usually symmetrical.

L21.1   Seborrheic infantile dermatitis

Seborrheic infantile dermatitis is very common in infants and is characterized by yellow, crusty, greasy scaling lesions affecting the head and trunk. The condition typically occurs during the first six weeks following birth and is self-limiting lasting only a few weeks, although in some cases it may last several months. The condition usually resolves on its own and does not require treatment.

L22   Diaper dermatitis

This common type of dermatitis is an irritation of the skin of the buttocks, groin, lower abdomen, and upper thighs. Diaper dermatitis is the result of irritation from contact with urine and feces, the introduction of new foods to the baby's diet, chafing, or due to skin sensitivity.

L23.-   Allergic contact dermatitis

Allergic contact dermatitis is a rash that results from an allergic reaction to something that has come in contact with the skin. Initially, the rash may be limited to the site of contact but may spread. Signs and symptoms of allergic contact dermatitis range from transient redness to severe swelling, itching, and vesiculation. In allergic dermatitis, patch testing may be performed to determine the allergen responsible for the skin inflammation and other symptoms.

> **Focus Point**
>
> With the use of history gathering and patch testing, a specific hypersensitivity and a probable cause of dermatitis can be identified in most cases of allergic contact dermatitis.

L23.0   Allergic contact dermatitis due to metals

Nickel, the chromates, and mercury are the most common causes of allergic contact metal dermatitis in the United States. Other metals associated with dermatitis are rhodium, platinum, cobalt, tungsten, cadmium, beryllium, vanadium, and zinc.

L23.81   Allergic contact dermatitis due to animal (cat) (dog) dander

Contact dermatitis is an allergic reaction of the skin characterized by a rash or hives. This is usually an immune reaction to a protein found in animal dander. This may be a result of direct contact with an animal or contact with fabric containing the animal dander.

L24.-   Irritant contact dermatitis

Irritant contact dermatitis is a rash that results from a substance that comes in contact with the skin. The resulting redness, inflammation, mild edema, and scaling is not due to an allergic reaction but is instead due to damage to the skin from the substance itself. Inflammation occurs in response to contact with an irritating substance, as a result of disruption of skin barriers, epidermal changes, and release of cytokines that cause inflammation. Irritant contact dermatitis can also coexist with allergic contact dermatitis.

L24.81   Irritant contact dermatitis due to metals

Nickel, the chromates, and mercury are the most common causes of irritant contact metal dermatitis in the United States. Other metals associated with dermatitis are rhodium, platinum, cobalt, tungsten, cadmium, beryllium, vanadium, and zinc.

L26   Exfoliative dermatitis

Also referred to as erythroderma, it involves most of the skin and is a condition where the normal cycling time of sloughing of the epidermal layer of the skin is decreased and more cells are lost causing erythema, scaling, and tightness. Etiology can be idiopathic although some causes are believed to be underlying systemic or cutaneous disease or drug reaction. Most often occurs in men and women older than age 40.

L27.-   Dermatitis due to substances taken internally

This type of dermatitis is due to the ingestion of drugs, chemicals, foodstuffs, or other substances. The condition usually manifests with an abrupt onset of diffuse, symmetric erythematous eruptions. The cause may be an allergic reaction, adverse effect, drug interaction, idiosyncratic reaction, or some other cause. The definition of dermatitis due to drugs and medicines taken internally is systemic erythematous inflammation of the skin, also known as dermatitis medicamentosa or drug eruption. The condition may mimic inflammatory skin conditions such as eczema, toxic erythema, and erythroderma. Onset may be sudden (e.g., urticaria or angioedema after penicillin) or delayed. Signs and symptoms of dermatitis due to drugs and medicines taken internally include mild rash to toxic epidermal microlysis, malaise, fever, arthralgia, and headache.

L27.1 Localized skin eruption due to drugs and medicaments taken internally

This code includes palmar-plantar erythrodysesthesia (PPE), also called hand-foot syndrome, which is a side effect of certain chemotherapy. It presents as a reddened, sunburn-like discoloration and can develop into numbness and tingling. Exposure to heat and friction can precipitate the condition as it increases the amount of drug leaking into the capillaries in the hands and feet, which is the cause of this condition.

L28.- Lichen simplex chronicus and prurigo

These two conditions are characterized by itching. Lichen simplex chronicus is an eczematous dermatitis, while prurigo has several different presentations with the most common being nodule formation.

L28.0 Lichen simplex chronicus

Lichen simplex chronicus is an eczematous dermatitis of the face, neck, extremities, scrotum, vulva, and perianal region due to repeated itching, rubbing, and scratching. It can occur spontaneously or evolve with other dermatoses. Chronic scratching in turn creates lichenification or thick, leathery, discolored, skin.

L28.1 Prurigo nodularis

Prurigo nodularis is characterized by itchy nodule formation on the extremities. The intense pruritus encourages scratching, which leads to skin thickening. Even though it is a relatively benign condition, it can negatively impact work and daily activities and can be a sign of an internal malignancy such as Hodgkin lymphoma. The etiology is unknown and most commonly affects middle aged and elderly.

L29.- Pruritus

Pruritus is characterized by an intense itching and/or burning sensation of the skin. Most cases of generalized pruritus are due to dry skin but other causes include a variety of dermatologic or systemic conditions. Therapies include elimination of soaps or detergents, cessation of all but necessary medications, the application of moisturizers while the skin is wet, tranquilizers in severe cases, and topical or systemic corticosteroids, as well as antihistamines and anti-serotonin drugs.

L30.- Other and unspecified dermatitis

This category includes a number of codes for specific types of dermatitis not classified elsewhere.

L30.0 Nummular dermatitis

Nummular dermatitis is typically characterized by itchy, oval, or coin-shaped lesions on the arms and legs. Cause is generally unknown, but the condition sometimes appears after a skin trauma such as a burn or insect bite or with use of certain medications. It can last for months and then resolve or become chronic with periods of exacerbation.

L30.2 Cutaneous autosensitization

Cutaneous autosensitization is a secondary dermatitis caused by an inflammatory response somewhere else in the body.

L30.5 Pityriasis alba

The name is derived from pityriasis meaning scaly and alba meaning white, as it presents with scaly patches that leave light, hypopigmented areas when they eventually subside. It is most common in children and young adults frequently on the cheek of the face but also on the upper limbs and torso. Etiology is unknown and it is not contagious.

Papulosquamous Disorders (L40-L45)

Papulosquamous refers to skin disorders that are scaly and present with papules or plaques.

The categories in this code block are as follows:

L40	Psoriasis
L41	Parapsoriasis
L42	Pityriasis rosea
L43	Lichen planus
L44	Other papulosquamous disorders
L45	Papulosquamous disorders in diseases classified elsewhere

L40.- Psoriasis

Psoriasis is an autoimmune disorder that affects the skin and, in some cases, the cartilage in the joints. The skin condition is characterized by patches of inflamed, red skin, covered by silvery scales. When the joints are involved, cartilage is destroyed causing painful swelling and stiffness of the joints, referred to as psoriatic arthritis. With psoriasis, new skin cells are produced 10 times faster than normal, but the rate at which old cells are shed is unchanged. Consequently, the stratum corneum becomes thickened with flaky, immature skin cells. Occurring predominantly over the elbows, knees, scalp, and trunk, psoriasis tends to run in families, affects men and women equally, and usually appears between the ages of 10 and 30. Therapies include moderate exposure to sunlight or phototherapy and the use of an emollient for mild cases, ointment containing coal tar or anthralin for moderate cases, and topical corticosteroids and oral methotrexate for severe cases. In recent years, biologics that target specific parts of the immune system have also been added to the list of drugs used to treat moderate to severe forms of psoriasis.

L40.0   Psoriasis vulgaris

Psoriasis vulgaris is the most common form of psoriasis, affecting 80 to 90 percent of all psoriasis diagnoses. Also known as plaque psoriasis, it presents as raised and inflamed red areas covered with silvery/white scaly skin. These areas are known as plaques and can be itchy and painful.

L40.1   Generalized pustular psoriasis

These conditions are characterized by white blisters of pus consisting of white blood cells surrounded by red skin. Primarily occurs in adults and can cover the entire body. This subcategory includes impetigo herpetiformis, which may occur in pregnancy.

Focus Point

One type of pustular psoriasis called Von Zumbusch can be life-threatening. It appears acutely with large areas of painful, red skin followed by the development of pustules that burst and dry leaving a glazed appearance on the skin. It often requires hospitalization for rehydration and systemic antibiotics.

L40.2   Acrodermatitis continua

Acrodermatitis continua is a form of pustular psoriasis that results in skin lesions on the ends of the fingers and toes. It is quite rare and is referred to by many different names, such as acropustulosis, acrodermatitis continua of Hallopeau, dermatitis repens, and pustular acrodermatitis. This condition tends to be resistant to common psoriasis treatment, so it can require more aggressive treatment even for what seems like a less serious form of psoriasis.

L40.3   Pustulosis palmaris et plantaris

Pustulosis palmaris et plantaris, or palmoplantar pustulosis (PPP), causes pustules specifically on the hands and feet, hence its name. It is a persistent condition, typically recurring over and over. Interestingly, it is suggested that patients with PPP refrain from smoking, as nicotine has been known to cause flare-ups.

L40.4   Guttate psoriasis

Guttate psoriasis is characterized by small red spots on the skin, as opposed to the large, scaly regions of other types of psoriasis. They are usually found on the upper body, specifically the trunk and upper limbs. It is predominantly found in adolescents and young adults and can be precipitated by many different types of illnesses, such as an upper respiratory infection, strep throat, tonsillitis, or even simply stress or the administration of certain drugs. It is important that this condition be treated so it does not become a more serious form of psoriasis in the future.

L40.5-   Arthropathic psoriasis

Arthropathic psoriasis is a form of inflammatory arthritis that affects patients with psoriasis. It causes joint inflammation but can also cause tendinitis, issues with the nails, and swelling of the digits. There are various forms of this condition, described by distinctive names. Many of these forms have been assigned different codes in the ICD-10-CM code set.

L40.51   Distal interphalangeal psoriatic arthropathy

Distal interphalangeal psoriatic arthropathy is arthropathic psoriasis characterized by inflammation in the distal portions of the fingers and toes. In this particular type of arthropathy, there are often changes noted in the nails as well, including pitting, discoloration, ridging, and thickening.

L40.52   Psoriatic arthritis mutilans

Psoriatic arthritis mutilans is a severe, deforming form of arthritis. It gets progressively worse over months or even years, causing resorption of bones and severe joint damage. It is not a common condition, affecting less than 5 percent of patients with arthropathic psoriasis.

L40.53   Psoriatic spondylitis

Psoriatic spondylitis is a type of arthropathic psoriasis that results in pain and stiffness of the spine and neck. This occurs predominantly in male patients. These patients may show unusual radiological features, such as paravertebral ossification.

L40.54   Psoriatic juvenile arthropathy

Psoriatic juvenile arthropathy is arthropathic psoriasis with onset in childhood. The average age of onset is 9 to 10 years, and it occurs predominantly in female patients. Luckily, the disease tends to be mild in children. Psoriatic juvenile arthropathy accounts for 8 to 20 percent of all childhood arthritis.

L41.-   Parapsoriasis

Parapsoriasis is a group of skin diseases that have a resemblance to psoriasis, however they are unrelated in development of the disease, the microscopic examination of the tissue (histopathology), and treatment response. Symptoms include redness and itching.

L41.0   Pityriasis lichenoides et varioliformis acuta

Pityriasis lichenoides et varioliformis acuta (PLEVA) is a serious disease involving the immune system. It is characterized mainly by rashes and small lesions on the skin, caused by the immune system inappropriately "fighting" the skin cells and causing damage. It is often misdiagnosed as various similar looking conditions, such as chicken pox or rosacea. Common treatment for the condition is a combination of pharmaceuticals and phototherapy. Localized wound care may be required for large ulcerations or infections.

Focus Point

Mucha Habermann disease is a synonym for PLEVA. It is rare and more often affects children and young adults. Febrile ulceronecrotic Mucha Habermann is a more severe form of this disease and can be life-threatening in adults. The etiology is unknown.

L41.1   Pityriasis lichenoides chronica

Pityriasis lichenoides chronica is the milder, chronic form of PLEVA. This condition is characterized by the gradual development of symptomless, small, scaling papules that spontaneously flatten and regress over a period of weeks or months. The patient may have lesions at various stages present at any one time. Patients with this condition often have exacerbations and relapses of the condition, which can last for months or years.

L41.3   Small plaque parapsoriasis

Small plaque parapsoriasis is a mild version of parapsoriasis, resulting in small skin lesions typically on the trunk. This condition often resolves on its own and rarely, if ever, progresses.

L41.4   Large plaque parapsoriasis

Large plaque parapsoriasis is a serious chronic inflammatory disorder that results in large skin lesions. This condition can be concerning, not because of the skin issues themselves, which are quite treatable, but because approximately 10 percent of patients with large plaque parapsoriasis progress to cutaneous T-cell lymphoma or mycosis fungoides, both serious conditions.

L41.5   Retiform parapsoriasis

Retiform parapsoriasis is a form of large plaque parapsoriasis. It causes large skin lesions that result in a netlike pattern on the body and can also cause the skin to atrophy. As is the case with all large plaque parapsoriasis, treatment is important in avoiding disease progression.

L42   Pityriasis rosea

Pityriasis rosea (PR), also called pityriasis circinata, is a mild skin condition characterized by scaly, pink, oval shaped papules. PR commonly begins as a rash with one main patch of affected skin usually on the chest or back that resembles ringworm and is 2 to 10 centimeters in size. A widespread rash develops within a week or two following the first lesion. The rash often forms a pattern over the back resembling a Christmas tree. In some cases, a more severe reaction with

persistent itching can occur, particularly if the patient becomes overheated (e.g., due to exercise or a hot bath). PR develops most often in the spring and the fall, and seems to occur more frequently in children and young adults. The normal duration is four to eight weeks.

L43.-   Lichen planus

Lichen planus is a group of papular skin diseases characterized by small lesions set close together. The condition gets its name from its appearance, which resembles that of lichens (mixture of fungi and algae) found in nature. Lichen planus is an inflammatory cutaneous and mucous membrane condition characterized by pruritic, violaceous, and flattop papules with fine white streaks and symmetric distribution. Signs and symptoms of lichen planus include chronic papules, acute lesions of the skin and mucous membranes, and severe itching. A biopsy is performed to diagnose the particular form of the disease; treatments include topical corticosteroids to reduce itching and induce regression of the lesions. Other therapies include intralesional and systemic steroids, antihistamines, psoralens plus long-wave ultraviolet light, and oral griseofulvin. Hyperpigmented areas may persist after the lesions have resolved.

Focus Point

Lichen sclerosus et atrophicus is an atrophic skin disorder that is classified in category L90 unless the condition affects the female or male genital organs. When lichen sclerosis affects female genital organs, report N90.4. When the condition affects male genital organs report N48.0.

L44.-   Other papulosquamous disorders

Papulosquamous refers to skin disorders that are scaly and with papules or plaques. This category includes skin diseases that are not appropriate for the previous codes but share similar attributes.

L44.0   Pityriasis rubra pilaris

Pityriasis rubra pilaris, also known as Devergie's disease or lichen ruber acuminatus, is a chronic skin condition resulting in reddish orange scaly plaques and keratotic papules of the follicles. It can also cause palmoplantar keratoderma, which is a thickening of the skin on the palms of the hands and the soles of the feet.

L44.1   Lichen nitidus

Lichen nitidus, also known as Pinkus' disease, is a chronic, inflammatory, asymptomatic skin disorder, characterized by numerous glistening, flat-topped, discrete, skin-colored micropapules most often on the penis, lower abdomen, inner thighs, wrists, forearms, breasts, and buttocks.

L44.4 Infantile papular acrodermatitis [Gianotti-Crosti]

Infantile papular acrodermatitis, also known as Gianotti-Crosti syndrome, is a skin condition in children caused by the body's reaction to a viral infection. It is typically characterized by pink to pale flesh-colored papules covering the buttocks, the extremities, and the face. Rarely are other areas of the body involved. Hepatitis B was one of the initial viruses thought to cause this condition, although it is now just one of many viruses seen as the root cause.

Urticaria and Erythema (L49-L54)

This code block describes conditions that involve hives, also known as urticaria, or skin redness, also known as erythema. It includes exfoliation of skin, various causes of urticaria, and types of erythema multiforme.

The categories in this code block are as follows:

L49	Exfoliation due to erythematous conditions according to extent of body surface involved
L50	Urticaria
L51	Erythema multiforme
L52	Erythema nodosum
L53	Other erythematous conditions
L54	Erythema in diseases classified elsewhere

L49.- Exfoliation due to erythematous conditions according to extent of body surface involved

This category classifies epidermal skin loss involving exfoliation or sloughing of the skin by body surface percentage. The fourth character of the code indicates the percentage of total body surface skin loss.

> **Focus Point**
>
> *Code first the erythematous condition causing the exfoliation.*

L50.- Urticaria

Urticaria is an eruption of itching edema of the skin and is more often referred to as hives. It may be due to hypersensitivity to a drug, food, or insect stings or bites, but can also be due to stimuli such as physical exercise, heat, cold, sunlight, anxiety, and tension. Most episodes are acute and self-limiting over a period of one to two weeks. Signs and symptoms of urticaria include pruritus (itching), wheals (raised reddened areas) that may remain small or may enlarge, rings of erythema, and edema. The fourth character indicates the specific cause or type of the urticaria (e.g., allergic, idiopathic, or due to cold or heat).

L50.3 Dermatographic urticaria

Dermagraphic urticaria is one of the more common types and is a hypersensitive response when the skin is stroked, scratched, or rubbed. Sometimes called "skin writing disease," the response can cause a wheal within minutes that can burn or itch and typically lasts 15 to 30 minutes.

L50.4 Vibratory urticaria

This rare type of urticaria is induced by strong vibrations such as operating a jackhammer or lawnmower. It has also been found to occur from jogging or vigorous rubbing. It appears in about two minutes after being exposed to the stimulus and lasts about an hour.

L50.5 Cholinergic urticaria

Cholinergic urticaria is triggered from a hypersensitive response to an increase in body temperature, sweating, a strong emotional response, stress, or even eating spicy foods or taking a hot shower.

L51.- Erythema multiforme

Erythema refers to redness of the skin and mucous membranes caused by increased blood flow and congestion of the capillaries. The term "erythema multiforme" (EM) refers to the "multiple forms" in which these conditions, characterized by redness of the skin, are manifest from the nature of symptoms and associated conditions to the variance in degrees of severity. Papules, plaques, and bulls eye (target) lesions are diagnostic of erythema multiforme. On mucous membranes, it begins as blisters and progresses to ulcers. Erythema multiforme is a hypersensitivity (allergic) reaction that can occur at any age but primarily affects children or young adults. It may occur in response to medications, infections, or illness. The causal agent induces damage to dermal blood vessels and tissues. Clinical presentation may range from a mild, self-limited rash (minor) to a more severe, life-threatening form involving mucous membranes. These erythematous conditions are characterized by the sudden onset of multiple, symmetrical pruritic (itching) skin lesions of the limbs and face that may spread and form blisters. Other associated symptoms include fever, malaise, and joint pain. Facial lesions are often associated with painful conjunctivitis, vision abnormalities, and buccal lesions.

> **Focus Point**
>
> *Clinical classifications for erythema multiforme are based on the pattern and distribution of cutaneous lesions. Different causes, characteristics, and risk factors exist between erythema multiforme, Stevens-Johnson syndrome, and toxic epidermal necrolysis.*

L51.1   Stevens-Johnson syndrome

Stevens-Johnson syndrome (SJS), a severe form of erythema multiforme, can be fatal. In SJS, the lesions are more extensive than those characteristic of other forms of erythema multiforme, and the systemic symptoms are more severe. Multiple body areas are usually involved, especially the mucous membranes. SJS is part of the same spectrum of disease as toxic epidermal necrolysis (TEN), although SJS generally involves a body surface area of less than 10 percent. SJS is associated with severe adverse drug reactions to certain medications that cause an extreme immunologically mediated abnormal metabolic reaction in sensitive people.

L51.2   Toxic epidermal necrolysis [Lyell]

Toxic epidermal necrolysis (TEN), also called Lyell's syndrome, involves multiple large blisters with exfoliation of all or most of the skin and mucous membranes, generally involving more than 30 percent of the body surface area. It is similar to the skin loss that occurs with a severe burn, necessitating treatment in a burn unit. TEN is associated with severe adverse drug reactions to certain medications that cause an extreme immunologically mediated abnormal metabolic reaction in sensitive people.

L51.3   Stevens-Johnson syndrome-toxic epidermal necrolysis overlap syndrome

The overlap form of Stevens-Johnson syndrome (SJS) and toxic epidermal necrolysis (TEN) refers to a level of severity that is less severe than SJS, but not as severe as TEN. An intermediate amount of body surface area is affected, usually between 10 to 30 percent. SJS-TEN overlap syndrome is associated with severe adverse drug reactions to certain medications that cause an extreme immunologically mediated abnormal metabolic reaction in sensitive people.

L51.9   Erythema multiforme, unspecified

The unspecified classification of erythema multiforme (EM) includes erythema multiforme documented as minor or major. The minor form is considered a self-limiting condition with papules, plaques, and bullseye lesions primarily on the limbs, not involving mucous membranes, and accounts for approximately 80 percent of EM cases. Erythema multiforme major is a severe form and can be life-threatening. The lesions have painful blisters in the centers, which tend to appear on the eye, inside the mouth, genitals, and trunk. They typically involve one or more mucous membranes and may occasionally involve the internal organs. It has been strongly associated with the herpes virus infection.

L52   Erythema nodosum

Erythema nodosum is an inflammation of the fat under the skin forming tender red lumps commonly on the shins and also on the thighs and forearms. It occurs most frequently in adults between ages 20 and 45 and is more prevalent in women than men. It can occur as an isolated condition or in conjunction with other conditions.

> **Focus Point**
>
> One cause of Erythema nodosum is Behçet's disease, which involves ulcerations in the mouth, genitals, and eyes and can cause inflammation in the joints, skin, and subcutaneous fat. This code is located in Chapter 13 Diseases of the Musculoskeletal System and Connective Tissue.

L53.-   Other erythematous conditions

This category includes figurate or gyrate erythemas, a group of skin conditions that present as annular or figurate erythematous papules and plaques with peripheral spreading and central clearing.

L53.1   Erythema annulare centrifugum

Erythema annulare centrifugum is considered a gyrate and figurate erythema with unknown etiology, although it has been linked to certain malignancies, chronic diseases, infections, and medications. It can appear at any age and typically starts as a red spot, enlarging to a ring shape, most often occurring on the legs but the lesion can appear elsewhere.

L53.2   Erythema marginatum

Erythema marginatum is often a symptom of rheumatic fever. It appears as red spots on the trunk, arms, and legs that evolve into ring-shaped lesions. The appearance can assist with early diagnosis of rheumatic fever.

Radiation-related Disorders of the Skin and Subcutaneous Tissue (L55-L59)

This category represents sunburns and various types of skin response to solar and other radiation.

The categories in this code block are as follows:

L55	Sunburn
L56	Other acute skin changes due to ultraviolet radiation
L57	Skin changes due to chronic exposure to nonionizing radiation
L58	Radiodermatitis
L59	Other disorders of skin and subcutaneous tissue related to radiation

L55.- Sunburn

ICD-10-CM codes use a fourth character to specify the degree of the sunburn. The degrees of burns are:

- **First-degree burns:** Also known as erythema, first degree burns are limited to tissue damage to the outer layer of the epidermis.

- **Second-degree burns:** Blistering with extension beyond the epidermis to partial thickness of the dermis.

- **Third-degree burns:** Full-thickness skin loss. Can be described as "with necrosis."

L56.- Other acute skin changes due to ultraviolet radiation

This category classifies skin changes caused by sun exposure or other ultraviolet radiation source. Some acute skin conditions are due to adverse reactions to a drug or chemical in combination with sun exposure.

L56.0 Drug phototoxic response

Phototoxic contact dermatitis is a nonimmunologic reaction that occurs within minutes to hours after the skin has been exposed to a photosensitizing agent and solar radiation. The clinical presentation is similar to sunburn.

L56.1 Drug photoallergic response

Photoallergic dermatitis is an allergic dermatitis caused by a photosensitizing substance, in this case a drug, plus sunlight in a sensitized person. The clinical presentation is similar to allergic contact dermatitis with symptoms ranging from transient redness to swelling, itching, and vesiculation.

L56.2 Photocontact dermatitis [berloque dermatitis]

This is an acute contact photosensitive reaction when certain chemicals are applied and exposed to solar radiation. Berloque (perfume) dermatitis is included in this code.

L56.3 Solar urticaria

Solar urticaria is a condition classified as hives or wheals caused specifically by exposure to the sun or UV radiation.

L56.4 Polymorphous light eruption

Polymorphous light eruption presents as inflammatory skin eruptions due to sunlight exposure in which the eruptions differ in size and shape.

L56.5 Disseminated superficial actinic porokeratosis (DSAP)

Characterized by superficial annular, keratotic, brownish-red spots or thickenings with depressed centers and sharp ridged borders, DSAP is an autosomal dominant skin condition occurring in skin that has been overexposed to the sun. DSAP may evolve into squamous cell carcinoma.

L56.8 Other specified acute skin changes due to ultraviolet radiation

Photodermatitis is included here.

L57.- Skin changes due to chronic exposure to nonionizing radiation

These skin changes are caused by long-term exposures to solar and other forms of ultraviolet radiation, such as tanning booths.

L57.0 Actinic keratosis

Also known as solar or senile keratosis, actinic keratosis is characterized by precancerous warty lesions caused by the cumulative effect of overexposure to sunlight. Actinic keratosis lesions may begin as rough spots, much like sandpaper, barely visible to the human eye but that can be felt. As lesions develop they may become erythematous, scaly plaques that may enlarge to several centimeters. Lesions may be light or dark, tan, pink, red, a combination of these, or the same color as the skin. They may itch or have a tender sensation, especially after sun exposure. Actinic keratosis occurs most frequently in fair-skinned patients. Common sites include areas of long-term sun exposure, such as the back, chest, ears, face, forearms, backs of the hands, legs, and scalp. The lesions may regress with sun avoidance, may persist unchanged for years, or may progress to invasive squamous cell carcinoma if they are not treated.

L57.1   Actinic reticuloid

A severe and chronic form of photosensitivity, actinic reticuloid usually affects males between the ages of 45 and 70. Actinic reticuloid requires complete avoidance of sunlight and other forms of ultraviolet radiation since it is resistant to treatment with sunscreens and steroids.

L57.5   Actinic granuloma

Actinic granuloma is a form of photosensitivity that results in granulomatous skin lesions. Actinic granuloma begins as papules and nodules. These lesions grow very slowly and eventually become annular. Persistent for years, actinic granuloma is believed to be due to defective repair of connective tissue damaged by sun and heat.

L58.-   Radiodermatitis

Radiodermatitis represents skin reactions caused by radioactive therapy for treatment of cancer or noncancerous conditions. The fourth character indicates whether the condition is acute, chronic, or unspecified.

Disorders of Skin Appendages (L60-L75)

Nails are hard, keratinized cells of epidermis that consist of a nail body, a free edge, and a nail root. Vascular tissue gives the visible nail body its pink color, except at the whitish lunula where the vascular tissue does not show through. The nail groove is between the nail fold and the nail bed, which is the epidermis beneath the nail. The cuticle, or eponychium, is a narrow band of epidermis that adheres to the nail wall. The thickened stratum corneum below the free edges is referred to as the hyponychium. The nail matrix, at the proximal end of the nail bed, promotes nail growth, which occurs when superficial cells of the matrix transform into nail cells. In the process, the harder layer is pushed forward over the stratum germinativum. The average growth rate for fingernails is about 1.0 millimeter per week; growth is slower for the toenails.

The primary function of hair is protection (e.g., eyebrows and eyelashes protect the eyes from foreign objects). Hair follicles (downgrowths into the dermis) develop during the third and fourth months of fetal life and by the sixth month the follicles produce lanugo, which is shed from the trunk prior to birth. Several months after birth, a coarser hair, vellus, develops and the remaining lanugo is shed from the eyebrows, eyelids, and scalp and replaced by terminal hairs. Terminal hairs also develop in the axillary and pubic regions and on the face at puberty.

The hair shaft, which projects above the surface of the skin, is made up of the inner medulla, which consists of cells containing eleidin and air spaces; the cortex, which contains pigment granules in dark hair but mostly are in white hair; and the cuticle, the outermost layer of the shaft. The root is the portion below the surface that penetrates into the dermis and, like the shaft, consists of a medulla, cortex, and cuticle. The color of hair is due primarily to melanin.

A sweat, or sudoriferous, gland is a type of exocrine gland that eliminates perspiration to cool the skin. The sweat glands are a simple cuboidal or columnar epithelium with pale-staining cells. The base of the sweat glands has a row of myoepithelial cells wrapped around the outside of the gland. Eccrine sweat glands are found in skin throughout the body, particularly on the forehead, scalp, axillae, palms, and soles and produce watery and neutral or slightly acidic sweat. Apocrine sweat glands are in the axilla, areola, and circumanal region and begin to function in puberty and produce viscid milky secretions in response to external stimuli. Apocrine glands accumulate secretory products at the outer margin of the cell and that portion pinches off to form the secretion; the remaining part of the cell repairs itself and repeats the process.

A sebaceous gland is one of several types of glands located in the skin and occurs most commonly in association with hair follicles (e.g., on the face and scalp and in the genital area). These glands produce sebum, a thick, slightly oily secretion that conditions the skin, which empties into the hair follicle.

The categories in this code block are as follows:

L60	Nail disorders
L62	Nail disorders in diseases classified elsewhere
L63	Alopecia areata
L64	Androgenic alopecia
L65	Other nonscarring hair loss
L66	Cicatricial alopecia [scarring hair loss]
L67	Hair color and hair shaft abnormalities
L68	Hypertrichosis
L70	Acne
L71	Rosacea
L72	Follicular cysts of skin and subcutaneous tissue
L73	Other follicular disorders
L74	Eccrine sweat disorders
L75	Apocrine sweat disorders

L60.-   Nail disorders

This category includes acquired deformities of the nails.

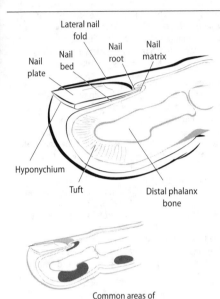

Lateral nail fold

Nail root

Nail matrix

Nail bed

Nail plate

Hyponychium

Tuft

Distal phalanx bone

Common areas of finger infection

Focus Point

Infection of the fingernail or toenail is reported with a code from category L03. Fungal infection of the nail, also called onychomycosis, is reported with B35.1. Codes for congenital anomalies of the nail are found in category Q84.

L60.0   Ingrowing nail

Onychocryptosis or ingrowing nail is a painful condition, usually of the big toe, in which one or both edges of the nail press into the adjacent skin, leading to infection and inflammation. Common causes include tight-fitting shoes and incorrect nail cutting. Therapies include soaking, antibiotics to control infection, and removal of the nail edge.

L60.1   Onycholysis

In onycholysis, the nail separates from the nail bed, typically starting at the distal free margin and separating proximally. It can occur for many reasons, including traumatic injuries, systemic diseases, and infections. Patients may be placed on medication to avoid a potential fungal infection related to this nail separation.

L60.2   Onychogryphosis

This condition also referred to as Rams horn nails is most common with the elderly who are unable to trim toenails. The toenails become long, thickened, yellow, and curved, looking claw-like and making them even more difficult to cut.

L60.3   Nail dystrophy

Nail dystrophy is a general term relating to malformation of the nail caused by some other condition or a drug or substance the patient has taken or been exposed to.

L60.4   Beau's lines

Beau's lines are horizontal depressions or lines across the nail bed. These lines grow out as the nail continues to grow. They can be caused by infections or trauma, or potentially even medication use.

L60.5   Yellow nail syndrome

Yellow nail syndrome is a rare condition characterized by yellow-tinted nails. The nails lack cuticles and can grow quite slowly. These patients are also typically affected by onycholysis.

L63.-   Alopecia areata

Alopecia is hair loss, localized or generalized, that is associated with dysfunction or destruction of the hair follicles. Alopecia areata is a fairly common autoimmune disease of the skin that can cause hair loss on the scalp, as well as on the body. Specific types of alopecia include alopecia totalis (complete loss of scalp hair) and alopecia universalis (complete loss of all body hair).

L63.0   Alopecia (capitis) totalis

Alopecia capitis totalis is total, typically permanent, hair loss on the scalp. Alopecia universalis is a total hair loss on the body, including eyebrows and eyelashes. Unlike alopecia totalis, however, the hair can grow back in some cases. Interestingly, there is no known cause for these conditions, as is the case for most forms of alopecia. Some researchers consider these conditions to be autoimmune disorders.

L63.2   Ophiasis

Patients with ophiasis typically have hair loss on the back of their head in the shape of a wave, near the nape of the neck. Outside of this specific pattern, there is no difference between ophiasis and other types of alopecia areata.

L64.-   Androgenic alopecia

Androgenic alopecia is a general term for the most common form of hair loss. It is often referred to as male or female pattern baldness. There are various causes of hair loss, including stress, abnormal hormone levels, and disease states. In most instances, people are genetically predisposed to certain types of hair loss.

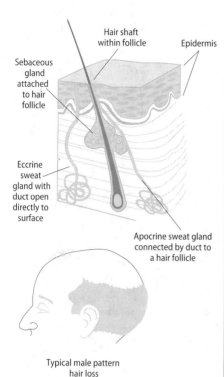

Hair shaft within follicle

Epidermis

Sebaceous gland attached to hair follicle

Eccrine sweat gland with duct open directly to surface

Apocrine sweat gland connected by duct to a hair follicle

Typical male pattern hair loss

L64.0   Drug-induced androgenic alopecia

Drug-induced androgenic alopecia is a hair loss condition in males and females caused by the ingestion of or exposure to some drug or substance. In many cases, this hair loss can be stopped by preventing exposure, and there is potential that the patient will have hair regrowth as well.

L65.-   Other nonscarring hair loss

Nonscarring hair loss is more common than the cicatricial or scarring types. These types typically do not destroy the hair follicle so hair regrowth is possible.

L65.0   Telogen effluvium

Telogen effluvium is the excessive loss of normal hairs despite the follicles themselves being normal. The condition is most often seen in females and is related to a stressful incident occurring six to 16 weeks prior to the hair loss. It may occur during the postpartum period, as well as after a fever, surgery, or trauma.

L65.1   Anagen effluvium

Anagen effluvium is hair loss that affects hair follicles specifically in the anagen stage of hair development. This hair loss most commonly occurs in patients undergoing radiation therapy or systemic chemotherapy treatments including Tamoxifen, but

can be caused by exposure to other pharmaceuticals or chemicals. Unfortunately, there is no treatment for the hair loss, but hair does typically regrow following conclusion of the therapies.

L65.2   Alopecia mucinosa

Alopecia mucinosa is characterized by patches of hair loss, as well as purulent papules and plaques. There is no known cause for this condition. Treatments can include topical medications and phototherapies, although these help with the papules and plaques more than they do hair loss. There is no standard treatment protocol for this condition, and it seems that in many cases the issue resolves on its own.

L66.-   Cicatricial alopecia [scarring hair loss]

These are rare disorders that cause destruction of the hair follicle causing permanent hair loss.

L66.0   Pseudopelade

Pseudopelade is a form of cicatricial alopecia. It is characterized by irregularly shaped, slightly depressed lesions of the scalp. Sometimes there are a few hairs remaining in the lesion; otherwise it is typically hypopigmented in appearance. Once these lesions have occurred, there is unfortunately no medical treatment available. However, the patient may take pharmaceuticals to avoid other lesions from occurring. In serious cases, skin grafts and hair transplants may be used to replace hair loss if the disease has stabilized.

L66.1   Lichen planopilaris

Typically affecting young women, Lichen planopilaris is a rare inflammatory disease that causes patchy, permanent hair loss. It appears as smooth, white patches on the scalp with scaly redness around the hair follicles at the edge of the patches. No cause is known and hair loss is slowly progressive and permanent.

L66.2   Folliculitis decalvans

Folliculitis decalvans is another form of scarring alopecia. This condition is characterized by recurrent waves of follicular pustules that cause the hair to fall out. Treatment for this condition is typically a combination of topical corticosteroids and oral tetracycline to control the infection and the hair loss.

L67.-   Hair color and hair shaft abnormalities

This category includes conditions that cause weakening or fragility of the hair shaft causing hair breakage. Hair color and hair shaft changes are sometimes symptoms of underlying conditions such as vitamin deficiencies, metabolic disorders, and endocrine disorders.

L67.0   Trichorrhexis nodosa

A common defect of the hair shaft is trichorrhexis nodosa, also called trichonodosis, where there is a breakdown of the cuticle that encloses and protects the cortex of the hair. The resulting exposure of the cortex weakens the hair, making it vulnerable to breakage. The condition may be acquired or congenital. The congenital type is quite rare and becomes evident at an early age. More often, the condition is acquired due to excess brushing or hair products (e.g., perms). The abnormal production of brittle hair may also be seen in metabolic disorders such as abnormal copper or zinc metabolism.

L67.1   Variations in hair color

Depending on the ethnicity of the individual, natural hair color can be black, brown, red, or blonde, and is genetically related to eye colors and skin tones. Melanocytes produce two types of melanin (pigments) that provide color to the hair: eumelanin and pheomelanin. Eumelanin, with the subtypes of black or brown, establishes the darkness of the hair. For instance, a low strength of brown eumelanin yields blonde hair, but a higher concentration results in brown hair. Black hair results from a high concentration of black eumelanin, while low strength results in gray hair. Pheomelanin colors hair red. As an individual ages, melanocyte activity starts to diminish, and gray hairs appear. Premature graying is when gray hairs occur during childhood. This may occur as the result of the child's genetic schedule or it may be due to rare conditions such as neurofibromatosis or tuberous sclerosis. There are, however, other conditions that can cause premature graying, including a deficiency of vitamin B12, anemia, vitiligo, hyperthyroidism, and Vogt-Koyanagi syndrome.

L68.-   Hypertrichosis

Hypertrichosis is excessive hair growth typically on parts of the body where heavy hair growth is not normally seen.

L68.0   Hirsutism

Hirsutism is excessive and increased male patterned hair growth in women in locations where the occurrence of terminal hair normally is minimal or absent (e.g., chest, face, abdomen, and back). It may occur from an excess of male hormones such as testosterone or it may be an inherited trait. Some known causes of hirsutism are polycystic ovary syndrome, Cushing's syndrome, tumors, or medications. Women of Mediterranean, Middle Eastern, or South Asian descent are more likely to develop hirsutism of unknown cause.

L70.-   Acne

Acne is an inflammatory skin condition characterized by superficial skin eruptions that occur when sebaceous glands within the hair follicles become plugged, because secretion occurs faster than the oil and skin cells can exit the follicle. If the plug ruptures the wall of the follicle, the oil, dead skin cells, and bacteria found on the surface of the skin can enter to form the infected pustules (e.g., pimples). The condition usually begins at puberty and affects 75 percent of all teenagers to some extent, probably due to hormonal changes that stimulate the sebaceous glands.

L70.0   Acne vulgaris

Acne vulgaris, also known as common acne, is a skin disorder faced by many adolescents who may deal with the disorder into adulthood. It is typically characterized by outbreaks of pimples, cysts, comedones, and inflammation. In youth, acne can have psychological effects, such as reduced self-esteem.

L70.1   Acne conglobata

Acne conglobata is a severe but somewhat rare form of acne that causes nodules on the skin, typically the trunk, upper arms, buttocks, thighs, and face. Also called cystic acne, these nodules create abscesses that become interconnected under the skin, creating a network of abscesses. This can cause significant scarring, to the point of disfigurement. It is typically treated with pharmaceuticals, but surgical excision may be required as well.

L70.2   Acne varioliformis

Acne varioliformis, also referred to as acne necrotica miliaris, is a rare inflammatory condition with papules and pustules typically on the forehead and temples caused by a pyogenic infection of the hair follicles.

L70.3   Acne tropica

Acne tropica, or tropical acne, is seen in tropical climates. The warm air and humidity cause this condition, especially when the body is not use to higher temperatures. Acne tropica is caused by a significant build-up of oil, dead skin cells, and bacteria in the pores, which causes a heat rash-like reaction. Perspiration from the hot and humid weather exacerbates the condition, causing a vicious cycle. Treatment for acne tropica is much like that for acne vulgaris. Most patients are advised to use an over-the-counter benzoyl peroxide or salicylic acid treatment.

L70.4   Infantile acne

Infantile acne affects infants, typically starting around 2 to 3 months of age. There is no specific explanation for this form of acne, although there is a hypothesis that it is genetic in nature. It typically affects the nose and cheeks of the infant, but can spread to the chin and forehead. It usually dissipates by 6 months of age, but some cases have lasted up to age 3.

L70.5   Acne excoriee

Acne excoriée, also known as excoriated acne or picker's acne, is characterized by comedones or pustules that have been excoriated, or "picked," leaving open wounds or scratch marks. In most instances, much of the acne resolves, but scarring and sores remain. Treatment for this condition varies, based on severity and the root cause of excoriation. In some cases, the excoriation can be caused by an underlying psychological condition, for which the patient may need to seek treatment. The acne itself can be treated with oral pharmaceuticals. In some cases, aggressive treatment to resolve the acne can curtail the patient's habitual picking, thus breaking the cycle.

L71.- Rosacea

Rosacea is a hereditary, chronic disorder characterized by groups of arterioles, capillaries, and venules that become dilated, resulting in small papules and pustules, especially around the nose, forehead, cheekbones, and chin.

L71.Ø Perioral dermatitis

Perioral dermatitis is not exclusively related to rosacea but is a condition afflicting many with rosacea. Perioral refers to the area around the mouth. This form of dermatitis typically results in redness of the skin, small bumps that can be pus-filled, and peeling of the skin on the chin, the sides of the mouth, and around the nose. There is usually a band of skin around the mouth that is spared. There are various treatments for this condition, but the most common is the use of oral antibiotics, such as tetracycline. Corticosteroid creams are used in some cases but have been known to cause additional flare-ups.

L71.1 Rhinophyma

Rhinophyma is the most recognizable condition related to rosacea. Although this condition isn't exclusive to rosacea, in most instances rosacea is involved. Rhinophyma results in the nose taking on a large, bulbous, distorted appearance, typically red in color. This distortion is caused over time by the hypertrophy of the sebaceous glands of the nose. It is often thought to be related to alcoholism, although there is no direct link. Heavy alcohol use, however, can aggravate the condition in patients with existing disease.

L72.- Follicular cysts of skin and subcutaneous tissue

Cysts of the skin and subcutaneous tissue are fibrous capsules that are filled with fluid and cells.

L72.Ø Epidermal cyst

Epidermal cysts are benign cysts of the skin resulting from any number of things, including a blocked pore or a traumatic injury. Such a cyst can be filled with pus or other purulent material and most likely needs to be removed surgically.

L72.11 Pilar cyst

Pilar cysts are common benign, keratinous lesions of the skin of the head or neck that form on or around the sheath of a hair follicle. Approximately 9Ø percent occur on the scalp. They contain keratinous material,

surrounded by a fibrous capsule that is encircled by epithelial cells and squamous epithelium. Causation is unknown, although some cases suggest an inherited component. Presenting symptoms may include swelling, tenderness, erythema, drainage, or pain. A patient may present with a solitary lesion or multiple lesions. Complications include cyst rupture or infection.

L72.12 Trichodermal cyst

Trichodermal cysts, also called trichilemmal cysts, are intradermal or subcutaneous lesions that are almost always benign. Like pilar cysts, they contain keratin and are surrounded by a fibrous capsule that is encircled by epithelial cells and squamous epithelium. A small percentage of trichilemmal cysts contain proliferating cells that cause tumors, in which case they are referred to as proliferating trichilemmal cysts. The proliferating form is characterized by a gradual increase in size sometimes becoming as large as 25 cm and these cysts have a tendency to ulcerate. In rare cases they may become locally aggressive, growing rapidly. While proliferating trichilemmal cysts are considered benign, in very rare cases they can transform into malignant lesions. Because of this, cells and tissue must be monitored for signs of atypia. If transformation occurs, the lesions require complete surgical removal and, in some cases, adjunct radiation or antineoplastic chemotherapy.

> **Focus Point**
>
> *Merkel cell carcinoma has been reported in association with trichilemmal cysts.*

L72.2 Steatocystoma multiplex

Steatocystoma multiplex is a condition typically described as congenital, causing multiple cysts over the body. These cysts, typically small and fluid filled, are usually found in areas with the highest concentration of sebaceous glands (chest, arms, axillae, and neck). Treatment includes excision of particularly large or disfiguring lesions and pharmaceuticals to help prevent complications.

L72.3 Sebaceous cyst

A sebaceous cyst is a slowly developing, benign cystic tumor of the skin containing follicular, keratinous, and sebaceous material. Frequently found on the scalp, ears, face, back, or scrotum, sebaceous cysts may grow very large and become infected by bacteria. An exam reveals a firm, globular, movable, and nontender mass.

L73.- Other follicular disorders

Most follicular disorders classified here affect the hair follicles, although one condition, hidradenitis suppurativa is a condition that affects the apocrine sweat glands.

L73.0 Acne keloid

Acne keloids are a form of keloid scarring that typically occurs at the base of the neck. It is associated with the occlusion of hair follicles in that area and is most often encountered in black and Asian men. The skin in the area becomes inflamed and bumpy, and it can be quite painful. Treatment varies, based on the severity of the condition. The use of antibiotics and steroid gels is common and, in more advanced cases, intralesional steroid injections may be required. Larger keloids may require surgical removal.

L73.1 Pseudofolliculitis barbae

Also called shaving bumps, this condition primarily affects African-American men, although it can be found in other racial and ethnic groups but is not as common. Papules and pustules form around the hair shaft after shaving and can lead to hyperpigmentation and scarring in chronic cases.

L73.2 Hidradenitis suppurativa

Hidradenitis suppurativa is inflammation of the apocrine sweat glands occurring in the axillae, anogenital regions, nipples, and under the female breast. The condition may produce chronic abscesses or sinus tract formation. In most cases, hidradenitis is caused by the obstruction of the apocrine sweat pores due to the application of underarm deodorants, irritant depilatories, or other topical ointments or creams. Signs and symptoms of hidradenitis include large painful abscesses resulting from double comedones and extensive deep dermal inflammation, local pain, and tenderness. Systemic symptoms may include weight loss, fever, and malaise.

L73.9 Follicular disorder, unspecified

Folliculitis (superficial) is included here. Folliculitis is a hair follicle infection most frequently seen in areas where there has been irritation or friction. It is manifested by the appearance of tiny white heads at the base of hair shafts, with a small red area around each pimple.

Focus Point

Sequence an additional code secondarily to identify the infective organism, typically Streptococcus or Staphylococcus.

L74.- Eccrine sweat disorders

Eccrine sweat glands are found in the skin throughout the body, particularly on the forehead, scalp, axillae, palms, and soles and produce watery and neutral or slightly acidic sweat. This category identifies different types of prickly heat/heat rash.

L74.0 Miliaria rubra

Miliaria rubra is the second most serious heat rash condition. It tends to affect adults in hot and humid conditions or neonates aged 1 to 3 weeks. It occurs deep within the epidermis and can cause pruritic papules across the body. The lesions tend to resolve quickly after the patients leave hot and humid climates.

L74.1 Miliaria crystallina

Miliaria crystallina is the mildest form of heat rash. It tends to affect adults with other conditions that may be causing a fever or neonates younger than 2 weeks. Some adults who have relocated to a significantly warmer climate may be affected by this condition as well. This form affects the most superficial layer of the skin, causing what almost looks like tiny beads of liquid on the skin. It tends to be asymptomatic and often disappears on its own within a few days.

L74.2 Miliaria profunda

Miliaria profunda is the most serious form of heat rash, caused by repeated episodes of miliaria rubra. This condition causes deep pustules to form at the dermal/epidermal junction. These pustules block the sweat glands and can make it impossible for the body to cool itself properly if widespread. In warm climates, patients with this condition are more likely to be predisposed to heat exhaustion.

L74.4 Anhidrosis

Anhidrosis, also called hypohidrosis, is the inability to sweat normally. When the body can't cool itself through perspiration it can lead to heatstroke, a life-threatening condition. It can occur in all or just part of the body. When only part of the body is affected the other areas can perspire profusely.

L74.5- Focal hyperhidrosis

Hyperhidrosis is the clinical disorder of excessive sweating, beyond what the body requires to maintain thermal control. Focal hyperhidrosis may be primary or secondary.

L74.51- Primary focal hyperhidrosis

Primary hyperhidrosis occurs in the absence of any underlying or causative condition, and is almost always confined to one or more specific areas of the body, like the axilla, the soles of the feet, the palms, or the face. Primary focal hyperhidrosis is first treated by a trial of topical medication applications with surgery as a final step. A sixth character indicates the site affected.

L74.52 Secondary focal hyperhidrosis

Secondary hyperhidrosis may occur as a focal condition, limited to one or more sites, but more often it is a generalized condition. Secondary hyperhidrosis occurs with another associated condition such as metabolic or endocrine disorder, malignancies, drugs, substance abuse, toxins, infections, cardiovascular disorders, or respiratory failure. Typically, secondary hyperhidrosis occurs focally at a single site when it is caused by a local condition or treatment, such as radiation therapy to a specific tumor location, spinal disease, or injury. Frey's syndrome is included in this category. It is an auriculotemporal syndrome due to a lesion on the parotid gland with characteristic redness and excessive sweating on the cheek in connection with eating.

L74.8   Other eccrine sweat disorders

This subcategory includes Granulosis rubra nasi, which is an idiopathic condition of children that manifests as redness and sweating around the nose, face, and chin and tends to end by puberty. Also included in this code is urhidrosis, which is described as the secretion of urinous substance, such as uric acid, in sweat and most commonly occurs in uremia.

L75.-   Apocrine sweat disorders

Apocrine sweat glands are in the axilla, areola, and circumanal region and begin to function in puberty and produce viscid milky secretions in response to external stimuli. Apocrine glands accumulate secretory products at the outer margin of the cell and that portion pinches off to form the secretion; the remaining part of the cell repairs itself and repeats the process.

L75.0   Bromhidrosis

Also known as excessive body odor, bromhidrosis is a chronic condition of foul-smelling axillary sweat due to decomposed bacteria. Although a common occurrence especially in postpubertal people, it can be pathological if excessive.

L75.1   Chromhidrosis

Chromhidrosis is a rare condition of apocrine gland secretion of yellow, green, blue, or black sweat. The color is from a higher concentration of lipofuscin pigment, which forms colors when oxidized in the apocrine glands.

L75.2   Apocrine miliaria

Also called Fox-Fordyce disease, apocrine miliaria is described as chronic, usually pruritic disease evidenced by small, follicular papular eruptions, especially in the axillary and pubic areas. It develops from the closure and rupture of the affected apocrine gland's intraepidermal portion of the ducts.

Intraoperative and Postprocedural Complications of Skin and Subcutaneous Tissue (L76)

There is a single category in this code block that reports intraoperative and postprocedural complications of skin and subcutaneous tissue that occur as a result of a dermatological procedure or a procedure performed on another body system.

L76.-   Intraoperative and postprocedural complications of skin and subcutaneous tissue

This category is further defined by whether the procedure performed was dermatological or another procedure, whether the injury/complication occurred during or after the procedure, and the type of complication or injury. The descriptions of these injury types are as follows:

- Hemorrhage is the rapid blood loss from vessels.

- Hematoma is a collection of blood clots within tissue or organ due to a broken blood vessel.

- Seroma is a fluid accumulation just under the skin surface, often forming after a surgery involving an incision or tissue extraction.

- Laceration is simply a torn wound.

- Puncture is a wound due to perforation or piercing.

Other Disorders of the Skin and Subcutaneous Tissue (L80-L99)

This code block includes a wide variety of conditions that do not fit well into more specific categories.

The categories in this code block are as follows:

L80	Vitiligo
L81	Other disorders of pigmentation
L82	Seborrheic keratosis
L83	Acanthosis nigricans
L84	Corns and callosities
L85	Other epidermal thickening
L86	Keratoderma in diseases classified elsewhere
L87	Transepidermal elimination disorders
L88	Pyoderma gangrenosum
L89	Pressure ulcer
L90	Atrophic disorders of skin
L91	Hypertrophic disorders of skin

L92	Granulomatous disorders of skin and subcutaneous tissue
L93	Lupus erythematosus
L94	Other localized connective tissue disorders
L95	Vasculitis limited to skin, not elsewhere classified
L97	Non-pressure chronic ulcer of lower limb, not elsewhere classified
L98	Other disorders of skin and subcutaneous tissue, not elsewhere classified
L99	Other disorders of skin and subcutaneous tissue in diseases classified elsewhere

L80   Vitiligo

Vitiligo is a condition of persistent, progressive development of nonpigmented white patches on otherwise normal skin.

L81.-   Other disorders of pigmentation

This category represents many conditions that occur from an excess amount of melanin, which produces hyperpigmentation conditions such as melasma, lentigo, café au lait spots, and freckles, or a lack of melanin.

L81.1   Chloasma

Commonly referred to as melasma or mask of pregnancy, this condition tends to occur in younger women who are pregnant or taking oral contraceptives or hormone replacement therapy. It appears as darker patches on the face and is exacerbated by sun exposure.

L81.4   Other melanin hyperpigmentation

This code includes lentigo, which is flat, darker oval spots commonly caused by chronic sun exposure. Sometimes called liver spots, they usually start to appear at middle age.

L81.5   Leukoderma, not elsewhere classified

This acquired condition refers to a localized loss of skin pigmentation.

> **Focus Point**
>
> *Albinism, a metabolic pigment condition, is not included in this chapter. It can be located in Chapter 4 Endocrine, Nutritional and Metabolic Diseases, at category E70.*

L82.-   Seborrheic keratosis

Seborrheic keratoses are superficial noninvasive tumors (usually multiple) originating in the epidermis. Also known as seborrheic warts or verrucae, these tumors are characterized by numerous yellow or brown, sharply marginated, oval raised lesions. Seborrheic keratoses typically produce no symptoms unless they become inflamed, which can then cause pain and itching. Inflammation may occur due to friction caused by skin surfaces or clothing rubbing on the lesion. They occur commonly in middle-aged or older patients. Therapies include shaving the lesions or destruction by cryotherapy or electrosurgery.

L83   Acanthosis nigricans

Acanthosis nigricans is a skin disorder characterized by hyperpigmented, thick, velvety skin in body folds and creases. Areas usually affected are the armpits, groin, and neck, although, less common, the lips, palms, and soles of the feet may also be affected. The skin changes appear slowly, sometimes over months or years. It is most commonly associated with conditions that increase insulin levels, such as Type 2 diabetes or obesity. It can also be seen in patients with polycystic ovarian disease or patients taking certain medications such as human growth hormone or oral contraceptives. Some cases are genetically inherited or may be linked to cancer. Skin changes are the only signs of this condition. One syndrome coded here is Gougerot-Carteaud syndrome or disease, which consists of benign, neoplasm producing, finger-like projections (papilla) from the epithelial surface in girls nearing puberty. The papilla-like lesions begin on the back and between the breasts, eventually spreading over the torso and throughout the body.

L84   Corns and callosities

Calluses and corns are knobs of hyperkeratotic tissue caused by pressure or friction, most commonly seen in the bony prominences of the feet or hands. Benign conditions, they can cause pain that requires treatment by a podiatrist or physician.

L85.-   Other epidermal thickening

These conditions involve thickening of the outer layer of the skin.

L85.0   Acquired ichthyosis

Derived from the Greek word fish, this condition of dry, scaly skin, when acquired, generally appears in adults and is often a sign of a systemic disease or from the use of certain medications.

L85.1   Acquired keratosis [keratoderma] palmaris et plantaris

This condition is characterized by thickening of the skin of the palms and soles and can be attributed to a multitude of causes.

> **Focus Point**
>
> *Inherited or congenital forms of ichthyosis and keratosis (PPK) are located in Chapter 17 Congenital Malformations, Deformations and Chromosomal Abnormalities.*

L87.- Transepidermal elimination disorders

Transepidermal elimination is a necessary function of the skin that allows removal of foreign or altered substances from the dermal layer of the skin through the epidermal layer to the external surface of the skin.

L87.0 Keratosis follicularis et parafollicularis in cutem penetrans

This condition includes Kyrle disease, which is a perforating skin condition. It is characterized by the appearance of widespread, large keratotic papules that contain a plug in the center that contains keratin and necrotic debris. It most commonly occurs with diabetes mellitus and chronic renal failure.

L87.1 Reactive perforating collagenosis

This condition represents a rare skin disorder of transepidermal elimination of altered collagen. It can be inherited or acquired and occurs most commonly in diabetics and chronic renal failure patients on dialysis, although other causes such as malignancies have been found. The lesions trigger severe itching causing scarring from scratching.

L87.2 Elastosis perforans serpiginosa

This rare skin disorder is characterized by the elimination of abnormal elastic skin fibers and other cellular debris from the papillary dermis through the epidermis. There are three categories of elastosis perforans serpiginosa: idiopathic, reactive, or drug induced. Small papules grouped together develop and erupt with a central core of fibrous material and debris. The reactive form is most often associated with Down syndrome.

L88 Pyoderma gangrenosum

This uncommon persistent debilitating skin disease is characterized by irregular, boggy, blue-red ulcerations, with central healing and undermined edges. Fifty percent of cases are associated with systemic diseases. It can subside if treated with immunosuppressive therapy, but may reoccur.

L89.- Pressure ulcer

A pressure ulcer, also known as a bedsore, decubitus ulcer, plaster ulcer, pressure area, or pressure sore, is a localized injury to the skin that may also affect underlying tissue that results from prolonged pressure. Pressure ulcers typically occur over bony prominences and are classified by location and stage. The pressure injury initially affects superficial tissues and, depending on the state of the patient's health and other circumstances, may progress to affect muscle and bone. Patients at risk for development of pressure ulcers include the bedridden, unconscious, or immobile, such as stroke patients or those with paralysis and limited motion. Intrinsic loss of pain and pressure sensations, disuse atrophy, malnutrition, anemia, and infection contribute to the formation and progression of pressure ulcers. In the early stages, the condition is reversible, but left untended, the pressure ulcer can become extensively infected, necrotic, and, ultimately, irreversible. Pressure ulcers are classified by site and stage. Stage describes the severity of the pressure injury to the skin and underlying tissues and specific descriptions of the extent of the pressure injury are listed in the inclusion notes under each code.

Pressure Ulcer Stages

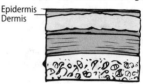

Stage 1
Persistent focal erythema

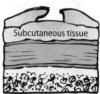

Stage 2
Abrasion, blister, partial thickness skin loss involving epidermis and/or dermis

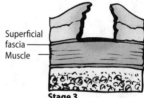

Stage 3
Full thickness skin loss involving damage or necrosis of subcutaneous tissue

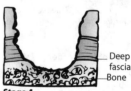

Stage 4
Necrosis of soft tissues through to underlying muscle, tendon, or bone

The ulcer stage is captured by the 5th or 6th character of each code. Descriptions of these stages follow:

0 *Unstageable: Used if pressure ulcer stage cannot be clinically determined. For example, the ulcer is obscured by eschar or has been previously treated with a graft or when only documented as deep tissue injury but not as due to trauma*

1 *Stage 1: Pre-ulcer skin changes limited to persistent focal edema*

2 *Stage 2: Abrasion, blister, partial thickness skin loss involving epidermis and/or dermis*

3 *Stage 3: Full thickness skin loss involving damage or necrosis of subcutaneous tissue*

4 *Stage 4: Necrosis of soft tissues through to underlying muscle, tendon, or bone*

9 *Unspecified stage: Only used when there is no documentation regarding the stage of the pressure ulcer; not to be confused with unstageable*

If the pressure ulcer is documented as healed, or completely healed, no code is assigned for the condition.

If the pressure ulcer is documented as "healing," the appropriate current pressure ulcer stage code should be used.

Two codes should be assigned for a pressure ulcer site that evolves from one stage to another during the admission. The first code should be the stage of the ulcer upon admission, and the second code should be the highest stage the ulcer progressed to during the admission.

L90.- Atrophic disorders of skin

Atrophic disorders of the skin are characterized by thinning of the upper layers of the skin, a process often associated with aging, but may also be due to some disease processes.

L90.0 Lichen sclerosus et atrophicus

This condition consists of white plaques associated with thinning of the epidermis along with thickened, hardened scarring most often in the genitals. This condition occurs more often in females than males.

L90.1 Anetoderma of Schweninger-Buzzi

This benign condition is characterized by noninflammatory lesions that result in loss of dermal elastic tissue and localized areas of herniated saclike skin. Etiology is unknown.

L90.2 Anetoderma of Jadassohn-Pellizzari

This benign condition is characterized by inflammatory lesions that result in loss of dermal elastic tissue and localized areas of herniated saclike skin. Etiology is unknown.

L90.3 Atrophoderma of Pasini and Pierini

Idiopathic atrophoderma of Pasini and Pierini (IAPP) is a form of dermal atrophy that presents as single or multiple sharply demarcated, dark patches marked by a slight indentation of the skin with a sharp edge. It usually appears on the backs of adolescents or young adults. Etiology is unknown.

L90.6 Striae atrophicae

This condition is described as bands of atrophic, depressed, wrinkled skin associated with stretching of skin from pregnancy, obesity, or rapid growth during puberty. The condition is also referred to as stretch marks.

L90.8 Other atrophic disorders of skin

A number of other atrophic skin disorders are classified here, including nephrogenic fibrosing dermopathy (NFD). NFD is a chronic, progressive, systemic condition associated with kidney disease. There is also a link between NFD and some patients who have had imaging studies (e.g., magnetic resonance angiography) with gadolinium contrast. NFD is reminiscent of, but distinct from, scleroderma or scleromyxedema. Characteristic dark plaque-like lesions appear on the skin of the limbs and torso, which may be accompanied by muscle weakness, tightening of skin, flexion contractures of the extremities, itching, burning, or pain at the affected sites. Treatments may include extracorporeal photopheresis (ECP), plasmapheresis, UV light therapy, intravenous immunoglobulin, or oral corticosteroid therapy.

L91.- Hypertrophic disorders of skin

Hypertrophy refers to an overgrowth or thickening of a tissue, in this case the skin.

L91.0 Hypertrophic scar

A hypertrophic scar consists of actively growing hypertrophic cutaneous scar tissue. Included in this code are keloid scars that act more like benign tumors of hypertrophic cutaneous tissue. The term hypertrophic scar is generally used when overgrowth of scar tissue lacks the characteristic tumor formation of keloids and does not grow beyond the margins of the original injury. Hypertrophic scars and keloids occur as a result of trauma or irritation such as burns, incisions, vaccinations, insect bites, and other stimuli. Ulcerated keloids are prone to carcinomatous transformation, but the majority behaves as benign neoplasms. Dark-skinned races are particularly susceptible to keloid formation. Signs and symptoms of keloid scar include a history of surgery or skin trauma, overreactive visible scar formation, itching, and burning. A skin biopsy may be performed to determine the histopathology.

Focus Point

In many cases, keloids and hypertrophic scars are residuals of previous trauma or surgery. If the etiology of the keloid or hypertrophic scar is known and described as a late effect or sequela, assign a secondary code describing the sequela.

L92.- Granulomatous disorders of skin and subcutaneous tissue

Granulomatous disorders are characterized by nodular inflammatory lesions of the skin and subcutaneous tissues.

L92.0 Granuloma annulare

There are several types of granuloma annulare, the most common of which is localized and the rarest is perforated. The localized type is benign and often asymptomatic and presents as cutaneous lesions or subcutaneous nodules commonly appearing in groups of papules often in the distal extremities. The generalized type may appear over multiple body regions. The perforated type presents as papules that evolve into pustular lesions that secrete a thick or viscous fluid, forming crusts and scales and eventually leaving scars.

L92.1 Necrobiosis lipoidica, not elsewhere classified

Most cases of necrobiosis lipoidica are related to diabetes, but this code encompasses all nondiabetic-related cases. This condition presents as shiny patches of red-brown plaques that are asymptomatic and enlarge over time. They can progress into ulcerations that can be painless because of cutaneous nerve damage or be painful and require long periods of wound care and eventually leave scarring. Despite extensive research, the etiologies of nondiabetic causes are uncertain.

L93.- Lupus erythematosus

Lupus erythematosus is a group of disorders brought on by an autoimmune disease in which the body's autoimmune system attacks healthy tissue. The types classified in this chapter manifest in the integumentary system. Lupus erythematosus can attack at any age and affects women more than men. The cause is not fully known but onset may be brought on by certain drugs or provoked by sun exposure. The condition tends to be more severe in smokers. Although no two cases are alike, many start with a butterfly shaped rash on the face on the bridge of the nose and spreading across the cheeks.

L93.0 Discoid lupus erythematosus

Discoid lupus erythematosus is a chronic disease that causes inflammation of the connective tissue of the skin only. Red plaques with an expanding inflammatory border and hypopigmented atrophic scarring are characteristic of discoid lupus erythematosus, which is not usually associated with systemic manifestations. Lesions are commonly found in areas exposed to sunlight, such as the face, ears, neck, and scalp. Occurring worldwide, this disease affects nine times as many women as men, usually those of childbearing age, and can lead to scarring and permanent disfigurement.

L94.- Other localized connective tissue disorders

Connective tissue disorders classified here are confined to a specific site or region.

L94.0 Localized scleroderma [morphea]

Localized scleroderma is an autoimmune disease in which an immune response causing inflammation triggers the production of excess collagen. It affects more women than men and is most common found in Caucasians. The word scleroderma means "hard skin" and morphea is the most common type. Localized morphea presents as a few patches of skin thickening with discoloration, generally only affecting the superficial layer.

L94.1 Linear scleroderma

Linear scleroderma appears as a band of skin thickening that may extend deep into the skin. These bands are most often on the limbs and can involve underlying muscle or cause stiffness when crossing over joints. One type of linear scleroderma called "en coup de sabre" appears as a line across the face. The name comes from the French meaning "cut from a sword." It can cause atrophy of the face and involve the tongue and mouth.

L94.5 Poikiloderma vasculare atrophicans

Poikiloderma vasculare atrophicans (PVA) is a condition characterized by hypopigmentation or hyperpigmentation of the skin, atrophy of the skin, and telangiectasia (dilated blood vessels) near the surface of the skin. These issues are often related to another condition, such as mycosis fungoides, other parapsoriasis, and other conditions that might cause the skin issues. Treatment for PVA is typically geared toward the underlying condition.

L97.- Non-pressure chronic ulcer of lower limb, not elsewhere classified

Non-pressure ulcers, unlike pressure ulcers, are not represented by specific stage numbers. However, they are still described based on site (character 5) and the description of the depth of the ulcer. Non-pressure ulcers may only involve skin breakdown, or the fat layer may be exposed. Deeper ulcers can involve muscle or even bone with or without necrosis of the muscle or bone. Code descriptions in this category specifically define these phases.

L98.- Other disorders of skin and subcutaneous tissue, not elsewhere classified

Conditions classified here generally do not fit into another category, or there may not be a more specific code available for the condition.

L98.0 Pyogenic granuloma

A pyogenic granuloma is a benign, rapidly growing, red skin lesion that may have an ulcerated appearance and may ooze or bleed. The lesion may be sessile or pedunculated. Although the cause is not known, it is believed this type of lesion forms when capillary vessels start growing rapidly as a reaction to skin trauma. Pyogenic granulomas are a common skin condition in children and young adults, generally appearing on the face, arms, and hands. Therapies include surgical excision, along with cauterizing the base of the lesion. Incomplete removal may result in a recurrent lesion. Occasionally a cluster of lesions may appear.

L98.2 Febrile neutrophilic dermatosis [Sweet]

Most commonly affecting women between 30 and 50 years of age, Sweet syndrome or febrile neutrophil dermatosis is marked by abrupt appearance of painful papules grouping together to form plaque-like lesions on the face, neck, and upper extremities. It can be accompanied by conjunctivitis, mucosal lesion, malaise, fever, and arthralgia. At times the condition occurs after a fever or upper respiratory infection, although it can manifest in response to other systemic factors such as infection, cancers, hematologic disease, or drug exposure.

L98.4- Non-pressure chronic ulcer of skin, not elsewhere classified

Non-pressure ulcers, unlike pressure ulcers, are not represented by specific stage numbers. However, they are still described based on site (character 5) and the description of the depth of the ulcer. Non-pressure

ulcers may only involve skin breakdown, or the fat layer may be exposed. Deeper ulcers can involve muscle or even bone with or without necrosis of the muscle or bone. Code descriptions in this category specifically define these phases. Body sites included here are buttocks, back, and other sites not specified elsewhere.

Focus Point

Non-pressure ulcers of the skin are most common in the lower extremities. Lower extremity non-pressure skin ulcers are classified in category L97.

L98.7 Excessive and redundant skin and subcutaneous tissue

Excessive skin and subcutaneous tissue is often the result of weight loss or bariatric surgery to assist in weight loss. The amount of redundant skin or tissue varies based on the patients' body, the fat distribution, and the total amount of weight reduction. The resulting excessive skin may lead to further problems such as infections within the skin folds.

Abdominoplasty is performed to reduce the amount of excessive skin and fat in the abdominal area and is often classified as cosmetic surgery. Other procedures may be performed in conjunction with the abdominoplasty to address other specific issues or to remove, reconstruct, or "lift" areas of concern.

Typically all procedures of this nature are considered cosmetic unless documentation supports some form of functional deficit due to the excess skin.

L98.8 Other specified disorders of the skin and subcutaneous tissue

This is the appropriate code for Bazex syndrome or paraneoplastic acrokeratosis, which is a rare condition that appears similarly to psoriasis and is more common in men than women. It generally begins with scaling in the fingers and toes, spreading to eruptions on the external ears and keratoderma on the hands and feet. It can eventually involve the limbs and trunk. In most cases it is caused by an underlying neoplasm.

Chapter 13: Diseases of the Musculoskeletal System and Connective Tissue (MØØ-M99)

This chapter classifies diseases and disorders of the bones, muscles, cartilage, fascia, ligaments, synovia, tendons, and bursa.

Connective tissue disorders classified to Chapter 13 are those primarily affecting the musculoskeletal system. Injuries and certain congenital disorders of the musculoskeletal system are classified elsewhere.

Many codes for the manifestation of musculoskeletal diseases due to specified infections and other diseases and disorders classified elsewhere are included in this chapter. Also included are many codes describing the residuals of previous diseases, disorders, and injuries classified as late effects. These codes often can be identified by the term "acquired" in the description.

The chapter is broken down into the following code blocks:

MØØ-MØ2 Infectious arthropathies

MØ4 Autoimmune syndromes

MØ5-M14 Inflammatory polyarthropathies

M15-M19 Osteoarthritis

M2Ø-M25 Other joint disorders

M26-M27 Dentofacial anomalies [including malocclusion] and other disorders of jaw

M3Ø-M36 Systemic connective tissue disorders

M4Ø-M43 Deforming dorsopathies

M45-M49 Spondylopathies

M5Ø-M54 Other dorsopathies

M6Ø-M63 Disorders of muscles

M65-M67 Disorders of synovium and tendon

M7Ø-M79 Other soft tissue disorders

M8Ø-M85 Disorders of bone density and structure

M86-M9Ø Other osteopathies

M91-M94 Chondropathies

M95 Other disorders of the musculoskeletal system and connective tissue

M96 Intraoperative and postprocedural complications and disorders of musculoskeletal system, not elsewhere classified

M99 Biomechanical lesions, not elsewhere classified

Infectious Arthropathies (MØØ-MØ2)

This category includes infections of the articular joints of bones, and must be differentiated from infections of the bones classifiable to osteomyelitis. Direct microbial contamination may cause a primary infection of the articular joints. The routes of infection include open fractures, surgical procedures, diagnostic needle aspirations, and therapeutic drug injections. Infectious arthropathies are due to an acute, destructive bacterial process in a joint following infection, usually occurring as acute monoarticular (single joint) arthritis. The knee and large joints are most often involved.

The categories in this code block are as follows:

MØØ Pyogenic arthritis

MØ1 Direct infections of joint in infectious and parasitic diseases classified elsewhere

MØ2 Postinfective and reactive arthropathies

MØØ.- Pyogenic arthritis

This category represents forms of arthritis due to an acute inflammation of the synovial membranes with purulent effusion into the joint specifically caused by a bacterial infection. It may also be referred to in the medical record documentation as suppurative or septic arthritis or suppurative synovitis. Signs and symptoms of pyogenic arthritis include fever, joint pain, decreased range of motion, and swelling and redness over the affected joint. Gross examination of aspirated synovial (joint) fluid confirms the presence of pus (pyarthrosis); a gram stain and culture may detect microorganisms and crystals. Pyogenic or septic arthritis has the potential to progress and become chronic resulting in sinus formation, osteomyelitis, and joint deformity. Septic arthritis is classified by bacterial organism, including staphylococcal, pneumonococcal, and streptococcal. All other bacterial causes of arthritis are included in the other bacterial subcategory. Conditions classified here are further specified by site and laterality.

Focus Point

It is important for appropriate coding to identify the presence or type of bacteria since the unspecified pyogenic arthritis code not only lacks specificity as to the cause, but also does not identify the site or laterality of the arthritis.

M01.- Direct infections of joint in infectious and parasitic diseases classified elsewhere

This subcategory refers to a direct infection within a joint that is secondary to an infectious process occurring elsewhere in the body. This includes bacterial infections and a wide variety of viral diseases, including viral hepatitis, mumps, infectious mononucleosis, lymphogranuloma venereum, or variola. They can also be associated with mycoses, which are caused by fungi. A variety of fungal organisms may lodge in the synovium and create suppurative or granulomatous lesions. The synovium usually is the primary site of joint involvement, but secondary infection can spread from the marrow cavity to the subchondral bone and into the articular tissues. Arthropathy associated with helminthiases or other parasitic infection is also included here.

M02.- Postinfective and reactive arthropathies

Occasionally, a joint is affected by an infection elsewhere in the body. Inflammation of a joint as a reaction to another disease is referred to as reactive arthropathy. Subcategories include cause of the arthropathy or inflammation such as postdysenteric, postimmunization, Reiter's disease, or other, in addition to specific sites and laterality.

Focus Point

Categories M01.- and M02.- require a code be assigned first for the underlying disease, such as leprosy, mycoses, or paratyphoid fever.

M02.1- Postdysenteric arthropathy

Postdysenteric arthropathies are rare enteropathic arthropathies due to a wide range of specific dysentery-causing organisms, Shigella, and typhoid fever.

M02.3- Reiter's disease

Reiter's disease is a seronegative reactive arthritis. Reactive arthritis occurs as a result of a bacterial infection in another site usually an infection of the gastrointestinal or genitourinary tract. Occurring predominantly in the joints of the lower extremities, Reiter's disease consists of a triad of nonspecific (nongonococcal or simple) urethritis, conjunctivitis (or sometimes uveitis), and arthritis, and sometimes appears with mucocutaneous lesions. There is a close correlation between this disease and the presence of the histocompatibility antigen HLA-B27. Treatment of Reiter's disease is directed at symptoms. The condition typically resolves within two to six months.

Autoinflammatory Syndromes (M04)

The autoinflammatory syndromes involve problems with immune system regulation with manifestations related to episodes of acute systemic inflammation. They were not well understood until fairly recently, due to advanced techniques in genetics. Symptoms include recurrent fever associated with rheumatologic symptoms involving joints, skin, muscles, and eyes. Although the syndromes are generally rare, treatment is directed toward decreasing the acute attacks of fever and involves a combination of drugs like nonsteroidal anti-inflammatory drugs (NSAIDs) and analgesics.

M04.1 Periodic fever syndromes

This code includes familial Mediterranean fever (FMF), which is characterized by attacks of recurrent high fevers accompanied by pain and inflammation in the lining of the chest and abdominal cavities, skin or joints, and blood vessels (vasculitis). Some but not all patients may also develop amyloid protein deposits in the kidneys that can destroy renal tissues. Onset of attacks usually occurs in childhood or adolescence. An attack can persist for 12 to 72 hours and vary in intensity. The intervals between attacks are unpredictable, occurring days or even months apart. Although the underlying cause is seemingly genetic, the catalyst for onset is unknown. However, stress, physical trauma, and exertion have been reported by patients as possible precipitates or contributive factors. Treatment for the attacks is usually a combination of nonsteroidal anti-inflammatory drugs (NSAIDs) and analgesics. Colchicine is also prescribed and greatly reduces the frequency and intensity of clinical attacks and prevents the development of renal amyloidosis.

M04.2 Cryopyrin-associated periodic syndromes

Cryopyrin-associated periodic syndrome (CAPS) is a genetic permutation of the cryopyrin protein, which manages inflammation within the body and can be passed via one copy of the gene from one parent. The specific conditions are diagnosed based on the severity and specific symptoms of the patient. CAPS encompasses the following three diseases, all related to the same gene defect:

- Neonatal onset multisystem inflammatory disease (NOMID) starts with a skin rash. Inflammation of the brain membrane causes symptoms of headache, vision and hearing loss, protuberance of the eyes, and vomiting leading to fever due to widespread systemic inflammation. Children with this condition often show signs of joint pain and inflammation in about 50 percent of the cases by the age of 1 year.

- Muckle-Wells syndrome shows sporadic, recurring symptoms of rash, blood-shot eyes, joint pain, headaches, and vomiting with durations from one to three days per episode. These episodes may lead to complete hearing loss by the time the patient reaches the teen years.

- Familial cold autoinflammatory syndrome triggers rash, fever, chills, nausea, headache, joint pain, and unquenchable thirst when the patient is exposed to cold and other external factors.

These conditions may be managed with medication such as interleukin-1, or methotrexate, physical therapy, and splints. In rare cases, surgery may correct any serious joint abnormalities.

M04.8   Other autoinflammatory syndromes

Several autoinflammatory syndromes are grouped in this subcategory, including some described below:

- Blau syndrome is an inflammatory condition affecting the skin, eyes, and joints with symptoms surfacing before a child turns 4 years old. The initial symptom is a rash on the skin of the body and extremities. Arthritis presents in the joints of hands, feet, wrist, and ankles. Inflammation occurs within the uvea of the eye but may also invade other parts of the eye, causing pain and light sensitivity that progresses to loss of vision. In rare cases, the inflammation may spread to internal organs such as the liver, kidneys, brain, vessels, and heart, leading to very serious complications. This condition is caused by an abnormality in the NOD2 gene, resulting in overproduction of protein and leading to an inflammatory response. It is inherited by one parent with the condition and requires just one copy of the abnormal gene in each cell to precipitate the condition.

- Deficiency of interleukin 1 receptor antagonist (DIRA) is a rare condition typically recognized within the first days of life and resembles an acute and serious systemic infection. Early diagnosis for treatment is essential to avoid death due to multiorgan failure. Although rare, this condition may affect nearly 25 percent of children when both parents carry the recessive genetic disorder. The condition is due to a permutation of the IL1RN gene or another deletion within the same group of chromosome 2. Common symptoms include fetal distress, rash, and lesions in the mouth, inflammation in the bones and joints with pain, and an enlarged liver and/or spleen. Patients are treated with daily injections of protein, which has shown a promising response; however, this treatment is lifelong.

- Those with Majeed syndrome present with frequent fevers with inflammation affecting the skin and bones. Chronic recurrent multifocal osteomyelitis (CRMO) starts when the patient is very young and may continue sporadically into the adult years with complications affecting growth and development and possibly contractures. Other complications may include congenital dyserythropoietic anemia, which presents with fatigue, pale appearance, and difficulty breathing, all of which vary in severity. Many patients with Majeed syndrome also manifest symptoms of Sweet syndrome, characterized by fever in addition to blisters on the face, neck, torso, and arms. This syndrome is caused by an abnormality within the LPIN2 gene that results in inadequate signals to the body to product protein. It is inherited when both parents are carriers of one copy of the abnormal gene.

- Periodic fever, aphthous stomatitis, pharyngitis, and adenopathy syndrome (PFAPA) is more common and classified as an idiopathic hereditary fever syndrome. It presents as recurrent fevers in children beginning between 2 and 5 years of age and is seen more often in males. These recurrent encounters last between three to six days and reappear in cycles of 28 days. Symptoms include fever, sore throat, ulcers, and lymphadenopathy. This condition does not affect growth, and patients are otherwise healthy between encounters. Treatment may include medications such as steroids, with patients typically outgrowing the condition with no lasting effects.

- Pyogenic arthritis, pyoderma gangrenosum, and acne syndrome (PAPA) is also referred to as familial recurrent arthritis and is inherited when one parent carries the abnormal gene or an inadvertent gene mutation leads to the condition. The gene abnormality is found in the PSTPIP1 gene, which causes inadequate function of the body's immune response process, leading to aggravation of symptoms following injury, trauma, or stress-related inflammation. Symptoms of arthritis with skin disorders are seen, and complications may lead to joint decomposition and scars from skin lesions.

Inflammatory Polyarthropathies (M05-M14)

Inflammatory polyarthropathies are a group of diseases that affect the joints, muscles, connective tissues, skin, and internal organs. Single or multiple sites may be affected. Rheumatoid arthritis is an autoimmune disorder that can affect the entire body. Rheumatoid arthritis and other types of arthritis with an onset during childhood are differentiated from inflammatory joint disease with onset later in life.

The categories in this code block are as follows:

M05	Rheumatoid arthritis with rheumatoid factor
M06	Other rheumatoid arthritis
M07	Enteropathic arthropathies
M08	Juvenile arthritis
M1A	Chronic gout
M10	Gout
M11	Other crystal arthropathies
M12	Other and unspecified arthropathy
M13	Other arthritis
M14	Arthropathies in other diseases classified elsewhere

M05.- Rheumatoid arthritis with rheumatoid factor

Rheumatoid arthritis, a chronic, systemic inflammatory disease, is an autoimmune disorder characterized by a variable but prolonged course with exacerbations and remissions of joint pain and swelling. In early stages, the disease attacks the joints of the hands and feet. As the disease progresses, more joints become involved. Also known as primary progressive arthritis and proliferative arthritis, the disease often leads to progressive deformities, which may develop rapidly and cause permanent disability. Clinical manifestations of rheumatoid arthritis are highly variable, particularly in the mode of onset, distribution, degree of severity, and rate of progression. Joint disease is the major manifestation; systemic involvement (spleen, liver, eyes, etc.) is rare. Rheumatic arthritis can affect multiple body systems and/or sites, including joints, muscles, connective tissues, skin, and internal organs. Single or multiple sites may be affected. Signs and symptoms of rheumatoid arthritis include articular inflammation, malaise, weight loss, paresthesia, Raynaud's phenomenon, periarticular pain and stiffness, symmetrical joint swelling and stiffness, warmth, and tenderness (most severe in the morning, somewhat subsiding during the day). Rheumatoid factor is an antibody that is detected in 80 percent of adults with RA, although it can also be detected in other normal adults or those with other autoimmune diseases. The presence of rheumatoid factor is considered to indicate a more aggressive disease. Rheumatoid arthritis subcategories specify whether or not there is involvement of any other body system or organ, such as the lungs, blood vessels, muscles, nerves, or heart, in addition to the site and laterality of the joints affected.

Focus Point

Rheumatoid arthritis can occur during childhood (called juvenile rheumatoid arthritis) or adulthood. Juvenile rheumatoid arthritis is classified in category M08.

M05.0- Felty's syndrome

Felty's syndrome is the association of rheumatoid arthritis with splenomegaly and leukopenia. Mild anemia and thrombocytopenia may accompany the variable severe neutropenia and skin and pulmonary infections are frequent complications. The subcategories identify the site and laterality of the rheumatoid arthritis.

M05.1- Rheumatoid lung disease with rheumatoid arthritis

Rheumatoid lung disease is a group of lung disorders associated with rheumatoid arthritis, including bronchiolitis obliterans, pleural effusion, pulmonary hypertension, lung nodules, and pulmonary fibrosis. Rheumatoid lung disease may present as chest pain, cough, and/or shortness of breath or there may be no symptoms. Caplan's syndrome, a syndrome of rheumatoid pneumoconiosis seen in patients with concomitant coal worker's pneumoconiosis, is included in this subcategory. The subcategories identify the site and laterality of the rheumatoid arthritis.

M05.2- Rheumatoid vasculitis with rheumatoid arthritis

Rheumatoid vasculitis affects only a small population of rheumatoid arthritis sufferers. It generally occurs in patients with severe rheumatoid arthritis of more than 10 years. Vasculitis is inflammation and stenosis of mostly arteries but also can affect veins. On rare occasions, it can cause ischemia and gangrene to body parts affected. The subcategories identify the site and laterality of the rheumatoid arthritis.

M06.- Other rheumatoid arthritis

This category includes rheumatoid arthritis without rheumatoid factor and adult-onset Still's disease.

M06.1 Adult-onset Still's disease

This inflammatory arthritis is similar to rheumatoid arthritis causing inflammation that can damage the affected joints, especially the wrist. It presents with sore throat, rash, and fever prior to the onset of joint pain. The cause is unknown but viral or bacterial infection is suspect. Still's disease can be an acute episode or become a chronic condition. It generally appears in ages 15 to 25 years or 36 to 46 years.

Focus Point

If the Still's disease is not documented as adult-onset, it is considered a juvenile rheumatoid arthritis and is located in subcategory MØ8.2-.

MØ6.2- Rheumatoid bursitis

This condition occurs when inflammation from rheumatoid arthritis causes increased fluid and redness of the bursa, which is the small sac of fluid that cushions the joint. The subcategories identify the site and laterality of the rheumatoid bursitis.

MØ6.3- Rheumatoid nodule

Rheumatoid nodules typically appear as firm lumps under the skin nearby affected joints, although they can also develop on lungs, heart, or other internal organs. They can be painful or asymptomatic and some can be moved around while others are immobile. Nodule development is almost always linked to the presence of rheumatoid factor. Cigarette smoking and the use of Methotrexate have also been linked to the increased risk of nodule development. The subcategories identify the site and laterality of the rheumatoid nodule.

MØ7.- Enteropathic arthropathies

The arthritis in this subcategory is an inflammatory joint reaction associated with an inflammatory bowel disease such as Crohn's or ulcerative colitis. The subcategories identify the site and laterality of the joints affected.

Focus Point

The codes at MØ2.1- Postdysenteric arthropathy, are differentiated from this subcategory by the presence of an infectious or parasitic etiology for the postdysenteric arthritis.

MØ8.- Juvenile arthritis

Juvenile arthritis contains subcategories for distinct forms of arthritis with onset during childhood (prior to age 17). This category includes juvenile ankylosing spondylitis, juvenile rheumatoid arthritis with systemic onset, juvenile rheumatoid polyarthritis, pauciarticular juvenile rheumatoid arthritis, as well as other and unspecified types.

Focus Point

The disease process for juvenile rheumatoid arthritis and polyarthritis is different genetically and immunologically from rheumatoid arthritis in adults. Juvenile rheumatoid arthritis has a much more favorable prognosis than adult-onset disease.

MØ8.Ø- Unspecified juvenile rheumatoid arthritis

Juvenile rheumatoid arthritis (JRA) is a group of related disorders characterized by inflammation of one or more joints that occurs in children with onset prior to age 17. The arthritis must be present for at least six weeks in a row in the same joint to be diagnosed as JRA. Children with JRA often outgrow the condition, which is different from adult rheumatoid arthritis that is chronic and lasts a lifetime. JRA may affect the bone development in a growing child and occurs in girls twice as often as boys. The cause of JRA is unknown, although it is known to be an autoimmune disorder, which means the immune system attacks the body's own tissues. Signs and symptoms include fever, joint swelling, limping, rash, stiffness, and reduced motion. Treatment includes NSAIDS, immunosuppressive agents, intraarticular steroid injections, and physical therapy. The subcategories identify the site and laterality of the juvenile rheumatoid arthritis.

MØ8.1 Juvenile ankylosing spondylitis

Juvenile ankylosing spondylitis is a form of arthritis that affects the vertebral joints of the spine and the sacroiliac joint of the pelvic girdle. The condition may also affect the intercostal joints between the ribs. Cartilage, muscles, tendons, and ligaments become inflamed causing pain and stiffness in the spine and sacroiliac joints. The inflammation may cause erosion of the vertebral and sacroiliac joints with formation of bony bridges that may fuse these joints limiting mobility. The causes of juvenile ankylosing spondylitis are not entirely known, but it is believed to be due to genetic and environmental factors. Juvenile ankylosing spondylitis has a later onset than most juvenile arthritis, with first symptoms typically appearing between the ages of 17 and 35, although onset may occur in early adolescence. Common symptoms are back pain, early morning stiffness, stooped posture adopted to relieve pain, and painful respiration when the intercostal joints are affected. There may also be joint pain at other sites, particularly in the lower extremities. Systemic symptoms are also common and include fever, anorexia, weight loss, fatigue. Other organ involvement is sometimes present with the most common organs affected being the eyes (conjunctivitis and sensitivity to light), lungs, heart, and kidneys. Treatment is aimed at reducing inflammation and maintaining mobility.

MØ8.2- Juvenile rheumatoid arthritis with systemic onset

Juvenile rheumatoid arthritis with systemic onset, also known as Still's disease, is characterized by systemic symptoms that include high fever, erythematous rash, anemia, generalized lymphadenopathy, and, in some cases, hepatosplenomegaly, iridocyclitis, and pericarditis. Juvenile rheumatoid arthritis (JRA) is a group of related disorders characterized by inflammation of one or more joints that occurs in children with onset prior to age 17. The arthritis must be present for at least six weeks in a row in the same joint to be diagnosed as JRA. Children with JRA often outgrow the condition, which is different from adult rheumatoid arthritis that is chronic and lasts a lifetime. JRA may affect the bone development in a growing child and occurs in girls twice as often as boys. The cause of JRA is unknown, although it is known to be an autoimmune disorder, which means the immune system attacks the body's own tissues. The subcategories identify the site and laterality of the juvenile rheumatoid arthritis.

M08.3 Juvenile rheumatoid polyarthritis (seronegative)

Polyarticular juvenile rheumatoid arthritis affects five or more joints in the first six months of onset. Unlike other forms of juvenile rheumatoid arthritis, children with the polyarticular form do not develop systemic symptoms along with joint inflammation. Typically the only symptom is joint inflammation that is often symmetric, meaning it affects the same joints on the right and left side. Polyarticular rheumatoid polyarthritis may be seronegative (blood tests are negative for rheumatoid factor[Rf]) or seropositive (blood tests are positive for Rf); the seropositive form affects only 5 percent of all children with the polyarticular form of juvenile rheumatoid arthritis. The seronegative form is characterized by periods of joint inflammation and remission, usually over a three to five year period, and then symptoms tend to diminish. The seropositive form is much more aggressive and symptoms may continue through adulthood.

Focus Point

Even though this code description has the term "seronegative" in parentheses, this code should be assigned for seronegative and seropositive forms of juvenile rheumatoid polyarthritis.

M08.4- Pauciarticular juvenile rheumatoid arthritis

Pauciarticular juvenile rheumatoid arthritis is a disease, also known as oligoarticular juvenile arthritis, affecting a small number of joints, usually two to five. This condition is often asymmetrical, meaning it does not affect the same joint on both sides of the body. It usually begins acutely but does not usually affect other parts of the body. It is usually a mild form of arthritis with resolution before adulthood. It is associated with chronic iridocyclitis in 25 to 30 percent of patients and, if not monitored and detected early, can lead to blindness. Monoarticular juvenile rheumatoid arthritis is juvenile arthritis limited to one joint and is also classified here. The subcategories identify the site and laterality of pauciarticular juvenile rheumatoid arthritis.

M1A.- Chronic gout

Gout is a disorder in which urate (uric acid) crystals are deposited in joints, synovial fluid, and soft tissues, causing inflammation and degenerative changes. Individuals at the highest risk include men older than age 40 and those who are overweight, have excessive alcohol intake, or regularly eat foods high in purines (e.g., meat and fish). Certain medications (e.g., antirejection drugs, diuretics) can increase a patient's risk of gout. Gout is characterized by hyperuricemia (excessive uric acid in the blood), although hyperuricemia does not always progress to gout. Uric acid is normally dissolved in the bloodstream and passes through the urinary system. However, if the body produces too much uric acid or the kidneys excrete too little uric acid, an abnormal accumulation occurs that can become deposited in the joints and surrounding tissues as abnormal urate crystals. Only chronic gout is reported with codes in this category. Chronic tophaceous gout, a stage of chronic gouty arthritis associated with accumulation of tophi (concentrated urate crystal deposits in and around joints and subcutaneous tissue) and characterized by tender and swollen joints, is included here. The subcategories identify the cause of the chronic gout, such as drug-induced, lead induced, induced by renal impairment, and idiopathic or secondary due to another cause, in addition to site and laterality. All codes in this category must include a seventh character identifying with or without tophus.

M10.- Gout

Gout is a disorder in which urate (uric acid) crystals are deposited in joints, synovial fluid, and soft tissues, causing inflammation and degenerative changes. Gout classified here may be described as acute or as a gout attack or flare. Acute gout is a recurrent condition in which excessive uric acid in the blood is deposited in the peripheral joints causing intermittent painful and sometimes debilitating inflammation. Symptoms commonly occur suddenly without warning and often at night. Common symptoms include an attack of pain, burning, swelling, redness, and stiffness in a joint. The first metatarsophalangeal joint (a.k.a., big toe) is often affected, but gout can occur in any joint—most commonly joints of the lower extremity (e.g., foot, ankle, and knee) or upper extremity (e.g., hand, wrist, or elbow). Attacks (flares) typically persist for three to 10 days on average and then subside for a period of months or perhaps years. Recurrent attacks are common if left untreated. Eventually, the urate deposits can cause debilitating damage to the joints, tendons, and other tissues. The subcategories identify the cause of the gout, such as drug-induced, lead induced, induced by renal impairment, idiopathic, or secondary due to another cause in addition to site and laterality.

M11.- Other crystal arthropathies

Use codes in this category to report hydroxyapatite deposition disease, familial and other types of chondrocalcinosis, and other crystal arthropathies excluding gout. The presence, and not the chemical composition, of crystals (apatite and hydroxyapatite, calcium pyrophosphate, calcium and dicalcium phosphate, calcium oxalate, and lipid crystals) act as irritants. The mechanisms of initial precipitation are unknown, but predisposing conditions such as degradation of the cartilage matrix may be involved. Once the crystals have accumulated, they are taken up by phagocytic cells, initiating the inflammatory sequence. This in turn causes additional damage to the affected tissues. The term chondrocalcinosis refers to calcification of articular cartilage. Articular chondrocalcinosis is also known as pseudogout since the disease is characterized by calcified deposits in the cartilage, but is free of the urate crystals found in gout. Aspiration and examination of synovial fluid allows precise diagnosis. Therapies include aspiration of the acutely inflamed joint; drugs such as corticosteroid injections; nonsteroidal, anti-inflammatory drugs; and intravenous colchicine.

M11.0- Hydroxyapatite deposition disease

Hydroxyapatite (HA) deposition disease is caused by the deposits of HA, which are calcium phosphate crystals located nearby the joints in the soft tissues (especially tendons) or in the joints. These calcifications can be mono or polyarticular and most commonly affect the shoulder, although they can affect any joint. Intraarticular crystals can cause destruction of the joint involved. The subcategories identify site and laterality of the affected area.

M11.1- Familial chondrocalcinosis

Familial chondrocalcinosis is characterized by deposits in the joint cartilage of calcium pyrophosphate dihydrate crystals (CPPD) with symptoms similar to gout. It is a rare inherited condition and is thought to be more severe in individuals who carry two of a pair of defective genes (homozygotes). It most often affects the knee joints although it can occur in any joint and cause damage to the joint. This disorder most often presents in ages 60 and older, but rare cases have been found in younger patients. The subcategories identify site and laterality of the affected area.

M11.8- Other specified crystal arthropathies

Other specified crystal arthropathies included here are due to lipid crystals, calcium oxalate, calcium phosphate, and other identifiable crystals not elsewhere classifiable. The subcategories identify site and laterality of the affected area.

M12.- Other and unspecified arthropathy

This category represents conditions such as chronic postrheumatic arthropathy, Kaschin-Beck disease, villonodular synovitis, palindromic rheumatism, intermittent hydrarthrosis, and traumatic and transient arthropathy.

M12.0- Chronic postrheumatic arthropathy [Jaccoud]

The definition of chronic postrheumatic arthropathy is a form of arthropathy of the hands and feet caused by repeated attacks of rheumatic arthritis. Also called Jaccoud's syndrome, this disease is characterized by flexion deformities, particularly of the metacarpophalangeal joints, and is associated with pronounced ulnar deviation of the fingers. Chronic rheumatoid nodular fibrositis is a variation of this disease characterized by the presence of subcutaneous nodules in the region of the previously involved joints. The subcategories identify site and laterality of the affected area.

M12.1- Kaschin-Beck disease

Also referred to as big bone disease, this disorder is a disabling degenerative disease of the peripheral joints and spine, causing necrosis of growth plates of bones and joint cartilage and leading to shortened limb length and stature. It is prevalent in eastern Siberia, northern China, and Korea and thought to be caused by ingestion of cereal grains infected with the fungus *Fusarium sporotrichiella*. The subcategories identify site and laterality of the affected area.

M12.2- Villonodular synovitis (pigmented)

Villonodular synovitis is a form of inflammation involving the synovial membranes of joints. There are two types of villonodular synovitis: pigmented and nonpigmented. Both types are reported here. Villonodular synovitis may be a form of benign neoplasm of the connective tissue of the synovium or be representative of granulomatous disease. Therapies include steroidal and nonsteroidal medication to reduce inflammation and synovectomy when nonoperative therapy fails. The subcategories identify site and laterality of the affected area.

> **Focus Point**
>
> The term "villonodular synovitis" is sometimes used to describe conditions such as xanthofibroma (tumor), giant cell tumor of tendon sheath, and benign synovioma, which are classified in Chapter 2 Neoplasms.

M12.3- Palindromic rheumatism

Palindromic rheumatism is sudden and recurring attacks of moderate to severe joint pain and swelling generally occurring in the hands or feet. After the attack subsides, the joints appear normal again. This condition is rare, with little research done, so the etiology is unknown, but the condition has been associated with irritants and allergic reactions with a possible genetic component. The subcategories identify site and laterality of the affected area.

M13.-   Other arthritis

This category includes nonspecific polyarthritis, affecting two or more joints or monoarthritis affecting only one site. The subcategories identify site and laterality of the affected area.

M13.8-   Other specified arthritis

This subcategory includes allergic arthritis. Allergic arthritis is associated with a hypersensitive state acquired through exposure to an allergen. The subcategories identify site and laterality of the affected area.

M14.-   Arthropathies in other diseases classified elsewhere

This category represents arthropathies such as Charcot's joint or in other diseases such as amyloidosis, sickle-cell, erythema nodosum, and erythema multiforme among others.

M14.6-   Charcot's joint

This disorder, also called neurogenic arthropathy, most commonly affects one joint, usually not more than three. Because of the neuropathy, patients often can't feel pain and aren't aware of the joint damage until it is advanced. Many diseases or injuries can cause nerve damage such as stroke, syphilis, and spinal cord disorders and injuries. The lack of pain sensation near the joint allows the joint to be damaged many times before the patient is aware of any permanent dysfunction. The subcategories identify site and laterality of the affected area.

Focus Point

Charcot joint that is due to a diabetic complication is not coded in this chapter. Diabetic combination codes located in Chapter 4 Endocrine, Nutritional and Metabolic Diseases, are used for diabetic Charcot joint.

Osteoarthritis (M15-M19)

The most common form of arthritis is osteoarthritis (OA). Physicians often call this form of arthritis by various terms including degenerative joint disease (DJD), osteoarthrosis, degenerative arthritis, and hypertrophic arthritis.

Osteoarthritis noted as generalized is a chronic noninflammatory arthritis that affects multiple sites. Commonly found in older patients, it is marked by degeneration of articular cartilage, enlargement of

bone, and pain and stiffness occurring with any type of activity but subsiding when the patient rests. Generalized disease is osteoarthrosis without any known preexisting abnormality.

Localized osteoarthrosis is disease confined to a limited number of sites, generally one or two of the larger weight-bearing joints, such as the hip or knee. There are several categories of localized osteoarthritis, including primary, secondary due to old traumatic injury, and secondary due to other causes.

Primary osteoarthritis, also known as idiopathic degenerative arthritis, commonly affects joints of the spine, hip, knee, and small joints of the hands and feet. Primary osteoarthrosis may also be due to some constitutional or genetic factor.

Secondary osteoarthrosis is due to some identifiable initiating factor. These factors include obesity, congenital malformations, superimposition of fibrosis and scarring from previous inflammatory disease or infection, foreign bodies, malalignment of joints, metabolic or circulatory bone diseases, and iatrogenic factors such as osteoarthrosis caused by continuous pressure on the joint surfaces during orthopedic treatment of congenital deformities. Secondary osteoarthroses may require a second code describing the causative injury, disorder, or disease.

Focus Point

Note that posttraumatic osteoarthritis now has distinct codes, separate from secondary osteoarthritis.

The categories in this code block are as follows:

M15	Polyosteoarthritis
M16	Osteoarthritis of hip
M17	Osteoarthritis of knee
M18	Osteoarthritis of first carpometacarpal joint
M19	Other and unspecified osteoarthritis

M15.-   Polyosteoarthritis

This category describes various types of generalized primary and secondary arthritis; generalized arthritis affects multiple joints. Included in this category are classic signs of hand osteoarthritis called Heberden's nodes, which are bony bumps on the distal interphalangeal joint, and Bouchard's nodes located on the middle interphalangeal joint. These nodes most often affect postmenopausal women. Another type of generalized arthritis captured in this category is erosive (osteo) arthritis, which is characterized by sudden pain and swelling from erosions of cartilage typically in the hands. This disorder also most commonly occurs in middle aged and postmenopausal women.

M16.- Osteoarthritis of hip

This category reports unilateral or bilateral osteoarthritis of the hip, including primary, secondary, and posttraumatic osteoarthritis. This category also includes unilateral or bilateral osteoarthritis resulting from hip dysplasia, a condition that occurs when the femoral head and the acetabular socket are incorrectly positioned or shaped causing increased force and excessive wear on the cartilage and labrum.

M17.- Osteoarthritis of knee

This category reports unilateral or bilateral osteoarthritis of the knee, including primary, secondary, and posttraumatic osteoarthritis.

M18.- Osteoarthritis of first carpometacarpal joint

This category reports unilateral or bilateral osteoarthritis of the carpometacarpal joint, including primary, secondary, and posttraumatic osteoarthritis. This joint, also called the trapeziometacarpal joint, is located at the base of the thumb and is often a site of osteoarthritis in postmenopausal women.

M19.- Other and unspecified osteoarthritis

This category captures codes for other sites (shoulder, elbow, wrist, hand, ankle, and foot) affected by primary, posttraumatic, or secondary osteoarthritis.

Other Joint Disorders (M20-M25)

This section includes nonarthritic disorders of joints and joint structures including acquired deformities, derangements, dislocations, contractures, and ankylosis. Other conditions of joints located in this category are hemarthrosis, fistulas, effusion, instability, stiffness, pain, and flail joints.

The categories in this code block are as follows:

M20	Acquired deformities of fingers and toes
M21	Other acquired deformities of limbs
M22	Disorder of patella
M23	Internal derangement of knee
M24	Other specific joint derangements
M25	Other joint disorder, not elsewhere classified

M20.- Acquired deformities of fingers and toes

This category includes non-congenital deformities of various sites and their lateralities.

M20.01- Mallet finger

Also referred to as hammer or drop finger, this deformity is characterized by the fixed flexion of the distal interphalangeal (DIP) joint caused by the disruption of the terminal extension tendon attachment to the DIP. Mallet finger is typically caused by injury and is common in athletes, although it can occur with activities as simple as pushing off a sock or forcefully tucking in bedsheets

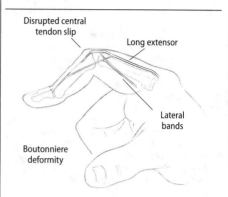

Disruption of the central tendon slip causes the finger to drop. Tension from the lateral bands causes the finger tip to be fully extended

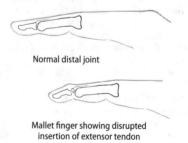

Mallet finger showing disrupted insertion of extensor tendon

M20.02- Boutonniere deformity

Also referred to as buttonhole deformity, this finger deformity occurs when the proximal interphalangeal (PIP) joint becomes flexed (bent) and the distal interphalangeal (DIP) joint is pulled into hyperextension. This happens when injury or prolonged inflammation from arthritis weakens or ruptures the extensor tendon attachment to the PIP.

M20.03- Swan-neck deformity

Opposite of the Boutonniere deformity, Swan-neck originates in the proximal interphalangeal (PIP) joint and is characterized by a hyperextended proximal interphalangeal (PIP) joint and a flexed distal interphalangeal (DIP) joint, forming a swan-neck. It occurs when chronic inflammation of the PIP joint stretches and weakens the volar plate, which is the ligament that normally keeps the PIP in place. It is most often caused by rheumatoid or other types of arthritis. This abnormal bending may become permanent causing significant disability.

M20.1-   Hallux valgus (acquired)

Hallux valgus is an acquired positional deformity of the first metatarsophalangeal joint. There are no muscles that originate on the first metatarsal to help stabilize the first metatarsophalangeal joint. Although the abductor and adductor hallucis muscles pass to the MTP joint, they are located closer to the plantar surface, which allows any pushing force to be relatively unrestrained. In most cases, these muscles can bounce back from the strain of movement, but in some instances the constant strain causes these tissues to rupture, allowing the bones to rotate and to become misaligned. Although the exact cause of this deformity is not clearly understood; genetic predisposition, abnormal anatomic foot structures or mechanics, and inflammatory joint disease are a few underlying etiologies that may individually or collectively predispose the patient to acquire a hallux valgus deformity.

Focus Point

Most podiatrists do not equate hallux valgus to bunion and consequently codes in subcategory M21.61- Bunion were created. It is not the deformity or movement of the foot and toe bones that characterize a bunion but the presence of soft tissue edema and bursitis along with hypertrophy of the medial condyle at the first metatarsal head. Therefore it is possible to have hallux valgus without also having a true bunion. Should the two conditions exist simultaneously, a code representing each condition would be appropriate.

M20.2-   Hallux rigidus

Hallux rigidus, also called stiff big toe, is a deformity where there is a limitation to normal movements of flexion and extension of the first metatarsal (big toe). It is the second most common toe disorder after hallux valgus. As it progresses, it causes pain and stiffness in the joint, and with time it gets increasingly harder to bend the toe. Hallux rigidus is actually a form of degenerative arthritis but can be brought on by injury or overuse in addition to rheumatoid or osteoarthritis.

M20.3-   Hallux varus (acquired)

Hallux varus is characterized by a medial deviation of the great toe. It most often occurs due to an overcorrection during a hallux valgus surgery. Unlike hallux valgus or rigidus, footwear tends to correct rather than exacerbate this deformity. This code also includes hallux malleus, not elsewhere classified.

Focus Point

Codes for congenital hallux rigidus, valgus, and varus are not located in this chapter. The appropriate codes for these conditions can be found in the Alphabetic Index and are located in Chapter 17 Congenital Malformations, Deformations and Chromosomal Abnormalities.

M21.-   Other acquired deformities of limbs

This category includes deformities such as valgus (inward) and varus (outward) deformities, wrist and foot drop, flat foot, and unequal limb lengths.

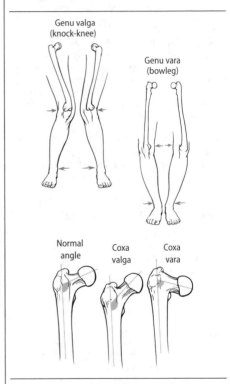

M21.0-   Valgus deformity, not elsewhere classified

A valgus deformity is characterized by the distal part of the limb, below the joint, deviating (bowing) more outwardly (laterally) from the proximal joint than it should be.

M21.02- Valgus deformity, not elsewhere classified, elbow

Also referred to as cubitus valgus, acquired, this deformity is characterized by the deviation of the elbow away from the body midline upon extension; it occurs when the palm is turning outward.

M21.05- Valgus deformity, not elsewhere classified, hip

Valgus deformity of the hip, also referred to as coxa valga (acquired), is a condition in which the angle formed by the head and neck of the femur and axis of the shaft is increased.

M21.06- Valgus deformity, not elsewhere classified, knee

Valgus deformity of the knee, also referred to as genu valgum or "knock knee," is a condition in which the knees are close together and the ankles are lateral from the knee or far apart.

M21.1- Varus deformity, not elsewhere classified

A varus deformity is characterized by the distal part of the limb, below the joint, deviating (bowing) more inwardly (medially) from the proximal joint than it should.

M21.12- Varus deformity, not elsewhere classified, elbow

A varus deformity of the elbow, also referred to as acquired cubitus varus, is a condition in which the elbow joint is displaced and angled laterally. When the forearm is extended, it deviates toward the midline of the body. It is also called "gun stock" deformity.

M21.15- Varus deformity, not elsewhere classified, hip

A varus deformity of the hip, also referred to as coxa vara (acquired), is a condition in which the angle formed by the head and neck of the femur and axis of the shaft is decreased.

M21.16- Varus deformity, not elsewhere classified, knee

A varus deformity of the knee, also referred to as genu varum or "bow leg," is a condition in which the knees are far apart and the ankles are medial from the knee or close together.

Focus Point

Genu recurvatum (acquired), knee, also called "back knee," is a hyperextension deformity of the knee and is not located in this subcategory; it is included in M21.86- Other specified acquired deformities of lower leg.

M21.33- Wrist drop (acquired)

This deformity is described as the inability to extend the hand at the wrist typically due to extensor muscle paralysis.

M21.4- Flat foot [pes planus] (acquired)

Flat feet have a low arch and leave a nearly complete imprint; there is only a slight inward curve where the arch should be. The stretching or tearing of the posterior tibial tendon, which supports the arch and helps lift the heel off the ground, can lead to an adult acquired flatfoot deformity. Causes include trauma, overuse, and medical conditions such as obesity, diabetes, previous surgery, and steroid injections. The condition progresses from pain, swelling, and weakness to the tendon to a rigid flattening of the foot and ankle pain. Treatment depends on the stage of progression at the time of examination. Early stages can be treated nonsurgically by rest and antiinflammatory drugs. Orthotics and minor tendon surgery can help in advanced states, while later stages may require reconstructive surgery to stabilize the foot and ankle.

M21.51- Acquired clawhand

A claw hand, also called intrinsic minus hand, is characterized by MCP hyperextension and PIP and DIP flexion causing curved or bent fingers, making the hand appear claw-like. Acquired claw develops as a consequence of nerve lesions, syringomyelia, leprosy, or compartment syndrome.

M21.52- Acquired clubhand

This condition is rarely acquired—it is generally congenital and not coded to this subcategory. On rare occasions it can be acquired as a result of osteomyelitis or other infections. It occurs when the axis of the forearm and hand don't coincide. Whereas congenital cases are associated with birth defects of absent bones, acquired is typically due to paralysis, nerve damage, or destruction by a disease of the arm or hand.

M21.53- Acquired clawfoot

Also called "main en griffe," acquired clawfoot is characterized by a high foot arch with hyperextended toes at the metatarsophalangeal joint and flexed toes at the distal joints.

M21.61- Bunion

A bunion is a localized friction-type bursitis located at the medial or dorsal aspect of the first metatarsophalangeal joint. Although malalignment of the foot bones, such as that seen with hallux valgus, may be present, it is not the malalignment that characterizes a bunion. It is actually the presence of hypertrophy of the medial condyle, soft tissue edema, and bursitis at the first metatarsal head. Bunions are more prevalent in women, often noted in family history, and aggravated, rather than brought on, by footwear.

Focus Point

The terms hallux valgus and bunion are often used interchangeably and until recently were classified to the same codes in subcategory M20.1- Hallux valgus (acquired). Although the two conditions can coexist, each is separate and distinct from the other, and consequently a separate subcategory was created specifically for bunion. Should the two conditions exist simultaneously, a code representing each condition would be appropriate.

M21.62- Bunionette

A bunionette (Tailor's bunion) is similar to a bunion but involves the outside of the foot where the small toe attaches to the foot. A hypertrophic lateral condyle of the fifth metatarsal head is present, with associated soft tissue edema and lateral bursitis.

M21.6X- Other acquired deformities of foot

This subcategory includes the following disorders: acquired equinus deformity, also referred to as tip-toe walking deformity, which is a plantar flexion defect that forces people to walk on their toes; acquired cavus deformity of the foot, which is characterized by an abnormally high arch; and acquired cavovarus deformity of the foot, which is the inward turning of the heel from the midline of the leg and an abnormally high longitudinal arch.

M21.86- Other specified acquired deformities of lower leg

This subcategory includes genu recurvatum, which is characterized by the hyperextension of the knees, also referred to as "back knee."

M22.- Disorder of patella

This category includes disorders of the kneecap and its supporting structures (cartilage, ligaments). It includes conditions such as recurrent dislocation (complete) or subluxation (incomplete) and chondromalacia.

M22.4- Chondromalacia patellae

This condition is the degeneration or softening of the articular cartilage of the patella.

M23.- Internal derangement of knee

Internal derangement of the knee refers to degeneration, spontaneous rupture, or other damaged structures that can be present within the knee, including old meniscal cartilage tears, ligament ruptures, or cysts or loose bodies in the knee. The subcategories represent the specific condition, site, and laterality.

Focus Point

This category does not report damage from an acute, current injury (S80-S89). This category represents derangements that are nontraumatic or are due to an old injury or tear.

M23.4- Loose body in knee

Loose body in the knee is also referred to as joint mice, rice bodies, and debris described as calcified cartilaginous (cartilage only), osseous (bony), osteocartilaginous, or fibrous particles. Osteochondritis dissecans is a common cause of loose bodies in the knee; other causes include synovial chondromatosis, osteophytes, fractured articular surfaces, and damaged menisci.

M24.- Other specific joint derangements

This category reports damage incurred to joints, cartilage, or ligaments that is not due to any current injury. This category includes conditions such as loose bodies and tears or instability due to old injuries of other joints and joint structures other than the knee, recurrent subluxations, pathological dislocations, contractures, and ankylosis of joints. Subcategories represent the specific condition, site, and laterality.

M24.0- Loose body in joint

Loose body in joint is also referred to as joint mice, rice bodies, and debris described as calcified cartilaginous (cartilage only, radiolucent on x-rays), osseous (bony), osteocartilaginous, or fibrous particles. This subcategory includes joints other than the knee.

M24.3- Pathological dislocation of joint, not elsewhere classified

Pathological dislocation is dislocation of an articular joint due to a disease process (e.g., poliomyelitis) rather than trauma.

M24.4- Recurrent dislocation of joint

Recurrent dislocation is chronic, subsequent, additional, and repeated dislocations or subluxations of a joint.

M24.5- Contracture of joint

Contracture of a joint is a disorder characterized by restriction of joint motion due to contraction of the muscles that articulate the joint. The condition may be due to tonic spasm, fibrosis, loss of musculature equilibrium, or disuse atrophy.

M24.6- Ankylosis of joint

Ankylosis is described as the immobility, solidification, or fixation of a joint. This condition can be due to a disease process or old injury.

M24.7 Protrusio acetabuli

This intrapelvic protrusion of the acetabulum, also referred to as Otto's pelvis, is characterized by the sinking of the floor of the acetabulum, causing the femoral head to protrude. It limits hip movement and is of unknown etiology.

M25.- Other joint disorder, not elsewhere classified

Disorders of joints located in this category include hemarthrosis, fistulas, effusion, instability, stiffness, pain, and flail joints.

M25.0- Hemarthrosis

Hemarthrosis is the presence of gross blood in the joint spaces, excluding that due to current injury or hemophilia. Nontraumatic causes can include osteoarthritis, degenerative tears of a meniscus, or neuropathy with impaired position sensation.

M25.2- Flail joint

Flail joint is characterized by a hinged joint that exhibits an abnormal or excessive degree of range and mobility.

M25.4- Effusion of joint

Effusion of a joint is the accumulation of fluid in the joint space, also referred to as hydrarthrosis. Effusion indicates synovial irritation that may be due to a current disease or an old traumatic injury.

Focus Point

Nontraumatic hemorrhagic effusion is from blood and is reported with a code from subcategory M25.0- Hemarthrosis. Intermittent hydrarthrosis is not included here. See subcategory M12.4-.

M25.46- Effusion, knee

Czerny's disease, which is a periodic joint effusion of the knee, is included here.

M25.5- Pain in joint

Pain in a joint, also called arthralgia, is a common complaint and a frequent reason for seeking medical care. Joint pain is a symptom with many causes. Until the cause of the joint pain is determined, this symptom code is reported.

M25.7- Osteophyte

Osteophyte is also referred to as bone spurs; however, unlike the name implies, an osteophyte is actually a bone or cartilage protrusion that is smooth and forms over a long period of time. They are a common condition with aging and can indicate degeneration of the structure involved.

Dentofacial Anomalies [Including Malocclusion] and Other Disorders of Jaw (M26-M27)

Malocclusion is an abnormal alignment of teeth and the way that the upper and lower teeth fit together (bite). It may cause problems with biting and chewing but can usually be corrected with a brace on the teeth and proper orthodontic care. Dentofacial anomalies classified in this chapter may be acquired or due to congenital anomalies.

Focus Point

While many dentofacial anomalies due to congenital conditions are classified here, there are a few that are classified to Chapter 17. Review the excludes notes and check the index under both the condition and the main term "Anomaly, anomalous" to ensure proper code assignment. If associated with a congenital anomaly and not an inherent part of the congenital anomaly, report both conditions and sequence in accordance with coding guidelines.

The categories in this code block are as follows:

M26	Dentofacial anomalies [including malocclusion]
M27	Other diseases of jaws

M26.- Dentofacial anomalies [including malocclusion]

Malocclusion is an abnormal alignment of teeth and the way that the upper and lower teeth fit together (bite). It may cause problems with biting and chewing but can usually be corrected with a brace on the teeth and proper orthodontic care.

M26.0- Major anomalies of jaw size

This subcategory classifies conditions affecting the size of the jaw, including hyperplasia, hypoplasia, macrogenia, and microgenia.

M26.01 Maxillary hyperplasia

This condition is an overgrowth or overdevelopment of the upper jawbone.

M26.02 Maxillary hypoplasia

This condition is an incomplete or underdeveloped upper jawbone.

M26.03 Mandibular hyperplasia

This condition is an overgrowth or overdevelopment of the lower jawbone.

M26.04 Mandibular hypoplasia

This condition is an incomplete or underdeveloped lower jawbone.

M26.05 Macrogenia

This is an enlarged jaw, especially chin, that affects bone, soft tissue, or both.

M26.06 Microgenia

This is an underdeveloped mandible, characterized by an extremely small chin.

M26.07 Excessive tuberosity of jaw

Tuberosity of the jaw is seen as an elongated, raised, or protruding area on the angle of the jawbone. Sometimes the tuberosity can be raised or uneven after tooth extraction. Surgical correction of the tuberosity can be performed to correct a defect.

M26.1- Anomalies of jaw-cranial base relationship

This subcategory classifies inequality in the size or shape of one side of the maxilla and/or mandible compared with the other, or a difference in placement or arrangement of one of the jawbones about the craniofacial axis. These anomalies include prognathism, retrognathism, and maxillary asymmetry.

M26.19 Other specified anomalies of jaw-cranial base relationship

This code includes prognathism and retrognathism. Prognathism is anterior protrusion of the mandible or maxilla beyond the projection of the forehead. Retrognathism is the location of the maxilla or mandible behind the frontal plane of the forehead; it also is used as a general term meaning underdevelopment of the maxilla or mandible.

M26.2- Anomalies of dental arch relationship

The dental arch is the curved structure of a line created by the buccal surfaces or the central grooves of all natural teeth and the residual ridge of missing teeth in the upper or lower jaw. Anomalies may occur as a malocclusion, including an abnormal contact line between the biting and chewing tooth surfaces of the upper or lower teeth, an overbite or overlapping of upper teeth over the lower when biting down, or inadequate or excessive interarch distances, which is the vertical space between the upper and lower alveolar or residual arches or ridges.

M26.21- Malocclusion, Angle's class

Angle's class I, also called a neutro-occlusion, is a malocclusion with a correct mesiodistal relationship of the first permanent molars. Angle's class II, also called a disto-occlusion, is a posterior malocclusion in which the lower jaw and its first permanent molar is positioned further back than the upper. Angle's class III, also called a mesio-occlusion, is a protrusive malocclusion in which the lower jaw is more forward than the upper and its first permanent molar is positioned nearer to the center line of the arch than

the upper. Returning the dental arch to proper positioning usually requires carefully planned orthodontic care, possibly concurrent with orthognathic surgery to reposition one or both jaws.

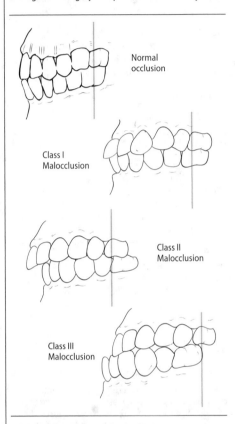

Normal occlusion

Class I Malocclusion

Class II Malocclusion

Class III Malocclusion

M26.3- Anomalies of tooth position of fully erupted tooth or teeth

This subcategory classifies anomalies of tooth position. Crowding occurs when teeth come in too close to one another and have no room for the normal spacing that should be present between the teeth. Crowding also causes overlapping and displacement of adjacent teeth in various directions. Excessive spacing is the opposite problem when a tooth is too far apart from its neighboring tooth, leaving an unfilled gap between them. Horizontal displacement may be seen as crowns and roots out of the normal line, including "tipping" in their position. Vertical displacement may present as supraeruption of a tooth in which it continues to grow out from the gingiva when the opposing tooth is missing in the other jaw, and may require replacing the missing tooth and adjusting the height of the other. Infra-eruption of a tooth occurs when it has not sufficiently erupted above the gum line. Tooth rotation is the malposition of a tooth that has turned about its own longitudinal axis. The interocclusal distance in teeth is determined from the biting/chewing contact surfaces of teeth in the maxilla (upper jaw) and the mandible (lower jaw) when the lower jaw is in the normal resting position. This natural space or clearance may be greater than normal or insufficient. These problems may require orthodontic care to move the teeth into proper position and/or the strategic removal of certain teeth.

M26.6- Temporomandibular joint disorders

This subcategory classifies temporomandibular joint disorders. The temporomandibular joints (TMJ) are located just in front of the ears and attach the mandible to the skull allowing the jaw to move. Symptoms of TMJ disorders include pain in the jaw, headache, stiffness in the jaw, earaches, and popping or clicking sounds when opening the mouth. Symptoms may often be alleviated with pain-relief medications, heat/cold, and other palliative measures. Oftentimes, TMJ problems resolve without intervention over time. In some instances, surgery is required to correct the problem.

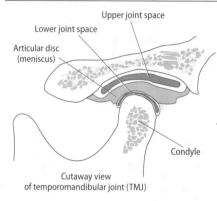

Cutaway view
of temporomandibular joint (TMJ)

TMJ syndrome is often related to stress and tooth-grinding; in other cases, arthritis, injury, poorly aligned teeth, or ill-fitting dentures may be the cause

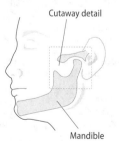

Cutaway detail

Mandible

Symptoms include facial pain and chewing problems; TMJ syndrome occurs more frequently in women

M26.61- Adhesions and ankylosis of temporomandibular joint

This condition is defined as stiffening or union of the temporomandibular joint due to a bony or fibrous union across the joint.

M26.62- Arthralgia of temporomandibular joint

This subcategory is used to report pain caused by arthritis in the jaw, specifically where the mandible meets the temporal bone in front of the ears on both sides of the face. There are several reasons for TMJ problems, with arthritis being the major cause reported in this subcategory of codes. Typical symptoms include pain, limited mobility, popping sounds when the joint is functioning, trouble with chewing, or swelling, among others. Most treatments remain simple in that relief is often found with hot/cold packs, a diet of soft foods to reduce the stress from chewing, or anti-inflammatory medications. When these basic remedies fail, the patient may seek care from a maxillofacial health care provider for arthrocentesis, arthroscopy, or open joint surgery, or alternative treatments, including transcutaneous electrical nerve stimulation, ultrasound or radiowave therapy, and trigger point injections.

M26.63- Articular disc disorder of temporomandibular joint

The most common type of internal temporomandibular joint derangement involves the anterior displacement or misalignment of the articular disc above the condyle. Popping on jaw movement and localized joint pain especially during mastication (chewing) are commonly associated with the disorder. Derangement may occur with or without spontaneous reduction, and either type may cause capsulitis or synovitis of the ligaments, tendons, connective tissue, and synovium surrounding the joint. Treatment includes analgesics, passive jaw-motion devices, corticosteroid injection for capsulitis, and if conservative treatment fails, surgery.

M26.7- Dental alveolar anomalies

This subcategory identifies anomalies of the dental alveoli and alveolar ridge, including hyperplasia and hypoplasia. Dental alveoli are the tooth sockets of the maxilla and mandible. The alveolar ridge is the bony process of the maxilla or mandible that contains the tooth sockets. Hyperplasia of the alveoli is an overgrowth or overdevelopment of bone and hypoplasia of the alveoli is an underdevelopment or agenesis of bone.

M26.79 Other specified alveolar anomalies

This code includes vertical displacement and occlusal plane deviation. A vertical displacement of the alveolus and teeth includes the extrusion or extended movement of the tooth and the root cavity or socket in the jawbone where the tooth is held, beyond the normal occlusal plane when the opposing occlusal force is missing. The occlusal plane is the hypothetical surface on which upper and lower teeth meet when biting or chewing. The plane appears as a straight line to the lateral view, even though it is actually a compound curved surface, and the planar reference points are taken from specific points within the dental arches. A structural aberration that results in canting or tipping of the occlusal plane is a deviation that may require orthopedic and/or orthodontic care to achieve the true horizontal and vertical references for the occlusal plane that are the optimal end-point of treatment for the best mandibular maxillary relationship.

M27.- Other diseases of jaws

This category includes developmental disorders of the jaw, giant cell granuloma, and alveolitis. It also represents complications from endodontic treatment (e.g., root canal). In a root canal, the pulp is removed and the root canals are cleaned, enlarged, and shaped into a form that can be filled. The pulp chamber and root canals are then filled and sealed, before a crown or other restorative material is placed over the tooth. Root canal fillings ideally fill the entire obliterated pulp space and provide a seal at the surface where the cementum and dentin of the tooth's root join (dentinocemental junction). Complications of various types of dental implants are also included in this category.

M27.5- Periradicular pathology associated with previous endodontic treatment

Endodontic treatment failure is related to perforations of the root canal occurring during root canal treatment, in which an opening is made into the pulp chamber. Two of the more frequently encountered problems include penetration of the pulp chamber floor in multirooted teeth during access and labial perforation during access through crowned anterior teeth. Overextension of filler or extrusion of sealer may act as chronic irritants, preventing the healing of periapical disease or causing apical breakdown in areas that were previously without pathology. Endodontic underfill is another complication of root canal treatment in which the pulp space is inadequately filled.

M27.6- Endosseous dental implant failure

There are two types of failures: pre-osseointegration and post-osseointegration. Pre-osseointegration failure can occur when the implant fails to join together with the surrounding bone and soft tissue. This type of failure is most often related to placement of the implant into poor-quality bone, which may include previously irradiated bone. Hemorrhagic complications and iatrogenic causes may also be the culprits in pre-osseointegration failure.

Post-osseointegration failures may be due to biological factors such as periodontal infection, lack of attached gingiva, or occlusal trauma caused by insufficient support. Mechanical failure in the form of fracture of the implant body itself may also cause post-osseointegration failure.

Systemic Connective Tissue Disorders (M30-M36)

This code block reports a group of diseases in which the primary lesion appears to be damage to collagen, a protein that is the major component of connective tissue. Collagen (rheumatoid) diseases are attributed largely to disorders of the immune complex mechanism.

The categories in this code block are as follows:

M30	Polyarteritis nodosa and related conditions
M31	Other necrotizing vasculopathies
M32	Systemic lupus erythematosus (SLE)
M33	Dermatopolymyositis
M34	Systemic sclerosis [scleroderma]
M35	Other systemic involvement of connective tissue
M36	Systemic disorders of connective tissue in diseases classified elsewhere

M30.- Polyarteritis nodosa and related conditions

Polyarteritis nodosa is a systemic disease characterized by segmental inflammation with infiltration and necrosis of medium-sized or small arteries. It is most common in males and produces symptoms related to involvement of arteries in the kidneys, muscles, gastrointestinal tract, and heart.

M30.0 Polyarteritis nodosa

Polyarteritis nodosa is characterized by inflammation of small and mid-size arteries. Symptoms are related to involved arteries in the kidneys, muscles, gastrointestinal tract, and heart. This condition results in tissue death.

M30.3 Mucocutaneous lymph node syndrome [Kawasaki]

Mucocutaneous lymph node syndrome (MCLS) is an acute febrile disease of children marked by erythema of conjunctiva and mucous membranes of the upper respiratory tract, skin eruptions, and edema.

M31.- Other necrotizing vasculopathies

Included in this category are various types of vasculitis that are characterized by necrosis. Some conditions include hypersensitivity angiitis, thrombotic microangiopathy, Wegener's granulomatosis, aortic arch syndrome (Takayasu), microscopic polyangiitis, and giant cell arteritis.

M31.0 Hypersensitivity angiitis

Also termed hypersensitivity vasculitis or allergic vasculitis, this is a systemic autoimmune disorder similar to polyarteritis nodosa but it tends to affect small vessels. Goodpasture syndrome is included in this code and is a condition in which the collagen in the glomeruli of the kidneys is attacked by a substance called antiglomerular basement membranes antibodies. This causes glomerulonephritis associated with hematuria that progresses rapidly and results in death from renal failure.

Focus Point

An additional code should be added to identify any renal disease occurring with hypersensitivity angiitis.

M31.1 Thrombotic microangiopathy

Thrombotic microangiopathy describes blockages due to hyaline deposits in the smallest arteries and arterioles. It includes Moschcowitz's syndrome and Baer-Schifrin disease. Symptoms include purpura and central nervous system disorders.

M31.2 Lethal midline granuloma

Lethal midline granuloma is characterized by a granulomatous lesion or tumor that begins midface, typically in the nose or paranasal sinuses. It occurs chiefly in males and is often fatal. It is also referred to as malignant granuloma of the face.

M31.3- Wegener's granulomatosis

Wegener's granulomatosis is a disease occurring mainly in men that is marked by necrotizing granulomas and ulceration of the upper respiratory tract. These are caused by a vasculitis affecting small vessels due to an immune disorder. The fifth character indicates the presence or absence of renal involvement.

M31.4 Aortic arch syndrome [Takayasu]

Aortic arch syndrome is a progressive obliterative arteritis of the brachiocephalic trunk, left subclavian, and left common carotid arteries above the aortic arch. It results in ischemia in the brain, heart, and arm. It typically occurs in younger women.

M31.5 Giant cell arteritis with polymyalgia rheumatica

M31.6 Other giant cell arteritis

Giant cell arteritis, also called temporal arteritis, is characterized by an inflammation of the head arteries, especially in the temple area due to giant cells affecting carotid artery branches, resulting in occlusion. Symptoms include fever, headache, and neurological problems and it typically occurs in people 50 years of age or older. It can often be associated with polymyalgia rheumatica, which presents with pain and stiffness in the muscles of the neck, shoulders, hips, and thighs.

M32.- Systemic lupus erythematosus (SLE)

Systemic lupus erythematosus (SLE) is an inflammatory autoimmune disorder that may affect multiple organ systems. The disease is usually chronic and the clinical course is mild to fulminating. Clinical exacerbations and remissions of manifestations involving the skin, serosal surfaces, central nervous system, kidneys, and blood cells are characteristic. Arthralgia, symmetrical arthritis, and inflammatory muscle involvement are common musculoskeletal features of acute systemic lupus erythematosus. The disease is most prevalent in women, particularly black women, of childbearing age. No single etiology for the disease has been discovered, but initiation and expression of the disease has been associated with hormonal influences, genetic factors, loss of tolerance to autoantigens, and certain viruses and drugs. The hands and wrist are two sites commonly affected by lupus arthritis. Signs and symptoms of systemic lupus erythematosus include fever, anorexia, malaise, weight loss, and skin lesions identical to chronic discoid lupus erythematosus, redness and edema affecting the nose and cheeks revealing a classic butterfly rash, photosensitivity and other ocular manifestations, and joint symptoms with or without acute synovitis.

M33.- Dermatopolymyositis

Dermatopolymyositis is a classification of diseases that involve nonsuppurative inflammation of the skin, subcutaneous tissues, and muscles with necrosis of muscle fibers. This family of diseases includes polymyositis, which does not include the skin, and dermatomyositis, which is differentiated from polymyositis by the presence of a characteristic rash of edema and erythema and a pinkish -purple discoloration particularly around the eyes. Physical exam reveals prominent proximal muscle weakness. Lab work shows elevated muscle enzymes. Electromyograph (EMG) reveals myopathic patterns and muscle biopsy reveals inflammatory infiltrates.

M33.0- Juvenile dermatomyositis

M33.1- Other dermatomyositis

Dermatomyositis is polymyositis (see description at M33.2-) with the addition of cutaneous involvement such as lesions and eruptions with erythremia or pruritus on face, hands, and thighs. Scaly scalp or hair loss may occur. Dermatomyositis affects both children and adults.

M33.2- Polymyositis

Polymyositis is an idiopathic inflammatory disease that predominantly affects muscles causing bilateral weakness affecting mainly younger and middle-aged adults. Inflammation may also be present in the blood vessels supplying blood to the muscles as well as in the muscles of the lungs causing respiratory problems. Most often affected are the muscles in the upper extremities, neck, hips, and thighs although systems such as the esophageal (dysphagia, reflux) and heart (cardiomyopathy, arrhythmias) muscle may be involved. Polymyositis does not involve skin lesions.

M34.- Systemic sclerosis [scleroderma]

Systemic sclerosis, also called scleroderma, is characterized by widespread small vessel obliteration and fibrotic thickening of the skin and multiple organs, including the alimentary tract, kidneys, lungs, muscles, joints, nerves, and heart. When localized to the face and extremities (with Raynaud's phenomena), it is called acrosclerosis. A distinct form of systemic sclerosis is CR(E)ST syndrome, which stands for subcutaneous Calcinosis, Raynaud's phenomenon, Esophageal motility dysfunction, Sclerodactyly, and Telangiectasia.

M35.- Other systemic involvement of connective tissue

This category identifies conditions of the connective tissue such as sicca syndrome, Behçet's disease, polymyalgia rheumatica, diffuse fasciitis, multifocal fibrosclerosis, relapsing panniculitis, and hypermobility syndrome.

M35.0- Sicca syndrome [Sjögren]

Sicca syndrome, also called Sjögren's syndrome, is an idiopathic, autoimmune disorder. Sjögren's syndrome is characterized by xerostomia (dry mouth), keratoconjunctivitis sicca (dry eyes), and parotid gland enlargement. Primary Sjögren's syndrome presents a wide variety of clinical manifestations due to a wider involvement of the exocrine glands. The organs involved may include the skin, lung, GI tract, kidney, muscles, nerves, spleen, and thyroid. Secondary Sjögren's syndrome is limited to symptoms of the lacrimal and salivary glands.

M35.2 Behçet's disease

Behçet's disease is a multisystem disorder of unknown etiology named after the Turkish dermatologist who first described it. Recurrent oral and genital ulcers, uveitis, seronegative arthritis, and central nervous system abnormalities characterize the syndrome. The arthritic component involves large and small joints with a nonspecific, self-limiting synovitis and, in more than two-thirds of the patients, commonly affects the knees and ankles. The arthritic changes resemble those of rheumatoid arthritis but are milder and lead only to shallow erosions of the articular cartilage in the more severe cases. Therapies include immunomodulating drugs and corticosteroids.

M35.3 Polymyalgia rheumatica

Polymyalgia rheumatica is a self-limiting disease of the elderly that often develops abruptly with joint and muscle pain and stiffness of the pelvis and shoulder girdle in association with fever, malaise, fatigue, weight loss, and anemia. The disease bears a close relationship with giant cell arteritis and the two conditions often occur concomitantly.

M35.8 Other specified systemic involvement of connective tissue

Eosinophilic myalgia syndrome (EMS) is reported here. This condition was first identified in 1989 and was associated with use of certain brands of L-tryptophan, an oral nutritional supplement of amino acids that were contaminated. However, a small percentage of EMS cases occur in the absence of L-tryptophan use. Three criteria must be met for a diagnosis of EMS, including incapacitating muscle pain (myalgia), elevated blood eosinophils of than more than 1000 cells/microliter, and no evidence of infection or neoplastic disease. Signs and symptoms of EMS include muscle and joint pain, weakness, swelling of the arms and legs, fever, and rash. Blood work shows increased circulating eosinophils.

Deforming Dorsopathies (M40-M43)

Deforming dorsopathies include curvature of the spine such as kyphosis, lordosis, and scoliosis.

The categories in this code block are as follows:

M40	Kyphosis and lordosis
M41	Scoliosis
M42	Spinal osteochondrosis
M43	Other deforming dorsopathies

M40.- Kyphosis and lordosis

Kyphosis is an abnormal increase in the thoracic convexity as viewed from the side. Lordosis, a swayback appearance, also called hollow or saddleback, is the anterior convexity of the cervical and lumbar spine as viewed from the side. Postural kyphosis or "round back" is kyphosis that is considered to be due to slouching or poor posture and occurs mostly in teens and young adults. Flat-back syndrome is when the spine loses its normal curve and becomes straight. It can occur from the loss of lordosis or kyphosis or a combination of both.

M41.- Scoliosis

Scoliosis is lateral curvature of the spine and kyphoscoliosis is a lateral curvature of the spine with extensive flexion. Spinal curvature from scoliosis may occur on either side of the spine or on both sides in different sections. The thoracic and lumbar spine may be affected. In 80 percent of the cases, scoliosis is idiopathic, meaning it has no known cause. Adolescents are the most common age group to have idiopathic scoliosis. It usually begins between the ages of 8 and 10. It occurs equally in boys and girls, although in girls scoliosis is much more likely to progress and require treatment. Scoliosis is usually asymptomatic until the spinal curve becomes large. Then the child may display physical deformities such as:

- Child appears to lean to one side
- Head does not look centered over the body
- One shoulder blade sticks out more than the other
- One shoulder or hip looks higher than the other
- Ribs look higher on one side when the child bends forward at the waist
- Waistline is flat on one side

Children may develop a compensatory curve that keeps the shoulders level and gives the appearance that the back is straight. Children may be at higher risk for developing scoliosis if they have another family member with scoliosis. The percentage of children that require treatment is low at 10 percent. The degree of curvature helps to determine the course of treatment. Treatment includes bracing or surgery. Scoliosis is most serious in young children who are still growing since the curve progresses as the child grows. For children with rapidly progressing curves, or with curves above 30 degrees, treatment is likely necessary.

Scoliosis

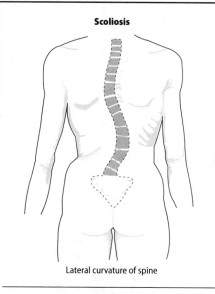

Lateral curvature of spine

M42.- Spinal osteochondrosis

Osteochondropathies are self-limiting disorders of unknown etiology that mostly affect children (juvenile osteochondrosis) 3 to 10 years of age. Four phases in the pathogenesis of the disease have been identified: necrosis, revascularization with bone deposition and resorption, bone healing, and bone deformity. The fourth phase often is associated with degenerative arthropathy. The subcategories distinguish between juvenile and adult osteochondrosis of the spine and the level affected.

M42.0- Juvenile osteochondrosis of spine

Also referred to as Scheuermann's disease, juvenile osteochondrosis of the spine is a deformity that occurs typically in teens. It occurs when the normal amount of kyphosis is increased because of a slower growth in the upper spine compared to the back of the spine, causing the vertebra to become wedge shaped. This creates a roundback appearance. It is most common in the thoracic spine generally from T7 to T9 although it can also occur in the lower back. The condition stops when the growth plates are complete but the deformity remains.

Focus Point

The difference between Scheuermann's and postural kyphosis (M40.0-) can be distinguished when lying down. The deformity goes away in postural kyphosis but remains with Scheuermann's kyphosis.

M43.- Other deforming dorsopathies

This category identifies conditions of the spine including spondylolysis, spondylolisthesis (forward slipping), fusion, recurrent dislocation, and torticollis.

M43.0- Spondylolysis

Spondylolysis is a defect in the connection between the vertebra, mainly in L5 or L4, which is a common cause of back pain in adolescent athletes. This can be hereditary and exacerbated by stress from sports, resulting in stress fractures.

M43.1- Spondylolisthesis

Acquired spondylolisthesis is forward slipping of one vertebral body (with the remainder of the spinal column above it) in relation to the vertebral segment immediately below, not due to congenital deformity or fracture. Acquired spondylolisthesis may be secondary to degenerative disk disease, a late effect of fracture, or due to spondylolysis (not qualified as congenital) or pathological weakness of bone.

M43.6 Torticollis

Torticollis is an involuntary position where the head is tilted to one side and/or turned in the opposite direction due to twisting or rotating of the neck. Also referred to as "wryneck," this condition may be congenital or acquired, although this code reports only the acquired, nonspasmodic form that is not due to a current acute injury. Acquired torticollis may result from an old injury or current inflammatory process.

Spondylopathies (M45-M49)

Spondylopathy is a medical term for any disease of the vertebra or spinal column.

The categories in this code block are as follows:

M45	Ankylosing spondylitis
M46	Other inflammatory spondylopathies
M47	Spondylosis
M48	Other spondylopathies
M49	Spondylopathies in diseases classified elsewhere

M45.- Ankylosing spondylitis

Ankylosing spondylitis is a form of chronic inflammation of the spine and the sacroiliac joints. Chronic inflammation in these areas causes pain and stiffness in and around the spine and can lead to a complete fusion of the vertebrae, a process called ankylosis. Ankylosis causes total loss of mobility of the spine. The disease is more common in males. Although ankylosing spondylitis can occur at any age, onset usually falls in the second and third decades; the cause is believed to be genetic. Common symptoms include back pain and stiffness over a period of weeks or months and lasting longer than three months; early morning stiffness improves by warm shower or light exercise. Subcategories identify specific levels of the spine.

Focus Point

Ankylosing spondylitis shares many features with other arthritic conditions, such as psoriatic arthritis, reactive arthritis, arthritis associated with Crohn's disease, and ulcerative colitis. The conditions are collectively referred to as spondyloarthropathies.

M46.- Other inflammatory spondylopathies

This category identifies diseases of the spinal vertebra or column involving inflammation.

M46.0- Spinal enthesopathy

This condition is characterized by inflammation of a tendon, ligament, or cartilage at its insertion into the vertebral bone.

M46.2- Osteomyelitis of vertebra

Osteomyelitis of vertebra is an inflammation of bone and bone marrow. The condition is commonly due to a pathogen such as bacteria, virus, protozoa, or fungus. Osteomyelitis may develop as an extension of a contiguous infection, particularly infections involving ischemic, diabetic, or neurotrophic ulcers.

M46.3- Infection of intervertebral disc (pyogenic)

M46.4- Discitis, unspecified

Discitis is inflammation of the intervertebral discs often caused by a viral or bacterial infection or autoimmune disorders that commonly occur along with osteomyelitis. When affecting children, it follows a more acute course with sudden symptoms and faster diagnosis. Symptoms in adults tend to come on more slowly, delaying diagnosis, and causing infection to spread.

M47.- Spondylosis

Spondylosis is a degenerative rather than inflammatory condition. Myelopathy (pinched spinal cord) is a qualifying term describing diseases and disturbances of the spinal cord and is indicative of neurologic deficits due to severe nerve compression that is affecting the entire spinal cord. Paresthesia, loss of sensation, and loss of sphincter control are among the most common forms of myelopathy. Radiculopathy (pinched nerve) is nerve dysfunction from compression on specific spinal nerve roots causing referred extremity pain, numbness, and muscle weakness. Subcategory combination codes identify whether the spondylosis includes specific complications and the specific vertebral level affected.

M48.- Other spondylopathies

Spondylopathies or disorders of the vertebra that are represented in this category include spinal stenosis, ankylosing hyperostosis, kissing spine, traumatic spondylopathy, fatigue or stress fracture, and collapsed vertebra.

M48.0- Spinal stenosis

Spinal stenosis is a narrowing of the spinal canal that most commonly occurs due to degenerative arthritis, formation of bone spurs, overgrowth of supportive structures (ligaments), or degenerative disc disease. These disease processes reduce the normal space available in the spinal canal, causing compression of structural and nerve tissue.

M48.06- Spinal stenosis, lumbar region

Spinal stenosis of the lumbar spine may be with or without neurogenic claudication. Neurogenic claudication (NC) describes a syndrome associated with compression of the cauda equina (lumbar nerve root) caused by significant lumbar spinal stenosis. It is neurological in origin and should be distinguished from the circulatory origins of vascular claudication. Symptoms of neurogenic claudication include unilateral or bilateral muscle cramping, fatigue and pain, and weakness or numbness in the buttocks and lower extremities. These symptoms are often exacerbated by extension of the lumbar spine during sitting or walking. Conversely, the patient experiences relief of symptoms while in the flexed, forward-bent position (e.g., sitting or leaning on objects for support). The presence of neurogenic claudication in spinal stenosis may indicate the need for surgical intervention to correct the condition causing the nerve compression and relieve the NC symptoms.

M48.1- Ankylosing hyperostosis [Forestier]

Diffuse idiopathic skeletal hyperostosis (DISH) or Forestier's disease is characterized by calcification of the ligaments that attach to the spine. Although the cause is unknown, it typically affects older (over 50) men and Type 2 diabetics. Ankylosing hyperostosis usually only causes mild pain and stiffness but with progression can increase risk of spinal fracture.

M48.2- Kissing spine

Also called Baastrup syndrome, this is a common condition that develops when the spinous processes of adjacent vertebrae come into contact with one another causing severe pain. Kissing spine most often occurs in the lumbar spine and can lead to a new joint forming between them. It is thought to be caused by loss of disk space.

M48.4- Fatigue fracture of vertebra

This fracture is also called a stress fracture because the etiology is from repetitive stress or "trivial" repeated trauma to an area. This code is not to be used for acute, traumatic fracture.

Focus Point

Fatigue fracture of vertebra does not include pathological fracture due to osteoarthritis (M80.-) or neoplasm (M84.58-).

Other Dorsopathies (M50-M54)

Included in this code block are disorders of the intervertebral discs. An intervertebral disc is the flexible plate that connects any two adjacent vertebrae in the spine; they cushion the spinal cord from the impact produced by the body's movements. Each disc is composed of a gelatinous material in the center, called the nucleus pulposus, surrounded by rings of a fibrous tissue. With age, these discs can degenerate and dry out and the fibers holding them in place can tear. Eventually, the disc torn from the tissue can rupture the fibrocartilaginous material, which releases the nucleus pulposus. Pressure may force the nucleus pulposus outward, placing pressure on the spinal cord and causing pain. Disc herniation most commonly affects the lumbar region between the fifth lumbar vertebra and the first sacral vertebra. However, disc herniation also occurs in the cervical spine.

The categories in this code block are as follows:

M50	Cervical disc disorders
M51	Thoracic, thoracolumbar, and lumbosacral intervertebral disc disorders
M53	Other and unspecified dorsopathies, not elsewhere classified
M54	Dorsalgia

M50.- Cervical disc disorders

Conditions of the cervical spine that are represented in this category include disc disorders with myelopathy and radiculopathy. Also included here are cervical disc displacement and degeneration.

Focus Point

The codes in this category distinguish between high cervical, midcervical, and cervicothoracic regions. When the condition affects overlapping sites, the instructional note directs users to code to the most superior level.

M50.0- Cervical disc disorder with myelopathy

Cervical disc disorder with myelopathy is a degenerative condition that includes myelopathy, which is the compression or pinching of the spinal cord causing pain and any neurological deficit related to the spinal cord. It is one of the most common causes of neck pain.

M50.1- Cervical disc disorder with radiculopathy

Radiculopathy (pinched nerve) is nerve dysfunction from compression on specific spinal nerve roots rather than the spinal cord itself (myelopathy). It causes referred extremity pain, numbness, and muscle weakness.

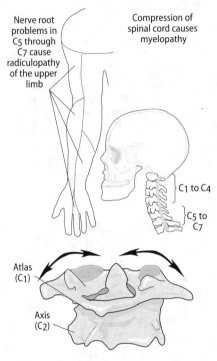

Nerve root problems in C5 through C7 cause radiculopathy of the upper limb

Compression of spinal cord causes myelopathy

C1 to C4

C5 to C7

Atlas (C1)

Axis (C2)

The specialized atlas allows for rotary motion, which turns the head

M51.- Thoracic, thoracolumbar, and lumbosacral intervertebral disc disorders

Conditions of the thoracic, lumbar, sacral spine, and overlapping sites that are represented in this category include disc disorders with myelopathy and radiculopathy. Also included here are intervertebral disc displacement and degeneration and Schmorl's nodes.

M51.0- Thoracic, thoracolumbar and lumbosacral intervertebral disc disorders with myelopathy

Intervertebral disc disorder with myelopathy is a degenerative condition that includes myelopathy, which is the compression or pinching of the spinal cord causing pain and any neurological deficit related to the spinal cord. It is one of the most common causes of back pain.

M51.1- Thoracic, thoracolumbar and lumbosacral intervertebral disc disorders with radiculopathy

Radiculopathy (pinched nerve) is nerve dysfunction from compression on specific spinal nerve roots rather than the spinal cord itself (myelopathy). It causes referred extremity pain, numbness, and muscle weakness.

M51.4- Schmorl's nodes

Schmorl's nodes describe the prolapse of the nucleus pulposus into an adjoining vertebra, as seen on x-rays of the spine.

M53.- Other and unspecified dorsopathies, not elsewhere classified

This category includes neurological disorders of the upper spine including cervicocranial and cervicobrachial syndrome.

M53.0 Cervicocranial syndrome

Also referred to as Barre-Lieou syndrome, this is a neurologic disorder of the upper cervical spine and nerve roots.

M53.1 Cervicobrachial syndrome

This is a complex of symptoms due to the scalenus anterior muscle compressing the brachial plexus; pain radiates from the shoulder to the arm or back of the neck.

M54.- Dorsalgia

This chapter represents various types of pain in the back such as panniculitis, radiculopathy, cervicalgia, sciatica, and lumbago, some with known causes and others from unknown causes.

M54.0- Panniculitis affecting regions of neck and back

Panniculitis is inflammation of the panniculus adiposus (subcutaneous fat) in the neck and back.

M54.1- Radiculopathy

Radiculopathy (pinched nerve) is nerve dysfunction from compression on specific spinal nerve roots rather than the spinal cord itself (myelopathy). It causes referred extremity pain, numbness, and muscle weakness. This symptom code is used when the cause is unknown.

M54.2 Cervicalgia

Cervicalgia is the general term for a pain in the neck or the cervical spine without radiation down the arm. It may be associated with trauma, an underlying condition (e.g., arthritis), or it may be positional or postural in nature. Straining and tension of the muscles of the neck are a common cause of the condition.

> **Focus Point**
>
> *The code for cervicalgia is reported when the underlying cause of the pain is not known. If the underlying cause is documented, such as cervical intervertebral disc disorder, the condition causing the neck pain is reported instead of the code for cervicalgia.*

M54.3- Sciatica

M54.4- Lumbago with sciatica

M54.5 Low back pain

Sciatica is a symptom that is characterized by leg pain that originates in the lower back and radiates down the buttock through the large sciatic nerve in the back of the leg. It can also cause numbness, tingling, and weakness. It is usually worse when sitting and occurs in one leg. Low back pain, sometimes called lumbar pain or lumbago, is reported when the underlying cause of the pain is not known.

Disorders of Muscles (M60-M63)

Muscle is an organ composed of one of three types of muscle tissue (skeletal, cardiac, or smooth) that is specialized for contraction to produce voluntary or involuntary movements. Ligament is dense, regularly arranged connective tissue that attaches bone to bone. The fascia is thin connective tissue covering, or separating, the muscles and internal organs of the body. It varies in thickness, density, elasticity, and composition. Fascia, muscles, and ligaments are normally exposed to stress throughout life. Damage occurs when the muscle or connective tissue is exposed to higher-than-usual stress levels, such as sudden excessive stress or the result of repetitive

stress. Whether damaged by repetitive overuse or by acute injury, treatment includes a brief period of relative rest, with length depending on the extent of injury, followed by gradual movement and activity.

The categories in this code block are as follows:

M60	Myositis
M61	Calcification and ossification of muscle
M62	Other disorders of muscle
M63	Disorders of muscle in diseases classified elsewhere

M60.- Myositis

Myositis means inflammation of the muscles. The codes in this category identify inflammation from sources such as infection, foreign bodies, and interstitial (fibrosa).

M60.0- Infective myositis

Infective myositis is inflammation of the voluntary muscles due to infection. It is usually secondary to osteomyelitis or a penetrating wound, but hematogenous infection can occur in debilitated patients or patients with suppressed immunity. Signs and symptoms of infective myositis include marked swelling and pain, usually confined to shoulder girdle and arms, but may affect any part of the body.

M60.1- Interstitial myositis

Also referred to as myositis fibrosa, it occurs due to a fibrous connective tissue formation within the muscle causing muscle stiffness.

M61.- Calcification and ossification of muscle

Ossification describes the formation of bone in soft tissue.

M61.0- Myositis ossificans traumatica

Myositis ossificans traumatica begins from a single blow causing a painful area in the muscle that eventually develops cartilage-like masses that progress to solid bone.

M61.1- Myositis ossificans progressiva

Also referred to as Munchmeyer syndrome or fibrodysplasia ossificans progressiva, this is a very rare condition characterized by recurrent, painful swelling of soft tissue that progresses to abnormal bone formation in the tissue.

M62.- Other disorders of muscle

Disorders of muscles identified in this category include nontraumatic muscle separation, rupture, or ischemic infarction. Also included are conditions of the muscles such as contracture, wasting and atrophy, weakness, spasm, and rhabdomyolysis.

M62.82 Rhabdomyolysis

Rhabdomyolysis ensues when the breakdown or necrosis of muscle tissue causes the tissue to dissolve, releasing toxic creatine phosphokinase (CK) and myoglobin into the bloodstream. It can progress to life-threatening renal failure.

M62.84 Sarcopenia

Sarcopenia was originally defined as the expected and nearly universal age-related loss of muscle mass, strength, and function. The current definition requires a clinically significant decrease in mobility and daily functions brought on by the combination of low muscle mass and weakness. Muscle mass loss measurements are made based on non-bone lean mass of the limbs, usually assessed by using dual-energy X-ray absorptiometry (DEXA). Various strength and functionality tests are also used to look for limitations in mobility or in performing activities of daily living. When patients are diagnosed with sarcopenia, interventions such as physical and occupational therapy, as well as nutritional counseling can be initiated. Individuals may be identified as high risk, and preventative measures can be developed to avert falls and future disability.

Disorders of Synovium and Tendon (M65-M67)

This section identifies disorders of the tendons that are dense, fibrous connective tissues that connect the muscle to the bone. Also represented are synovial disorders that refer to the fluid-filled cavity separating and cushioning the bones it joins. This cavity is called the synovial cavity and the fluid is synovial fluid. The joint cavity is surrounded by a two-layer capsule called the articular capsule. The external layer of the capsule is a dense connective tissue that is contiguous with the periosteum of the related bones. The internal layer is a synovial membrane that covers all surfaces within the joint cavity except for the opposing bone surfaces.

The categories in this code block are as follows:

M65	Synovitis and tenosynovitis
M66	Spontaneous rupture of synovium and tendon
M67	Other disorders of synovium and tendon

M65.- Synovitis and tenosynovitis

Synovitis is inflammation of a synovial membrane, especially the synovium that lines articular joints. In a normal synovial joint, the smooth and reciprocally shaped cartilaginous opposing surfaces permit a fluid, frictionless, and painless articulation. Irregularities, disease, and damage to the articular surfaces lead to progressive degenerative changes resulting in pain and limitation of movement. The joint capsule is particularly sensitive to stretching and increased fluid pressure. Tenosynovitis is the inflammation of a tendon and its synovial sheath, also known as tendosynovitis, tendovaginitis, tenontothecitis, tenontolemmitis, and vaginal or tendinous synovitis. At the site of friction, the tendon is enveloped by a sheath consisting of a visceral and parietal layer of synovial membrane and is lubricated by a synovial-like fluid containing hyaluronate. The synovial sheath is in turn covered by a dense, fibrous tissue sheath. Irregularities, disease, and damage to the tendon's attachment to the articular joints may lead to progressive degenerative changes with resultant limitation of movement and pain. The synovial membranes of tendon sheaths and bursae are capable of the same inflammatory reactions to abnormal conditions as the synovial membranes of joints.

M65.2- Calcific tendinitis

This condition is the buildup of macroscopic deposits of hydroxyapatite (crystalline calcium phosphate) in the tendon. In contrast to degenerative tendinitis, calcific may resolve with the tendon healing spontaneously.

> **Focus Point**
>
> *Even though there is a choice for upper arm in this subcategory, it is not the appropriate code for calcific tendinitis of the shoulder, which is the most commonly affected site. The correct code for calcific tendinitis of the shoulder is located at M75.3-.*

M65.3- Trigger finger

This subcategory refers to acquired trigger finger. The space within the tendon sheath narrows from inflammation causing stenosing tenosynovitis or nodule in flexor tendon. This creates cessation of flexion or extension movement in the finger, followed by snapping into place.

M66.- Spontaneous rupture of synovium and tendon

Rupture of tendon, nontraumatic, is a rupture due to pathology rather than trauma or injury. A normal tendon seldom ruptures even with strenuous activity, but if it has become damaged by disease (e.g., secondary to tenosynovitis) or degenerated due to the fraying caused by friction (e.g., due to bony erosion), it may rupture even with normal activity. Degeneration occurs in rheumatic arthritis, lupus erythematosus, hyperparathyroidism, and systemic steroid use, or when steroids are injected directly into a tendon. Therapies include reconstructive surgery to repair or replace the abnormal part of the ruptured tendon.

M66.0 Rupture of popliteal cyst

Synovial cysts of the popliteal space are Baker's cysts, sometimes called popliteal cysts. In children, Baker's cysts are common but usually are asymptomatic and regress spontaneously. In adults, Baker's cysts, in conjunction with synovial effusion due to rheumatoid arthritis or degenerative joint disease, may produce significant impairment. When a Baker's cyst interferes with normal knee function, surgical exploration and excision of the cyst is indicated. The cysts usually communicate with the knee joint through a long and tortuous duct, allowing the cyst to become distended by any synovial effusion and possibly extend down as far as the midcalf.

M66.1-   Rupture of synovium

Rupture of tendon, nontraumatic, is a rupture due to pathology rather than trauma or injury. A normal tendon seldom ruptures even with strenuous activity, but if it has become damaged by disease (e.g., secondary to tenosynovitis) or degenerated due to the fraying caused by friction (e.g., due to bony erosion), it may rupture even with normal activity. Degeneration occurs from rheumatic arthritis, lupus erythematosus, hyperparathyroidism, and systemic steroid use or when steroids are injected directly into a tendon. Therapies include reconstructive surgery to repair or replace the abnormal part of the ruptured tendon.

M67.-   Other disorders of synovium and tendon

Conditions represented in this category include acquired short Achilles tendon, synovial hypertrophy, transient synovitis, toxic synovitis, ganglion, and plica syndrome.

M67.4-   Ganglion

A ganglion of synovium, tendon, and bursa is a thin-walled cystic lesion of unknown etiology containing thick, clear, mucinous fluid, possibly due to mucoid degeneration. Arising in relation to periarticular tissues, joint capsules, and tendon sheaths, ganglia are typically in the hands and feet and are most common in the dorsum of the wrist. Depending on the size, cysts may feel firm or spongy. Usually a single cyst appears, although on occasion multiple cysts may develop. They may have a common stalk within the deeper tissue connecting them. They rarely exceed 2 cm in diameter. Ganglion cysts are generally asymptomatic or minimally symptomatic. Signs and symptoms include limitation of motion, pain, paresthesias, and weakness. Treatment may not be necessary as many ganglions spontaneously resolve over time. Others may need to be aspirated or surgical excision may be required due to pain or limited motion. Ganglions have a high rate of recurrence.

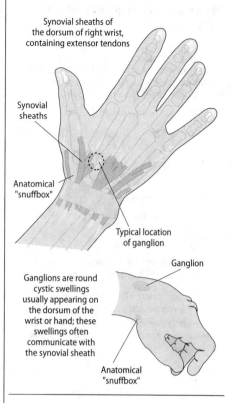

Synovial sheaths of the dorsum of right wrist, containing extensor tendons

Synovial sheaths

Anatomical "snuffbox"

Typical location of ganglion

Ganglion

Ganglions are round cystic swellings usually appearing on the dorsum of the wrist or hand; these swellings often communicate with the synovial sheath

Anatomical "snuffbox"

M67.5-   Plica syndrome

Synovial plica refers to a fold in the synovial tissue formed before birth, creating a septum or membrane between two pockets of synovial tissue. The most common are the medial patellar plica and the suprapatellar plica. Plica syndrome, or plica knee, refers to symptomatic plica from irritation and inflammation.

Other Soft Tissue Disorders (M70-M79)

This section represents other disorders of bursa, which is the fluid-filled sac located between articulating surfaces that reduce friction from the moving parts. Also located here are various other disorders of tendons, synovium, and generalized soft tissue.

The categories in this code block are as follows:

M70	Soft tissue disorders related to use, overuse and pressure
M71	Other bursopathies
M72	Fibroblastic disorders
M75	Shoulder lesions
M76	Enthesopathies, lower limb, excluding foot
M77	Other enthesopathies
M79	Other and unspecified soft tissue disorders, not elsewhere classified

M70.- Soft tissue disorders related to use, overuse and pressure

This category represents bursitis and other soft tissue disorders that are only specifically due to use, overuse, or pressure, and not due to other causes.

M70.1- Bursitis of hand

M70.2- Olecranon bursitis

M70.3- Other bursitis of elbow

M70.4- Prepatellar bursitis

M70.5- Other bursitis of knee

M70.6- Trochanteric bursitis

M70.7- Other bursitis of hip

Bursitis is inflammation of the bursae that cushion the bones, tendons, and muscles near the joints. It can be painful and most often affects joints that perform repetitive movements like shoulder, hip, and elbow. These codes are specific to bursitis that is caused by use, overuse, or pressure.

> **Focus Point**
>
> Bursitis NOS is not coded here. The appropriate code for bursitis NOS is M71.9 Bursopathy, unspecified.

M71.- Other bursopathies

This category identifies conditions of the bursa, such as abscess, infection, cysts, calcium deposits, and synovial cysts.

M71.2- Synovial cyst of popliteal space [Baker]

A synovial cyst of the popliteal space may also be called a Baker's cyst or popliteal cyst. In children, Baker's cysts are common but are usually asymptomatic and regress spontaneously. In adults, Baker's cysts, in conjunction with synovial effusion due to rheumatoid arthritis or degenerative joint disease, may produce significant impairment. When a Baker's cyst interferes with normal knee function, surgical exploration and excision of the cyst is indicated.

M72.- Fibroblastic disorders

Fibroblasts are the main cells that make the extracellular matrix and collagen that forms the fiber of the connective soft tissue. This category includes conditions such as Dupuytren, knuckle pads, plantar fascial fibromatosis, pseudosarcomatous fibromatosis, and necrotizing fasciitis.

M72.0 Palmar fascial fibromatosis [Dupuytren]

This condition occurs when the type of cell (fibroblast) that is responsible for making the extracellular matrix and collagen creates an excess, causing benign nodules and pain of the hands; not associated with contractures.

M72.1 Knuckle pads

Knuckle pads are pea-size nodules on the dorsal surface of the interphalangeal joints with new growth of fibrous tissue with thickened dermis and epidermis.

M72.2 Plantar fascial fibromatosis

This condition occurs when the fibroblast cell—the type of cell that is responsible for making the extracellular matrix and collagen—creates an excess, causing benign nodules and pain of the foot; not associated with contractures. This code also includes plantar fasciitis, an inflammation and irritation of the plantar fascia, which is the large band of fascia that supports the arch. Repetitive stretching and tension creates small tears to the fascia causing pain in the heel.

M72.6 Necrotizing fasciitis

This condition occurs when a bacterial, fulminating infection of the fascia spreads to deep fascia and causes thrombosis of subcutaneous vessels and gangrene of underlying tissue. It is rapidly progressing and moves along the fascial plane.

M75.- Shoulder lesions

This category identifies conditions of the soft tissue of the shoulder such as adhesive capsulitis, nontraumatic rotator cuff tear or rupture, tendinitis, impingement syndrome, and bursitis.

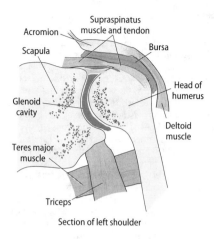

Section of left shoulder

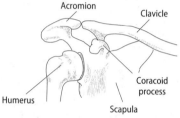

The fibrous capsule enclosing the shoulder is thin and loose to allow freedom of movement; four rotator cuff muscles (supraspinatus, infraspinatus, teres minor, and scapularis) work together to hold the head of the humerus in the glenoid cavity

M75.0- Adhesive capsulitis of shoulder

Adhesive capsulitis of the shoulder, also called frozen shoulder syndrome and Duplay's bursitis or periarthritis, is characterized by development of diffuse inflammation of the glenohumeral joint capsule with subsequent adherence of the inflamed capsule to the humeral head. Contracture due to the shrunken, adherent capsule prevents motion in the glenohumeral joint; that is, the joint is "frozen" in one position. Therapies include arthroscopic lavage, distension, and instillation of cortisone.

M75.1- Rotator cuff tear or rupture, not specified as traumatic

Rotator cuff tear or rupture is a disorder of the ligamentous or muscular attachments of the shoulder joint involving the rotator cuff. The rotator cuff is a musculotendinous structure that blends with the joint capsule and is attached to the humerus. The supraspinatus is the major muscle that contributes to the formation of the rotator cuff. The rotator cuff is comprised of four muscles and several tendons that form a covering around the humeral head and stabilize it within the shoulder joint, while enabling the arms to

rotate. Nontraumatic rotator cuff tears are often the result of years of cumulative overuse, and are often associated with other chronic shoulder conditions, such as arthritis and bone spur. As such, nontraumatic rotator cuff tear is prevalent in persons 40 years or older, whereas traumatic rotator cuff tear most commonly affects a younger population. People who engage in repetitive overhead motions, such as baseball, tennis, rowing, and weight lifting, are at an increased risk for overuse injury.

M75.11- Incomplete rotator cuff tear or rupture not specified as traumatic

An incomplete or partial rotator cuff tear involves an area of damage to the rotator cuff tendons that appears as a fraying of an otherwise intact tendon.

M75.12- Complete rotator cuff tear or rupture not specified as traumatic

A complete rotator cuff tear is a through-and-through hole or tear that may remain attached to the humeral head or may involve partial or complete detachment of the tendon from the bone. Consequently, the degree of attachment often corresponds to the level of impairment.

> **Focus Point**
>
> *A rotator cuff tear can be traumatic, degenerative, or nontraumatic in nature. Only rotator cuff tears that are degenerative or nontraumatic in nature are reported here. Current acute rotator cuff tears are reported with codes from Chapter 19.*

M75.3- Calcific tendinitis of shoulder

This condition is the buildup of macroscopic deposits of hydroxyapatite (crystalline calcium phosphate) in the tendon of the shoulder. In contrast to degenerative tendinitis, calcific may resolve and the tendon may heal spontaneously.

M75.5- Bursitis of shoulder

Bursitis is an inflammation of the bursae that cushion the bones, tendons, and muscles near the joints. It can be painful and most often affects joints that perform repetitive movements like the shoulder.

M76.- Enthesopathies, lower limb, excluding foot

Enthesopathies are diseases or disorders that affect the enthesis of the joint. The enthesis is the site in the joint where ligaments, tendons and muscles, the joint capsule, and bones join. It also refers to the nearby structures such as bursae, surrounding adipose tissue, and bone where the structures meet. This category includes inflammations, tendinitis, bursitis, and bone spurs of the enthesis of the hip and leg structures.

M77.- Other enthesopathies

Enthesopathy is a disorder of the tendon, muscle, or ligament insertions to bone. It also refers to the nearby structures such as bursae, surrounding adipose tissue, and bone where the structures meet. This category classifies enthesopathies affecting the elbow (medial and lateral epicondylitis), wrist (periarthritis), heel (calcaneal spur), metatarsals (metatarsalgia), and other enthesopathies affecting other sites in the foot.

M79.- Other and unspecified soft tissue disorders, not elsewhere classified

This category identifies many conditions of the soft tissue that involve pain such as rheumatism, myalgia, neuralgia, panniculitis, pain, and fibromyalgia. Fibromyalgia is a chronic disorder that presents as widespread body pain and tenderness in addition to fatigue and issues with memory, mood, and sleep disturbance. Other conditions located in this category are residual foreign body, hypertrophy of (infrapatellar) fat pad, and nontraumatic compartment syndrome.

M79.1 Myalgia

Myalgia refers to muscle aches and pain that can involve ligaments, tendons, and fascia, the soft tissues that connect muscles, bones, and organs. Myalgia may be temporary or chronic and is often a symptom of another underlying condition. Report this code only when the cause of the myalgia is not known. Treatment includes ibuprofen, acetaminophen, massage, and alternating heat and cold packs to alleviate pain.

Focus Point

When myalgia is due to trauma, such as a muscle strain or another documented condition such as influenza, the myalgia is considered a symptom and is not reported additionally.

M79.2 Neuralgia and neuritis, unspecified

Neuralgia is defined as paroxysmal pain along a nerve. Symptoms include brief pain and tenderness at the point in which the nerve exits. Neuritis is inflamed nerves. Symptoms include paresthesia, paralysis, and loss of reflexes at the nerve site.

M79.3 Panniculitis, unspecified

Panniculitis, unspecified, is inflammation of subcutaneous fat. The term often is used solely to refer to an inflammation of the panniculus adiposa of the abdominal wall.

Focus Point

Many variations of panniculitis, such as erythema nodosum (tuberculous and nontuberculous) and erythema pernio, are classified elsewhere.

M79.A- Nontraumatic compartment syndrome

Compartment syndrome occurs when swelling of the muscle within the muscle compartment causes pressure to increase constricting the muscles, blood vessels, and nerves. Muscle groups in the arms and legs are separated by fascia or thick layers of tissue. Inside each layer of fascia is a compartment, a limited space containing muscle tissue, nerves, and blood vessels. Fascia does not expand; therefore, any swelling within a compartment results in increased pressure. Sufficiently high pressure blocks blood flow to the compartment, potentially leading to permanent injury to the muscle and nerves. If the pressure persists, the limb may become necrotic and require amputation. Nontraumatic compartment syndrome can have numerous underlying causes. Most often occurring in the lower leg or forearm, compartment syndrome may also occur in other sites such as the hand, foot, thigh, upper arm, abdomen, or buttock. Repetitive activities such as running or other forms of vigorous exercise or sports can result in a form of compartment syndrome known as exertional compartment syndrome. Prognosis for compartment syndrome depends largely on the underlying cause. If the condition is diagnosed and treated promptly, there is an excellent chance of recovery of the muscles and nerves within the compartment. However, delayed diagnosis can result in permanent nerve injury and loss of muscle function; this can occur after 12 to 24 hours of compression. In the most severe cases, amputation may be required.

Disorders of Bone Density and Structure (M80-M85)

The composition of bone consists mainly of collagen fibers and an inorganic bone mineral in the form of small crystals. A bone consists of two tissue types, the difference between which is seen only microscopically. Compact bone, also known as cortical bone, is tightly packed tissue with minimal gaps and spaces. Spongy or cancellous bone looks disorganized with what appears to be random gaps and holes in the tissue. The bones also produce and house a highly specialized connective tissue called bone marrow. There are two types of bone marrow: yellow and red. Yellow bone marrow stores fat for the body and is found mainly in the hollow spaces in the long bones of adults. Blood cell formation occurs in red bone marrow, which is primarily stored in spongy bone. Bones can be classified into five major categories: long, short, flat, irregular, and sesamoid.

The external surfaces of all bone types have visible bulges, depressions, and holes for various physiological purposes, including providing sites for muscle, ligament, and tendon attachment to passageways for blood vessels and nerves. Some of the more commonly referred to markings for the purposes of coding are:

- **Condyle**: Rounded process that articulates with another bone.

- **Epicondyle**: Raised area on or above a condyle.

- **Facet**: Smooth surface that articulates with another bone.

- **Foramen**: Round opening through a bone.

- **Process**: Prominent projection.

- **Trochanter**: Very large, blunt process (found only on the femurs).

- **Tubercle**: Small rounded process.

- **Tuberosity**: Large rounded process.

The categories in this code block are as follows:

M80	Osteoporosis with current pathological fracture
M81	Osteoporosis without current pathological fracture
M83	Adult osteomalacia
M84	Disorder of continuity of bone
M85	Other disorders of bone density and structure

M80.- Osteoporosis with current pathological fracture

Osteoporosis is generalized bone disease characterized by decreased osteoblastic formation of matrix combined with increased osteoclastic resorption of bone, resulting in a marked decrease in bone mass. Osteoporosis often presents with osteopenia, which is a decrease in bone mineralization. A pathological fracture occurs at a site weakened by preexisting disease in this case due to osteoporosis. These fractures are often differentiated from traumatic fractures by clinically assessing the magnitude of the trauma or stress causing the fracture. A relatively minor trauma or stress can cause a pathological fracture in bones diseased by osteoporosis.

Focus Point

Osteopenia is reported with codes in subcategory M85.8-.

M81.- Osteoporosis without current pathological fracture

Osteoporosis is generalized bone disease characterized by decreased osteoblastic formation of matrix combined with increased osteoclastic resorption of bone, resulting in a marked decrease in bone mass. Osteoporosis often presents with osteopenia, which is a decrease in bone mineralization. Signs and symptoms of osteoporosis include chronic and intermittent back pain (due to vertebral microfractures), skeletal remodeling such as dorsal kyphosis, or loss of height. Radiographs and bone scans determine the extent and severity of osteoporosis and osteopenia and may reveal fresh or old evidence of pathological fractures. Quantitative computed tomography (CT) and single and dual energy x-ray absorptiometry (DEXA) measure bone density, and bone biopsy occasionally is done for histological studies. The fourth character identifies whether the osteoporosis is age-related, localized, or another form, including drug induced, posttraumatic, post-oophorectomy, or postsurgical malabsorption osteoporosis.

Focus Point

Osteopenia is reported with codes in subcategory M85.8-.

M83.- Adult osteomalacia

Osteomalacia is characterized by the softening of bones usually by the lack of or inability to absorb vitamin D and phosphates. The bone building process can be disrupted by certain gastro-surgeries, diseases, drugs, or disorders of the kidney or liver, all of which can hinder the absorption of vitamin D or certain minerals necessary to complete the bone building process. The main causes of osteomalacia are differentiated by subcategories identifying whether the osteomalacia is puerperal, senile, or due to malabsorption or malnutrition. The subcategories also include less common causes of aluminum toxicity or other drug induced. Other and unspecified codes are also included.

Focus Point

Even though osteomalacia and osteoporosis can lead to bone fractures, osteomalacia is the result of dysfunction in the bone development process while osteoporosis is the weakening of previously fully-developed bone.

M84.- Disorder of continuity of bone

This category identifies stress fractures and pathological fractures. It is important to differentiate between them. Pathological fractures occur when the bone is weakened by a specific disease process, such as neoplasm or osteoporosis with minimal or even no trauma involved. Stress fractures are incurred on healthy bones weakened by repetitive stress or repeated trauma to the same location.

Focus Point

Combination codes for pathological fractures due to osteoporosis are located in category M80 Osteoporosis with current pathological fracture. This category identifies pathological fractures due to other disease processes.

M84.3- Stress fracture

Also called a fatigue fracture, the etiology is from repetitive stress or "trivial" repeated trauma to an area. This code should not be used for acute, traumatic fracture. This subcategory also includes the "march fracture," which is a stress fracture of the distal metatarsals, common in the military from repetitive stress, but also occurs in any profession that requires excessive standing.

M84.4- Pathological fracture, not elsewhere classified

M84.5- Pathological fracture in neoplastic disease

M84.6- Pathological fracture in other disease

A pathological fracture can occur at a site weakened by preexisting disease. These fractures are often differentiated from traumatic fractures by clinically assessing the magnitude of the trauma or stress causing the fracture. A relatively minor trauma or stress can cause a pathological fracture in bones diseased by metabolic bone disease, disseminated bone disorders, inflammatory bone diseases, Paget's disease, neoplasms, or any other condition that can compromise bone strength and integrity. Pathologic fractures are also referred to as chronic fractures due to the chronic nature of the underlying disease processes.

Focus Point

Excluded from these pathological fracture codes are pathological fractures due to osteoporosis (M84.3-) and stress fractures that are from repetitive stress.

M84.7- Nontraumatic fracture, not elsewhere classified

Atypical femoral fractures are currently the only fractures classified at this subcategory. Although they resemble stress or pathological fractures, the unique mechanics and characteristics of atypical femoral fractures do not clearly identify them as one or the other.

M84.75- Atypical femoral fracture

The diagnosis of atypical femoral fracture (AFF) is one of "exclusion," meaning that the fracture *cannot* be high-trauma, of the femoral neck, intertrochanteric with spiral subtrochanteric extension, associated with primary or metastatic bone tumors, or periprosthetic. Studies are underway to evaluate the relationship between these distinct fractures and the use of bisphosphonate (BP) therapy.

The American Society for Bone and Mineral Research (ASBMR) has described specific features that distinguish femoral fractures as atypical. The list consists of prominent characteristics that must all be present to classify the fracture as an AFF and minor characteristics that are not required but are regularly associated with this type of fracture. The prominent characteristics include:

- Fracture location at any point between the lesser trochanter and the supracondylar flare

- Fracture configuration of a transverse or short oblique nature

- Fracture that is noncomminuted

- Fracture that is nontraumatic

- Complete fracture traversing both cortices versus incomplete fracture traversing only the lateral cortex

The codes in this subcategory embody a good majority of the characteristics described above with specific codes created for complete transverse, complete oblique, and incomplete fracture presentations.

M85.- Other disorders of bone density and structure

This category identifies conditions related to the structure and density of bone such as fibrous dysplasia, skeletal fluorosis, osteitis condensans, hyperostosis of skull, and bone cysts.

M85.0- Fibrous dysplasia (monostotic)

Fibrous dysplasia is a bone disorder that occurs when bone is replaced by a fibrous tissue that can weaken or deform the affected bone. It typically affects a single bone and is a genetic disorder affecting children and young adults.

M85.1- Skeletal fluorosis

Skeletal fluorosis is bone damage, weakness, and pain caused by prolonged or excessive exposure to fluoride, which can accumulate in the bones.

M85.2 Hyperostosis of skull

Also referred to as hyperostosis interna frontalis or Leontiasis ossium, this is an abnormal bone growth on the inner aspect of the cranial bones.

M85.3- Osteitis condensans

Also referred to as piriform sclerosis of ilium, this is an idiopathic condition marked by low back pain; it is associated with oval or triangular sclerotic, opaque bone next to the sacroiliac joints in the ilium.

M85.5- Aneurysmal bone cyst

An aneurysmal bone cyst is a solitary bone lesion that bulges into the periosteum and is marked by a calcified rim.

Other Osteopathies (M86-M90)

This section represents various disease processes and disorders of the bones, both of an infectious and noninfective nature.

The categories in this code block are as follows:

M86	Osteomyelitis
M87	Osteonecrosis
M88	Osteitis deformans [Paget's disease of bone]
M89	Other disorders of bone
M90	Osteopathies in diseases classified elsewhere

M86.- Osteomyelitis

Osteomyelitis, periostitis, and other infections involving bone is a broad spectrum of bone infections. Osteomyelitis is an inflammation of bone and bone marrow. The condition is commonly due to a pathogen such as bacteria, virus, protozoa, or fungus. Periostitis is an inflammation of the periosteum, the thick fibrous membrane covering all of the surfaces of bones except at the articular cartilage. The combination of osteomyelitis and periostitis is periosteomyelitis. Signs and symptoms of osteomyelitis, periostitis, and other infections involving bone include pain and unwillingness to move the affected area and, occasionally, malaise, fever, chills, and anorexia. Sometimes the site of infection closest to the surface may be detected by palpation. Therapies include long-term antibiotic therapy and surgery to incise and drain the involved area and remove necrotic debris in severe acute cases. Other surgery includes sequestrectomy, excision of multiple sinus tracts, craterization, saucerization, partial excision of bone, and bone grafting for chronic osteomyelitis. Periostitis is included in the osteomyelitis codes.

M86.0- Acute hematogenous osteomyelitis

Hematogenous osteomyelitis (acute) is a form of osteomyelitis common to children where blood-borne organisms settle in the metaphyseal vascular bed of the rapidly developing long bones.

M86.9 Osteomyelitis, unspecified

This is the appropriate code to use for periostitis that occurs without osteomyelitis. Periostitis is an inflammation of the periosteum, the thick fibrous membrane covering all of the surfaces of bones except at the articular cartilage.

M87.- Osteonecrosis

Osteonecrosis can be used to describe a wide variety of disorders, infectious and noninfectious, resulting in the death of bone tissue or bone infarction. The cause may be undetermined (idiopathic) or due to specific noninfectious etiologies, such as fractures (avascular necrosis due to fracture), ischemic disorders, and immunosuppressive agents such as corticosteroids following renal transplants.

M87.180 Osteonecrosis due to drugs, jaw

Osteonecrosis of the jaw (ONJ) is defined by the American Association of Oral and Maxillofacial Surgeons (AAOMS) as "any patient who has not received radiation therapy to the oral cavity or neck, and who has exposed bone in the maxillofacial area that occurred spontaneously or following dental surgery and has no evidence of healing for more than three to six weeks after appropriate care." A potential relationship between osteonecrosis of the jaw (ONJ) and the use of bisphosphonates and other medications is being studied in the oral and maxillofacial surgery (OMS) patient population. Common bisphosphonates include Fosamax, Zometa, Aredia, Actonel, and Boniva.

Focus Point

Osteonecrosis differs from osteoradionecrosis (M27.2), which is caused by radiation therapy.

M88.- Osteitis deformans [Paget's disease of bone]

Osteitis deformans is a disseminated bone disorder also known as Paget's disease. Characterized by slow and progressive enlargement and deformity of multiple bones, Paget's disease is associated with unexplained acceleration of deposition and resorption of bone. During the early (osteolytic) phase of the disease, resorption exceeds deposition, and the bone, although enlarged, becomes sponge-like, weakened, and deformed. The second (osteosclerotic) phase is marked by deposition exceeding resorption resulting in the bones becoming thick and dense. The disease sometimes is associated with an invariably fatal form of malignant osteogenic sarcoma as a result of hyperactive osteoblast activity. Etiology is unknown, but there is some evidence that it may be triggered by a "slow virus" that affects primarily the osteoclasts.

M89.- Other disorders of bone

This chapter represents conditions of the bone such algoneurodystrophy, physial arrest, hypertrophy, osteolysis, osteopathy after poliomyelitis, and major osseous defect.

M89.0- Algoneurodystrophy

This condition, also referred to as shoulder-hand syndrome, is a result of a dysfunction related to the sympathetic nerve supply. Shoulder-hand syndrome involves a painful, red, swollen hand and forearm along with a stiff and painful shoulder. Eventually the pain subsides but the muscles atrophy and severe osteoporosis sets in. Left untreated, the hand becomes functionally useless and cyanotic.

M89.5- Osteolysis

Osteolysis is characterized by bone that is thin, weak, and suffering from bone erosion by the resorption of bone by osteoclasts faster than it can be replaced or repaired. It can be caused by excessive use or can be associated with other bone or joint diseases and disorders.

Focus Point

Osteolysis is becoming a common complication of joint replacements. The appropriate code for this complication (T84.05-) is located in Chapter 19 Injury, Poisoning and Certain Other Consequences of External Causes.

M89.7- Major osseous defect

Major osseous defects are conditions that occur as a result of extensive bone loss. Underlying causes for osseous defects are varied. They may or may not be associated with previous joint replacement, and may include osteomyelitis, osteoporosis, pathological fractures, trauma, or benign or malignant neoplasms. One of the most common causes of major osseous defect, however, is periprosthetic osteolysis from a previous joint replacement.

Chondropathies (M91-M94)

Chondropathies are diseases or conditions that affect the cartilage. Cartilage is tough, but flexible connective tissue with no nerves or blood vessels that covers joints and bones and gives structure to other areas of the body like nose and ears. There are three types: hyaline, the most common and weakest is made from fine collagen fibers and found in ribs, nose, trachea and larynx; fibro, the strongest is found in joint capsules, ligaments, and intervertebral discs; and elastic, which is found in the external ear, larynx, and epiglottis.

The categories in this code block are as follows:

M91	Juvenile osteochondrosis of hip and pelvis
M92	Other juvenile osteochondrosis
M93	Other osteochondropathies
M94	Other disorders of cartilage

M91.- Juvenile osteochondrosis of hip and pelvis

This category breaks down various deformities due to juvenile osteochondrosis that affect the hip and pelvic bones. It includes coxa plana, which is a flattening of the head of the femur, and coxa magna, which is an abnormal widening of the head and neck of the femur.

M91.1- Juvenile osteochondrosis of head of femur [Legg-Calve-Perthes]

This hip disorder is due to an interruption of the blood supply to the growing femoral head (avascular necrosis). Indications can include coxa magna and/or coxa plana, arrest of physial growth, short femoral neck, and collapse or fragmentation of femoral epiphysis. It occurs in children between ages 4 and 8, affecting boys more than girls. The etiology for the interruption is unknown. Children with this condition are at higher risk of developing arthritis at a young age unless treated early.

M92.- Other juvenile osteochondrosis

Osteochondrosis is a group of disorders that directly affect bone and cartilage growth of children and adolescents.

M92.4- Juvenile osteochondrosis of patella

Also called Sinding-Larsen-Johansson, this self-limiting, inflammatory condition occurs at the inferior pole of the patella. It is a common cause of knee pain usually affecting children between 10 and 13 years of age, most of whom are involved in athletic activities. It is exacerbated by jumping and direct pressure.

M92.5- Juvenile osteochondrosis of tibia and fibula

Also called Osgood-Schlatter, this condition is an inflammatory disorder found in children and a common cause of anterior knee pain exacerbated by kneeling or activities causing stress or direct pressure to the patellar tendon on the tibial tubercle.

M93.- Other osteochondropathies

This category includes disorders such as slipped epiphysis, Kienböck's disease, and osteochondritis dissecans.

M93.2- Osteochondritis dissecans

Osteochondritis dissecans is a form of osteochondropathy in which the convex surfaces of certain pressure epiphyses are susceptible to avascular necrosis. When a small tangential segment of subchondral bone becomes separated or "dissected" from the remaining portion of the epiphysis by reactive fibrous and granulation tissue, it is designated as osteochondritis or osteochondrosis dissecans.

M94.-   Other disorders of cartilage

This category represents conditions affecting the cartilage, including chondrocostal junction syndrome (Tietze), relapsing polychondritis, chondromalacia, and chondrolysis.

M94.0   Chondrocostal junction syndrome [Tietze]

Costochondral junction syndrome, also called Tietze's disease, is a rare, inflammatory disorder, characterized by chest pain radiating to the arms or shoulder and a localized swelling at the junction of the ribs and sternum. Tietze's disease generally has a sudden onset without any preceding respiratory illness or any history of minor trauma. The condition typically lasts for several months.

M94.2-   Chondromalacia

This condition is described as deterioration or softening of cartilage.

M94.26-   Chondromalacia, knee

Also known as runner's knee, this is the most common site of chondromalacia and occurs when the cartilage on the underside of the patella that cushions the knee begins to deteriorate. It is common in young athletes or older adults with knee arthritis.

Other Disorders of the Musculoskeletal System and Connective Tissue (M95)

This code block includes the codes for acquired deformity of nose, head, neck, chest, rib, pelvis, and other acquired deformities of the musculoskeletal system.

Periprosthetic Fracture Around Internal Prosthetic Joint (M97)

A periprosthetic fracture is one that occurs at or near the site of a joint prosthesis. Periprosthetic fractures may be the result of trauma or may occur due to underlying bone disease such as osteoporosis or tumor. While the fractures may occur around any prosthesis, they are most commonly seen at joint replacement sites of the hip, knee, ankle, shoulder, or elbow. Most cases require surgical correction and may utilize a new prosthetic device.

Biomechanical Lesions, Not Elsewhere Classified (M99)

"Biomechanical lesions" is the term used to describe conditions treated by osteopathic and chiropractic physicians. The biomechanical lesions category includes musculoskeletal conditions such as segmental and somatic dysfunction, chiropractic subluxation (misalignment) and subluxation complex, and certain types of neural canal and intervertebral foramina stenosis, as well as other and unspecified biomechanical lesions that cannot be more appropriately classified to a more specific code. The chiropractic definition of subluxation refers to a misalignment and differs from the medical definition classified elsewhere. This terminology often describes an altered anatomical state occurring within the musculoskeletal system, such as structural deviations, misalignments, or certain stenoses. The bones, muscles, fascia, ligaments, discs, related nerves, and vessels may be affected, resulting in impaired function. Associated symptoms may include pain, inflammation, tenderness, muscle spasms, rigidity, and tension. These conditions may or may not be readily identified upon diagnostic imaging; however, the mechanical nature of the associated dysfunction and manifestations in the body often require further assessment or diagnosis.

Chapter 14: Diseases of the Genitourinary System (NØØ-N99)

This chapter classifies diseases and disorders of the reproductive system and the urinary system, collectively known as the genitourinary system. The urinary system is comprised of two kidneys, two ureters, the bladder, two sphincter muscles, and the urethra. The reproductive system is a series of organs found around the pelvic region, primarily outside the body in males and primarily inside the body in females, as well as the male and female breasts. Although the organs and structures differ between the male and female reproductive systems, their collective purpose is for sexual reproduction.

The chapter is broken down into the following code blocks:

NØØ-NØ8   Glomerular diseases

N10-N16   Renal tubulo-interstitial diseases

N17-N19   Acute kidney failure and chronic kidney disease

N20-N23   Urolithiasis

N25-N29   Other disorders of kidney and ureter

N30-N39   Other diseases of the urinary system

N40-N53   Diseases of male genital organs

N60-N65   Disorders of breast

N70-N77   Inflammatory diseases of female pelvic organs

N80-N98   Noninflammatory disorders of female genital tract

N99   Intraoperative and postprocedural complications and disorders of genitourinary system, not elsewhere classified

Glomerular Diseases (NØØ-NØ8)

Glomeruli are clusters of microscopic blood vessels located within the kidneys containing small pores through which waste products are filtered from the blood and urine is formed. A large number of conditions within the urinary system affect the glomeruli and hinder the filtering efficacy of the kidneys. The most common conditions that affect the glomeruli are two very similar sounding syndromes: nephritic syndrome and nephrotic syndrome. While both syndromes result from damage to the glomeruli, the primary symptoms characterizing the two syndromes are different.

Nephritic syndrome is characterized by blood in the urine (hematuria); reduced urine output (oliguria); elevated blood urea nitrogen (BUN) and elevated serum creatinine levels, collectively called azotemia; and elevated blood pressure (hypertension).

Nephrotic syndrome is characterized by massive amounts of protein in the urine (proteinuria), low blood protein levels (hypoalbuminemia), excessive fluid in body tissues (edema), and elevated blood cholesterol and triglyceride levels (hyperlipidemia).

The categories in this code block are as follows:

NØØ   Acute nephritic syndrome

NØ1   Rapidly progressive nephritic syndrome

NØ2   Recurrent and persistent hematuria

NØ3   Chronic nephritic syndrome

NØ4   Nephrotic syndrome

NØ5   Unspecified nephritic syndrome

NØ6   Isolated proteinuria with specified morphological lesion

NØ7   Hereditary nephropathy, not elsewhere classified

NØ8   Glomerular disorders in diseases classified elsewhere

With the exception of category NØ8, each 4th character in this code block identifies the specific type of glomerulonephritis based on the structural or morphological changes occurring in the glomeruli. The applicable 4th characters and their definitions are as follows:

Ø   minor glomerular abnormality

Minor glomerular abnormality, also referred to as minimal change disease, is a diagnosis that is typically based on abnormal laboratory values such as an increase in lipids and proteins in the urine while microscopic examination shows no visible changes or very subtle changes to the glomeruli.

1   focal and segmental glomerular lesions

Focal and segmental glomerular lesions, also referred to as focal and segmental glomerulosclerosis (FSGS), refers to scar tissue (sclerosis) that has formed in the glomeruli. Focal indicates that only some of the glomeruli are involved. Segmental indicates that only a part of an individual glomerulus has been damaged.

2   diffuse membranous glomerulonephritis

Diffuse membranous glomerulonephritis (GN) is the result of widespread thickening of the glomerular basement membrane caused by immune complex formation in the glomeruli. As the basement membrane thickens it loses its filtering capacity, which results in an increase in protein lost in the urine. As this condition progresses, the kidneys degenerate (waste away). Typically, this specific type of manifestation is associated with cancer, but it also can arise spontaneously without any known cause.

3   diffuse mesangial proliferative glomerulonephritis

Mesangial proliferative glomerulonephritis, also called diffuse mesangial proliferation, is a rare form of GN. Characteristics of this manifestation include blood in the urine caused by a particular type of inflammation inside the kidneys. Abnormalities within the immune system can lead to abnormal immune deposits in the mesangial cells, which are specialized cells of smooth muscle origin that surround and support the capillaries inside the kidneys. As a result, the mesangial cells become bigger and their numbers increase.

4   diffuse endocapillary proliferative glomerulonephritis

Diffuse endocapillary proliferative GN occurs when there is an overproduction of mesangial, endothelial, and inflammatory cells. Along with the cellular proliferation, edema of the endothelial cells also occurs, which results in occlusion or blockage of capillary lumens.

5   diffuse mesangiocapillary glomerulonephritis

Mesangiocapillary GN or membranoproliferative GN occurs when there is an increase in mesangial cells in the glomeruli along with thickening of the capillary walls.

6   dense deposit disease

This pattern of glomerular injury is characterized by thick or closely packed endothelial cells in the glomerular basement membrane. A key player in the development of dense deposit disease (DDD) is nephritic factor; however, the exact pathogenesis of DDD is not yet understood.

7   diffuse crescentic glomerulonephritis

The crescentic description is attributed to pathological findings, after biopsy, of extensive glomerular injury accompanied by crescent shaped scars. This characteristic is due to extracapillary proliferation of the epithelial cells in the Bowman's space. This may also be documented as extracapillary proliferative GN.

8   other morphologic changes

This 4th character identifies morphological changes to the glomeruli that cannot be classified to a more specific 4th-character subclassification.

9   unspecified morphologic changes

This 4th character identifies glomeruli changes that are not better defined in the documentation or cannot be classified to one of the more specific 4th characters above.

N00.-   Acute nephritic syndrome

Acute nephritic syndrome, also called acute glomerulonephritis (AGN), is a grouping of renal diseases caused by a number of immunologic reactions that cause inflammation and proliferation of glomerular tissue. Proliferation is defined as a rapid reproduction of tissue. This condition often presents with the sudden onset of blood or protein in the urine, known as hematuria or proteinuria, respectively, along with red blood cells. Hypertension, edema (swelling due to fluid retention), and impaired renal function are also characteristic symptoms. In AGN, the disease process involves deposition of immune complexes in the glomeruli. Immune complexes are clusters of antigens and antibodies that are locked together. Basically antibodies attach directly to the kidney cells or to antigens outside of the kidney and are then carried to the kidney through the bloodstream. The antigens get trapped in the glomeruli, causing inflammation. When enough of the glomeruli are damaged, blood filtering is decreased and waste products build up in the blood. Scarring may develop, which also impairs filtering. As a result, the kidneys become enlarged and may increase to twice the size of normal kidneys.

> **Focus Point**
>
> *When acute glomerulonephritis does not heal within one to two years or when it progresses to chronic renal failure or chronic renal insufficiency, it is designated as chronic glomerulonephritis.*

N01.- Rapidly progressive nephritic syndrome

As the name implies, rapidly progressive nephritic syndrome is characterized by rapid deterioration of kidney function, usually a few weeks to a few months. Most patients who survive this condition develop chronic renal failure within two years.

N02.- Recurrent and persistent hematuria

Hematuria defined in this category is due to a glomerular cause but without specific nephritic syndrome characteristics. Hematuria is the presence of blood in the urine, which may be described as gross hematuria meaning visible blood in the urine or microscopic hematuria meaning the red blood cells are only visible under microscopy. Common characteristics of glomerular-related hematuria include gross hematuria with brown or cola-colored urine, proteinuria, and misshapen RBCs upon examination.

N03.- Chronic nephritic syndrome

Chronic nephritic syndrome is a slowly progressing disease characterized by chronic inflammation of the glomeruli resulting in sclerosis, scarring, and eventual chronic renal failure. Although any form of acute nephritic syndrome has the potential to progress to chronic, in some cases the disease may be progressing silently, over many years, before signs or symptoms appear.

N04.- Nephrotic syndrome

Nephrotic syndrome is caused by damage to the glomeruli, which results in massive amounts of protein being excreted in the urine accompanied by the accumulation of fluid in the body, low levels of protein albumin, and high levels of fats in the blood. Nephrotic syndrome can be congenital, primary (affecting only the kidneys), or secondary (caused by a disease process that affects other parts of the body such as diabetes mellitus or system lupus erythematosus). It may also be caused by viral infections or glomerulonephritis.

> **Focus Point**
>
> *Nephrotic syndrome that is congenital or hereditary is reported with codes in category N07 or with more specific codes in Chapter 17 Congenital Malformations, Deformations, and Chromosomal Abnormalities.*
>
> *Nephrotic syndrome that is secondary to another disease process is reported with codes in category N08 or with more specific codes for the underlying disease.*

N06.- Isolated proteinuria with specified morphological lesion

Proteinuria is defined by urinary protein excretion of greater than 150 mg per day. Proteinuria classified to this category is related to glomerular disease, its most common cause, but is lacking the pathophysiological characteristics to categorize it as a nephritic or nephrotic syndrome.

N07.- Hereditary nephropathy, not elsewhere classified

Nephropathy resulting from damage to glomeruli that is due to a congenital or hereditary disease is classified here.

N08 Glomerular disorders in diseases classified elsewhere

Glomerular disorders that are due to an underlying disease are classified here. Conditions that can cause glomerular disorders include acute and chronic conditions and range from systemic infections to blood disorders to malignant neoplasms.

Renal Tubulo-interstitial Diseases (N10-N16)

When kidney disease involves structures outside the glomerulus, it is broadly referred to as tubulointerstitial. A tubule is a small, fluid-filled collecting tube at the end of each glomerulus. The glomerulus and tubule unit combined is called a nephron, which is the functional unit of the kidneys. Each kidney contains approximately one million nephrons. The interstitial tissue is found around the tubules. Tubulointerstitial kidney disease can present as acute or chronic and has a number of different causes.

The categories in this code block are as follows:

N10	Acute pyelonephritis
N11	Chronic tubulo-interstitial nephritis
N12	Tubulo-interstitial nephritis, not specified as acute or chronic
N13	Obstructive and reflux uropathy
N14	Drug- and heavy-metal-induced tubulo-interstitial and tubular conditions
N15	Other renal tubulo-interstitial diseases
N16	Renal tubulo-interstitial disorders in diseases classified elsewhere

N10 Acute pyelonephritis

Acute pyelonephritis or acute tubulointerstitial nephritis (ATIN) is an inflammatory process that involves the tubules and interstitial tissue of the kidney. The acute condition is sudden in onset and may be triggered by bacterial infections such as streptococcus, staphylococcus, and salmonella; viral infections such as Epstein Barr, cytomegalovirus (CMV), and human immunodeficiency virus (HIV); and allergic reactions to medications or other substances. ATIN may lead to acute renal failure.

> **Focus Point**
>
> *Acute renal failure associated with acute pyelonephritis should be reported additionally with a code from category N17.*

N11.-   Chronic tubulo-interstitial nephritis

Chronic tubulointerstitial nephritis (CTIN) is most likely caused by repeated injuries to the tubules resulting in chronic inflammation of the tubules and interstitial tissue. CTIN is characterized by gradual interstitial infiltration and fibrosis, tubular atrophy and dysfunction, and a gradual deterioration of renal function, usually over years. Glomerular involvement (glomerulosclerosis) is also characteristic of the chronic forms of the disease. CTIN can be attributed to a number of causes, including hereditary renal diseases, exogenous or metabolic toxins, autoimmune disorders, infection, and neoplastic disorders.

N13.-   Obstructive and reflux uropathy

Obstructive uropathy is a blockage in a ureter that prevents urine from draining into the bladder. Because urine is prevented from draining into the bladder by the blockage, the kidney swells with urine, a condition referred to as hydronephrosis. The cause of obstructive uropathy may be intraluminal (within the ureter) or extraluminal (outside of the ureter). Reflux uropathy is the backward flow of urine which may involve reflux from the ureters to the kidneys and/or reflux from the bladder to the ureters. When reflux from the bladder to the ureters occurs, it is called vesicoureteral reflux. Reflux uropathy can cause swelling, scarring, and infection in the ureters and/or kidneys.

N13.0   Hydronephrosis with ureteropelvic junction obstruction

Ureteropelvic junction (UPJ) obstruction involves the blockage of urine passing from the kidney to the ureter, the most common site of the obstruction being at the renal pelvis. The obstruction may be due to a congenital abnormality, other related urinary disorders or previous surgery. When urine is blocked and held in the kidney over time, it can result in hydronephrosis, an enlargement of the renal pelvis, which carries a significant risk for long-term kidney damage. Treatment ranges from antibiotics for UTI prevention and close follow-up to pyeloplasty.

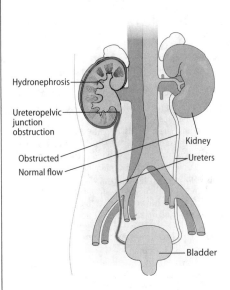

Hydronephrosis

Hydronephrosis

Ureteropelvic junction obstruction

Obstructed

Normal flow

Kidney

Ureters

Bladder

N13.1   Hydronephrosis with ureteral stricture, not elsewhere classified

A ureteral stricture is a narrowing of the ureter. The ureters are tubes that connect the kidneys to the bladder. This narrowing reduces the amount of urine that can flow into the bladder, leading reflux of urine from the ureter to the kidneys, which can cause swelling (hydronephrosis) of the kidneys. Scar formation, within the ureter itself or structures in the vicinity of the ureters, is the most common cause of ureteral stricture.

> **Focus Point**
>
> *Although a calculus (stone) does narrow the lumen of the ureter at the site of the calculus and may cause partial or complete obstruction of the ureter, the code for a ureteral stricture would only be used if there is damage to the ureter causing stricture following passage of the calculus.*

N13.2   Hydronephrosis with renal and ureteral calculous obstruction

A calculus or stone contained within the kidney or ureter can partially or completely obstruct the flow of urine. Most urinary tract calculi are composed of calcium salts or magnesium/ammonium phosphate and are idiopathic. Other calculi may be composed of cystine or uric acid, and are a result of a defect in urinary acidification. When the flow of urine is obstructed, the kidney can become distended with urine, a condition known as hydronephrosis.

N13.4   Hydroureter

Hydroureter is distension of the ureter with urine.

N13.5   Crossing vessel and stricture of ureter without hydronephrosis

Abnormally configured blood vessels adjacent to the ureter sometimes cross the ureter causing compression and narrowing of the ureter where the blood vessels cross. When this occurs without complete obstruction, urine is still able to drain from the kidneys, through the ureter, and into the bladder, although drainage of urine may be associated with pain. The patient may also note blood in the urine and may experience repeated urinary tract infections. This code reports narrowing of the ureter without distension of the kidney.

N13.6   Pyonephrosis

Pyonephrosis is an infection of the kidney, which in this case is associated with narrowing or obstruction of the ureter that impedes drainage of urine from the kidneys and ureters into the bladder. The infection may occur with or without distension of the kidney (hydronephrosis).

N13.7-   Vesicoureteral-reflux

Vesicoureteral-reflux (VUR) describes a condition in which urine flows backward from the bladder into one or both ureters. The normal flow of urine is one directional from the kidneys to the ureters to the bladder. Normally when the bladder is full, muscles contract to push the urine into the urethra to be expelled and a one-way valve at the junction of the ureters and bladder prevents reflux of urine back into the ureters. In reflux uropathy when the bladder muscles contract to expel urine, some urine is also pushed back into the ureters and/or kidneys due to an abnormality at the junction of the ureters and bladder. VUR is usually due to an abnormality at the junction of the ureters and bladder. Either the ureters do not tunnel through the bladder wall properly or the one-way valve does not function properly allowing reflux of urine.

Vesicoureteral Reflux

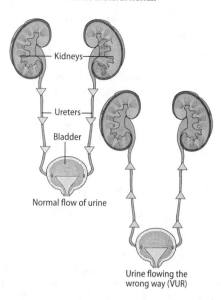

Normal flow of urine

Urine flowing the wrong way (VUR)

N13.71   Vesicoureteral-reflux without reflux nephropathy

Vesicoureteral-reflux (VUR) without associated damage or scarring to the kidneys caused by reflux of urine into the kidneys is captured by this code.

N13.72-   Vesicoureteral-reflux with reflux nephropathy without hydroureter

N13.73-   Vesicoureteral-reflux with reflux nephropathy with hydroureter

Vesicoureteral-reflux (VUR) may cause damage or scarring to the kidneys referred to as reflux nephropathy. Hydroureter is distention of the ureter with urine due to blockage or obstruction. VUR is classified as with or without hydroureter. It is also classified based on whether one (unilateral) or both (bilateral) ureters and kidneys are affected.

Acute Kidney Failure and Chronic Kidney Disease (N17-N19)

Acute kidney failure and chronic kidney disease (CKD) are not necessarily chronological conditions. Those who acquire acute kidney failure may have full recovery without permanent damage leading to a chronic renal condition. Likewise, CKD may not be preceded by a notable acute phase, with damage to the kidneys going unnoticed until other conditions, including some not associated with the kidneys, appear.

The categories in this code block are as follows:

N17   Acute kidney failure

N18   Chronic kidney disease (CKD)

N19   Unspecified kidney failure

N17.-   Acute kidney failure

Acute kidney (renal) failure is sudden interruption of renal function following any one of a variety of conditions that insult the normal kidney. Although usually reversible with treatment, acute kidney failure may progress to chronic renal insufficiency, chronic renal failure, or death. The causes of acute kidney failure are classified to prerenal, intrinsic (renal), or postrenal. Prerenal failure is due to diminished blood flow to the kidneys. Intrinsic failure results from diseases and disorders of the kidneys themselves. Postrenal failure is due to problems moving urine out of the kidneys.

N17.0   Acute kidney failure with tubular necrosis

Acute tubular necrosis is the most common intrinsic cause of acute renal failure. The tubules are structures within the kidney that filter waste and other products from the blood. Tubular necrosis occurs when cells that make up the tubules became irreversibly damaged and die, resulting in decreased function and less waste being filtered. Etiologies may involve vascular issues, glomerular conditions, and systemic diseases.

N17.1   Acute kidney failure with acute cortical necrosis

The renal cortex is the light red, smooth-textured, outer part of the kidney. Necrosis of the cortex occurs when small arteries that supply blood to the cortex are blocked causing ischemic lesions. Kidney function is often severely reduced but recovery can occur depending on the extent of the lesions. It is often seen as a complication in pregnancy.

N17.2   Acute kidney failure with medullary necrosis

The renal medulla is the darker reddish brown area found just inside the cortex of the kidney. It is made up of multiple cone-shaped renal pyramids. The base or wider end of each pyramid faces the renal cortex and its apex, also called the renal papillary, and the narrower portion points toward the renal hilum. Medullary or papillary necrosis occurs when the blood supply to these pyramids are blocked resulting in tissue death.

N18.-   Chronic kidney disease (CKD)

Chronic kidney (renal) disease is a multisystem disease due to a progressive loss of kidney function. It usually develops gradually as a consequence of a wide spectrum of diseases. Kidney function is primarily measured through the glomerular filtration rate (GFR) with lower numeric values representing more severe CKD. This measurement takes into account the patient's age, weight, sex, and race in combination with serum creatinine. Although a single GFR measurement at one point in time can indicate a disease process, the measurement is more effective in identifying the presence of kidney disease if measurements are taken on several occasions over an extended period of time. This establishes what is called a patient's baseline, a specific measurement for that patient that can be monitored regularly to determine whether the GFR is staying at the baseline or whether there are changes indicating rapid or slowly progressive decline in kidney function.

N18.1   Chronic kidney disease, stage 1

Stage 1 CKD involves some kidney damage but with normal or slightly increased GFR (>90).

N18.2   Chronic kidney disease, stage 2 (mild)

Stage 2 CKD involves a mild decrease in renal function. The GFR value is usually 60 to 89.

N18.3   Chronic kidney disease, stage 3 (moderate)

Stage 3 CKD is defined by a GFR value of 30 to 59.

N18.4   Chronic kidney disease, stage 4 (severe)

Stage 4 CKD is characterized by a GFR value of 15 to 29. At this stage, a nephrologist is required to manage the disease.

N18.5   Chronic kidney disease, stage 5

Stage 5 CKD is defined by a GFR value of less than 15. Management of the disease is not to the point of dialysis or transplant but the conversation and preparation for renal replacement therapies is starting and nephrologist intervention is essential.

N18.6   End stage renal disease

In the last stage of CKD, the kidneys can no longer function and a patient will not survive without dialysis or transplantation.

Urolithiasis (N20-N23)

Urolithiasis is the presence of a calculus or kidney stone in the urinary tract. Codes are specific to the site of the calculus, which may be located in the kidney (nephro-), ureter (uretero-), bladder (cysto-), or urethra. Most urinary tract calculi are composed of calcium salts or magnesium/ammonium phosphate and are idiopathic. Other calculi may be composed of cystine or uric acid and are a result of a defect in urinary acidification.

The categories in this code block are as follows:

N20	Calculus of kidney and ureter
N21	Calculus of lower urinary tract
N22	Calculus of urinary tract in diseases classified elsewhere
N23	Unspecified renal colic

N21.-   Calculus of lower urinary tract

The lower urinary tract includes the bladder, which stores the urine, and the urethra, a tube that transports the urine out of the body.

N21.0   Calculus in bladder

Bladder stones are usually the result of another urologic problem, such as a urinary tract infection, bladder diverticulum, neurogenic bladder, or an enlarged prostate. Approximately 95 percent of all bladder stones occur in men. Bladder stones can cause irritation and damage inside the urinary tract, and chronic irritation with bladder calculi predisposes the bladder to cancer.

Other Disorders of Kidney and Ureter (N25-N29)

The balance of fluid and chemicals in the body is largely dependent upon kidney function. The kidneys filter the blood, reabsorbing nutrients such as potassium, calcium, and hormones that are essential for healthy organ function and eliminate waste products contained in urine from the body. The ureters assist the kidneys in this process by draining urine and waste products into the bladder so that they can be expelled from the body.

The categories in this code block are as follows:

| N25 | Disorders resulting from impaired renal tubular function |

N26	Unspecified contracted kidney
N27	Small kidney of unknown cause
N28	Other disorders of kidney and ureter, not elsewhere classified
N29	Other disorders of kidney and ureter in diseases classified elsewhere

N25.-   Disorders resulting from impaired renal tubular function

The primary function of the renal tubules is to transport substances in and out of the blood. This is done through reabsorption, moving substances from the tubules into the bloodstream, and secretion, moving substances from the tubules into the urine. When tubular function is impaired there may be too little or too much of a particular substance in the blood disrupting the delicate balance of these substances in the body. Some of the substances the tubules regulate include vitamins, glucose, and water.

N25.0   Renal osteodystrophy

Renal osteodystrophy is actually a bone (osteo-) disease that develops when the kidneys cannot maintain the appropriate blood levels of calcium, phosphorus, or vitamin D. The balance of these minerals in the body is essential in maintaining normal calcium levels needed for healthy bone mass and structure. When the calcium levels in the blood decrease beyond a certain level, the body pulls calcium from the bones to compensate. Eventually, if the loss of calcium is prolonged or excessive, the bones weaken. Children are more severely affected by loss of calcium from the bones because it disrupts the normal growth and development of the bones causing deformities.

N25.1   Nephrogenic diabetes insipidus

Nephrogenic diabetes insipidus is caused by the failure of the kidneys to regulate water filtration from the blood. The tubules in the kidneys need a hormone called antidiuretic hormone (ADH) to identify how much water should be secreted into the urine or reabsorbed into the blood. In nephrogenic diabetes insipidus, the communication between ADH and the tubules is defective resulting in too much water lost to the urine. Dehydration, fatigue, rapid pulse, and low blood pressure are common symptoms accompanied by excessive thirst and excessive urination.

N25.8-   Other disorders resulting from impaired renal tubular function

The renal tubules are the filtering site for the kidneys, regulating the absorption and secretion of certain nutrients and hormones and removing waste. Impaired function can alter when and/or where certain nutrients get absorbed, which can result in other body chemicals being under or overproduced in response.

N25.81 Secondary hyperparathyroidism of renal origin

Hyperparathyroidism is over activation of the parathyroid glands. One cause of hyperparathyroidism is chronic kidney disease. The kidneys are the primary regulator of calcium in the bloodstream. When the kidneys do not function properly, calcium blood levels can drop. Lowered calcium blood levels activate the parathyroid glands to produce a hormone called PTH or parathyroid hormone. PTH helps regulate the levels of calcium in the blood by prompting the release of calcium from bone, regulating the amount of calcium taken from food, and increasing the intestinal absorption of calcium. If the renal condition is not reversed, the constant activity of the parathyroid glands also cannot be reversed and the production of PTH continues, even when calcium blood levels are normal or high. The constant PTH production leads to excess calcium being removed from bones.

Focus Point

Although secondary hyperparathyroidism develops due to low calcium levels in the blood (hypocalcemia), hypercalcemia, or increased levels of calcium in the blood, is a common sign of hyperparathyroidism. The overactive parathyroid glands constantly produce PTH hormone, which results in calcium being pulled from the bones, sometimes even when the body currently has normal blood levels of calcium. The elevated blood calcium levels accompanied by a concurrent increase in the level of PTH hormone signals a disruption in parathyroid function.

N26.- Unspecified contracted kidney

A contracted kidney is one that is reduced in size due to scarring, atrophy, or other disease processes.

N26.2 Page kidney

Page kidney results from a subcapsular mass or collection of fluid that compresses the renal parenchyma causing hypertension. The renal capsule consists of tough fibrous tissue that does not expand. When a tumor, mass, or fluid collection from a hematoma, seroma, or urinoma occurs beneath the renal capsule it puts pressure on the renal parenchyma causing obstruction to blood flow and resultant hypertension.

N28.- Other disorders of kidney and ureter, not elsewhere classified

The balance of fluid and chemicals in the body is largely dependent upon the appropriate function of the kidneys. The kidneys filter the blood while the ureters take any wastes from the filtering process and move them into the bladder.

N28.0 Ischemia and infarction of kidney

Infarction can be defined as an area of necrosis in tissue, in this case the kidney, due to ischemia from lack of circulation. The lack of normal blood flow may be reduced to just part of the kidney or to the whole kidney. Etiologies may include embolism or thrombosis of the renal artery, renal trauma, and renal artery dissection.

Other Diseases of the Urinary System (N30-N39)

The urinary system is a collection of various organs, tubes, muscles, and nerves whose function is to create, store, and transport urine out of the body. Infection, abscess, strictures, and changes in the nerve or muscle function of urinary organs are just a few of the conditions captured in this code block.

The categories in this code block are as follows:

N30	Cystitis
N31	Neuromuscular dysfunction of bladder, not elsewhere classified
N32	Other disorders of bladder
N33	Bladder disorders in diseases classified elsewhere
N34	Urethritis and urethral syndrome
N35	Urethral stricture
N36	Other disorders of urethra
N37	Urethral disorders in diseases classified elsewhere
N39	Other disorders of urinary system

N30.- Cystitis

This category reports inflammation of the bladder, with the most common cause being a bacterial infection. Bacteria are normally removed from the bladder during urination. However, when there is rapid growth of the bacteria before urination or when there is retention of urine in the bladder, bacterial infection can occur. Codes in this category are classified by the type or site of cystitis and whether or not it is complicated by hematuria. Hematuria is the presence of blood in the urine, which can be seen with the naked eye (gross hematuria) or can only be seen upon microscopic exam (microscopic hematuria).

N30.1- Interstitial cystitis (chronic)

This chronic bladder inflammation of unknown etiology is characterized by bladder pressure and pain in the bladder or pelvic area. Patients feel they need to urinate often even when only small amounts of urine are present in the bladder.

N30.3-   Trigonitis

The trigone is a smooth, triangular shaped area on the back wall of the bladder. This area, along with the rest of the urinary tract, is lined with tissue called urothelium. Trigonitis develops as a result of benign changes in the cells of the urothelium. This condition is most often seen in women of childbearing age and rarely in men or children.

N31.-   Neuromuscular dysfunction of bladder, not elsewhere classified

The nervous system plays an important role in the control of bladder function. Damage to the brain, spinal cord, or nerves can cause a disruption in the signals needed to control the muscles of the bladder leading to urinary incontinence, which is an inability to hold urine in, or urinary retention, which is an inability to get urine out.

N31.0   Uninhibited neuropathic bladder, not elsewhere classified

An uninhibited neuropathic bladder is a condition that disrupts the normal inhibitory control of the detrusor muscle function by the central nervous system. A patient with this condition often does not realize the bladder has filled until urine begins to involuntarily empty from it.

N31.1   Reflex neuropathic bladder, not elsewhere classified

Reflex neuropathic bladder is an interruption in the sensory and motor nerve pathways of the bladder occurring just above the sacral segments in the spinal cord. Bladder sensations are absent leading to spontaneous contraction of the detrusor muscle and complete relaxation of the sphincter muscle, resulting in incontinence. This condition is often associated with spinal cord injuries.

N31.8   Other neuromuscular dysfunction of bladder

Hypertonicity or hypertony of the bladder is included here and refers to excessive muscle tone or tension of the bladder muscles.

Focus Point

Hypertonic bladder (N31.8) is often used synonymously with overactive bladder (N32.81). However, ICD-10-CM considers these two conditions as separate disease processes. Although urinary urgency is a defining characteristic of both conditions, the distinction is made in their etiology. Hypertonicity is considered to be a neuromuscular dysfunction of the bladder, related to a brain, spinal, or nerve abnormality, while overactive bladder is from a nonneurogenic origin.

N32.-   Other disorders of bladder

The urinary bladder is a triangular or pear-shaped, expandable hollow organ located in the pelvic area. Disorders of the bladder included here range from fistula formation to overactive bladder.

N32.0   Bladder-neck obstruction

The bladder-neck is the narrowed distal portion of the bladder that connects to the urethra. It is composed of a group of muscles that contract and relax, regulating the passage of urine into the urethra. An obstruction in this area prevents the muscles from opening completely and limits the flow of urine out of the bladder. This can lead to difficulty urinating, incontinence, diverticula, and even kidney damage. It can occur in either sex but is primarily seen in men as a consequence of benign prostatic hypertrophy or prostatic cancer.

N35.-   Urethral stricture

A urethral stricture is a narrowing of the urethra, the tube that moves urine from the bladder to outside the body. This category encompasses urethral strictures that are the result of previous trauma, infection, or other specified causes that are unrelated to postsurgical states.

N36.-   Other disorders of urethra

The urethra is the tube through which urine is drained from the bladder. The flow of urine through the urethra is controlled by two sphincters: the internal sphincter, where the urethra meets the bladder, and the external sphincter, which surrounds the urethra at the pelvic floor. Fistula formation, diverticulum, and sphincter dyssynergy are just a few conditions captured in this category.

N36.4-   Urethral functional and muscular disorders

This subcategory identifies problems associated with the internal and external sphincter muscles and other functional disorders that may alter the way urine is passed through the urethra.

N36.41   Hypermobility of urethra

Urethral hypermobility refers to inferior and posterior motion of the urethra into the potential space of the vagina due to a loss of urethral supporting and backing structures of the pelvis and pelvic floor. Urethral hypermobility is associated with pathologies such as vaginal prolapse and cystoceles and is commonly seen in females with urinary stress incontinence.

N36.42   Intrinsic sphincter deficiency (ISD)

Intrinsic (urethral) sphincter deficiency (ISD) is due to intrinsic sphincteric damage in which the urethra is well supported but the sphincter muscle is weak and cannot close properly.

N36.44 Muscular disorders of urethra

Detrusor sphincter dyssynergia, also known as bladder neck dyssynergia, is included here. Normal micturition (urination) involves the coordination between two muscle groups: the bladder detrusor muscles and the external urethral sphincter muscles. When the detrusor muscles contract, the urethral sphincter muscles should relax to allow the flow of urine out of the bladder. With detrusor sphincter dyssynergia, the signals to the muscles get mixed up and the urethral sphincter muscles contract at the same time as the detrusor muscles interrupting the flow of urine. Spinal cord injuries and neurological conditions are common causes.

N39.- Other disorders of urinary system

Disorders included here are unspecified site urinary tract infections and incontinence.

N39.0 Urinary tract infection, site not specified

This code reports the presence of infectious microorganisms in an unspecified part of the urinary tract.

Focus Point

"UTI" is commonly used as a synonym for acute cystitis or acute urethritis although the site of the infection has not been clearly established. Before assigning the more specific code, be sure the specific site is supported with the necessary documentation.

N39.3 Stress incontinence (female) (male)

Urine leakage is referred to as stress incontinence when it is caused by physical forces such as exercise or heavy lifting putting pressure on the bladder. This can also occur from more benign exertions, such as coughing, sneezing, or even laughing.

N39.4- Other specified urinary incontinence

Urinary incontinence is the inability to control urination or lack of bladder control. The symptoms may range from leaking when the patient coughs or sneezes to sudden urges that cause leakage before the patient can make it to the restroom. This subcategory identifies several forms of incontinence.

N39.41 Urge incontinence

Urge incontinence is the abrupt need to urinate, followed by leaking, with increased frequency at any hour of the day or night. The typical causes can be some form of infection or more severe comorbidities like diabetes or neurological abnormalities.

N39.42 Incontinence without sensory awareness

Sensory awareness means the body sends out signals alerting the patient to tension or muscle reaction; in the case of incontinence, the patient is not aware of the need to urinate.

N39.43 Post-void dribbling

Post-void dribbling is the evacuation of small amounts of urine right after the patient has just urinated. This is typically seen as a symptom of an enlarged prostate and generally occurs after a male patient is 40 years old.

N39.44 Nocturnal enuresis

Nocturnal enuresis is leakage of urine only during the night and is typical in children with "bed-wetting" problems. It may be due to some genetic anomaly or a functional bladder disorder. Although once thought to be psychologically induced, nocturnal enuresis is now known to be most often familial based with children inheriting the trait from one or both parents. Treatment may include training, hypnosis, and biofeedback. In some cases, certain medications have been beneficial.

N39.45 Continuous leakage

Continuous leakage may sometimes be referred to as "true" incontinence, caused by a fistula between the vagina and ureter, bladder, or urethra.

N39.46 Mixed incontinence

Mixed incontinence simply describes a patient who displays more than one form of the disorder, such as urgency and leakage with exertion.

N39.49- Other specified urinary incontinence

This subcategory captures conditions specified as urinary incontinence but not classified elsewhere.

N39.490 Overflow incontinence

Overflow incontinence describes symptoms of recurrent urine leakage because of the patient's inability to completely empty the bladder.

N39.491 Coital incontinence

Coital incontinence affects women during intercourse and/or at arousal or orgasm and is often connected to pelvic floor disorders or malfunctions such as stress incontinence. Medical treatment may include physical or nerve therapy, prescription drugs, or surgery.

N39.492 Postural (urinary) incontinence

Postural incontinence is urinary incontinence that occurs when changing body positions, particularly moving from a seated or lying down position. Various forms of treatment may focus on the lower urinary tract symptoms in the form of rehabilitation, electrical stimulation, or catheterization.

Diseases of Male Genital Organs (N4Ø-N53)

The male reproductive system includes the two testes that produce spermatozoa (sperm) and male hormones. A system of ducts conveys sperm to the exterior of the body. This includes the epididymis and vas deferens, the seminal vesicles (glands that contribute secretions to semen), and the external genitalia (scrotum and penis). The primary function of the male genital system is sexual intercourse and propagation of the species.

The categories in this code block are as follows:

N4Ø	Benign prostatic hyperplasia
N41	Inflammatory diseases of prostate
N42	Other and unspecified disorders of prostate
N43	Hydrocele and spermatocele
N44	Noninflammatory disorders of testis
N45	Orchitis and epididymitis
N46	Male infertility
N47	Disorders of prepuce
N48	Other disorders of penis
N49	Inflammatory disorders of male genital organs, not elsewhere classified
N5Ø	Other and unspecified disorders of male genital organs
N51	Disorders of male genital organs in diseases classified elsewhere
N52	Male erectile dysfunction
N53	Other male sexual dysfunction

N4Ø.- Benign prostatic hyperplasia

The normal healthy prostate gland is comparable in size to a walnut. It is located below the urinary bladder, in front of the rectum, and surrounds the neck of the bladder and urethra. It consists of three lobes: right, left, and middle. Enlargement of the prostate can occur as a result of a number of disease processes.

N4Ø.Ø	Benign prostatic hyperplasia without lower urinary tract symptoms
N4Ø.1	Benign prostatic hyperplasia with lower urinary tract symptoms
N4Ø.2	Nodular prostate without lower urinary tract symptoms
N4Ø.3	Nodular prostate with lower urinary tract symptoms

An enlarged prostate, also referred to as benign prostatic hypertrophy or hyperplasia (BPH) is overgrowth of the prostate gland. It is believed to be caused by a combination of hormone changes and abnormal cell growth. Typically seen in men older than age 50, it is considered a normal consequence of aging. A nodular prostate is also an overgrowth of the prostate gland, but in addition the prostate has distinct raised areas (nodules) that are palpable on digital rectal exam. Both conditions are classified based on the presence or absence of lower urinary tract symptoms or LUTS. With continued growth of the prostate and/or development of nodules, the urethra can be pinched or compressed causing the bladder to work extra hard to void urine through the urethra. If prolonged, the bladder becomes weak resulting in symptoms such as urinary frequency and urgency, nocturia, urinary retention, and urinary incontinence. Having just one of these LUTS is enough to classify the enlarged prostate or a nodular prostate as "with lower urinary tract symptoms."

N42.- Other and unspecified disorders of prostate

The prostate is a three lobed gland located below the urinary bladder. This category classifies calculus, hemorrhage, and dysplasia of the prostate, as well as syndromes such as prostatodynia and prostatosis.

N42.3- Dysplasia of prostate

Dysplasia is an abnormality or alteration in the size, shape, and organization of cells from their normal pattern of development. In the prostate it is the cells of the epithelium lining that are altered, with cells dividing more rapidly than normal epithelium.

N42.31 Prostatic intraepithelial neoplasia

Prostatic intraepithelial neoplasia (PIN) is classified into three grades: high (PIN III), medium (PIN II), and low (PIN I). Each grade represents the extent of cellular change that is taking place within the prostate cells. The higher the grade, the more pronounced the cellular abnormalities. Although the presence of prostatic intraepithelial neoplasia is thought to be a precursor to prostate cancer, not all men actually go on to develop cancer. This is true regardless of the stage.

N42.32 Atypical small acinar proliferation of prostate

Atypical small acinar proliferation (ASAP) may mimic cancer but does not constitute a cancer diagnosis; however, the cause and effect of ASAP may be either benign reactive atrophy of the acini or acini prostate cancer. Initial biopsy may not be enough to determine a specific diagnosis, as ASAP is diagnosed in fewer than 2 percent of biopsies. However, reports have indicated that 30 percent to 40 percent of these ASAP-diagnosed patients eventually develop cancer of the prostate. For that reason, a second biopsy is recommended within three to six months. Given the uncertainty of initial biopsies, it is suggested that an initial ASAP diagnosis be considered "suspicious" for cancer to indicate the need for follow-up. This initial specimen generally does not possess all characteristics or sufficient quantity to suggest either a benign disease process or be cause to proceed with prostatectomy. Active surveillance or additional biopsies are almost always required to determine a specific diagnosis.

N44.- Noninflammatory disorders of testis

The testes are two small oval glands contained in the scrotum. Both are suspended in the scrotal sac by scrotal tissue and the spermatic cords.

N44.0- Torsion of testis

Testicular torsion refers to a twisting of the testicle or spermatic cord structures within the scrotal sac, which can cut off the blood supply to the testis. This is an emergent condition because of the risk of ischemia or testicular necrosis due to the interrupted circulation of blood and oxygen to the testis. The most common symptom associated with torsion is sudden pain and tenderness in the scrotum or iliac fossa. The pain can present unilaterally or bilaterally or spread into the groin, abdomen, or flank.

N44.01 Extravaginal torsion of spermatic cord

Extravaginal torsion involves twisting of the spermatic cord in an area where the tunica vaginalis and the spermatic cord are still attached. Both the spermatic cord and the tunica vaginalis are twisted, unlike intravaginal torsion where the tunica vaginalis is not involved. This type usually manifests in the neonatal period and can develop in utero.

N44.02 Intravaginal torsion of spermatic cord

Intravaginal torsion is most often associated with a condition called bell clapper deformity. Normally the testicles are attached to the scrotum, limiting testicular movement. In a bell clapper deformity, the testicle is not attached and is able to twist within the scrotum.

N44.03 Torsion of appendix testis

N44.04 Torsion of appendix epididymis

The appendix testis and appendix epididymis are small appendages (projections of tissue) found on the upper portion of the testis and the top of the epididymis respectively. Although both of these appendages have no physiological function, torsion or twisting of these appendages is symptomatic, with the most common symptom being pain. In some cases, torsion of the appendix testis cannot easily be differentiated from the more serious testicular torsion.

N46.- Male infertility

Infertility is defined as the inability or decreased ability to produce offspring. Male infertility is the primary factor in roughly a third of the couples having problems conceiving a child. In order for an egg to be fertilized the sperm must be healthy, mobile, numerous, and be able to move from the testicles and into the semen. Various conditions can alter any of these factors, decreasing the chances of conception.

N46.0- Azoospermia

Azoospermia is a condition in which there is total absence of sperm in the ejaculate fluid. Primarily this is an issue with production and/or transport: either there is inadequate production of sperm or production of sperm is normal but the sperm are inhibited in some way in reaching the semen.

N46.02- Azoospermia due to extratesticular causes

Extratesticular or acquired causes of azoospermia are outside forces or factors that alter the structures or organs that transport the sperm or inhibit sperm production.

N46.1- Oligospermia

Oligospermia, or low sperm count, occurs when semen contains fewer sperm than normal. Abnormal sperm count is defined as fewer than 15 million sperm per milliliter of semen. In some cases oligospermia may be temporary.

N46.12- Oligospermia due to extratesticular causes

Extratesticular causes of oligospermia are outside forces or factors that alter the structures or organs that transport the sperm or inhibit sperm production.

N47.- Disorders of prepuce

The prepuce, also called foreskin, is the double-layered sheath of skin covering the glans. The foreskin and glans are fused at birth by a shared membrane. This membrane eventually dissolves and the foreskin separates from the glans.

N47.1   Phimosis

Phimosis is a constriction or tightening of the prepuce that prevents retraction (pulling back) of the foreskin behind the glans or tip of the penis. This condition may be congenital but is most often the result of chronic infection of the foreskin.

N47.2   Paraphimosis

Paraphimosis occurs when the foreskin retracts and tightens below the glans. This compromises lymphatic drainage and causes glans to swell, which in turn inhibits blood flow to the distal aspect of the penis and glans. This condition is considered a urological emergency because the reduced blood flow to the penis can lead to necrosis or tissue death.

N48.-   Other disorders of penis

As part of the urinary system, the penis is the external organ that transports urine and semen out of the body via the urethra. Disorders captured here range from painful erection to lichen sclerosus to torsion of the penis.

N48.0   Leukoplakia of penis

Leukoplakia is characterized by abnormal white spots or lesions that occur on the penis most often at the head of the penis near the urethral opening. These white spots are a risk indicator for future development of squamous cell carcinoma. Balanitis xerotica obliterans (BXO), also called penile lichen sclerosis, is included here. BXO is characterized by a whitish colored, hardened ring of tissue near the tip of the penis. Although it can be managed, BXO is a chronic condition that can lead to more serious complications, such as stricture of the urethra.

N48.1   Balanitis

Balanitis is inflammation of the glans penis. The most common etiology is poor hygiene, especially in males who have not been circumcised. Balanitis can also be caused by injury, medications, and in rare cases diseases such as reactive arthritis or diabetes.

Focus Point

Balanitis, as defined above, should not be confused with a condition called balanitis xerotica obliterans (BXO) which is reported with code N48.0 Leukoplakia of penis. BXO is a dermatological condition characterized by a whitish colored, hardened ring of tissue near the tip of the penis. Although it can be managed, BXO is a chronic condition that can lead to more serious complications.

N48.6   Induration penis plastica

Induration penis plastica (IPP), also known as Peyronie's disease, is a rare disorder of the penis that is characterized by plaque formation on the upper or lower side of the penis in the layers containing erectile tissue. It begins as a localized inflammation and can develop into hardened scar tissue. The cause is not known but suspected causes include chronic inflammation and microtrauma. Symptoms include pain and abnormal bending or curvature of the penis during erection. The pain typically decreases over time, but the bend in the penis may remain a problem, making sexual intercourse difficult. In a small percentage of patients with the milder form of the disease, inflammation may resolve without pain or bending.

N50.8-   Other specified disorders of male genital organs

This subcategory includes symptoms specific to the male genitourinary system, including pain in the testes or scrotum as well as a number of other conditions that do not have a more specific code.

N50.89   Other specified disorders of the male genital organs

A male patient may present with a variety of genital-related signs and symptoms. These symptoms may be related to more specific underlying conditions or may resolve spontaneously. Codes in this subcategory should be assigned when no underlying condition causing the symptom is found at the conclusion of the visit. Examples include chylocele of tunica vaginalis, which is a collection of chylous fluid in the testis; edema (swelling) of the scrotum, seminal vesicle, spermatic cord, testis, tunica vaginalis, or vas deferens.

N52.-   Male erectile dysfunction

A man's inability to get an erection to start sex or inability to keep an erection to finish sex is known as erectile dysfunction (ED). ED has many causes, including diabetes, heart disease, injuries to the spinal cord or brain, or corollary to surgery or radiation therapy.

N52.3-   Postprocedural erectile dysfunction

Potentially any procedure on the prostate or male genital organs can result in postprocedural erectile dysfunction (ED), including major invasive procedures, such as radical prostatectomy, to less invasive procedures of ablative, interstitial seed, or other radiation therapy treatment. Damage to the nerves and/or vascular structures from these procedures is typically the root cause. Treatment for post-procedural ED is similar to treatments used for ED due to other conditions. Medications include Viagra, Levitra, or Cialis; or phosphodiesterase-5 inhibitors, which are designed to support an erection by increasing blood flow to the penis. A vacuum erection device may also be used to passively supply blood to the penile erectile tissue, aiding in healing and stretching the tissues to prevent scarring or fibrosis.

Disorders of Breast (N60-N65)

The female breast is comprised of four major structures: lobules or glands, milk ducts, fat, and connective tissue. A grouping of lobules form a larger unit called a lobe. Each breast contains approximately 15 to 20 lobes, emanating from the nipple and areolar area and arranged in what appears to be a wheel-spoke pattern. The lobes empty into milk ducts that course through the breast toward the nipple/areolar region, converging into about six to 10 larger ducts called collecting ducts. These collecting ducts enter at the base of the nipple and connect to the outside of the body.

The nipple is located near the tip of each breast, surrounded by a circular area of pigmented and irregular surfaced skin called the areola.

The mammary glands are accessory organs of the female reproductive system and are contained within the breast. The function of the mammary gland is lactation, which is the secretion of colostrum and subsequently milk for the nourishment of newborn infants.

The male breast is almost identical in structure to the female breast with one exception. The male breast does not have lobules, which are the structures in the female breast that are necessary for lactation and storage of milk. The male breast does however have glandular tissue, but this glandular tissue does not enlarge and develop as it does in females during puberty because males lack the necessary levels of estrogen needed for breast development. Male breast development only occurs when there is an endocrine disorder.

The categories in this code block are as follows:

N60	Benign mammary dysplasia
N61	Inflammatory disorders of breast
N62	Hypertrophy of breast
N63	Unspecified lump in breast
N64	Other disorders of breast
N65	Deformity and disproportion of reconstructed breast

N60.- Benign mammary dysplasia

Benign mammary dysplasia refers to changes in the breast tissue due to a nonmalignant disease process. This broad category includes conditions such as solitary cysts, diffuse cystic mastopathy, fibroadenoma, fibrosclerosis, and mammary duct ectasia.

N60.1- Diffuse cystic mastopathy

Diffuse cystic mastopathy, also called fibrocystic breast disease, is a condition characterized by changes in the breast tissue. It is a common condition found in normal breasts and is believed to be a normal tissue variant as opposed to a disease. Changes that occur in diffuse cystic mastopathy may affect the appearance and texture of the breast and include a dense, irregular, and bumpy consistency, especially in the outer upper quadrants. Symptoms include mild to severe breast discomfort that often coincides with the patient's menstrual cycle with symptoms typically peaking just before each menstrual period and improving immediately after the menstrual period.

N60.4- Mammary duct ectasia

Ectasia is a pathological expansion, dilation, or distension of a hollow or tubular anatomic organ or structure. In mammary duct ectasia, the milk duct widens and its walls thicken. This in turn can lead to fluid build-up and blockage of the milk duct. The incidence of this condition increases with age and often with no symptoms. Those patients that do exhibit symptoms may experience tenderness of the breast and a sticky, thick discharge from the nipple.

N60.9- Unspecified benign mammary dysplasia

A condition included here is atypical ductal hyperplasia (ADH). ADH is the development of abnormal cell growth in the breast tissue that resembles carcinoma in situ. Although associated with an increased risk for developing breast cancer, ADH is a nonmalignant condition. ADH cannot be found on mammography or felt during a breast exam. It can only be identified on microscopic review of a biopsy sample.

N61.- Inflammatory disorders of breast

The breast contains a variety of tissue types, from those that support lactation—the ducts, lobules, and nipple—to blood vessels, fat cells, connective tissue, and lymph nodes. Any of these structures may become inflamed, causing various disorders. This category specifically categorizes mastitis and abscess of the breast not related to pregnancy (puerperal) or lactation. The distinction between mastitis and frank abscess is very important because the management of these two conditions varies significantly.

N61.0 Mastitis without abscess

N61.1 Abscess of the breast and nipple

Nonpuerperal mastitis, or inflammation of breast tissue, can be classified as simple or periductal, meaning involving the breast ducts beneath the nipple. Hormonal imbalances, ruptured cysts, duct obstruction, and bacterial invasion are common etiologies.

Current research shows a link between smoking and periductal mastitis, 90 percent of which occurs in smokers as compared with 38 percent in nonsmokers. This may be due to smoking's either directly or indirectly damaging the wall of the subareolar breast ducts, making them vulnerable to infections. The incidence of nonpuerperal mastitis has also increased in recent years due to increasing numbers of women undergoing nipple piercing.

An abscess is a pocket of purulent material that forms in response to infection, in this case forming within the breast tissue. Breast abscess can be a complication of mastitis or be secondary to other disease processes such as diabetes or trauma. Drainage of the abscess is almost always necessary and recurrence is high.

Focus Point

When an inflammatory breast disorder occurs during pregnancy or the puerperium or involves lactation, the condition should be classified to category O91 Infections of breast associated with pregnancy, the puerperium and lactation, in chapter 15, "Pregnancy, Childbirth and the Puerperium."

N62   Hypertrophy of breast

Hypertrophy of the breast is the relative enlargement of one or both breasts when compared to overall body size and frame. Hypertrophy is typically used to describe enlargement of breast tissue in women while the term gynecomastia is used to describe breast enlargement in men. Gynecomastia is a benign condition in which excess amounts of firm breast tissue forms in males typically as a result of hormone imbalances. Another cause of gynecomastia is obesity.

N63.-   Unspecified lump in breast

Lumps found in the breast without a specific diagnosis are classified here with specific codes to describe the location of the lump including the laterality and the quadrant involved.

Female Breast

Upper outer quadrant

Upper inner quadrant

Midline

Areola

Axillary tail

Nipple

Mammary gland

Lower outer quadrant

Lower inner quadrant

Right Breast

N64.-   Other disorders of breast

This category classifies other disorders of native breasts.

N64.81   Ptosis of breast

Breast ptosis may be defined as drooping breasts. In general, it is a naturally occurring process of aging in which loosening of the skin and suspensory ligaments causes the breast to sag. Additional factors influencing the development of ptosis include tobacco use, number of pregnancies, and weight changes.

N64.82   Hypoplasia of breast

Breast hypoplasia or micromastia refers to postpubertal underdevelopment of breast tissue. In most cases this is subjective, based on the patient's body perception. The size of the breast does not necessarily indicate abnormal development although some congenital or traumatic conditions may contribute to a smaller breast size.

N65.-   Deformity and disproportion of reconstructed breast

Breast reconstruction procedures are performed to correct defects resulting from prior surgery or trauma to the breast. Attaining symmetry and aesthetic balance with the natural breast can pose a challenge for the surgeon. Postmastectomy, circulation, and healing of breast tissue may be compromised resulting in an unfavorable anatomic appearance of the reconstructed breast. Codes in this category report deformity of the reconstructed breast and disproportion of the reconstructed breast when compared with the native breast and establish medical necessity of additional procedures on the reconstructed or native breast.

Focus Point

Capsular contracture of breast implants occurs due to an abnormal response of the immune system to the artificial implant. This is considered a complication of a breast implant and is reported with a code from Chapter 19 Injury, Poisoning and Certain Other Consequences of External Causes.

Inflammatory Diseases of Female Pelvic Organs (N70-N77)

The female pelvic organs include the vulva and vagina, cervix, uterus, broad ligament, Bartholin's gland, ovaries, and fallopian tubes. Inflammatory diseases of some structures adjacent to or surrounding these organs are also included here, such as the peritoneum. In addition to capturing inflammation that may occur at these sites, codes in this code block also capture abscess, cyst, and ulcer formation.

The categories in this code block are as follows:

N70 Salpingitis and oophoritis

N71 Inflammatory disease of uterus, except cervix

N72 Inflammatory disease of cervix uteri

N73 Other female pelvic inflammatory diseases

N74 Female pelvic inflammatory disorders in diseases classified elsewhere

N75 Diseases of Bartholin's gland

N76 Other inflammation of vagina and vulva

N77 Vulvovaginal ulceration and inflammation in diseases classified elsewhere

N70.- Salpingitis and oophoritis

Infection and inflammation involving just the fallopian tubes is called salpingitis; when just the ovaries are involved, the term is oophoritis. These conditions are categorized based on chronicity and whether just the fallopian tubes, just the ovaries, or both are affected.

N73.- Other female pelvic inflammatory diseases

This category identifies conditions related to infection and/or inflammation of pelvic structures adjacent to the organs of the female genital tract. Adhesions or scar tissue of female pelvic organs is also coded here except when the condition is related to a previous procedure.

N73.0 Acute parametritis and pelvic cellulitis

N73.1 Chronic parametritis and pelvic cellulitis

N73.2 Unspecified parametritis and pelvic cellulitis

The parametrium is the fibrous fascial layer of tissue that covers the outer surface of the upper aspect of the cervix and separates it from the bladder. Parametritis is an inflammation or infection of this tissue. Pelvic cellulitis is inflammation or infection of all the internal structures of the female reproductive tract, along with the surrounding structures and pelvic peritoneum. This condition is sometimes referred to as female pelvic inflammatory disease or PID. Parametritis and pelvic cellulitis may both lead to abscess formation, which is included in these codes. Codes are assigned based on chronicity. The acute condition is characterized by sudden onset and more severe symptoms including

fever, pain, and vaginal discharge with or without bleeding, while the chronic condition is characterized by less severe symptoms that persist over a long period of time.

> **Focus Point**
>
> *Parametritis is most often seen after a complicated birth or abortion and when it is associated with these conditions it is reported with a code from Chapter 15 Pregnancy, childbirth and the Puerperium.*
>
> *Female pelvic inflammatory disease due to gonococcal infection is reported with code A54.24; when due to chlamydial infection, it is reported with A56.11.*

N73.3 Female acute pelvic peritonitis

N73.4 Female chronic pelvic peritonitis

N73.5 Female pelvic peritonitis, unspecified

Peritonitis is infection or inflammation of the peritoneum, a thin membrane that lines the abdominal wall. In this case, the infection or inflammation is limited to a region of the peritoneum surrounding the internal structures of the female reproductive tract. The condition may be acute or chronic. The acute condition is characterized by sudden onset and more severe symptoms including fever and pelvic pain, while the chronic condition is characterized by less severe symptoms that persist over a long period of time.

N75.- Diseases of Bartholin's gland

The Bartholin's gland is one of two mucous-producing glands found on each side of the opening of the vagina. The glands are connected to the Bartholin ducts that take the mucous produced by the gland to the vaginal surface.

N75.0 Cyst of Bartholin's gland

A Bartholin gland cyst occurs when the Bartholin duct is blocked causing fluid to buildup in the gland. Cyst formation may be caused by inflammation, infection, or trauma to the area around the duct. Symptoms such as localized pain or painful intercourse (dyspareunia) may be present, although Bartholin gland cysts are often asymptomatic and resolve on their own.

N75.1 Abscess of Bartholin's gland

An abscess occurs when the Bartholin's gland becomes infected. This can occur in relation to cyst development in the duct or as a result of direct invasion of infectious organisms from the vaginal area. Vulvar pain is a common symptom and may be accompanied by redness and swelling.

N76.- Other inflammation of vagina and vulva

The vulva is an external genital organ with many anatomical structures, including the labia minora and majora, the mons pubis, and the clitoris. The vagina is a tubular, internal genital organ that connects the vulva to the uterus.

N76.0 Acute vaginitis

N76.1 Subacute and chronic vaginitis

Vaginitis is an infectious or a noninfectious inflammation of the vagina. Symptoms may include swelling, itching, and burning in the vagina, often accompanied by an abnormal discharge. Vulvovaginitis, infection or inflammation of both the vulva and the vagina, is also included here. The condition may be acute, occurring suddenly often with more severe symptoms but also resolving quickly; subacute with a more gradual onset and less severe symptoms; or chronic, persisting over a long period of time.

N76.8- Other specified inflammation of vagina and vulva

Inflammation is the body's response to damaged cells, irritants, pathogens, and other harmful stimuli.

N76.81 Mucositis (ulcerative) of vagina and vulva

The cells of the mucosal tissues are especially vulnerable to damage by antineoplastic or immunosuppressive drugs used during chemotherapy and damage from radiological procedures and radiation therapy. Mucositis of female genital sites such as the vagina and vulva presents with signs of inflammation, redness, pseudomembrane formation, bleeding, or open sores (ulcers).

N76.89 Other specified inflammation of vagina and vulva

Included here is female Fournier disease or gangrene. Fournier gangrene is a type of necrotizing fasciitis that occurs in the external genitalia and perineum. The condition results from an infectious process usually from multiple organisms. The initiating infection may occur anywhere around the genital area. Pain is often the first symptom and may occur before any changes in the tissue are noted; however, pain is typically followed by rapid progression to necrosis of surrounding tissue that may lead to organ failure and death. Predisposing factors include an immunocompromised state, diabetes, and chronic alcohol use.

Noninflammatory Disorders of Female Genital Tract (N80-N98)

The female genital tract includes the vulva and vagina, cervix, uterus, broad ligament, Bartholin's gland, ovaries, and fallopian tubes. Noninflammatory conditions captured in this code block include dysplasia of various female genital organs, menstruation problems, infertility, and polyp or cyst formation.

The categories in this code block are as follows:

N80	Endometriosis
N81	Female genital prolapse
N82	Fistulae involving female genital tract
N83	Noninflammatory disorders of ovary, fallopian tube and broad ligament
N84	Polyp of female genital tract
N85	Other noninflammatory disorders of uterus, except cervix
N86	Erosion and ectropion of cervix uteri
N87	Dysplasia of cervix uteri
N88	Other noninflammatory disorders of cervix uteri
N89	Other noninflammatory disorders of vagina
N90	Other noninflammatory disorders of vulva and perineum
N91	Absent, scanty and rare menstruation
N92	Excessive, frequent and irregular menstruation
N93	Other abnormal uterine and vaginal bleeding
N94	Pain and other conditions associated with female genital organs and menstrual cycle
N95	Menopausal and other perimenopausal disorders
N96	Recurrent pregnancy loss
N97	Female infertility
N98	Complications associated with artificial fertilization

N80.- Endometriosis

Endometriosis is the presence of endometrial tissue (functioning endometrial cells) outside of its normal location (lining the uterine cavity). Pain is the most common symptom and universal to almost all patients affected, regardless of the site of endometrial growth. The endometrial tissue growing on sites outside the uterus behaves the same way normal intrauterine endometrium behaves during the monthly menstrual cycle, growing and bleeding in response to hormonal changes. When endometrial tissue is present outside of the uterus it can cause obstruction, trapped blood can cause cysts, and scar tissue can form. Endometriosis is classified by site.

N81.- Female genital prolapse

Genital prolapse is the protrusion or projection of pelvic organs into or outside the vaginal opening, often caused by weakening or damaged support structures. There are a number of contributing factors that can cause genital prolapse, including pregnancy and childbirth, menopause, raised pressure in the abdomen, and genetic predisposition.

N81.Ø Urethrocele

Urethrocele occurs when the urethra descends and presses into the vagina. This is due to stretching or weakness of the muscle and tissue that surround the urethra. These supporting structures can weaken with age but are most often damaged from childbirth.

N81.1- Cystocele

Cystocele occurs when tissues supporting the wall between the bladder and the vagina weaken, allowing a portion of the bladder to descend and protrude into the vagina.

N81.10 Cystocele, unspecified

N81.11 Cystocele, midline

N81.12 Cystocele, lateral

A cystocele, also referred to as a bladder prolapse, may occur in a midline or lateral location and, in some cases, there are coexisting defects of both sites. A midline or central defect is caused by overstretching or fascial tear in the middle of the vaginal wall. A lateral or paravaginal defect indicates a weakness or tearing in the connective tissue that attaches the vagina to the pelvic sidewall. This defect commonly develops as a result of childbirth.

Focus Point

These codes are also used to report a cystocele associated with prolapse of the urethra or what is known as a cystourethrocele.

N81.2 Incomplete uterovaginal prolapse

N81.3 Complete uterovaginal prolapse

N81.4 Uterovaginal prolapse, unspecified

Uterine prolapse refers to descent of the uterus and cervix down into the vaginal canal due to weak or damaged pelvic support structures. The extent of the prolapse is described by the terms incomplete and complete. An incomplete prolapse identifies a sagging uterus but without portions of the cervix or uterus falling outside of the vagina. Complete prolapse occurs

when the uterus falls so far down that all or a portion of the uterus protrudes outside the vagina. The extent of uterine prolapse is sometimes described in terms of degree, grade, or stage using the numerical values Ø to 4. The numerical value Ø describes a normally positioned uterus with no prolapse, values 1 and 2 an incomplete prolapse, and values 3 and 4 a complete prolapse.

N81.5 Vaginal enterocele

Enterocele refers to herniation of a portion of intestine with protrusion into the vagina.

N81.6 Rectocele

Rectocele occurs when tissues supporting the wall between the vagina and the rectum weaken allowing the rectum to descend and protrude into the vagina.

N81.8- Other female genital prolapse

Prolapse is the protrusion or sagging of an anatomical structure into a space it doesn't belong usually due to weakening of muscles and connective tissue that normally support the anatomical structure.

N81.81 Perineocele

A perineocele in the female is a hernia in the perineum occurring between the rectum and the vagina.

N81.85 Cervical stump prolapse

Following a partial hysterectomy, the portion of the cervix left in situ, called the cervical stump, may collapse and descend into the vaginal vault, resulting in tears of the fascial points of attachment. This can also occur when the cervical stump is pushed out of the vaginal vault by loops of small intestine.

N82.- Fistulae involving female genital tract

A fistula is an abnormal tube-like passage between two body cavities or organs or from an organ to the exterior surface of the body. This category represents various fistula formations between the vagina and other female genital tract organs to gastrointestinal, urinary, and external body sites.

N83.- Noninflammatory disorders of ovary, fallopian tube and broad ligament

The conditions in this category include various types of ovarian cysts; atrophy, hernia, prolapse and torsion of the ovary and fallopian tube; and hematosalpinx, a condition of bleeding into the fallopian tube.

N83.0- Follicular cyst of ovary

N83.1- Corpus luteum cyst

Ovarian cysts are quite common, particularly those designated as functional, meaning that they develop during or after ovulation from the sac that held the ovum before it was released. Follicular cysts, which are common among women of child-bearing age, develop when a follicle does not rupture or release its ova and instead grows and fills with fluid.

Corpus luteum cysts develop when ovum follicles become sealed off after releasing the ova and become filled with fluid. The fertility drug clomiphene (Clomid, Serophene), used to induce ovulation, increases the risk of corpus luteum cyst development. Most functional ovarian cysts are harmless and painless and disappear within two or three menstrual cycles.

N83.3- Acquired atrophy of ovary and fallopian tube

Atrophy, a degenerative breakdown of tissue, can affect the ovaries and fallopian tubes. An atrophied ovary generally means a decrease in the ovarian tissue volume and in some cases the inability to generate or produce healthy eggs; it may also be a sign of early menopause.

N83.51- Torsion of ovary and ovarian pedicle

N83.52- Torsion of fallopian tube

N83.53 Torsion of ovary, ovarian pedicle and fallopian tube

Torsion is the twisting of an organ. Twisting of the ovary or fallopian tube affects the blood flow and causes severe pain. Patients with ovarian cysts and/or tumors (either benign or malignant) are three times more likely to develop torsion, and most cases involve both the ovary and the fallopian tube. Because the presenting symptoms (lower abdominal pain) may mimic other conditions, most patients with torsion have a delayed diagnosis. Ultrasonography with color Doppler analysis can most easily confirm the diagnosis and help determine the best way to manage it.

N84.- Polyp of female genital tract

A polyp is an abnormal tissue growth originating in a mucous membrane. Polyps may be described as pedunculated or sessile. Pedunculated polyps are attached to the mucous membrane with a narrow stalk at the base, while sessile polyps have a flat base and are directly attached to the mucous membrane. Polyps can be found almost anywhere along the female genital tract. Code selection under this category is based on the specific location of the polyp.

N85.- Other noninflammatory disorders of uterus, except cervix

The uterus is a hollow, pear-shaped organ with two parts: the cervix or lower portion and the corpus or main body. Only noninflammatory conditions of the corpus uteri are classified here.

N85.0- Endometrial hyperplasia

Endometrial hyperplasia is an abnormal thickening of the tissue that lines the uterus due to an increase in the number of endometrial cells that make up the endometrial tissue. In most cases, endometrial hyperplasia is caused by a hormonal imbalance of estrogen and progesterone. These hormones are normally activated at different times during the menstrual cycle to signal certain uterine activities. Estrogen is released by the ovaries during the first half of the menstrual cycle signaling the uterine lining to grow in preparation for pregnancy. Release of the egg causes levels of progesterone to increase, which is necessary for implantation and nourishment of a fertilized egg. If the egg has not been fertilized, levels of estrogen and progesterone decrease and the thickened uterine lining is shed. It is the decrease in progesterone that signals the uterus to shed. However, if excess levels of estrogen are produced in the absence of progesterone, the endometrial lining of the uterus grows but shedding of the endometrial lining will not occur resulting in crowding and abnormal growth patterns of the endometrial cells. Endometrial hyperplasia is clinically classified into benign endometrial hyperplasia and a premalignant condition called endometrial intraepithelial neoplasia (EIN). These designations are based on the histologic behavior of the abnormal tissue. An important distinction between the two conditions is that EIN lesions have initiated the first step of the carcinogenesis process by clonal expansion of a mutated cell, whereas benign endometrial hyperplasia has not.

N85.01 Benign endometrial hyperplasia

Benign endometrial hyperplasia is synonymous with the simple or complex hyperplasia without atypia. Both simple and complex types have the characteristic increased thickness of the endometrium but differ in the type of cell and gland abnormalities that are seen. The simple type rarely progresses to cancer while the complex type without atypia has a greater potential for becoming malignant especially without treatment.

N85.02 Endometrial intraepithelial neoplasia [EIN]

Endometrial intraepithelial neoplasia (EIN) refers to abnormal neoplastic changes (i.e., genetically mutated monoclonals) of the endometrial glands that are prone to malignant transformation. Although EIN is a premalignant lesion requiring a distinct classification due to the associated cancer risk, not all EIN lesions progress to carcinoma in situ; some lesions spontaneously resolve. The progression of EIN to carcinoma in situ occurs through acquisition of certain genetic mutations that precipitate local tissue invasion and metastatic growth. This condition may also be referred to as complex hyperplasia with atypia.

N85.3 Subinvolution of uterus

Uterine subinvolution is failure of the uterus to return to normal size after physiological hypertrophy following an infection or other disease process.

N87.- Dysplasia of cervix uteri

When abnormal changes to cells on the surface of the cervix are observed this is called cervical dysplasia or cervical intraepithelial dysplasia (CIN). The cells, although abnormal, are not cancerous but may have the potential to transform and become cancerous (malignant). Cytological and histological studies are used to determine the extent of change in the dysplastic cells. Based on these changes dysplasia is classified into three severity levels, two of which are coded to this category: CIN I or mild dysplasia and CIN II or moderate dysplasia. CIN grades are defined based on the depth of epithelial tissue involvement.

N87.0 Mild cervical dysplasia

Mild cervical dysplasia is defined as involving up to a third of the thickness of the cell layer overlying the cervix and is considered to be a low-grade lesion. The mild form is typically monitored and has the potential to resolve on its own without any intervention.

N87.1 Moderate cervical dysplasia

Moderate cervical dysplasia is defined as involvement of up to two-thirds of the cell layer and is considered a high-grade lesion. Intervention is essential in moderate cervical dysplasia as there is the potential for development of a malignancy.

N89.- Other noninflammatory disorders of vagina

The vagina is the internal tubular structure that connects the uterus to the vulva.

N89.0 Mild vaginal dysplasia

N89.1 Moderate vaginal dysplasia

N89.3 Dysplasia of vagina, unspecified

Dysplasia describes abnormal changes in the cells found on the surface of the vagina. It is categorized by three stages: mild (VAIN grade I), moderate (VAIN grade II), and severe (VAIN grade III), but only the mild and moderate varieties are coded here. VAIN grades are defined based on the depth of epithelial tissue involvement. Mild vaginal dysplasia is defined as involving up to a third of the thickness of the cell layer overlying the vagina and is the most common form. Moderate vaginal dysplasia is defined as involvement of up to two-thirds of the cell layer. Intervention is essential in moderate vaginal dysplasia as there is the potential for development of a malignancy. The mild form is typically monitored and has the potential to resolve on its own without any intervention.

N90.- Other noninflammatory disorders of vulva and perineum

The vulva is an external female genital organ composed of several structures, including the labia majora and minora and the clitoris. In females, the perineum is the area between the vulva and the anus.

N90.0 Mild vulvar dysplasia

N90.1 Moderate vulvar dysplasia

N90.3 Dysplasia of vulva, unspecified

Vulvar intraepithelial neoplasia (VIN) refers to abnormal (dysplastic) changes to cells on the surface of the vulva. While these cellular changes are not cancerous or malignant, some forms of VIN if left untreated can transform into squamous cell carcinoma, so VIN is considered a precancerous or premalignant condition. VIN is relatively rare and the mild and moderate forms are thought to be associated with a history of infection with certain strains of human papilloma virus (HPV).

N90.6- Hypertrophy of vulva

Hypertrophy of an organ is when enlargement of component cells causes the volume of the organ or tissue to increase. The vulva consists of the external genital organs of a female and includes the mons pubis, labia majora and minora, clitoris, and the urethral and vaginal openings.

N90.61 Childhood asymmetric labium majus enlargement

Childhood asymmetric labium majus enlargement (CALME) is a condition that appears in girls that are prepubescent or in early puberty. One side of the labia majora, the fatty tissue covering the vagina, is increased in size as a result of excess growth of the vaginal tissue on that side. Beyond the abnormal color and texture of the growth and the asymmetrical appearance, symptoms are minimal with only minor irritation or discomfort in certain clothing. Surgical removal is recommended with good results, but recurrence is possible.

N91.- Absent, scanty and rare menstruation

Menstruation is the part of the menstrual cycle when the inner lining of the uterus is shed. During the normal reproductive years, each woman's menstrual cycle may differ in timing, length, and associated symptoms, but rarely is it absent. Menstruation that has stopped or slowed prior to perimenopause or menopause may be the result of hormonal changes, scarring in the uterus, certain medical conditions, and stress.

N91.0 Primary amenorrhea

N91.1 Secondary amenorrhea

N91.2 Amenorrhea, unspecified

Amenorrhea is the absence of menstruation. One cause of amenorrhea is an imbalance of hormones in the body. Menstrual cycles are controlled by hormones so if there is an abnormality in the release or use of these hormones, a problem with the menstrual cycle results. Occasionally an increase in activity, stress, or medications can cause a change in the body's hormones and result in amenorrhea. There are two classifications of amenorrhea: primary and secondary. Primary amenorrhea is defined as failure to start menstruating by age 16 or within three years after the first signs of puberty. Primary amenorrhea can be caused by a genetic abnormality, pituitary disease, a hormonal imbalance, or a structural problem. Secondary amenorrhea is absence of menstruation for three cycles after having had a menstrual period for longer than two years. Eating disorders, stress, and drastic weight loss can also disrupt the menstrual cycle, as can certain types of medication, such as antidepressants, chemotherapy medicine, and antipsychotics.

N91.3 Primary oligomenorrhea

N91.4 Secondary oligomenorrhea

N91.5 Oligomenorrhea, unspecified

Scanty or infrequent menstruation is termed oligomenorrhea. It is loosely defined as menstrual periods at greater than 35 day intervals or no more than nine periods a year. Oligomenorrhea may be caused by heavy exercise regimes and eating disorders.

Focus Point

Oligomenorrhea associated with conditions that cause hormonal changes such as polycystic ovary syndrome are reported with codes from Chapter 4 Endocrine, Nutritional, and Metabolic Disorders.

N93.- Other abnormal uterine and vaginal bleeding

Abnormal uterine bleeding, also referred to as dysfunctional uterine bleeding (DUB), is defined as any additional bleeding other than during menses or anovulatory bleeding (AUB). This can happen for any number of reasons: hyperprolactinemia, pituitary lesion, bleeding disorder, polyps, fibroids, thyroid disorder, endometrial cancer, or infection. However, it most often is due to hormonal irregularity, and further classification relies on the age of the patient.

N93.0 Postcoital and contact bleeding

Postcoital bleeding (PCB) is unrelated to menses and occurs immediately after intercourse. This is simply a symptom of an unknown condition that requires further evaluation. Potential causes of PCB include:

- Infection
- Cervical ectropion
- Polyps
- Cancer
- Injury

Upon examination, treatment is related to the underlying cause

N93.1 Pre-pubertal vaginal bleeding

Prepubertal vaginal bleeding is a rare complaint for girls under 10 years of age and is typically a benign condition; however, it does not preclude a more serious condition requiring further evaluation. One published study of over 80 girls found that just over 54 percent were found to have localized lesions with just over 18 percent due to hormonal issues while the remainder had uncertain etiology. Additional possibilities for underlying conditions creating this symptom may include an endocrine or congenital disorder. Careful examination is required to evaluate and treat the bleeding, particularly if abuse is thought to trigger the injury.

Focus Point

Due to the many potential causes of prepubertal vaginal bleeding, care must be taken to report this condition from the proper chapter. Some endocrine conditions such as precocious menstruation, precocious pseudopuberty, and precocious or central precocious puberty are classified to chapter 4, "Endocrine, Nutritional and Metabolic Diseases." A similar presenting congenital condition called McCune-Albright syndrome is reported with a code from chapter 17, "Congenital Malformations, Deformations and Chromosomal Abnormalities."

N94.- Pain and other conditions associated with female genital organs and menstrual cycle

Pain during the menstrual cycle most often occurs during menstruation and in most cases is mild. Pain that is severe during menstruation or occurs at other times of the menstrual cycle is not as common and may be a sign of another underlying condition.

N94.0 Mittelschmerz

Mittelschmerz (German for "middle pain") is defined as abdominal pain that presents halfway through the typical 28-day menstrual cycle. Typically, this does not require medical intervention since over-the-counter medications treat the symptoms. It is recommended that patients seek medical treatment if the condition worsens, such as intense pain in conjunction with nausea and fever, which may indicate a more serious condition.

N94.1- Dyspareunia

Dyspareunia is the term for painful intercourse, which may occur before, during, or after sex with treatment focused on the cause of this symptom. The physician may narrow down the cause examination in addition to addressing when the pain occurs. This subcategory classifies physiological dyspareunia involving several factors that may lead to this pain:

- Inadequate lubrication
- Injury
- Inflammatory disorder
- Vaginal wall muscle spasms
- Congenital malformation
- Complications from previous surgery

Treatment depends on the underlying cause and may include oral or topical medications and home remedies such as using lubricant, changing positions, and longer foreplay.

> **Focus Point**
>
> *Dyspareunia may also be related to psychogenic causes, which are reported in chapter 5, "Mental, Behavioral and Neurodevelopmental Disorders."*

N94.2 Vaginismus

This term identifies vaginal wall muscle spasms in reaction to something entering the vagina. The spasms can range from irritating to painful and typically subside upon withdrawal. The exact cause is unclear, but it may be due to anxiety or some underlying physical condition, and the medical provider must further evaluate the patient to determine all factors associated with the pain. This subcategory includes only physiological vaginismus caused by physical forces such as infections, malignancies, injuries, pelvic

surgeries, menopause, or other disease conditions. Typical treatment depends on the underlying cause and may include medication, Kegel exercises, or dilation therapy.

> **Focus Point**
>
> *Vaginismus may also be related to psychogenic causes such as anxiety, stress, or emotional fear, which are reported in Chapter 5, "Mental, Behavioral and Neurodevelopmental Disorders."*

N94.3 Premenstrual tension syndrome

Premenstrual tension syndrome (PMT) is the same thing as premenstrual syndrome (PMS), which describes the changes women's bodies go through during their monthly menstrual cycle, with about one in every three women complaining of symptoms associated with the condition. The hormonal changes that occur before menstruation are typically the cause of these physical symptoms, such as painful breasts, cramps, headaches, fatigue, bloating, acne, plus many emotional symptoms. Some women appear more sensitive to the changes than others. Treatment depends on contributing factors and the severity of symptoms. While some benefit from antidepressants or the contraceptive pill, others may find relief in simple things such as exercise, healthy diet, relaxation techniques, and/or supplements.

> **Focus Point**
>
> *Some women experience premenstrual headaches or migraines as part of PMT, which need to be additionally reported with codes from subcategory G43.8- in chapter 6, "Diseases of the Nervous System."*

N94.4 Primary dysmenorrhea

N94.5 Secondary dysmenorrhea

N94.6 Dysmenorrhea, unspecified

Dysmenorrhea is a menstrual condition characterized by menstrual cramps and pain associated with menstruation. Dysmenorrhea is one of the most common gynecologic complaints in adolescent girls and young women. There are two classifications of dysmenorrhea: primary or secondary. Primary dysmenorrhea is a term used when there is not a disease or other underlying condition causing menstrual pain. In primary dysmenorrhea, the severe cramping and abnormal uterine contractions are a result of a chemical imbalance in the body due to prostaglandin and arachidonic acid, chemicals that control the contractions of the uterus. Primary dysmenorrhea typically begins in the first few years after menarche.

Secondary dysmenorrhea is menstrual pain as a result of an underlying condition, such as endometriosis or pelvic inflammatory disease.

N94.81- Vulvodynia

Vulvodynia is persistent vulvar pain.

N94.810 Vulvar vestibulitis

The area surrounding the entrance to the vagina is called the vulvar vestibule. Vulvar vestibulitis is pain or a burning sensation at the vestibule that comes only after touch or pressure to the area. Sexual intercourse, inserting a tampon, or even tight fitting clothing can provoke vestibular pain and as a result can impact the patient's quality of life.

N94.818 Other vulvodynia

N94.819 Vulvodynia, unspecified

Vulvodynia is pain in the vulvar area that occurs with varying presentations. Some experience pain in only one specific area of the vulva while others experience pain in multiple areas. The pain can be constant or sporadic and although touch or pressure may exacerbate the pain, it often does not provoke the pain. Vulvodynia documented as a specific type or with a specific presentation is reported as other vulvodynia, while unspecified vulvodynia is reported when there are no qualifiers describing the location or type of pain.

N94.89 Other specified conditions associated with female genital organs and menstrual cycle

Pelvic congestion syndrome is classified here. This condition is caused by varicose veins in the pelvis. These veins become distended and engorged, resulting in an excessive accumulation of blood in these vessels, especially when standing. Pelvic congestion syndrome is often a diagnosis of exclusion but may be suspected if related pain is noncyclical with a duration of six months or more and is exacerbated when standing, during intercourse, or just before menses.

N95.- Menopausal and other perimenopausal disorders

Menopause refers to a natural biological process occurring in a female's reproductive life. Physically, this process has four stages: premenopause, perimenopause, menopause, and postmenopause. Premenopause refers to the cusp of menopause. Menstrual cycles may be irregular, but there are no classic menopausal symptoms such as hot flashes or vaginal dryness. Perimenopause refers to the onset of symptoms, such as erratic periods, hot flashes, and vaginal dryness, which correlate with a drop in estrogen and progesterone. This stage lasts about four years, covering the roughly two years before and after the last menstrual period. Decreased levels of estrogen affect REM sleep, which precipitates the stress, depression, and anxiety associated with menopause.

Menopause refers to the one-year period that follows the last menses. Postmenopause begins one year following the last menstrual period and lasts until the end of life.

N95.0 Postmenopausal bleeding

Bleeding from the female reproductive tract, including any bleeding from the vagina, after a year without a menstrual period is defined as postmenopausal bleeding. Postmenopausal bleeding may be entirely benign or it may signify the presence of a malignancy or other medical condition.

N96 Recurrent pregnancy loss

Recurrent pregnancy loss, also referred to as habitual spontaneous abortion or recurrent miscarriage status, is typically defined as the loss of two or more consecutive pregnancies. Multiple causes can be attributed to recurrent miscarriage ranging from uterine or cervical conditions to chromosomal disorders to lifestyle issues.

N97.- Female infertility

Female infertility is defined as the failure to conceive despite regular intercourse and in the absence of contraceptive measures for at least a one-year period. In order for a female to become pregnant, several things need to occur: an egg needs to be produced, the sperm and egg need to meet, and the fertilized egg needs to implant into the uterus to grow. Various chemical processes also play a role throughout each of these steps. Female infertility occurs when one or more of these processes are in some way disrupted.

Code selection in this category is based on etiology behind the infertility. These can include anatomical abnormalities, like a blocked fallopian tube, or functional abnormalities, like a hormonal imbalance.

N97.0 Female infertility associated with anovulation

Anovulation is when a mature ovum (egg) is not released by the ovaries during a menstrual cycle. Each woman has anovulatory cycles but unless chronic it rarely impacts fertility. Typically a female patient still experiences regular menstruation (monthly periods) and may not suspect that she is not producing eggs until trying to conceive. The most common etiology is a hormonal or chemical imbalance, which has been linked to problems with the pituitary gland, hypothalamus, thyroid, and even anorexia or obesity. Far less common are problems that may stem from the ovaries themselves: the egg may not be produced at all by the ovary, the ovary may produce a mature egg but is unable to release it, and/or the ovary may be damaged.

N97.1   Female infertility of tubal origin

Infertility related to the fallopian tubes is largely due to a blocked or damaged tube. When the tube is blocked, the egg cannot travel down the tube to be fertilized by the sperm. Common etiologies include scar tissue from previous infection or surgery, pelvic inflammatory disease (PID), and endometriosis.

N97.2   Female infertility of uterine origin

The uterus is the implantation site of the fertilized egg. If the fertilized ovum cannot implant into the uterus it cannot mature into a fetus. The shape of the uterus, narrowing of the cervix, the presence of tumors or polyps in the uterus, as well as scarring from a previous surgery or endometriosis are a few conditions that may interfere with implantation of the egg into the uterine wall.

Intraoperative and Postprocedural Complications and Disorders of Genitourinary System, Not Elsewhere Classified (N99)

Intraoperative and postprocedural complications can range from stricture formation to adhesions to hemorrhage and hematoma. Complications of artificial openings to the urinary tract (stomas) are also included here.

The categories in this code block are as follows:

N99   Intraoperative and postprocedural complications and disorders of genitourinary system, not elsewhere classified

N99.1-   Postprocedural urethral stricture

This category defines complications of procedures specific to narrowing of the urethra. The urethra is a small tube lined with mucous membrane that leads from the bladder to the exterior of the body. In the male, it is approximately 20 cm long and passes through the prostate gland just below the bladder, where it joins the ejaculatory ducts. Urine is prevented from mixing with semen during ejaculation by the reflex closure of the sphincter muscles guarding the opening into the bladder. In the female, the urethra lies directly behind the symphysis pubis and in front of the vagina and is only about 3 cm long.

N99.11-   Postprocedural urethral stricture, male

In the male patient, strictures may occur within the posterior urethra (initial 1 to 2 inches of the urethra, including the neck of the bladder, prostatic urethra, membranous urethra, and external urinary sphincter) or the anterior urethra (final 9 to 10 inches of the urethra, including the bulbar urethra, penile urethra, and meatus). Men are more likely to develop these kinds of complications due to the length of the urethra. Typical symptoms leading to diagnosis of such a stricture include blood in urine or semen, abnormal urine stream, pain during urination, infection, inability to control bladder, and/or swelling of the penis. Treatment depends on the extent of the stricture and if scar tissue forms and how much but may include dilation, urethrotomy, stent insertion, or open surgery to repair the damage.

Specific codes are assigned based on locations of the stenosis identified in this subcategory.

N99.110   Postprocedural urethral stricture, male, meatal

This type of stricture occurs where the urethra exits the body at the end of the penis.

N99.111   Postprocedural bulbous urethral stricture, male

This type of postprocedural stricture occurs in the portion of urethra from proximal back through the membranous urethra.

N99.112   Postprocedural membranous urethral stricture, male

This type of postprocedural stricture occurs in the small portion of the urethra beginning with the proximal bulbar urethra through the area of the ejaculatory ducts through the point where the sperm enters the urethra.

N99.113   Postprocedural anterior bulbous urethral stricture, male

This type of postprocedural stricture occurs in the front portion of the bulbous urethra situated within the perineum and scrotum.

N99.115   Postprocedural fossa navicularis urethral stricture

This type of postprocedural stricture occurs in the portion of the urethra proximal to the meatus through the distal muscle.

N99.12   Postprocedural urethral stricture, female

The symptoms for postprocedural urethral stricture in women are similar to those for men with the exception of anatomical differences and less frequent occurrence than in men. Further complications may occur if not treated in both men and women, such as urinary retention leading to possible kidney damage. Treatment may include cystoscopy to enlarge the urethra, catheter placement, urinary diversion procedures, or surgery to repair the damage if extensive. Early diagnosis and treatment are the keys to recovery and, in some instances, several procedures may be required to eliminate scar tissue formation.

N99.3   Prolapse of vaginal vault after hysterectomy

Vaginal vault prolapse is a complication most often seen after total hysterectomies that can be attributed to many factors related to the procedure. One part of the equation is the vaginal vault itself. Not part of the normal female anatomy, the vaginal vault is a surgically created structure where the top of the vagina is sewn closed after the removal of the uterus and cervix. This alters the elasticity of the vaginal tissue, which over time can weaken allowing the top of the vagina to sag. Another factor is the interconnected relationship of the pelvic organs and their supporting structures. When the uterus is removed, ligaments and muscles that also support the vagina are severed. If not reattached properly or if the repair does not hold, the vaginal vault sags or droops into the vaginal opening.

Chapter 15: Pregnancy, Childbirth and the Puerperium (O00-O9A)

This chapter classifies diseases and disorders that occur during pregnancy, childbirth, and the six weeks immediately following childbirth (puerperium).

Pregnancy or gestation is the time it takes to grow one or more fetuses from conception until the birth of the child, roughly 40 weeks. It is broken down into three phases or trimesters, starting from the first day of the last menstrual period. Some conditions related to pregnancy may occur in only one specific trimester, more than one trimester, or may not be related to any trimester. As a result, the options for reporting an applicable trimester are tailored to each condition. The trimesters are defined as follows:

1st trimester: Less than 14 weeks 0 days

2nd trimester: 14 weeks 0 days to less than 28 weeks 0 days

3rd trimester: 28 weeks 0 days until delivery

Childbirth is the conclusion of pregnancy. Also described as labor or delivery, it also has phases or stages. The first stage is divided into two parts—latent phase and active phase—and is collectively defined by regular uterine contractions, passage of the mucous plug, and dilation of the cervix. The second stage is the expulsion of the child after the cervix has fully dilated. The delivery of the placenta, which is the sac that surrounds the fetus, is the third and final stage of childbirth.

Puerperium is the six-week period of time, starting immediately following the birth of the child, where the mother's body returns to a nonpregnant state.

The chapter is broken down into the following code blocks:

O00-O08 Pregnancy with abortive outcome

O09 Supervision of high risk pregnancy

O10-O16 Edema, proteinuria and hypertensive disorders in pregnancy, childbirth and the puerperium

O20-O29 Other maternal disorders predominantly related to pregnancy

O30-O48 Maternal care related to the fetus and amniotic cavity and possible delivery problems

O60-O77 Complications of labor and delivery

O80-O82 Encounter for delivery

O85-O92 Complications predominantly related to the puerperium

O94-O9A Other obstetric conditions, not elsewhere classified

There are select codes within this chapter that may need a 7th-character designation to identify the fetus to which a specific condition applies. The selection of the appropriate fetus should come from documentation in the record only. Seventh characters 1 through 5 and 9 are used in multiple gestation pregnancies. A 7th character of 0 is typically used for a single gestation; however, it can also be used with multiple gestations when the affected fetus is not specified in the documentation.

> **Focus Point**
>
> *Some physicians may identify each fetus in a multiple gestation with an alphabetical character (A, B, C) instead of a numerical character (1, 2, 3). For coding purposes and appropriate selection of the 7th character, A is equivalent to 1, B is equivalent to 2, and so forth.*

Pregnancy with Abortive Outcome (O00-O08)

A pregnancy with abortive outcome is one in which the fetus does not survive beyond 20 weeks gestation due to natural or spontaneous causes or elective termination.

The categories in this code block are as follows:

O00 Ectopic pregnancy

O01 Hydatidiform mole

O02 Other abnormal products of conception

O03 Spontaneous abortion

O04 Complications following (induced) termination of pregnancy

O07 Failed attempted termination of pregnancy

O08 Complications following ectopic and molar pregnancy

> **Focus Point**
>
> *According to guideline I.C.21.c.11, Encounters for Obstetrical and Reproductive Services, category Z3A codes should not be assigned for pregnancies with abortive-outcomes (categories O00-O08), elective termination of pregnancy (code Z33.32), or postpartum conditions, as category Z3A is not applicable to these conditions.*

O00.- Ectopic pregnancy

An ectopic pregnancy is the implantation of a fertilized egg (ovum) in an anatomic location other than the uterus. Although some of the associated symptoms mimic those that would be present with a normal intrauterine pregnancy, additional abnormal symptoms may also occur, such as abdominal pain and abnormal vaginal bleeding. One serious complication associated with ectopic pregnancies is a rupture at the site of implantation, leading to internal hemorrhaging.

All ectopic pregnancies, regardless of the site, can occur simultaneously with an intrauterine pregnancy. The classification allows the coder to capture this fact with code options for "with intrauterine pregnancy" or "without intrauterine pregnancy" for each ectopic pregnancy site.

Ectopic Pregnancy

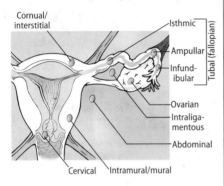

O00.0- Abdominal pregnancy

An abdominal pregnancy occurs when a fertilized egg attaches to abdominal tissue somewhere outside the uterus. This may result from the sperm and egg actually meeting in the abdomen or as a result of a tubal pregnancy that has since migrated to the abdomen. Unlike other ectopic pregnancies, the fetus in abdominal pregnancy may mature for some time undetected and it is not uncommon for a fetus to remain viable until it can be delivered.

O00.1- Tubal pregnancy

Tubal pregnancy is the implantation of a fertilized ovum in the fallopian tube, more often in the right than in the left. In a majority of cases, tubal pregnancy is a result of damage to the fallopian tube, such as inflammation or scar tissue formation, obstructing the passage of the fertilized egg through the tube and into the uterus. It can also simply be the result of abnormally shaped tubes. A tubal pregnancy may occur in conjunction with an intrauterine pregnancy.

O00.2- Ovarian pregnancy

Typically in order for an egg to be fertilized it must first be released into the fallopian tube. The sperm released in the vagina move their way up into the fallopian tubes where they meet the egg and fertilization takes place. Ovarian pregnancy occurs when the egg is not released into the fallopian tube but instead is fertilized inside the ovary. Implantation occurs within the ovary and the embryo starts to develop. An ovarian pregnancy may occur in conjunction with an intrauterine pregnancy.

O00.8- Other ectopic pregnancy

This code reports implantation of a fertilized ovum in other specified sites such as the cervix, the uterine musculature (mesometric), uterine cornu (horn), and the broad ligament.

O01.- Hydatidiform mole

Hydatidiform mole is abnormal mass or tissue growth occurring in the placenta. It is a direct result of abnormal genetic material found in the fertilized egg. The fertilized egg primarily produces two sets of cells: trophoblasts, which develop into and attach the placenta to the uterine wall, and cells that develop into the embryo. Due to abnormal or absent genetic material, there is extensive trophoblast proliferation with little or no embryonic development resulting in an abnormal mass of tissue. Because it is the trophoblasts that take over, this condition is often called gestational trophoblastic disease.

> **Focus Point**
>
> *Although rare, some hydatidiform moles develop into a malignant tumor called choriocarcinoma or malignant hydatidiform mole. This condition is classified to category D39 in the neoplasms chapter.*

O01.0 Classical hydatidiform mole

Classical hydatidiform mole, also called a complete hydatidiform mole, occurs when a fertilized egg is not carrying any female chromosomal material. Without two sets of chromosomes within the egg (one set from the male, one set from the female), an embryo cannot develop. The trophoblasts are essentially free to grow into the space where the embryo would have been, proliferating without inhibition. A complete hydatidiform mole has no fetal tissue found within the abnormal placental tissue mass.

O01.1 Incomplete and partial hydatidiform mole

An incomplete hydatidiform mole most often occurs when two sperm fertilize one normal egg. Only one set of chromosomes from the male and female are necessary to develop the embryo; when two male sets exist, there is too much genetic material. The result is an excess of trophoblastic cells growing into the space the embryo needs to grow limiting the development of the fetus. Because some fetal development occurs in partial hydatidiform moles, fetal tissue is often found in the abnormal placental mass.

O02.- Other abnormal products of conception

Products of conception refers to tissue that is formed when the egg and the sperm unite, including fetal tissue and the placenta. In early miscarriage, a pathologist may have to examine the tissue in order to identify whether or not products of conception are present.

O02.1 Missed abortion

For coding purposes, a missed abortion is a fetal death occurring before 20 weeks gestation with the retention of the fetus. Signs and symptoms may be minimal and the patient may be unaware of the fetal loss; however, clinical evaluation shows the disappearance of normal signs of pregnancy, such as abnormal levels of hCG, no embryo in the uterus, or the fetus has no heartbeat.

O03.- Spontaneous abortion

The definition of spontaneous abortion, or what is often referred to as miscarriage, is complete or incomplete expulsion of the products of conception before completion of 20 weeks of gestation. Vaginal bleeding, abdominal cramping, and passage of tissue from the vagina are common signs and symptoms. In most cases, the cause of the miscarriage is unknown but certain viruses, uterine abnormalities such as fibroids, environmental toxins, and chromosomal anomalies in the embryo are just a few of the linked etiologies. The codes in this category are classified based on three factors: whether or not there is a complication associated with the spontaneous abortion, the specific complication when a complication is present, and whether the abortion is complete or incomplete.

Focus Point

There is a hierarchy for infections, shock, and sepsis codes related to abortion, whether spontaneous or induced. The sepsis code trumps the infection (genital tract and pelvis) and shock codes and only the sepsis code needs be reported.

O03.3- Other and unspecified complications following incomplete spontaneous abortion

Incomplete spontaneous abortion is expulsion of only part of the products of conception. In an incomplete abortion, the amniotic sac and fetus may be expelled without the chorion and decidua, only the embryo may be expelled, or the amniotic sac may rupture with passage of the fetus alone. Incomplete abortion requires evacuation of the remaining tissue.

O03.31 Shock following incomplete spontaneous abortion

Maternal shock is an acute peripheral circulatory failure due to an aberration of circulatory control or loss of circulating fluid. In most cases, it is related to excessive bleeding. Signs and symptoms of shock can include hypotension, coldness of skin, tachycardia, anxiety, or loss of consciousness.

O03.37 Sepsis following incomplete spontaneous abortion

Sepsis is a systemic (body wide) inflammatory response to the presence of toxins or microorganisms in the bloodstream. Risk of infection is high after an abortion, especially when products of conception are retained as occurs with incomplete abortions. Sepsis following incomplete spontaneous abortion is evidenced by an infection, along with symptoms that may include fever, foul smelling vaginal discharge, abdominal pain or cramping, and heavy vaginal bleeding. Localized infections that may lead to sepsis include endometritis and sexually transmitted diseases.

O03.8- Other and unspecified complications following complete or unspecified spontaneous abortion

Complete spontaneous abortion is the expulsion of the entire products of conception. In general, complications are less likely to occur with a complete abortion and treatment is often not necessary.

O03.81 Shock following complete or unspecified spontaneous abortion

Maternal shock is an acute peripheral circulatory failure due to an aberration of circulatory control or loss of circulating fluid. In most cases it is related to excessive bleeding. Signs and symptoms of shock can include hypotension, coldness of skin, tachycardia, anxiety, or loss of consciousness.

O03.87 Sepsis following complete or unspecified spontaneous abortion

Sepsis is a systemic (body wide) inflammatory response to the presence of toxins or microorganisms in the bloodstream. Risk of infection is high after an abortion, especially when products of conception are retained as occurs with incomplete abortions. Sepsis following complete spontaneous abortion is evidenced by an infection, along with symptoms that may include fever, foul smelling vaginal discharge, abdominal pain or cramping, and heavy vaginal bleeding. Localized infections that may lead to sepsis include endometritis and sexually transmitted diseases.

O08.-   Complications following ectopic and molar pregnancy

Codes from this category are reported in addition to a code from categories O00-O02 to identify any associated complications of ectopic pregnancies (O00), hydatidiform moles (O01), or other abnormal products of conception (O02). The codes are further classified by the type of complication ranging from shock to metabolic disorders to urinary tract infections.

O08.0   Genital tract and pelvic infection following ectopic and molar pregnancy

Genital tract and pelvic infection following an ectopic or molar pregnancy may be caused by aerobic or anaerobic organisms. The infection may be localized to the products of conception or it may result in endometritis, parametritis, oophoritis, salpingitis, salpingo-oophoritis, or pelvic peritonitis. Signs and symptoms of genital tract and pelvic infection include pain, bleeding, fever, and vaginal discharge.

Supervision of High Risk Pregnancy (O09)

A high-risk pregnancy is loosely defined as one with the potential to give rise to complications or that increases the mortality risk to the mother or baby.

The categories in this code block are as follows:

O09   Supervision of high risk pregnancy

O09.-   Supervision of high risk pregnancy

A high-risk pregnancy is loosely defined as one with the potential to give rise to complications or that increases the mortality risk to the mother or baby.

Focus Point

A high-risk pregnancy can pose problems for the maternal patient before, during, or after delivery (puerperium). However, the codes in category O09 are to be used only for the prenatal period. Should complications arise during labor or the postpartum period, a specific obstetric code for the complication should be used instead of a code from category O09.

O09.A-   Supervision of pregnancy with history of molar pregnancy

A molar pregnancy (also known as hydatidiform mole) occurs when tissue that would normally develop into a fetus instead becomes an abnormal growth of tissue or large number of cysts that can resemble a cluster of grapes. It is thought that the underlying cause is related to a problem with the genetic information from the egg or sperm. A patient with a personal history of molar pregnancy is considered at high risk because she is much more likely to develop a subsequent molar pregnancy.

O09.5-   Supervision of elderly primigravida and multigravida

A pregnant woman is considered "elderly" if she will be 35 years of age or older at expected date of delivery. A primigravida is a first pregnancy while a multigravida is a second or greater pregnancy.

O09.51-   Supervision of elderly primigravida

O09.52-   Supervision of elderly multigravida

One of these codes should be used even if the pregnancy is normal in all other respects because elderly primigravida and multigravida women have higher risk pregnancies, deliveries, and puerperal periods simply due to age. The risk of complications is even greater for first time "elderly" mothers. Associated complications may include hypertension, gestational diabetes, prolonged labor, malpresentation, and the need for cesarean section. Fetal chromosomal abnormalities have also been linked to "elderly" patients; the older the maternal age the greater the risks.

O09.6-   Supervision of young primigravida and multigravida

Pregnant patients that are 16 years old or younger are classified here. A primigravida is a first pregnancy while a multigravida is a second or greater pregnancy.

O09.61-   Supervision of young primigravida

O09.62-   Supervision of young multigravida

There are various risks to the baby and the mother when pregnancy occurs in or before the teenage years. These are largely related to little or no prenatal care. Complications include premature birth, high blood pressure that can lead to preeclampsia, anemia, and a low birth weight baby. The risk of postpartum depression is also much greater in pregnant teens.

Edema, Proteinuria and Hypertensive Disorders in Pregnancy, Childbirth and the Puerperium (O10-O16)

Edema is swelling due to fluid accumulation in the intercellular spaces. During pregnancy, slight swelling of the extremities is normal as the blood and body fluid production has increased to support the baby and get the body ready for delivery. However edema can also be a sign of preeclampsia, which is a more serious complication. Proteinuria is abnormal quantities of serum proteins present in the urine. The threshold levels of these serum proteins are different between a pregnant and nonpregnant patient as it is normal for protein levels to increase during pregnancy. Proteinuria, like edema, is clinically important because proteinuria that is above the normal threshold for a pregnant patient can be indicative of a serious pregnancy related condition called preeclampsia. Hypertension is abnormally increased arterial blood pressure. Hypertensive disorders in pregnancy range from those associated with heart disease and/or chronic kidney disease to eclampsia to those brought on by the pregnancy (gestational hypertension).

The categories in this code block are as follows:

O10	Pre-existing hypertension complicating pregnancy, childbirth and the puerperium
O11	Pre-existing hypertension with pre-eclampsia
O12	Gestational [pregnancy-induced] edema and proteinuria without hypertension
O13	Gestational [pregnancy-induced] hypertension without significant proteinuria
O14	Pre-eclampsia
O15	Eclampsia
O16	Unspecified maternal hypertension

O10.- Pre-existing hypertension complicating pregnancy, childbirth and the puerperium

Hypertension is followed closely in pregnant patients due to worrisome complications that can be associated with the condition. These complications may include stroke, placental abruption, and superimposed pre-eclampsia.

O10.0- Pre-existing essential hypertension complicating pregnancy, childbirth and the puerperium

Pre-existing essential hypertension is persistent blood pressure of 140/90 or greater diagnosed before the onset of pregnancy or within the first trimester. Examination reveals elevated blood pressure without proteinuria or nondependent edema.

O10.1- Pre-existing hypertensive heart disease complicating pregnancy, childbirth and the puerperium

Hypertension (high blood pressure) causes the heart stress because the heart has to work harder to pump blood against the high pressure in the blood vessels. If prolonged, it can eventually cause changes to the conduction system, the myocardium, and/or the coronary vessels, manifested as arrhythmias, infarctions, and angina. When circulatory changes that occur as part of pregnancy are added to the equation, the demand on the maternal cardiovascular system is compounded.

O10.2- Pre-existing hypertensive chronic kidney disease complicating pregnancy, childbirth and the puerperium

The relationship between hypertension and kidney disease is cyclical. Hypertension damages the filtering units of the kidneys, reducing the effectiveness of the kidneys in removing excess waste and excess fluid from the blood. The excess fluid in the blood makes it harder for the heart to move the blood, thereby increasing blood pressure. Even in the absence of pre-existing disease, a maternal patient can experience blood pressure and renal function changes related to pregnancy. The effect the pregnancy has on the maternal patient's existing renal function depends largely on the stage of CKD: the more advanced the disease, the greater the risk for complications to the mother and/or the fetus.

O10.3- Pre-existing hypertensive heart and chronic kidney disease complicating pregnancy, childbirth and the puerperium

Hypertension (high blood pressure) causes the heart stress because the heart has to work harder to pump blood against the high pressure in the blood vessels. If prolonged, it can eventually cause changes to the conduction system, the myocardium, and/or the coronary vessels, manifested as arrhythmias, infarctions, and angina.

Prolonged elevated blood pressure damages the filtering units of the kidneys, reducing the effectiveness of the kidneys in removing excess waste and excess fluid from the blood. The excess fluid in the blood makes it harder for the heart to move the blood, which in turn elevates the blood pressure.

Although hypertension is the initiating cause of damage to the heart and kidneys, the interrelationship between these two organs also plays a role; for example, reduced kidney function can lead to cardiovascular dysfunction and vice versa. Careful management during and after pregnancy is critical for maternal patients with pre-existing hypertensive heart and chronic kidney disease.

O10.4- Pre-existing secondary hypertension complicating pregnancy, childbirth and the puerperium

Pre-existing secondary hypertension is a chronic hypertensive condition that was brought on by another underlying disorder, such as renovascular disease or endocrine disorders. Management of the underlying disorder often is enough to keep the hypertension under control.

O11.- Pre-existing hypertension with pre-eclampsia

Pre-eclampsia is a complication of pregnancy that is most often characterized by hypertension and proteinuria with or without edema of the extremities. Other symptoms that may be seen are vision changes, oliguria, pulmonary edema, and evidence of organ dysfunction, such as impaired liver function. Pre-eclampsia typically presents during the second or third trimester, usually when the pregnancy is at or beyond 20 weeks of gestation, but when the patient has pre-existing hypertension, pre-eclampsia may present during the first trimester. With pre-existing hypertension and pre-eclampsia, the patient may present with high blood pressure that is not able to be controlled with medication that was previously effective.

O12.- Gestational [pregnancy-induced] edema and proteinuria without hypertension

Edema and proteinuria may occur during pregnancy and in many cases appear together. Edema (swelling) may affect several different body sites, most commonly the legs and feet, but some patients have edema symptoms of the hands, face, or labia. Proteinuria is defined as more than 300 mg of protein in a 24-hour urine sample. Patients with either of these symptoms are monitored closely to ensure that the condition does not progress to pre-eclampsia.

O13.- Gestational [pregnancy-induced] hypertension without significant proteinuria

Gestational hypertension is a clinical diagnosis defined by the new onset of hypertension (systolic blood pressure >= 140 mmHg and/or diastolic blood pressure >= 90 mmHg) at >= 20 weeks of gestation and in the absence of proteinuria or new signs of end-organ dysfunction. The blood pressure readings should be documented on at least two occasions at least four hours apart. Gestational hypertension is severe when systolic blood pressure is >= 160 mmHg and/or diastolic blood pressure is >= 110 mmHg. Patients with gestational hypertension are monitored to ensure that the condition does not progress to pre-eclampsia.

O14.- Pre-eclampsia

The underlying etiology of pre-eclampsia, although not completely understood, is predominantly thought to be related to placental dysfunction. Other causes may include immunological, dietary, and environmental factors. Pre-eclampsia presents during the second or third trimester, usually when the pregnancy is at or beyond 20 weeks of gestation, and even into the postpartum period. It is characterized by a blood pressure of 140/90 or higher accompanied by abnormal liver or kidney function, proteinuria, visual disturbances, or decreased blood platelets. The patient can recover from pre-eclampsia after the baby is born; however, depending on the extent of related organ damage, some organs may be permanently affected.

O14.0- Mild to moderate pre-eclampsia

O14.1- Severe pre-eclampsia

The diagnosis of pre-eclampsia alone, regardless of the severity, usually begins with an elevated blood pressure of 140/90. The higher the blood pressure goes and the time period for which it persists increases the severity level. Severity level is also measured based on associated features. Usually mild to moderate pre-eclampsia only exhibits proteinuria in addition to the high blood pressure. Patients with severe pre-eclampsia will have proteinuria but also exhibit other organ damage, such as abnormal liver or kidney function, changes in vision, and fluid in the lungs (edema).

O14.2- HELLP syndrome

HELLP syndrome, which stands for Hemolysis, Elevated Liver enzymes, and Low Platelet count, is a very severe type of pre-eclampsia that can lead to internal bleeding from the liver. This condition is a medical emergency with potential for associated lifelong health problems or even death.

O15.- Eclampsia

Eclampsia is a complication of pregnancy characterized by the onset of grand mal seizures and/or unexplained coma. It is considered a complication of severe pre-eclampsia. Edema, proteinuria, and hypertension are clinical manifestations of pre-eclampsia that when detected early can reduce the chances of the pregnant patient progressing to an eclamptic event. The majority of these cases occur during the third trimester, with about 80 percent of them during delivery or within the first 48 hours postpartum. Patients frequently experience neurologic symptoms such as headache before eclamptic seizures.

Ruling out eclampsia in an obstetric patient who has been involved in an unexplained trauma is important, because the trauma may actually have been preceded by a seizure.

Other Maternal Disorders Predominantly Related to Pregnancy (O20-O29)

A majority of the conditions included in this code block largely occur as a direct result of being pregnant. Many changes in the maternal body, including changes in hormone and other chemical levels, are necessary to provide an adequate environment for the fetus. When the maternal body cannot adjust to these changes certain conditions may result, ranging from endocrine disorders to vascular complications.

This code block also identifies conditions that may arise as a result of anesthesia and abnormalities found on antenatal screening that may predispose a patient to problems during pregnancy.

The categories in this code block are as follows:

O20	Hemorrhage in early pregnancy
O21	Excessive vomiting in pregnancy
O22	Venous complications and hemorrhoids in pregnancy
O23	Infections of genitourinary tract in pregnancy
O24	Diabetes mellitus in pregnancy, childbirth, and the puerperium
O25	Malnutrition in pregnancy, childbirth and the puerperium
O26	Maternal care for other conditions predominantly related to pregnancy
O28	Abnormal findings on antenatal screening of mother
O29	Complications of anesthesia during pregnancy

O20.- Hemorrhage in early pregnancy

Early pregnancy is defined as before the completion of 20 weeks gestation.

O20.0 Threatened abortion

A threatened abortion is characterized by vaginal bleeding and/or abdominal pain or cramping with no associated cervical dilation and no passage of tissue. Threatened abortion may suggest an increased risk for miscarriage, although symptoms may also resolve with the pregnancy developing to full term.

O22.- Venous complications and hemorrhoids in pregnancy

Venous complications that arise during pregnancy can range from thrombus formation to varicose veins.

O22.0- Varicose veins of lower extremity in pregnancy

During pregnancy many changes in the body can influence the development of varicose or dilated veins. The first is the increase in blood volume. The veins in the legs are already working against gravity to push the blood to the heart; the greater volume is an additional burden. As the uterus grows, pressure is placed on the pelvic blood vessels, again causing the lower extremity vessels to push harder to get the blood through the veins. Finally, the hormone levels of progesterone rise, causing the blood vessels to dilate. In most instances varicose veins are harmless and resolve quickly after pregnancy. When symptoms are present they may include night cramps, localized pain, edema, and inflammation often exacerbated by standing.

O22.1- Genital varices in pregnancy

Some women develop varices, dilated veins, of the vulvar region during pregnancy. Often genital varices are asymptomatic, but in some cases they may cause swelling, pressure, and discomfort.

O22.2- Superficial thrombophlebitis in pregnancy

Thrombophlebitis is inflammation of a vein (phlebitis) due to a blood clot (thrombus). Thrombophlebitis typically affects the lower extremities and is classified by the depth of the vein in which it is found: superficial or deep. The veins located near the surface of the skin are considered superficial. Superficial veins in the legs include the greater and lesser saphenous veins.

O22.3- Deep phlebothrombosis in pregnancy

Phlebothrombosis occurs when a thrombus develops in a vein, in this case the deep veins. Inflammation of the vein (phlebitis) can occur but is rarely associated with deep vein thrombosis. This condition primarily affects the deep veins of the lower extremities, which include the iliac, femoral, popliteal, and tibial veins. The risk of developing a deep vein thrombosis (DVT) increases with pregnancy due to changing hormones, clotting factors that make the blood clot more easily, and decreased blood flow to the lower extremity arteries due to compression from the uterus and growing baby. DVTs carry a risk of blocking the blood flow of the affected vein completely or breaking free and moving to other areas in the body, like the heart or lung, which can be fatal.

O22.4- Hemorrhoids in pregnancy

Hemorrhoids are dilated veins of the hemorrhoidal plexus in the lower rectum and are a common complaint during pregnancy. Hemorrhoids are typically caused by straining related to constipation and pressure on the veins in the rectum and perineum. They can be painful and itchy, but are not usually a serious medical condition. External hemorrhoids occur in the region of the external anal sphincter and are covered by the skin of the anal canal. Internal hemorrhoids occur in the rectum and are covered with rectal mucosa; these typically cannot be seen or felt unless they prolapse through the anal canal.

O23.- Infections of genitourinary tract in pregnancy

This category identifies infections related to, but not limited to, the following organs found in the female genitourinary tract: kidneys, bladder, urethra, cervix, ovaries, and fallopian tubes.

O23.1- Infections of bladder in pregnancy

Bladder infections are a common complication of pregnancy. Most bladder infections are caused by bacteria. Bacteria are normally removed from the bladder during urination. During pregnancy the growing uterus, which sits directly above the bladder, can block the passage of urine. The bacteria that are not passed can proliferate, causing an infection.

O24.- Diabetes mellitus in pregnancy, childbirth, and the puerperium

Diabetes mellitus (DM) is a metabolic disorder that is a product of inadequate insulin production by the pancreas or the body not responding to the insulin that is produced. Diabetes can be a pre-existing condition or brought on by the pregnancy itself (gestational) and can increase the potential for adverse health conditions in the mother and the neonate. The codes in this category are classified based on the type of diabetes (e.g., Type 1, Type 2, gestational) and by the timing of the diabetes (e.g., during a pregnancy, childbirth, or postpartum).

Focus Point

The link between diabetes mellitus and pre-eclampsia can be a two-way street. Pregnant patients with any form of diabetes during pregnancy have an increased risk of also developing pre-eclampsia and those patients who have had pre-eclampsia during pregnancy but without a history of diabetes are at an increased risk of developing diabetes during or after pregnancy.

O26.- Maternal care for other conditions predominantly related to pregnancy

This category includes a myriad of maternal conditions from liver and biliary tract disorders to renal disease to recurrent pregnancy loss that may complicate the management of a pregnant patient.

O26.8- Other specified pregnancy related conditions

This subcategory includes conditions such as renal disease, exhaustion and fatigue, and peripheral neuritis that may occur during the course of the pregnancy.

O26.84- Uterine size-date discrepancy complicating pregnancy

Uterine size and expected date of delivery can be difficult to estimate. Although not an exact science, typically the fundal height (centimeters above the pubic symphysis) should correspond to the gestational age. If the subjective estimation of the last menstrual period does not correspond with the fundal height measurement, an ultrasonography is performed to gain an accurate, objective assessment. Fetal viability, development, and health are also assessed during the ultrasonogram. Many things can contribute to a discrepancy between the gestational date compared to the uterine size, including too little (oligohydramnios) or too much (polyhydramnios) amniotic fluid, intrauterine growth retardation, and multiple gestations.

O26.85- Spotting complicating pregnancy

Spotting is very light bleeding that can vary in color from pink to red to brown. Some spotting is normal during pregnancy needing only to be monitored. However, it can also be a sign of a potentially serious complication or condition that may need prompt treatment. Therefore, it's often necessary for the obstetrician to investigate and rule out possible problems, such as threatened spontaneous abortion, ectopic pregnancy, infection, or early labor.

Focus Point

Spotting should not be confused with hemorrhage in early pregnancy (O20) or hemorrhage associated with conditions such as placenta previa (O44.-), abruptio placenta (O45.-), or other antepartum hemorrhage (O46.-).

O26.86 Pruritic urticarial papules and plaques of pregnancy (PUPPP)

PUPPP is an itchy, harmless, rash-like skin disorder. The true etiology is unknown but it is thought that it is related to the stretching of the skin, as it typically doesn't appear until late in the third trimester and is more commonly seen in those women with multiple fetus pregnancies. The characteristic papules and plaques start on the abdomen and spread to other areas, primarily the legs, arms, chest and neck. This condition is typically seen in a first time mother only, rarely occurring in subsequent pregnancies.

O26.87-   Cervical shortening

The cervix is the lower part of the uterus that extends into the vagina. Cervical length is defined as the length of the closed endocervical canal and usually measures around 3 to 3.5 cm around the end of the second trimester. This cervical length decreases and the cervix softens and opens as the pregnancy progresses into the latter part of the third trimester. If the cervical length starts to decrease too soon, before the end of the second trimester, it can result in preterm labor and premature birth. The cause of preterm labor may be multifactorial, but a short cervix may exacerbate these causes and increase the risk of preterm labor.

Focus Point

Cervical shortening and cervical incompetence (insufficiency) should not be used interchangeably. Classic cervical incompetence is a diagnosis based on an obstetric history of recurrent second or early third trimester fetal loss, following painless cervical dilatation, prolapse or rupture of the membranes, and expulsion of a live fetus despite minimal uterine activity. In contrast to cervical incompetence, cervical shortening may pose a risk factor for premature birth, and may alter the course of treatment and management of the pregnancy, yet the patient may carry the fetus to term. For treatment of cervical incompetence during pregnancy, see subcategory O34.3.- Maternal care for cervical incompetence.

Maternal Care Related to the Fetus and Amniotic Cavity and Possible Delivery Problems (O30-O48)

The amniotic cavity or sac, as it is sometimes referred to, is just that, a sac that surrounds the fetus. It is composed of a thin membrane called amnion that holds the amniotic fluid and the fetus.

Amniotic fluid is the fluid found within the amniotic sac. This fluid brings important nutrients to the fetus, cushions the fetus, regulates temperature, and is essential in the development of the fetal lungs and gastrointestinal tract.

The placenta is a flat, disc-shaped organ formed from cells of the fertilized egg. The placenta is attached to the uterine wall and the umbilical cord is attached to the placenta, creating a transfer site between the mother and the baby, without the maternal and fetal blood mixing. Nutrients and oxygen can be transferred to the baby and waste products and carbon dioxide can be transferred to the mother.

Around the tenth week of gestation, the fertilized egg or embryo enters the fetal stage of development, which lasts until the baby's birth. Although most of the organs and structures are formed, differentiation and growth of these organs and structures continues throughout the fetal stage.

Codes found in the categories classified here report issues with the fetus, pelvic organs, placenta, and other conditions that may complicate the management of the pregnancy or the delivery.

The categories in this code block are as follows:

O30	Multiple gestation
O31	Complications specific to multiple gestation
O32	Maternal care for malpresentation of fetus
O33	Maternal care for disproportion
O34	Maternal care for abnormality of pelvic organs
O35	Maternal care for known or suspected fetal abnormality and damage
O36	Maternal care for other fetal problems
O40	Polyhydramnios
O41	Other disorders of amniotic fluid and membranes
O42	Premature rupture of membranes
O43	Placental disorders
O44	Placenta previa
O45	Premature separation of placenta [abruptio placentae]
O46	Antepartum hemorrhage, not elsewhere classified
O47	False labor
O48	Late pregnancy

O30.-   Multiple gestation

Multiple gestation is two or more fetuses in one pregnant patient. The possibility of developing complications that can affect both the mother and the babies increases with multiple gestations.

O30.02- Conjoined twin pregnancy

Conjoined twins are identical (monozygotic) twins that fail to completely separate into two individuals. They are most often joined at the head, chest, or pelvis and may share one or more internal organs. Conjoined twins pose significant risks during pregnancy with vaginal delivery rarely possible.

Chapter 15: Pregnancy, Childbirth and the Puerperium (O00–O9A)

Focus Point

Approximately half of conjoined twins develop excessive amniotic fluid (polyhydramnios), which increases the risk of premature rupture of the membranes, problems with the umbilical cord, and stillbirth. Polyhydramnios is reported with codes from category O40. Another possible complication is twin-to-twin transfusion syndrome (TTTS), which is considered a placental complication and is reported with a code from category O43.

O31.- Complications specific to multiple gestation

The complications classified in this category are primarily related to the loss of one or more fetuses with continuation of the pregnancy for those viable fetuses remaining. In some cases, the termination of a fetus may be the patient's choice or one or more of the fetuses may spontaneously abort or die.

O31.0- Papyraceous fetus

Papyraceous fetus is a rare complication in a multiple gestation pregnancy where a fetus has died but remains in utero. As the other viable fetus grows, the dead fetus gets compressed until it is compacted and mummified, with skin resembling parchment. A papyraceous fetus can increase the risk of infection and hemorrhage and, depending on its position in the uterus, can obstruct a vaginal delivery necessitating a cesarean section.

Focus Point

Vanishing twin or vanishing twin syndrome is when one fetus from a multiple gestation dies but is reabsorbed (partially or completely) by the other fetus. When the fetus is not fully absorbed it can result in a papyraceous fetus.

O32.- Maternal care for malpresentation of fetus

Presentation is the position of the fetus when entering the birth canal and is described by the anatomical part that enters the canal first. The most common presentation, vertex, is when the top or crown of the head is the first to enter. Malpresentation describes any position other than vertex. Because the position of the baby influences how easy or difficult the delivery will be, the position of the fetus becomes increasingly important the closer the patient gets to delivery. Malpresentation can cause the baby to essentially get stuck in the birth canal, thus obstructing the labor process, which can prolong labor and/or require a cesarean section.

Fetal Malposition

Breech — Mother's pelvis

Shoulder (arm prolapse)

Face (mentum)

Oblique

Compound (extremity together with head)

Focus Point

Codes from this category should be used only for observations, hospitalization, or other obstetric care or cesarean delivery that occurs before the onset of labor. According to the Excludes 1 note, any malpresentation of fetus with obstructed labor is reported with a code from category O64.-.

O32.0- Maternal care for unstable lie

An "unstable lie" occurs when the fetus continues to change positions in the late stages of pregnancy, from 37 weeks and beyond. In earlier pregnancy, the changing of fetal positions is generally considered normal and not a significant concern. However flipping from head-down position to transverse, oblique, or breech persisting into late-term pregnancy may require extra management to avoid cord compression and other risks of malposition at delivery. Causes can include placenta previa, uterine malformations or fibroids, oligohydramnios, and fetal macrosomia, among others. Management may include elective cesarean, hospital management, or daily examinations with the goal of ensuring that spontaneous rupture of membranes (SROM) does not occur while the fetus is in a malpresentation and obstructive state.

O32.1- Maternal care for breech presentation

In breech presentation, the buttocks present first. There are several types of breech presentation, but only two types of breech presentation are included here: frank breech in which the hips are flexed and the legs are straight, extending over the abdomen and thorax so that the feet lie beside the face, and complete breech, where the hips and knees are flexed and the legs are crossed.

O32.2- Maternal care for transverse and oblique lie

Transverse lie describes the presentation of the fetus before the onset of labor that is sideways across the uterus, perpendicular to the birth canal with the head on one side and the bottom across the abdomen on the other side. Less common is oblique lie, which means the fetus is at a diagonal angle with the head in the mother's hip. Both are normal positions in the earlier term up through the 31st week, but the mother should be checked to rule out placental previa. Both are complications for vaginal delivery if the fetus does not turn before the onset of labor, in which case external version or cesarean delivery is performed.

O32.3- Maternal care for face, brow and chin presentation

These presentations can occur in concurrence with a large fetal head or the premature rupture of membranes. They are characterized by head and neck hyperextension rather than the tucked chin that is present in the normal cephalic position. This often corrects itself before the pushing phase of labor begins, and the baby can still be delivered vaginally unless the labor is arrested, at which time a cesarean section may be necessary.

O32.6- Maternal care for compound presentation

Compound is a relatively rare presentation that involves the baby's arm and leg prolapsing into the birth canal alongside the head. Most commonly involved is the hand or arm, and often the extremity retracts on its own as labor progresses or reacts, and reflexively moves away in response to a slight stimulus such as a pinch. Normal vaginal delivery is frequently possible, but excessive pressure on the limb is not recommended. If the labor is prolonged, blood supply can be cut off, in which case cesarean delivery may be necessary.

O32.8- Maternal care for other malpresentation of fetus

This code includes two types of breech presentation: footling and incomplete. For both types, although the buttocks are still close to the birth canal, typically one foot (incomplete) or both feet (footling) present before the buttocks.

O33.- Maternal care for disproportion

Disproportion refers to maternal and/or fetal structural abnormalities or disproportions that interfere with normal delivery. There are two general terms used to describe disproportion: cephalopelvic disproportion and fetopelvic disproportion. Codes in this category are specific to whether the disproportion is due to a maternal factor, mixed maternal and fetal factors, or fetal factors alone. Possible maternal factors include deformity of the pelvic bones, generally contracted pelvis, inlet contraction, and outlet contraction. Possible fetal factors include unusually large fetus, hydrocephalic fetus, and fetal hydrops.

O34.- Maternal care for abnormality of pelvic organs

The female pelvic organs represented in this category include the uterus, cervix, vagina, vulva, and perineum.

> **Focus Point**
>
> *Codes from this category should be used only for observations, hospitalization, or other obstetric care or cesarean delivery that occurs before the onset of labor. When obstructed labor is associated with one of these conditions, code first O65.5 Obstructed labor due to abnormality of maternal pelvic organs.*

O34.0- Maternal care for congenital malformation of uterus

This code includes congenital conditions such as double or bicornis uterus. Double uterus occurs in female fetal development when the two small tubes (Müllerian ducts) that normally merge together to create one uterus instead develop their own separate uterus. There may be only one cervix (opening) in the vagina or each uterus may have its own cervix, divided by a thin vaginal septum. A bicornate uterus is also due to an incomplete fusing of the paramesonephric (Müllerian) ducts and appears externally as only one uterus but is divided into two lateral horns, referred to as heart-shaped uterus. Both conditions carry a higher risk of miscarriage or premature delivery.

O34.2- Maternal care due to uterine scar from previous surgery

Previous uterine surgery is an indication for a higher level of supervision as it can carry increased risk during pregnancy. An incisional scar from a prior uterine surgery raises the risk of uterine rupture along the scar line is higher as well as the risk of issues with the placenta.

O34.21- Maternal care for scar from previous cesarean delivery

Previous cesarean sections carry a higher risk of placental problems and uterine tears or rupture along the previous scar. Despite this higher risk, according to the American Pregnancy Association, 90 percent of all vaginal births after cesarean (VBAC) are successful.

O34.211 Maternal care for low transverse scar from previous cesarean delivery

Low transverse incisions are the most commonly used and include various types, including Pfannenstiel and Joel-Cohen techniques. This incision leaves a small, horizontal scar directly above the pubis. This is typically a stronger scar with faster healing than other incisions.

O34.212 Maternal care for vertical scar from previous cesarean delivery

A small, low vertical incision is sometimes used for malpositioned infants. This code is also used to report previous classical incisions, which are larger, midline vertical incisions generally performed only in emergent or preterm deliveries.

O34.29 Maternal care due to uterine scar from other previous surgery

Other previous surgeries, such as transmural incision of the uterine wall to remove uterine fibroids or tumors, leave scars that can also pose a risk during pregnancy. They are reported with this code.

O34.3- Maternal care for cervical incompetence

The cervix is the opening at the bottom of the uterus that extends into the vagina. At the beginning of a pregnancy the cervix is firm and closed in order to support the growing baby. As the pregnancy reaches the end of the last trimester, the cervix begins to soften and open. Cervical incompetence, sometimes called insufficient cervix, occurs when the cervical tissue is not strong enough to support the growing baby to full term, opening up before the baby is able to survive outside the womb. It is often diagnosed based on an obstetric history of recurrent second or early third trimester fetal loss, following painless cervical dilatation, prolapse or rupture of the membranes, and expulsion of a live fetus despite minimal uterine activity. The etiology may be congenital or due to acquired causes such as previous surgical dilation, conization, or other trauma of delivery.

O35.- Maternal care for known or suspected fetal abnormality and damage

This category identifies confirmed or suspected damage to the fetus that alters the management of the mother. Drugs and/or alcohol consumed by the mother, medical procedures on the fetus in utero, and congenital conditions that cause malformations or abnormalities in the fetus are some but not all of the conditions included here.

O35.7- Maternal care for (suspected) damage to fetus by other medical procedures

Medical procedures performed on the mother or fetus pose a risk of damage to the fetus. This subcategory covers a wide range of medical procedures, from surgeries on the uterus to diagnostic amniocentesis to a relatively new surgical specialty, fetal surgery.

> **Focus Point**
>
> Although the fetus is also affected by the in utero surgery it is not appropriate to assign a code from the perinatal chapter (chapter 16). The maternal record should never include a perinatal code.

O36.- Maternal care for other fetal problems

Fetal abnormalities can have a significant impact on the mother, in some cases necessitating the termination of the pregnancy. Incompatibilities between the mother and baby's blood and abnormalities in the development of the fetus are a few of the conditions represented here.

O36.2- Maternal care for hydrops fetalis

Hydrops fetalis is abnormal fluid buildup in at least two of the following fetal organ spaces: the skin (edema), abdomen (ascites), around the heart (pericardia effusion), and around the lung (pleural effusion). Fluid accumulation may also occur in the mother as polyhydramnios and edema of the placenta. There are two types of hydrops fetalis: immune and nonimmune. The nonimmune type, which is coded here, occurs when fluid levels are not properly regulated due to another underlying condition. Fetal conditions such as severe anemia, heart conditions, or birth defects are just a few of the related causes. Mortality rates can be high if the underlying condition cannot be determined or effectively treated.

O36.8- Maternal care for other specified fetal problems

This subcategory identifies fetal abnormalities that alter the care for the pregnant patient, such as decreased fetal movements.

O36.82- Fetal anemia and thrombocytopenia

Fetal anemia is the result of inadequate production or quality of red blood cells (RBC) needed in the fetal circulatory system to carry oxygen to fetal organs. Causal conditions include maternal-fetal incompatibility, maternal viral infection, or blood loss from fetal circulation. If anemia is diagnosed or suspected, the pregnancy requires close observation, as it can be fatal for the fetus. Fetal thrombocytopenia is a potentially fatal condition whereby the fetus' platelet (blood clotting) cell count is abnormally low or deficient. As with fetal anemia, this can occur when there is an incompatibility between maternal and fetal blood or as a result of maternal viral infections.

O36.83- Maternal care for abnormalities of the fetal heart rate or rhythm

The average normal fetal heart rate is between 110 and 160 beats per minute, but can vary by 5 to 25 beats per minute. The fetal heart rate may change in response to conditions in the uterus. An abnormal fetal heart rate may be transient and benign, or may mean that the fetus is not getting enough oxygen or has other problems.

This subcategory was created to report abnormal fetal heart rate or rhythm as an indication for maternal care or intervention related to pregnancy, labor, and delivery. Codes from this category are reported on the mother's record. A pregnant woman may be seen at any time during the first, second, or third trimester and evaluated for nonreassuring fetal heart rate heart rate or rhythm. Therapies may include administration of oxygen to the mother or medication given to the mother to help regulate the baby's heart rate.

Focus Point

Codes from category O36 Maternal care for other fetal problems, are assigned only when the fetal condition is actually responsible for modifying the management of the mother, i.e., by requiring diagnostic studies, additional observation, special care, or termination of pregnancy. The fact that the fetal condition exists does not justify assigning a code from this series to the mother's record.

O40.- Polyhydramnios

Polyhydramnios is excess amniotic fluid surrounding the fetus. It may be related to a maternal condition like diabetes or it could indicate a fetal abnormality, such as a fetal lung or gastrointestinal disorder or fetal anemia. Although often asymptomatic, in very severe cases of polyhydramnios the pregnant patient may experience lower extremity swelling, shortness of breath, and/or decreased production of urine.

O41.- Other disorders of amniotic fluid and membranes

There are two important membranous layers that surround the fetus: the chorion and amnion. The chorion is the outermost membrane and the amnion is the innermost membrane closest to the fetus. Collectively these two membranes provide protection to the fetus and are a critical point of exchange for nutrients and fluid between mother and baby. The placenta is a flat, disc-shaped organ that attaches the chorion/amniotic sac to the uterine wall. It is the point at which nutrients and oxygen from the mother's blood can be passed to the fetal blood and carbon dioxide and waste products can move from the fetal blood back to the mother to process. A large part of this category classifies infection related to the amniotic fluid and/or membranes.

O41.0- Oligohydramnios

Oligohydramnios is an abnormally low level of amniotic fluid surrounding the fetus. Amniotic fluid is important for proper development of the lungs and the gastrointestinal tract, it allows the baby to move promoting muscle and limb development, and it provides cushioning. Low amniotic fluid may indicate a fetal abnormality such as kidney or urinary tract defects or it may indicate a maternal issue such as a placental problem, dehydration, or a chronic condition like diabetes. The earlier in the pregnancy oligohydramnios occurs the more serious the potential complications will be.

O43.- Placental disorders

The placenta is the lifeline between the fetus and the mother. Not only does it act as a transfer site for nutrients, fluids, and waste, it also helps keep the mother's blood from mixing with the fetal blood and vice versa. Without proper placental placement and adherence to the uterine wall or proper placental development, both the mother and the fetus can be adversely affected.

O43.0- Placental transfusion syndromes

Placental transfusion syndromes occur as a result of abnormal blood circulation secondary to placental abnormalities. Circulation between the mother and fetus may be affected or between fetuses when there is a multiple gestation.

O43.02- Fetus-to-fetus placental transfusion syndrome

A pregnancy complicated by fetus-to-fetus placental transfusion syndrome, also called twin-to-twin transfusion syndrome (TTTS), carries significant risk of severe disabilities or death of one or both twins. TTTS occurs when monozygotic (identical) twins or higher multiple gestation fetuses share the same placenta and blood vessels resulting in an intrauterine blood transfusion from one fetus to the other. The fetus receiving the extra blood has an increased risk for heart failure due to the strain on the heart to pump extra blood; the donor fetus has a decreased blood volume, slowing growth, and urine production.

Twin-to-Twin Transfusion Syndrome (TTTS)

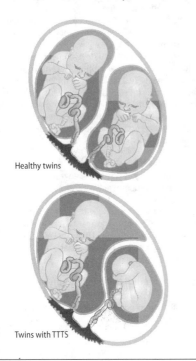

Healthy twins

Twins with TTTS

Focus Point

Although not in the Alphabetic Index, documentation in the record may identify twin-to-twin transfusion syndrome (TTTS) as TOPS or twin oligohydramnios-polyhydramnios sequence. This name relates the discrepancy in the amniotic fluid levels contained in each amniotic sac. The twin receiving the blood often has excess amniotic fluid (polyhydramnios) due to increased urine production while the donor fetus has a low level of amniotic fluid (oligohydramnios) because urine production is decreased due to a reduced blood volume.

O43.2-   Morbidly adherent placenta

It is normal for the placenta to be attached to the uterine wall; in fact, it is essential for the passage of nutrients and oxygen between mother and fetus. Adherent placenta describes a condition where the placenta attaches too deeply into the uterus. The following subcategories relate the depth and severity of the placental attachment. No matter the severity, all adherent placenta cases result in some degree of retained placenta necessitating surgical removal. Severe maternal hemorrhaging is the greatest risk factor and hysterectomy (removal of the uterus) may be the only way to stop the bleeding.

O43.21- Placenta accreta

This condition is the most commonly seen and least severe form of the adherent placenta conditions. Although placental adherence is deep, there is minimal penetration into the uterine muscle (myometrium).

O43.22- Placenta increta

In placenta increta, there is considerably more penetration into the uterine muscle.

O43.23- Placenta percreta

Placenta percreta is the rarest form but the most severe. Placental adherence goes beyond the uterine wall and muscle extending to the outer covering of the uterus and sometimes even invading adjacent organs.

O44.-   Placenta previa

In a normal pregnancy the placenta attaches at the sides or top of the uterus. Placenta previa is implantation of the placenta in the lower portion of the uterus over or near the opening of the cervix. The condition can be diagnosed in any trimester but is most often identified during the second trimester. Placenta previa diagnosed early in pregnancy may resolve as the uterus expands and grows during pregnancy. Placenta previa diagnosed later in pregnancy or persisting into the third trimester is unlikely to resolve and can cause bleeding or other complications that can become severe to the point of being life-threatening. Although bleeding may occur during any trimester, it is more common later in pregnancy.

O44.Ø-   Complete placenta previa NOS or without hemorrhage

O44.1-   Complete placenta previa with hemorrhage

If the placenta completely covers the internal cervical os, it is designated as a complete placenta previa. Many patients have third-trimester bleeding, as the lower uterine segment thins in preparation for the onset of labor. The presence of complete placenta previa puts the patient at higher risk for significant hemorrhage, preterm delivery, placental abruption, need for blood transfusion, and an increased incidence of postpartum endometritis. Cesarean delivery is customarily the only option with complete placenta previa.

O44.2- Partial placenta previa without hemorrhage

O44.3- Partial placenta previa with hemorrhage

A placenta that only partially covers the internal cervical os is classified as a partial placenta previa. Treatment includes bed rest and limitation of movement. Trial of labor is an option for partial placenta previa although this depends greatly on how much of the cervical os is covered by the placenta.

O44.4- Low lying placenta NOS or without hemorrhage

O44.5- Low lying placenta with hemorrhage

If the placenta is positioned at the edge of the cervix but not covering the cervix, it is considered a low-lying placenta. Complications are low with low-lying placenta, but close observation throughout the pregnancy is warranted. In many cases, a low-lying placenta migrates upwards as the uterus expands with the pregnancy.

O45.- Premature separation of placenta [abruptio placentae]

Premature separation of the placenta is separation of the placenta from the site of uterine implantation and can occur at any time after 20 weeks gestation but before delivery of the fetus. The risk of associated complications to the mother and the baby are dependent on the degree and timing of the placental separation. Bleeding and coagulation defects are the greatest risks to the mother.

O45.8- Other premature separation of placenta

Other codes in the O45 category link a specific coagulation defect with the premature separation of the placenta. This subcategory captures conditions or manifestations besides coagulation defects that may occur as a result of early placental separation. Included under this subcategory is a potential life-threatening condition called Couvelaire uterus or uteroplacental apoplexy. This condition occurs when blood forms and gets trapped between the placenta and uterus. Having no place to go, the blood is forced into and/or through the uterine wall. Rupture of the myometrium (the muscular wall of the uterus) and internal bleeding into the peritoneal cavity may result.

O47.- False labor

False labor is the experience of contractions, mild or severe, without cervical changes. False labor contractions are irregular. They vary in intensity, length, and pattern and, in most cases, subside with position changes or activity. This condition is commonly referred to as Braxton Hicks contractions.

False labor is often felt later in the pregnancy, typically late in the third trimester. The codes in this category identify whether the false labor was experienced before or after 37 completed weeks of gestation.

O48.- Late pregnancy

Late pregnancy refers to any pregnancy beyond 40 completed weeks of gestation, with specific codes identifying whether the pregnancy is postterm or prolonged. Both types are treated by careful fetal monitoring with no intervention until there are indications that the fetus is at risk.

O48.0 Post-term pregnancy

Any pregnancy with a gestational period of 40 completed weeks to 42 completed weeks is considered a postterm pregnancy.

O48.1 Prolonged pregnancy

Any pregnancy that goes beyond 42 completed weeks of gestation is considered a prolonged pregnancy.

> **Focus Point**
>
> The term "completed" does not mean that the patient has to be on the seventh day of a particular gestational week. If the patient is anywhere within the 42-week timeframe (42 1/7 or 42 7/7), the code for postterm pregnancy is applied. In order for the prolonged pregnancy code to be applied, the patient has to be in week 43 or greater.

Complications of Labor and Delivery (O60-O77)

Labor is a staged process the maternal body goes through in order to expel the baby from the uterus. Delivery is the final stage of labor when the fetus and placenta are completely expelled from the uterus. Problems in labor can greatly increase the likelihood of problems with delivery if not managed appropriately. The list of possible complications that can occur during or as a result of labor or delivery is extensive, ranging from obstructed labor to complications with anesthesia.

The categories in this code block are as follows:

O60	Preterm labor
O61	Failed induction of labor
O62	Abnormalities of forces of labor
O63	Long labor
O64	Obstructed labor due to malposition and malpresentation of fetus
O65	Obstructed labor due to maternal pelvic abnormality
O66	Other obstructed labor

O67	Labor and delivery complicated by intrapartum hemorrhage, not elsewhere classified
O68	Labor and delivery complicated by abnormality of fetal acid-base balance
O69	Labor and delivery complicated by umbilical cord complications
O70	Perineal laceration during delivery
O71	Other obstetric trauma
O72	Postpartum hemorrhage
O73	Retained placenta and membranes, without hemorrhage
O74	Complications of anesthesia during labor and delivery
O75	Other complications of labor and delivery, not elsewhere classified
O76	Abnormality in fetal heart rate and rhythm complicating labor and delivery
O77	Other fetal stress complicating labor and delivery

O60.- Preterm labor

Preterm labor is regular, painful uterine contractions with effacement or dilation of the cervix occurring before completion of 37 weeks gestation. It may or may not result in the birth of the baby. Codes are classified into three major subcategories: one subcategory for preterm labor only with no associated delivery and two subcategories for preterm labor with delivery of the baby, preterm or at term.

O62.- Abnormalities of forces of labor

Labor is the period of time from the start of uterine contractions to the delivery of the placenta and is divided into three stages. The first stage is the period from the onset of labor until the cervix is fully dilated to 10 cm and is the longest of the three stages. The first stage has two phases: early and active. In the early (latent) phase, contractions start and are mild and cervical dilation begins and progresses slowly to roughly 3 to 4 centimeters. In the active phase, contractions come in regular increasing intervals, are stronger and last longer, and cervical dilation speeds up until fully dilated to 10 cm. Often the pregnant patient does not present to the hospital until the first stage of labor has progressed to the active phase. The second stage of labor is the period from full dilation of the cervix (10 cm) to delivery of the fetus. The third stage is delivery of the placenta. Abnormal forces of labor are defined as changes in one or more of the stages above.

O62.0 Primary inadequate contractions

Contractions are the force needed to not only push the baby into the birth canal but also help efface (shorten) and dilate (open) the mother's cervix. If the strength, duration, or frequency of the contractions is not adequate during the beginning of the first stage of labor, what is called the latent phase, the cervix fails to dilate.

O62.1 Secondary uterine inertia

Secondary uterine inertia occurs during the active phase of the first stage of labor, meaning the cervix has already dilated to at least 3 or 4 cm. With secondary uterine inertia, contractions that were once strong and coming in regular intervals become less intense and/or slow down. As a result, cervical dilation also slows.

O63.- Long labor

Labor is described in stages and each stage takes a certain amount of time to complete. The first stage is usually the longest and the third stage the shortest. Typically labor stages take longer for a first time mother and take less time with each subsequent pregnancy. However, each pregnancy and each pregnant patient is different and therefore the amount of time it takes one patient to get through one particular stage of labor may be more or less than what it may take the next patient.

O63.0 Prolonged first stage (of labor)

The first stage of labor is the longest of the three stages, beginning with regular uterine contractions and ending when the cervix has fully dilated. There is conflicting guidance on what is considered a prolonged first stage and often the timing is based on the latent phase of the first stage rather than the entire first stage as a whole. That being said, on average the first stage of labor is considered to be prolonged if the early (latent) phase takes more than 20 hours for a first time mother and more than 14 hours for a woman with previous deliveries. Weak uterine contractions, malposition, and surgical scars may contribute to a prolonged first stage.

O63.1 Prolonged second stage (of labor)

The second stage of labor begins with complete dilation of the cervix to 10 cm and ends with the delivery of the baby. A second stage is considered prolonged when it takes more than three hours for a first time mother and more than two hours for a woman with previous deliveries to deliver the baby. Causes may include cephalopelvic disproportion, malpresentation, and medications.

O64.- Obstructed labor due to malposition and malpresentation of fetus

In a typical delivery, the baby presents head-down with the top of the head first or what is considered vertex presentation. The baby's head is tucked into the chest and the back of the baby's head (occiput) is positioned toward the front of the mother with the face toward the spine, what is known as occiput anterior (OA) position. Malposition refers to anything other than occiput anterior and malpresentation refers to anything other than vertex. Obstructed labor is the failure of the baby to move down the birth canal even with strong uterine contractions. Any malposition or malpresentation can cause obstructed labor, although some are potentially more serious than others.

Focus Point

Codes from category O64.- should be used when the condition causes obstruction during labor. Encounters for malpresentation without obstruction during observations, hospitalization, or other obstetric care or cesarean delivery that occur before the onset of labor are reported with codes from category O32-.

Fetal Malpositions

Breech Mother's pelvis

Shoulder (arm prolapse)

Face (mentum)

Oblique

Compound (extremity together with head)

O64.0-   Obstructed labor due to incomplete rotation of fetal head

This code includes transverse presentation arrest and various occipital presentations only when they result in obstructed labor. Transverse lie describes the presentation of a fetus that is sideways across the uterus, perpendicular to the birth canal with the head on one side and bottom across the abdomen on the other side. Less common is oblique presentation, which means the fetus is at a diagonal angle with the head in the mother's hip, although other forms of

occipital presentations such as occipitoposterior or occipitosacral are included here. All are complications for vaginal delivery if the fetus does not turn before the onset of labor, in which case external version or cesarean delivery is performed.

O64.1-   Obstructed labor due to breech presentation

This code includes obstruction from breech or buttock first presentations. There are several types of breech presentations but only frank and complete breech is represented here. Frank breech occurs when the legs are flexed only at the hips, and the legs extend over the abdomen and thorax so that the feet lie beside the face. Complete breech occurs when the legs are flexed at both the hips and the knees, and the legs are crossed.

O64.2-   Obstructed labor due to face presentation

O64.3-   Obstructed labor due to brow presentation

These presentations can occur in concurrence with a large fetal head or the premature rupture of membranes. They are characterized by head and neck hyperextension rather than the tucked chin of the normal cephalic position. The condition may resolve on its own before the pushing stage of labor; this category is used if the presentation causes obstructed labor. If the labor is obstructed or arrested, a cesarean section delivery may be necessary.

O64.5-   Obstructed labor due to compound presentation

Compound is a relatively rare presentation that involves the baby's arm and leg prolapsing into the birth canal alongside the head. Most commonly the hand or arm and often the extremity retracts on its own as labor progresses or reacts and reflexively moves away in response to a slight stimulus such as a pinch. Normal vaginal delivery is frequently possible, but excessive pressure on the limb is not recommended. If the labor is prolonged, blood supply can be cut off, in which case cesarean delivery may be necessary. This code is reported when the compound presentation causes obstructed labor and/or delivery.

O64.8-   Obstructed labor due to other malposition and malpresentation

There are two types of breech presentation included under this code that may result in obstructed labor: footling and incomplete breech. In both of these breech presentations, although the buttocks are still closer to the birth canal than the head, it is one foot (incomplete) or both feet (footling) that present into the birth canal first.

O65.- Obstructed labor due to maternal pelvic abnormality

In some cases it is the maternal pelvic anatomy itself that precludes the fetus from entering into the birth canal. This may be due to a deformity of the pelvic bones, an abnormality of one of the pelvic organs (i.e., cervix, uterus), or some type of contracted pelvis.

O66.- Other obstructed labor

Most of the codes in this category identify a variety of fetal abnormalities that may result in the fetus getting stuck in the birth canal, halting the progression of labor. In some instances these conditions may result in the need for cesarean delivery.

O66.0 Obstructed labor due to shoulder dystocia

Shoulder dystocia is when the baby's head has been delivered but the shoulders get stuck and hinder any further advancement of the baby out of the birth canal.

O68 Labor and delivery complicated by abnormality of fetal acid-base balance

Abnormality of fetal acid-base balance refers to metabolic abnormalities in the fetus causing fetal distress. Maintenance of a normal fetal acid-base balance is dependent on the ability of the fetus to buffer acids produced during normal fetal metabolic activities. Normally as long as blood supply to the placenta is adequate and the fetus is well oxygenated, the fetus is able to maintain optimal acid-base ratios. However, if blood supply to the placenta and in turn to the fetus is compromised, fetal hypoxia occurs and fetal metabolism is impaired, which prevents complete metabolism of carbohydrates, causes a buildup of organic acids that the fetus is unable to metabolize or excrete, and leads to an acid-base imbalance. Relatively small variations in the acid-base ratio can result in an imbalance, most often acidosis, which can adversely affect the function of the central nervous system, cardiovascular system, and other organ systems.

O69.- Labor and delivery complicated by umbilical cord complications

The umbilical cord is a tube that connects the fetus to the placenta. The placenta is a sort of neutral zone between the mother's circulatory system and the fetal circulatory system allowing nutrients, oxygen, and waste to transfer from mother to baby and baby to mother without the mixing of fetal blood with the maternal blood. The cord typically has one umbilical vein that carries blood that is full of oxygen and nutrients from the placenta to the fetus and two umbilical arteries that carry blood that is depleted of nutrients and oxygen from the fetus back to the placenta.

O69.0- Labor and delivery complicated by prolapse of cord

Cord prolapse occurs when the cord presents in the birth canal before the baby. As the baby goes through the canal it can compress the cord, effectively cutting off the oxygen supply to the fetus. It most commonly occurs spontaneously with breech presentation but also occurs with vertex presentation, particularly when membranes are ruptured and the presenting part is not engaged.

O69.4- Labor and delivery complicated by vasa previa

Vasa previa is when the umbilical vessels run across the cervical opening. During pregnancy the location of these vessels is of little concern and poses no risk to the development of the fetus. It does become a concern when it comes time to deliver. As labor progresses, the cervix thins out and opens up to allow the baby to pass through the birth canal. The membranes are now exposed through the opening and the pressure from the baby on the membranes and low lying vessels can compress the vessels or cause them to rupture when the membranes rupture. This condition may be related to a low lying placenta, bilobed placenta, multiple pregnancy, or velamentous umbilical cord insertion. Although the pregnant patient in most cases has to have a cesarean section, this condition is not normally dangerous to the mother.

O70.- Perineal laceration during delivery

The perineum is defined as the area between a women's vagina and anus. During a vaginal birth, the tissues around the vaginal opening are subjected to extreme stretching as the baby exits the mother's body. Sometimes the tissues get stretched to the point that they tear. The codes in this category are classified by the severity of the laceration.

O70.0 First degree perineal laceration during delivery

In most cases only the skin of the perineum is torn. No muscle tissue is involved and rarely is it necessary to stitch up the tear. Documentation in the record may also describe this as a tear of the vagina, vulva, labia, or fourchette.

O70.1 Second degree perineal laceration during delivery

A second-degree perineal laceration involves underlying muscle tissue. The tear may be described as involving the pelvic floor, perineal muscles, or vaginal muscles.

O70.2- Third degree perineal laceration during delivery

A perineal laceration considered third degree extends into the anal sphincter. The anal sphincter comprises two muscles, the internal and external anal sphincter. The type of treatment and potential complications vary depending on the extent of the tear; that is, whether it went through just one or both sphincter muscles. Third-degree perineal lacerations have therefore been classified into three levels: IIIa, IIIb, and IIIc. The levels are defined as follows:

IIIa   Tear involves the external anal sphincter only

      Tear involves less than 50 percent of the muscle

IIIb   Tear involves the external anal sphincter only

      Tear involves greater than 50 percent of the muscle

IIIc   Tear involves the external anal sphincter AND the internal anal sphincter

O70.3 Fourth degree perineal laceration during delivery

A fourth-degree laceration of the perineum is one that goes beyond the anal sphincter muscle extending into the anal and/or rectal mucosa underneath.

O70.4 Anal sphincter tear complicating delivery, not associated with third degree laceration

An anal sphincter tear can occur independently of a perineal laceration. These tears are hard to identify and it may not be recognized until it complicates a subsequent delivery.

O71.- Other obstetric trauma

Obstetrical trauma is not limited to the perineum but can occur in any of the pelvic organs. Injuries related to the uterus, cervix, bladder or urethra, joints and ligaments of the pelvis, and other specified obstetric traumas are included in this category.

O72.- Postpartum hemorrhage

Postpartum hemorrhage is excessive vaginal bleeding that occurs after the baby has been delivered. Of the four codes classified to this category, three codes identify the timing of the postpartum bleeding: during the third stage of labor, in the immediate postpartum period, or after the first 24 hours following delivery of the placenta. The fourth code identifies coagulation defects, such as fibrinolysis, that may have developed secondary to the hemorrhaging. In general, the majority of the cases of hemorrhaging are related to retained products of conception, in which all or pieces of placenta or other membranes are still attached to the uterine wall.

O73.- Retained placenta and membranes, without hemorrhage

The third stage of labor is the expulsion of the placenta. In a normal delivery this usually occurs spontaneously and within 30 minutes of delivering the baby. If the placenta does not deliver spontaneously or it appears that some but not all of the placenta delivered, the practitioner may attempt manual extraction of the placenta. In some cases, the uterus needs to be suctioned or scraped to remove residual tissues. Even without associated hemorrhaging, retained placenta poses a high risk of maternal death if left untreated.

O74.- Complications of anesthesia during labor and delivery

The use of anesthesia during labor and delivery poses the same risk of complications to an obstetric patient as it does nonobstetric patients needing anesthetic medications. The codes are categorized based on the specific complication that occurred as a result of the anesthesia, including but not limited to pulmonary and cardiac complications, toxic reactions, and anesthesia-induced headaches.

O75.- Other complications of labor and delivery, not elsewhere classified

Labor is a staged process the maternal body goes through in order to expel the baby from the uterus. Delivery is the final stage of labor when the fetus and placenta are completely expelled from the uterus. Problems in labor can greatly increase the likelihood of problems with delivery if not managed appropriately. Maternal distress, infection, fever, and pulmonary or cardiac complications are a few conditions included in this category.

O75.3 Other infection during labor

This code includes sepsis that develops during labor.

O75.8- Other specified complications of labor and delivery

This subcategory captures complications that do not fit into previous categories identifying labor and delivery complications.

O75.82 Onset (spontaneous) of labor after 37 completed weeks of gestation but before 39 completed weeks gestation, with delivery by (planned) cesarean section

The American College of Obstetricians and Gynecologists (ACOG) and the American Academy of Pediatrics (AAP) recommend that elective cesarean deliveries not be planned before 39 completed weeks of gestation, to ensure full development of the fetus. However, if labor begins prior to 39 completed weeks of gestation but after 37 completed weeks of gestation, the onset of labor is an indication for performance of the planned cesarean section even though the obstetric patient has not yet reached the recommended gestational period set by ACOG and AAP standards.

This code is reported secondarily along with the code indicating the reason for the planned cesarean (i.e., previous C-section) to support medical necessity for the cesarean section prior to 39 completed weeks of gestation.

Focus Point

Recent quality reporting requirements have necessitated that hospitals review criteria for elective inductions and cesarean sections, primarily regarding the timing of the procedures. Research indicates that infants delivered prior to 39 completed weeks of gestation suffer a higher incidence of complications than those who gestate to full term, beyond 39 weeks. Based on this research, both ACOG and AAP standards require a gestation of 39 completed weeks prior to elective delivery.

O77.-   Other fetal stress complicating labor and delivery

Management of the mother during labor can change if the fetus is not responding favorably to the forces of labor. Signs of fetal stress may be evidenced by electrocardiogram, ultrasound, or changes in the amniotic fluid.

O77.Ø   Labor and delivery complicated by meconium in amniotic fluid

The first feces the baby passes is a dark green tarry looking substance called meconium. Normally, meconium passage does not occur until after the baby is born but occasionally the baby passes it before or during delivery. Once in the amniotic fluid, the meconium may be aspirated or inhaled by the baby. The more meconium inhaled, the greater the risk for associated complications such as cyanosis, limpness, respiratory distress, and other breathing problems.

Focus Point

Code O77.Ø may be assigned when documentation only states meconium stained fluid even if there is no documentation of related fetal stress.

Encounter for Delivery (O8Ø-O82)

This code block not only captures an uncomplicated vaginal delivery but also identifies those rare instances where a cesarean delivery occurred but without any indication as to why it was necessary (i.e., obstructed labor).

The categories in this code block are as follows:

O8Ø	Encounter for full-term uncomplicated delivery
O82	Encounter for cesarean delivery without indication

O8Ø   Encounter for full-term uncomplicated delivery

The following criteria must be met in order for this code to be assigned:

- Single, full term and live born baby (Full term is 37 weeks to 4Ø weeks gestation)

- Head first (cephalic) presentation

- Little to no assistance during delivery (Episiotomy does not affect code assignment)

- No current antepartum or postpartum complications

Focus Point

Code O8Ø is always the principal diagnosis and is never reported with other codes from chapter 15. However, conditions from other chapters that are unrelated to the pregnancy and that in no way complicate the pregnancy may be reported additionally when present.

Complications Predominantly Related to the Puerperium (O85-O92)

The puerperium is the six-week period of time following the delivery of the placenta. This is typically the time it takes for the maternal body to return to a prepregnancy or nonpregnant state.

The categories in this code block are as follows:

O85	Puerperal sepsis
O86	Other puerperal infections
O87	Venous complications and hemorrhoids in the puerperium
O88	Obstetric embolism
O89	Complications of anesthesia during the puerperium
O9Ø	Complications of the puerperium, not elsewhere classified

O91   Infections of breast associated with pregnancy, the puerperium and lactation

O92   Other disorders of breast and disorders of lactation associated with pregnancy and the puerperium

O85   Puerperal sepsis

Sepsis is a complication of a localized infection caused by a systemic inflammatory response to the infectious agent. Puerperal sepsis is when the systemic inflammatory response is triggered during the postpartum period, a six-week period following the birth of the baby.

O86.-   Other puerperal infections

Puerperal infection refers to a localized, bacterial infection following childbirth. The infection may be related to an obstetrical surgical wound or related to the genital or urinary tract. Although symptoms vary depending on the site and nature of the infection, often the first and most common sign of a puerperal infection is fever. If left untreated, the infection could spread to other parts of the body and potentially be fatal.

O86.1-   Other infection of genital tract following delivery

Specific sites of infection that are included in this subcategory include the cervix, endometrium, ovaries, fallopian tubes, and vagina.

O86.12   Endometritis following delivery

Among puerperal infections, the genital tract is the most commonly infected site. Endometritis is the most prominent of these infections, resulting in inflammation of the inner uterine lining, also known as the endometrium. Etiologies may include prolonged labor or cesarean section, lower genital tract colonization, and introduction of internal instruments (fetal monitoring) during labor or delivery.

O86.8-   Other specified puerperal infections

Puerperal infections occur directly after and up to six weeks following the delivery of the placenta.

O86.81   Puerperal septic thrombophlebitis

Septic thrombophlebitis is inflammation of a vein (phlebitis) due to an infected blood clot (thrombus). Puerperal septic thrombophlebitis is when the infected thrombus develops during the postpartum period. In most cases, these occur as a complication from a puerperal infection (e.g., endometritis). Septic embolism is a potential complication.

O87.-   Venous complications and hemorrhoids in the puerperium

It takes time for a maternal body to return to a prepregnancy state, both chemically and physically. Because of this circulatory issues that may or may not have been present during the pregnancy can still occur in the postpartum, particularly venous complications. The conditions included here are also used to report venous complications during labor and delivery although the incidence of this is rare.

O87.0   Superficial thrombophlebitis in the puerperium

The threat of a blood clot (thrombus) forming and causing inflammation of a vein (phlebitis) is as great a risk after delivery as it is during pregnancy. It is primarily the superficial veins in the lower extremities, the greater and lesser saphenous veins, that are affected.

O87.1   Deep phlebothrombosis in the puerperium

Deep phlebothrombosis occurs when a thrombus develops in a deep vein. During the postpartum period it is most often the deep veins of the lower extremities that are affected, including the iliac, femoral, popliteal, and tibial veins. Inflammation of the vein (phlebitis) may also be present but is rarely associated with deep vein thrombosis. The risk of developing a deep vein thrombosis (DVT) is often the greatest following delivery as pressure and/or damage to the blood vessels during the delivery in addition to the still elevated hormone and clotting factor levels expedite clot formation. DVTs carry a risk of blocking the blood flow of the affected vein completely and are also at risk of breaking free and moving to other areas in the body, like the heart or lung, which can be fatal.

O88.-   Obstetric embolism

An embolism is the obstruction of a blood vessel due to a blockage from a moving particle or substance. The most common cause of an embolism is a blood clot that has dislodged from its site of origin, like in a lower extremity vein, moving to another location, most often the pulmonary arteries.

O88.1-   Amniotic fluid embolism

This is a rare but life-threatening condition that occurs when amniotic fluid or other fetal material enters the mother's circulation. The complete pathophysiology is not yet understood but it is thought that one or both of the following occur: a massive allergic response is triggered and/or the complement pathway (immune response) is initiated. Regardless of etiology the results are the same: severe cardiorespiratory complications, including cardiac arrest and hypoxia; neurological changes, such as seizures and loss of consciousness; all followed by excessive hemorrhaging and coagulopathy usually in the form of disseminated intravascular coagulation (DIC). This condition is essentially untreatable due to its unpredictable nature making mortality rates for mother and baby extremely high.

O88.3- Obstetric pyemic and septic embolism

Septic and pyemic embolisms cause a twofold insult: obstruction of a vessel and seeding of an infectious agent. Septic and pyemic embolism occur when an infected piece of tissue, blood clot (thrombus), or other substance travels from its site of origin to other parts of the body. The infected embolus gets trapped, clogging the vessel and disrupting the flow of blood and oxygen to areas beyond the clot. In addition, microorganisms carried by the embolus provoke abscess formation at the site where it is now lodged. The most common sites for an embolus to get trapped are the pulmonary and coronary arteries. Septic thrombophlebitis (infected blood clot) is often the greatest risk factor for pyemic or septic embolism in an obstetric patient.

O90.- Complications of the puerperium, not elsewhere classified

The puerperium is defined as a six-week time period following the delivery of the placenta. Complications classified here include various conditions from acute kidney failure to complications of obstetrical wounds.

O90.3 Peripartum cardiomyopathy

Cardiomyopathy is a disease of the heart muscle that results in an enlarged and very weak heart. A weak heart cannot pump as much blood, which limits the amount of oxygen getting to other organs in the body.

Peripartum cardiomyopathy is a rare complication of pregnancy. Severity may range from mild to severe. Mild cardiomyopathy manifests as slight edema (swelling) of the legs and mild shortness of breath. When these mild symptoms occur during the last month of pregnancy they may be overlooked because slight edema and shortness of breath are common in late pregnancy. Severe cardiomyopathy is more easily diagnosed because the patient experiences symptoms of severe shortness of breath, pulmonary edema, and significant edema of the lower extremities.

O91.- Infections of breast associated with pregnancy, the puerperium and lactation

This category identifies infection and/or abscess formation in the breast during pregnancy, during the postpartum period, or when the maternal patient is lactating.

O91.2- Nonpurulent mastitis associated with pregnancy, the puerperium and lactation

Breast tissue that becomes infected is termed mastitis. Mastitis is a common complication of pregnancy and, although it can occur early in the pregnancy, it is most often seen in the postpartum period when the mother is breastfeeding. Etiologies can range from a blocked milk duct to introduction of a microorganism from the baby's mouth.

O92.- Other disorders of breast and disorders of lactation associated with pregnancy and the puerperium

Lactation is the production and secretion of milk from the mammary glands. When a baby is fed the secreted milk directly from the breast, this action is called breastfeeding. Abnormalities of the breast, more often the nipple, and/or problems with the production of milk can alter whether or not a mother can successfully breastfeed.

O92.3 Agalactia

This condition is the inability of the mother to produce breast milk. Causes may include nutrient deficiencies, dehydration, medications, or injury.

O92.4 Hypogalactia

In hypogalactia, breast milk is produced but in less than normal amounts.

O92.5 Suppressed lactation

Suppressed lactation is a decision made by the mother to try and stop milk production or lactation. Although this occurs spontaneously without intervention, some mothers may want it stopped sooner. There are several methods that have been used to suppress milk production including binding of the breasts, birth control pills, and other pharmacological aids. Currently there are no medications that are FDA approved specifically for lactation suppression.

Other Obstetric Conditions, Not Elsewhere Classified (O94-O9A)

Most of the codes classified here are conditions that typically are found outside the obstetric chapter but are currently complicating the pregnancy, are exacerbated by the pregnancy, or are the reason for obstetric care.

The categories in this code block are as follows:

O94	Sequelae of complication of pregnancy, childbirth, and the puerperium
O98	Maternal infectious and parasitic diseases classifiable elsewhere but complicating pregnancy, childbirth and the puerperium
O99	Other maternal diseases classifiable elsewhere but complicating pregnancy, childbirth and the puerperium
O9A	Maternal malignant neoplasms, traumatic injuries and abuse classifiable elsewhere but complicating pregnancy, childbirth and the puerperium

O98.- Maternal infectious and parasitic diseases classifiable elsewhere but complicating pregnancy, childbirth and the puerperium

This category includes conditions that in a nonpregnant patient would normally be coded in Chapter 1. Certain Infectious and Parasitic Diseases. Although the majority of the codes in this category do identify the specific infectious condition, the code may not give all of the necessary information, such as the site or chronicity, therefore an additional code from Chapter 1 is recommended. Some specific infectious and parasitic diseases identified in this category include tuberculosis, HIV, viral hepatitis, protozoal diseases, and other sexually transmitted diseases.

O99.- Other maternal diseases classifiable elsewhere but complicating pregnancy, childbirth and the puerperium

This category captures diseases from the endocrine, nervous, circulatory, respiratory, and digestive system chapters, the blood disorders chapter, mental/behavioral disorders chapters, and some infectious and postsurgical state conditions that are currently affecting the management of the pregnant patient.

O99.0- Anemia complicating pregnancy, childbirth and the puerperium

Anemia is a common complication of pregnancy, childbirth, and the puerperium. During pregnancy the body must increase the volume of blood to support the pregnancy. If the number of circulating red blood cells does not increase along with blood volume, anemia occurs. Nutritional deficiencies or malabsorption of vitamins and minerals needed to produce healthy red blood cells, such as iron, folate (folic acid), or vitamin B12, is often the cause. Signs and symptoms of anemia include fatigue, palpitations, tachycardia, dyspnea, and pallor.

O99.1- Other diseases of the blood and blood-forming organs and certain disorders involving the immune mechanism complicating pregnancy, childbirth and the puerperium

Coagulation disorders are a group of the conditions included here. Depending on the type of coagulation defect, transfusion or other management may be indicated. Because transfusions during pregnancy pose significant risks, increased monitoring of blood coagulation factors are often necessary to adequately manage the patient. Some conditions seen are as follows:

- Complicating factors such as hypertension or preeclampsia can result in a hypercoagulable state that can precipitate thromboembolism formation.

- Disseminated intravascular coagulation (DIC) is a serious condition that can result in tissue damage and abnormal bleeding when physiological complications cause material from the inside of the womb to get into the mother's bloodstream.

- Inherited diseases such as von Willebrand disease and hemophilia put patients at a high risk of bleeding problems early in pregnancy and in the puerperium. In some cases, this can result in first trimester bleeding and miscarriage. Patients with this inherited coagulopathy have increased rates of postabortal anemia and hemorrhage. The inheritability of these conditions also poses significant risk to the offspring, necessitating genetic testing.

- Certain medications are contraindicated in pregnancy because they can cause coagulation defects. For example, aspirin and other nonsteroidal antiinflammatory drugs (NSAID) should be avoided in late pregnancy. These drugs can adversely affect maternal platelet function and increase the risk of antepartum and postpartum hemorrhage, as well as cause premature closure of the fetal ductus arteriosus, delaying labor and birth.

- Antiphospholipid syndrome (APS) is a disorder that causes a hypercoagulable state that predisposes the patient to recurrent vascular thromboses, which can result in recurrent spontaneous abortions. APS can be primary in nature or secondary to an autoimmune or rheumatic disorder. During pregnancy, management may necessitate treatment with subcutaneous heparin injection or low doses of aspirin antepartum or postpartum, although contraindicated at the time of delivery.

Focus Point

Coagulation defects may be the direct result of obstetrical-related hemorrhaging, in the antepartum (O45.- and O46.0-), intrapartum (O67.0), or postpartum (O72.3) period. This can occur in addition to or exacerbate a coagulation disorder the patient already has.

O99.2- Endocrine, nutritional and metabolic diseases complicating pregnancy, childbirth and the puerperium

Any condition classified to the endocrine chapter, except diabetes mellitus, malnutrition, and postpartum thyroiditis, is included here.

O99.21- Obesity complicating pregnancy, childbirth, and the puerperium

Research has shown that obesity in pregnancy (BMI of 30 or higher) poses significant risks to the mother and baby. These may include:

- Labor and delivery complications, such as shoulder dystocia

- Thromboembolism

- Delivery of large-for-gestational-age (LGA) infants; macrosomia

- Increased need for cesarean section

- Maternal hypertension or preeclampsia

- Gestational diabetes

- Birth defects, especially neural tube defects

While weight loss is not encouraged during pregnancy, it is recommended that obese women limit the weight that is gained during pregnancy. Nutrition and exercise counseling is also recommended to ensure the fetus is being supplied with the necessary nutrients.

Focus Point

Codes in this subcategory are assigned for pre-existing obesity complicating pregnancy, childbirth, and the puerperium. Excessive weight gain during pregnancy is assigned to subcategory O26.0-.

O99.3- Mental disorders and diseases of the nervous system complicating pregnancy, childbirth and the puerperium

Any condition classified to Chapter 5. Mental, Behavioral, and Neurodevelopmental Disorders, or Chapter 6. Diseases of the Nervous System, that is complicating the management of the obstetric patient is coded to this subcategory.

O99.33- Tobacco use disorder complicating pregnancy, childbirth, and the puerperium

Women who smoke during pregnancy are at greater risk of having a miscarriage or a low-birth-weight baby. Additional risks to the mother include:

- Preterm birth

- Ectopic pregnancy

- Miscarriage

- Placenta previa and abruption

- Intrauterine growth restriction

Risks to the fetus and newborn include:

- Sudden infant death syndrome (SIDS)

- Permanent physical impairment

- Childhood asthma

- Upper respiratory and ear infections

O99.35- Diseases of the nervous system complicating pregnancy, childbirth, and the puerperium

Epilepsy is a group of neurological conditions that cause a predisposition to unprovoked and recurrent seizures. For many pregnant women, pregnancy can alter this disease due to the associated hormonal changes that occur during pregnancy, increasing seizures in some and decreasing seizures in others. The coordination of the hormonal process and seizure management with antiepileptic drugs during pregnancy pose special challenges. Many antiepileptic drugs pose significant risk when taken during pregnancy; however, so do epileptic seizures. For many patients, to simply stop taking their medication is ill-advised. Some recommendations for minimizing the risks to the mother include getting seizures under control and staying consistent with the lowest dosage possible of the single most effective medication, and having the medication levels regularly monitored. Fortunately, despite these challenges, approximately 90 percent of pregnant women who have epilepsy deliver healthy babies.

O99.8- Other specified diseases and conditions complicating pregnancy, childbirth and the puerperium

This subcategory captures obstetric patients with abnormal glucose levels, but no specific documentation of a diabetic condition, who are currently carriers of an infectious disease and patients with a history of bariatric surgery.

O99.84- Bariatric surgery status complicating pregnancy, childbirth and the puerperium

Bariatric surgery, also called weight loss surgery, is performed on morbidly obese individuals to reduce the size of the stomach, limiting the amount of food that can be eaten and the amount of calories that can be absorbed. Women who have had bariatric surgery and then become pregnant must be carefully monitored for medical and surgical complications related to the bariatric surgery status. Fertility generally increases postsurgery for obese patients who previously experienced infertility, because the dramatic weight loss often results in the spontaneous return of normal ovulation. However, the demands on the patient's body to adjust to the reduced size of the stomach and the absorption of nutrients are contrary to that needed for the normal growth and development of a fetus. For these reasons, patients are advised to use birth control during the rapid weight loss that follows the surgery. Once the body has adjusted to surgery and its metabolism has stabilized, pregnancy is no longer contraindicated, as it was in the past. Generally it is recommended that patients wait for 12 to 18 months status post-bariatric surgery to become pregnant. Prenatal care with adequate nutritional support and supplementation is advised.

This may involve the patient's obstetrician working as a team with the bariatric surgeon and a nutritionist. The most common medical complications associated with bariatric surgery status during pregnancy include dumping syndrome, malabsorption, hypoglycemia, and hyperinsulinemia.

Chapter 16: Certain Conditions Originating in the Perinatal Period (PØØ-P96)

Codes in this chapter are assigned for conditions that have their origin in the fetal or perinatal period, which is defined as the period before birth through the first 28 days after birth. While the condition must originate in the perinatal period, morbidity due to the perinatal condition may occur at any time after the first 28 days of life and when diagnosed or treated after the perinatal period, would still be reported with codes from this chapter, no matter the patient's age.

The chapter is broken down into the following code blocks:

PØØ-PØ4	Newborn affected by maternal factors and by complications of pregnancy, labor, and delivery
PØ5-PØ8	Disorders of newborn related to length of gestation and fetal growth
PØ9	Abnormal findings on neonatal screening
P1Ø-P15	Birth trauma
P19-P29	Respiratory and cardiovascular disorders specific to the perinatal period
P35-P39	Infections specific to the perinatal period
P5Ø-P61	Hemorrhagic and hematological disorders of newborn
P7Ø-P74	Transitory endocrine and metabolic disorders specific to newborn
P76-P78	Digestive system disorders of newborn
P8Ø-P83	Conditions involving the integument and temperature regulation of newborn
P84	Other problems with newborn
P9Ø-P96	Other disorders originating in the perinatal period

Newborn Affected by Maternal Factors and by Complications of Pregnancy, Labor, and Delivery (PØØ-PØ4)

Maternal conditions, both preexisting and those arising during the pregnancy, that have the potential to affect the health of the fetus or newborn are represented by the categories in this code block.

The categories in this code block are as follows:

PØØ	Newborn affected by maternal conditions that may be unrelated to present pregnancy
PØ1	Newborn affected by maternal complications of pregnancy
PØ2	Newborn affected by complications of placenta, cord and membranes
PØ3	Newborn affected by other complications of labor and delivery
PØ4	Newborn affected by noxious substances transmitted via placenta or breast milk

PØØ.- Newborn affected by maternal conditions that may be unrelated to present pregnancy

The mother's overall health status has the potential to affect the health of the newborn, including preexisting conditions from hypertension to periodontal disease to surgical or medical procedures performed directly on the mother. When the maternal condition is currently affecting the health of the newborn, it is reported with a code from this category.

PØØ.Ø Newborn affected by maternal hypertensive disorders

Hypertensive disorders in the mother include preexisting or gestational hypertension, preeclampsia, and eclampsia. The fetus or infant of a mother with hypertension has a 25 to 3Ø percent risk of prematurity and a 1Ø to 15 percent chance of being small for gestational age (SGA). These risks are largely associated with a reduction of blood flow to the placenta, which limits oxygen and nutrient transport from the mother to the baby. The more severe the hypertensive condition the greater the risk for associated adverse conditions in the newborn.

PØØ.2 Newborn affected by maternal infectious and parasitic diseases

Maternal infectious and parasitic diseases may affect the health of the fetus or newborn even when the infectious or parasitic disease is not currently manifesting symptoms in the fetus or newborn.

P00.6 Newborn affected by surgical procedure on mother

This code covers surgical procedures on the mother performed to diagnose or treat maternal conditions, as well as diagnostic procedures such as diagnostic amniocentesis that have affected the health of the fetus or newborn.

Focus Point

This code is for procedures performed on the mother that could impact the fetus; it does not classify procedures performed directly on the fetus while still in utero. When a fetal complication arises from an in utero procedure, it is reported with code P96.5 Complication to newborn due to (fetal) intrauterine procedure.

P01.- Newborn affected by maternal complications of pregnancy

This category identifies conditions related to the mother's pregnancy, and not the labor or delivery process, that affected the health and well-being of the newborn. These may include abnormal amniotic fluid levels, multiple gestations, and malpresentation.

P01.2 Newborn affected by oligohydramnios

Oligohydramnios is an abnormally low level of amniotic fluid surrounding the fetus. Amniotic fluid is important for proper development of the fetal lungs and gastrointestinal tract, it allows the baby to move promoting muscle and limb development, and it provides cushioning. If the amniotic fluid level is too low, these organs and structures cannot develop as they should.

P01.3 Newborn affected by polyhydramnios

Polyhydramnios is excess amniotic fluid surrounding the fetus. Polyhydramnios can be a symptom of a maternal condition, such as diabetes, or it can indicate a fetal abnormality, such as a fetal lung or gastrointestinal disorder or fetal anemia. In some cases, however, polyhydramnios can occur in the absence of a maternal disease or a fetal abnormality and to which a cause cannot be identified.

P02.- Newborn affected by complications of placenta, cord and membranes

The placenta is a flat, disc-shaped organ that attaches to the uterine wall. The umbilical cord attaches the placenta to the fetus creating a transfer site between the mother and the baby, without the maternal and fetal blood mixing. There are two membranes that surround and contain the fetus and amniotic fluid: amnion and chorion. This category captures abnormalities of these structures that are currently causing adverse health conditions in the newborn.

P02.0 Newborn affected by placenta previa

Placenta previa is implantation of the placenta over or near the internal os of the cervix. There are two forms of placental previa: complete, in which the placenta covers the entire internal cervical os; and partial, in which the placenta covers a portion of the internal cervical os. Placenta previa often results in a fetus being delivered prior to term.

P03.- Newborn affected by other complications of labor and delivery

Labor is the period of time from the start of uterine contractions to the delivery of the placenta. Delivery is the exiting of the fetus from the mother. The forces associated with labor can be extremely distressing to the fetus; the faster the delivery occurs, the less impact labor has on the fetus. Delivering the fetus, however, can be complicated by the position of the fetus, making it difficult for labor to progress and necessitating the need for alternate methods of delivery, including a cesarean section. This category captures delivery or labor complications that are affecting the health of the newborn.

P03.8- Newborn affected by other specified complications of labor and delivery

This subcategory captures conditions related to the newborn that are the result of complications not better defined in the previous categories. These may range from failed induction of labor to maternal distress or exhaustion due to the labor process.

P03.82 Meconium passage during delivery

Meconium is dark green fecal material present in the fetal intestines that may be discharged shortly before or during birth. Nearly 20 percent of newborns pass meconium during labor and delivery.

Focus Point

Meconium passage is not synonymous with meconium staining. Meconium staining indicates passage of meconium in utero, which is typically indicative of fetal stress prior to birth. Meconium staining without documented aspiration is reported with P96.83. Documented meconium aspiration with or without associated respiratory symptoms is reported with a code from subcategory P24.0-.

P04.- Newborn affected by noxious substances transmitted via placenta or breast milk

Many substances, including therapeutic drugs, analgesics, anesthetics, tobacco, alcohol, and other drugs of addiction, have the potential to affect the newborn. The mode of transmission for most substances is via the placenta, either after the maternal patient has directly ingested the substance or after being exposed to chemicals and/or noxious substances via the respiratory system, digestive tract, or skin. After birth, human breast milk can also be a source of noxious substances. Ingestion or other types of exposure to drugs and chemicals by the mother may result in these substances entering the bloodstream and from the bloodstream entering the breast milk. Contamination of breast milk may also be due to environmental pollutants and chemicals that are stored in the fatty tissues of the mother and released when this fatty tissue is broken down to produce breast milk. The specific effects on the fetus or newborn depend on the type of noxious substance.

P04.1 Newborn affected by other maternal medication

All prescribed and over-the-counter medications, other than anesthetics and analgesics used during labor and delivery, are included here. Antibiotics and antiseizure medications are examples of medications that may affect the newborn and should be reported when the newborn has suffered adverse effects from the medication or has documented conditions related to maternal use of these medications. Some antibiotics that have been associated with birth defects include sulfonamides, metronidazole, and tetracycline, as well as antibiotics that inhibit deoxyribonucleic acid (DNA) or ribonucleic acid (RNA) synthesis such as actinomycin D, mitomycin C, adenine arabinoside, and idoxuridine. Examples of types of birth defects seen with antibiotics include nerve damage, inhibition of bone growth, discoloration of teeth due to demineralization of enamel, and connective tissue defects. Many antiseizure medications are teratogenic, which means they are known to cause physical defects in the developing fetus when exposed in utero.

P04.3 Newborn affected by maternal use of alcohol

It is not known how much alcohol can be consumed safely during pregnancy. Mothers who consume alcohol especially during the first three months of pregnancy are at a greater risk for adverse effects of alcohol on the fetus. Alcohol enters the bloodstream and reaches the developing fetus by crossing the placenta. Since a fetus metabolizes alcohol more slowly than the mother, the blood alcohol concentrations in the fetus are higher. The presence of alcohol also impairs optimal nutrition for a baby's developing tissues and organs and can damage brain cells.

> **Focus Point**
>
> *Fetal alcohol syndrome, even when documented as suspected, is not reported with P04.3 but instead should be coded to Q86.0.*

P04.4- Newborn affected by maternal use of drugs of addiction

Drugs of addiction include both prescription and recreational or street drugs. Common prescription drugs that have the potential to cause addiction include oxycodone, morphine, codeine, papaverine, Demerol, methadone, and ADHD drugs. Common recreational or street drugs that have addiction potential include cocaine and methamphetamines.

> **Focus Point**
>
> *Maternal drug use can result in a newborn experiencing acute intoxication as well as withdrawal symptoms during the same admission. When both conditions are documented, the appropriate code from subcategory P04.4- should be coded along with P96.1 Neonatal withdrawal symptoms from maternal use of drugs of addiction.*

P04.41 Newborn affected by maternal use of cocaine

Two scenarios may present in newborns born to cocaine-addicted mothers. The newborn may exhibit no manifestations of the drug but test positive for cocaine or the newborn may exhibit physiopathological effects of the drug. Both scenarios are reported with this code. Signs and symptoms displayed in a newborn affected by maternal use of cocaine include hyperactivity, hyperthermia, tachycardia, dilated pupils, and, in severe cases, convulsions, coma, and circulatory collapse. Cocaine use by the mother is known to put the newborn at risk for renal system anomalies, central nervous system anomalies, and sudden infant death syndrome (SIDS).

Disorders of Newborn Related to Length of Gestation and Fetal Growth (P05-P08)

Length of gestation is the period of time from the mother's last menstrual cycle to when the newborn is delivered. As the fetus grows in the uterus it is measured in weeks referred to as the gestational age. Each week of gestation is associated with certain development milestones that allow the newborn to thrive outside of the womb. Certain adverse health conditions may arise if the newborn is born too early or is delivered past the average delivery age of 40 weeks.

Fetal growth is a relationship between the size (small or large) and weight (light or heavy) of the fetus at a particular gestational age. Typically a fetus grows proportionally in relation to the gestational age until about the 37th week, to which growth commonly plateaus. When a fetus is not the typical size at a particular gestational week it may be an indicator of an underlying condition.

The categories in this code block are as follows:

P05	Disorders of newborn related to slow fetal growth and fetal malnutrition
P07	Disorders of newborn related to short gestation and low birth weight, not elsewhere classified
P08	Disorders of newborn related to long gestation and high birth weight

P05.- Disorders of newborn related to slow fetal growth and fetal malnutrition

A newborn described as light or small for gestational age is one that is below the normal weight for a newborn typically seen at that gestational age at the time of delivery. Slow fetal growth may be related to many factors including multiple pregnancies, placenta previa, maternal drug use, or a genetic disorder. The diagnosis of fetal malnutrition has no bearing on the size or weight of the fetus or the gestational age but is solely dependent on evidence of subcutaneous tissue, fat, and muscle wasting. Malnutrition in a fetus may be due to defective assimilation or utilization of nutrients by the fetus or due to a maternal diet that is unbalanced or insufficient.

P05.9 Newborn affected by slow intrauterine growth, unspecified

Intrauterine growth retardation (IUGR) is included here. IUGR is a nonspecific term sometimes used to describe slow fetal growth.

P07.- Disorders of newborn related to short gestation and low birth weight, not elsewhere classified

The codes in this category relate the weight and/or the gestational age of the newborn at delivery. For these codes, the weight and gestational age are independent of each other and do not reflect any sort of relationship.

P07.0- Extremely low birth weight newborn

P07.1- Other low birth weight newborn

Codes that classify low birth weight are unrelated to gestational age and identify only that the newborn was born at a weight less than 2,500 grams.

Focus Point

Low birth weight is not synonymous with small or light for gestational age. For example, a newborn may be 2,250 grams at delivery, which is below the 2,500 gram marker for a normal newborn weight and as such the newborn is considered a low birth weight newborn. However, the newborn was delivered at 35 weeks gestation and 2,250 grams at 35 weeks gestation is in the range of a normal weight for that gestational age and therefore would not be considered small or light for gestational age.

P07.2- Extreme immaturity of newborn

P07.3- Preterm [premature] newborn [other]

Prematurity is differentiated as extreme immaturity, which is defined as less than 28 completed weeks of gestation, and preterm, which is defined as a gestational age of between 28 completed weeks but less than 37 completed weeks. Multiple births are about six times more likely to be premature than single birth babies. Prematurity by itself is not an illness; however, it puts the newborn at risk for many complications, including fetal lung immaturity, respiratory distress syndrome, inadequate or erratic brain perfusion, hypotension, blood pressure peaks, and infections including meningitis and sepsis.

P08.- Disorders of newborn related to long gestation and high birth weight

Newborn conditions classified here relate to gestational age beyond 40 weeks and/or a birth weight greater than 4,000 grams.

P08.0 Exceptionally large newborn baby

P08.1 Other heavy for gestational age newborn

Newborns may be heavy for gestational age, which is a birth weight of 4,000 to 4,499 grams, or exceptionally large, which is generally defined as a birth weight of 4,500 grams.

P08.21 Post-term newborn

P08.22 Prolonged gestation of newborn

Late newborn pregnancies are differentiated as postterm, which is a gestation over 40 weeks but less than 42 completed weeks, and prolonged gestation, which is a gestation of more than 42 completed weeks.

Abnormal Findings on Neonatal Screening (P09)

Neonatal screening is performed on all newborns regardless of how healthy they appear after birth. Every state has its own regulations on the conditions a newborn should be screened for, with some state programs more rigorous then others. However, a core panel of conditions is recommended and typically includes conditions such as sickle-cell disorders, thyroid disorders, hearing loss, and cystic fibrosis.

The categories in this code block are as follows:

| P09 | Abnormal findings on neonatal screening |

P09   Abnormal findings on neonatal screening

This code provides a method of reporting nonspecific yet abnormal findings on neonatal screening. Abnormal findings on neonatal screening may be transitory, posing no threat to the overall health of the neonate, or they may be early indicators of a condition or disease process that requires further work-up before a specific diagnosis can be made. This code should be used in conjunction with any signs, symptoms, and conditions that were revealed during the screening.

Birth Trauma (P10-P15)

The definition of birth trauma is injury to the fetus during delivery. Several factors may increase the risk of an injury during the birthing process, including maternal conditions (e.g., deformity of pelvic bones), fetal abnormalities (e.g., malpresentation or multiple gestations), and/or the use of obstetric instrumentation.

The categories in this code block are as follows:

P10	Intracranial laceration and hemorrhage due to birth injury
P11	Other birth injuries to central nervous system
P12	Birth injury to scalp
P13	Birth injury to skeleton
P14	Birth injury to peripheral nervous system

P12.-   Birth injury to scalp

Birth injuries to the scalp range from relatively minor bruising or laceration to severe and potentially life-threatening injuries such as epicranial subaponeurotic hemorrhage. These injuries are often associated with prolonged engagement in the birth canal or by instrumentation such as vacuum extractors, forceps, or fetal monitoring equipment.

Birth Scalp Injury

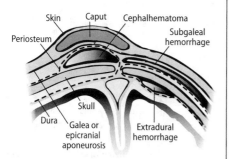

P12.0   Cephalhematoma due to birth injury

Cephalhematoma in a neonate is typically caused by prolonged labor or trauma due to instrument assisted delivery (e.g., forceps, vacuum extraction), although in rare circumstances, cephalhematoma may indicate a linear skull fracture with intracranial hemorrhage. Cephalhematoma occurs when blood vessels between the skull and periosteum rupture and blood collects in the subperiosteal space (below the periosteum). The condition is characterized by a well demarcated, undulating swelling, most commonly over the parietal bone. There is seldom skin discoloration and the swelling does not cross suture lines. A cephalhematoma appears within two to three days of birth and although it typically resolves without intervention in some instances, the hematoma may calcify resulting in a skull deformity. Other complications related to cephalhematoma include anemia, hypotension, and infection.

P12.1   Chignon (from vacuum extraction) due to birth injury

A chignon is an artificial caput succedaneum and occurs when a collection of interstitial fluid and blood forms in the area of the scalp to which the suction cup was applied during a vacuum assisted delivery. The swelling has a firm consistency and may cross the suture lines. It is a temporary condition, usually resolving within 24 hours, and is not a sign of serious injury.

P12.2   Epicranial subaponeurotic hemorrhage due to birth injury

Epicranial subaponeurotic hemorrhage, also called subgaleal hemorrhage, is a rare, but potentially fatal birth injury. The galeal aponeurosis is a layer of fibrous tissue, lying just below the skin of the scalp and just above the periosteum, and provides an attachment site to muscles in the front and back of the head. Hemorrhage occurs when the emissary veins rupture resulting in blood accumulation in the subgaleal space, which has the potential to hold as much as 50 percent of a newborns blood supply. As such, moderate to severe epicranial subaponeurotic hemorrhages are potentially life-threatening as they can lead to hypovolemia (decreased blood volume in the body); newborns often require treatment in an intensive care unit.

> **Focus Point**
>
> *The severity of a subaponeurotic hemorrhage over a cephalhematoma is related to the area to which the blood can accumulate. A cephalhematoma occurs below the periosteum, a membrane covering each bone of the skull, which therefore limits the spread of the blood to vast areas of the head. In contrast, subaponeurotic hemorrhage occurs above the periosteum and is not inhibited by periosteum boundaries and allows more blood to accumulate.*

P12.81 Caput succedaneum

A caput succedaneum is a swelling of the scalp. The swelling is a result of pressure being exerted on the head from the vaginal walls, uterus, or instrumentation used in assisting a delivery (e.g., vacuum). Although it can occur early in the third trimester, secondary to low amniotic fluid, it typically occurs when labor and delivery is prolonged. It is characterized by a soft, fluctuant swelling in the presenting area of the head, which may be accompanied by swelling across suture lines, bruising, and discoloration of the skin. No treatment is necessary and the condition resolves spontaneously within a few days.

P14.- Birth injury to peripheral nervous system

The peripheral nervous system includes the brachial plexus nerves that emerge from the cervical spinal cord and continue to the shoulder, arm, and hand; and the sacral plexus nerves that emerge from the lumbar/sacral spine and continue to the lower extremities. Peripheral nerve damage occurs when the presenting fetal part encounters mechanical forces such as compression, contortion, torque, or traction. Large fetal size, maternal pelvic size/shape, abnormal presentation (e.g., breech, face, and shoulder), use of forceps and/or vacuum extractor, and neurologic immaturity can all lead to nerve damage. The following identifies different types of nerve damage, listed from most severe to least severe:

- Avulsion is the complete dislocation of the nerve from the spinal cord

- Neurotmesis is complete division of a nerve at any point except the spinal cord

- Axonotmesis occurs when the axons of the nerve are severed

- Rupture involves stretching and partial tearing of a nerve anywhere but at the spine

- Neurapraxia involves stretching or compression of the nerve without tearing of the nerve fibers

Complications related to peripheral nerve injury include progressive bony deformities, muscle atrophy, joint contractures, impaired limb growth, and weakness of the extremity.

P14.0 Erb's paralysis due to birth injury

Erb's palsy or paralysis is the most common type of brachial plexus (peripheral nerve) injury in a neonate and involves nerve damage at the level of C5-C6. Symptoms include loss of shoulder motion and the inability to flex the elbow. Moro, biceps, and radial reflexes are absent on the affected side and, in severe cases, there may be an ipsilateral paralysis of the diaphragm due to phrenic nerve damage. Hyperabduction or subluxation of the cervical spine

due to excessive force applied to the newborn, as well as other obstacles encountered during deliver such as shoulder dystocia or breech presentation, may all result in this type of paralysis.

P14.1 Klumpke's paralysis due to birth injury

Klumpke's paralysis is a rare brachial plexus (peripheral nerve) injury that involves nerve damage at the level of the eighth cervical and first thoracic vertebra. It is characterized by muscle weakness and loss of motor function and/or sensory signaling to the forearm and hand. The palmer grasp reflex is absent on the affected side. Typically this condition is caused by pulling on the extended arm of the newborn to extract the newborn from the birth canal.

P14.2 Phrenic nerve paralysis due to birth injury

Phrenic nerve palsy (paralysis) in a newborn is rare and results from a stretch injury caused by lateral hyperextension of the neck during delivery. It can occur with breech and vertex presentations and is often seen with forceps use. The most common site of injury is where the phrenic nerve crosses the brachial plexus and as such brachial plexus injuries (e.g., Erb's palsy, Klumpke's paralysis) often accompany a phrenic nerve injury. The phrenic nerve controls the diaphragm, a dome-shaped muscle that separates the thoracic and abdominal cavities and is involved in respiration (breathing). Damage to the phrenic nerve causes ipsilateral paralysis of the diaphragm. Symptoms of diaphragmatic paralysis can include chest asymmetry, decreased breath sounds on the affected side, and respiratory distress. The infant may require intubation and mechanical ventilation and is at risk for respiratory infection.

Respiratory and Cardiovascular Disorders Specific to the Perinatal Period (P19-P29)

Respiratory and cardiovascular disorders included in this code block capture abnormalities in the function and/or structure of the neonatal respiratory system, heart, and/or circulation.

The categories in this code block are as follows:

P19	Metabolic acidemia in newborn
P22	Respiratory distress of newborn
P23	Congenital pneumonia
P24	Neonatal aspiration
P25	Interstitial emphysema and related conditions originating in the perinatal period
P26	Pulmonary hemorrhage originating in the perinatal period

P27   Chronic respiratory disease originating in the perinatal period

P28   Other respiratory conditions originating in the perinatal period

P29   Cardiovascular disorders originating in the perinatal period

P19.-   Metabolic acidemia in newborn

Metabolic acidemia in the newborn is a biochemical acid-base disorder of the blood with onset occurring directly before, during, or after delivery. The condition is typically the result of early respiratory issues, such as asphyxia. Symptoms may include tachypnea, tachycardia, myocardial depression, seizures, poor tissue perfusion (shock), and multiorgan failure.

Focus Point

Codes from this category are limited to the period immediately prior to, during, and immediately after birth. Code P74.0 is used for late metabolic acidosis and is related to abnormal kidney function that generally is not evident until the newborn is two or three weeks old.

P22.-   Respiratory distress of newborn

Common symptoms among respiratory distress conditions include nasal flaring, cyanosis, chest wall retractions, grunting, and/or tachypnea, all of which indicate that the newborn is working very hard to breath. How these symptoms manifest is dependent on the specific condition causing the respiratory distress.

P22.0   Respiratory distress syndrome of newborn

Also known as hyaline membrane disease and respiratory distress syndrome (RDS) Type 1, this condition occurs primarily in premature infants (before completion of 37 weeks of gestation) or infants whose mothers are diabetic. In most instances, the etiology related to RDS is a reduction of surfactant in the lungs, a phospholipid mixture important in alveoli inflation and stability. The resultant alveolar collapse leads to atelectasis and hypoxemia with symptoms of respiratory distress apparent immediately following the birth of the newborn.

P22.1   Transient tachypnea of newborn

Transient tachypnea of the newborn (TTN) is a self-limited condition that occurs in 1 percent of newborns. Normally newborns expel fluid during birth due to pressure imposed on the newborn when passing through the birth canal. Upon their initial breaths, the lungs fill with air forcing additional fluid out. Absorption of the fluid into the bloodstream and lymphatic system eventually removes any remaining fluid left in the lungs. When not enough fluid is expelled from the lungs during the birth process or if

there is slow absorption of the fluid out of the lungs, it can result in TTN. This condition usually resolves within a few days with improvement of pulmonary status as the retained lung fluid is eventually absorbed.

P23.-   Congenital pneumonia

Congenital pneumonia occurs when an infectious agent is passed from the mother to the baby, resulting in inflammation of the newborn's lungs. The infectious agent is typically acquired via transplacental transmission or by picking up the pathogens when exiting the birth canal.

Focus Point

Aspiration of infected amniotic or other fluids by the newborn can also occur in utero or during the delivery process. Although an aspiration event may not always lead to respiratory complications, pneumonia can sometimes result and is not considered a congenital condition. Review the documentation carefully as pneumonia that is secondary to aspiration is coded from category P24 Neonatal aspiration.

P23.1   Congenital pneumonia due to Chlamydia

Chlamydia trachomatis is the most common sexually transmitted disease in the United States. *C. trachomatis* infects the columnar epithelium of the mucous membranes of the genitourinary tract and the infection can be transmitted to the newborn during passage through the birth canal. The infection is initially asymptomatic with respiratory symptoms usually occurring sometime after two weeks of age.

P23.2   Congenital pneumonia due to staphylococcus

Staphylococcus aureus is a bacterium that causes a wide spectrum of infectious diseases, including congenital pneumonia. In recent years, some *S. aureus* strains have become resistant to a number of antibiotics and *S. aureus* is now differentiated based on susceptibility or resistance to beta lactam antibiotics. The term methicillin-susceptible *Staphylococcus aureus* (MSSA) identifies strains of *S. aureus* that are susceptible or treatable with the traditional beta lactam class of antibiotics, such as penicillin, methicillin, and cephalosporins. Methicillin-resistant *Staphylococcus aureus* (MRSA) is a variant form of the bacterium that is resistant to the traditional beta lactam class of antibiotics such as penicillin, methicillin, and cephalosporins.

P23.3   Congenital pneumonia due to streptococcus, group B

Streptococcus is one of the more common causes of infectious disease. It is a spherical, gram positive, nonmotile bacterium that clusters together to form chains. *Streptococcus*, *S. agalactiae*, also called group B *Streptococcus*, used to be a common cause of congenital pneumonia in newborns because about 25 percent of all women are asymptomatic carriers of Group B strep in the vaginal and rectal regions. Even though these women do not display signs or symptoms of infection, they can pass the bacteria on to a newborn during the birth process. For this reason, women are screened for the presence of Group B strep between the 35th and 37th weeks of pregnancy. If the results are positive, antibiotics are given during labor to help prevent passage of the bacteria to the newborn.

P23.4 Congenital pneumonia due to Escherichia coli

Escherichia coli (*E. coli*) are a large and diverse group of bacteria that range from the relatively harmless to those which cause serious, life-threatening illness. Because *E. coli* inhabit the maternal intestinal tract, including the rectal and anal regions, newborns may be infected during the birth process. One of the more common manifestations, particularly in premature and low birth weight newborns, is congenital pneumonia.

P24.- Neonatal aspiration

Aspiration in a newborn occurs when a substance such as meconium, amniotic fluid, mucus, blood, or milk is inhaled into the trachea, bronchi, or lungs. Inhalation of a foreign substance into the lower respiratory tract can cause pneumonia, pneumonitis, or other respiratory complications. The presence of respiratory complications is dependent on the amount and how deeply the substance is inhaled.

P24.0- Meconium aspiration

Meconium is dark green fecal material present in the fetal intestines that may be discharged shortly before or during birth. In a distressed state, intestinal activity of the fetus or newborn increases, relaxing the anal sphincter and allowing passage of the first bowel movement. Nearly 20 percent of infants pass meconium prior to or during delivery and 20 to 30 percent of newborns who pass meconium inhale it while still in utero or at delivery. Depending on the amount aspirated, the viscosity, and how deeply inhaled, the newborn's lungs can become blocked, initiating an inflammatory response and causing severe lung problems. Aspiration does not necessarily develop into respiratory problems or meconium aspiration syndrome, but when respiratory symptoms are present they may include rapid, labored, or suspended breathing; cyanosis; or limpness, resulting in a low Apgar score.

P27.- Chronic respiratory disease originating in the perinatal period

This category reports respiratory disease arising in the perinatal period that is persistent or prolonged in duration. In some cases, the chronic respiratory disease resolves with appropriate medical care, but in others the respiratory disease may persist, causing long-term health issues in infancy, childhood, or even into adulthood.

P27.0 Wilson-Mikity syndrome

Wilson-Mikity syndrome is a rare type of chronic lung disease that affects very low birth weight, premature infants and is associated with significant morbidity. The disease is characterized by alveolar air leak, coarse infiltrates, and pulmonary inflammation induced by cystic interstitial air (emphysema), which leads to progressive respiratory distress and the need for aggressive mechanical ventilation and oxygen therapy.

> **Focus Point**
>
> *Wilson-Mikity syndrome has similar characteristics to bronchopulmonary dysplasia (BPD). It is important to understand however, that BPD occurs as a direct result of ventilatory support while Wilson-Mikity syndrome occurs despite the newborn ever having received ventilation of any kind.*

P27.1 Bronchopulmonary dysplasia originating in the perinatal period

Bronchopulmonary dysplasia (BPD) is a chronic lung disease found in premature infants that results from injury to the lungs due to the use of ventilation procedures used to treat respiratory issues. In premature infants, immature lungs can be injured when the air sacs are overstretched by the ventilator or when they are exposed to high oxygen levels over time. Consequently, the lungs become inflamed, and additional fluid accumulates within the lungs. Premature infants (less than 2.2 pounds or 1,000 grams), infants with breathing problems at birth, or those who need long-term breathing support and oxygen are the highest risk for developing BPD. Full-term newborns that have lung disorders (e.g., pneumonia) may also develop BPD. Most infants recover with limited symptoms. In rare cases, complications occur and this condition can be fatal. Infants with BPD are prone to an increased incidence of infection, as well as asthma during the first two years of life.

P28.- Other respiratory conditions originating in the perinatal period

Respiratory conditions classified here include some fairly common respiratory symptoms such as cyanotic attacks, as well as less common conditions such as respiratory failure and respiratory arrest.

P28.0   Primary atelectasis of newborn

Primary atelectasis of the newborn is the failure of the lungs to expand after birth causing a reduction or absence of gas exchange (oxygen, carbon dioxide) at the alveoli level. The condition is common in premature infants who lack the strength to inflate the lungs and may also have decreased levels of surfactant in the air sacs (alveoli). Other causes can include obstruction of the airway from mucus plugs, aspirated meconium stool, amniotic fluid or blood, respiratory depression from maternal anesthesia, and congenital respiratory malformation.

P28.11   Resorption atelectasis without respiratory distress syndrome

Resorption atelectasis without respiratory distress syndrome occurs when there is an obstruction in the trachea and a slow partial collapse of the air sacs (alveoli) occurs in the lung distal to the obstruction. The infant is able to compensate with the functioning lung lobe(s) and does not require supplemental oxygen or ventilator support.

P28.19   Other atelectasis of newborn

Secondary atelectasis and partial atelectasis are other types of atelectasis that can occur in a newborn. Secondary atelectasis manifests after the lungs have fully inflated and the newborn experiences subsequent impairment of lung expansion. This can be due to respiratory distress syndrome (RDS), aspiration, or pressure on the lung tissue from an outside force such as pneumothorax, pleural effusion, or diaphragmatic hernia. Partial atelectasis also occurs after lungs have inflated and is primarily due to obstruction. A portion of the alveoli, a lung segment, or an entire lobe of the lung may collapse as the residual gases are absorbed.

P28.2   Cyanotic attacks of newborn

Cyanosis is a bluish discoloration of the nail beds, skin, and/or mucus membranes due to low hemoglobin levels in the capillary beds and is a fairly common finding in a newborn. Cyanotic attacks are defined as a sudden manifestation of this bluish discoloration in a newborn with previously normal skin color. The episodes usually last less than 30 minutes with the infant's color returning to normal without intervention. Cyanosis may be further defined as central or peripheral. Central cyanosis is commonly experienced by infants directly after birth, but when the condition persists, it may be indicative of a more serious underlying condition. Peripheral or acrocyanosis is usually observed in the extremities as a response to hypothermia. The mechanism of acrocyanosis is an arteriovenous oxygen difference that manifests with a blue discoloration of tissue due to the slow transit of blood through the capillary beds.

P28.3   Primary sleep apnea of newborn

Primary sleep apnea of the newborn is when an infant stops breathing for short periods of time. These episodes typically last for more than 20 seconds and commonly occur in infants born prematurely. The episodes usually become evident on the second or third day after birth and can last for two or three months. As the infant matures, episodes of apnea occur less frequently. In premature infants, the part of the brain that controls breathing is not fully developed so they experience irregular breathing, alternating between normal breathing and brief pauses in breathing, also referred to as central sleep apnea. In severely premature infants, apnea may be a result of an obstruction of the pharynx due to lack of muscle tone or a bending forward of the neck (obstructive apnea). Apnea may lower the amount of oxygen in the blood, resulting in a decreased heart rate, which may cause cyanosis. Infants may also appear limp and breathing may be noisy. The infant may start breathing again or require stimulation to help resume breathing. There are several factors that can contribute to the severity of apnea, including infection, heart or lung problems, anemia, low oxygen levels, feeding problems, thermoregulation, and overstimulation. Premature infants are usually in the hospital's neonatal intensive care unit (NICU) where they are monitored closely for episodes of apnea in order to receive immediate treatment.

P28.81   Respiratory arrest of newborn

Apnea is the absence of spontaneous breathing from any cause. Prolonged apnea, also known as respiratory arrest, is a life-threatening condition that requires immediate medical intervention. Respiratory arrest in newborns is often a result of prematurity, although other contributing factors may include congenital abnormalities, birth injury, or genetic factors.

P29.-   Cardiovascular disorders originating in the perinatal period

The cardiovascular (CV) system is a complex network of blood vessels, arteries, and veins, moving blood to and from the heart, the major organ of the CV system. The heart is a muscle that assists in blood circulation, by pumping oxygenated and deoxygenated blood to the body and lungs respectively. When the function or structure of the heart or blood vessels is compromised, it is captured with a code from this category.

P29.0   Neonatal cardiac failure

Cardiac failure in the neonate (newborn infant) is characterized by tachypnea, tachycardia, feeding difficulties, pulmonary rales and rhonchi, liver enlargement, and cardiomegaly.

When cardiac failure occurs in the perinatal period (birth through the 28th day following birth), it is often due to structural congenital heart disease. It may also be secondary to arrhythmia, respiratory or central nervous system disease, severe anemia, systemic or pulmonary hypertension, or sepsis.

Treatment options include diuretics and other cardiac support medications as well as ventilation and nasogastric feeding. Surgery may be indicated in cases of structural congenital heart disease.

P29.1-   Neonatal cardiac dysrhythmia

Neonatal cardiac dysrhythmias such as tachycardia and bradycardia are relatively common occurrences with supraventricular tachycardia the most common, but unless they are sustained, they are rarely serious. Most of these dysrhythmias are asymptomatic or have nonspecific symptoms. Some causes are hypoxia, metabolic disturbances, sepsis, atrial lesions or structural heart disease, or there is no clear underlying pathology. Treatment is dependent on the underlying cause, with echocardiographic evaluation to exclude underlying structural heart disease.

P29.2   Neonatal hypertension

Neonatal hypertension is defined as elevated systolic BP which is more than 95% for infants of similar gestational and postnatal age, gender, height, and birth weight. Common causes are thromboembolisms secondary to umbilical artery catheterization, congenital renal structural malformation or disease, aortic coarctation, acute kidney injury, and medications. Diagnostic evaluation must be performed to identify the underlying cause, with treatment options depending on the severity and the underlying cause.

P29.3-   Persistent fetal circulation

Persistent fetal circulation includes pulmonary hypertension of newborn also referred to as persistent pulmonary hypertension of newborn, and other disorders of persistent fetal circulation such as delayed closure of ductus arteriosus.

P29.30   Pulmonary hypertension of newborn

A life-threatening condition, persistent pulmonary hypertension of the newborn (PPHN) is reported with this code. PPHN is defined as the failure of the normal circulatory transition that occurs in the blood vessels to the lungs after birth. It usually occurs in full-term or post-term babies who have had a difficult birth or infections, and is characterized by marked high blood pressure in the arteries leading to the lungs and heart, which decreases blood flow into the lungs and in turn, reduced oxygen supply to the body. This causes breathing problems such as rapid or slow breathing,

grunting, and retractions, with hypoxemia secondary to right-to-left shunting of blood. The ductus arterious remains open, thus the pressure in the lungs stays high and the blood is directed away from the lungs.

P29.38   Other persistent fetal circulation

Included here is delayed closure of ductus arteriosus. The ductus arteriosus is a normal component of fetal circulation consisting of a short duct that allows fetal blood to be shunted away from the pulmonary artery and pulmonary circulation and returned directly to the aorta. Normally, in a full term birth, within 12–24 hours, the ductus arteriosus closes so that oxygen-depleted blood from the systemic circulation can be routed to the pulmonary circulation where it can be oxygenated and returned to the heart. In delayed closure of the patent ductus arteriosus (PDA), generally found in premature births, the duct between the pulmonary arteries and the aorta does not close immediately after birth.

> **Focus Point**
>
> *A persistent PDA results in reversed blood flow from the aorta into the pulmonary artery and can cause pulmonary overload and congestive heart failure. Patent ductus arteriosus that does not close more than a few days after birth is reported from Chapter 17 Congenital malformations, deformations and chromosomal abnormalities with code Q25.0 Patent ductus arteriosus.*

P29.4   Transient myocardial ischemia in newborn

Transient myocardial ischemia (TMI) of the newborn is a form of severe cardiorespiratory distress in full-term infants, usually due to birth asphyxia caused by impaired myocardial perfusion from increased demand. It is frequently present without anatomic heart disease. Symptoms vary from severe cardiogenic shock, respiratory distress, congestive cardiac failure, and systolic murmur. This type of myocardial ischemia is transient and depending on the severity of symptoms, the baby can recover without sequelae.

P29.8-   Other cardiovascular disorders originating in the perinatal period

This subcategory can be used to identify circulatory and cardiovascular collapse or failure in a newborn, including cardiac arrest, a complete loss of heart function.

P29.81   Cardiac arrest of newborn

Cardiac arrest is defined as the cessation of cardiac mechanical activity, manifested by the inability to detect a central pulse, unresponsiveness, and apnea. Newborn cardiac arrest can be caused by multiple factors, including the use of beta-adrenergic antagonists for the control of high blood pressure in the mother, trauma, and congenital abnormalities.

Infections Specific to the Perinatal Period (P35-P39)

An infection occurs when a pathogen, introduced or native to the individual, invades and/or multiplies within the host's body. Perinatal infections occur when the pathogens are transmitted from the mother to the newborn while in the uterus or during delivery, or the pathogen may be acquired from the extrauterine environment.

The categories in this code block are as follows:

P35   Congenital viral diseases

P36   Bacterial sepsis of newborn

P37   Other congenital infectious and parasitic diseases

P38   Omphalitis of newborn

P39   Other infections specific to the perinatal period

P35.-   Congenital viral diseases

A number of viruses contracted by the mother during pregnancy have the potential to cause complications in the fetus and newborn, including life-threatening anomalies, malformations, and other disease processes.

P35.Ø   Congenital rubella syndrome

Maternal rubella infection with the rubella virus, also called German measles, that is contracted within a month before conception and through the second trimester is often associated with newborn disease with the greatest risk during the first trimester. Common congenital defects seen in newborns with congenital rubella syndrome include cataracts, congenital heart disease, hearing impairment, and developmental delay. Most newborns have more than one defect. Of those newborns presenting with a single defect, hearing impairment is the most common.

P36.-   Bacterial sepsis of newborn

Sepsis is a systemic or body wide response to an infection with the majority of sepsis cases being due to a bacterial infection. The systemic response is characterized by certain changes in body temperature, heart rate, respiratory rate or arterial blood gases, and white blood cell count. More specifically, these include elevated body temperature (usually above 1Ø1 degrees Fahrenheit) or subnormal body temperature (usually below 96.8 degrees Fahrenheit), elevated heart rate (usually above 9Ø beats per minute), elevated respiratory rate (usually above 2Ø breaths per minute) or arterial blood gases reflecting a reduced partial pressure of carbon dioxide PACO2, and an abnormal white blood cell count above 12,ØØØ cells/microliter or below 4,ØØØ cells/microliter or greater than 1Ø bands (immature white blood cell). Two or more of these indications and a suspected or known infection are indicative of sepsis.

P36.Ø   Sepsis of newborn due to streptococcus, group B

Streptococcus is one of the more common causes of infectious disease. It is a spherical, gram positive, nonmotile bacterium that clusters together to form chains. Streptococcus, S. agalactiae, also called group B Streptococcus, used to be a common cause of sepsis in newborns because about 25 percent of all women are asymptomatic carriers of Group B strep in the vaginal and rectal regions. Even though these women do not display signs or symptoms of infection, they can pass the bacteria on to a newborn during the birth process. For this reason, women are screened for the presence of Group B strep in the vagina between the 35th and 37th weeks of pregnancy. If the results are positive, antibiotics are given during labor to help prevent passage of the bacteria to the newborn. While the use of antibiotics during labor does reduce the incidence of Group B strep infection in newborns, some infants do develop infections and are at risk for developing sepsis.

P36.19   Sepsis of newborn due to other streptococci

Streptococcus is one of the more common causes of infectious disease. It is a spherical, gram positive, nonmotile bacterium that clusters together to form chains. The two most common pathogenic species reported here are S. pyogenes, also called group A, and S. pneumoniae.

P36.2   Sepsis of newborn due to Staphylococcus aureus

Staphylococcus aureus is a bacterium that causes a wide spectrum of infectious diseases, including newborn sepsis. In recent years, some S. aureus strains have become resistant to a number of antibiotics complicating the management of a newborn with this type of pathogen. S. aureus species that are resistant to traditional beta lactam antibiotics, such as penicillin, methicillin, and cephalosporins, are termed methicillin-resistant Staphylococcus aureus (MRSA) and those that are susceptible or treatable with the beta lactam class of antibiotics are termed methicillin-susceptible Staphylococcus aureus (MSSA).

P36.39   Sepsis of newborn due to other staphylococci

This classification includes coagulase negative staphylococcus species, including S. hominis and S. epidermidis, which inhabit the skin, and S. saprophyticus found in the vaginal tract. When confined to these sites, these species are typically not pathogenic. However, they can cause sepsis if they are introduced into the bloodstream secondary to infection.

P38.- Omphalitis of newborn

Infection and inflammation of the umbilical stump, most often due to bacteria, is termed omphalitis. In most cases, the source of the infection is a combination of aerobic and anaerobic organisms. Spread of the infection beyond the umbilical stump to the fascia, muscle, or even the umbilical vessels can occur. Signs and symptoms include purulent drainage, edema, tenderness, and erythema.

Hemorrhagic and Hematological Disorders of Newborn (P50-P61)

When something is wrong with a newborn's blood or blood constituents, it may be categorized as a hematological or hemorrhagic disorder. More specifically, hemorrhaging is excessive loss of blood while a hematological disorder relates to an abnormality with the blood itself.

The categories in this code block are as follows:

P50	Newborn affected by intrauterine (fetal) blood loss
P51	Umbilical hemorrhage of newborn
P52	Intracranial nontraumatic hemorrhage of newborn
P53	Hemorrhagic disease of newborn
P54	Other neonatal hemorrhages
P55	Hemolytic disease of newborn
P56	Hydrops fetalis due to hemolytic disease
P57	Kernicterus
P58	Neonatal jaundice due to other excessive hemolysis
P59	Neonatal jaundice from other and unspecified causes
P60	Disseminated intravascular coagulation of newborn
P61	Other perinatal hematological disorders

P55.- Hemolytic disease of newborn

Hemolytic disease refers to the premature destruction of red blood cells. This category includes newborn hemolytic disease due to isoimmunization. In isoimmunization, the mother develops antibodies against an antigen derived from a genetically dissimilar fetus. Symptoms of hemolytic disease range from mild to severe. Common symptoms seen in a newborn with hemolytic disease include jaundice and anemia.

> **Focus Point**
>
> *Hemolytic disease of the newborn can cause severe and even life-threatening conditions, such as hydrops fetalis and kernicterus. For these complications of hemolytic disease, see categories P56 and P57.*

P55.0 Rh isoimmunization of newborn

Rh factor is a protein found on the surface of red blood cells in some individuals. Individuals with Rh factor on the surface of their red blood cells are Rh-positive, while those without Rh factor are Rh-negative. Rh isoimmunization occurs when an Rh-negative mother carries an Rh-positive fetus and the fetal blood crosses the placenta entering the mother's bloodstream. The mother then makes antibodies to the Rh factor, which is identified as a foreign protein in the mother's blood. If these antibodies cross the placenta and enter the fetal blood, they damage and destroy the fetal red blood cells causing Rh isoimmunization.

P55.1 ABO isoimmunization of newborn

There are four blood types: A, B, AB and O. ABO isoimmunization may occur when a mother with one blood type carries a fetus with an incompatible blood type. If blood from a fetus with an incompatible blood type crosses the placenta and enters the mother's bloodstream, the mother's body makes antibodies to the foreign blood type. If these antibodies cross the placenta and enter the fetal blood, they can damage and destroy the fetal red blood cells resulting in ABO isoimmunization.

P56.- Hydrops fetalis due to hemolytic disease

Hemolytic disease causes abnormal destruction of the red blood cells (RBC), which results in anemia. If the production of new red blood cells is increased effectively and compensates for the loss of RBCs, the anemia may be mild. However, in some instances the RBC producing organs cannot compensate for the amount of RBCs being destroyed. This leads to organ failure and fluid buildup in various areas of the newborn's body, typically the skin, abdominal cavity, pleural space, and pericardial sac. When two or more of these body sites are affected it results in hydrops fetalis.

P57.- Kernicterus

Kernicterus is a significantly large accumulation of bilirubin in the brain that may result in brain damage.

P59.- Neonatal jaundice from other and unspecified causes

This category classifies jaundice due to conditions other than excessive hemolysis.

P59.9 Neonatal jaundice, unspecified

Hyperbilirubinemia, also called physiologic jaundice, refers to excess bilirubin in the blood. Bilirubin is a yellow byproduct of red blood cell destruction, removed from the body through the intestines after being processed by the liver. Prior to birth, the placenta removes the bilirubin from the infant so that it can be processed by the mother's liver. However, at birth, the baby's liver begins to perform this function and may not be able to process as much bilirubin as necessary. Physiological jaundice seen soon after the birth of an infant is not abnormal. It can cause the infant's skin and whites of the eyes to look yellow, with discoloration beginning in the face and then moving down to the trunk, legs, and soles of the feet. This type of jaundice usually causes no problems, appearing on the second or third day of life and resolving within two weeks.

Transitory Endocrine and Metabolic Disorders Specific to Newborn (P70-P74)

Only temporary endocrine and metabolic disorders occurring during the perinatal period are included in this code block. Endocrine and metabolic disorders classified here are due to maternal conditions that temporarily impact the newborn or relate to the newborn's adjustment to the environment outside of the uterus.

The categories in this code block are as follows:

P70	Transitory disorders of carbohydrate metabolism specific to newborn
P71	Transitory neonatal disorders of calcium and magnesium metabolism
P72	Other transitory neonatal endocrine disorders
P74	Other transitory neonatal electrolyte and metabolic disturbances

P70.- Transitory disorders of carbohydrate metabolism specific to newborn

Transitory metabolic disorders classified here manifest primarily as hyperglycemia or hypoglycemia.

P70.0 Syndrome of infant of mother with gestational diabetes

Gestational diabetes is a condition in which the placenta produces antiinsulin hormones that cause the mother's blood glucose levels (BGL) to rise. The extra glucose crosses the placenta to nourish the fetus. In turn, the fetus produces more insulin to metabolize the extra glucose, which is then stored as fat. The infant of a mother with gestational diabetes often presents with macrosomia (large for gestational age); unstable BGL (hypoglycemia); enlarged liver, heart, and adrenal glands; red skin color caused by polycythemia (increased red blood cells); and an imbalance of calcium and magnesium. Complications can include respiratory distress, jaundice, and feeding problems.

P70.1 Syndrome of infant of a diabetic mother

An infant born to a mother with preexisting diabetes may have similar characteristics to an infant of a mother who did not develop diabetes until she became pregnant (gestational diabetes). In preexisting diabetes, the placenta is not producing antiinsulin hormones but the fetus is subjected to fluctuations in maternal blood glucose levels (BGL) due to dietary intake and use of exogenous insulin. The infant of a mother with diabetes is at increased risk of being born prematurely or being large for gestational age (macrosomic) or small for gestational age (impaired fetal growth). Blood glucose instability (hypoglycemia) is common, as well as low calcium, magnesium, and iron levels and hyperviscosity due to polycythemia (increased red blood cells). Other complications may include respiratory distress syndrome (RDS) and hyperbilirubinemia (neonatal jaundice). Congenital abnormalities occur more frequently in infants of mothers with preexisting diabetes, particularly brain, central nervous system, and heart defects.

P70.2 Neonatal diabetes mellitus

Neonatal diabetes mellitus (NDM) is caused by a rare single gene (monogenic) mutation that impairs insulin production by the pancreas. Insulin is required by the body to transport glucose into cells for use as energy. NDM is often recognized within the first six months of life and may be permanent (PNDM) or transient (TNDM). NDM infants are typically small for gestational age (SGA) due to intrauterine growth restriction (IUGR). Symptoms include elevated blood glucose levels (hyperglycemia), glucosuria (glucose in the urine) which causes polyuria (excessive urination), dehydration, and excessive thirst. An infant with NDM frequently has feeding problems and poor weight gain (failure to thrive) due to an underdeveloped pancreas and decreased production of digestive enzymes. Ketoacidosis is a serious, life-threatening condition that may develop if hyperglycemia is not treated and neurological problems including seizures and developmental delays are common.

P74.- Other transitory neonatal electrolyte and metabolic disturbances

Temporary electrolyte and metabolic disturbances classified here include dehydration, temporarily elevated or decreased levels of electrolytes such as sodium and potassium, and disorders of amino acid metabolism.

P74.0   Late metabolic acidosis of newborn

Late metabolic acidosis of the newborn is associated with a renal system dysfunction that typically affects low birth weight and/or premature infants during the second or third week of life. These infants are unable to excrete acids (hydrogen ions, H+) via the kidneys due to renal immaturity leading to excess H+ accumulation in the blood and a lowered pH level. The condition usually resolves spontaneously as the renal system develops. Excessive protein intake has also been associated with late metabolic acidosis and the infant's protein intake, especially when being fed formula, should be closely monitored and adjusted should the infant begin to show signs of the condition. Impaired weight gain is the most common symptom of late metabolic acidosis.

Focus Point

Metabolic acidosis may also occur as a result of respiratory issues, with onset right before or after delivery. This type is referred to as early metabolic acidosis and is coded to category P19.

Digestive System Disorders of Newborn (P76-P78)

Starting at the mouth and ending at the anus, the digestive system works to turn food consumed into energy. Most of the organs that make up the digestive tract are hollow tubes to which the food passes through, with additional organs—pancreas, gallbladder, and liver—also assisting in digestion.

The categories in this code block are as follows:

P76	Other intestinal obstruction of newborn
P77	Necrotizing enterocolitis of newborn
P78	Other perinatal digestive system disorders

P76.-   Other intestinal obstruction of newborn

Intestinal obstruction is one of the more common digestive tract complications seen in newborns. There are some common indicators of newborn intestinal obstruction regardless of the specific cause, including maternal polyhydramnios, vomiting of bile, failure to pass meconium during the first 24 hours following birth, and abdominal distension.

P76.0   Meconium plug syndrome

Meconium is dark green fecal material present in the fetal intestines that is usually passed within 24 hours after birth. Meconium plug syndrome, also referred to as meconium ileus or meconium obstruction, occurs when the meconium in the digestive tract fails to pass resulting in the obstruction of the intestine. The primary symptom of meconium plug syndrome is abdominal distention.

P77.-   Necrotizing enterocolitis of newborn

Necrotizing enterocolitis is a major cause of morbidity and mortality in premature infants. It is a serious gastrointestinal illness seen mainly in very low birth weight (VLBW) infants. In necrotizing enterocolitis, the lining of the intestinal wall dies and the tissue sloughs off. The cause for this disorder is unknown, but it is thought that a decrease in blood flow to the bowel keeps the bowel from producing mucus that protects the gastrointestinal tract. Bacteria in the intestine may also be a contributing factor. Necrotizing enterocolitis of the newborn is classified by stage. In stage 1, necrotizing enterocolitis is suspected but there are no signs of pneumatosis or perforation. Pneumatosis is the presence of gas in the bowel wall while a perforation is a break or tears in the bowel. Stage 2 represents definitive necrotizing enterocolitis and presents with absent bowel sounds and radiological studies that show intestinal dilation, ileus, and pneumatosis. Ascites may also be present. Stage 3 is advanced necrotizing enterocolitis with pneumatosis and/or perforation of the intestine and systemic symptoms such as hypotension or shock, acute respiratory distress, and peritonitis.

P78.-   Other perinatal digestive system disorders

This category classifies certain other specific perinatal digestive system disorders such as neonatal peritonitis and diarrhea as well as congenital liver cirrhosis, peptic ulcer of newborn, newborn/neonatal esophageal reflux, and gestational alloimmune liver disease (GALD).

P78.84   Gestational alloimmune liver disease

Gestational alloimmune liver disease (GALD) is a unique disease presenting as severe hepatic injury in newborn infants. Its onset is during fetal development and manifestations of the disease begin during fetal life. It is caused by maternal antibodies to fetal hepatic cells (hepatocytes) that cross the placenta into the fetal circulation, causing hepatic cell necrosis. Fetal liver injury often results in systemic iron overload, and this condition was previously referred to as neonatal hemochromatosis (NH). GALD is poorly responsive to medical or surgical management in the neonate, and there is a high morbidity and mortality rate associated with this condition. However, it is preventable if diagnosed antepartum with maternal intravenous administration of immunoglobulin.

Conditions Involving the Integument and Temperature Regulation of Newborn (P80-P83)

Temperature regulation is included here because one of the primary functions of the skin is to help maintain body temperature. Newborns have only a limited ability to control body temperature. While adults are able to maintain a relatively constant body temperature regardless of the surrounding air temperature, the immature thermoregulatory response in newborns does not allow them to effectively maintain a relatively constant body temperature making newborns more susceptible to hypothermia and hyperthermia.

The categories in this code block are as follows:

P80	Hypothermia of newborn
P81	Other disturbances of temperature regulation of newborn
P83	Other conditions of integument specific to newborn

P80.-   Hypothermia of newborn

Hypothermia of the newborn is a temperature less than 36.5°C (97.7°F). In utero, the fetus has no independent thermoregulation and maintains a body temperature approximately 0.5°C higher than the mother. Rapid cooling occurs following delivery as the newborn loses heat through evaporation of amniotic fluid from the skin, conduction from contact with cold surfaces, convection as air currents move around the room, and radiation to colder solid surfaces in the room. Newborns are at risk for hypothermia because of their larger ratio of surface area to body weight, thin skin with blood vessels close to the surface, and a limited amount of subcutaneous and brown fat. Brown fat is located around the adrenal glands and kidneys, nape of neck, interscapular area, axilla, and mediastinum. Heat is transported to areas of the newborn's body when blood that flows through the brown fat is warmed. Symptoms of hypothermia may include mottled skin, peripheral cyanosis (acrocyanosis) or central cyanosis, hypotonia, hypoglycemia, restlessness, bradycardia, tachypnea, apnea, lethargy, and restlessness.

P80.0   Cold injury syndrome

Sclerema neonatorum or cold injury syndrome (CIS) of the newborn is most common during the cold seasons of the year. The condition can manifest in premature infants at any time but usually affects full-term neonates in the first three days of life. Infants are at risk for cold injury because of the immaturity of their temperature regulation system, large body surface area, decreased subcutaneous fat, limited energy stores, and an inability to use shivering for thermogenesis and heat production primarily from brown fat metabolism. CIS is caused by cold stress, which leads to lowered body temperature, scleredema, and can progress to multiple organ dysfunctions (MOD). The mechanism of onset is a cold environment leading to infant heat loss and lowered body temperature. Peripheral vasoconstriction occurs with subsequent dysfunction of microcirculation. Left untreated, this can then lead to anoxia, metabolic disturbances, acidosis, and finally MOD (cardiovascular, hepatic, immunological, and hematological). Symptoms include lethargy, poor feeding, decreased urine output, edema, bradycardia, apnea, hypoglycemia, acidosis, and red discoloration of the hands, feet, and face. Morbidity is very high with CIS and neurodevelopmental delays occur frequently in infants who do survive.

P83.-   Other conditions of integument specific to newborn

Conditions classified here involve disorders of the skin occurring during the perinatal period.

P83.2   Hydrops fetalis not due to hemolytic disease

Fluid buildup in two or more compartments of a newborn's body, primarily the skin, abdominal cavity, pleural space, and pericardial sac, characterize hydrops fetalis. The nonimmune form of hydrops fetalis has many etiologies, from heart failure in the neonate to congenital conditions, including infection. The infant mortality rate is very high, particularly with premature infants.

P83.5   Congenital hydrocele

A congenital hydrocele is a collection of fluid in the tunica vaginalis of the testicle or along the spermatic cord that is present at birth. During normal development the testes move from the abdomen into the scrotum where they are walled off with any peritoneal fluid that flowed into the scrotum eventually getting absorbed back into the body. A congenital hydrocele occurs when the opening stays slightly patent, allowing fluid to move from the peritoneum into the scrotum. This is termed a communicating hydrocele. Almost all congenital hydroceles are communicating. In a noncommunicating hydrocele, the scrotum opening between the peritoneum and scrotum closes normally but the fluid that came with the testes as it descended is slow to absorb out of the scrotal sac. In a majority of the cases, the hydrocele, whether communicating or noncommunicating, spontaneously resolves. However, persistent congenital hydroceles, those present beyond age 12 months, may require surgical correction.

P83.8-   Other specified conditions of integument specific to newborn

This subcategory classifies certain other specific conditions of the integument (skin) specific to newborn infants not captured elsewhere such as umbilical granuloma, scleroderma, urticaria, or bronze baby syndrome.

P83.81   Umbilical granuloma

An umbilical granuloma is a common condition affecting approximately 1 in 500 newborns that presents as a small, red, round growth, sometimes on a stalk, in the center of the navel after the umbilical cord has fallen off. It is usually not painful but can ooze fluid and become irritated. Without treatment, the granuloma will usually grow in size and can become an entry point for umbilical infections. Routine treatment is the application of a silver nitrate stick, usually repeated two or three times over a number of clinic visits.

P83.88   Other specified conditions of integument specific to newborn

Bronze baby syndrome is a rare neonatal complication of phototherapy treatment for hyperbilirubinemia characterized by development of a dark gray-brown pigmentation of the skin, mucous membrane, and urine within a week of phototherapy treatment. No treatment is generally required for bronze baby syndrome as the pigmentation slowly disappears after cessation of phototherapy.

Neonatal scleroderma is a rare neonatal autoimmune disease involving the interaction between maternal antibodies and fetal/neonatal antigens resulting in areas of the skin becoming hard and thick.

Urticaria neonatorum, often documented as erythema toxicum neonatorum (ETN), is a common transient, urticaria-like rash characterized by small papular reddened lesions with white or yellow pustules in the center, which manifests in the first few days of the perinatal period. It generally disappears spontaneously.

Other Problems with Newborn (P84)

This code block is comprised of a single code that captures many nonspecific conditions of the newborn, such as electrolyte abnormalities described only as academia or acidosis and respiratory conditions described only as anoxia, asphyxia, hypercapnia, hypoxemia, or hypoxia.

The categories in this code block are as follows:

P84	Other problems with newborn

Focus Point

More specific codes exist for many of the conditions associated with code P84. For example, metabolic acidemia, when documented around the time of birth, is reported with a code from category P19, while electrolyte and metabolic disturbances described as transient are reported with codes in category P74. All documentation should be carefully reviewed prior to assignment of code P84 to ensure that there is not a more specific code for the newborn condition.

Other Disorders Originating in the Perinatal Period (P90-P96)

Some of the codes in this code block are ill-defined conditions that often require testing and monitoring to establish etiology. For example, vomiting is a nonspecific complaint with many possible causal conditions. Certain types of vomiting can be indicative of very serious conditions, requiring a more extensive evaluation.

Also classified here are certain congenital conditions in the newborn, consequences of drug administration to the newborn, and conditions that specifically relate abnormalities in the function of the newborn's brain.

The categories in this code block are as follows:

P90	Convulsions of newborn
P91	Other disturbances of cerebral status of newborn
P92	Feeding problems of newborn
P93	Reactions and intoxications due to drugs administered to newborn
P94	Disorders of muscle tone of newborn
P95	Stillbirth
P96	Other conditions originating in the perinatal period

P91.-   Other disturbances of cerebral status of newborn

This category identifies alterations in the functionality of a newborn's brain (cerebral status). Disturbances in brain function can manifest in a variety of ways depending on the etiology of the disturbance, including abnormalities in consciousness, tone and reflexes, and/or seizures, and may or may not result in permanent neurologic impairment.

P91.6- Hypoxic ischemic encephalopathy [HIE]

Hypoxic ischemic encephalopathy (HIE), also referred to as intrapartum asphyxia, occurs when not enough oxygen reaches the newborn's brain. This lack of oxygen may be secondary to severe systemic hypoxia (not enough oxygen available to the newborn) and/or reduced cerebral blood flow (not enough oxygenated blood getting to the brain). Criteria for diagnosing HIE includes a profound metabolic or mixed acidemia with an arterial cord blood pH < 7.0, an Apgar score of 0 to 3 for > 5 minutes, hypotonia, seizures, coma, and multiple system involvement (renal, pulmonary, hepatic, cardiac, gastrointestinal).

P91.61 Mild hypoxic ischemic encephalopathy [HIE]

An infant with mild HIE may have slightly increased muscle tone with brisk deep tendon reflexes that manifest in the first few days of life. Transient abnormal behaviors may be present including poor feeding, irritability, or alternating fussiness and sleepiness. Symptoms may resolve within 24 hours.

P91.62 Moderate hypoxic ischemic encephalopathy [HIE]

An infant with moderate HIE may have symptoms that include significant hypotonia and decreased deep tendon reflexes, lethargy, slow or absent neonatal reflexes (grasp, suck, Moro), decreased respiratory effort, and/or apnea and seizures within 24 hours of birth. Severity of central nervous system complications secondary to moderate HIE is dependent on the recovery time of the infant, with more favorable outcomes in those infants that recover within one to two weeks.

P91.63 Severe hypoxic ischemic encephalopathy [HIE]

Severe HIE is characterized by delayed and often treatment-resistant seizures. The infant often exhibits irregular respirations and may require ventilator support. Muscle tone is decreased (hypotonia) with decreased deep tendon reflexes. Neonatal reflexes (grasp, suck, Moro) may be completely absent. Disturbances of ocular motion (nystagmus, bobbing, dolls eyes) may be present and pupils may be dilated, fixed, or have a sluggish response to light. Cardiac arrhythmias and blood pressure instability can manifest as the infant's level of consciousness progresses into a stupor or coma.

P91.81- Neonatal encephalopathy

Neonatal encephalopathy (NE) is clinically defined by signs and symptoms of abnormal neurological function in the first few days of life in a term infant. This subcategory is used to report cases of neonatal encephalopathy other than hypoxic ischemic encephalopathy. When neonatal encephalopathy occurs in conjunction with congenital cirrhosis of the liver, intracranial nontraumatic hemorrhage of the newborn, or kernicterus, the underlying condition is reported first.

P92.- Feeding problems of newborn

Nutritional intake is vital to the growth and development of the newborn. When feeding problems occur, it may herald a more serious underlying condition. Some feeding problems resolve spontaneously, but others require medical attention. Certain problems (e.g., poor latching, spitting up, and weak suck) can be alleviated with feeding techniques. An oral sensorimotor feeding evaluation and barium swallow assists in identifying or ruling out any underlying pathology.

P92.0- Vomiting of newborn

Vomiting is a nonspecific complaint with many possible causal conditions. Certain types of vomiting can be indicative of very serious conditions.

P92.01 Bilious vomiting of newborn

Bile-stained vomitus in a newborn is most commonly a sign of intestinal obstruction and should be taken seriously. Diagnostic radiographic testing can confirm possible causal conditions such as intestinal malrotation, Hirschsprung's disease, or necrotizing enterocolitis. If a bowel obstruction is confirmed, treatment is dependent upon the nature of the causal condition. Premature infants are at high risk for necrotizing enterocolitis; however, some premature infants may suffer self-limiting bilious emesis due to an immature digestive system.

P92.6 Failure to thrive in newborn

Failure to thrive (FTT) is indicative of an inability to receive, retain, or properly utilize nutrition to grow and develop as expected. It is important to determine whether it is due to environmental factors (e.g., neglect) or underlying medical issues. FTT is a form of arrested growth that can affect long-term health and emotional development. The most common causes include feeding difficulties, gastroesophageal reflux, infection, and congenital metabolic or digestive disorders (e.g., malabsorption syndrome) although many other congenital systemic or structural anomalies can cause failure to thrive. Diagnostic workup to determine the cause of FTT is recommended for any infant that has not regained its birth weight within seven weeks with lactation and nutritional support.

P93.- Reactions and intoxications due to drugs administered to newborn

Toxic conditions and adverse drug reactions in neonates, especially premature infants, are often caused by the body's immature detoxification and excretion mechanisms.

P93.0   Grey baby syndrome

Grey baby syndrome is a condition caused by an infant's inability to efficiently conjugate and eliminate the antibiotic chloramphenicol. Newborns, particularly premature newborns, lack the necessary liver enzymes to metabolize chloramphenicol. The inability to metabolize and eliminate chloramphenicol results in a syndrome that is characterized by a potentially life-threatening drop in blood pressure (hypotension) and cyanosis as evidenced by blueness in the lips, nailbeds, and skin due to a lack of oxygen. Because of the potential for a life-threatening adverse reaction to chloramphenicol, it is now rarely administered to newborns.

P94.-   Disorders of muscle tone of newborn

Disorders of muscle tone may manifest as weakness or flaccidity of the muscles or as rigid or tense muscles.

P94.0   Transient neonatal myasthenia gravis

Myasthenia gravis is an autoimmune disease where antibodies develop against specific receptors at the neuromuscular junction, altering the signals between the nerve and the muscle. Infants whose mothers have myasthenia gravis (MG) may acquire the abnormal antibodies via the placenta during gestation, manifesting as weak suck, swallow, and poor respiratory effort. The condition usually resolves spontaneously in a few weeks as the infants body produces normal antibodies to replace the abnormal ones received from the mother.

P94.1   Congenital hypertonia

Congenital hypertonia is a neurological disorder characterized by increased tone in the skeletal muscles. Common characteristics include prolonged episodes of muscular tightness/rigidity, feeding problems due to dysphagia and laryngospasm, and apneic episodes do to respiratory muscle spasms.

P94.2   Congenital hypotonia

Congenital hypotonia is a neurological disorder characterized by decreased tone in the skeletal muscles and may be accompanied by decreased muscle strength. The problem can occur anywhere along the nerve pathway that controls muscle movement, including the brain, spinal cord, peripheral nerve, or the muscle. Symptoms include floppiness appearance (rag doll), delayed acquisition of fine and gross motor skills (sitting, crawling), feeding problems (weak suck), underactive gag reflex, and shallow respirations. Congenital hypotonia is a symptom associated with a large number of syndromes caused by gene mutations including Down syndrome, Prader-Willi, Tay-Sachs disease, and diseases such as congenital hypothyroidism, congenital cerebellar ataxia, and achondroplasia.

P95   Stillbirth

A stillbirth is an infant born after 20 weeks of gestation that does not show any signs of life at the time of birth. The death may have occurred in utero prior to labor, during labor, or during delivery.

P96.-   Other conditions originating in the perinatal period

Other conditions occurring or originating in the perinatal period that do not fit well into more specific categories are included here.

P96.1   Neonatal withdrawal symptoms from maternal use of drugs of addiction

This code reports withdrawal symptoms in newborns caused by maternal use of addictive drugs. Narcotics, cocaine, and coca plant derivatives are the most frequently abused drugs capable of causing withdrawal symptoms in the newborn, but barbiturates, other tranquilizers, amphetamines, other stimulants, and other addictive substances can also cause the syndrome. Signs and symptoms of drug withdrawal syndrome in the newborn include irritability, tremulousness, tachypnea, vomiting or diarrhea, fever, and convulsions. Toxicology tests of blood or urine identify the drug. Therapies include close monitoring for seizure activity or arrhythmias, detoxification tailored for the drug of dependence, drugs such as phenytoin sodium (Dilantin) or phenobarbital for seizures, and, in some cases, exchange transfusions in life-threatening emergencies.

P96.5   Complication to newborn due to (fetal) intrauterine procedure

In utero interventional procedures provide alternatives to improve outcomes for pregnancies complicated by fetal conditions not previously amenable to treatment. However, these interventional procedures are not without risk for the fetus. The types of complications to the newborn depend on the specific procedure, but the primary risk for the newborn is premature birth or injury as a result of a procedural intervention during the pregnancy. Premature infants face an increased risk of potentially serious complications and typically require neonatal intensive care unit (NICU) care.

P96.83   Meconium staining

Meconium is dark green fecal material present in the fetal intestines that may be discharged shortly before or during birth. Depending on the timing of the fecal excretion, evidence of meconium staining may include dark green streaks or colored stains in the amniotic fluid or coating the newborn or discoloration of the newborn's skin, fingernails, and toenails may occur.

Focus Point

Meconium staining is not synonymous with meconium passage. Meconium passage typically occurs at the time of labor and delivery and does not typically indicate fetal stress. Meconium passage is reported with code P03.82.

Chapter 17: Congenital Malformations, Deformations and Chromosomal Abnormalities (Q00-Q99)

Congenital malformation, deformation, and chromosomal abnormalities may be the result of genetic factors (chromosomes), teratogens (agents causing physical defects in the embryo), or both. Congenital abnormalities may be apparent at birth or identified sometime after birth. Code blocks in this chapter are organized by the organ system except in the case of cleft lip and cleft palate, which have their own code block, and chromosomal abnormalities, which often affect multiple organ systems. Most of the codes categorized to these code blocks identify the principal or defining defect rather than the cause, chromosome abnormalities being an exception.

The chapter is broken down into the following code blocks:

Q00-Q07	Congenital malformations of the nervous system
Q10-Q18	Congenital malformations of eye, ear, face and neck
Q20-Q28	Congenital malformations of the circulatory system
Q30-Q34	Congenital malformations of the respiratory system
Q35-Q37	Cleft lip and cleft palate
Q38-Q45	Other congenital malformations of the digestive system
Q50-Q56	Congenital malformations of genital organs
Q60-Q64	Congenital malformations of the urinary system
Q65-Q79	Congenital malformations and deformations of the musculoskeletal system
Q80-Q89	Other congenital malformations
Q90-Q99	Chromosomal abnormalities, not elsewhere classified

Congenital Malformations of the Nervous System (Q00-Q07)

Congenital malformations can occur in the development of the brain (encephalon), the spinal cord, the membranes that cover the brain and spinal cord (meninges), as well as in the peripheral nervous system.

The categories in this code block are as follows:

Q00	Anencephaly and similar malformations
Q01	Encephalocele
Q02	Microcephaly
Q03	Congenital hydrocephalus
Q04	Other congenital malformations of brain
Q05	Spina bifida
Q06	Other congenital malformations of spinal cord
Q07	Other congenital malformations of nervous system

Q00.-   Anencephaly and similar malformations

Conditions classified here are severe often fatal malformations of the brain, including failure of part or all of the brain to fully develop and failure of the skull to fully develop resulting in exposure of brain tissue.

Q00.0   Anencephaly

Anencephaly is a usually fatal brain defect of the newborn caused by a closure of the neural groove early in the first trimester of pregnancy. It can present in several forms: the cranial vault may be absent, the cerebral hemispheres may be missing or exist as masses attached to the base of the skull, or the brain may be abnormally shaped. When part or the entire skull is absent, the term acrania is used to describe the anencephaly. Amyelencephalus is the absence of the brain and spinal cord. Hemianencephaly is absence of half the brain. Hemicephaly is absence of one of the brain hemispheres.

Q01.- Encephalocele

An encephalocele is a neural herniation of brain parenchyma and meninges that protrudes through a cranial defect. Encephalocele is also known as cranium bifidum with encephalocele, hydrencephalocele, and hydrencephalomeningocele. Lesions may occur in the occipital region or anywhere in the cranial vault.

Q02 Microcephaly

In microcephaly, the head circumference is more than two standard deviations below the mean for age, sex, race, and gestation. Anomalous development, such as a chromosomal disorder or maternal phenylketonuria, during the first seven months of gestation causes primary microcephaly. Secondary microcephaly results from an insult, such as infection, trauma, anoxia, or metabolic disorders, during the last two months of gestation or during the perinatal period.

Q03.- Congenital hydrocephalus

Ventricular enlargement, abundant cerebral spinal fluid (CSF), and, in most cases, increasing intracranial pressure are present in congenital hydrocephalus. CSF cushions the brain and protects it from injury. It also carries nutrients to and removes waste products from the brain and spinal cord. An imbalance of CSF may be due to excess production of fluid by the brain, obstruction between the ventricles, or impaired absorption into the thin tissue surrounding the brain and spinal cord. Causes can include bleeding in the brain during fetal development, infections passed from mother to fetus (syphilis), or inherited genetic defects. Symptoms may include large head size (macrocephaly), bulging fontanelles, wide separation of cranial sutures, irritability, sleepiness/lethargy, vomiting and/or poor feeding. With complete blockage, symptoms usually appear early in childhood. When the blockage is incomplete, an individual may be asymptomatic until adulthood.

Congenital Hydrocephalus

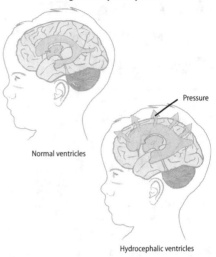

Pressure

Normal ventricles

Hydrocephalic ventricles

Focus Point

Neural tube defects, such as spina bifida, that have associated hydrocephalus are captured under category Q05. Hydrocephalus secondary to maternal toxoplasmosis (congenital toxoplasmosis) is captured with code P37.1.

Q03.0 Malformations of aqueduct of Sylvius

The aqueduct of Sylvius is a narrow channel that passes through the midbrain and connects the third and fourth ventricles. Malformation of this channel is the most common cause of congenital hydrocephalus. Malformations include a general narrowing of the channel or small webs or rings of tissue that stretch across the channel causing an increased volume of cerebral spinal fluid (CSF) in the other ventricles and pressure on the cortex of the brain.

Q03.1 Atresia of foramina of Magendie and Luschka

Atresia of foramina of Magendie and Luschka is a congenital anomaly of the skull and brain caused by a developmental failure of these structures during fetal development. The foramen of Magendie is a large opening in the roof of the fourth ventricle of the brain that drains cerebral fluid into the cisterna magna. The foramen of Luschka is a lateral opening in the fourth ventricle that drains cerebral fluid into the subarachnoid space. Failure of these structures to form leads to fluid accumulation and enlargement of the fourth ventricle. This causes malformation of other structures of the brain and hydrocephalus. Symptoms include projection of the occipital bone, increased head size (macrocephaly) with a bulging anterior fontanelle, swelling of the optic disc due to the increased intracranial pressure, lack of muscle coordination and movement disorders, a type of involuntary eye movement called nystagmus, and cognitive delays. Dandy-Walker is a syndrome that is classified here and is a type of noncommunicating hydrocephalus attributed to atresia of the Magendie and Luschka foramen. Dandy-Walker syndrome is characterized by failure of development of the cerebellum, hydrocephalus, and cyst formation in the back of the brain in the region of the brain stem and cerebellum.

Q04.-   Other congenital malformations of brain

Codes in this category capture other congenital malformations of the brain that may involve failure of portions of the brain to form, congenital cerebral cysts, as well as other conditions.

Q04.6   Congenital cerebral cysts

The cerebrum is the largest part of the brain and is located in the upper and anterior portion of the skull. It is comprised of two halves or hemispheres. Congenital cerebral cysts, also called arachnoid cysts, are fluid filled regions that form between the arachnoid membrane and the brain. Etiology may be due to disturbances in blood flow during fetal development, cerebral degeneration or atrophy, maternal infection, or genetic defects/mutations. Porencephaly is a rare type of congenital cerebral anomaly characterized by fluid filled cysts or cavities in the cerebral hemisphere. An individual may have only minor neurological problems with normal intelligence or severe physical and cognitive disabilities. Schizencephaly is another rare congenital anomaly of the cerebral hemisphere characterized by abnormal clefts or slits. The condition can be unilateral or bilateral. Symptoms of unilateral schizencephaly include paralysis on one side of the body but often intellectual development is normal. Bilateral schizencephaly is most commonly accompanied by speech/language delays, poor muscle tone, and seizures.

Q05.-   Spina bifida

Spina bifida, a defect in the vertebral column, may present in conjunction with other anomalies or it may occur as a solitary anomaly. Prognosis depends on the number and severity of anomalies and on the size and location of the vertebral defect. Paralysis at the level below of the defect is always present when the cord or spinal nerve roots are involved. Defects at the lumbosacral level can cause bladder and rectal problems. Spina bifida is classified by site with the presence or absence of hydrocephalus being the second axis of code assignment. In hydrocephalus, the circulation of the cerebrospinal fluid (CSF) is impeded. When hydrocephalus occurs with spina bifida, it is the spinal malformation that causes CSF fluid accumulation in the cranial vault resulting in increased intracranial pressure on the brain.

Q06.-   Other congenital malformations of spinal cord

This category captures additional congenital malformations of the spinal cord not easily classified to the other categories.

Q06.0   Amyelia

Amyelia is the absence of the spinal cord.

Q06.1   Hypoplasia and dysplasia of spinal cord

Myelodysplasia and myelatelia are synonymous terms describing a defective spinal cord. Atelomyelia is an incompletely developed cord.

Q06.2   Diastematomyelia

Diastematomyelia is a longitudinal fissure in the spinal cord that results in gait disturbance, muscular atrophy, and lack of sphincter control.

Q06.4   Hydromyelia

Hydromyelia reports a dilated spinal canal.

Q07.-   Other congenital malformations of nervous system

This category includes Type II Arnold Chiari syndrome and other congenital anomalies of the peripheral nervous system nerves and other nervous system structures.

Q07.0-   Arnold-Chiari syndrome

Type II is the most serious of the four types of malformations found in Arnold-Chiari or Chiari disease and the only type assigned to this code. In this variation, the inferior poles of the cerebellum and the medulla protrude through the foramen magnum into the spinal canal. It is commonly associated and code classification is based on whether other anomalies, such as spina bifida and/or hydrocephalus, are also present. Spina bifida is a neural tube defect affecting the spinal cord. There are varying severities of spina bifida. It may occur as a closed defect with few symptoms; with a meningocele, which involves protrusion of the meninges and a collection of spinal fluid through the defect; or with a myelomeningocele, which is the protrusion of the meninges and spinal cord through the defect. Hydrocephalus is a brain malformation characterized by ventricular enlargement, abundant cerebral spinal fluid (CSF), and, in most cases, increasing intracranial pressure.

Congenital Malformations of Eye, Ear, Face and Neck (Q10-Q18)

Any structure or organ of the body is subject to a failure or deviation in development. Congenital anomalies of the eye, ear, face, and neck are classified according to the specific site affected and the type of defect.

The categories in this code block are as follows:

Q10	Congenital malformations of eyelid, lacrimal apparatus and orbit
Q11	Anophthalmos, microphthalmos and macrophthalmos
Q12	Congenital lens malformations
Q13	Congenital malformations of anterior segment of eye
Q14	Congenital malformations of posterior segment of eye
Q15	Other congenital malformations of eye
Q16	Congenital malformations of ear causing impairment of hearing
Q17	Other congenital malformations of ear
Q18	Other congenital malformations of face and neck

Q10.- Congenital malformations of eyelid, lacrimal apparatus and orbit

The structures of the eye, which include structures of the ball or globe, are differentiated from its supporting structures, which are ocular adnexa and bony orbit. The globe of the eye rests in fatty tissue in the bony orbit of the skull where it is protected from jarring actions. The external structures of the eye, which include the eyelids, lacrimal system, and ocular muscles, together make up the ocular adnexa. The lacrimal system of each eye, also called the lacrimal apparatus, consists of the lacrimal gland, ducts, canaliculi, and the nasolacrimal sac.

Q10.1 Congenital ectropion

Ectropion is the eversion of the lower eyelid.

Q10.2 Congenital entropion

Entropion is inversion of the lower eyelid. This condition requires surgical correction since rubbing caused by the displacement often scars the cornea.

Q10.3 Other congenital malformations of eyelid

Ablepharon, the congenital absence of an eyelid, seldom appears as a solitary variant, which is typical of agenesis anomalies. An accessory eyelid, which is also coded here, is an additional eyelid.

Q11.- Anophthalmos, microphthalmos and macrophthalmos

Conditions included in this category classify congenital abnormalities of the eye.

Q11.0 Cystic eyeball

Congenital cystic eyeball (CCE) is a failure of the optic vesicle to develop, resulting in formation of a cyst instead of the eye. Causal factors are unknown. The birth defect is thought to occur early in the first trimester, at approximately 35 days gestation, when invagination of the vesicle fails. The ocular vesicles are early embryonic neurologic tissues from which the eyes begin to develop. Treatment may include enucleation of rudimentary tissues followed by ocular prosthetic insertion.

Q11.1 Other anophthalmos

Anophthalmos is the complete absence of the eyes or the presence of vestigial (rudimentary) eyes. It is a congenital condition in which the ocular tissue is completely missing inside the orbit, often due to underdevelopment of the optic vessel. This disorder can lead to serious problems not only from the lack of vision for that eye, but also from the abnormal development of the orbit, eyelid, and/or eye socket. Causal factors include dominant/recessive inheritance, chromosome deletion, and maternal exposure to environmental toxins and/or maternal infections during the course of pregnancy.

Q11.2 Microphthalmos

Microphthalmos is a congenital condition of abnormally small eyeballs. The condition may be unilateral or bilateral. Simple microphthalmos is abnormally small eyeballs that are essentially normal in function. However, microphthalmos is often associated with other ocular abnormalities such as opacities of the cornea and lens or scarring of the choroid and retina, causing significant vision impairment. Cryptophthalmos, also reported here, is an abnormal continuous skin growth over the eyeball that usually occurs bilaterally. It is associated with a malformation of the globe. Incomplete cryptophthalmos is an abnormal fusion of the skin to the middle globe area, with presence of the lateral eyelid. Failure of eyelid separation may be associated with other ocular abnormalities.

Q12.- Congenital lens malformations

The lens of the eye is a nearly transparent (crystalline) biconvex structure that is suspended behind the iris. The function of the lens of the eye is to focus rays of light onto the retina.

Q12.0 Congenital cataract

Congenital cataract is an opacification of the lens of the eye, present at birth, that can give rise to disturbances in the field of vision. Causal conditions include hereditary factors, maternal infections, and certain metabolic disorders.

Q12.1 Congenital displaced lens

A displaced lens, also called an ectopic lens, is one that is in an abnormal position.

Q12.2 Coloboma of lens

A coloboma describes a part that is missing from the eye, in this case the lens. The condition is usually due to a chromosomal defect

---

Coloboma

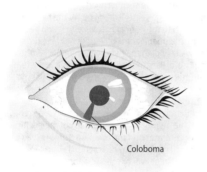

Coloboma

Coloboma

Q12.3 Congenital aphakia

Congenital aphakia is absence of the lens occurring at birth.

Q12.4 Spherophakia

Spherophakia is a congenital anomaly related to the shape of the lens, which in this case is sphere shaped.

Q12.8 Other congenital lens malformations

Microphakia, an abnormally small lens that is present at birth, is classified here.

Q13.- Congenital malformations of anterior segment of eye

The anterior segment of the eye includes the iris, cornea, and sclera. These structures are surrounded by fluid called aqueous humor.

Q13.0 Coloboma of iris

Coloboma of the iris is an ocular tissue defect associated with incomplete fusion of the fetal intraocular fissure. This anomaly may present as a black hole in or around the iris at the edge of the pupil

or a split from the pupil to the edge of the iris. The condition is usually due to a chromosomal defect. Coloboma may increase the risk of iridial tearing and often includes iris and choroid defects.

> **Focus Point**
>
> *Coloboma of the iris is typically associated with CHARGE syndrome (C = coloboma; H = heart; A = atresia of choanae, R = retarded growth and development, G = genital hypoplasia, E = ear anomalies).*

Q13.1 Absence of iris

This condition, also called aniridia or congenital hyperplasia of the iris, is hereditary and usually occurs with additional ocular defects. It is characterized by vision loss of varying severity. Typically aniridia is bilateral and gives the appearance of black irises, though it is the pupil and not the iris that is dark. If caused by an autosomal dominant or autosomal recessive trait, it is associated with additional health or developmental problems.

Q13.2 Other congenital malformations of iris

This code includes other specified anomalies of the iris and ciliary body, such as congenital anisocoria, atresia of the pupil, and corectopia. Anisocoria is an unequal pupil size. When not associated with other deformities, it is typically caused by a defect within the nerve pathway controlling the pupil. Atresia of the pupil, also known as atretopsia, is the congenital absence of the papillary opening. Corectopia is a displacement of the pupil from its normal location. In corectopia, the pupil is asymmetrically placed in the iris.

Q13.81 Rieger's anomaly

Rieger's anomaly affects the anterior chamber and related structures. This anomaly presents with bilateral opaque rings around the corneal margin with iris strand attachment, widened trabecular meshwork, large iridial bands, and glaucoma. In addition, other characteristics include iris atrophy, pupil distortion, and associated dental, craniofacial, and skeletal anomalies.

Q14.- Congenital malformations of posterior segment of eye

Structures of the posterior segment of the eye include the retina, optic disc, and choroid. The structures of the posterior segment are surrounded by fluid called vitreous humor.

Q15.- Other congenital malformations of eye

This category includes a specific code for congenital glaucoma and two other codes for other specified and unspecified malformations of the eye.

Q15.0 Congenital glaucoma

Congenital glaucoma is present at birth and is usually diagnosed within the first year of life. The most common symptom is epiphora, a functional defect that causes an excessive amount of tearing. Buphthalmos, also termed hydrophthalmos, is a distended, abnormally enlarged eyeball as a result of increased intraocular pressure of congenital glaucoma. The increase in intraocular pressure can lead to corneal tear, optic nerve cupping, and vision loss. Cupping of the optic disk is a distinguishing feature of the disease, and occurs early, assisting in diagnosis. Megalocornea is a clouding of the cornea. Congenital glaucoma causes the eye to stretch abnormally and may result in rupture. Early diagnosis and treatment are essential to optimal outcomes, as blindness often occurs early.

Q18.- Other congenital malformations of face and neck

This category includes congenital malformations of the structures of the face and neck other than the eye and ocular adnexa, ear, skull, and facial bones.

Q18.0 Sinus, fistula and cyst of branchial cleft

Branchial cleft relates to embryonic development of the external auricle, the external auditory meatus, and the tympanic membrane. A sinus is a blind ending tract. A fistula is an open-ended tract.

Q18.3 Webbing of neck

Pterygium colli is a webbed effect produced by an anomalous band of fascia extending from the mastoid process to the clavicle.

Congenital Malformations of the Circulatory System (Q20-Q28)

Cardiac anomalies may involve the heart chambers, the septa that separate the chambers, the heart valves, or other areas of the heart. One percent of all births have a cardiac anomaly. There may also be malformations of the aorta or pulmonary artery, the vena cava or pulmonary vein, the cerebral or precerebral vessels, or the peripheral vascular system.

The categories in this code block are as follows:

Q20	Congenital malformations of cardiac chambers and connections
Q21	Congenital malformations of cardiac septa
Q22	Congenital malformations of pulmonary and tricuspid valves
Q23	Congenital malformations of aortic and mitral valves
Q24	Other congenital malformations of heart
Q25	Congenital malformations of great arteries
Q26	Congenital malformations of great veins
Q27	Other congenital malformations of peripheral vascular system
Q28	Other congenital malformations of circulatory system

Q20.- Congenital malformations of cardiac chambers and connections

This category covers malformations of the atria and ventricles, as well as malformations of the aorta and pulmonary vessels involving the connection of these vessels to the heart.

Q20.0 Common arterial trunk

Common arterial trunk, also called persistent truncus arteriosus, is a congenital heart defect where there is only one large vessel leading out of the heart as opposed to the normal two vessels exiting each lower heart chamber (ventricle). Additionally, a portion of the wall dividing the two lower chambers of the heart is missing. Persistent truncus arteriosus is the failure of the fetal aorticopulmonary trunk to divide at the correct developmental stage. This is a rare defect that causes oxygen-poor blood returning from the peripheral circulation and oxygen-rich blood returning from the pulmonary circulation to combine within the lower ventricles and the common trunk instead of being channeled from each ventricle into separate vessels that deliver oxygen-poor blood to the main trunk of the pulmonary artery and oxygen rich blood to the aorta. An infant born with this condition may develop congestive heart failure due to the effects of the abnormally increased pulmonary artery blood flow.

Q20.1 Double outlet right ventricle

Double outlet right ventricle is a congenital condition in which the connection of the aorta rises from the right ventricle instead of from the left. In this case, the pulmonary artery and the aorta are attached to the same chamber with no arterial vessels connected to the left ventricle. This condition usually includes some form of ventricular septal defect, which may be helpful in allowing some of the oxygen-rich blood to flow into the right chamber of the heart.

Q20.3 Discordant ventriculoarterial connection

Discordant ventriculoarterial connection represents a complete transposition of the great vessels, meaning that the positions of the aorta and pulmonary artery are reversed. The aorta arises from the right ventricle instead of the left, and the pulmonary artery arises from the left ventricle instead of the right. This results in oxygen deficient blood being pumped out to the body causing organ malfunction. The survival rate of individuals born with transposed vessels depends on several things but most important is whether or not there is mixing of oxygenated blood with nonoxygenated blood. Often atrial or ventricular septal defects (holes in the septum) are also present concomitantly with the transposition of the vessels. These defects allow oxygen-poor blood to mix with oxygen-rich blood resulting in at least a modicum of oxygen reaching body tissues. If mixing of the blood is not occurring or is limited, surgery may be performed to create a hole in the septum or make the hole bigger.

Q20.4   Double inlet ventricle

This common ventricle anomaly occurs when a single ventricle arises from the absence of a ventricular septum. Infants born with this condition have only one functional lower chamber (ventricle) of the heart. This disorder causes oxygen-rich blood to mix with oxygen-poor blood, which is distributed into the lungs and throughout the body depriving the body of adequate amounts of oxygen. This disorder affects about 10 in every 100,000 infants and while it usually develops during pregnancy, the exact cause is unknown.

Q20.5   Discordant atrioventricular connection

Discordant atrioventricular connection, also called corrected transposition of the great vessels, is a congenital condition in which two separate defects actually correct the circulation problem. In this disorder, the ventricles of the heart are reversed and the aorta and pulmonary artery arise from the wrong heart chamber. However, circulation is still flowing in the right direction due to the reversal of the heart chambers. This disorder is very uncommon and reported in less than 1 percent of the population. It is seen more frequently in males than females.

Q21.-   Congenital malformations of cardiac septa

The cardiac septa are the walls within the heart that separate the heart chambers into the right and left atria in the upper aspect of the heart and the right and left ventricle in the lower aspect of the heart.

Q21.0   Ventricular septal defect

A ventricular septal defect (VSD) is a hole in the wall between the ventricles. The size of the hole relates directly to the seriousness of the condition. In minor cases, the defect may close on its own; in more serious cases, surgery or cardiac catheterization may be required. When the defect is large, excess blood is pumped into the lungs, which can cause heart failure due to the excess pressure on the heart to function properly. Without treatment, pulmonary hypertension and ventricular hypertrophy occur. The cause of this disorder is unknown and, in many cases, other

congenital defects are present. VSD may involve the membrane and muscular portions of the ventricles, although about 80 percent occur within the membranous septum.

Ventricular Septal Defect

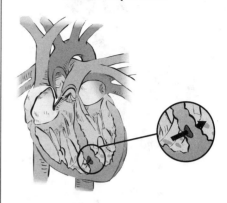

Q21.1   Atrial septal defect

An atrial septal defect (ASD) is a hole in the wall between the upper chambers of the heart. Ostium secundum is a specific type of ASD included here and is characterized by an abnormal opening in the atrial septum caused by lack of fusion between the septum secundum and endocardial cushions with an additional rim of septum encompassing the defect. Ostium secundum accounts for 90 percent of all ASDs. Minor defects may close as the infant develops. Larger defects need surgical closure. If left untreated, a large defect may lead to permanent heart and lung damage due to the excess blood being pumped into the lungs and the stress placed on the heart. Additionally, the right side of the heart becomes enlarged and weak and pulmonary hypertension occurs. Patent foramen ovale is seen when a portion of the channel between the atria does not close after birth; about one in three infants present with this condition.

Atrial Septal Defect

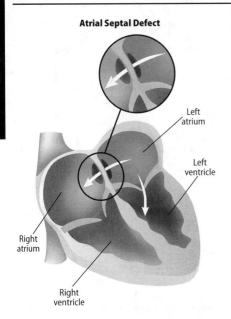

Atrioventricular Septal Defect

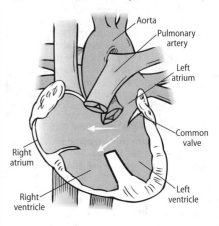

Q21.2   Atrioventricular septal defect

An atrioventricular septal defect (AVSD), also called endocardial cushion defect, occurs when there are defects in the atrial septum between the two upper chambers of the heart and the ventricular septum between the two lower chambers of the heart. AVSDs may be complete or incomplete/partial and both types are reported here. Complete defects are characterized by a large opening near the center of the heart that encompasses the atrial septum and ventricular septum. In addition, there is a single valve between the upper and lower chambers of the heart instead of the two valves (tricuspid and mitral) that normally regulate blood flow between the upper (atria) and lower (ventricles) chambers of the heart. The central defect allows blood to flow between all four chambers instead of from one chamber to another through the tricuspid and mitral valves. In an incomplete/partial defect there is usually a hole near the center of the heart that affects the atria or ventricles and there are two valves, but the mitral valve is typically defective. Incomplete/partial defects are more common than complete defects.

Q21.3   Tetralogy of Fallot

Tetralogy of Fallot is a rare congenital heart defect that involves four separate defects: ventricular septal defect, pulmonary stenosis, right ventricular hypertrophy, and an aorta that arises from both ventricles as opposed to just the left ventricle. A ventricular septal defect occurs when there is a hole in the wall separating the right and left ventricle of the heart. Pulmonary stenosis is an abnormally narrow passageway between the heart and lungs. Right ventricular hypertrophy is a thickened wall within the muscle of the right ventricle. A right aortic arch, abnormal origin of coronary arteries, a left superior vena cava, and an enlarged bronchial artery are characteristic. Symptoms of tetralogy of Fallot typically present by 6 months of age. Palliative repairs are performed in the early years, with definitive repair reserved until the child is 5 to 7 years old. This condition is reported in about five out of every 10,000 infants and affects both genders. Infants with this defect are more likely to have other nonheart-related defects.

Q22.-   Congenital malformations of pulmonary and tricuspid valves

The pulmonary valve separates the right ventricle from the pulmonary artery, which delivers blood to the lungs. The tricuspid valve regulates blood flow from the right atrium to the right ventricle.

Q22.0   Pulmonary valve atresia

Pulmonary valve atresia is a very rare condition where the valve is replaced by solid tissue preventing blood flow from the heart to the lungs where the blood would normally be oxygenated. This condition may also be described as congenital absence of the pulmonary valve.

Q22.1   Congenital pulmonary valve stenosis

Pulmonary valve stenosis is a congenital condition where the blood flow is blocked due to malformation of the valve between the right ventricle and the pulmonary artery. This condition is rare, occurring in about 10 percent of infants with congenital heart defects.

Q22.4   Congenital tricuspid stenosis

Congenital tricuspid stenosis describes a malformation in the ability of the valve to open properly forcing the heart to work harder in order to push the blood through. Tricuspid atresia is also reported here and occurs when the valve between heart chambers is absent; instead solid tissue separates the chambers. This prevents blood flow between the heart and lungs, making it difficult for the rest of the body to get the oxygen needed to function properly.

Q22.5   Ebstein's anomaly

Ebstein's anomaly is an uncommon congenital heart defect in which the valve between the lower and upper heart chambers does not function normally, is not formed properly, or is positioned incorrectly. A portion of the right ventricle (RV) is atrialized (i.e., positioned above the valve) and is also thinned and dysplastic. The tricuspid annulus and right atrium (RA) are dilated. Of the four classifications, "D" is the most severe, manifesting with nearly total atrialization of the RV and other cardiac anomalies such as atrial septal defect (ASD) and Wolff-Parkinson-White syndrome. These malformations result in the backflow of blood making the heart work harder to function properly with consequential fluid accumulation within the lungs and liver.

Q23.-   Congenital malformations of aortic and mitral valves

The aortic valve regulates blood flow from the left ventricle to aorta. The mitral valve regulates blood flow from the right ventricle to the left ventricle.

Q23.0   Congenital stenosis of aortic valve

Congenital aortic valve stenosis occurs when infants are born with an abnormal narrowing of the valve between the left ventricle and the aorta. Since this passageway is abnormally narrow, the left ventricle has to work harder to force the blood into the aorta causing enlargement (hypertrophy) of the left ventricle. In addition to the narrowing, the valve may not have all three leaflets and there may be a malformation within the shape of the canal. This condition may not be initially diagnosed due to lack of symptoms. However, as the infant matures, the body's need for adequate blood supply increases causing increased symptoms. This condition appears in 7 percent of congenital heart defects, affecting males more often than females.

Q23.1   Congenital insufficiency of aortic valve

Congenital insufficiency of the aortic valve describes conditions where blood flows back into the left ventricle from the aorta due to a weak valve that does not close completely. Over time, this condition causes the ventricle to become abnormally enlarged, making it difficult for the heart to pump blood into the aorta.

Q23.2   Congenital mitral stenosis

Congenital mitral stenosis is a narrowing of the valve that regulates blood flow from the left atrium to the left ventricle, resulting in restriction of blood flow into the left ventricle. Because blood flow into the left ventricle is restricted, there is not enough blood available to the body. In addition, the increased pressure in the left atrium leads to enlargement and may also cause backflow of blood into the lungs resulting in pulmonary edema.

Q23.3   Congenital mitral insufficiency

Congenital mitral insufficiency is a defect in the mitral valve inhibiting the ability to close, causing blood to flow from the left ventricle back into the left atrium. Oftentimes this birth defect is associated with a more complex congenital disorder. This insufficiency causes stress on the heart because it has to work harder to force the blood out to the rest of the body as necessary for proper function.

Q23.4   Hypoplastic left heart syndrome

The left side of the heart pumps blood to the systemic circulation and supplies oxygen-rich blood to the organs and tissues of the body. In hypoplastic left heart syndrome, the structures of the left side of the heart (aorta, aortic valve, left ventricle, mitral valve) are underdeveloped and in some cases the mitral and aortic valves may be absent. Because these structures are smaller than normal, the heart is unable to pump sufficient quantities of oxygen-rich blood to the systemic circulation and therefore cannot meet the oxygen and nutrient needs of the organs and tissues of the body. Symptoms of hypoplastic left heart syndrome may not become apparent until 24 to 48 hours after birth when two fetal heart structures, the foramen ovale and ductus arteriosus, close. These fetal heart structures temporarily allow communication between the left and right sides of the heart, and this also allows the oxygen-rich blood from the pulmonary circulation to bypass the left side of the heart relying on the right side of the heart to pump blood to the lungs and the rest of the body. However, once these structures close, the inability of the left heart to pump blood to the body becomes evident resulting in respiratory distress, pounding heart and heart murmur, weak peripheral pulses, and cyanosis of lips and skin. Hypoplastic left heart syndrome is a life-threatening congenital malformation that requires prompt diagnosis and multiple staged surgical procedures to restore and maintain blood flow to the body.

Q24.- Other congenital malformations of heart

Malposition of heart and cardiac apexes are included in this category and are conditions where the position of the heart and cardiac apex are not in the proper location within the chest cavity. The three most common types of malposition include dextrocardia, levocardia, and ectopic cordis.

Q24.Ø Dextrocardia

In dextrocardia, the heart is situated on the right side of the chest as opposed to the left. There are several types of dextrocardia, including dextroposition and dextroversion. In dextroposition, extrinsic factors cause the heart to shift to the right, leading to hypoplastic right lung, a partial anomaly of the pulmonary venous connection to the inferior vena cava, and right-sided pulmonary collaterals. In dextroversion, abnormal rotation of the cardiac loops in embryological development leads to atrioventricular or ventricular discordance, or a single ventricle, which may be part of Cantrell syndrome (omphalocele or other midline defect, lower sternal defect, anterior inferior diaphragmatic defect, pericardial and intracardiac defects).

Focus Point

Ventriculoatrial situs inversus, which is a type of dextrocardia, is reported with code Q89.3. This condition is associated with tetralogy of Fallot and Kartagener's syndrome.

Q24.1 Levocardia

The normal position of the heart is slightly to the left of the mediastinum, but in this malformation, also called levoposition, the heart is shifted further to the left than is normal due to dysgenesis of the left lung or other malformations in the thoracic cavity. Severe heart defects usually accompany levocardia including transposition of the great vessels, along with abnormalities of the spleen such as asplenia or polysplenia.

Focus Point

Levocardia may also occur with situs inversus. In this condition, the heart is situated to the left of the mediastinum but the position of other thoracic organs and often other abdominal organs is reversed. Levocardia with situs inversus is reported with code Q89.3.

Q24.2 Cor triatriatum

Cor triatriatum, or heart with three atria (triatrial heart), is a congenital defect that occurs when either the right atrium (cor triatriatum dextrum) or the left atrium (cor triatriatum sinistrum) splits into two chambers separated by a membrane of varying size and shape. The more common and more threatening cor triatriatum sinistrum of the left atrium usually consists of a small extra chamber above the left atrium(LA) that receives the blood from the pulmonary vein that empties into the mitral valve. This extra chamber hampers the force of the blood entering the LA, which could cause congestive heart failure. Cor triatriatum dextrum is extremely rare with mild septation asymptomatic and seen only incidentally. More severe cases are thought to cause right heart failure. This code captures both anomalies.

Q24.3 Pulmonary infundibular stenosis

Infundibular (subvalvular) pulmonic stenosis is a congenital defect where narrowing occurs within the outflow tract of the right ventricle due to thickening of the muscle below the pulmonary valve in the infundibulum. The condition is due to a fibrous diaphragm or to a long, narrow fibromuscular channel.

Q24.4 Congenital subaortic stenosis

Subaortic stenosis is narrowing of the left ventricle below the aortic valve that obstructs blood flow from the left ventricle into the aorta. The left ventricle must work harder to force blood past the narrowed area. This extra work puts pressure on the heart increasing the risk of aortic valve damage due to the elevated pressure of the blood flow and also causes enlargement of the ventricle that may lead to left heart failure. This is a rare cardiac anomaly that is typically seen in children who have additional cardiac anomalies. Males are twice as likely to be affected by this defect as females.

Q24.5 Malformation of coronary vessels

Coronary artery anomalies occur when there is a malformation related to the origin or termination of the coronary artery, as well as anomalies of the coronary vessels and collateral vessels. Variations may occur anywhere within the coronary artery and can affect the shape and size of the vessel. Deviations from normal coronary anatomy that occur frequently are considered normal variants. In spite of this condition being congenital, it often goes undiagnosed until later in life when symptoms occur. This abnormality may inhibit oxygenated blood flow to the heart muscle and over time can cause a myocardial infarction and even sudden death. Surgery to revascularize the heart is often utilized.

Q24.6   Congenital heart block

Congenital heart block refers to any conduction disorder of the heart. Even though the very definition of a congenital condition is a condition present at birth, diagnosis of a congenital conduction disorder may be made prior to birth, during labor and delivery, or after birth—usually within the first 28 days or in some cases even later. Conduction disorders are caused by disruption of electrical impulses within the heart that result in an irregular heart rate and rhythm. These electrical impulses originate in the upper chambers (atria) and are conducted from the atria to the atrioventricular (AV) node and from the AV node to the additional electrical fibers in the lower chambers (ventricles) of the heart. These electrical impulses stimulate the heart muscle to expand and contract. When these signals are blocked, the normal rhythmic contractions and the rate of contraction are affected. This condition may appear as a sole variant or as part of a syndrome of congenital abnormalities.

Q24.8   Other specified congenital malformations of heart

Coded here is ectopic cordis, a rare malformation in which the heart is located partially or completely outside the thoracic cavity. The heart may be adjacent to the thoracic cavity in which case the sternum is split and the heart protrudes from the thoracic cavity. Alternatively, the heart may be displaced to the abdomen or neck. Ectopic cordis is typically associated with other congenital anomalies and rarely does the fetus survive.

Q25.-   Congenital malformations of great arteries

Congenital malformations classified here involve the aorta and pulmonary artery.

Q25.0   Patent ductus arteriosus

The ductus arteriosus is a normal component of fetal circulation consisting of a short duct that allows fetal blood to be shunted away from the pulmonary artery and pulmonary circulation and returned directly to the aorta. Shortly after birth the ductus arteriosus closes so that oxygen depleted blood from the systemic circulation can be routed to the pulmonary circulation where it can be oxygenated and returned to the heart. In patent ductus arteriosus (PDA), the duct between the pulmonary arteries and the aorta does not close after birth. A persistent PDA results in reversed blood flow from the aorta into the pulmonary artery and can cause pulmonary overload and congestive heart failure

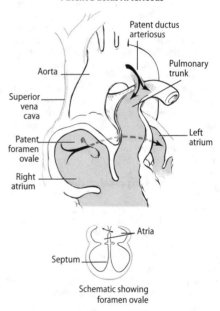

Patent Ductus Arteriosus

Patent ductus arteriosus

Aorta

Pulmonary trunk

Superior vena cava

Left atrium

Patent foramen ovale

Right atrium

Atria

Septum

Schematic showing foramen ovale

Q25.1   Coarctation of aorta

In coarctation of the aorta, there is a narrowing in the vessel leaving the heart (aorta) that distributes blood to the rest of the body. The narrowing is usually located distal to the origin of the left subclavian artery. The terms "preductal" and "postductal" are sometimes used to describe the location of the narrowing and indicate the location of the coarctation in relation to the ductus arteriosus. Another term describing location is "juxtaductal" meaning near the ductus arteriosus. When the aorta is narrowed, the left ventricle, which pumps blood into the aorta, and the systemic circulation must work harder to get adequate blood supply through the narrowed vessel. This may lead to congestive heart failure and/or an inadequate blood supply to organs and tissues in the body.

Q25.2-   Atresia of aorta

Atresia of the aorta, also called interruption of aortic arch (IAA), is a rare condition that is usually related to other anomalies of the heart and great vessels.

Q25.3   Supravalvular aortic stenosis

Supravalvular aortic stenosis (SVAS) is a narrowing of the aorta located just above the aortic valve. SVAS is an inherited anomaly caused by genetic mutation that affects the production of a protein called tropoelastin. Tropoelastin is needed to form the protein elastin, which is a key component in elastic fibers found in connective tissue, including those that form the walls of blood vessels. The gene mutation that causes SVAS results in reduction in the production of tropoelastin, which in turn decreases the amount of elastin available to form elastic fibers. This results in a thinning of the aortic wall. This thinning of the aortic wall is compensated for by the increased production of smooth muscle cells in the lining of the aorta, making the aorta thicker and narrowing the lumen in the region above the aortic valve. The heart must work harder to pump blood through the narrowed lumen resulting in symptoms of shortness of breath and chest pain, which can eventually lead to congestive heart failure.

Q25.4-   Other congenital malformations of aorta

Anomalies of the aortic arch include a wide range of conditions, including double aortic arch, anomalous arch arteries, and persistent right aortic arch.

Q25.41   Absence and aplasia of aorta

The congenital absence of the aortic arch is rare and typically found in conjunction with an interventricular septum defect and patent ductus arteriosus.

Q25.42   Hypoplasia of aorta

Hypoplasia of the thoracic and abdominal aorta refers to a smaller and more elongated than normal aorta, which causes narrowing, similar to coarctation of aorta. Aortic hypoplasia is a more critical condition, however, as it affects a larger segment of the aorta. This rare defect generally presents prior to age 30 with life-threatening symptoms of severe hypertension and lower extremity or abdominal ischemia requiring treatment such as bypass grafting.

Q25.43   Congenital aneurysm of aorta

Congenital abdominal aortic aneurysms (AAA) in newborns are rare and idiopathic with a high mortality rate unless identified and treated early. Aneurysm of the aortic root, which houses the sinus of Valsalva, is located in the thoracic aorta and may not be apparent

until adulthood. Congenital heart defects such as tetralogy of Fallot and bicuspid aortic valve (BAV) are associated with congenital aortic dilation, which becomes aneurysmal as it enlarges. Since dissection is a high mortality risk for this condition, AAA requires close monitoring or prophylactic surgery.

Q25.44   Congenital dilation of aorta

Although not a lot is known about this condition, current research shows that patients born with bicuspid aortic valve (BAV) have a vastly higher incidence of dilated aorta. Research has indicated that these BAV patients have a larger and faster growing ascending aortic diameter that may be found as early as infancy or may not present until mid-life. Since dissection is a high mortality risk for this condition, those with aortic dilation require close monitoring or prophylactic surgery.

Q25.45   Double aortic arch

In double aortic arch, normal embryonic development of the aorta does not occur, resulting in persistence of the right and left aortic arches. In one of the variations of this condition, the arches can encircle the trachea or the esophagus in a vascular ring. This leads to tracheal compression and repeated respiratory infections.

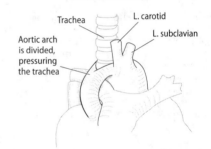

Double Aortic Arch

Trachea

L. carotid

L. subclavian

Aortic arch is divided, pressuring the trachea

Q25.46   Tortuous aortic arch

A tortuous aorta is described as twists, turns, or kinks in the aortic path, which distort the normal straight pathway. This distortion causes elevated blood pressure and loss of circulation to the organs. The condition is sometimes referred to as persistent aortic convulsions. This limiting of blood supply can cause the formation of plaque and atherosclerosis. Surgery may remove the affected area; if the aorta lacks the sufficient length for anastomosis, a graft may be used. In some cases, a balloon angioplasty may be the treatment of choice for placement of a stent.

Q25.47 Right aortic arch

The aortic arch is located on the left side during normal fetal development. In rare cases, an anomaly develops, especially when tetralogy of Fallot is present, wherein the aortic arch is on the right side with or without an aberrant left subclavian artery or a retro esophageal segment. Depending on the presence of other associated abnormalities, this condition can create a vacular ring around the esophagus and trachea, which can result in compression. Symptoms of respiratory impairment and swallowing difficulties usually present later in life. Outcomes of surgical intervention to divide the vascular ring, which can be performed with an open or a video-assisted thorascopic approach, are excellent.

Q25.48 Anomalous origin of subclavian artery

An anomalous subclavian artery is one that develops from an abnormal origin. Rather than following a normal course posterior to the esophagus, it may run between the esophagus and trachea or anteriorly to the trachea. One common example that does not usually produce symptoms and is seen only incidentally is the right subclavian originating from the last branch of the aortic arch.

Q25.6 Stenosis of pulmonary artery

The pulmonary artery is the large artery that takes the blood from the right ventricle of the heart to the lungs to become oxygenized. This code for congenital pulmonary artery stenosis is reported for narrowing of the artery, not the pulmonary valve. It is often present in conjunction with other heart birth defects such as tetralogy of Fallot, truncus arteriosus, pulmonary valve stenosis, or patent ductus arteriosus. This congenital defect can also be caused during pregnancy by infection or by a genetic anomaly. This narrowing can make the heart work harder, causing cardiomyopathy or high blood pressure. This defect is often detected by a heart murmur. In most cases, this condition is managed by balloon angioplasty and stent insertion; however, in more severe cases involving extensive stenosis, surgery may be necessary.

Q25.72 Congenital pulmonary arteriovenous malformation

A pulmonary arteriovenous malformation (PAVM) is an abnormal vascular communication between pulmonary arteries and pulmonary veins. PAVM may also be identified as pulmonary arteriovenous aneurysms or pulmonary arteriovenous fistulae. This is described by the classic whooshing sound detected by stethoscope that is due to the abnormal connection between the higher pressure arteries to the lower pressure veins. The circulating desaturated (improperly oxygenated) blood manifests systemically as dyspnea and cyanosis. Hemoglobin and hematocrit rise proportionately in compensation. Additionally, when the PAVMs are concentrated in the lower lobes of the lung, gravity may cause the deoxygenation of blood to eventually become more pronounced when someone is upright. PAVMs may lie quiescent until adulthood, when physiological manifestations and associated complications begin to appear as the PAVMs enlarge. Cardiorespiratory symptoms include dyspnea, cyanosis, heart failure, and respiratory failure. Other circulatory symptoms include stroke and hemorrhage caused by stress on the weakened, compromised vasculature, such as epistaxis or GI bleeding. While certain effects of PAVM may be managed medically, definitive therapy requires therapeutic embolization or surgical resection.

Focus Point

A rare congenital defect called scimitar syndrome combines pulmonary hypoplasia, which is an incomplete development of or abnormally small lungs, with partial anomalous pulmonary venous return (PAPVR). In this return, the blood from the lung is abnormally drained by the PAPVR into the systemic venous system, commonly the inferior vena cava rather than to the left atrium. This condition is captured in code Q26.8 Other congenital malformations of great veins.

Q26.- Congenital malformations of great veins

These codes describe congenital conditions that result in malformation of the great veins, including the superior and inferior vena cava, the pulmonary veins, and the coronary sinus. The superior and inferior vena cava and the coronary sinus connect to the right atrium in the normal heart. The pulmonary veins connect to the left atrium.

Q26.0 Congenital stenosis of vena cava

This code includes stenosis, narrowing, interruption, or coarctation of a congenital nature of either the superior or inferior vena cava. The superior vena cava is the vein that returns the blood from the upper body—including the head, neck, and upper limbs—back to the heart. The inferior vena cava is the vein that takes the blood from the lower body and limbs back to the heart. This is a rare anomaly that may occur with other congenital heart defects and is often asymptomatic due to the development of other veins as collaterals such as the azygos/hemiazygos veins.

Focus Point

Congenital complete or partial absence, or agenesis, of either superior or inferior vena cava is included in code Q26.8 Other congenital malformations of great veins.

Q26.1 Persistent left superior vena cava

Persistent left superior vena cava (LSVC), the most common thoracic venous anomaly, is a remnant of a structure that normally disappears during embryological development and, if a solitary variant, is seldom symptomatic or significant. It is often discovered incidentally during a central venous catheter insertion as it can cause malposition of the catheter. It is considerably more prevalent in populations with other congenital heart defects.

Q26.2 Total anomalous pulmonary venous connection

Total anomalous pulmonary venous connection (TAPVC) or return is a congenital malformation in which all four of the pulmonary veins are connected to the right atrium instead of the left. When this happens, blood simply circulates from the lungs to the heart and back again without being pumped to the rest of the body. In order for an infant to survive with this condition, there must be an atrial septal defect (ASD) or canal between the left and right atrium to let the oxygenated blood pass to the left side of the heart so that it can be pumped to the rest of the body.

Q26.3 Partial anomalous pulmonary venous connection

In partial anomalous pulmonary venous connection (PAPVC), there is still some appropriate connection to the left atrium, but one or more pulmonary veins are connected to the right atrium or to the superior or inferior vena cava, which are the two main vessels that carry oxygen-depleted blood from the body to the right atrium. Most often, only one pulmonary vein is anomalous. However, in PAPVC there can be a range of pulmonary anomalous venous connection configurations.

Q26.6 Portal vein-hepatic artery fistula

Often referred to as congenital hepatic shunts, this is an abnormal connection between the portal vein and hepatic artery, both part of the hepatic (liver) venous system. These arterio-portal fistulas (APFs) may be formed by congenital arteriovenous malformations (AVMs), or they can be associated with other congenital disorders such as biliary atresia, Ehlers-Danlos syndrome, or other hereditary diseases. APF can cause an increase in pressure in the portal venous system, leading to a rapid onset of severe portal hypertension. Interventional radiology procedures are the treatment of choice.

Q27.- Other congenital malformations of peripheral vascular system

The peripheral vascular system includes all of the blood vessels in the arterial system (those vessels that supply the organs and tissues of the body with oxygen and nutrient rich blood) and all of the blood vessels in the venous system (those vessels that return oxygen poor blood to the heart).

Q27.3- Arteriovenous malformation (peripheral)

Arteriovenous (A-V) malformations are anomalous communications between a vein and an artery that are congenital in nature. Congenital A-V malformations are caused by persistent embryonic vessels that fail to differentiate into veins and arteries.

Q27.39 Arteriovenous malformation, other site

A-V malformation of the spinal vessels is reported here. Spinal dural A-V malformations are the most common type seen in adults. These lesions may result in progressive sensory motor symptoms ranging from painful paraparesis to acute quadriplegia.

Q27.4 Congenital phlebectasia

Congenital phlebectasia is a very rare defect that is described as vascular malformation lesions of the skin. Also called cutis marmorata telangiectatica congenita (CMTC), the condition is characterized by abnormally dilated large veins and capillaries near the surface of the skin. Most often visible in newborns, the appearance of the dilated vessels spontaneously fades with age.

Q28.0 Arteriovenous malformation of precerebral vessels

Arteriovenous (A-V) malformations are congenital lesions created by anomalous communications between a vein and an artery that are connected by fistulae, causing a mass or tangle of vessels. Congenital A-V malformations can be idiopathic or caused by persistent embryonic vessels that fail to differentiate into veins and arteries. This code includes only the precerebral vessels, which are arteries that lead to the cerebrum such as the common carotid, vertebral, or basilar arteries. Medical intervention may be necessary for younger patients at risk for rupture, while older patients with little to no risk of rupture may be treated with medication focused on the symptoms.

Q28.2 Arteriovenous malformation of cerebral vessels

Arteriovenous (A-V) malformations are congenital lesions created by anomalous communications between a vein and an artery that are connected by fistulae, causing a mass or tangle of vessels. Congenital A-V malformations can be idiopathic or caused by persistent embryonic vessels that fail to differentiate into veins and arteries. This code classifies the AVMs of the cerebral vessels, which most commonly present in younger adults with symptoms such as severe headaches, seizures, hemorrhage, or neurological deficits. In infants the condition may manifest as prominent veins showing in the scalp or macrocephaly. Medical intervention may be necessary for younger patients at risk for rupture, while older patients with little to no risk of rupture may be treated with medication focused on the symptoms.

Congenital Malformations of the Respiratory System (Q30–Q34)

This code block classifies congenital malformations of the two main parts of the respiratory system: the upper respiratory tract and the lower respiratory tract. The upper respiratory tract contains the nose (external, nasal cavity), sinuses (frontal, ethmoid, sphenoid, maxillary), pharynx (nasopharynx, oropharynx), larynx (true and false vocal cords, glottis), and trachea. The lower respiratory tract contains the bronchi (left, right, main, carina) and lungs (intrapulmonary bronchi, bronchioli, lobes, alveoli, pleura).

The categories in this code block are as follows:

Q30	Congenital malformations of nose
Q31	Congenital malformations of larynx
Q32	Congenital malformations of trachea and bronchus
Q33	Congenital malformations of lung
Q34	Other congenital malformations of respiratory system

Q32.- Congenital malformations of trachea and bronchus

The trachea is the tube that forms the connection between the larynx and the main bronchus. The main bronchus divides into the right and left bronchi that connect with the smaller airways in the lungs.

Q32.0 Congenital tracheomalacia

The trachea is formed by rings of cartilage connected to each other by muscle and connective tissue and lined with a mucosal membrane. Tracheomalacia is a structural malformation of the cartilage that results in softening of the cartilage. This results in a tendency for the trachea to collapse, particularly when an infant is crying or feeding, obstructing the flow of air into the lungs. This condition is usually temporary, resolving as the cartilage matures and becomes stronger usually between 6 and 12 months of age.

Cleft Lip and Cleft Palate (Q35–Q37)

The hard and soft palates are the structures that comprise the roof of the mouth—the hard palate forming the anterior portion and the soft palate the posterior portion. During normal fetal development, the right and left sides of the lip and the roof of the mouth grow together. In this condition, the tissue that forms the upper lip and roof of the mouth (palate) does not develop correctly leaving a gap (cleft) in the lip and palate.

The categories in this code block are as follows:

Q35	Cleft palate
Q36	Cleft lip
Q37	Cleft palate with cleft lip

Q35.- Cleft palate

A cleft palate is caused when the roof of the mouth (palate) does not form correctly during pregnancy, leaving a gap (cleft) that may extend as far as the nasal cavity. A cleft palate may involve any parts of the palate, including the hard palate and/or soft palate, or the uvula. It may appear by itself or along with other birth defects of the face and skull, most commonly with a cleft lip.

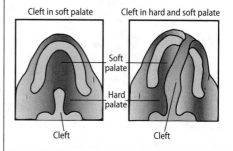

Cleft Palate

Cleft in soft palate   Cleft in hard and soft palate

Soft palate

Hard palate

Cleft   Cleft

Q36.- Cleft lip

A cleft lip is a congenital malformation of the tissues of the upper lip, due to failure of the tissues of the upper lip to connect during fetal development. This deformity can extend to the nose, which may be described as a complete cleft lip. Although rare, the lower lip may also be involved. Cleft lip is classified based on whether it is unilateral or bilateral or whether it occurs in the median.

Cleft Lip

Unilateral incomplete

Unilateral complete

Bilateral complete

Q37.- Cleft palate with cleft lip

Cleft lip and cleft palate are facial and oral congenital deformities that occur during the early weeks of development. During normal fetal development, the right and left sides of the lip and the roof of the mouth grow together. In this condition, the tissue that forms the upper lip and roof of the mouth (palate) do not develop correctly, leaving a gap (cleft) in the lip and palate. When these two malformations occur together, they can occur in multiple configurations, such as cleft of the hard palate only with a unilateral or bilateral cleft lip, cleft of the soft palate only with a unilateral or bilateral cleft lip, or a cleft involving both the hard and soft palate with a unilateral or bilateral cleft lip.

Other Congenital Malformations of the Digestive System (Q38-Q45)

This code block classifies congenital malformations of the organs comprising the alimentary (digestive) tract, which is the long, muscular tube that begins at the mouth and ends at the anus. The major digestive organs include the pharynx, esophagus, stomach, and intestines. Supporting structures include the salivary and parotid glands, jaw, teeth, tongue, biliary tract, and peritoneum.

Congenital malformations of accessory organs or structures that support the digestive process from outside this continuous tube are also included in this code block: gallbladder, pancreas, and liver. These organs provide secretions that are critical to the breakdown of food and absorption and use of nutrients by the body.

The categories in this code block are as follows:

Q38	Other congenital malformations of tongue, mouth and pharynx
Q39	Congenital malformations of esophagus
Q40	Other congenital malformations of upper alimentary tract
Q41	Congenital absence, atresia and stenosis of small intestine
Q42	Congenital absence, atresia and stenosis of large intestine
Q43	Other congenital malformations of intestine
Q44	Congenital malformations of gallbladder, bile ducts and liver
Q45	Other congenital malformations of digestive system

Q38.- Other congenital malformations of tongue, mouth and pharynx

Congenital malformations classified here cover many structures that make up or are contained in the oral cavity including the lips (excluding cleft lip), tongue, salivary glands and ducts, and palate (excluding cleft palate). Also classified here are malformations of the throat or pharynx.

Q38.1 Ankyloglossia

Ankyloglossia, also known as tongue tie, identifies conditions ranging in severity from a malposition of the frenulum on the underside of the tongue to partial or total fusion of the tongue to the floor of the mouth. The lingual frenulum is a narrow fold of mucous membrane midway on the underside of the tongue that attaches to the back portion of the tongue, securing it to the floor of the mouth without impeding the movement of the tip of the tongue. When the frenulum is too short or attaches close to the tip of the tongue, it restricts the movement of the tongue. This may lead to problems with feeding, tooth development, and speech.

Q38.2 Macroglossia

Macroglossia is an abnormally large tongue.

Q38.3 Other congenital malformations of tongue

This code is used to report aglossia, bifid tongue, and microglossia. Aglossia is absence of the tongue. Bifid tongue occurs when the tongue buds fail to develop normally resulting in a longitudinal cleft at the tip of the tongue, which gives the tongue a forked appearance. Microglossia is an abnormally small tongue.

Q39.- Congenital malformations of esophagus

The esophagus is a muscular, tubular structure that serves as a conduit for the passage of food and water from the pharynx to the stomach. Transportation of food and fluids from the mouth to the stomach is accomplished by a combination of gravity and peristaltic waves in the esophagus. The esophagus is equipped with two sphincters: the pharyngeal-esophageal sphincter located at the level of the cricoid cartilage and the gastroesophageal sphincter (also known as the lower esophageal sphincter) located at the level of the esophageal hiatus of the diaphragm.

Q39.0 Atresia of esophagus without fistula

Q39.1 Atresia of esophagus with tracheo-esophageal fistula

Q39.2 Congenital tracheo-esophageal fistula without atresia

In esophageal atresia, the esophagus ends in a blind pouch. A tracheoesophageal fistula, which is an abnormal opening between the trachea and the esophagus, must be repaired immediately after birth.

Q39.3 Congenital stenosis and stricture of esophagus

Esophageal stenosis is an abnormally narrowed lumen of the esophagus associated with vomiting and dysphagia.

Q39.5 Congenital dilatation of esophagus

This code includes cardiospasm. Cardiospasm is the failure of the cardiac sphincter to relax. The cardiac sphincter is a valve between the lower end of the esophagus and the cardia of the stomach that helps prevent stomach contents from refluxing into the esophagus.

Q40.- Other congenital malformations of upper alimentary tract

Congenital malformations classified to this category include malformations that involve the stomach, such as the pyloric sphincter, which controls passage of food into the small intestine.

Q40.0 Congenital hypertrophic pyloric stenosis

Hypertrophic pyloric stenosis is the most common cause of surgery in the young infant, excluding hernia surgery. In this condition, the outlet to the intestines becomes blocked, leading to projectile vomiting, electrolyte imbalances, and dehydration. The condition is often diagnosed between 2 and 4 weeks of age.

Q40.1 Congenital hiatus hernia

A hiatal hernia is an upward displacement of the stomach through the esophageal hiatus into the mediastinal cavity, and can lead to esophageal reflux disease.

Q40.2 Other specified congenital malformations of stomach

In hourglass stomach, fibrous bands pinch in the stomach, giving it an hourglass appearance. When the stomach is transposed, it lies on the right side of the abdomen. Megalogastria is an abnormally large stomach and microgastria is an abnormally small stomach.

Q41.- Congenital absence, atresia and stenosis of small intestine

Obstruction or complete blockage of an intestine secondary to a birth defect is termed atresia. The jejunum and/or ileum are the two most common sites for congenital small intestine blockages, followed by the duodenum, and finally the pylorus to which congenital obstructions rarely occur. While congenital atresia is complete blockage of the intestine due to a birth defect, congenital stenosis is a partial blockage of the small intestine due to a birth defect, typically due to narrowing of the lumen.

Q43.- Other congenital malformations of intestine

Congenital malformations of the small and large intestines are included here, with the exception of absence, atresia, and stenosis, which have their own categories.

Q43.0 Meckel's diverticulum (displaced) (hypertrophic)

Meckel's diverticulum is a sacculation of the distal ileum caused by failure of the vitelline duct to atrophy. It is the most frequently occurring digestive malformation and usually presents with massive dark red rectal bleeding, which is often painless to the child. Strangulation or intussusception of the intestines can occur as a result of this malformation.

Q43.1 Hirschsprung's disease

Hirschsprung's disease is an extensive distention of the colon with associated inability to defecate due to lack of innervation of the affected portion of the colon. It has familial associations and is more commonly seen in males. The condition is often diagnosed about 48 hours after birth, as the infant is unable to pass meconium, and treatment is immediate to prevent the onset of enterocolitis.

Q43.3 Congenital malformations of intestinal fixation

Categorized to this code are malrotation, adhesions, and anomalous fixation of the colon. During normal fetal development, the intestines migrate, rotate, and are then secured within the abdominal cavity. If any part of this development is interrupted, it can result in nonrotation or incomplete rotation of the intestine (malrotation), displaced or mobile colon, or abnormal bands (adhesions). Risks associated with these malformations include obstruction of the intestine and volvulus.

Q43.7 Persistent cloaca

A persistent cloaca is the third level of a developmental anomaly involving the persistence of a urogenital sinus. In this condition, there is a single orifice behind the clitoris and agenesis of the anus and vagina. Treatment is delayed until the child is at least 1 year of age. A colostomy is performed after birth as a temporary measure and the infant is catheterized intermittently until corrective surgery is performed.

Q43.8 Other specified congenital malformations of intestine

Dolichocolon and volvulus are two intestinal malformations that are included here. Dolichocolon is an abnormally long colon. Volvulus is twisting of the intestine resulting in obstruction of the intestine and/or a reduction in blood available to the intestinal tissue. Although it is typically seen as a complication of malrotation of the intestine, this is not always the case.

Q44.- Congenital malformations of gallbladder, bile ducts and liver

The gallbladder, bile ducts, and liver are accessory organs and structures that support the digestive process from outside the alimentary tract. These organs provide secretions that are critical to food absorption and use of nutrients by the body.

Q44.2 Atresia of bile ducts

Biliary atresia is the lack of patency of the extrahepatic ducts thought to be an obliterative process rather than a developmental anomaly. It is a serious condition, which may lead to cirrhosis of the liver. Approximately 10 percent of the cases are associated with multiple malformations, the most common being polysplenia (multiple right-sided spleens, a midline liver, a preduodenal portal vein, and cardiac malformations).

Q44.6 Cystic disease of liver

Congenital polycystic disease of the liver involves the formation of numerous cysts that block the drainage of bile.

Q45.- Other congenital malformations of digestive system

Congenital anomalies of the pancreas, an accessory organ that supports the digestive process from outside the alimentary tract, are coded here. This category also includes malposition and duplication of digestive system organs.

Q45.0 Agenesis, aplasia and hypoplasia of pancreas

If the pancreas does not develop (agenesis) or is extremely underdeveloped (hypoplasia), intrauterine growth is retarded due to the lack of insulin that would normally be secreted by the pancreas.

Congenital Malformations of Genital Organs (Q50-Q56)

There are a wide range of congenital malformations that can affect the genital organs ranging from agenesis, which is a failure of an organ or structure to develop, to duplication of genital organs to indeterminate sex and ambiguous genitalia.

The categories in this code block are as follows:

Q50	Congenital malformations of ovaries, fallopian tubes and broad ligaments
Q51	Congenital malformations of uterus and cervix
Q52	Other congenital malformations of female genitalia
Q53	Undescended and ectopic testicle
Q54	Hypospadias
Q55	Other congenital malformations of male genital organs
Q56	Indeterminate sex and pseudohermaphroditism

Q51.- Congenital malformations of uterus and cervix

Müllerian ducts are present in the embryo of both sexes. In males, they degenerate due to the presence of anti-Müllerian hormone (AMH). In female embryogenesis, the absence of anti-Müllerian hormone (AMH) allows for the development of female reproductive organs. The Müllerian ducts develop into the upper vagina, cervix, uterus, and oviducts. This transformative process is highly complex, consisting of cellular differentiation, migration, fusion, and canalization. Any failures or disruptions in this system can result in various malformations, including various stages of agenesis, fusion, malpresentation, malformation, and duplication. Müllerian malformations may be associated with certain skeletal and renal anomalies due to their proximity and relational development. Depending on the nature and severity of the anomaly, women with Müllerian malformations may remain asymptomatic until complications of menstruation, conception, or pregnancy occur. Ovarian development occurs independently of Müllerian duct transformation; therefore, Müllerian duct anomalies are often present in women with normal, functional ovaries. Congenital malformations of the uterus and cervix range from failure of these structures to form, a condition referred to agenesis or aplasia, to duplication of part or all of the uterus or cervix to abnormal underdevelopment of these structures.

Q51.10   Doubling of uterus with doubling of cervix and vagina without obstruction

Q51.11   Doubling of uterus with doubling of cervix and vagina with obstruction

Doubling of the uterus (didelphys) is a congenital anomaly caused by failure of the Müllerian ducts, two tubular structures, to fuse together during embryonic development. This results in two uteruses, each uterus having a single horn with a fallopian tube and ovary. Often coinciding with this type of doubling is the development of two cervixes and two vaginas. There may be two patent vaginal openings allowing menstrual blood to flow out of the body without obstruction or a single vaginal opening with obstruction of menstrual blood flow causing pain and an abdominal mass on the affected side. Pregnancy is possible but is associated with an increased risk of preterm delivery and malpresentation. The condition may be associated with congenital malformation of the kidneys and/or the urinary tract and the skeleton.

Q51.2   Other doubling of uterus

Septate uterus is a malformation characterized by a longitudinal septum or partition in the middle of a normal shaped uterus. It occurs with partial or complete failure of the uterovaginal septum to be absorbed after fusion of the Müllerian ducts. Fibrous tissue usually makes up the septum, but in some cases it may be composed of muscle tissue. When a partial septum is present, only the uterine cavity is divided by fibrous or muscle tissue. A complete septum involves the uterine cavity with the septum extending into the cervix. In some cases, there is doubling of the cervix and vagina as a result of the septum. Septate uterus is largely asymptomatic and pregnancy is possible, although pregnancy is associated with increased risk of miscarriage, preterm delivery, and malpresentation.

Q51.3   Bicornate uterus

Like other uterine malformations, bicornate uterus occurs when the Müllerian ducts fail to fuse properly, in this case resulting in a partial septum in the upper portion of the uterus between two widely separated horns with a depression at the top and a normally configured lower uterine segment. This gives the uterus a heart-shaped appearance. Bicornate uterus is largely asymptomatic and pregnancy is possible, but is associated with an increased risk of cervical incompetence, miscarriage, preterm delivery, and malpresentation.

Q51.4   Unicornate uterus

A unicornate uterus is comprised of only one lateral half of a normal uterus with only one horn and commonly with only one fallopian tube. The condition occurs when one Müllerian duct fails to elongate and the other develops normally. In some women, a second rudimentary horn develops that may or may not communicate with the uterus. Unicornate uterus is usually asymptomatic. Even with a single fallopian tube and ovary, there is typically normal menstruation. However, there is a high rate of infertility with this malformation and when pregnancy does occur, miscarriage is more common. Other pregnancy complications may include preterm delivery and malpresentation. When a communicating rudimentary horn containing endometrial tissue is present, an embryo may implant there, creating a high risk for uterine rupture.

Q51.810 Arcuate uterus

Arcuate uterus is often considered to be a normal variant in the structure of the uterus. It differs from the normal uterus in that the uterovaginal septum present during fetal development almost completely resorbs except for a small portion at the top of the uterus, which results in a small indentation in the lining of the uterus. The condition is rarely associated with other congenital malformations or problems with conception or pregnancy.

Q52.-   Other congenital malformations of female genitalia

Congenital malformations classified here include those affecting the vagina, hymen, labia, clitoris, and vulva.

Q52.11   Transverse vaginal septum

A transverse vaginal septum is a partition of tissue that separates the vagina into two vaginal cavities, one upper and one lower. This is a rare Müllerian duct development malfunction causing a sideways septum across the vagina. A transverse septum may be symptomatic only if it obstructs the menstrual flow and can be removed with surgery. Without surgery, the blood can flow backwards, leaking into the body cavity through the fallopian tubes and resulting in endometriosis and infertility.

Q52.12- Longitudinal vaginal septum

This defect occurs when a partition of tissue or septum, created by the incomplete fusion of the Müllerian, ducts divides the vagina into two lengthwise pathways. It often occurs with other congenital conditions involving the female reproductive system organs. This condition may go unnoticed until leakage during menstruation despite the use of a tampon or when sexual intercourse is painful. Infertility and miscarriage are risks most often occurring with other anomalies such as double uterus or cervix. Once the specific anomaly is identified, multiple surgical options are available. Advances in assisted reproductive technologies have improved fertility and obstetric outcomes for these patients.

Focus Point

Codes in the longitudinal vaginal septum subcategory specify laterality and whether the septum is obstructing, nonobstructing, microperforated, or partially obstructing.

Q52.4 Other congenital malformations of vagina

A Gartner's duct cyst is a benign, tumor-like cyst of the vagina that develops from the embryonic remnants of the Gartner's duct, which is part of the mesonephros that develops into the reproductive organs.

Q53.- Undescended and ectopic testicle

During fetal development, the testes form in the abdominal cavity and move down into the scrotal sacs during the latter part of the pregnancy. Movement of the testes into the scrotal sacs results from the production of androgens, which are male sex hormones. There are a number of health risks associated with undescended and ectopic testes, including infertility, testicular cancer, and trauma or torsion that can potentially obstruct blood supply leading to infarction. In some cases of undescended or ectopic testicle, the testes are also small and underdeveloped or severely malformed.

Q53.0- Ectopic testis

During fetal development, the testes are located in the retroperitoneum near the kidney. Late in pregnancy they move down to the inguinal ring and through the inguinal canal to the scrotum. An ectopic testis begins descending along this path but becomes misdirected usually at the external inguinal ring. The testis then continues to descend into an abnormal location such as the skin of the thigh or even into the opposite scrotal sac.

Focus Point

Ectopic perineal testis is reported with code Q53.12 or Q53.22 depending on whether the condition affects one or both testis.

Q53.1- Undescended testicle, unilateral

Q53.2- Undescended testicle, bilateral

An undescended testicle occurs when the testicle fails to drop into the scrotal sac prior to birth. The condition may affect one or both testicles and the condition is classified based on the location of the undescended testicle (e.g., abdominal or perineal). Perineal ectopic testicle is rare and occurs when the testicle descends into the region between a ridge of tissue at the top of the scrotum and the skin overlying the perineum. Perineal testicle typically presents as a mass in the perineum.

Intra-abdominal testes is the most common type of cryptorchidism (undescended testes) most often occurring in premature births because the testes are not located in their appropriate position until approximately the seventh month. The end location can depend on the time of birth as the testes develop intra-abdominally and normally travel down through the inguinal canal into the high scrotal sac and finally down into the scrotal sac at about 30 weeks. Unique codes in this subcategory specify the final position. Other conditions that can affect development include intrauterine growth retardation, use of alcohol or tobacco, gestational diabetes, or rare congenital syndromes. Left untreated, cryptorchidism can lead to complications such as malignant seminoma testicular cancer, ischemia, or infertility.

Q54.- Hypospadias

Hypospadias is a male developmental defect in the penis in which the urethral opening (meatus) is not located at the tip of the penis (glans). Hypospadias can occur anywhere along the urethral groove located on the underside (ventral aspect) of the penis.

Q54.0 Hypospadias, balanic

In balanic hypospadias, also called first-degree or glanular hypospadias, the urethral opening is on the underside of the glans between the tip (head) of the penis and the penile shaft. The foreskin often has a dorsal hood that leaves the tip of the penis exposed.

Q54.1 Hypospadias, penile

Penile hypospadias, also called second-degree, distal penile, or mid-shaft hypospadias, presents with a urethral opening proximal to the glans but distal to the scrotum.

Q54.2 Hypospadias, penoscrotal

Q54.3 Hypospadias, perineal

These two types of hypospadias are known as third-degree or proximal hypospadias. In penoscrotal hypospadias, the urethral opening is on the proximal penile shaft, close to or in the scrotum. In perineal hypospadias, the urethral opening is located behind the scrotum distal to the anal opening.

Q54.4 Congenital chordee

Congenital chordee is an abnormal downward curvature of the erect penis that is present from birth. The condition can occur with or without hypospadias. It is most likely due to a defect of fascial tissue and/or corpus spongiosum along the penile shaft with more elastic tissue developing on the top half of the penis. Chordee may cause erectile dysfunction and/or pain with sexual intercourse. The condition often goes undetected until late childhood or early adulthood, especially when hypospadias is not present.

Q55.- Other congenital malformations of male genital organs

A wide range of congenital malformations of the male genital organs are included here, such as failure of the male reproductive organs to form, a condition known as aplasia; hypoplasia or underdevelopment; abnormal curvature or twisting of the penis; and congenital fistula between the vas and the skin.

Q55.22 Retractile testis

A retractile testicle descends normally but moves freely between the scrotal sac and the groin. The testicle is easily guided back into a normal position without pain or discomfort. The testicle usually descends and remains fixed in the scrotum around puberty.

Q55.5 Congenital absence and aplasia of penis

Congenital failure of the penis to develop, a condition called penile agenesis, is so rare that it occurs in one out of 30 million births. In most cases of penis agenesis, the scrotum is normal, though the testicles are undescended.

Q55.62 Hypoplasia of penis

Micropenis, a form of ambiguous genitalia, is caused by a lack of endocrine output during fetal life, specifically lack of testosterone. This condition is due to the developmental failure of the penis caused by failure of testosterone to stimulate the tissues or failure of the tissues to respond to testosterone stimulation. Typically the penis, though small, is normal in function. Testosterone shots administered in infancy allow the penis to obtain normal size.

Q55.63 Congenital torsion of penis

In torsion of the penis, the rotation is typically to the left.

Q55.69 Other congenital malformation of penis

Penile duplication presents as a bifid penis with two corpora cavernosa and two hemialgias and may range from the glans only to duplication of the entire urogenital tract.

Q56.- Indeterminate sex and pseudohermaphroditism

Conditions classified here involve failure of the male or female genitalia to develop normally during fetal development in spite of having normal XX and XY chromosomes.

Q56.1 Male pseudohermaphroditism, not elsewhere classified

Male pseudohermaphroditism (MPH) is the incomplete masculinization of external genitalia in a person with normal 46 XY karyotype. The condition may go undetected until puberty or adulthood. Causes can include exposure to teratogenic compounds or defects in testosterone biosynthesis or androgen action.

Q56.2 Female pseudohermaphroditism, not elsewhere classified

Female pseudohermaphroditism (FPH) is the masculinization of external genitalia in a person with normal 46 XX karyotype. Ovaries are present and the uterus and fallopian tubes are usually normal; however, the labia are fused and the clitoris is enlarged. FPH is due to exposure of the female fetus to elevated levels of male hormones (primarily testosterone) during gestation. The most common cause is congenital adrenal hyperplasia; however, the condition may also occur with maternal intake or exposure to male hormones, presence of a male-hormone producing tumor in the mother, or an aromatase enzyme deficiency.

Congenital Malformations of the Urinary System (Q60-Q64)

There are a number of congenital malformations that can affect the kidneys, ureters, bladder, and urethra. Malformations of the kidneys include agenesis (absence) of the kidney, small hypoplastic kidney, and cystic kidney disease. The renal pelvis and ureters may be affected by malformations that result in occlusion or obstruction of the flow of urine. There also may be malposition of the ureter in the bladder causing reflux of urine. A congenital diverticulum of the bladder may be present. There may be malposition of the urethral opening, duplication of the urethra, or the presence of posterior urethral valves. These and other congenital malformations of the urinary system are found in this code block.

The categories in this code block are as follows:

Q60	Renal agenesis and other reduction defects of kidney	
Q61	Cystic kidney disease	
Q62	Congenital obstructive defects of renal pelvis and congenital malformations of ureter	

| Q63 | Other congenital malformations of kidney |
| Q64 | Other congenital malformations of urinary system |

Q61.- Cystic kidney disease

Cystic kidney disease may present as single or multiple cysts. In some cases, the cause is unknown but one form, polycystic kidney disease, is an inherited disorder that presents in childhood if it is autosomal-recessive or in adulthood if it is autosomal-dominant.

Q61.01 Congenital single renal cyst

Q61.02 Congenital multiple renal cysts

A congenital renal cyst is present at birth. The condition may affect one or both kidneys as an isolated congenital anomaly or as part of a syndrome. Congenital cysts are usually benign and no treatment is necessary unless they enlarge and cause pain.

Q61.1- Polycystic kidney, infantile type

This type of kidney disease may be referred to as autosomal recessive polycystic kidney disease (ARPKD). It results from a mutation of the PKHD1 gene, which is found on chromosome 6. Presentation varies significantly. Symptoms may manifest prior to birth, at birth, during infancy, or during early childhood. This type of PKD results in multiple cysts in the kidneys, collecting ducts, and liver, leading to failure of both organs. Generally when symptoms occur earlier in life they correlate with more severe kidney and liver disease.

Q61.5 Medullary cystic kidney

Medullary cystic kidney disease (MCKD) is a genetic disorder that prompts cyst formation in the medulla, the inner layer of the kidney. This area contains tubules that help filter blood and produce urine. Secondary to the formation of the cysts, these tubules become damaged and the filtering process malfunctions causing the kidneys to work extra hard to eliminate waste products from the body, which can eventually lead to kidney failure. Nephronophthisis is a similar condition to medullary cystic kidney disease, with almost identical symptoms and kidney damage. Age of onset is the distinguishing factor between these two conditions: nephronophthisis typically occurs before age 20 and MCKD occurs later into adulthood.

Q62.- Congenital obstructive defects of renal pelvis and congenital malformations of ureter

The renal pelvis collects urine and delivers it into the ureters. The ureters then move the urine down into the bladder.

Q62.11 Congenital occlusion of ureteropelvic junction

Congenital obstruction of the ureteropelvic junction is the most common urinary tract anomaly. The condition occurs when the kidney and ureter do not develop normally during gestation and a blockage forms in the area of the renal pelvis and the proximal ureter. The flow of urine from the renal pelvis is obstructed and causes back pressure into the kidney, which may lead to progressive renal damage or dysfunction. Its appearance is associated with other anomalies of the urinary tract, such as horseshoe kidney, ectopic kidney, multicystic, and dysplastic kidney. The condition may be diagnosed antenatally and is corrected within the first few months of life.

Q62.12 Congenital occlusion of ureterovesical orifice

Congenital occlusion of the ureterovesical orifice is a renal anomaly that is present at birth. The obstruction occurs at the junction of the ureter and the bladder. The ureter normally propels urine from the kidney to the bladder with rhythmic muscle action. When the ureter is blocked, the urine backs up causing the ureter and/or the kidney to dilate or swell, a condition called hydronephrosis. This can lead to progressive renal damage or dysfunction. Symptoms include pain in the abdomen, flank, or side and urinary tract infection.

Q62.5 Duplication of ureter

Congenital duplication of the ureter is one of the more common congenital anomalies of the urinary system. There may be two ureters arising from the kidney that join before reaching the bladder (this is called a bifid ureter) or there are two ureters arising from the kidney that each implant separately in the bladder. The condition may occur unilaterally or bilaterally. In some cases, there is also duplication of the kidney on the affected side. Because many individuals are completely asymptomatic, diagnosis is typically made only when complications occur, such as vesicoureteral reflux, ureteral obstruction, ureterocele, or urinary tract infection.

Q63.- Other congenital malformations of kidney

Congenital malformations included here are those that do not fit well into the more specific categories for kidney anomalies.

Q63.1 Lobulated, fused and horseshoe kidney

Horseshoe and discoid kidneys are the products of fusion anomalies. A discoid kidney is fused medially at both poles, while a horseshoe kidney is fused at the lower poles. Horseshoe kidney may be associated with Wilms' tumor and anomalies of a number of body systems.

Q64.- Other congenital malformations of urinary system

Congenital malformations of the bladder and urethra are included here.

Q64.0 Epispadias

This condition is a partial or complete dorsal fusion anomaly of the urethra. It may appear in male and female patients, but is typically seen in males. As a male defect, it is marked by the urethral opening on the dorsal surface of the penis; in females, it appears as a slit in the upper wall of the urethra.

Q64.4 Malformation of urachus

An urachal cyst presents as an extraperitoneal mass near the umbilicus. It may become infected or rupture, possibly causing peritonitis if it drains into the peritoneum rather than through the umbilicus.

Q64.6 Congenital diverticulum of bladder

Congenital diverticulum of the bladder, also known as Hutch diverticulum, is when a portion of the bladder wall protrudes (herniates) through a weakened portion of the bladder muscle. Although often asymptomatic, some instances of bladder diverticulum can lead to urinary tract infections, reflux of urine back up into the ureters, and/or bladder stones.

Congenital Malformations and Deformations of the Musculoskeletal System (Q65-Q79)

This code block classifies congenital malformations and deformations of the bones, muscles, cartilage, fascia, ligaments, synovia, tendons, and bursa.

The categories in this code block are as follows:

Q65	Congenital deformities of hip
Q66	Congenital deformities of feet
Q67	Congenital musculoskeletal deformities of head, face, spine and chest
Q68	Other congenital musculoskeletal deformities
Q69	Polydactyly
Q70	Syndactyly
Q71	Reduction defects of upper limb
Q72	Reduction defects of lower limb
Q73	Reduction defects of unspecified limb
Q74	Other congenital malformations of limb(s)
Q75	Other congenital malformations of skull and face bones
Q76	Congenital malformations of spine and bony thorax
Q77	Osteochondrodysplasia with defects of growth of tubular bones and spine
Q78	Other osteochondrodysplasias
Q79	Congenital malformations of musculoskeletal system, not elsewhere classified

Q65.- Congenital deformities of hip

Dislocation and subluxation of the hip occur in conjunction with ligamentous laxity of the hip joint capsules. Females are affected nine times out of 10 and there is a 30 to 50 percent incidence among breech births. Osteoarthritis, gait abnormalities, pain, and unequal leg length may result if left untreated.

Q65.81 Congenital coxa valga

Q65.82 Congenital coxa vara

The angle between the long axes of the neck and shaft of the femur is 120 to 125 degrees in the normal individual. When this angle is increased, it results in coxa valga. When it is decreased, it results in coxa vara. In coxa valga, this angle is increased to approximately 140 degrees, creating extreme adduction with the possibility of a superior dislocation in the immature hip. In coxa vara, this angle is abnormally decreased, creating an extreme abduction. Coxa vara is much more common than coxa valga.

Q66.- Congenital deformities of feet

There are a number of congenital deformities that can affect the feet causing difficulties with standing and walking.

Q66.0 Congenital talipes equinovarus

Often referred to as club foot, in talipes equinovarus the foot rotates inward. Although it can occur in just one foot, both feet are affected in more than half the patients who are born with this congenital deformity.

Q66.1 Congenital talipes calcaneovarus

This deformity is displayed by toe up position, meaning the foot is flexed with the toes up by the shin and the sole facing out and the foot turned slightly toward the outside of the knee.

Q66.21 Congenital metatarsus primus varus

Metatarsus primus varus is a congenital deviation between the first and second metatarsal bones, where the first metatarsal is angled more toward the midline than the second metatarsal.

Q66.22 Congenital metatarsus adductus

Metatarsus (adductus) varus is a toeing-in deformity where the forefoot bones (metatarsals) angle in toward the midline while the hindfoot bones are in a normal position.

Q66.4 Congenital talipes calcaneovalgus

In talipes calcaneovalgus, the foot deviates up toward the leg; in some cases, the top of the foot is almost in direct contact with the shin. The arch of the foot is often flat and the heel is turned out, away from the body.

Q66.7 Congenital pes cavus

A very high arch is the characteristic presentation of pes cavus or talipes cavus.

Q67.- Congenital musculoskeletal deformities of head, face, spine and chest

Congenital deformities of the head and face are collectively referred to as craniofacial malformations. Also included here are deformities of the spine and chest.

> **Focus Point**
>
> *Some craniofacial malformations are part of syndromes that affect multiple body systems; these syndromes are reported with codes from category Q87.*
>
> *Potter's facies is a congenital facial malformation characterized by deep folds under the eyes. The folds are caused by oligohydramnios related to agenesis of the kidneys, what is collectively known as Potter's syndrome. When documentation supports Potter's facies and/or Potter's syndrome, code Q60.6 should be used.*

Q67.2 Dolichocephaly

Dolichocephaly is a skull that is long in relation to the anterior/posterior axis.

Q67.3 Plagiocephaly

Plagiocephaly is a lopsided and twisted skull.

Q67.6 Pectus excavatum

Pectus excavatum is a congenital chest wall deformity that produces a deep indentation in the chest at the level of the sternum and costal cartilages. The exact cause of pectus excavatum is unknown, although children with a family history of the condition may be more likely to develop it. A mild deformity may be noted at birth and often worsens as the child grows, particularly at puberty. The condition varies in severity from very mild to severe with the chest being so depressed that the sternum nearly touches the spine.

Q67.7 Pectus carinatum

Pectus carinatum is a congenital condition that causes the chest to curve outward like a pigeon's breast. The overgrowth of cartilage and forward buckling onto the sternum and secondary pressures can cause pain, exertional dyspnea, tachypnea, and fatigue, although most children are asymptomatic. The exact cause of pectus carinatum is unknown; children with a family history of the condition may be more likely to develop it. A mild deformity may be noted at birth and often worsens as the child grows, particularly at puberty. The severity of the deformity generally stabilizes as the child reaches adulthood.

Q68.- Other congenital musculoskeletal deformities

Congenital deformities included here are conditions that do not fit well in more specific anatomical categories, such as deformity of the sternocleidomastoid, congenital bowing of the long bones, some deformities of the hand and fingers, and deformities of the knee joint and meniscus.

Q68.0 Congenital deformity of sternocleidomastoid muscle

Sternocleidomastoid torticollis is apparent after birth. Because there are other non-muscular causes of congenital torticollis, the pediatrician must ascertain the cause. If it is muscular, the child should be checked for hip dysplasia, as it is frequently associated with muscular torticollis. Treatment involves daily stretching for the first year of life. If torticollis persists, surgery is necessary to correct the asymmetrical tilt to the face.

Q69.- Polydactyly

Polydactyly is a condition in which there are accessory thumbs, fingers, or toes. The condition may be genetic and may present as a solitary congenital malformation or be a part of a specific syndrome. The accessory (supernumerary) digits may be rudimentary or normally formed.

Q70.- Syndactyly

Syndactyly is a genetically-linked disorder and may appear in conjunction with other syndromes. Syndactyly involves fusion or webbing of the digits and is one of the more common musculoskeletal malformations. Fusion involves the bones of the digits as well as the soft tissues, while webbing involves only the soft tissues. When the webbing occurs in the fingers and is confined to the skin, surgery is generally performed early in childhood to allow normal digit development. The corrective operation involves splitting the webbing and applying skin grafts. When the bones are fused, the situation is more complex and surgery may not be able to provide optimal function, particularly when all five bones are involved.

Q71.- Reduction defects of upper limb

Reduction defects are the incomplete development or formation of all or part of a limb, in this case the upper arm, forearm, hand, and/or fingers. These defects may be due to teratogenic factors or related to congenital amputation of part or the entire upper limb due to constriction by fibrous amniotic bands.

Q71.0- Congenital complete absence of upper limb

Amelia of the upper limb refers to the congenital absence of the entire limb: upper/lower arm, hand, and fingers.

Q71.1- Congenital absence of upper arm and forearm with hand present

This condition is also referred to as phocomelia. In complete phocomelia, the hands are attached to the trunk. In incomplete phocomelia, there may be a rudimentary long bone.

Q71.6- Lobster-claw hand

Lobster-claw hand, a rare disorder, affects the phalanges of the middle finger. The corresponding metacarpal may be absent and the hand is separated into medial and lateral sections by a deep cleft giving the hand the appearance of a lobster-claw.

Q72.- Reduction defects of lower limb

Reduction defects are the incomplete development or formation of all or part of a limb, in this case the thigh, lower leg, foot, and/or toes. These defects may be due to teratogenic factors or related to congenital amputation of part or the entire upper limb due to constriction by fibrous amniotic bands.

Q72.0- Congenital complete absence of lower limb

Amelia of the lower limb refers to the congenital absence of the entire limb: thigh, lower leg, foot, and toes.

Q72.1- Congenital absence of thigh and lower leg with foot present

This condition is also referred to as phocomelia. In complete phocomelia, the feet are attached to the trunk. In incomplete phocomelia, there may be a rudimentary long bone.

Q74.- Other congenital malformations of limb(s)

A variety of congenital malformations of the limbs that do not fit well into more specific categories are classified here.

Q74.0 Other congenital malformations of upper limb(s), including shoulder girdle

Coded to this subcategory are Madelung's deformity and cleidocranial dysostosis. Madelung's deformity is a dysplasia of the radius involving an exaggerated radial inclination, a short forearm, dorsal dislocation of the ulnar head, and a "V" shaped proximal carpal row. The condition may arise from an abnormal fibrous band tethering the sigmoid notch of the radius proximally to the ulna. Cleidocranial dysostosis, or Scheuthauer-Marie-Sainton syndrome, is a genetic disease most often characterized by the absence or hypoplastic development of the collarbone, in association with anomalies of the facial bones, altered tooth eruption patterns, and supernumerary teeth.

Q74.1 Congenital malformation of knee

This code includes genu valgum and genu varum. Genu valgum, also called knock-knee, is an abnormal angling in at the knees. In some cases, it is a normal part of development; however, the condition may require surgical intervention if it persists beyond 10 or 12 years of age and if there are more than three inches between the ankles. Genu varum is an abnormal bowing or angling out at the knees.

Q74.8 Other specified congenital malformations of limb(s)

Larsen's syndrome is included here and is a genetic, multi-system disorder that presents with multiple dislocations and other bony irregularities, as well as cylindrical fingers and unusual facies. Other symptoms include intellectual disabilities, short stature, and cardiac abnormalities.

Q75.- Other congenital malformations of skull and face bones

This category includes congenital malformations of the skull and face bone that do not fit well into more specific categories.

Q75.0 Craniosynostosis

Craniosynostosis is the premature closure of one or more of the cranial sutures resulting in abnormalities of the cranial contour. The cranial sutures are fibrous tissues that connect the skull bones together while still providing the skull bones a finite amount of movement to allow for easier access through the birth canal and to allow the brain to grow within the skull. Typically these sutures do not fuse until an infant is months to years old, depending on the specific sutures. When the cranial sutures fuse prematurely, the brain has to move into areas of the skull that will accommodate its growth. In some cases, the consequence is a misshapen head with possible facial abnormalities but in severe cases, intracranial pressure may be imposed on the brain leading to problems with mental development, visual losses, and other adverse conditions.

Q76.- Congenital malformations of spine and bony thorax

Congenital malformations classified here involve the vertebrae, ribs, and sternum.

Q76.0 Spina bifida occulta

Spina bifida occulta is a benign form of spina bifida where proper formation of one or more of the vertebral segments has not occurred, leaving an opening to which the spinal cord could potentially protrude. However, in this case the opening is so small that the spinal cord stays in place with only minor skin changes, if any, observed in the area of defect, such as abnormal hair growth or an indentation.

Q76.1   Klippel-Feil syndrome

A short neck caused by the fusion of existing cervical vertebrae and the absence of at least one cervical vertebra characterize Klippel-Feil syndrome. It has a high rate of associated malformations or syndromes and affects females.

Q76.3   Congenital scoliosis due to congenital bony malformation

Congenital scoliosis, an anterior/posterior plane vertebral malformation, may appear in three variants. It can be an isolated deformity or be associated with other multisystem deformities. Approximately 2Ø percent of the cases include genitourinary malformations, while another 2Ø percent show coexistent cord defects.

Q76.42- Congenital lordosis

Lordosis is an exaggerated inward curve in the low back.

Q76.5   Cervical rib

A cervical rib is a supernumerary rib in the cervical region, which can lead to thoracic outlet syndrome.

Q78.-   Other osteochondrodysplasias

Osteochondrodysplasia is any abnormality affecting the bones and/or cartilage.

Q78.Ø   Osteogenesis imperfecta

Osteogenesis imperfecta is a genetically inherited disorder that primarily affects bone tissue making the bones extremely fragile and subject to fractures, spontaneously or with only mild trauma. Fractures may even occur prior to birth. Four gene mutations have been identified as the cause of osteogenesis imperfecta, all of which affect the production of a form of collagen that is necessary for the development of healthy bone structure. Osteogenesis imperfecta varies significantly in presentation with eight forms currently identified and classified as Types I to VIII with Type I being the least severe form and Type II the most severe. In the least severe forms, fractures following mild trauma occur in childhood and adolescence. In the most severe forms, spontaneous fractures occur in utero and continue throughout life.

Q78.1   Polyostotic fibrous dysplasia

Polyostotic fibrous dysplasia is a congenital abnormality characterized by replacement of normal healthy bone with fibrous tissue. This condition usually becomes symptomatic in childhood with slow-growing fibrous lesions appearing around the age of 8. The condition usually leads to fractures and deformities of the legs, arms, and skull. Symptoms

include bone pain or tenderness and swelling in affected bones, most commonly in the femur, tibia, pelvis, and foot and less commonly in the ribs, skull, and upper extremities. Polyostotic fibrous dysplasia is associated with Albright-McCune-Sternberg syndrome, which is also classified here. Other symptoms of this syndrome include a pigmentation disorder called café-au-lait and hormonal disturbances resulting in premature sexual development.

Q78.2   Osteopetrosis

Osteopetrosis is a genetically inherited disease characterized by increased bone density. The condition occurs when osteoclasts fail to reabsorb bone, impairing bone modeling and remodeling. Albers-Schonberg syndrome, also called autosomal dominant osteopetrosis (ADO), is the mildest form of osteopetrosis. As this form is often asymptomatic, it is often discovered accidentally during the course of an unrelated illness. More severe forms of osteopetrosis, such as autosomal recessive osteopetrosis (ARO) and intermediate autosomal osteopetrosis (IAO), are symptomatic with the most distinguishing feature being bones that are easily fractured, along with other symptoms that begin in infancy or early childhood.

Q78.6   Multiple congenital exostoses

Multiple congenital exostoses is a condition in which benign bone tumors, called osteochondromas, form in the cartilage at the end of the long bones and on the flat bones due to an autosomal dominant inherited genetic disorder. The condition usually presents by the age of 3 and rarely is newly diagnosed beyond the age of 12. The severity of the condition varies significantly with some individuals having only a few small tumors and others having a severe disabling disease. Symptoms include limb length discrepancies, hip dysplasia, gait disturbances, limited range of motion in the joints, pain from pressure on nerves, blood vessels and/or spinal cord, and premature osteoarthritis. There is an increased risk of developing a bone malignancy later in life.

Q79.-   Congenital malformations of musculoskeletal system, not elsewhere classified

Congenital malformations classified here are primarily those affecting the muscles and tendons.

Q79.2   Exomphalos

An exomphalos, also called an omphalocele, is a congenital defect where intestine or abdominal organs protrude outside of the abdomen through an opening in the abdominal muscles at the umbilicus. The omphalocele is usually covered by the peritoneum, which is a very thin membrane. The size of the omphalocele may vary. It may be small, with only a portion of the intestine protruding outside the abdominal cavity, or large, with the intestine, liver, and spleen protruding outside of the abdominal cavity.

During normal fetal development, the intestines grow more rapidly than the abdominal cavity. Consequently, there is a period of time where there is a portion of the intestines that are outside of the abdomen in a sac within the umbilical cord. Normally, abdominal muscles close before birth but in some infants that does not occur. An omphalocele occurs when the abdominal organs do not return to the abdominal cavity.

Omphalocele

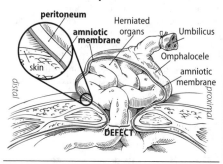

Q79.3   Gastroschisis

Gastroschisis is a congenital abdominal fusion defect that results in herniation of the intestines due to an opening in the abdominal cavity muscles. This defect usually occurs on the right side of the umbilicus. In gastroschisis there is no membrane around the herniated small and large intestines, leaving them exposed to amniotic fluid during development, which can cause them to swell and shorten.

Gastroschisis

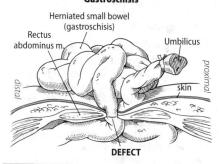

Q79.4   Prune belly syndrome

Prune belly syndrome, also known as Eagle-Barrett syndrome, is named as such due to the prune or wrinkly appearance of the abdominal skin after birth. In general, there are typically three manifestations associated with this syndrome: the absence of the lower rectus abdominis and the medial portions of the oblique muscles, abnormalities or malformations of the urinary tract, and undescended testes.

Q79.6   Ehlers-Danlos syndrome

Ehlers-Danlos syndrome, a genetic collagen disorder, causes hyperelasticity of the skin, hypermobility of the joints, and fragility of blood vessels. Wound healing is impaired.

Other Congenital Malformations (Q80-Q89)

Congenital malformations classified in this code block are those affecting the skin, breast, hair, nails, or multiple tissues; certain syndromes caused by drugs or alcohol; and syndromes affecting multiple body systems.

The categories in this code block are as follows:

Q80	Congenital ichthyosis
Q81	Epidermolysis bullosa
Q82	Other congenital malformations of skin
Q83	Congenital malformations of breast
Q84	Other congenital malformations of integument
Q85	Phakomatoses, not elsewhere classified
Q86	Congenital malformation syndromes due to known exogenous causes, not elsewhere classified
Q87	Other specified congenital malformation syndromes affecting multiple systems
Q89	Other congenital malformations, not elsewhere classified

Q82.-   Other congenital malformations of skin

Congenital malformations of the skin classified here are those that do not fit well into more specific categories.

Q82.0   Hereditary lymphedema

Hereditary lymphedema is a disorder of the lymph drainage system affecting the legs. Infection is a constant threat.

Q82.4   Ectodermal dysplasia (anhidrotic)

Congenital ectodermal dysplasia, or hidrotic ED, is an inherited disorder primarily affecting the French. The nails are thick, there is thick skin on the palms and soles, and dark skin on the elbows and knees.

Q82.5   Congenital non-neoplastic nevus

Included here is port wine stain, or nevus flammeus, a red, flat area on the skin that is present at birth, and which can thicken over time.

Q85.- Phakomatoses, not elsewhere classified

Phakomatoses are congenital malformations composed of multiple tissues that resemble neoplasms.

Q85.0- Neurofibromatosis (nonmalignant)

Neurofibromatosis (NF) is a genetic disorder characterized by abnormal growth of tumors along various nerves. Genetic mutations prevent normal protein synthesis required to control cell production, thereby resulting in uncontrolled cell growth manifesting as tumors. Ongoing clinical research focuses on identifying mechanisms that control key proteins in order to suppress tumor growth. NF tumors arise from the connective and supportive cells that comprise the nerve and myelin sheath, not the impulse-transmitting neurons (nerve cells). The type of cell-supporting tissues involved determines the type of neurofibromatosis. NF has been clinically categorized into three genetically distinct groups: Type 1 (NF1), Type 2 (NF2), and schwannomatosis.

Q85.03 Schwannomatosis

Schwannomatosis is a rare form of NF where patients do not manifest the neurofibromas characteristic of NF1 and NF2 but instead the genetic mutation exclusively affects the cells that make up the myeline sheath (Schwann cells). As a result, multiple tumors develop along cranial, spinal, and peripheral nerves, with the exception being the vestibular nerve. As these patients do not develop vestibular tumors, deafness is not associated with schwannomatosis. Dominant neurological symptoms include paresthesia, weakness, and severe debilitating pain.

Q85.1 Tuberous sclerosis

Tuberous sclerosis promotes benign tumors in the vital organs, as well as in the eyes and skin, and affects both sexes. This condition can cause epileptic seizures and developmental delays and may be referred to as Bourneville's disease, Epiloia, Bourneville-Pringle syndrome, or Pringle's disease.

Q87.- Other specified congenital malformation syndromes affecting multiple systems

There are a number of syndromes that affect multiple body systems and many of these are classified here under a single fairly general code that describes the primary body structures involved.

Q87.0 Congenital malformation syndromes predominantly affecting facial appearance

Apert's syndrome is a congenital malformation syndrome that primarily affects facial appearance. In this syndrome, there is premature fusing of the cranial sutures, asymmetrical facies, webbed hands, and progressive calcification and fusion of the bones of the hands, feet, and cervical spine.

Q87.4- Marfan's syndrome

Marfan's syndrome is caused by an autosomal dominant genetic mutation on the FBNY1 gene that is responsible for instructing a protein (fibrillin-1) to form microfibrils. This leads to overgrowth and instability of the body's connective tissue, affecting the long limbs, fingers, and toes. Characteristic features of the disorder, including skeletal, ocular, and cardiovascular manifestations, may appear in early infancy or not until adulthood.

Q87.410 Marfan's syndrome with aortic dilation

Q87.418 Marfan's syndrome with other cardiovascular manifestations

The mutated fibrillin found in Marfan's syndrome does not bind efficiently to transforming growth factor-beta (TGF-β) in the heart valves and aorta causing it to accumulate in the vascular smooth muscle leading to decreased integrity of the extracellular matrix. In the aorta, particularly the descending aorta, this can lead to dilation (aneurysm). It can also weaken the heart valves, particularly the mitral and aortic valves, leading to mitral valve prolapse and/or aortic valve regurgitation. Typical symptoms with cardiovascular changes include fatigue, shortness of breath, arrhythmias, chest pain (angina), cold hands and feet, and heart murmur.

Q87.42 Marfan's syndrome with ocular manifestations

Ocular manifestations seen in Marfan's syndrome are a result of overgrowth and instability of connective tissues in the eye. Partial lens dislocation is caused by weakness in the ciliary zonules, a type of connective tissue in the eye responsible for suspending and anchoring the lens. Myopia (nearsightedness), retinal detachment, early onset cataract, and open angle glaucoma are also commonly found with Marfan's syndrome.

Q87.43 Marfan's syndrome with skeletal manifestation

Some of the most definitive characteristics of Marfan's syndrome involve the skeletal system. Individuals with Marfan's syndrome are usually tall and thin with long fingers and toes and arm span often exceeds height. Weak wrists, flat feet, and hammer toes are also characteristic features. Distinctive facial features include a narrow face with sharp features and a small jaw. A high palate and crowded teeth are also common. The chest may be deformed manifesting as pectus excavatum or carinatum. There may be spine abnormalities (scoliosis, kyphosis) and abnormal joint flexibility. Symptoms commonly associated with this syndrome include joint and muscle pain, speech problems, early osteoarthritis, and unexplained stretch marks.

Q87.81   Alport syndrome

Alport syndrome is a genetically inherited disorder characterized by progressive loss of kidney function, abnormalities of the inner ear with sensorineural hearing loss, and abnormalities of the eye specifically the lens and retina. Symptoms include hematuria and proteinuria, which are precursors to chronic kidney disease eventually leading to kidney failure. In most cases of Alport syndrome, the mutation occurs on the COL4A5 gene located on the X chromosome in an X-linked inheritance pattern. Because males receive only one copy of the X chromosome, they are more severely affected than females who receive a copy from each parent. Males with the defective gene typically experience kidney failure, hearing loss, and eye conditions while females often experience only hematuria that does not progress to kidney failure. In about 15 percent of cases, mutations occur on the COL4A3 or COL4A4 genes in an autosomal recessive pattern. Both parents must be carriers of these mutations to pass the condition to their children. The autosomal recessive pattern tends to cause less severe kidney disease with basement membrane nephropathy and hematuria being the primary symptoms. In about 5 percent of cases, mutations in COL4A3 or COL4A4 genes express themselves in an autosomal dominant pattern and in this case a defective gene from one parent causes symptoms associated with Alport syndrome. The autosomal dominant mutation may result in all features associated with Alport syndrome or may only cause basement membrane nephropathy.

Q87.82   Arterial tortuosity syndrome

Arterial tortuosity syndrome (ATS) is a rare genetic disorder that affects the connective tissue, the tissue that provides flexibility and strength to structures within the body. The most prominent features of ATS are elongated arteries that become tortuous. The twisting and distortion of the arteries make them more susceptible to stenosis and aneurysm formation, the complications of which are the greatest concern. Aneurysms that have ruptured or arterial dissection can lead to blood loss, and poor blood flow through the stenotic or twisted arteries can lead to heart failure. Although certain surgical interventions have been successful, there is not an established standardized treatment regime, surgical or otherwise, and most treatment efforts focus on symptomatic

relief. Symptoms are often present in body systems outside the circulatory system and can include soft, stretchy skin, hypermobile joints, arachnodactyly, pectus deformities, and contractures.

Q89.-   Other congenital malformations, not elsewhere classified

This category is the catch-all for remaining congenital malformations that are not classified elsewhere. Congenital malformations of the endocrine glands, a malformation called situs inversus that affects the heart and other organs of the thorax and abdomen, and conjoined twins are some of the malformations classified here.

Q89.2   Congenital malformations of other endocrine glands

Included under this code is thyroglossal duct cyst. During embryological development, the thyroglossal duct extends from the tongue base to the thyroid and later disappears during fetal development. When all or a portion of the duct does not disappear, pockets can form in the persistent duct, which can fill with fluid. A mass or lump in the neck may be the extent of the effects on the individual, although there can be associated swallowing or breathing difficulties or increased risk of infection in severe cases.

Q89.3   Situs inversus

Situs inversus (situs inversus totalis) is an autosomal recessive or X-linked congenital genetic disorder characterized by the inverted position of organs in the thoracic and abdominal cavities (mirror image of normal). The heart is located on the right side along with a bilobed lung and a trilobed lung on the left side. The stomach and spleen are located on the right side and the liver and gallbladder on the left side. In the absence of congenital heart defects, the individual is considered to be phenotypically normal. In 5 percent to 10 percent of cases, congenital heart defects are present, most commonly transposition of the great vessels. In 25 percent of cases, situs inversus is accompanied by primary ciliary dyskinesia (PCD) and the condition is referred to as Kartagener syndrome.

Q89.4   Conjoined twins

Conjoined twins are born from a single ovum and a shared single placenta. They are always identical. The incidence is one in every 50,000 to 80,000 births, with the highest incidence in Africa and India. The twins can be joined at various sites, the most common being the thoracopagus arrangement where the twins are joined at the chest and share a heart, followed by omphalopagus, an anterior union at the midtrunk. Most conjoined twins miscarry or are stillborn.

Chromosomal Abnormalities, Not Elsewhere Classified (Q90-Q99)

Chromosomes are divided into two types: autosomes and sex-linked. Of the 23 pairs, only one pair, the 23rd, is related to sex and is distributed as XX in girls and XY in boys. The other 22 pairs are called autosomes. The conditions in this code block involve anomalies in the sex chromosome or autosome arrangements.

The categories in this code block are as follows:

Q90 Down syndrome

Q91 Trisomy 18 and Trisomy 13

Q92 Other trisomies and partial trisomies of the autosomes, not elsewhere classified

Q93 Monosomies and deletions from the autosomes, not elsewhere classified

Q95 Balanced rearrangements and structural markers, not elsewhere classified

Q96 Turner's syndrome

Q97 Other sex chromosome abnormalities, female phenotype, not elsewhere classified

Q98 Other sex chromosome abnormalities, male phenotype, not elsewhere classified

Q99 Other chromosome abnormalities, not elsewhere classified

Q90.- Down syndrome

Down syndrome (DS) is the result of an extra chromosome (trisomy) on the 21st pair of chromosomes. At the time of conception, a fetus normally receives 46 chromosomes, 23 from each parent. In DS, an additional chromosome 21 is produced for a total of 47 chromosomes. This genetic anomaly causes delays in the way a child develops, mentally and physically. Signs and symptoms include a flat hypoplastic face with a short nose, prominent epicanthic skin folds, hearing loss due to the angle of the ear canals, delay in language skills, and some degree of mental retardation. Medical problems and physical characteristics can vary from child to child. Children with DS have a higher risk for developing conditions such as leukemia and Alzheimer's disease, and nearly half of these children have congenital cardiac conditions. The mutation can occur by meiotic nondisjunction (nonmosaicism), mitotic nondisjunction (mosaicism), or by translocation. Trisomy 21 is classified based on how the genetic mutation occurs.

Q90.0 Trisomy 21, nonmosaicism (meiotic nondisjunction)

In nonmosaic trisomy 21 Down syndrome, an extra copy of chromosome 21 is present in all body cells. Either the sperm cell or egg cell contained an extra copy of the chromosome resulting in 47 total chromosomes.

Q90.1 Trisomy 21, mosaicism (mitotic nondisjunction)

In mosaic Trisomy 21 Down syndrome, an extra copy of chromosome 21 is present in some but not all body cells. Characteristics of Down syndrome are milder in mosaicism but common features include dysmorphic facial features, cardiac anomalies, fetal edema (hydrops fetalis), and duodenal atresia.

Q90.2 Trisomy 21, translocation

In translocation Trisomy 21 Down syndrome, part of chromosome 21 attaches to another chromosome during early fetal development. This results in two (normal) copies of chromosome 21 and extra genetic material from chromosome 21 in all body cells.

Q91.- Trisomy 18 and Trisomy 13

Characteristics of Trisomy 18, also known as Edwards syndrome, include delays in growth and the respiratory system, craniofacial malformations, skeletal defects, webbing (clenched fists with overlapping fingers), and intellectual disabilities. There is a high rate of miscarriage (fetal loss) and infants that are carried to term often have intrauterine growth restriction (IUGR), low birth weight, and cardiac (or other organ) defects. Trisomy 13 or Patau's syndrome is a trisomic condition involving the 13th pair of autosomes. The brain's failure to divide into lobes is a primary characteristic of Patau's syndrome affecting the senses of sight, smell, and hearing. Lip and palate (typically cleft) anomalies may be present. Other characteristics of the disorder include severe intellectual disabilities and physical anomalies such as heart defects, spinal cord abnormalities, extra digits (fingers, toes), and small poorly developed eyes (microphthalmia). The physical anomalies often cause miscarriage (fetal loss) and early neonatal death is common when the pregnancy is carried to term.

Q91.0 Trisomy 18, nonmosaicism (meiotic nondisjunction)

Nonmosaic Trisomy 18 is a genetic disorder that is not usually inherited from a parent with Trisomy 18 but occurs as a random event in cell division (nondisjunction) during the formation of egg and sperm reproductive cells. The egg or sperm cell has an extra copy of chromosome 18 and the embryo that forms has 47 chromosomes in all body cells.

Q91.1 Trisomy 18, mosaicism (mitotic nondisjunction)

Mosaic Trisomy 18 is a genetic disorder that is not usually inherited from a parent with Trisomy 18 but occurs as a random event in cell division during early embryonic life. Not all cells have an extra copy of the chromosome. Individuals with Trisomy 18 mosaicism may have no physical features or intellectual impairment or both physical features and intellectual development may be severely affected.

Q91.2 Trisomy 18, translocation

Translocation Trisomy 18 is a genetic disorder that can be inherited from a parent with balanced Trisomy 18 or it may occur as a random event in cell division (nondisjunction) during the formation of egg and sperm reproductive cells or in early embryonic division. The egg and sperm cells have a normal copy of chromosome 18 and an extra part of chromosome 18, usually the q arm, attached to another chromosome. The characteristics of an individual with Trisomy 18 translocation can vary widely depending upon how much genetic material is repeated. Partial q arm translocation is less severe than full q arm translocation, which usually manifests with the same characteristics as nonmosaicism.

Q91.4 Trisomy 13, nonmosaicism (meiotic nondisjunction)

Nonmosaic Trisomy 13 is a genetic disorder that is not usually inherited from a parent with Trisomy 13 but occurs as a random event in cell division (nondisjunction) during the formation of egg and sperm reproductive cells. The egg or sperm cell has an extra copy of chromosome 13 and the embryo that forms has 47 chromosomes in all body cells.

Q91.5 Trisomy 13, mosaicism (mitotic nondisjunction)

Mosaic Trisomy 13 is a genetic disorder that is not usually inherited from a parent with Trisomy 13 but occurs as a random event in cell division during early embryonic life. Not all cells have an extra copy of the chromosome. The severity of symptoms in individuals with Trisomy 13 mosaicism depends on the type and number of cells that contain the extra copy of the chromosome.

Q91.6 Trisomy 13, translocation

Translocation Trisomy 13 is a genetic disorder that can be inherited from a parent with balanced Trisomy 13 or it may occur as a random event in cell division (nondisjunction) during the formation of egg and sperm reproductive cells or in early embryonic division. The egg and sperm cells have a normal copy of chromosome 13 with an extra part of chromosome 13 located on an entirely different chromosome. The characteristics of an individual with Trisomy 13 translocation can vary widely depending upon how much genetic material is repeated.

Q93.- Monosomies and deletions from the autosomes, not elsewhere classified

Normally individuals inherit 23 chromosomes from each parent. These 23 chromosome pairs make up the normal configuration of 46 chromosomes. A monosomy is a condition where one chromosome in a pair is missing. A deletion is when part of a chromosome is missing. Both monosomies and deletions result in birth defects.

Q93.4 Deletion of short arm of chromosome 5

Cri-du-chat syndrome, also called cat's cry syndrome, results from a deletion of the short arm of the fifth chromosome and may vary from a tiny deletion of one band to the entire small arm. Incidence makes it one of the most common autosomal deletions with variability between one in 20,000 to 50,000 births. Children with cri-du-chat present with an abnormally small head (microcephaly), with accompanying small jaw and chin (micrognathia), low set ears, wide set eyes (hypertelorism), and profound or severe intellectual disabilities and psychomotor problems. The identifying characteristic diagnosed in infants is the unusual, high-pitched, cat cry.

Q93.81 Velo-cardio-facial syndrome

Velo-cardio-facial syndrome (VCFS) refers to the palate, the heart, and the face, where the most common, identifying signs and symptoms of this syndrome are often manifested. These manifestations are characterized as cleft palate, heart defects, an elongated face with almond-shaped eyes, a wide nose, and small ears. VCFS is caused by the deletion of genes on a specific part of the 22nd chromosome. There is still great variation in the presentation of this disease—up to 30 different problems have been related to it, including feeding problems, weak immune systems, weak musculature, hypothyroidism, short stature, and scoliosis.

Q93.88 Other microdeletions

Microdeletion, such as Miller-Dieker and Smith-Magenis syndromes, are included here. Miller-Dieker syndrome is seen when there is a deletion from the short arm of chromosome 17, sometimes in combination with duplication of the long arm. Also known as agyria (lack of sulci and gyri) and lissencephaly (smooth surface of the brain), it causes death in infancy or early childhood with an array of problems from the multiple developmental defects and abnormalities of the brain that it produces: retarded mental, speech, and motor development; neurological complications; and multiple abnormalities affecting the kidneys, heart, gastrointestinal tract, and other organs. Smith-Magenis syndrome is also due to a deletion in a certain area of chromosome 17 that results in craniofacial changes, speech delay, hoarse voice, hearing loss in many, and behavioral problems, such as self-destructive head banging, wrist biting, and tearing at nails.

Q96.- Turner's syndrome

Turner's syndrome, also known as XO syndrome, affects females. It is sex chromosome linked, occurring once every 2,500 births. Characteristics include short stature, ovarian dysgenesis, and associated heart, kidney, and thyroid disorders. Growth hormone and estrogen are used to treat the symptoms.

Q98.- Other sex chromosome abnormalities, male phenotype, not elsewhere classified

Phenotype refers to the outward expression of a person's genes combined with environmental factors. In these sex chromosome abnormalities, the outward expression of the person's genotype is male.

Q98.0 Klinefelter syndrome karyotype 47, XXY

Q98.1 Klinefelter syndrome, male with more than two X chromosomes

Q98.3 Other male with 46, XX karyotype

Q98.4 Klinefelter syndrome, unspecified

Klinefelter's syndrome affects only males and involves one or more additional X chromosomes, creating varying patterns of the X and Y chromosomes instead of the normal XY, such as XXY, XX YY, or XXXXY. The signs and symptoms associated with Klinefelter's syndrome vary significantly from one individual to the next; however, in most cases there are physical and cognitive manifestations. Because of the presence of one or more additional X chromosome, there is often a shortage of testosterone that if untreated by testosterone injections at puberty causes breast development and lack of facial hair, as well as infertility. There may be other anomalies of the genitalia affecting the testicles, penis, and the location of the urethra. Learning disabilities are common, as is delayed speech and language development. A risk during adulthood is the development of breast cancer; males with Klinefelter's syndrome have 20 times the risk when compared with non-Klinefelter males and there is also an increased incidence of mediastinal germ cell cancer.

Q99.- Other chromosome abnormalities, not elsewhere classified

A few, very rare chromosome abnormalities are included here.

Q99.0 Chimera 46, XX/46, XY

Chimera 46, XX/46, XY is a very rare genetic condition that can occur in a number of ways such as fusion of two separate oocytes (egg cells) that have been fertilized by two separate sperm cells into a single embryo; fertilization of both an ovum and its polar body; and fertilization of each of two ova contained within a single binucleated follicle. If any of these things occur at fertilization and during the zygote stage of development, the result is that some cells in the body have XY chromosomes and other cells have XX chromosomes from the genetically distinct zygotes. Due to the mix of XX and XY chromosomes in various cells and tissue, the individual may have normal male or normal female genitalia or a mix of both. The condition occurs more commonly with advanced maternal age and medically assisted reproduction.

Q99.1 46, XX true hermaphrodite

This rare genetic condition 46, XX true hermaphrodite is an ovotesticular disorder in which the individual has ovarian follicle tissue and testicular tissue including the presence of seminiferous tubules. A definitive characteristic is the presence of ovaries and testes. Some true hermaphrodites have a unilateral or bilateral fused ovary and testis. Others have an ovary on one side and a testis on the other. Other reproductive organs often present are a uterus, one or two fallopian tubes, a vas deferens, and an epididymis. The appearance of the external genitalia varies greatly and is dependent on the influence of the Y chromosome, although typically the genitalia do not have the normal distinctive male or female characteristics. Breast development and menstruation usually occur at puberty.

Q99.2 Fragile X chromosome

Fragile X chromosome or syndrome is a genetically inherited X-linked dominant disorder characterized by learning disabilities and cognitive impairment. Males are more severely impacted because they have only one X chromosome. The mutation occurs on the FMR1 gene, which instructs a protein called fragile X mental retardation protein (FMRP) that functions in nerve cell synapses and is required for normal brain development. In Fragile X syndrome, the mutation causes a specific segment, called CGG triplet, to repeat in the FMR1 gene more times than it would normally repeat in a person without this mutation. The severity of the condition varies based on how many times the CGG triplet repeats. Individuals with fragile X chromosome may have delayed speech and language acquisition. Both males and females typically have some intellectual impairment but in males this impairment is typically more significant ranging from mild to severe. Mental and behavioral conditions such as anxiety, hyperactivity, attention deficit disorder (ADD), and autism spectrum disorders and neurological disorders such as seizures may also be present. Certain physical characteristics are associated with fragile X and become more pronounced with age, including long narrow face, large ears, prominent forehead and jaw, hyper-flexible joints particularly in the fingers, flat feet, and males may have enlarged testicles after puberty.

Chapter 18: Symptoms, Signs and Abnormal Clinical and Laboratory Findings, Not Elsewhere Classified (RØØ-R99)

This chapter includes symptoms, signs, and abnormal results of laboratory or other investigative procedures, as well as ill-defined conditions for which there are no other, more specific diagnoses classifiable elsewhere.

In general, codes from this chapter are used to report symptoms, signs, and ill-defined conditions that point with equal suspicion to two or more diagnoses or represent important problems in medical care that may affect management of the patient. In addition, this chapter provides codes to classify abnormal findings that are reported without a corresponding definitive diagnosis. Codes for such findings can be located in the Alphabetic Index under such terms as "Abnormal, abnormality, abnormalities," "Decrease, decreased," "Elevation," and "Findings, abnormal, inconclusive, without diagnosis."

Codes from this chapter also are used to report symptoms and signs that existed on initial encounter but proved to be transient and without a specified cause. Also included are provisional diagnoses for patients who fail to return for further investigation, cases referred elsewhere for further investigation before being diagnosed, and cases in which a more definitive diagnosis was not available for other reasons.

Do not assign a code from this chapter when the symptoms, signs, and abnormal findings pertain to a definitive diagnosis. For example, a patient with acute appendicitis would not need additional codes for abdominal pain and abdominal rigidity. These signs and symptoms are integral to acute appendicitis and add no pertinent information regarding the patient's condition and do not alter the course of treatment for acute appendicitis.

However, a code from this chapter may be used to report symptoms, signs, and abnormal findings that pertain to a particular clinical diagnosis if they represent important problems in medical care. Such problems may be useful to record because they may affect length of stay or level of nursing care and/or monitoring. Such problems also may require additional diagnostic or clinical evaluation or may affect treatment plans. In these cases, list the definitive condition as the principal or first-listed diagnosis and the symptoms secondarily.

List as a secondary diagnosis any symptoms, signs, and abnormal findings that are not integral to the principal diagnosis but provide important clinical information. For example, a patient with benign prostatic hypertrophy admitted in acute urinary retention might have acute urinary retention listed as a secondary diagnosis. Acute urinary retention is not integral to the disease process for benign prostatic hypertrophy, and it may alter the course of treatment. Acute urinary retention can be viewed as an "important medical problem" when the medical record documentation shows the need for clinical evaluation or diagnostic procedures to rule out pathology other than benign prostatic hypertrophy as the etiology. Therapeutic treatment may also be affected by the acute urinary retention.

The chapter is broken down into the following code blocks:

RØØ-RØ9	Symptoms and signs involving the circulatory and respiratory systems
R1Ø-R19	Symptoms and signs involving the digestive system and abdomen
R2Ø-R23	Symptoms and signs involving the skin and subcutaneous tissue
R25-R29	Symptoms and signs involving the nervous and musculoskeletal systems
R3Ø-R39	Symptoms and signs involving the genitourinary system
R4Ø-R46	Symptoms and signs involving cognition, perception, emotional state and behavior
R47-R49	Symptoms and signs involving speech and voice
R5Ø-R69	General symptoms and signs
R7Ø-R79	Abnormal findings on examination of blood, without diagnosis
R8Ø-R82	Abnormal findings on examination of urine, without diagnosis
R83-R89	Abnormal findings on examination of other body fluids, substances and tissues, without diagnosis
R9Ø-R94	Abnormal findings on diagnostic imaging and in function studies, without diagnosis
R97	Abnormal tumor markers
R99	Ill-defined and unknown cause of mortality

Symptoms and Signs Involving the Circulatory and Respiratory Systems (R00-R09)

Symptoms associated with the circulatory system may be associated with the conduction system that regulates heart rate, the heart muscle (myocardium) and the strength of muscle contractions, the heart valves, and blood pressure within the blood vessels. Symptoms associated with the respiratory system include the rate, rhythm, and abnormal sounds associated with breathing; levels of oxygen available to the organs and tissues of the body; and respiratory secretions. Pain symptoms centered in the throat and chest are also classified here.

The categories in this code block are as follows:

R00	Abnormalities of heart beat
R01	Cardiac murmurs and other cardiac sounds
R03	Abnormal blood-pressure reading, without diagnosis
R04	Hemorrhage from respiratory passages
R05	Cough
R06	Abnormalities of breathing
R07	Pain in throat and chest
R09	Other symptoms and signs involving the circulatory and respiratory system

R00.- Abnormalities of heart beat

Symptoms classified here are associated with heart rate and rhythm.

R00.0 Tachycardia, unspecified

Tachycardia is a heart rate greater than 100 beats per minute, which is caused by the heart making an effort to deliver more oxygen to the body tissues by increasing the rate at which blood passes through the vessels. Usually the patient complains of palpitations or racing of the heart. Tachycardia may be the result of excitement, exercise, pain, or fever, as well as the use of caffeine and tobacco. However, it may be an early sign of a life-threatening disorder such as cardiogenic or septic shock.

R00.1 Bradycardia, unspecified

A normal heart rate is 60 to 100 beats per minute. Bradycardia is an abnormally slow heart rate. When the heart rate is abnormally slow, it may adversely affect the amount of oxygen-rich blood available to the organs and tissues of the body, although some individuals do not experience any adverse effects from a slow heart rate. Symptoms indicating that a slow heart rate is adversely affecting the availability of oxygen-rich blood to the body include light-headedness, generalized fatigue or fatigue caused by low levels of activity, shortness of breath, chest pains, and mental confusion.

R00.2 Palpitations

Palpitations are described as the feeling that the heart is "fluttering" or "skipping a beat." The sensation can also be described as the heart pounding or racing. The heart's rhythm may be normal or abnormal. Palpitations may be felt in the chest, throat, or neck and generally are very short in duration lasting only a few seconds to minutes. Palpitations may have many triggers, including exercise, anxiety, caffeine drinks, medication, panic attacks, and hyperventilation. Health conditions may also cause palpitations, such as cardiac arrhythmias, anemia, fever, and hyperthyroidism.

R01.- Cardiac murmurs and other cardiac sounds

The heart makes certain sounds as the heart beats and blood moves from one cardiac chamber to another. Abnormal sounds that are heard on auscultation with a stethoscope may indicate an abnormality with the heart, particularly the heart valves, although some abnormal sounds do not impact overall health.

R01.0 Benign and innocent cardiac murmurs

The most common type of heart murmur is a benign, innocent, functional murmur. This is a murmur that is heard in a normal healthy heart. It is a common finding in infants and young children and usually resolves on its own as the child matures.

R03.- Abnormal blood-pressure reading, without diagnosis

Blood pressure measurements are taken to determine the force and amount of blood flowing through the arteries as the heart pumps and also to evaluate the size and flexibility of the arteries. Blood pressure readings can be affected by level of activity, temperature, diet, emotions, medication use, and posture, which is why blood pressure is typically done while sitting with the arm resting at the level of the heart. The systolic reading indicates the highest pressure during contraction of the heart, while the diastolic reading indicates the pressure during the resting phase. A normal reading for an adult should be below 120 (systolic)/80 (diastolic) mmHg. Abnormal blood pressure readings are those that are higher or significantly lower than normal.

R03.0 Elevated blood-pressure reading, without diagnosis of hypertension

Also known as transient hypertension, elevated blood pressure reading without a diagnosis of hypertension is reported only when there is no documented diagnosis of hypertension or when the elevated blood pressure is an isolated incidental finding.

R03.1 Nonspecific low blood-pressure reading

Some individuals normally have and experience no ill-effects from lower than normal blood-pressure. This code is assigned when the blood-pressure reading is lower than normal but does not constitute a health threat to the patient.

R04.- Hemorrhage from respiratory passages

This category is used to report bleeding from the nose, throat, or lungs and blood identified in the sputum from the lungs.

R04.0 Epistaxis

Epistaxis is the medical term for nosebleed. Typically occurring unilaterally, epistaxis may be spontaneous or induced and may occur at any site in the front or back of the nose. Most often bleeding occurs within the anterior-inferior nasal septum (Kiesselbach's plexus) or at the point where the inferior turbinates meet the nasopharynx.

R04.2 Hemoptysis

Hemoptysis is coughing up or spitting out of blood or bloody sputum from the lungs or tracheobronchial tree. Bleeding into the respiratory tract by bronchial or pulmonary vessels causes hemoptysis, which reflects changes in the vascular walls and blood-clotting mechanisms.

R04.8- Hemorrhage from other sites in respiratory passages

This subcategory identifies bleeding from sites other than the nose and throat, and bleeding described as hemoptysis.

R04.81 Acute idiopathic pulmonary hemorrhage in infants

Clinically confirmed acute idiopathic pulmonary hemorrhage in infants (AIPHI) is defined as a pulmonary hemorrhage in a previously healthy infant older than 28 days with no prior history of medical problems that could cause pulmonary hemorrhage. This is a relatively rare condition. AIPHI is characterized by an abrupt onset of bleeding or blood in the airway accompanied by acute respiratory distress or respiratory failure. It is an acute, severe condition requiring hospitalization in a pediatric intensive care unit with intubation or mechanical respiration.

R05 Cough

Coughing is a reflex that clears the throat and lungs and helps the body to heal and protect itself. Coughing is a frequent symptom that generally occurs with an upper respiratory infection, although it can be a sign of a more serious disorder, especially if it is accompanied by difficulty breathing. A cough can be acute or chronic. Acute coughing begins suddenly, usually occurs with an infection, and lasts two to three weeks. Chronic coughing lasts longer than acute coughing. Only a cough for which the underlying cause is not known is reported here.

R06.- Abnormalities of breathing

Abnormalities in breathing include dyspnea (difficulty breathing), abnormal sounds made during inspiration and expiration, respiratory rates that are slower or faster than normal, and respiratory rhythm that is intermittent.

R06.0- Dyspnea

Dyspnea can be defined as breathlessness, shortness of breath, and difficult or labored breathing. Causes typically relate to cardiac or pulmonary issues.

R06.01 Orthopnea

Orthopnea is difficulty breathing when lying down. Patients with orthopnea require elevation of the head to ease difficulty breathing. Orthopnea is a common symptom in people with heart or lung problems.

R06.02 Shortness of breath

Shortness of breath is an inability to take in enough air or oxygen. This can be a result of something simple, such as an upper respiratory infection or strenuous activity, or due to a more serious disease, such as asthma, emphysema, or pneumonia. The exact sensation that accompanies shortness of breath may differ for individuals experiencing this condition, but the sensation is often described as tightness or constriction of the chest or a feeling of suffocation.

R06.1 Stridor

Stridor is a high-pitched sound that occurs during breathing. It is caused by the airway being blocked by an object, swelling of the tissues of the throat or upper airway, or spasm of the airways or the vocal cords. Stridor may be inspiratory, expiratory, and may differ in sound depending on the location of the obstruction. Stridor is usually a symptom of an underlying condition, such as laryngomalacia, subglottic stenosis, vocal cord dysfunction, and subglottic hemangioma. The condition can also be caused by infections, injuries, anaphylaxis, and foreign body aspiration.

R06.2 Wheezing

Wheezing is a high-pitched sound heard while breathing caused by narrowing of breathing passages. The sound often originates from the bronchial tubes but may also be heard in other airways.

R06.3 Periodic breathing

Periodic breathing is an abnormal breathing pattern characterized by changes in respiratory rate and depth of inspiration.

Cheyne-Stokes respiration is a type of periodic breathing where breathing is first shallow and infrequent and then increases gradually to abnormally deep and rapid before fading away completely for about five to 30 seconds. This cycle then repeats itself beginning again with shallow infrequent breaths. Cheyne-Stokes respiration is often accompanied by changes in the level of consciousness; it most commonly occurs in seriously ill patients with brain or heart disorders. It may occur during sleep.

R06.4 Hyperventilation

Hyperventilation is faster than normal breathing that can occur during times of anxiety or panic. Hyperventilation can lead to symptoms of dizziness, dry mouth, and palpitations due to a decreased amount of carbon dioxide in the blood.

R06.6 Hiccough

A hiccough, or hiccups, is repetitive, involuntary, spasmodic contractions of the diaphragm. Hiccups are a symptom not a disease. Hiccups involve the diaphragm (large, thin muscle that separates the chest from the abdomen) and phrenic nerve (nerve that connects the diaphragm to the brain). Hiccups are caused by an irritation of nerves that control breathing muscles, especially the diaphragm. Almost everybody gets hiccups, even a fetus in a mother's womb. There is no known prevention for hiccups. Most episodes of hiccups resolve on their own, although prolonged episodes may require medical or surgical intervention.

R06.8- Other abnormalities of breathing

Hypercapnia, hypoventilation, narcosis, irregular breathing, and even yawning are additional breathing abnormalities that may be captured in this subcategory.

R06.81 Apnea, not elsewhere classified

Apnea is a pause or brief cessation of breathing. Brief pauses may be completely normal; however, extended and frequent pauses in breathing result in an abnormal pattern that can reduce the amount of oxygen entering the body.

R06.82 Tachypnea, not elsewhere classified

Tachypnea is an abnormally rapid respiratory rate with a shallow breathing pattern. Tachypnea can be associated with asthma, chronic obstructive pulmonary disease, or pulmonary embolism.

Focus Point

Neuroendocrine cell hyperplasia of infancy (NEHI), also known as persistent tachypnea of infancy and chronic bronchiolitis, is a diffuse lung disease of children that presents with symptoms of tachypnea, hypoxia, and retractions. Use code J84.841 to report NEHI.

R07.- Pain in throat and chest

Pain in the throat or chest due to an unknown cause or condition is reported here.

R07.1 Chest pain on breathing

Use this code to report chest pain due to painful inhalation, expiration, or both. It may be due to pain in the chest wall (rib cage and sternum), pleura, or accessory muscles of respiration.

R07.2 Precordial pain

Precordial pain is pain felt in the anterior (front) chest wall over the region of the heart. This type of pain is generally felt slightly to the left of the sternum, but may also extend into the surrounding chest wall region.

R07.8- Other chest pain

Included under this subcategory is pain in the chest that may be described as discomfort, pressure, pleuritic, or atypical.

R07.81 Pleurodynia

Pleurodynia is sudden onset attacks of chest pain. The quality of the pain is typically described as severe or lancinating. The severe pain may last for seconds to minutes and is followed by pain resolution for a few minutes or hours and then another more severe pain attack. Pain is usually localized in the lower aspect of the rib cage and is most often unilateral, but pain can also occur over the anterior chest, posterior chest, or in the substernal region. The periodic attacks of severe pain usually occur over three to five days but may continue for as much as a month. A continuous dull aching pain is common between the severe pain attacks. Pleurodynia is often associated with other symptoms of inflammation of the upper respiratory tract, such as rhinitis and pharyngitis, and gastrointestinal symptoms, such as abdominal pain, nausea, vomiting, and diarrhea.

R07.9   Chest pain, unspecified

This code reports discomfort occurring in the chest that cannot be localized to a more specific site, such as the precordial or intercostal region, or to a specific action, such as breathing. Among possible etiologies are acute myocardial infarction, angina, chest trauma, and peptic ulcer disease.

R09.-   Other symptoms and signs involving the circulatory and respiratory system

Symptoms and signs classified here range from life-threatening conditions such as respiratory arrest to more benign symptoms, such as nasal congestion and postnasal drip.

R09.0-   Asphyxia and hypoxemia

Asphyxia is a condition caused by the inadequate intake of oxygen. Hypoxemia is below normal oxygen content in the arterial blood that impairs tissue perfusion. Hypoxia, reported with the same code as hypoxemia, is a reduction in the supply of oxygen reaching tissues and low oxygen levels in the blood from reduced oxygen intake during inspiration. Adequate tissue perfusion by the blood may still be present with hypoxia.

R09.1   Pleurisy

Pleurisy, also called pleuritic chest pain, is inflammation of the pleural membrane that lines the chest cavity and contains the lung. Most cases are caused by infection and many are associated with pneumonia in the underlying lung. Some cases are caused by viral infections or it may occur in other diseases such as tuberculosis, systemic lupus erythematosus, rheumatic fever, and kidney failure. Pleurisy may develop in conjunction with a blood clot on the lung; it may also be associated with the development of fluid in the pleural space between the chest wall and the lung. Sharp pain brought on by breathing and coughing is the most common symptom.

R09.2   Respiratory arrest

This code is used to report a cessation of breathing, which may be primary or secondary. Primary respiratory arrest may be due to airway obstruction, decreased respiratory drive, or respiratory muscle weakness. Secondary respiratory arrest may be a result of cardiac arrest.

R09.8-   Other specified symptoms and signs involving the circulatory and respiratory systems

A majority of the codes in this subcategory identify more benign symptoms related to the circulatory and respiratory system that typically are not life-threatening, such as rales, scratchy throat, and labile blood pressure.

R09.82   Postnasal drip

Postnasal drip is the symptom of excess fluid or mucous dripping down the back of the throat. Patients with postnasal drip may complain of a variety of symptoms, including constant clearing of the throat, excessive swallowing, sore throat, nasal or sinus congestion, chronic cough, bad breath and a sour taste in mouth, and white or yellow coating on the tongue.

R09.89   Other specified symptoms and signs involving the circulatory and respiratory systems

One symptom/sign classified here is abnormal chest sounds. Abnormal chest sounds can be heard in auscultation with a stethoscope. Two common abnormal chest sounds are bruits and rales.

A bruit is a blowing sound heard via a stethoscope during auscultation that is caused by obstructed blood flow within an artery. People with bruits may be at increased risk of myocardial infarction, especially if they have additional risk factors. Diagnosing and treating bruits is dependent on the location and the degree of the underlying stenosis.

Rales are clicking, crackling, or bubbling sounds heard during the inhalation phase of breathing that are believed to occur when air opens the smaller air passages. It is characterized as dry or moist to indicate whether or not fluid is trapped within the airway.

Symptoms and Signs Involving the Digestive System and Abdomen (R10-R19)

The most common symptoms/signs associated with the digestive system and abdomen classified to this code block are pain and nausea and vomiting. Also classified here are symptoms related to swallowing function, gas in the digestive tract, fecal incontinence, and nonspecific abnormalities or symptoms related to the liver and spleen.

The categories in this code block are as follows:

R10	Abdominal and pelvic pain
R11	Nausea and vomiting
R12	Heartburn
R13	Aphagia and dysphagia
R14	Flatulence and related conditions
R15	Fecal incontinence
R16	Hepatomegaly and splenomegaly, not elsewhere classified
R17	Unspecified jaundice
R18	Ascites
R19	Other symptoms and signs involving the digestive system and abdomen

R10.-   Abdominal and pelvic pain

This category classifies localized pain or discomfort affecting the abdominal and pelvic regions. The abdomen contains many organs and pain can come from any one of them. Abdominal pain may be characterized in many different ways. It can be acute (short lived) or chronic (present for a period of weeks or months), dull, sharp, or crampy. Each type of pain and its location in the abdomen may be associated with a different cause. Abdominal pain is commonly caused by infections and often associated with diarrhea and vomiting. It may also be caused by food allergies, food poisoning, excess food ingestion, a reaction to a medication, lactose intolerance, constipation, inflammatory bowel disease, ulcer disease, gastritis, gynecologic problems, or stress.

R10.0   Acute abdomen

Acute abdomen is a sudden, severe bout of abdominal pain that may be accompanied by abdominal rigidity (tense, contracted muscles), guarding (involuntary contraction of muscles), and fever. When abdominal pain comes on suddenly and is severe it requires immediate medical evaluation as this type of pain is often indicative of a serious condition affecting the organs of the digestive tract or genitourinary tract.

R10.8-   Other abdominal pain

Codes in this subcategory classify tenderness of the abdomen, colic, and generalized abdominal pain.

R10.81-   Abdominal tenderness

The feeling of pain when pressure is applied to the abdominal wall is referred to as abdominal tenderness. Pressure applied in the left lower abdomen but felt in the right lower abdomen is called Rovsing's sign and can indicate appendicitis. Additional diagnostic signs of appendicitis are pain upon pressure to McBurney's point, which is in the lower right abdomen over the cecum, or referred pain in the epigastric area.

R10.82-   Rebound abdominal tenderness

Pain felt upon the removal of pressure on the abdomen instead of the application of pressure is considered rebound abdominal tenderness. This type of pain, also referred to as Blumberg's sign, can suggest peritonitis.

R10.83   Colic

Colic is a common condition seen in infants that is characterized by periods of crying and distress. A general definition is crying for more than three hours a day, three or more days a week, and for more than three weeks in an otherwise well-fed, healthy baby. Colic is associated with intense, inconsolable crying that occurs in predictable episodes—nearly the same time every day, typically late afternoon or evening. The duration of these episodes may range from a few minutes to three hours or more. Posture changes are common in colic episodes. The infant appear tenses with a rigid abdomen, clenched fists, or curled-up legs. Colic generally affects newborns and infants between 3 and 12 weeks of age. Although it is distressing to parents, it is a benign condition and typically ends by nine months of age. The underlying cause is largely unknown, yet is thought to include allergies, lactose intolerance, immature digestive system, or other environmental stressors. In an otherwise healthy baby in whom underlying pathology has been ruled out, colic is treated palliatively and the focus is on soothing the baby and providing support to the parents.

R11.-   Nausea and vomiting

Nausea and vomiting are nonspecific complaints with many possible causal conditions.

R11.0   Nausea

Nausea is an unsettled feeling in the stomach.

R11.1-   Vomiting

Vomiting (emesis) is voluntary or involuntary forceful expulsion of the contents of the stomach, which may include undigested food, mucus, or bile. Certain types of vomiting can be indicative of very serious conditions, requiring a more extensive evaluation.

R11.14   Bilious vomiting

Bilious vomiting refers to emesis, which contains bile that has been regurgitated from the duodenum, usually indicating ileus or obstruction distal to the junction of the duodenum and common bile duct.

R12   Heartburn

Heartburn is a burning sensation in the throat or chest. The burning is due to stomach acid that backs up into the esophagus. Heartburn that occurs more frequently than twice a week may be an indication of gastroesophageal reflux disease (GERD). Heartburn can also occur during pregnancy or be brought on by certain foods and/or medications.

R13.-   Aphagia and dysphagia

Aphagia and dysphagia are symptoms related to the swallowing function.

R13.1-   Dysphagia

Dysphagia is difficulty in swallowing. Since dysphagia is a dynamic disorder, the symptoms vary significantly depending on the affected phase of swallow. Swallowing is divided into four phases: oral, oropharyngeal, pharyngeal, and pharyngoesophageal. Dysphagia is classified based on which phase the swallowing difficulty occurs.

Swallowing Phases

Oral phase

Oropharyngeal phase

Pharyngeal phase

Pharyngoesophageal phase

R13.11 Dysphagia, oral phase

Oral-phase dysphagia typically results from impaired tongue control. It affects sucking, chewing, and moving food or liquid to the throat (pharynx) where it can be swallowed.

R13.12 Dysphagia, oropharyngeal phase

The oropharynx is the middle region of the throat that begins just below the soft palate and extends to the superior aspect of the epiglottis and is involved in voluntary and involuntary swallowing functions. Dysphagia at the oropharyngeal phase may involve the inability to initiate swallowing, the inability of pharyngeal muscles to propel food through the oropharyngeal region, or the inability to close the epiglottis and prevent food or liquids from entering the esophagus.

R13.13 Dysphagia, pharyngeal phase

Dysphagia that occurs at the pharyngeal phase primarily involves the distal third of the pharynx (laryngopharynx), which is located below the superior aspect of the epiglottis and extends to the pharyngoesophageal junction. The pharyngeal phase involves involuntary swallowing functions including closure of the epiglottis, pharyngeal muscle contraction, and relaxation of the sphincter between the pharynx and esophagus to allow passage of the bolus into the esophagus.

R13.14 Dysphagia, pharyngoesophageal phase

Impairment of esophageal function may cause food and liquid to be retained in the esophagus after swallowing. This can result from mechanical obstruction, motility disorder, or impaired opening of the lower esophageal sphincter. Pharyngoesophageal phase dysphagia is the most common symptom of esophageal disorders, and dysphagia localized to this region is subclassified as phase one, two, or three.

Phase one of pharyngoesophageal dysphagia is the transfer phase and typically results from a neuromuscular disorder. The transport phase is phase two and is often caused by esophageal spasm or carcinoma. Phase three is the entrance phase and typically results from lower esophageal narrowing by diverticula, esophagitis, and other disorders.

R14.- Flatulence and related conditions

This category includes codes for abdominal pain, distension or bloating due to excess gas, flatulence described as emission of excess of gas in the stomach or intestines through the anus, and eructation, which means belching or burping.

R15.- Fecal incontinence

Fecal incontinence is the inability to control bowel movements, resulting in stool leakage from the rectum with subsequent soiling. Normal defecation requires physical and mental capability to respond to the urge to pass stool. Therefore, persons with mental or cognitive disorders, mobility problems, paralysis, or other muscle or nervous system damage or disease may be at risk for fecal incontinence. Causation may include rectocele, rectal muscle damage, bowel cancer, hemorrhoids, anal sphincter dysfunction, childbirth trauma, chronic constipation, or nerve damage due to injury or neurological disease.

R16.- Hepatomegaly and splenomegaly, not elsewhere classified

Hepatomegaly is an enlargement of the liver and splenomegaly is enlargement of the spleen. Both of these symptoms can be caused by a number of conditions and often prompt further clinical workup.

R17 Unspecified jaundice

Jaundice is a yellow discoloration of the skin and/or mucous membranes due to excessive levels of bilirubin in the blood. Pruritus, dark urine, and clay-colored stools commonly accompany jaundice. Etiologies for jaundice include congestive heart failure, carcinoma of the papilla of Vater or pancreas, cholecystitis and cholelithiasis, Kaye or Byler cholestasis, Laennec's or primary cirrhosis of the liver, liver abscess, hepatitis, acute or chronic pancreatitis, Dubin-Johnson syndrome, hemolytic anemia, glucose-6-phosphate dehydrogenase (G6PD) deficiency, and drug-induced hepatic insult.

R18.- Ascites

Ascites is accumulation of serous fluid in the peritoneal cavity. Signs and symptoms of ascites include abdominal discomfort, distention, and dyspnea. On examination, abdominal percussion transmits a fluid wave and reveals shifting dullness. Ascites is classified based on whether the condition is due to a malignant neoplasm or whether it is due to another disease process.

R18.Ø   Malignant ascites

Malignant ascites is caused by the presence of cells from a malignant neoplasm in the peritoneal cavity and is most often seen in patients with primary ovarian, endometrial, breast, colon, gastric, and pancreatic cancer with metastases to the peritoneum. Management of malignant ascites can include systemic chemotherapy, instillation of radioisotopes or chemotherapeutic drugs into the peritoneal cavity, and peritoneal-venous shunting procedures.

R18.8   Other ascites

Ascites due to conditions other than malignancy are classified here. Associated nonmalignant conditions include chronic or subacute liver disease (most commonly cirrhosis from alcoholism), chronic active hepatitis, severe alcoholic hepatitis without cirrhosis, hepatic vein obstruction, systemic disease (heart failure, nephrotic syndrome), and tubercular peritonitis.

R19.-   Other symptoms and signs involving the digestive system and abdomen

General symptoms in the abdominal region include generalized swelling, mass or lumps felt on palpation, abnormal bowel sounds heard on auscultation with a stethoscope, abdominal rigidity, and changes in bowel function.

R19.2   Visible peristalsis

Peristalsis is the muscular contractions along the digestive tract that move the food downward from esophagus to rectum. Certain conditions, such as obstructions, may increase the strength and frequency of peristaltic waves, making them more visible across the abdomen. This is also referred to as hyperperistalsis.

R19.6   Halitosis

Halitosis, also referred to as fetor oris, is a medical term for bad breath, which is most commonly caused by poor dental hygiene but can be symptomatic of other disease processes such as infection, gastroesophageal reflux disease (GERD), liver failure, or even some cancers.

R19.7   Diarrhea, unspecified

Diarrhea is an increase in the number of stools per day and/or an increase in the looseness of stools (usually more than three times in one day). Diarrhea commonly is associated with cramps, bloating, nausea, and a sense of urgency to have a bowel movement. Acute diarrhea typically lasts no more than one week and generally is a self-limited problem. Most cases do not require treatment. While diarrhea can be caused by a variety of pathogens and conditions including bacteria, viruses or parasites, certain medicines (e.g.,

antibiotics), food intolerances, food poisoning, food allergies, stress, and diseases that affect the stomach, small intestine, or colon, in many cases, the cause is unknown.

Symptoms and Signs Involving the Skin and Subcutaneous Tissue (R2Ø-R23)

Symptoms and signs affecting the skin and subcutaneous tissue that do not point to a specific diagnosis are included here.

The categories in this code block are as follows:

R2Ø	Disturbances of skin sensation
R21	Rash and other nonspecific skin eruption
R22	Localized swelling, mass and lump of skin and subcutaneous tissue
R23	Other skin changes

R2Ø.-   Disturbances of skin sensation

This category describes various skin sensations such as anesthesia, hypoesthesia, and paraesthesia.

R2Ø.Ø   Anesthesia of skin

Anesthesia of skin is described as a numbness or lack of feeling.

R2Ø.1   Hypoesthesia of skin

Hypoesthesia is a reduced sensation of touch.

R2Ø.2   Paresthesia of skin

Paresthesia is the sensation of "pins and needles" or falling asleep.

R2Ø.3   Hyperesthesia

Hyperesthesia is an increased sensation of touch.

R23.-   Other skin changes

Conditions classified here include changes in the color of the skin and skin texture.

R23.Ø   Cyanosis

Cyanosis is a bluish discoloration of the skin and mucous membranes caused by low oxygen levels in the blood.

R23.3   Spontaneous ecchymoses

Ecchymosis is a purplish, flat bruise that occurs when blood leaks out into the top layers of skin; the bruise is not raised but may be irregular in shape. Spontaneous ecchymosis is often a symptom of a coagulation disorder.

Symptoms and Signs Involving the Nervous and Musculoskeletal Systems (R25-R29)

Common symptoms and signs classified here relate to abnormal movement that may be involuntary or voluntary, lack of coordination, and weakness that are associated with disorders of the nervous or musculoskeletal system.

The categories in this code block are as follows:

R25	Abnormal involuntary movements
R26	Abnormalities of gait and mobility
R27	Other lack of coordination
R29	Other symptoms and signs involving the nervous and musculoskeletal systems

R25.-   Abnormal involuntary movements

Conditions classified to codes in this category of abnormal involuntary movements (AIMs) are also referred to as dyskinesias and include only those that do not have a specific diagnosis or cause. Uncontrollable abnormal head movement, unspecified tremors, and cramps or spasms not found elsewhere are included. Fasciculation, or twitching, is also classified here. Fasciculations are generally weak, rapid movements of muscle fibers that are visible to the clinician. They commonly affect the eyelid muscles of normal, healthy individuals.

Focus Point

Unspecified tremors are included in this category. Note that codes for essential or intention tremors are located in the Diseases of the Central Nervous System chapter and hysterical tremor is found in the Mental, Behavioral and Neurodevelopmental Disorders chapter.

R26.-   Abnormalities of gait and mobility

Gait abnormalities include paralytic or ataxic. Paralytic gait, also referred to as spastic or crisscrossing gait, presents as stiffness, extension or adduction, and bilateral scissoring. Ataxic or staggering gait is characterized by wide stance, staggering, or hesitation.

Difficulty in walking, dysbasia, unsteadiness on feet, and imbalance are other gait or mobility issues that can be classified to this category.

R27.-   Other lack of coordination

This category includes ataxia that is not specified as ataxic gait or caused by vertigo, CVA, or hereditary conditions or for which no other diagnosis classified elsewhere has been assigned. Ataxia is a lack of coordination, balance, or movement that is controlled by the nervous system. Ataxia can be due to injuries, infections, or degeneration of the nervous system.

Focus Point

The ICD-10-CM alphabetic index should be consulted before reporting a code from category R27 as many types and forms of ataxia are specified using codes from other chapters.

R29.-   Other symptoms and signs involving the nervous and musculoskeletal systems

Symptoms and signs classified here involve some types of muscle contractions and muscle weakness, abnormal sounds, such as clicking hip that may indicate a joint condition, transient paralysis, repeated falls, as well as others.

R29.0   Tetany

Tetany is a type of cramp that causes the muscles of the hands and feet to cramp rhythmically. It may also manifest as spasms of the larynx that may be accompanied by difficulty in breathing, nausea, vomiting, convulsions, and considerable pain. Tetany often stems from a mineral imbalance, such as a lack of calcium, potassium, or magnesium, or an acid or alkaline condition of the body.

R29.7-   National Institutes of Health Stroke Scale (NIHSS) score

The National Institutes of Health Stroke Scale (NIHSS) is used to evaluate neurologic outcome and degree of recovery for patients with strokes. It was designed by a group of stroke research neurologists to document the baseline severity of neurologic deficits in acute stroke patients and assesses 11 items—consciousness, horizontal eye movement, vision-field loss, facial palsy, leg and arm motor function (i.e. drift), limb coordination (ataxia), sensory loss, language and speech deficits, and finally extinction/inattention. The scores (and corresponding codes) range from 0 to 42, with 42 being the highest severity stroke. Studies have demonstrated that the NIHSS can reliably represent stroke severity and can also help identify clinical findings that may indicate complications, such as dysphagia following dysarthria and facial weakness. The patient is assessed and assigned points for each item, which are then added together to determine the final score. The following is a general classification of the stroke severity based on the final score:

0	No symptoms of stroke
1-4	Mild stroke
5-15	Moderate stroke
16-20	Moderate-severe stroke
21-42	Severe stroke

In addition, the scale may also be useful in predicting stroke outcomes and helping neurologic researchers assess the efficacy of certain stroke treatments. For example, 80 percent of stroke survivors with scores of less than 5 are discharged home, while those with scores of between 6 and 13 typically require acute inpatient rehabilitation, and those with scores greater than 14 frequently require long-term skilled care.

Symptoms and Signs Involving the Genitourinary System (R30-R39)

Most of the symptoms and signs included here relate to the process of urination. Symptoms such as pain, blood in the urine, urinary retention, passing urine in smaller or larger amounts than expected, and other difficulties related to the passage of urine are all classified here.

The categories in this code block are as follows:

R30	Pain associated with micturition
R31	Hematuria
R32	Unspecified urinary incontinence
R33	Retention of urine
R34	Anuria and oliguria
R35	Polyuria
R36	Urethral discharge
R37	Sexual dysfunction, unspecified
R39	Other and unspecified symptoms and signs involving the genitourinary system

R30.- Pain associated with micturition

Micturition is simply the passage of urine and conditions classified here relate to pain during the passage of urine.

R30.0 Dysuria

Dysuria is pain or a burning sensation during urination. Dysuria is commonly caused by bacterial infections of the urinary tract. It can also be a symptom of other conditions, including cystitis, pyelonephritis, urethritis, vaginitis, and vulvovaginitis.

R30.1 Vesical tenesmus

Vesical tenesmus is the feeling the bladder is full even when there is little or no urine in the bladder. This may be caused by irritation or inflammation of the bladder wall or external pressure on the bladder from other organs or structures in the lower abdomen. Vesical tenesmus may or may not be accompanied by pain.

R31.- Hematuria

Hematuria is the presence of blood in the urine.

R31.0 Gross hematuria

Gross hematuria identifies blood in the urine that is visible to the human eye.

R31.1 Benign essential microscopic hematuria

This condition, also referred to as benign familial hematuria, begins in childhood. The primary finding is the presence of red blood cells in the urine, typically present only in small amounts that are not visible to the human eye. The urine may have a cloudy appearance. Benign essential microscopic hematuria is associated with abnormalities in the glomeruli, which are the small clusters of blood vessels that filter the blood passing through the kidneys. The membrane that supports the glomeruli is abnormally thin allowing passage of small numbers of red blood cells into the urine. This condition is typically caused by an inherited genetic trait.

R31.2- Other microscopic hematuria

Microscopic hematuria is blood in the urine that is not visible to the human eye.

R32 Unspecified urinary incontinence

Urinary incontinence, also referred to as enuresis, is the involuntary loss of urine after the age at which bladder control should have been established.

R33.- Retention of urine

Retention of urine is the accumulation of urine in the bladder due to the inability to void.

R34 Anuria and oliguria

Normal urine output per day is approximately one to two liters. Oliguria is a diminished urinary output of less than 400 ml in a 24-hour period that can be related to dehydration, obstructions, hypovolemic shock, impaired renal function, or other conditions. Anuria or absence of urine is extreme oliguria with less than 100 ml per day of urinary secretion.

R35.- Polyuria

Polyuria is a condition in which large amounts of urine are produced with an increase in urinary frequency. Polyuria may be accompanied with thirst and these two symptoms are common first signs of diabetes.

R35.0 Frequency of micturition

Urinary frequency is the need to urinate many times during the day but in normal or less than normal volumes.

R35.1 Nocturia

Nocturia is the need to urinate many times during the night. It commonly occurs as a result of aging but may also signify the presence of another underlying condition such as infection, diabetes, and cancer of the bladder or prostate.

R36.-   Urethral discharge

Urethral discharge includes any abnormal fluid loss from the urethra that is not urine or semen or semen fluid that is not normal. It is most often related to an infection, such as urethritis, or to a sexually transmitted disease.

R36.0   Urethral discharge without blood

Urethral or penile discharge without blood in males is often a sign of a sexually transmitted disease.

R36.1   Hematospermia

Hematospermia means there is blood in the semen and is a common and generally self-limited condition of unknown cause.

R39.-   Other and unspecified symptoms and signs involving the genitourinary system

Most of the symptoms and signs classified here relate to urination (micturition), such as hesitancy, weak or splitting of stream, urgency, straining, or the feeling of incomplete bladder emptying.

R39.0   Extravasation of urine

Extravasation of urine is where a defect or injury in the urethra allows urine to exit the urethra into other cavities in the body, including the penis, scrotum, and lower abdominal wall.

R39.1-   Other difficulties with micturition

Micturition disorders involve problems related to either bladder storage function or urine elimination function. Many of these disorders are considered lower urinary tract symptoms (LUTS). LUTS are commonly associated with various types of obstructive uropathies. However, these symptoms can herald various other possible etiologies depending on other clinical factors. Symptoms in this subcategory include hesitancy of micturition, straining or urgency of urination, poor or splitting of urinary stream, and the feeling of incomplete bladder emptying, in addition to other symptoms. In male patients, LUTS including both urinary hesitancy and straining on urination are common symptoms associated with an enlarged prostate, bladder outlet obstruction (BOO), calculi, and other obstructive or functional uropathies. In female patients, LUTS can be due to conditions such as hormonal changes, reduction or loss of estrogen, obstructive pelvic mass, inverted uterus, cystocele, urethral diverticulum, or neuromuscular disease.

R39.19-   Other difficulties with micturition

Codes in this subcategory of voiding dysfunction (VD) symptoms are further divided based on the need to immediately re-void or micturition (urination) that is position-dependent.

R39.191   Need to immediately re-void

The sensation that the bladder is not empty after micturition is a common symptom of voiding dysfunction (VD) along with many other voiding symptoms. All of these symptoms can coexist, making diagnosing the cause of dysfunction difficult.

R39.192   Position dependent micturition

This voiding dysfunction (VD) symptom is described as having to be in a specific position to micturate and adequately empty the bladder. This can coexist along with many other voiding symptoms, making diagnosing the cause of dysfunction difficult.

R39.8-   Other symptoms and signs involving the genitourinary system

Incontinence related to cognitive function, passage of air with urine (pneumaturia), and urethral pain (urethralgia) are a few conditions classified to this subcategory.

R39.81   Functional urinary incontinence

Functional urinary incontinence (FUI) is leakage of urine related to impairment of cognitive functioning or other disability that inhibits the control of bladder function. FUI may be a temporary or permanent condition depending on the underlying cause and contributing factors. Patients with FUI may suffer constant leaking of urine, the inability to hold urine, and impairment of sensation related to urination. FUI is common among the elderly population, particularly those who suffer from dementia or mobility issues. Precipitating causes include stroke, neurological deficits (Parkinson's, Alzheimer's), severe depression, and effects of medication or musculoskeletal deconditioning due to aging. This type of incontinence varies in progression, approaches to treatment, and expected outcomes, which are linked to underlying causal conditions.

R39.82   Chronic bladder pain

Chronic bladder pain, or painful bladder syndrome, typically includes recurrent discomfort and pain in the bladder and surrounding pelvic areas. It can include many symptoms and range in intensity from mild discomfort, tenderness, or pressure, to frequency, urgency, and major debilitating pelvic pain. This pain may change during or before urination, and in women it may increase during the menstrual period. Diagnosis is made based on ruling out other conditions such as urinary tract infections, bladder stones, interstitial cystitis, and malignancy. Cystoscopy or urodynamic studies may be performed to aid in diagnosis.

R39.83 Unilateral non-palpable testicle

R39.84 Bilateral non-palpable testicles

In certain cases one or both testicles may not be located or palpated and may appear to be missing. These codes are reported when one or both testicles cannot be felt (palpated) and no diagnosis has been determined. A patient may require further evaluation to determine the location and presence/absence of that testicle.

Focus Point

Codes for signs and symptoms may be assigned when a definitive diagnosis has not been established. If a patient is found to have an undescended or ectopic (in an abnormal place or position) testicle, report the appropriate code from category Q53 Undescended and ectopic testicle, depending on the location.

Symptoms and Signs Involving Cognition, Perception, Emotional State and Behavior (R40-R46)

Symptoms and signs included in this code block relate to impaired consciousness due to dysfunction of the cerebral hemispheres, the upper brainstem, or both. These codes include coma, transient alteration of awareness, persistent vegetative state, and other alterations in cognition or perception such as drowsiness, somnolence, stupor, or suppressed or impaired awareness or unconsciousness. Symptoms and signs related to general sensations and perceptions include those related to vision, hearing, smell, and taste. Emotional symptoms and signs include conditions such as nervousness, anger, hostility, low self-esteem, emotional lability, and other conditions that may be indicative of a mental health disorder that requires additional work-up before a definitive diagnosis can be determined.

The categories in this code block are as follows:

R40	Somnolence, stupor and coma
R41	Other symptoms and signs involving cognitive functions and awareness
R42	Dizziness and giddiness
R43	Disturbances of smell and taste
R44	Other symptoms and signs involving general sensations and perceptions
R45	Symptoms and signs involving emotional state
R46	Symptoms and signs involving appearance and behavior

R40.- Somnolence, stupor and coma

Somnolence, stupor, and coma are symptoms and signs that all relate to a level of consciousness.

R40.2- Coma

Coma is a state of profound stupor or unconsciousness from which the patient cannot be aroused by external stimuli. The etiology may be trauma, intracranial neoplasm, infection and toxic reaction to infection, poisoning and adverse effects of drugs and chemicals, hypertensive and atherosclerotic cerebrovascular disease, or thrombosis.

R40.20 Unspecified coma

This code is used when detailed information about the coma, such as specific coma scale scores, is unknown.

R40.21- Coma scale, eyes open

R40.211- Coma scale, eyes open, never

R40.212- Coma scale, eyes open, to pain

R40.213- Coma scale, eyes open, to sound

R40.214- Coma scale, eyes open, spontaneous

R40.22- Coma scale, best verbal response

R40.221- Coma scale, best verbal response, none

R40.222- Coma scale, best verbal response, incomprehensible words

R40.223- Coma scale, best verbal response, inappropriate words

R40.224- Coma scale, best verbal response, confused conversation

R40.225- Coma scale, best verbal response, oriented

R40.23- Coma scale, best motor response

R40.231- Coma scale, best motor response, none

R40.232- Coma scale, best motor response, extension

R40.233- Coma scale, best motor response, abnormal

R40.234- Coma scale, best motor response, flexion withdrawal

R40.235- Coma scale, best motor response, localizes pain

R40.236- Coma scale, best motor response, obeys commands

Code classifications for coma have been expanded to reflect clinical severity in accordance with the Glasgow clinical coma scaling used in assessing trauma. One code from each R40.2- subcategory—eyes open, best verbal response, and best motor response—is required to report coma. Instructional notations have been included to direct the coder to sequence first the associated trauma or fracture. It is appropriate to determine the Glasgow coma score based on prehospital reports and EMT and other nonphysician documentation. If the score is broken into categories such as E3V3M4 = GCS 10 (Eyes 3 Verbal 3 Motor 4 = Glasgow coma scale total score 10), then the individual scores can be used, on the condition that all three categories were documented at the same time during the same encounter. If a score of 3 is given for the eye category, the appropriate code would then be the third code in the eye category – R40.213 – coma scale, eyes open, to sound. To be a valid code, the seventh character must be added to identify the encounter. Seventh characters describe the point in time during the health care encounter that the coma scale was recorded. These seventh characters must match for all three subcategory R40.2- codes.

Focus Point

In addition to the narratives provided within the codes, instructional notes are provided specifically for pediatric verbal and motor response. These descriptions are differentiated by age – one for two through five years of age and another for under two years old. These descriptors use sounds, words, and movements more appropriate to the pediatric population such as cooing, screaming, grunting, crying, and others.

R40.24- Glasgow coma scale, total score

Total scores for coma severity range from 3 (worst) to 15 (best) based on points assigned in three different categories: eyes open response (1 to 4 points), best verbal response (1 to 5 points), and best motor response (1 to 6 points). A total score code is only used when the total score is documented and the three individual scores are not documented or only partially documented.

R40.244- Other coma, without documented Glasgow coma scale score, or with partial score reported

Report this code when there is incomplete documentation of the Glasgow coma scale scores and/ or the total score is not documented.

R40.4 Transient alteration of awareness

Transient alteration of awareness refers to a temporary lack of mental presence and/or the inability to recall events or actions for a period of time. The ability to perform some routine tasks may not be impaired during the alteration of awareness, but the ability to recall the episode and memory related to the event is often impaired. Transient alteration of awareness may be caused by a variety of conditions, such as a nonconvulsive seizure disorder or temporary reduced blood flow to the brain, but until the cause is determined, the most appropriate diagnosis is the symptom.

R41.- Other symptoms and signs involving cognitive functions and awareness

Cognition refers to all mental activities related to thinking. Symptoms and signs related to cognition may affect the ability to understand, learn, or remember things.

R41.8- Other symptoms and signs involving cognitive functions and awareness

The term "cognitive deficits" is a general, inclusive term used to describe symptoms associated with a variety of thought processes, including perception, memory, learning, concentration, attention, communication, and executive function. Multiple underlying conditions can cause cognitive deficits, including metabolic disorders, poisoning, toxic exposures, neoplasm, circulatory disease (e.g., stroke), neurologic disease (e.g., multiple sclerosis), mental disorders (e.g., depression), anoxia, and adverse effects of medications. The most common causes of cognitive impairments include senile or age-related decline (e.g., memory loss, dementia) and those due to traumatic brain injury. Depending on the underlying cause, cognitive deficits may develop over variable time periods. Presentation varies in severity.

R41.81 Age-related cognitive decline

Age-related cognitive decline is not considered a dementia, but a normal part of the aging process. All humans, as they age, develop some degree of cognitive decline with slower processing of information and mild forgetfulness. As the brain ages, there is often a decrease in volume and loss of neurons. The extent of decline is not the same for all, with the rate and severity linked to many factors, including amount of chronic low-level inflammation, declining hormone levels, excess body weight, inadequate nutrition, poor lifestyle habits, social network, and chronic medical conditions. Not all factors are yet fully understood, but progress is being made through a variety of research studies.

R41.82 Altered mental status, unspecified

Significant changes in mental status can occur without the patient losing consciousness. These changes often include various degrees of cognitive impairment. Many conditions initially manifest with a change in mental status as the primary symptom. Depending on the age and general health of the patient, there are a wide variety of potential underlying causes of this symptom. In pediatric populations, neurological disorders, trauma, shock, metabolic disorders, poisoning, and CNS infections are most common. In the elderly, mental status changes are common effects of medication, electrolyte imbalances, or infection.

A change in mental status is most often noticed by family or caregivers, with the patient unaware or reluctant to seek care. Altered mental status is reportable when it cannot be attributed to an underlying cause, or if there is no other diagnosis or condition for which mental status changes are an integral part of the disease process.

R42   Dizziness and giddiness

The term dizziness is often used interchangeably with lightheadedness and vertigo, which may also be described as a feeling of losing one's balance, an illusion of movement, or a feeling of unsteadiness. Dizziness usually resolves by itself or is easily treated, although it can be a symptom of an underlying illness. Ear infections, medications, and motion sickness can cause the condition.

Lightheadedness may also be described as feeling faint and may be associated with nausea or vomiting. This condition is often caused by a momentary drop in blood pressure and blood flow to the head. Lightheadedness has many causes, including allergies, anxiety and stress, illnesses (such as the flu or colds), dehydration, heavy menstrual bleeding, hyperventilation, and from the use of tobacco, alcohol, or illegal drugs. Lightheadedness can be a symptom of a more serious illness, such as intestinal bleeding.

Vertigo is a perception of spinning or that surrounding objects are moving. Vertigo is different from dizziness because patients with vertigo have an illusion of movement. There are many things that may cause this condition, such as a sudden head movement or moving the head in a certain direction, inner ear disorders, injury to the ear or head, vertebrobasilar insufficiency, migraine headaches, and cholesteatomas. More serious conditions may cause vertigo, such as multiple sclerosis, cerebellar hemorrhage, and tumors. The duration of symptoms can be from minutes to hours, and symptoms can be constant or episodic. Severe vertigo may be accompanied by nausea and vomiting.

R43.-   Disturbances of smell and taste

Sight and taste are important senses for humans as they can alert us to potential dangers such as fire, fumes, or food that is spoiled. Infections, polyps, dental problems, and medications are just a few underlying conditions that can alter these two senses. In some cases, the person may even have been born with the disturbance.

R43.0   Anosmia

This is a disturbance in the sense of smell where the person is unable to detect odors.

R43.1   Parosmia

Parosmia is an altered sense of smell, making most all odors unpleasant.

R43.2   Parageusia

Parageusia is defined as having a bad taste in the mouth. The most common taste described in parageusia is a metallic taste of food.

R43.8   Other disturbances of smell and taste

Hyposmia is a decrease in the ability to smell.

Phantosmia is when the patient detects an odor when none is present.

Ageusia or hypogeusia is the inability or decreased ability to taste.

R44.-   Other symptoms and signs involving general sensations and perceptions

Symptoms and signs classified here involve hallucinations and other nonspecific sensations and perceptions with an unknown cause. Hallucinations are sensory perceptions of an object or event without corresponding external stimuli. The two most common types of hallucinations are auditory and visual but hallucinations may involve smell, taste, or touch as well.

R44.0   Auditory hallucinations

Auditory refers to the sense of hearing and auditory hallucinations involve the perception of nonexistent voices or sounds.

R44.1   Visual hallucinations

Visual refers to the sense of sight, and visual hallucinations involve the perception of nonexistent people, places, or other visual stimuli such as flashes of light. Visual hallucinations have many causes but can be generally linked to disturbances in brain structure, disturbances in brain biochemistry, or disturbances in consciousness, primarily due to emergence from unconsciousness to a conscious state. The underlying cause may be due to a psychiatric condition, such as schizophrenia, or a physiological disorder, such as Lewy body dementia, neoplasms of the brain, or even an organic sleep disorder. Visual hallucinations are sometimes related to seizure disorders or migraines, and may also occur as an adverse effect of a medication.

R44.2   Other hallucinations

Olfactory, gustatory, and tactile hallucinations are specific types of hallucinations that are classified here.

Olfactory refers to the sense of smell and olfactory hallucinations involve the perception of nonexistent odors.

Gustatory refers to the sense of taste and gustatory hallucinations involve the perception of nonexistent, usually unpleasant tastes.

Tactile refers to the sense of touch and tactile hallucinations refer to the perception of nonexistent contact stimuli such as crawling insects on skin.

Symptoms and Signs Involving Speech and Voice (R47-R49)

Speech conditions classified here include symptoms and signs that may be indicative of a more pervasive medical disorder but need additional work-up before a more definitive diagnosis can be made. Other symptoms and signs related to speech include general symptoms related to function such as hoarseness, loss of voice, or changes in the pitch of the voice.

The categories in this code block are as follows:

R47   Speech disturbances, not elsewhere classified

R48   Dyslexia and other symbolic dysfunctions, not elsewhere classified

R49   Voice and resonance disorders

R47.-   Speech disturbances, not elsewhere classified

Speech disturbances classified here are those that cannot be assigned to a more specific condition often because causality has not yet been determined. In some cases, the condition may be transitory and resolve on its own.

R47.0-   Dysphasia and aphasia

A difficulty with language and communication is the underlying definition of dysphasia and aphasia. The difference is in the severity of the two with aphasia being the most severe.

R47.01   Aphasia

Aphasia is impaired expression or comprehension of written or spoken language due to disease or injury of one or more of the brain's language centers: Broca's area, Wernicke's area, or arcuate fasciculus. Broca's area controls the muscle for speech (expressive aphasia). Wernicke's area controls the auditory and visual comprehension for speech (receptive aphasia). The arcuate fasciculus aids in control of the content of speech and enables repetition.

R47.1   Dysarthria and anarthria

Dysarthria is a speech disorder due to disturbances of neuromuscular control (e.g., paralysis, spasticity), often caused by damage to the central or peripheral nervous system by illness or injury. It is characterized by a difficulty expressing certain words or sounds, often resulting in slurring or interrupted rhythm of speech. In severe cases, distortion of vowel sound may be significantly impaired. Speech intelligibility varies on the severity of presentation and extent of neurological damage.

Anarthria is the inability to verbalize words even though the words are clearly defined and remembered by the brain.

R47.8-   Other speech disturbances

Problems related to voice production (slurred speech) and fluency disorder that are a consequence of an underlying condition is included in this subcategory.

R47.82   Fluency disorder in conditions classified elsewhere

Fluency disorder may be described as a condition in which the flow of speech is interrupted, impairing communication. Stuttering is a common fluency disorder characterized by uncontrolled interruption of the normal rate and pattern of speech. Fluency disorders classified here are associated with specific diseases that are classified elsewhere such as certain neurological conditions.

R48.-   Dyslexia and other symbolic dysfunctions, not elsewhere classified

Symbolic dysfunctions can range from communication difficulties, such as understanding written words, to the inability of the brain to recognize colors and sounds.

R48.0   Dyslexia and alexia

Developmental dyslexia is one of the most common of all learning disabilities and is often a congenital or genetic condition affecting up to 8 percent of the school aged population. Dyslexia can also be caused by brain injury or hormonal issues. It is described as difficulty in reading and often involves reversal of letters and numbers or the inability of the brain to translate images and comprehend written words.

Alexia, or the inability to read, is an acquired condition usually due to brain damage from injury or stroke where patients are unable to read written words or even recognize single letters. Often people with this disability can still write but cannot read the words they've written.

R48.1   Agnosia

Agnosia is characterized by the inability to recognize common things such as faces, objects, smells, or voices.

R48.2   Apraxia

Apraxia is a poorly understood neurological condition relating to the inability to make or coordinate voluntary movements.

R49.- Voice and resonance disorders

This category includes various disorders of voice production (phonation) and resonance. Phonation disorders include hoarseness and loss of voice. Resonance disorders manifest as changes in the tone or pitch of the voice.

R49.0 Dysphonia

Dysphonia is a disorder of phonation (voice production). Phonation occurs when air is expelled from the lungs through the glottis, creating a pressure drop across the larynx causing the vocal folds of the larynx to vibrate. When the vocal folds fail to vibrate, the vocal noises are not produced. This may be due to reduced or excessive tension or if the pressure gradient across the larynx is insufficient. Dysphonia is often a symptom of a laryngeal disorder affecting the structure and/or function of the larynx.

R49.2- Hypernasality and hyponasality

Hyper- and hyponasality are disorders of resonance that are often associated with an impairment affecting the structure and/or function of the oral cavity, nasal airway, and/or the velopharyngeal port. These disorders affect vibratory characteristics in amplitude and change the tone and pitch of the voice. Common causes of resonance disorders are impaired airway flow, reduced orolaryngeal pressure, and compensatory articulation. Structural anomalies or deficits (cleft palate), certain neurological disorders (cerebral palsy), and poor voice hygiene (improper learning) are often primary causes of voice resonance disorders.

R49.21 Hypernasality

Hypernasality is often caused by a dysfunction of the velopharyngeal mechanism, the soft palate (velum) and related musculature used to close the nasopharynx, which separates the oral and nasal cavities.

R49.22 Hyponasality

Hyponasality is often associated with certain types of velopharyngeal incompetence (VPI) in which the nasopharynx is obstructed and cannot open sufficiently to produce certain consonant sounds. Causal conditions include hypertrophied adenoids or other structural abnormalities.

General Symptoms and Signs (R50-R69)

General symptoms and signs are those that are not associated with a specific body system.

The categories in this code block are as follows:

R50	Fever of other and unknown origin
R51	Headache
R52	Pain, unspecified
R53	Malaise and fatigue
R54	Age-related physical debility
R55	Syncope and collapse
R56	Convulsions, not elsewhere classified
R57	Shock, not elsewhere classified
R58	Hemorrhage, not elsewhere classified
R59	Enlarged lymph nodes
R60	Edema, not elsewhere classified
R61	Generalized hyperhidrosis
R62	Lack of expected normal physiological development in childhood and adults
R63	Symptoms and signs concerning food and fluid intake
R64	Cachexia
R65	Symptoms and signs specifically associated with systemic inflammation and infection
R68	Other general symptoms and signs
R69	Illness, unspecified

R50.- Fever of other and unknown origin

Fever is an abnormal elevation of body temperature (at least 38.3 C or 101 F). Fever is often a symptom of a diagnosed condition and in most instances is not reported separately. Codes classified here represent fever that cannot be explained by an underlying etiology and those that are found to be related to certain procedures.

R50.8- Other specified fever

There are certain instances when a fever may require additional work-up or the fever is affecting the course of treatment. These may include fevers in the postoperative period and those that are secondary to a separate disease process.

R50.81 Fever presenting with conditions classified elsewhere

While inherent in a number of conditions, fever is considered a significant complication when associated with many chronic conditions, such as leukemia and sickle cell disease. In these chronic conditions, the presence of a fever may be a warning sign that the disease is being exacerbated or that a complicating infectious or inflammatory process is occurring in the body.

R50.84   Febrile nonhemolytic transfusion reaction

A febrile nonhemolytic transfusion reaction (FNHTR) is a self-limiting, responsive fever occurring one to six hours after blood transfusion, which may persist for eight to 12 hours. The fever may be accompanied by headache, tachycardia, chills, rigors, or minor dyspnea. The two most commonly described mechanisms of the reaction are passively transfused cytokines and a reaction between recipient antibodies and transfused leukocytes. Fever is the most common adverse blood transfusion reaction, occurring in approximately 3 percent to 4 percent of all transfusions. Clinical presentation is generally benign in the absence of hemolysis or anaphylaxis, with no lasting side effects. Recognition of FNHTR is important, however, as a febrile reaction may be an initial indication of a developing septic or hemolytic condition.

R51   Headache

Headaches appear to be caused by blood vessels that overreact to various triggers, such as stress, or an allergic reaction that cause a vasoconstrictive spasm. The spasm reduces blood flow to the brain, decreasing oxygen supply to the brain. In response, vasodilation occurs, triggering the release of pain-producing substances called prostaglandins. Headache may occur on one or both sides of the head, it may be isolated to a certain site, or radiate across the head. The result is a dull, aching, or throbbing pain in the head.

R52   Pain, unspecified

This code captures generalized pain, which is pain that cannot be attributed to a specific anatomic site or type or that has overlapping or multiple characteristics. Usually, a diagnosis of generalized pain or pain NOS is applied only until underlying cause or more specific diagnosis is made. Generalized pain can vary in nature as stabbing, tingling, dull, or cramping or it may exhibit one or more of these features. The generalized term typically refers to pain of multiple anatomic sites or all-over "aching." Treatment can be as difficult as defining the pain; effective treatment is based on obtaining an underlying diagnosis and addressing the root cause.

R53.-   Malaise and fatigue

Malaise is characterized by a generalized feeling of illness or just not feeling well without more specific symptoms that can be attributed to specific etiology.

Fatigue is a feeling of tiredness usually beyond what would be considered normal based on a patient's age and state of health.

R53.2   Functional quadriplegia

Functional quadriplegia is the inability to move due to another severe physiological condition such as severe contractures or arthritis. Functionally, the patient is the same as a paralyzed person. The individual is completely unable to move and perform routine daily tasks and care for him/herself. This state poses certain associated health risks such as pressure ulcers or pneumonia. The amount and type of care required to attend to these patients is greater than that of a patient with a similar state of health who is more mobile or has a greater degree of physical function.

R53.8-   Other malaise and fatigue

Other less specific symptoms related to a generalized feeling of illness, malaise, or feeling of tiredness are categorized here.

R53.82   Chronic fatigue, unspecified

Chronic fatigue syndrome (CFS) NOS is marked by unrelenting exhaustion, muscle pain, cognitive disorders that patients call "brain fog," and a profound weakness that does not go away with a few good nights of sleep. There is no known cause. CFS may begin after a bout with a cold, bronchitis, hepatitis, or an intestinal bug. For some, it follows a bout of infectious mononucleosis or a period of high stress. Unlike flu symptoms, CFS symptoms, such as a chronic headache, muscle and joint aches, and fatigue, hang-on or come and go frequently for more than six months. Some patients are bedridden since any exertion typically worsens symptoms; others can work or attend school at least part time.

R55   Syncope and collapse

Syncope is a transient loss of consciousness due to inadequate blood flow to the brain. The patient experiences generalized weakness, an inability to continue standing, and loss of consciousness. It can last anywhere from a few seconds to as long as 30 minutes.

Vasovagal syncope, which is included here, is a condition that results from a drop in blood pressure due to failure of peripheral resistance in the blood vessels with concomitant reduced venous return. It may also be due to slowing of the heart, emotional stress, pain, acute loss of blood, or assuming an upright position after having been supine for a prolonged period. It is not uncommon for patients who have just donated blood to experience this form of syncope.

Syncope and collapse symptoms include motionlessness, paleness, diaphoresis, weak pulse, and shallow breathing.

R56.- Convulsions, not elsewhere classified

Convulsions are a series of jerking movements of the face, trunk, or extremities, with involuntary contracture of voluntary muscles. Etiology is an acute focal or generalized disturbance in cerebral function. A small focus of diseased tissue in the cerebrum discharges abnormally in response to certain endogenous or exogenous stimuli. Spread of the discharge to other portions of the cerebrum results in convulsive activity and loss of consciousness.

R56.0- Febrile convulsions

Febrile convulsions usually begin with contraction or spasms of muscles. A distinctive cry or moan may result from the force of these spasms. The individual also may fall, vomit, or urinate as he or she loses voluntary muscle control. The individual may cease breathing until the muscles begin to periodically relax and contract again, which results in rhythmic jerking movements. Febrile seizures are thought to be triggered by the sudden stimulation of many brain cells at once. Both the severity of fever and the onset or rapidity of rise in temperature may be factors in initiating seizure. Fevers higher than 103 degrees Fahrenheit pose the greatest risk for seizure. These seizures often occur within the first 24 hours of an illness or infection, such as an upper respiratory infection or otitis media. Febrile seizures may run in families, especially if underlying neurologic problems or a history of epilepsy is also present.

R56.00 Simple febrile convulsions

Simple febrile convulsions typically last for 15 minutes or less and are generalized clonic or tonic-clonic type. Simple febrile seizures are also not associated with an illness affecting the brain, such as meningitis or encephalitis. Clonic seizures are characterized by rapid contraction and relaxation of the muscles of the extremities. A tonic-clonic seizure begins with the tonic phase that includes stiffening of the muscles and loss of consciousness. This is followed by the clonic phase where the arms, and often the legs as well, jerk rapidly as the muscles contract and relax. This typically lasts for only a few minutes with the jerking motions first slowing and then stopping and then consciousness returns; however, the individual may be drowsy, confused, or agitated for a period of time following the tonic-clonic seizure.

R56.01 Complex febrile convulsions

Complex (also atypical or complicated) febrile convulsions can be defined as focal or prolonged seizures that are associated with fever. Focal seizures are also called partial seizures because the abnormal electrical brain activity is limited to a single region of the brain. Prolonged seizures are those lasting more than 15 minutes or seizures that recur within 24 hours of initial onset. Although not limited exclusively to the pediatric population, complex febrile seizures most commonly occur in children between 6 months and 5 years of age. Complex febrile seizures may indicate a more serious problem, such as meningitis, abscess, or encephalitis. Also, fever as a reaction to DTP or MMR vaccines is sometimes an underlying cause of complex febrile seizures.

R56.1 Post traumatic seizures

Posttraumatic seizures (PTS) are acute, symptomatic seizures following a traumatic brain injury (TBI) and can be considered "reactive seizures." PTS is differentiated from posttraumatic epilepsy (PTE), a chronic condition of repeated seizures as sequelae of trauma. The risk of PTS progressively decreases as time passes following the injury. PTS that begins weeks to years after the trauma increases the likelihood of the patient developing PTE. Some studies suggest that the greatest risk factor for PTS is penetrating head trauma. Seizures that follow acute head trauma complicate management, requiring anticonvulsant therapy and diagnostic imaging surveillance to assess and prevent further complications or permanent brain damage. Acute head injury causes physiologic alterations in the normal circulation and metabolism of the central nervous system. A traumatic reduction in adequate oxygenation may alter the normal neurochemistry of the brain, causing a serious and potentially fatal excess in intracranial pressure.

R57.- Shock, not elsewhere classified

Cardiogenic, hypovolemic, other shock, and unspecified shock are classified here.

Focus Point

Shock due to other specific causes (e.g., anaphylactic shock) is classified in other chapters or in other categories in this chapter (e.g., septic shock).

R57.0 Cardiogenic shock

Cardiogenic shock results from decreased cardiac output usually associated with severe forms of heart disease, such as an acute myocardial infarction. When cardiac output is decreased, the heart cannot deliver an adequate volume of oxygenated blood to the organs and tissues that are supplied by the systemic circulation.

R57.1 Hypovolemic shock

Hypovolemic shock occurs when there is severe loss of blood or other body fluids that affects the volume of blood available to the organs and tissues of the body. Blood volume can decrease when too many fluids are lost through diarrhea, vomiting, bleeding, or burns. When blood loss reaches one-fifth of normal blood volume, hypovolemic shock occurs. Severity of hypovolemic shock is related to the amount of blood lost, the rate at which it is lost, the type of injury or illness responsible for the blood loss, and the presence of underlying medical conditions. Complications of hypovolemic shock include organ and tissue damage, including brain damage. Loss of blood volume can also cause myocardial infarction. Emergent medical care is required to prevent death from hypovolemic shock.

R59.- Enlarged lymph nodes

Lymph nodes are part of the immune system and are distributed throughout the body. Enlargement typically occurs due to viral or bacterial infection of a site near the affected nodes. A less common cause of lymph node enlargement is a malignancy. Typically sudden onset of enlarged lymph nodes with associated pain is attributed to injury or infection, while a gradual onset may indicate cancer or other malignant neoplasm. Treatment for this condition depends on the underlying cause.

R60.- Edema, not elsewhere classified

Edema is the accumulation of excessive amounts of fluid (water and sodium) in the intercellular tissue spaces of the body. Edema results when the balance of the lymphatic system, which normally transports excess interstitial fluid back to the intravascular space, is compromised. Pitting edema is characterized by indentation produced by the application of pressure that forces fluid into the underlying tissues. Nonpitting edema is a type of edema that leaves no indentation when pressure is applied because fluid has coagulated in the tissues. Edema may occur at any site of the body, indicating different causes.

R61 Generalized hyperhidrosis

Excessive sweating is a disorder that can be induced by a metabolic disorder, fevers, medication use, chronic alcoholism, or secondary to another disease process such as a malignancy. Menopause is also a common cause of secondary generalized hyperhidrosis.

Focus Point

Hyperhidrosis documented as focal or localized is a form of hyperhidrosis that mainly affects feet, hands, face, head, and underarms and usually starts in childhood and is a lifelong complaint. Cause is unknown, although may be hereditary. This diagnosis is not included in this symptom category but is located in Chapter 12 Diseases of the Skin and Subcutaneous Tissue, subcategory L74.5-.

R62.- Lack of expected normal physiological development in childhood and adults

Conditions classified here are nonspecific symptoms and signs associated with failure of physiological development to progress as one would normally expect.

R62.5- Other and unspecified lack of expected normal physiological development in childhood

In children, lack of physiological development may be evident when age-related milestones for speech, walking, weight gain, or growth are not reached.

R62.51 Failure to thrive (child)

Failure to thrive (FTT) describes a child that is not gaining weight normally. Children with FTT generally have a weight that is below the third or fifth percentile for their age and a decreasing growth velocity (not gaining weight as expected) and/or a downward change in growth percentiles. There are two types of failure to thrive. Nonorganic or psychosocial failure to thrive occurs in a child who has no known medical condition that causes poor growth. Organic failure to thrive is when the poor growth is caused by an underlying medical condition.

R62.52 Short stature (child)

Short stature describes a child who is significantly below the average height of peers, specifically, the shortest third to fifth percentile on the growth chart for height. There are different types of short stature. One is familial or genetic; children with a family history of short stature may be more likely to develop it. These children have an age-appropriate bone age, normal growth velocity (growth of two and a half inches a year), and calculated adult height in line with the familial pattern.

Constitutional growth delay is another type of short stature. In this condition, children are small for their age and are growing at a normal rate. These children are asymptomatic. They are usually below the third percentile for their age, they have delayed bone age, but their growth velocity is normal. They normally achieve puberty at a later age than peers and continue to grow at an older age. They eventually catch up with peers in height. Children with this condition usually have a family history of the condition. In some cases, short stature may be a result of a chronic disease, including Down's syndrome, growth hormone deficiency, hypothyroidism, precocious puberty, delayed puberty, and Turner syndrome.

R63.- Symptoms and signs concerning food and fluid intake

Loss of appetite, excessive thirst, excessive eating, and feeding difficulties are classified here, along with abnormal weight loss or gain and underweight.

R63.0   Anorexia

Anorexia refers to a loss of appetite. This is a common symptom of gastrointestinal (GI) and endocrine disorders, as well as psychological disturbances. Associated conditions include hypopituitarism, hypothyroidism, ketoacidosis, appendicitis, cirrhosis, Crohn's disease, gastritis, hepatitis, chronic renal failure, pernicious anemia, alcoholism, and cancer.

Focus Point

Anorexia nervosa is an eating disorder characterized by anorexia but in the context of a negatively perceived body image that is so extreme that the patient purposely restricts food intake, exercises excessively, and/or purges food that is consumed so as not to gain weight. It is exhibited by an extremely low and unhealthy body weight. Anorexia nervosa is captured in subcategory F50.0- in the Mental, Behavioral and Neurodevelopmental Disorders chapter.

R63.2   Polyphagia

Polyphagia refers to eating to the point of being focused only on eating (or excessive eating) before feeling full. This can be a symptom of various disorders. It can be intermittent or persistent and depending on the cause, it may or may not result in weight gain. Common causes include anxiety, premenstrual syndrome, bulimia, diabetes mellitus, gestational diabetes, Graves' disease, hyperthyroidism, hypoglycemia, and drugs such as corticosteroids, cyproheptadine, and tricyclic antidepressants.

R64   Cachexia

The protein-wasting syndrome called cachexia most commonly occurs with lung, pancreatic, stomach, bowel, and prostate cancers, and less often with breast cancer. It also affects people with AIDS, uncontrolled rheumatoid arthritis, severe infections, chronic lung and bowel disease, and heart failure. Cachexia associated with cancer is usually related to liver metastasis with resulting pain and loss of appetite. Sometimes the cause is mechanical, such as when a tumor grows into the stomach or blocks the intestine. Undiagnosed and untreated cachexia is life-threatening. It can decrease the effectiveness of cancer treatments, such as chemotherapy and radiation therapy, and magnify their side effects.

R65.-   Symptoms and signs specifically associated with systemic inflammation and infection

Systemic inflammatory response syndrome (SIRS) due to a noninfectious disease process is classified here along with severe sepsis, which is a systemic response to an infectious process with associated organ dysfunction.

R65.1-   Systemic inflammatory response syndrome (SIRS) of non-infectious origin

Unlike sepsis, which is a clinical response due to infection, SIRS is an inflammatory response due only to a noninfectious origin such as trauma, ischemia, inflammation (e.g., pancreatitis), heatstroke, neoplasm, or other noninfectious disease processes. SIRS is characterized by two or more of the following conditions: fever, tachycardia, tachypnea, and abnormal white blood cell count. More specifically, these include elevated body temperature (usually above 101 degrees Fahrenheit) or subnormal body temperature (usually below 96.8 degrees Fahrenheit), elevated heart rate (usually above 90 beats per minute), elevated respiratory rate (usually above 20 breaths per minute) or an abnormal white blood cell count above 12,000 cells/microliter or below 4,000 cells/microliter or greater than 10 percent bands (immature white blood cell).

R65.10   Systemic inflammatory response syndrome (SIRS) of non-infectious origin without acute organ dysfunction

R65.11   Systemic inflammatory response syndrome (SIRS) of non-infectious origin with acute organ dysfunction

Codes for SIRS of noninfectious origin are classified based on associated acute organ dysfunction. Some inclusions of acute organ dysfunction are acute respiratory failure, acute kidney or liver failure, disseminated intravascular coagulopathy (DIC), encephalopathy, critical illness myopathy, or polyneuropathy.

Code first the noninfectious causal condition followed by the appropriate code from R65.1-. Add any codes identifying specific acute organ dysfunction if applicable.

Focus Point

If documentation states SIRS with an infection such as pneumonia, only the pneumonia (infection) can be coded. There is no separate code or index entry in ICD-10-CM for SIRS due to an infectious process. If the record supports sepsis criteria, the physician must be queried for clarification of sepsis due to infection.

R65.2-   Severe sepsis

Severe sepsis is a system-wide response to an infectious process that includes acute organ dysfunction. Some inclusions of acute organ dysfunction are acute respiratory failure, acute kidney or liver failure, disseminated intravascular coagulopathy (DIC), encephalopathy, critical illness myopathy, or polyneuropathy. Severe sepsis is classified by the presence or absence of septic shock.

R65.20   Severe sepsis without septic shock

If severe sepsis occurs with no septic shock, additional codes are still required for the other specified acute organ dysfunction. Code first the underlying systemic sepsis infection, followed by any localized infection such as pneumonia, UTI, or cellulitis (if applicable), then code the severe sepsis without septic shock, and finally add all applicable acute organ dysfunction codes.

R65.21   Severe sepsis with septic shock

Septic shock refers to circulatory failure and is a form of organ dysfunction associated with sepsis and cannot occur in the absence of severe sepsis. Severe sepsis with shock involves persistent hypotension with a systolic blood pressure < 90 mmHg or a 40 mmHg drop in previous blood pressure, with no response to adequate fluid resuscitation. Severe sepsis with septic shock requires a minimum of two codes, including the underlying systemic sepsis infection, followed by the severe sepsis with septic shock. Add any other specified organ dysfunction codes as applicable.

Focus Point

Typical first coded, underlying systemic septic infections include sepsis NOS, Streptococcal sepsis, MRSA sepsis, sepsis due to E coli, etc. Other underlying infectious conditions that would be sequenced first include infections following a procedure or following infusions, transfusions, or therapeutic injection. Also coded first is sepsis following ectopic or molar pregnancy, spontaneous abortion or induced terminated pregnancy, and puerperal sepsis.

R68.-   Other general symptoms and signs

A variety of general symptoms and signs that do not fit well into other chapters, code blocks, or categories are included here.

R68.1-   Nonspecific symptoms peculiar to infancy

General symptoms and signs that may be exhibited by a newborn/infant are categorized here.

R68.13   Apparent life threatening event in infant (ALTE)

The term apparent life-threatening event (ALTE) describes a clinical syndrome in which a variety of symptoms may occur, possibly as a result of identifiable diseases or conditions (e.g., gastroesophageal reflux, respiratory disease, or seizures). Due to the wide variety of possible causal conditions, work-up may be extensive. In approximately one half of the cases, despite extensive workup, no cause for the episode is identified. These events can occur during sleep, wakefulness, or feeding, although over half of the episodes reported have occurred when the infant was awake. An ALTE event may manifest with cyanosis and apnea as predominant presenting symptoms, accompanied by syncope, altered or loss of consciousness, difficulty breathing, pallor, stiffness, floppiness, choking, red face, limb jerking, and vomiting. Once an underlying etiology is identified, further testing may not be indicated unless ALTEs continue or a risk for future ALTEs is established.

Focus Point

This may also be documented as a BRUE (brief resolved unexplained event) and also coded with R68.13.

R68.8-   Other general symptoms and signs

General symptoms and signs that do not fit well into the previous categories are included here.

R68.84   Jaw pain

Jaw pain is a general symptom describing pain or discomfort of the upper or lower jaw. Various conditions can cause jaw pain including temporomandibular joint disease, arthritis, bruxism (teeth grinding), malalignment of the jaw, dental abscess, or tumor. Jaw pain can also be referred from another site, such as that associated with coronary artery disease or quiescent myocardial infarction, whereby the chest pain radiates to the jaw area. It is appropriate to report the symptom of jaw pain until the underlying cause of the pain has been established.

Abnormal Findings on Examination of Blood, Without Diagnosis (R70-R79)

Abnormal findings classified here involve abnormalities of blood cell counts, blood sugar levels, and enzyme levels; the presence of elevated antibody titers and nonspecific immunological findings; abnormalities of proteins found in the blood; the presence of drugs or toxic substances in the blood; and abnormal blood chemistry.

The categories in this code block are as follows:

R70	Elevated erythrocyte sedimentation rate and abnormality of plasma viscosity
R71	Abnormality of red blood cells
R73	Elevated blood glucose level
R74	Abnormal serum enzyme levels
R75	Inconclusive laboratory evidence of human immunodeficiency virus [HIV]
R76	Other abnormal immunological findings in serum
R77	Other abnormalities of plasma proteins

R78   Findings of drugs and other substances, not normally found in blood

R79   Other abnormal findings of blood chemistry

R70.-   Elevated erythrocyte sedimentation rate and abnormality of plasma viscosity

Elevated erythrocyte sedimentation rate (ESR) ("sed rate") and plasma viscosity are both indicators of inflammation in the body that can be caused by many conditions including infections, abscesses, arthritis, MI, and neoplastic diseases. The plasma viscosity test is more sensitive but more difficult to perform and less commonly used than the ESR test.

R73.-   Elevated blood glucose level

Glucose is a form of sugar and an important energy source for humans. Any elevation in blood sugar is potentially dangerous and monitoring blood sugar levels is important for early detection of diseases like tumors in the pancreas, overactive thyroid, and diabetes.

R73.0-   Abnormal glucose

Two significant risk factors associated with but not yet diagnostic for diabetes are impaired fasting glucose and impaired glucose tolerance. An impaired glucose tolerance indicates a much higher risk for diabetes than the impaired fasting glucose and may also point to several risk factors related to cardiovascular disease.

R73.01   Impaired fasting glucose

Impaired fasting glucose is defined as glucose levels of 100 to 125 mg per dL in fasting patients.

R73.02   Impaired glucose tolerance (oral)

Impaired glucose tolerance is defined as two-hour glucose levels of 140 to 199 mg per dL on the 75-g oral glucose tolerance test.

R73.03   Prediabetes

Prediabetes is an interim diagnosis used to describe an elevated blood glucose level that is higher than normal but not yet high enough to be considered Type 2 diabetes. With no intervention, the condition is expected to become Type 2 diabetes within 10 years. A fasting blood glucose level of 100 to 125 mg/dL typically warrants a diagnosis of prediabetes, and the patient is counseled to adjust diet and exercise patterns to prevent the progression to Type 2 diabetes.

R74.-   Abnormal serum enzyme levels

Serum is the clear, pale yellow colored liquid component of blood. Serum contains enzymes and changes in enzyme levels are sometimes indicative of a disease process.

R74.0   Nonspecific elevation of levels of transaminase and lactic acid dehydrogenase [LDH]

Elevated transaminase in the bloodstream may indicate liver damage. The liver holds transaminases to break down amino acid with the normal concentration in the bloodstream being low so if the liver is damaged, these can escape into the bloodstream. There are two variations measured: alanine transaminase (ALT) and aspartate transaminase (AST), often referred to as liver enzymes.

Lactic acid dehydrogenase (LDH) is an enzyme contributing to the production of energy and is found in most of the tissues throughout the body. An elevated LDH may indicate cell damage and is measured by withdrawal of blood from a vein. Oftentimes this test is done to assist in diagnosis of lung disorders, lymphoma, anemia, and liver disease, as well as evaluating how chemotherapy treatment is working.

R75   Inconclusive laboratory evidence of human immunodeficiency virus [HIV]

An inconclusive HIV test can occur for a number of reasons. Conditions such as hypergammaglobulinemia, autoimmune disease, pregnancy, and other infections of the immune system such as human T-cell lymphotropic virus (HTLV), produce proteins or antibodies that can cross react with the antigen used to test for HIV. These proteins and antibodies cause a nonspecific reaction that may also occur in a patient with the presence of HIV antibodies. Inconclusive HIV test results require retesting and the second test is usually performed by a different technique.

R76.-   Other abnormal immunological findings in serum

Immunological laboratory tests are performed to identify antibodies to specific infectious organisms and increased levels of immunoglobulins that are produced in response to infection, inflammation, and other disease processes.

R76.1-   Nonspecific reaction to test for tuberculosis

Persons who have been infected with tuberculosis may not show signs or symptoms of active disease but may still be able to spread the bacteria. Skin tests and blood tests are used to identify the presence of the tuberculin bacteria so that further investigation into whether the patient has latent or active TB can be pursued.

R76.12 Nonspecific reaction to cell mediated immunity measurement of gamma interferon antigen response without active tuberculosis

Interferon gamma release assay (IGRA) is a blood test performed to aid in the diagnosis of *M. tuberculosis* (TB) infection. This test cannot differentiate between latent or inactive TB and active TB, but it does allow detection of the presence of *M. tuberculosis* bacteria. There are three possible test results:

- Negative: Infection is unlikely

- Indeterminate or borderline: There is an uncertain likelihood of infection

- Positive: Infection, latent or active, is likely

This code reports a nonspecific reaction without the presence of an active TB infection. There are two tests approved by the FDA for IGRA testing. These include QuantiFERON®-TB Gold In-Tube test, also called QFT-GIT, and T-SPOT®TB test, also called T-Spot.

R77.- Other abnormalities of plasma proteins

Plasma proteins, also known as serum proteins, are found in the blood plasma and provide transportation for important compounds and help to regulate certain body functions. The largest component is albumin, assisting in the transport of lipids and steroid hormones. Globulins and fibrinogen are involved in the immune process and blood clotting process respectively. Unspecified abnormalities of these proteins are represented in this category.

R77.0 Abnormality of albumin

A blood test with low albumin can indicate liver or kidney disease but also can occur after bariatric surgery, with Crohn's disease, or from a low protein diet.

R77.2 Abnormality of alphafetoprotein

Blood tests obtained of this protein primarily look to see if high levels exist, which can be an indicator for hepatocellular carcinoma, cancer of ovaries or testes, or metastatic cancer to the liver.

R78.- Findings of drugs and other substances, not normally found in blood

This category classifies the presence of drugs, toxic substances, and bacteria that although present are not adversely affecting the patient.

R78.8- Finding of other specified substances, not normally found in blood

Bacteria and lithium, as well as other specified substances that cannot be better classified into the other R78.- subcategories, are included here.

R78.81 Bacteremia

Bacteremia is the presence of live bacteria circulating in the bloodstream. Bacteremia frequently results from surgical procedures (e.g., incision and drainage of an abscess or dental extractions). It also may result from colonization of indwelling urinary catheters or other invasive apparatus.

R79.- Other abnormal findings of blood chemistry

Blood chemistry tests measure levels of certain substances in the blood, such as minerals, blood clotting factors, and blood gases. Abnormal findings classified here do not fit well into the more specific categories in the code block.

R79.8- Other specified abnormal findings of blood chemistry

Acetonemia, azotemia, melanemia, nonspecific abnormality of liver function test, C-reactive protein levels, and blood gas levels are blood chemistry findings that would be classified to this subcategory.

R79.82 Elevated C-reactive protein (CRP)

Elevated C-reactive protein is recognized as a risk factor in cardiovascular disease and stroke. Elevated C-reactive protein (CRP) found in blood is a marker for inflammation occurring anywhere in the body including arterial walls. The presence of inflammation in an arterial wall has been found to contribute to plaque rupture and artery obstruction and is a contributing factor to heart attacks and strokes, even in the absence of other classic risk factors, such as elevated cholesterol and triglycerides. Patients screened for CRP level may come from several different patient groupings, including those with hypothyroidism and/or progressive thyroid failure, premature atherosclerosis, those undergoing peritoneal dialysis, middle aged men and women with and without other risk factors, and those with periodontal disease. Patients presenting with periodontal disease, especially, are at risk for cardiovascular problems. The inflammation from periodontal disease allows oral bacteria to enter the bloodstream, and causes the liver to produce proteins, such as CRP, that inflame arteries and promote blood clot formation.

Abnormal Findings on Examination of Urine, Without Diagnosis (R80-R82)

Abnormal findings in urine include the presence of protein, which is often indicative of kidney disease; glucose, which may be indicative of diabetes; and other substances not normally found in the urine such as ketone, drugs, bacteria, cells, and casts.

The categories in this code block are as follows:

R80	Proteinuria
R81	Glycosuria
R82	Other and unspecified abnormal findings in urine

R80.- Proteinuria

Proteinuria can be an early sign of kidney disease, and is defined as urinary protein excretion of greater than 150 mg per day. The etiology of protein excretion may be related to a glomerular, tubular, or overflow problem.

Glomerular disease is the most common cause, resulting in urinary loss of albumin and immunoglobulins.

Tubular proteinuria occurs when tubulointerstitial disease prevents the proximal tubule from reabsorbing low-molecular-weight proteins. Tubular diseases include hypertensive nephrosclerosis and tubulointerstitial nephropathy caused by nonsteroidal antiinflammatory drugs.

In overflow proteinuria, low-molecular-weight proteins inhibit the reabsorption of filtered proteins.

R81 Glycosuria

Glycosuria is the presence of glucose, a sugar, in the urine. Normally there is no glucose in the urine because the kidneys are able to retrieve all glucose filtered out of the urine and return it to the circulation. Glucose is typically only present in the urine when there are excessive levels of glucose in the blood, an indication of diabetes mellitus, or when there is a dysfunction of glucose reabsorption by the kidneys, a condition called renal glycosuria. Frequent urination and excessive thirst are symptoms of glycosuria.

R82.- Other and unspecified abnormal findings in urine

Findings identified in this category include abnormalities in the urine such as heavy metals, ketones, and other chromosome abnormalities.

R82.0 Chyluria

Chyle is a bodily fluid containing lymph and fats. Urine that is of a milky white appearance indicates the presence of chyle. Chyluria is a sign of blocked lymph channels, and although it is typically self-limiting, it can lead to complications.

R82.1 Myoglobinuria

Myoglobin in the urine is characteristic of rhabdomyolysis or other muscle breakdown.

R82.2 Biliuria

Biliuria is bile in the urine, which can indicate liver or bile duct obstruction.

R82.3 Hemoglobinuria

Hemoglobinuria is hemoglobin, the protein found inside red blood cells, in the urine. The presence of hemoglobin can give urine a purple color and may be an indication of several disease processes from renal cancer to hemolytic anemia.

R82.71 Bacteriuria

Bacteriuria is the presence of bacteria in the urine. Asymptomatic bacteriuria is somewhat common in several types of patients and may not warrant any treatment. However, a urinary tract infection is a significant concern. Antibiotic treatment is avoided except in high-risk patients, such as those with a history of kidney transplant, pregnant women, and patients with suppressed immune systems.

Abnormal Findings on Examination of Other Body Fluids, Substances and Tissues, Without Diagnosis (R83-R89)

Abnormal findings in other body fluids such as cerebrospinal fluid, sputum, pleural fluid, saliva, peritoneal fluid, and seminal fluid are included here along with abnormal findings on examination of cells (cytological specimens) and tissue (histological) specimens.

The categories in this code block are as follows:

R83   Abnormal findings in cerebrospinal fluid

R84   Abnormal findings in specimens from respiratory organs and thorax

R85   Abnormal findings in specimens from digestive organs and abdominal cavity

R86   Abnormal findings in specimens from male genital organs

R87   Abnormal findings in specimens from female genital organs

R88   Abnormal findings in other body fluids and substances

R89   Abnormal findings in specimens from other organs, systems and tissues

R83.-   Abnormal findings in cerebrospinal fluid

Cerebrospinal fluid analysis looks at various components that may be found in the fluid such as protein, sugar, and other chemicals. A spinal tap is typically used to withdraw fluid for testing. Abnormal findings may indicate the following conditions:

- Alzheimer disease
- Amyotrophic lateral sclerosis
- Anthrax
- Cancer
- Encephalitis
- Encephalopathy
- Epilepsy
- Hydrocephalus
- Infection
- Inflammation
- Meningitis
- Multiple sclerosis
- Reye syndrome
- Tumor

Abnormal enzymes within the CSF can be linked to neurological conditions such as cerebral infarction, brain tumors, central nervous system infections, and acute brain injury. Immunological findings may be evidence of damage within the central nervous system due to inflammation, deterioration, or the development of antibodies.

R85.-   Abnormal findings in specimens from digestive organs and abdominal cavity

Digestive system organs include the mouth, throat, esophagus, stomach, small and large intestine, rectum, and anus. Most of these organs are located within the abdominal cavity, the largest of the human body cavities. When a specific condition or disease is not definitively linked to the abnormal findings related to digestive organs and the abdominal cavity, codes from this category should be used.

R85.6-   Abnormal cytological findings in specimens from digestive organs and abdominal cavity

Dysplastic changes in squamous intraepithelial tissue are the result of human papillomavirus (HPV) infection and anorectal cytology samples are some of the more common tests performed to determine the presence of dysplastic changes and the extent of the changes.

R85.61-   Abnormal cytologic smear of anus

The correlation between abnormal cytologic smears and the risk of dysplasia and carcinoma is the same for the anus as it is for the cervix; there are many pathophysiological parallels between cervical-vaginal and anal-rectal screening. Cytology samples are routinely collected under direct visualization, although a small anoscope may be utilized to introduce the collection device. The histological and immunological cell changes reported with the Bethesda system are determined by cytology studies of the cell samples obtained by smear tests.

> **Focus Point**
>
> *When a cytologic smear of the anus indicates the presence of human papillomavirus (HPV), additional DNA testing is performed to classify the type of HPV as high or low risk. Codes from subcategory R85.8- are used to report findings on HPV DNA test results taken from the anus.*

R85.610   Atypical squamous cells of undetermined significance on cytologic smear of anus (ASC-US)

ASC-US reflects minor changes of the thin, flat surface cells due to unknown causes.

R85.611 Atypical squamous cells cannot exclude high grade squamous intraepithelial lesion on cytologic smear of anus (ASC-H)

This code classifies the presence of atypical squamous cells that are at higher risk for an underlying high-grade neoplastic lesion. This code is used when the cells are more indicative of a high-grade squamous intraepithelial lesion (HGSIL) than those classified as undetermined significance, but the changes cannot be definitively described as representing HGSIL.

R85.612 Low grade squamous intraepithelial lesion on cytologic smear of anus (LGSIL)

LGSIL reflects minor cellular changes that are unlikely to progress to cancer but may be indicative of changes attributable to human papillomavirus (HPV) infection, such as mild dysplasia or anal intraepithelial neoplasia I (AIN I).

R85.613 High grade squamous intraepithelial lesion on cytologic smear of anus (HGSIL)

HGSIL reflects cellular changes that have a higher likelihood of progressing to cancer and that indicate but are not conclusive of moderate to severe dysplasia, carcinoma in situ (CIS), AIN 2 and AIN 3, or invasive cancer.

R85.614 Cytologic evidence of malignancy on smear of anus

This Bethesda classification reflects the presence of malignant cells identified on the cytologic smear.

R85.615 Unsatisfactory cytologic smear of anus

An unsatisfactory smear represents an inadequate cell sample that cannot be evaluated for squamous cell intraepithelial lesion. This finding requires that a new cytologic smear be obtained in order to evaluate cytological changes of anal cells.

R85.616 Satisfactory anal smear but lacking transformation zone

The transformation (transitional) zone in the anus refers to the area between the rectum where goblet cells are present and the anus where stratus squamous epithelium is found. This transformation zone contains transitional epithelium and is the zone where nearly all anal cancers develop, so it is important to obtain a cytological sample from these specific tissues. Cellular analysis of transformation zone cells provides valuable information in diagnosis and classification of the specific nature of the dysplastic changes.

R87.- Abnormal findings in specimens from female genital organs

When a specific condition or disease is not definitively linked to abnormal findings found in specimens from the female genital organs, codes from this category should be used. The most common female genital sites of which specimens are taken are the vagina, vulva, and cervix.

R87.6- Abnormal cytological findings in specimens from female genital organs

Cytology samples are obtained from the female genital organs to screen for changes in the cells and identify the presence of atypical cells, dysplastic changes (e.g., intraepithelial neoplasia), or malignancy. Cytological smears are specifically designed to detect dysplastic changes in squamous epithelial cells and squamous cell carcinoma (cancer). Codes in this category also report unsatisfactory cytologic smears that cannot be evaluated for cytologic changes. Cytology samples are routinely collected under direct visualization, although colposcopy may be utilized to introduce the collection device.

R87.61- Abnormal cytological findings in specimens from cervix uteri

The histological and immunological cell changes reported with the Bethesda system are determined by cytology studies of the cell samples obtained by smear tests. A pathologist interprets the findings and classifies abnormal findings and unsatisfactory smears.

> **Focus Point**
>
> *If human papillomavirus (HPV) infection is identified, cytologic testing may be followed up with DNA testing of the female genital organ to identify the type of HPV infection as low risk or high risk. HPV test results are classified in subcategory R87.8-.*

R87.610 Atypical squamous cells of undetermined significance on cytologic smear of cervix (ASC-US)

ASC-US reflects minor changes of the thin, flat surface cells due to unknown causes.

R87.611 Atypical squamous cells cannot exclude high grade squamous intraepithelial lesion on cytologic smear of cervix (ASC-H)

This code classifies the presence of atypical squamous cells that are at higher risk for an underlying high-grade neoplastic lesion. This code is used when the cells are more indicative of a high grade squamous intraepithelial lesion (HGSIL) than those classified as undetermined significance, but the changes cannot be definitively described as representing HGSIL.

R87.612 Low grade squamous intraepithelial lesion on cytologic smear of cervix (LGSIL)

LGSIL reflects minor cellular changes that are unlikely to progress to cancer but may indicate changes related to human papillomavirus (HPV) infection, such as mild dysplasia or cervical intraepithelial neoplasia I (CIN I).

R87.613 High grade squamous intraepithelial lesion on cytologic smear of cervix (HGSIL)

HGSIL reflects cellular changes that have a higher likelihood of progressing to cancer and may indicate, but are not conclusive of, moderate to severe dysplasia, carcinoma in situ (CIS), CIN 2 and CIN 3, or invasive cancer.

R87.614 Cytologic evidence of malignancy on smear of cervix

This Bethesda classification reflects the presence of malignant cells identified on the cytologic smear.

R87.615 Unsatisfactory cytologic smear of cervix

An unsatisfactory smear represents an inadequate cell sample that cannot be evaluated for squamous cell intraepithelial lesion. This finding requires that a new cytologic smear be obtained in order to evaluate cytological changes of cervical cells.

R87.616 Satisfactory cervical smear but lacking transformation zone

The transformation zone refers to the area between the keratinized and nonkeratinized epithelia. It is important to obtain a cytological sample from these specific tissues. Transformational zone tissue samples contain squamous metaplastic cells. Cellular analysis of transformation zone cells provides valuable information in diagnosis and classification of the specific nature of the dysplastic changes.

R87.618 Other abnormal cytological findings on specimens from cervix uteri

This code is used to report the presence of normal or benign appearing (non-atypical) endometrial cells found in cytologic smears of the cervix. When non-atypical glandular cells of endometrial origin are found on cytologic smears, there is a higher risk for the presence of endometrial adenocarcinoma and endometrial hyperplasia, particularly in women older than age 45.

R87.619 Unspecified abnormal cytological findings in specimens from cervix uteri

The current Bethesda system has a designation for atypical glandular cells (AGC) and a pathological finding of AGC is reported here.

Focus Point

In older systems for classifying abnormal cytological findings of the cervix, there was a classification for atypical glandular cells of undetermined significance (AGUS). This terminology was replaced to avoid confusion with the new classification of ASC-US. The term atypical glandular cells (AGC) is now used and laboratories are encouraged to identify the origin of the atypical glandular cells, which may originate from the endometrium or endocervix, or unqualified.

R87.8- Other abnormal findings in specimens from female genital organs

Abnormal findings classified here include positive DNA tests for high- and low-risk human papillomavirus (HVP). DNA tests are performed to identify the presence of HPV and to determine whether the specific type of HPV puts the patient at greater risk for developing cervical cancer. This subcategory also captures other abnormal laboratory findings that do not have a more specific code, such as abnormal chromosomal findings.

Abnormal Findings on Diagnostic Imaging and in Function Studies, Without Diagnosis (R90-R94)

Diagnostic imaging includes traditional x-ray exams, CT scans, MRI scans, PET scans, thermography, and ultrasonography. Function studies include nervous system studies such as electroencephalogram (EEG), electromyography (EMG), electro-oculogram (EOG), visually evoked potential (VEP), auditory and vestibular function studies; pulmonary function studies; cardiovascular function studies such as electrocardiogram (ECG) and intracardiac electrophysiological studies (EPS); and kidney, liver, thyroid, and other organ or body system specific function studies.

The categories in this code block are as follows:

R90	Abnormal findings on diagnostic imaging of central nervous system
R91	Abnormal findings on diagnostic imaging of lung
R92	Abnormal and inconclusive findings on diagnostic imaging of breast
R93	Abnormal findings on diagnostic imaging of other body structures
R94	Abnormal results of function studies

R90.-   Abnormal findings on diagnostic imaging of central nervous system

An echoencephalogram uses sound-reflecting surfaces within the skull to detect deviations of the brain tissue that can be caused by conditions such as a tumor or hemorrhage or other displacements of brain matter.

Included in this category is unspecified white matter disease (myelin) of the brain or spinal cord. The myelin is the insulation of the nerve fibers that form the connections between the nerve cells. MRIs or other imaging may detect damage of the white matter that interferes with the conduction impulses and can hamper brain function.

R91.-   Abnormal findings on diagnostic imaging of lung

The most common abnormal findings on diagnostic imaging of the lung are the presence of nodules, lesions, masses, shadows, and infiltrates in the lung tissue or lung space.

R91.1   Solitary pulmonary nodule

The finding of a single pulmonary nodule (SPN) typically involves a round or oval spot (lesion) in the lungs, which is commonly located deep within the lung tissue, embedded in the lung parenchyma, or in a subsegmental branch of the bronchial tree. Findings of SPN may be detected by x-ray or enhanced, high-frequency imaging, such as computed tomography (CT) and positron emission tomography (PET). Traditionally, if repeat x-rays over a period of two to three years failed to show significant change, the nodule was considered benign. Early detection and histological identification assists in early detection of potentially malignant lesions, which can significantly improve the patient's prognosis. Tissue biopsy is necessary to determine the histology of the lesion and establish a definitive diagnosis. Technological improvements that facilitate lung cancer screening and investigate those with SPN present an opportunity to provide early treatment and thereby reduce the incidence of mortality due to lung cancer.

R92.-   Abnormal and inconclusive findings on diagnostic imaging of breast

Abnormal and inconclusive findings on diagnostic imaging of the breast include microcalcifications, calcifications, and dense breasts.

R92.2   Inconclusive mammogram

A routine mammogram may be deemed inconclusive due to a finding documented as "dense breasts." This type of breast tissue is common in younger women, and poses certain mammographic challenges, because the density of the breast tissue can hide a tumor. This is not considered an abnormal condition, but one that requires further testing to confirm that no malignant condition exists. Digital mammography may be able to detect suspicious lesions in dense breast tissue by offering enhanced magnification and alternative viewing capabilities.

R93.-   Abnormal findings on diagnostic imaging of other body structures

This category classifies abnormal findings on diagnostic imaging of other body structures by site.

R93.4-   Abnormal findings on diagnostic imaging of urinary organs

Diagnostic imaging of the urinary system can be divided into two major groups: that with ionizing and that with nonionizing radiation (no radiation) techniques. Intravascular ultrasound, X-rays, CT scans, and radionuclide imaging are all considered ionizing radiation tests, while nonionizing radiation tests include ultrasound and magnetic resonance imaging (MRI). Cumulative radiation exposure is a significant danger to the pediatric population, particularly in patients with chronic health disorders requiring long-term follow-up and repeated imaging. Codes in this subcategory should be assigned when abnormalities are noted on a diagnostic imaging report but no firm diagnosis has been made.

R93.9   Diagnostic imaging inconclusive due to excess body fat of patient

Radiologists have reported that the prevalence of obesity in the patient population has resulted in an increased occurrence of inconclusive imaging test results due to excessive body fat. Unsatisfactory imaging due to excessive body fat can seriously impede the efficacy of imaging technologies to appropriately diagnose and treat an illness, trauma, or other condition. X-rays, CT scans, ultrasound, and magnetic resonance imaging equipment require accommodation by the patient; the patient has to be able to fit into or onto the examining table or machine. The patient's size or large body habitus (LBH) may preclude proper positioning. If the equipment can accommodate the patient, imaging may still be unsuccessful or unsatisfactory due to decreased visualization through the fatty tissues of the body. The x-ray or other imaging beam of light cannot penetrate the layers of fat to obtain a crisp image of its target internal organ or structure. When this occurs, it can be difficult or impossible to get a clear picture of the organs or any abnormality. Fatty tissue can obscure conditions such as diseased organs, obstructions, vascular compromise, abnormal tissues or tumors, and problems with fetal growth and development.

Abnormal Tumor Markers (R97)

The term "tumor markers" describes the presence of certain molecules (including antigens, hormones, and proteins) occurring in blood or tissue that are associated with the cancer. Identification and measurement of tumor markers helps clinical management by:

- Providing a screening mechanism for healthy and high-risk populations for the presence of cancer

- Assisting in the diagnosis of cancer or of a specific type of cancer

- Providing a measurement to evaluate the prognosis in a patient

- Providing a means of monitoring a patient in remission or the response to treatment in patients who have undergone treatment using surgery, radiation, or chemotherapy

The categories in this code block are as follows:

R97   Abnormal tumor markers

R97.-   Abnormal tumor markers

Tumor markers, also called tumor associated antigens (TAA) and tumor specific antigens (TSA), help in the diagnosis and follow-up of certain types of cancer. Tumor-associated antigens (TAA) are closely associated with the presence of tumor cells, and tumor-specific antigens (TSA) are unique identifiers of tumor cells. The presence of TSA is especially beneficial in diagnosing and following many types of cancer. There are many different types of TAA and TSA tests, many of which are specific to certain cancers, such as tests for elevated prostate-specific antigens (PSA) for prostate cancer, alpha-fetoprotein for hepatocellular cancer, and CA-19 for gastrointestinal and pancreatic cancer.

R97.0   Elevated carcinoembryonic antigen [CEA]

Elevated carcinoembryonic antigen (CEA) levels in the blood are used to help diagnose certain benign and malignant neoplasms and other diseases. CEA tests are primarily used to monitor patients with colorectal and advanced breast cancer; however, elevated CEA levels can also be present in other types of cancer such as pancreatic, gastric, and lung. Other diseases in which CEA may be elevated include cirrhosis, inflammatory bowel disease, chronic lung disease, and pancreatitis.

R97.2-   Elevated prostate specific antigen [PSA]

Elevated prostate specific antigen (PSA) levels can be an indication for both cancerous (prostate cancer being of primary concern) and noncancerous conditions in male patients. In addition, research has now indicated that a rising PSA level following completed definitive treatment (biochemical recurrence), rising to 0.4 ng per ml or more, may be an indicator of recurrent disease. There are two codes in this subcategory: the one describing a diagnosis of elevated prostate specific antigen (PSA) is assigned before a confirmed cancer or benign prostatic condition has been diagnosed, while the one for a diagnosis of rising PSA following treatment for malignant neoplasm of prostate is assigned only if the patient has elevated PSA after having undergone and completed treatment for a previous prostatic malignancy.

Ill-Defined and Unknown Cause of Mortality (R99)

This code block contains a single code that classifies death due to an ill-defined or unknown cause.

R99   Ill-defined and unknown cause of mortality

Sudden infant death syndrome (SIDS), also labeled cot or crib death, is classified here and is defined as the sudden death of an infant, usually younger than 1 year of age, that remains unexplained after a thorough case investigation, including performance of a complete autopsy, examination of the death scene, and review of the clinical history. According to the National SIDS Resource Center, most researchers now believe that babies who die of SIDS are born with one or more conditions that make them especially vulnerable to stresses that occur in the normal life of an infant, including internal and external influences. Maternal risk factors include cigarette smoking during pregnancy, maternal age under 20 years, poor prenatal care, low weight gain during pregnancy, anemia, use of illegal drugs, and a history of sexually transmitted disease or urinary tract infection. Most deaths from SIDS occur by the end of the sixth month, with the greatest number occurring between 2 and 4 months of age. A SIDS death occurs quickly and is often associated with sleep, with no signs of suffering. More deaths are reported in the fall and winter (in both the Northern and Southern Hemispheres) and there is a 60 to 40 percent male-to-female ratio. A death is diagnosed as SIDS only after all other alternatives have been eliminated.

Chapter 19: Injury, Poisoning and Certain Other Consequences of External Causes (SØØ-T88)

This chapter is divided into two sections. Section S covers different types of injuries related to single body regions, excluding foreign bodies in natural orifices, burns, and corrosions. Types of injuries in the S section range from minor injuries, such as contusions, cuts, and abrasions, to more severe injuries, such as fractures and penetrating wounds, to life-threatening injuries, such as brain and spinal cord injuries and injuries to internal organs. Section T covers injuries to unspecified body parts; foreign bodies in natural orifices; burns and corrosions; poisoning, adverse effects, and underdosing of drugs, medicaments, and biological substances; toxic effects; effects of external causes, such as radiation, heat, light, cold, asphyxiation, and other external causes; and complications of medical care.

S Codes

Injuries are classified first into code blocks by general anatomic site or region. Within each code block injuries are classified by type, such as open wound, fracture, dislocation, nerve injury, blood vessel injury, and amputation. Each type of injury is subclassified more specifically as to type and site. Some injuries such as fractures are classified based on multiple factors related to the injury.

Fractures

A fracture is a break in a bone resulting from two possible causes: the direct or indirect application of undue force against the bone and pathological changes resulting in spontaneous fractures. This chapter includes only those fractures that have arisen as a result of an injury. It includes delayed healing and nonunions of fractured bones. In the case of a fracture, the type of fracture (e.g., displaced or nondisplaced, open or closed) and the episode of care are components of the code.

Closed fractures are contained beneath the skin, while open or compound fractures connote an associated open wound. Open fractures are always compound, with a wound leading to the fracture or the broken bone ends protruding through the skin. There is a high risk of infection with open fractures since the tissues are exposed to contaminants.

Specific terminology is used to describe fractures that pertain to bones in a particular part of the body. Those terms are defined in their respective subcategories.

The following fracture types and definitions are used across many areas of the body, especially the extremities:

Comminuted:	Bone is fractured, splintered, or shattered into multiple pieces, contains small bone fragments, usually caused by severe force
Greenstick:	Incomplete fracture, bone bends and cracks, common in young, flexible bones of children
Oblique:	Fracture at a diagonal angle across the bone shaft
Physeal:	Pediatric fractures of the growth plate or physis. Salter-Harris classification system is a method of describing the involvement of the physis, metaphysis, and epiphysis of the fracture
Segmental:	Bone is broken in two places leaving at least one segment unattached to the body of bone
Spiral:	Also called a torsion fracture, caused by a twisting force resulting in a diagonal fracture around and through the bone
Transverse:	Fracture straight across the bone at a right angle to the long axis of the bone

The codes for fractures capture the type of encounter and whether the fracture is open or closed; open fractures are broken down further by the type of fracture based on the Gustilo classification. The Gustilo classification describes the severity of open fracture and soft tissue injury. Following are the definitions for open fractures as defined by the Gustilo classification:

Type I:	Low energy injury, clean wound less than 1 cm
Type II:	Wound is more than 1 cm with moderate soft tissue damage
Type III:	High energy wound, greater than 1 cm with extensive soft tissue damage, and subclassified to IIIA, IIIB, and IIIC

Type IIIA:	Adequate soft tissue coverage despite extensive soft tissue damage
Type IIIB:	Inadequate soft tissue coverage usually with severe wound contamination
Type IIIC:	Type III open fracture associated with arterial injury

Fracture Types

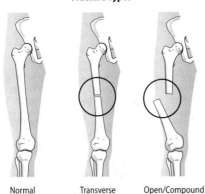

Normal	Transverse	Open/Compound

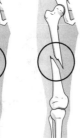

Oblique	Oblique displaced	Comminuted

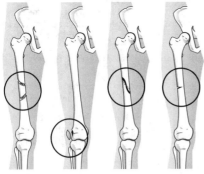

Segmental	Avulsed	Spiral	Greenstick

Focus Point

Many subcategories identify whether the fracture is displaced or nondisplaced. A fracture not indicated as nondisplaced or displaced should be classified to displaced.

The seventh character for an initial encounter specifies whether the fracture is open or closed. If unspecified, the default is closed.

The majority of codes in this chapter require seventh-character extensions. When consulting the Alphabetic Index, it is imperative to confirm each code in the Tabular List. Refer back to the beginning of the code category, where necessary, for the definitions of each applicable seventh character. For the most current, detailed information regarding the use of the seventh characters for this chapter, consult ICD-10-CM Coding Guideline: I.C.19.a.

T Codes

Section T begins with several codes for other and unspecified injuries that would rarely be used due to the lack of specificity as to the site and nature of the injury.

The next section reports foreign bodies that enter the body through a natural orifice; these codes are differentiated from foreign bodies in a superficial or penetrating wound, which are classified using S codes based on the body site.

The third section reports burns and corrosions. Burns are the result of a thermal or heat source, such as fire or a hot appliance, while corrosions are due to chemicals. Burns and corrosions of external surfaces (skin) are classified by site, depth, and extent. The burn section is followed by a short section related to frostbite.

The next two sections report poisoning, adverse effects, and underdosing of drugs, medicaments, and biological substances and toxic effects of nonmedicinal substances. Codes in these two sections are combination codes that include the external cause.

The next section relates to effects of external causes, such as radiation, heat, light, cold, asphyxiation, and other external causes.

The final section relates to certain complications of surgical and medical care that are not classified in the body system chapters.

The chapter is broken down into the following code blocks:

S00–S09	Injuries to the head
S10–S19	Injuries to the neck
S20–S29	Injuries to the thorax

S30-S39	Injuries to the abdomen, lower back, lumbar spine, pelvis and external genitals
S40-S49	Injuries to the shoulder and upper arm
S50-S59	Injuries to the elbow and forearm
S60-S69	Injuries to the wrist, hand and fingers
S70-S79	Injuries to the hip and thigh
S80-S89	Injuries to the knee and lower leg
S90-S99	Injuries to the ankle and foot
T07	Injuries involving multiple body regions
T14	Injury of unspecified body region
T15-T19	Effects of foreign body entering through natural orifice
T20-T25	Burns and corrosions of external body surface, specified by site
T26-T28	Burns and corrosions confined to eye and internal organs
T30-T32	Burns and corrosions of multiple and unspecified body regions
T33-T34	Frostbite
T36-T50	Poisoning by, adverse effect of and underdosing of drugs, medicaments and biological substances
T51-T65	Toxic effects of substances chiefly nonmedicinal as to source
T66-T78	Other and unspecified effects of external causes
T79	Certain early complications of trauma
T80-T88	Complications of surgical and medical care, not elsewhere classified

Injuries to the Head (S00-S09)

Head injuries described in this code block range from minor injuries such as abrasions and contusions to life-threatening conditions such as skull fractures and brain injuries.

The categories in this code block are as follows:

S00	Superficial injury of head
S01	Open wound of head
S02	Fracture of skull and facial bones
S03	Dislocation and sprain of joints and ligaments of head
S04	Injury of cranial nerve
S05	Injury of eye and orbit
S06	Intracranial injury
S07	Crushing injury of head
S08	Avulsion and traumatic amputation of part of head
S09	Other and unspecified injuries of head

S02.-   Fracture of skull and facial bones

A skull fracture is a break in one of the eight bones that encases the brain. These eight bones are collectively referred to as the cranium or cranial bones and include the frontal bone, two parietal bones, two temporal bones, the ethmoid bone, sphenoid bone, and occipital bone. Facial bones include the nasal bones, bones of the orbital floor, and bones of the upper and lower jaw. Traumatic fractures occur as a result of direct or indirect application of undue force against the bone. Closed fractures are contained beneath the skin, while open or compound fractures connote an associated open wound. Open fractures are always compound, with a wound leading to the fracture or the broken bone ends protruding through the skin. There is a high risk of infection with open fractures since the tissues are exposed to contaminants. In the case of skull fractures, this is a particular concern because open fractures expose the brain to these contaminants.

Focus Point

Fractures of the skull may be accompanied by an intracranial injury, such as a concussion, cerebral edema, diffuse brain injury, cerebral contusion or laceration, or a subarachnoid, subdural, or epidural (extradural) hemorrhage. These intracranial injuries are reported additionally with a code from category S06.

S02.0-   Fracture of vault of skull

The vault of the skull is composed of three bones: the frontal bone and two parietal bones. A fracture of any bone comprising the skull vault is classified here. Types of fractures include those described as simple or closed, open or compound, and depressed. A depressed fracture is one that is concave with the bone fractures pushed inward toward the brain.

S02.1-   Fracture of base of skull

There are five bones that comprise the skull base: the occipital bone, two temporal bones, the ethmoid bone, and the sphenoid bone.

S02.11-   Fracture of occiput

Fractures of the occiput are subdivided based on morphology, mechanism of injury, and laterality. The occiput is the bone at the base of the skull that contains the foramen magnum, the opening in the bone that allows the spinal cord to join the brain.

There are three common fracture types. The least common, Type I, is considered a stable injury due to minimal fragment displacement into the foramen magnum. It is an impaction fracture caused by an axial compression.

Type II is the most common fracture and is due to a direct blow to the skull. It is a basilar skull fracture that also involves one or both occipital condyles. It is considered a stable injury because the alar ligament and tectorial membrane are preserved.

Caused by forced contralateral bending and rotation, a Type III fracture can potentially become an unstable injury because of the craniocervical disruption. It is characterized as an avulsion injury of the condyle in the region of the alar ligament attachment.

S02.19- Other fracture of base of skull

Fractures of temporal bones and sphenoid or ethmoid bones are included here. The two temporal bones are located on the lateral aspect of the skull and adjoin the parietal, sphenoid, and occipital bones. The sphenoid bone is the large bone containing the sphenoid sinus, forming part of the back of the orbit. The ethmoid bone is situated in front of the sphenoid bone above the nasal cavity and between the orbits; it separates the nasal cavities from the brain. Basal skull fractures include orbital roof fractures. The orbital roof is comprised of the orbital process of the frontal bone and the lesser wing of the sphenoid bone. Sometimes fractures of the base of the skull are described as involving the cranial fossae. There are three fossae—anterior, middle, and posterior—that form the floor of the cranial cavity (on the superior aspect of the base of the skull) and provide a surface to support the various lobes of the brain. The frontal lobes rest on the anterior fossa, the temporal lobes on the middle fossa, and the pons and medulla oblongata are contained within the posterior fossa, with the cerebellum expanding over the medulla oblongata.

S02.2- Fracture of nasal bones

The nasal bone adjoins the frontal bone to form the superior aspect of the nose and the vomer provides inferior and interior support for nasal conchae.

S02.3- Fracture of orbital floor

The orbits, which surround the eyes, are complex structures formed by multiple bones of the skull and face. The frontal, mandible, lacrimal, orbital plate, zygomatic, and sphenoid bones fit together to support and protect the eyeball. The orbital floor is comprised of the orbital plates of the maxilla, zygoma, and palatine bones.

S02.4- Fracture of malar, maxillary and zygoma bones

The maxilla forms the upper jawbone. The zygomatic bones, also called the malar bones, are the two bones under the eye that form the prominence of the upper aspect of the cheek.

S02.41- LeFort fracture

Named for Rene Le Fort, these fractures describe different combinations of multiple fractures that occur from significant force to the midface. A common denominator in all three types of LeFort fractures is fracturing of the pterygoid processes, which are two bony plates resembling wings that extend downward from the sphenoid bone.

S02.411- LeFort I fracture

LeFort I is a horizontal fracture that separates the upper teeth from the upper face, crossing the nasal floor. It includes fractures of the pterygoid plates and the walls of the maxillary sinuses.

S02.412- LeFort II fracture

LeFort II is a triangular-shaped fracture with the teeth at the base and the nasofrontal suture at the top of the triangle. Fractures include the pterygoid plates, posterior and lateral walls of the maxillary sinus, inferior orbital rim, orbital floor, and medial wall of orbit.

S02.413- LeFort III fracture

LeFort III is a fractured line dividing the facial bones from the rest of the skull. Fractures include pterygoid plates, upper posterior margins of maxillary sinuses, zygomatic arch, lateral and medial orbital wall, orbital rim, sphenoid bone, and across the nasofrontal suture.

S02.6- Fracture of mandible

Mandible fractures are common due to the mandible's protuberance and decreased support of surrounding structures. It is the only moveable bone of the facial bones and is necessary for chewing action. In utero, the mandible originally comprises two U-shaped bones that fuse to form one bone in early childhood. This single bone is identified by specific sites, such as the condylar and subcondylar process, coronoid process, ramus, angle, symphysis, and alveolus. This subcategory contains specific codes to report these individual sites and, when applicable, identifies the laterality.

S02.61- Fracture of condylar process of mandible

This is the articular, uppermost portion of the mandible superior to the ramus on both sides and the most common of all mandibular fractures. Condylar fractures occur at the head of the bone and are considered intracapsular. The condylar process also includes the pterygoid fovea.

S02.62- Fracture of subcondylar process of mandible

Located below the condylar, the subcondylar is a separate classification of a fracture of the condylar indicating the break in the inferior portion of the bone, also considered extracapsular. This area also includes a break within the condylar neck.

S02.63- Fracture of coronoid process of mandible

The coronoid processes are bilateral triangular bony projections located above and situated anterior to the ramus. They are the insertion point for the temporalis muscle and are among the least common fractures of the mandible as they are protected by the zygomatic arch.

Focus Point

If a fracture of the coronoid process is documented, look for a fracture of the zygomatic arch, which is reported separately with a code from subcategory S02.4- Fracture of malar, maxillary and zygoma bones.

S02.64- Fracture of ramus of mandible

This quadrilateral area behind the back teeth runs vertically from the border of the angled portion of the jaw to the cheeks on each side. It contains the mandibular canal, which houses the inferior alveolar vessels and nerve. Ramus fractures are less common than other mandibular fractures.

Focus Point

Although the upper border of the ramus includes the coronoid and condylar processes, separate, more specific codes in this subcategory are reported for fractures in those particular sites of the ramus.

S02.65- Fracture of angle of mandible

The angle of the mandible is the triangular portion of the jaw just below the ramus and ending at the base of the back, bottom teeth. It is one of the more common fracture sites of the mandible, usually as a result of motor vehicle or sporting accidents as well as assault.

S02.66- Fracture of symphysis of mandible

The symphysis begins in utero as a fibrocartilage unification of the two halves of the mandible, which is fused typically during the first year of life, leaving only a midline ridge. In this case, the fracture occurs below the incisors at the inferior border of the mandible. Motor vehicle accidents and assaults typically account for these more common mandibular fractures.

S02.67- Fracture of alveolus of mandible

The alveolus is the area of the mandible that houses the teeth. Fractures of this site are unusual, accounting for only 1 percent to 5 percent of mandibular fractures.

S03.- Dislocation and sprain of joints and ligaments of head

Dislocations and sprains are injuries to the joint structures and tissues surrounding the joints.

S03.4- Sprain of jaw

S03.8- Sprain of joints and ligaments of other parts of head

S03.9- Sprain of joints and ligaments of unspecified parts of head

A sprain is an injury to the ligaments, which are the tough fibrous tissues that bind bones together at joints. Sprains are graded. A Type I sprain denotes minor ligamentous injury; Type II is an incomplete ligamentous injury; and Type III describes a complete disruption of the ligament. The more ligaments involved in the sprain, the more serious the injury. Sprains manifest with swelling, pain, and limited mobility. A mild sprain may heal in two to six weeks, while a severe sprain may require eight weeks to 10 months to heal. A sprain of the jaw involves the ligaments of the temporomandibular joints.

Focus Point

A sprain is not identical to a strain and the two terms should not be used synonymously. A strain is an injury to the muscles or tendons. Codes for strains at the head level are located in category S09.

S06.- Intracranial injury

One of the great problems associated with head trauma is that the brain sustains a double blow: the initial blow causes the brain to travel to the opposite side of the skull where the brain sustains a second blow when it smites the interior skull with significant force. This second blow is called contrecoup. Such force applied to the brain causes swelling and increased intracranial pressure that is very dangerous. Serious head trauma has a high mortality rate, nearly 50 percent. Patients who have survived severe head trauma often deal with posttraumatic epilepsy and other sequelae of the injury for many years.

S06.0- Concussion

A concussion is a traumatic brain injury caused by a blow to the head or a jarring or shaking injury to another part of the body that causes the brain to sustain trauma as it moves within the skull. One diagnostic symptom of a concussion is loss of consciousness, but it is possible to sustain a concussion without any loss of consciousness. Common symptoms include headache or painless sense of pressure within the skull, loss of memory particularly surrounding the event that caused the concussion, confusion, feeling stunned or dazed, dizziness, ringing in the ears, nausea, and vomiting.

Focus Point

When the patient is treated for the symptoms of a concussion within 24 to 48 hours and the diagnosis is identified as "postconcussion syndrome," verify with the physician whether the concussion is still in the current stage and should be reported with a code from subcategory S06.0-. If the concussion is not in the current stage, use code F07.81 Postconcussional syndrome.

S06.1-   Traumatic cerebral edema

Traumatic cerebral edema, also referred to as brain swelling or elevated intracranial pressure, can occur in one (focal) or several (diffuse) locations in the brain. As the brain swells, there is increased pressure against the skull that obstructs blood flow. It also blocks fluids from leaving the brain, increasing the swelling and causing cell damage and death.

S06.2-   Diffuse traumatic brain injury

Diffuse traumatic brain injury is damage that occurs in a more widespread area than the focal injury, including diffuse axonal brain injury, which happens as a result of the brain moving back and forth in the skull from acceleration, deceleration, or rotational injuries. This movement disrupts the part of the nerve cell (axons) that allow neurons to send messages between them. It also causes brain cells to die, which causes swelling. Diffuse axonal injury can include shearing injury, which occurs when the tissues slide over each other, causing unconsciousness and releasing chemicals that aggravate and further damage the brain. Diffuse axonal brain injury typically shows up on radiology as many white-matter lesions and is a leading cause of persistent vegetative state or death in traumatic brain injuries.

S06.3-   Focal traumatic brain injury

Focal brain injuries are limited to a specific area or region of the brain, most often caused by the head striking or being struck by an object. Focal brain injuries may also result from penetrating trauma such as a bullet wound. Focal injuries may result in contusion, laceration, or hemorrhage. Codes in this category are specific to the type of focal brain injury and the site of the injury.

S06.31-   Contusion and laceration of right cerebrum

S06.32-   Contusion and laceration of left cerebrum

S06.33-   Contusion and laceration of cerebrum, unspecified

These subcategories report a contusions or lacerations to the cerebrum, which is the largest part of the brain, consisting of two hemispheres: left and right. Also referred to as the cortex, it is responsible for higher functions such as thoughts, speech, or movement. The four lobes—frontal, parietal, occipital, and temporal—are located in the cerebrum. A brain contusion is a bruise of the brain tissue and a laceration is a cut or tear of the brain tissue. Both result in structural damage to the brain and represent more serious injuries than a concussion without structural damage.

Focus Point

Hematoma of the brain is included in the hemorrhage codes NOT the contusion codes.

S06.34-   Traumatic hemorrhage of right cerebrum

S06.35-   Traumatic hemorrhage of left cerebrum

S06.36-   Traumatic hemorrhage of cerebrum, unspecified

Bleeding within the brain due to trauma includes hemorrhage and hematoma and may also be called intracerebral hemorrhage or hematoma. Traumatic brain hemorrhage may be due to blunt or penetrating head injuries. A collection of blood within the brain tissue can compress adjacent brain structures and cause the brain to swell resulting in an increase in intracranial pressure and further damage to the brain. The cerebrum is the largest part of the brain, consisting of two hemispheres: left and right. Also referred to as the cortex, it is responsible for higher functions, such as thoughts, speech, or movement. The four lobes—frontal, parietal, occipital, and temporal—are located in the cerebrum.

S06.37-   Contusion, laceration, and hemorrhage of cerebellum

This subcategory includes any contusion, bruising, laceration, hemorrhage, or hematoma due to trauma of the cerebellum. The cerebellum, referred to as the little brain, is the smaller area in the back of the brain responsible for coordination of movement, balance, and posture. The thalamus, hypothalamus, amygdala, and hippocampus, which comprise the limbic system where many hormonal responses are generated, are located within the cerebellum. A brain contusion is a bruise of the brain tissue and a laceration is a cut or tear of the brain tissue. Both result in structural damage to the brain and represent more serious injuries than a concussion without structural damage. Bleeding within the brain due to trauma includes hemorrhage and hematoma. Traumatic brain hemorrhage may be due to blunt or penetrating head injuries. A collection of blood within the brain tissue can compress adjacent brain structures and cause the brain to swell resulting in an increase in intracranial pressure and further damage to the brain.

S06.38- Contusion, laceration, and hemorrhage of brainstem

This subcategory includes any contusion, bruising, laceration, hemorrhage, or hematoma due to trauma of the brainstem, which is responsible for all vital body functions. The brainstem is located between the spinal cord and the rest of the brain and is comprised of the midbrain (movement, vision, hearing), pons (posture, movement, sleep), and medulla (heart rate, breathing). A brainstem contusion is a bruise of the brainstem tissue and a laceration is a cut or tear of the brainstem tissue. Both result in structural damage to the brainstem and represent more serious injuries than a concussion without structural damage. Bleeding within the brainstem due to trauma includes hemorrhage and hematoma. Traumatic brainstem hemorrhage may be due to blunt or penetrating head injuries. While traumatic brainstem hemorrhage is rare, it represents a life-threatening injury because of the many vital functions controlled by the brainstem.

S06.4- Epidural hemorrhage

An epidural hemorrhage is bleeding within the epidural space. The epidural space is the potential space between the endosteum of the cranium (skull) and the dura mater, the outermost layer of a three-layer membrane that covers the brain. Another term used to refer to the epidural space is extradural space, which is nearly synonymous except that the term epidural implies bleeding in immediate proximity to the dura mater while extradural implies bleeding that may be unconnected to the membrane itself, such as hemorrhage from the skull vessels. Hemorrhage within the epidural space occurs due to an injury of the dural vessels, which include the middle meningeal artery branches, dural veins, dural venous sinuses, and skull vessels.

Focus Point

Even though the epidural hemorrhage code does not contain the word traumatic, hemorrhage of the epidural or extradural space that is due to a nontraumatic cause is not coded here. The appropriate code is I62.1 Nontraumatic extradural hemorrhage, which also includes nontraumatic epidural hemorrhage.

S06.5- Traumatic subdural hemorrhage

A subdural hemorrhage is bleeding into the subdural space and is the most common site of hemorrhage and hematoma due to head trauma. The subdural space is the potential space that results from the separation of the arachnoid mater from the dura mater as a result of trauma, pathologic process, or the absence of cerebrospinal fluid.

S06.6- Traumatic subarachnoid hemorrhage

A subarachnoid hemorrhage is bleeding into the subarachnoid space. The subarachnoid space is the space between the arachnoid membrane and the pia mater. This space contains cerebrospinal fluid.

S07.- Crushing injury of head

A crushing injury occurs when a body part is subjected to a high degree of force or pressure, typically after being pressed between two heavy or motionless objects. Damage related to crush injuries can include lacerations, fractures, bleeding, bruising, and compartment syndrome. Severe crush injuries cause extensive damage to skin, muscle, nerves, and bone. There may be bleeding, internally and/or externally, or blood supply may be cut off. Plasma may leak from the blood vessels into the damaged tissues, causing swelling and shock. When the crushed part is released, toxic chemicals produced by damaged muscles get into general circulation, which can cause kidney failure in severe cases.

Injuries to the Neck (S10-S19)

Injuries to the neck region described in this code block range from minor injuries, such as abrasions and contusions, to life-threatening conditions, such as cervical vertebrae fractures and spinal cord injuries.

The vertebral column forms a protective shield around the spinal column, much as the cranium protects the brain. In the neck, the cervical vertebrae allow movement through articulation. Each vertebra has a body and a neural arch that encase the spinal cord. Each vertebra has several prominent aspects called processes for the attachment of muscles, tendons, and other soft tissues. The two transverse processes of the cervical vertebrae have a small foramen, the foramen transversarium, through which the vertebral artery and vein and a plexus of sympathetic nerves travel. The first cervical vertebra is called the atlas and supports the globe of the head. It has no vertebral body; instead, the part of the vertebra that would have been the body is fused with the second cervical vertebra to form an osseous pivot around which the head turns. The second cervical vertebra is called the axis.

The spinal cord, protected by the vertebral column, shares the three meningeal layers—the dura, arachnoid, and pia maters—with the brain. It is described anatomically in relation to the vertebrae at each level, but the cord is not identical to the column. In addition to nerve tracts to the brain enclosed within the column, the spinal nerves exit the column to innervate specific muscle groups bilaterally, according to their level on the vertebral column.

Similar to the brain, the cord has gray and white matter. Hemorrhage into the gray matter is known as hematomyelia. Its symptoms, which are often permanent, include muscle wasting, diminished tendon reflexes, and muscle weakness.

Focus Point

The appropriate code for traumatic hematomyelia is currently indexed to nonspecific code T14.8 Other injury of unspecified body region.

The categories in this code block are as follows:

S10	Superficial injury of neck
S11	Open wound of neck
S12	Fracture of cervical vertebra and other parts of neck
S13	Dislocation and sprain of joints and ligaments at neck level
S14	Injury of nerves and spinal cord at neck level
S15	Injury of blood vessels at neck level
S16	Injury of muscle, fascia and tendon at neck level
S17	Crushing injury of neck
S19	Other specified and unspecified injuries of neck

S12.- Fracture of cervical vertebra and other parts of neck

A fracture is a break in a bone resulting from two possible causes: the direct or indirect application of undue force against the bone and pathological changes resulting in spontaneous fractures. This category includes only those fractures that have arisen as a result of an injury. It includes delayed healing and nonunions of fractured bones. Closed fractures are contained beneath the skin, while open or compound fractures connote an associated open wound. Open fractures are always compound, with a wound leading to the fracture or the broken bone ends protruding through the skin. There is a high risk of infection with open fractures since the tissues are exposed to contaminants.

Focus Point

Subcategories identify whether the fracture is displaced or nondisplaced. A fracture not indicated as nondisplaced or displaced should be classified to displaced. The seventh character for an initial encounter specifies whether the fracture is open or closed. If unspecified, the default is closed.

S12.0- Fracture of first cervical vertebra

The first cervical vertebra, also called the atlas, has a unique structure as it supports the "globe" of the head and is comprised of a ring that rotates around the second cervical vertebra allowing most of the head's ability to move from side to side.

S12.01- Stable burst fracture of first cervical vertebra

S12.02- Unstable burst fracture of first cervical vertebra

Also called Jefferson's fracture, this fracture of the atlas is generally caused by downward, axial-loading force on the occiput of the head, such as diving in shallow water striking the head. It usually involves fracture of bilateral sides of the anterior and posterior arch of C1 for a total of four fractures sites, although it can involve only two or three. The stable form of this fracture does not typically cause neurologic deficits, as cord compression is limited by the widening of the C1 ring.

S12.03- Posterior arch fracture of first cervical vertebra

The weak posterior arch can fracture when the head is hyperextended and the posterior arch is compressed between the occiput and the prominent spinous process of C2. It does not involve the anterior arch or transverse ligament of C1 making it different from the burst fracture. A posterior arch fracture is considered a stable fracture.

S12.04- Lateral mass fracture of first cervical vertebra

The lateral masses are the two articular facets that allow most of the flexion and extension of the head. This fracture occurs when it extends into these lateral masses. This type of fracture is considered unstable.

Anatomy C₁ and C₂

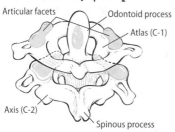

Anatomy C₁ and C₂

S12.1-   Fracture of second cervical vertebra

C2 is also known as the Axis or epistropheus vertebra. Part of C2, called the odontoid process (dens), forms the pivot that the atlas rotates on. The odontoid process lies just posterior to the anterior C1 arch and is attached by ligaments to the skull base and moves with C1. The transverse ligament of the atlas, together with the odontoid process, act as a protective restraint against horizontal displacement of the atlas. Other ligaments of the odontoid process provide rotational stability.

S12.11-   Type II dens fracture

This is a fracture at the base of the odontoid (dens) where it attaches to the body of C2. This is the most common of the dens fractures.

S12.12-   Other dens fracture

This subcategory includes Type I dens fracture, which is the least common. It involves the upper part of the odontoid process, is usually an avulsion injury to the tip, and is stable; however, it is occasionally associated with instability. Also included is the Type III dens, which occurs when the fracture extends through the body of C2.

S12.13-   Unspecified traumatic spondylolisthesis of second cervical vertebra

S12.14-   Type III traumatic spondylolisthesis of second cervical vertebra

S12.15-   Other traumatic spondylolisthesis of second cervical vertebra

Traumatic spondylolisthesis of C2 is one of the most common types of fractures seen in fatal motor vehicle accidents (MVA). They are categorized into four types. Type I consists of small bilateral pedicle fractures with little displacement and no angulation. If the anterior longitudinal ligament (ALL) and posterior longitudinal ligament (PLL) are intact, it is considered a stable injury. Type II fractures are considered unstable and are characterized by significant displacement and angulation, including bilateral pedicle fractures with

small disruption of the ALL and significant disruption of the PLL, with disruption to the intervertebral disc of C2 and C3. Type IIA, also unstable, is similar but less common than Type II, with only posterior displacement but severe angulation. It includes bilateral pedicle fractures with disruption of C2/C3 disc and some amount of PLL disruption. Type III includes severe displacement and severe angulation with bilateral pedicle fractures, disruption of C2/C3 disc, varying degrees of injury to the ALL and PLL, and dislocations of one or both sides of the C2/C3 facets. This is considered an unstable injury. Type III traumatic spondylolisthesis has a specific code. Type I, II, and IIA are included in the other specified subcategory.

S13.-   Dislocation and sprain of joints and ligaments at neck level

This subcategory includes subluxations, dislocations, and sprains of the cervical spine and neck. A subluxation refers to a partial dislocation. A sprain is an injury to the ligaments, which are the tough fibrous tissues that bind bones together at joints.

> **Focus Point**
>
> *A sprain is not identical to a strain and the two terms should not be used synonymously. A strain is an injury to the muscles or tendons. The code for a strain at the neck level is S16.1.*

S13.1-   Subluxation and dislocation of cervical vertebrae

Luxation is another term used to describe a complete dislocation, one that has separated the articulating surfaces of the joint. An incomplete dislocation, or subluxation, is one in which the joint surfaces maintain some articulation. A simple dislocation is a closed injury without a penetrating or communicating wound. An uncomplicated dislocation is not associated with other significant injuries.

S13.2-   Dislocation of other and unspecified parts of neck

Luxation is another term used to describe a complete dislocation, one that has separated the articulating surfaces of the joint. A simple dislocation is a closed injury without a penetrating or communicating wound. An uncomplicated dislocation is not associated with other significant injuries. Specific sites captured by the other specified code in this subcategory include dislocation of cricoarytenoid articulation, cricothyroid articulation, or thyroid cartilage.

S13.4-   Sprain of ligaments of cervical spine

S13.5-   Sprain of thyroid region

S13.8-   Sprain of joints and ligaments of other parts of neck

S13.9-   Sprain of joints and ligaments of unspecified parts of neck

A sprain is an injury to the ligaments, which are the tough fibrous tissues that bind bones together at joints. Sprains are graded. A Type I sprain denotes minor ligamentous injury; Type II is an incomplete ligamentous injury; and Type III describes a complete disruption of the ligament. The more ligaments involved in the sprain, the more serious the injury. Sprains manifest with swelling, pain, and limited mobility. A mild sprain may heal in two to six weeks, while a severe sprain may require eight weeks to 10 months to heal.

Focus Point

A sprain is not identical to a strain and the two terms should not be used synonymously. A strain is an injury to the muscles or tendons. Codes for strains at the neck level are located in category S16. Whiplash is a sprain of the ligaments of the neck caused by the sudden and forceful extension and flexion of the neck and is reported with a code in subcategory S13.4-.

S14.-   Injury of nerves and spinal cord at neck level

Nervous system injuries at the neck level may involve the spinal cord, one of the eight pairs of cervical nerve roots or nerves, the brachial plexus, the peripheral nerves of the neck, or the cervical sympathetic nerves. A plexus or ganglion is a bundle of nerves that serves a particular region of the body. A plexus lies relatively deep in the body as opposed to superficial nerves, which are close to the surface of the skin. Sympathetic nerves along with parasympathetic nerves are part of the autonomic nervous system. The autonomic system is considered to be involuntary, regulating body processes such as breathing, heartbeat, digestion, and orientation in space. The parasympathetic nervous system regulates everyday body processes that restore the body and conserve energy. In contrast, the sympathetic nervous system responds to emergency situations by activating the flight or fight response when there is a perception of danger or harm.

S14.0-   Concussion and edema of cervical spinal cord

A concussion of the spinal cord is a mild traumatic injury to the spinal cord that results in temporary neurological deficits at the level of the spinal cord injury with full recovery within 72 hours of the

occurrence. Spinal cord concussion typically results from a severe blow or jarring injury. Edema is swelling of the spinal cord that can also compromise neurological function.

S14.11-   Complete lesion of cervical spinal cord

A complete lesion of the spinal cord causes immediate total paralysis and sensory loss below the level of the injury. It is sometimes referred to as a complete injury or transverse cord injury. Depending on the site of injury, outcomes vary, ranging from respiratory paralysis (injury above C5 level); quadriplegia, which is paralysis of four limbs (C4-C5); and paralysis of the legs and partial paralysis of the arms, with abduction and flexion of the arms as movement potentials (C5-C6). A complete lesion of C6-C7 allows shoulder movement and elbow flexion, though the lower limbs are paralyzed.

S14.12-   Central cord syndrome of cervical spinal cord

This is an incomplete injury caused mainly by a hyperextension injury with anterior and posterior compression of the spinal cord. It causes weakness and motor impairment in upper extremities more than lower extremities and often includes bladder dysfunction (urinary retention). In older adults, central cord injury is more likely to occur in those already with cervical spondylosis when even a minor fall can cause central cord syndrome. In younger people it results from more major trauma.

S14.13-   Anterior cord syndrome of cervical spinal cord

Also known as Beck's syndrome, anterior cord syndrome is an injury that involves the anterior two-thirds of the spinal cord. This is caused by an ischemic insult to the cord from an injury to the anterior spinal artery or a flexion-compression type of injury to the spinal cord. It is characterized by paralysis below the injury level, autonomic dysfunction, orthostatic hypotension, and bladder and bowel dysfunction. It has the most dismal prognosis of incomplete spinal cord injuries with poor recovery of motor skills and coordination.

S14.14-   Brown-Sequard syndrome of cervical spinal cord

This is a rare condition typically caused by damage to one side (hemisection) of the spinal cord, such as a knife or gunshot wound, and is classified as an incomplete spinal cord lesion. It causes upper motor neuron paralysis to the injured side, as well as loss of pain and temperature sensation on the opposite side. Deficits can range from mild to severe.

S14.15- Other incomplete lesions of cervical spinal cord

Posterior cord syndrome is an incomplete injury resulting in motor paralysis and loss of posterior spinal column sensory function below the level of the injury. It typically results from a penetrating wound or from a hyperextension injury with fracture of the vertebral arch.

S15.- Injury of blood vessels at neck level

Vascular trauma may result from penetrating or blunt injury. Arterial blood loss manifests as profuse and bright red, while venous loss is steady and dark. Injury to the arteries at the neck level poses an extreme risk as this may cause loss of blood supply to the brain.

> **Focus Point**
>
> *Traumatic aneurysms are reported with codes for injury to blood vessels. An aneurysm is a weakening in the arterial wall that bulges with the pumping of the blood, posing the threat of rupture. When aneurysms are part of a disease process and not due to trauma, they are reported with codes from Chapter 9 Diseases of the Circulatory System.*

S16.- Injury of muscle, fascia and tendon at neck level

Strain injuries and lacerations of muscle, fascia, or tendon are classified here. Strains occur when the muscle, fascia, or tendon is stretched or subjected to a level of force beyond its stretching or strength capabilities. A tear of a muscle, fascia, or tendon is classified as a strain. A pulled muscle is also classified as a strain. Symptoms of strains include swelling, bruising, pain at rest and with activity, weakness in the strained muscle, and inability to use the affected body part. A laceration is a deep cut through the soft tissue and into the fascia, muscle, and/or tendon.

> **Focus Point**
>
> *A strain injury should not be confused with a sprain injury. A sprain is an injury to the ligaments, which are the tough fibrous tissues that bind bones together at joints. Sprains of the cervical spine and neck region are located in category S13.*

S17.- Crushing injury of neck

A crushing injury occurs when a body part is subjected to a high degree of force or pressure, typically after being pressed between two heavy or motionless objects. Damage related to crush injuries can include lacerations, fractures, bleeding, bruising, and compartment syndrome. Severe crush injuries cause extensive damage to skin, muscle, nerves, bone, and internal organs. There may be bleeding, internally and/or externally, or blood supply may be cut off. Plasma may leak from the blood vessels into the damaged tissues, causing swelling and shock. When the crushed part is released, toxic chemicals produced by damaged muscles get into the general circulation, which can cause kidney failure in severe cases.

Injuries to the Thorax (S20-S29)

Injuries to the thorax range from superficial injuries, such as contusions, abrasions, superficial foreign bodies, and insect bites, to deeper injuries involving the soft tissues to fractures, spinal cord injuries, and injuries of organs contained within the thoracic cavity, such as the heart, lungs, and great vessels.

Twelve pairs of ribs form the thoracic cage, which protect the critical organs in the thorax and abdomen. The true ribs are the first eight ribs and the false ribs are the last four ribs. The floating ribs are the last two of the false ribs.

All of the ribs, except the floating ribs, are connected to the sternum (the breastbone) with costal cartilage.

The categories in this code block are as follows:

S20	Superficial injury of thorax
S21	Open wound of thorax
S22	Fracture of rib(s), sternum and thoracic spine
S23	Dislocation and sprain of joints and ligaments of thorax
S24	Injury of nerves and spinal cord at thorax level
S25	Injury of blood vessels of thorax
S26	Injury of heart
S27	Injury of other and unspecified intrathoracic organs
S28	Crushing injury of thorax, and traumatic amputation of part of thorax
S29	Other and unspecified injuries of thorax

S22.- Fracture of rib(s), sternum and thoracic spine

A fracture is a break in a bone resulting from two possible causes: the direct or indirect application of undue force against the bone and pathological changes resulting in spontaneous fractures. This chapter includes only those fractures that have arisen as a result of an injury. It also includes delayed healing and nonunions of fractured bones. Closed fractures are contained beneath the skin, while open or compound fractures connote an associated open wound. Open fractures are always compound, with a wound leading to the fracture or the broken bone ends protruding through the skin. There is a very high risk of infection with open fractures since the tissues are exposed to contaminants.

Focus Point

Rib fracture is a common risk associated with cardiopulmonary resuscitation (CPR) and is not considered a complication of the procedure. Assign the appropriate rib fracture and external cause codes.

S22.0-   Fracture of thoracic vertebra

When diagnosing fractures, the spine is divided into the anterior, middle, and posterior column. A wedge compression fracture occurs when a force such as a fall or heavy weight crushes the anterior of the vertebra, forming a wedge shape. In contrast, a burst fracture happens when the force of the compression crushes the vertebra body in all directions fracturing two or three of the columns. Typically when only the anterior column is fractured, such as with the wedge fracture, it is considered to be stable. Fractures in both the anterior and middle column can be considered unstable or stable and fractures in all three columns are generally considered unstable.

S22.5-   Flail chest

Flail chest is one of the most dangerous thoracic injuries, resulting from an injury causing at least four fractured ribs in two locations and pulmonary contusion, leading to hypoventilation. In flail chest, a portion of the rib cage separates from the rest of the chest wall resulting in the loss of the ability of the separated area to perform necessary lung expansion for breathing. Generally, flail chest injuries carry a high mortality risk, with death attributed to hypoxemia, hypovolemia, or myocardial failure.

S23.-   Dislocation and sprain of joints and ligaments of thorax

This subcategory includes subluxations, dislocations, and sprains of the thoracic spine, ribs, and sternum. A subluxation refers to a partial dislocation. A sprain is an injury to the ligaments, which are the tough fibrous tissues that bind bones together at joints.

S23.1-   Subluxation and dislocation of thoracic vertebra

Luxation is another term used to describe a complete dislocation, one that has separated the articulating surfaces of the joint. An incomplete dislocation, or subluxation, is one in which the joint surfaces maintain some articulation. A simple dislocation is a closed injury without a penetrating or communicating wound. An uncomplicated dislocation is not associated with other significant injuries. Open dislocations are those with an open wound at the site of the joint. Open injuries, also called compound dislocations, are subject to infection. Reduction of a dislocation or subluxation is by manipulation, open or closed.

S23.3-   Sprain of ligaments of thoracic spine

A sprain is an injury to the ligaments, which are the tough fibrous tissues that bind bones together at joints. Sprains are graded. A Type I sprain denotes minor ligamentous injury, Type II is an incomplete ligamentous injury, and Type III describes a complete disruption of the ligament. The more ligaments involved in the sprain, the more serious the injury. Sprains manifest with swelling, pain, and limited mobility. A mild sprain may heal in two to six weeks, while a severe sprain may require eight weeks to 10 months to heal.

Focus Point

A sprain is not identical to a strain and the two terms should not be used synonymously. A strain is an injury to the muscles or tendons. Strains of the thorax are reported with codes in category S29.

S23.4-   Sprain of ribs and sternum

A sprain is an injury to the ligaments, which are the tough fibrous tissues that bind bones together at joints. Sprains are graded. A Type I sprain denotes minor ligamentous injury, Type II is an incomplete ligamentous injury, and Type III describes a complete disruption of the ligament. The more ligaments involved in the sprain, the more serious the injury. Sprains manifest with swelling, pain, and limited mobility. A mild sprain may heal in two to six weeks, while a severe sprain may require eight weeks to 10 months to heal.

Focus Point

A sprain is not identical to a strain and the two terms should not be used synonymously. A strain is an injury to the muscles or tendons. Codes for strains in the thoracic region are located in category S29.

S24.-   Injury of nerves and spinal cord at thorax level

Injuries classified here include those involving the spinal cord, nerve roots, peripheral nerves, and sympathetic nerves, including nerve plexuses and ganglions located in the region of the thoracic spine and chest. A plexus or ganglion is a bundle of nerves that serves a particular region of the body. A plexus lies relatively deep in the body as opposed to superficial nerves, which are close to the surface of the skin. Sympathetic nerves along with parasympathetic nerves are part of the autonomic nervous system. The autonomic system is considered to be involuntary, regulating body processes such as breathing, heartbeat, digestion, and orientation in space. The parasympathetic nervous system regulates everyday body processes that restore the body and conserve energy. In contrast, the sympathetic nervous system responds to emergency situations by activating the flight or fight response when there is a perception of danger or harm.

S24.0- Concussion and edema of thoracic spinal cord

A concussion of the spinal cord is a mild traumatic injury to the spinal cord that results in temporary neurological deficits at the level of the spinal cord injury with full recovery within 72 hours of the occurrence. Spinal cord concussions typically result from a very severe blow or jarring injury. Edema is swelling of the spinal cord that can also compromise neurological function.

S24.11- Complete lesion of thoracic spinal cord

A complete lesion of the spinal cord causes immediate total paralysis and sensory loss below the level of the injury. It is sometimes referred to as a complete injury or transverse cord injury. With injuries at the higher thoracic level, arm and hand movement is usually intact; paraplegia generally affects the legs and trunk. Lower thoracic injury usually maintains upper body movement but results in lower limb paraplegia and loss of bowel or bladder control.

S24.13- Anterior cord syndrome of thoracic spinal cord

This injury involves the anterior two thirds of the spinal cord. It is characterized by loss of motor function and pain or temperature sensation but limbs maintain normal movement because the sensory input from muscles and tendons are still intact.

S24.14- Brown-Sequard syndrome of thoracic spinal cord

This is a rare condition typically caused by damage to one side (hemisection) of the spinal cord, such as a knife or gunshot wound, and is classified as an incomplete spinal cord lesion. It causes upper motor neuron paralysis to the injured side, as well as loss of pain and temperature sensation on the opposite side. Deficits can range from mild to severe.

S24.15- Other incomplete lesions of thoracic spinal cord

Posterior cord syndrome is an incomplete injury resulting in motor paralysis and loss of posterior spinal column sensory function below the level of the injury.

S25.- Injury of blood vessels of thorax

Vascular trauma may result from penetrating or blunt injury. Arterial blood loss manifests as profuse and bright red, while venous loss is steady and dark. Injuries to the great vessels that enter and leave the heart are life-threatening as are injuries to most arteries in the thorax.

Focus Point

Traumatic aneurysms are reported with codes for injury to blood vessels. An aneurysm is a weakening in the arterial wall that bulges with the pumping of the blood, posing the threat of rupture. When aneurysms are part of a disease process and not due to trauma, they are reported with codes from Chapter 9 Diseases of the Circulatory System.

S27.- Injury of other and unspecified intrathoracic organs

Injuries classified here are those involving the pleura, lungs, bronchi, thoracic trachea, diaphragm, and esophagus. Some of the injuries included in this category are contusions, lacerations, and blast injuries.

A blast injury causes damage to organs or tissues caused solely by the direct effect of a blast wave pressure, called overpressurization shockwave, from high order explosives. These injuries are due to anatomical and physiological changes incurred upon the body from the direct or reflected impact of the overpressurization force. The force can emanate from a bomb, gas leak, or any other explosion. Blast injuries are graded as primary, secondary, tertiary, and miscellaneous. A primary blast injury affects air-filled organs, such as the lungs, ears, and bowel. If the tympanic membrane is ruptured, the physician automatically assumes serious organ damage. Secondary injury results from injuries associated with flying objects. Tertiary injuries may result from striking objects while airborne. Morbidity and mortality are greatest if the explosion occurs within a confined space or underwater.

Focus Point

Only primary blast injuries are reported in this category. Secondary and tertiary blast injuries are reported with codes describing the specific injuries sustained.

S27.0- Traumatic pneumothorax

S27.1- Traumatic hemothorax

S27.2- Traumatic hemopneumothorax

Pneumothorax is free air trapped in the pleural space with lung collapse on the affected side, in this case due to a traumatic closed or open injury to the chest. Common causes include falls, bicycle or motor vehicle accidents, and penetrating wounds. Hemothorax is blood in the pleural space that can be from the chest wall, lung, heart, or blood vessels and is a result of a blunt or penetrating trauma. Hemopneumothorax is the concurrent presence of air and blood.

Focus Point

When pneumothorax is caused by a medical procedure (iatrogenic), the appropriate code is J95.811 Postprocedural pneumothorax.

S28.-   Crushing injury of thorax, and traumatic amputation of part of thorax

This category reports crushed chest injury, as well as traumatic partial or complete amputation of the breast or other parts of the thorax.

S28.0-   Crushed chest

A crushing injury occurs when a body part is subjected to a high degree of force or pressure, typically after being pressed between two heavy or motionless objects. Damage related to crush injuries can include lacerations, fractures, bleeding, bruising, and compartment syndrome. Severe crush injuries cause extensive damage to skin, muscle, nerves, bone, and internal organs of the thorax. There may be bleeding, internally and/or externally, or blood supply may be cut off. Plasma may leak from the blood vessels into the damaged tissues, causing swelling and shock. When the crushed part is released, toxic chemicals produced by damaged muscles get into general circulation, which can cause kidney failure in severe cases.

S29.-   Other and unspecified injuries of thorax

Strain injuries and lacerations of muscle and tendon are classified here. Strains occur when the muscle, fascia, or tendon is stretched or subjected to a level of force beyond its stretching or strength capabilities. A tear of a muscle, fascia, or tendon is classified as a strain. A pulled muscle is also classified as a strain. Symptoms of strains include swelling, bruising, pain at rest and with activity, weakness in the strained muscle, and inability to use the affected body part. A laceration is a deep cut through the soft tissue and into the fascia, muscle, and/or tendon.

Focus Point

A sprain injury should not be confused with a strain injury. A sprain is an injury to the ligaments, which are the tough fibrous tissues that bind bones together at joints. Sprains of the thoracic spine, ribs, and sternum are located in category S23.

Injuries to the Abdomen, Lower Back, Lumbar Spine, Pelvis and External Genitals (S30-S39)

Injuries classified here range from minor injuries, such as contusions, abrasions, superficial foreign bodies, and insect bites, to more severe injuries involving the soft tissues, fractures, spinal cord injuries, and injuries of organs contained within the abdominal cavity.

The lumbar vertebrae are the largest of the moveable vertebrae or true vertebrae. The spinal cord, protected by the vertebral column, shares the three meningeal layers—the dura mater, arachnoid, and pia mater—with the brain. The spinal cord is described anatomically in relation to the vertebrae at each level, but the cord is not identical to the column. In addition to nerve tracts to the brain, enclosed within the column are the spinal nerves that exit the column to innervate specific muscle groups bilaterally, according to their level on the vertebral column. The part of the cord that extends below the lumbar level resembled a horse's tail to early anatomists, which is where it got its name cauda equina.

The pelvis includes the ilium, the ischium, the pubis, and the sacrum, which form a bony circle to protect the pelvic contents, provide stability for the vertebral column (sacrum), and provide an appropriate surface for femoral articulation for ambulation.

The innominate bone, or hipbone, refers to the three bones making up the hip: the pubis, ilium, and ischium. The acetabulum is the socket for the femoral head and is found anterior to the rings of the ischium on the lateral inferior surface of the ilium.

The categories in this code block are as follows:

S30	Superficial injury of abdomen, lower back, pelvis and external genitals
S31	Open wound of abdomen, lower back, pelvis and external genitals
S32	Fracture of lumbar spine and pelvis
S33	Dislocation and sprain of joints and ligaments of lumbar spine and pelvis
S34	Injury of lumbar and sacral spinal cord and nerves at abdomen, lower back and pelvis level
S35	Injury of blood vessels at abdomen, lower back and pelvis level
S36	Injury of intra-abdominal organs
S37	Injury of urinary and pelvic organs
S38	Crushing injury and traumatic amputation of abdomen, lower back, pelvis and external genitals

S39   Other and unspecified injuries of abdomen, lower back, pelvis and external genitals

S32.-   Fracture of lumbar spine and pelvis

A lumbar spine fracture involves any of the vertebrae that make up the lumbar spine. Pelvic fractures involve any of the bones that make up the pelvis. Pelvic fractures range in severity from minor fractures of individual bones in which the pelvic ring alignment remains intact to severe, displaced fractures of multiple pelvic bones in which the pelvic ring suffers significant displacement. Treatment is dependent upon the severity of the fracture, ranging from bedrest for nondisplaced fracture to open surgical reduction and fixation for unstable, displaced fractures. Likewise, outcome is dependent upon fracture severity, associated injuries, age, and health status of the patient. Closed pelvic fractures without pelvic circle disruption are associated with the most favorable outcome, as the pelvic organs remain uncompromised and mobility is likely to be reestablished upon healing. However, in some cases, distortion of the ring results in long-term pain and debility. Open pelvic fractures and those with pelvic circle disruption pose the highest risk for complications, which include organ damage, hemorrhage, and sepsis. Open fractures of the pelvis have a high mortality rate, in some estimates, up to 20 percent. In general, fractures of the pelvic circle pose significant mortality risk to the patient, due to the hemorrhagic capability of cancellous bone and risk of injury to the major blood vessels and organs housed within the pelvis. This category includes only those fractures that have arisen as a result of an injury. It includes delayed healing and nonunions of fractured bones.

S32.0-   Fracture of lumbar vertebra

When diagnosing fractures, the spine is divided into the anterior, middle, and posterior column. A wedge compression fracture occurs when a force such as a fall or heavy weight crushes the anterior aspect of the vertebra, forming a wedge shape. In contrast, a burst fracture happens when the force of the compression crushes the vertebral body in all directions fracturing two or three of the columns. Typically when only the anterior column is fractured, such as with the wedge fracture, it is considered to be stable. Fractures in both the anterior and middle column can be considered unstable or stable and fractures in all three columns are generally considered unstable.

S32.4-   Fracture of acetabulum

The acetabulum is the socket for the femoral head and is found anterior to the rings of the ischium on the lateral inferior surface of the ilium. When the acetabulum is fractured, the head of the femur functions as a hammer striking against its socket with undue force. Acetabular fractures are classified by wall (anterior or posterior), column (anterior or posterior),

and transverse fractures. Some fractures involve two sites such as transverse with posterior wall. Posterior wall fractures occur more often than anterior wall and can be in conjunction with posterior column and transverse fractures. Acetabular fractures typically involve both columns; it is rare to have one column fracture without the other. Column fractures divide the acetabulum into front and back halves while transverse fractures divide the acetabulum into top and bottom halves. The medial wall fracture, also called a T-shaped fracture, is a transverse fracture with the addition of a fracture of the acetabular medial wall. Dome fractures are fractures through the superior aspect or roof, the weight-bearing part of the acetabulum. Any of these fractures can be specified as displaced or nondisplaced; if unspecified, the default is displaced.

> **Focus Point**
>
> Note that the term hip fracture, which is often used to describe a fracture of the acetabulum, excludes the femur. A fracture of the shaft of the femur, or of the head of the femur, is anatomically distinct from acetabular fractures. Fractures of the femur are reported with codes from category S72.

S32.81-   Multiple fractures of pelvis with disruption of pelvic ring

S32.82-   Multiple fractures of pelvis without disruption of pelvic ring

The pelvis includes the ilium, the ischium, the pubis, and the sacrum, which form a bony circle (ring) to protect the pelvic contents, provide stability for the vertebral column (sacrum), and provide an appropriate surface for femoral articulation for ambulation. Closed pelvic fractures without pelvic circle disruption are associated with the most favorable outcome, as the pelvic organs remain uncompromised and mobility is likely to be reestablished upon healing. However, in some cases, distortion of the ring results in long-term pain and debility. Open pelvic fractures and those with pelvic circle disruption pose the highest risk for complications, which include organ damage, hemorrhage, and sepsis. In general, fractures of the pelvic circle pose significant mortality risk to the patient, due to the hemorrhagic capability of cancellous bone and risk of injury to the major blood vessels and organs housed within the pelvis.

S33.-   Dislocation and sprain of joints and ligaments of lumbar spine and pelvis

This category includes subluxations, dislocations, and sprains of the lumbar spine and pelvic region. A subluxation refers to a partial dislocation. A sprain is an injury to the ligaments, which are the tough fibrous tissues that bind bones together at joints.

S33.1- Subluxation and dislocation of lumbar vertebra

Luxation is another term used to describe a complete dislocation, one that has separated the articulating surfaces of the joint. An incomplete dislocation, or subluxation, is one in which the joint surfaces maintain some articulation. A simple dislocation is a closed injury without a penetrating or communicating wound. An uncomplicated dislocation is not associated with other significant injuries. Open dislocations are those with an open wound at the site of the joint. Open injuries, also called compound dislocations, are subject to infection. Reduction of a dislocation or subluxation is by manipulation, open or closed.

S33.2- Dislocation of sacroiliac and sacrococcygeal joint

S33.3- Dislocation of other and unspecified parts of lumbar spine and pelvis

Luxation is another term used to describe a complete dislocation, one that has separated the articulating surfaces of the joint. A simple dislocation is a closed injury without a penetrating or communicating wound. An uncomplicated dislocation is not associated with other significant injuries. Open dislocations are those with an open wound at the site of the joint. Open injuries, also called compound dislocations, are subject to infection.

S33.5- Sprain of ligaments of lumbar spine

S33.6- Sprain of sacroiliac joint

S33.8- Sprain of other parts of lumbar spine and pelvis

S33.9- Sprain of unspecified parts of lumbar spine and pelvis

A sprain is an injury to the ligaments, which are the tough fibrous tissues that bind bones together at joints. Sprains are graded. A Type I sprain denotes minor ligamentous injury, Type II is an incomplete ligamentous injury, and Type III describes a complete disruption of the ligament. The more ligaments involved in the sprain, the more serious the injury. Sprains manifest with swelling, pain, and limited mobility. A mild sprain may heal in two to six weeks, while a severe sprain may require eight weeks to 10 months to heal.

Focus Point

A sprain is not identical to a strain and the two terms should not be used synonymously. A strain is an injury to the muscles or tendons. Codes for strains in the abdomen, lower back, and pelvis are located in category S39.

S34.- Injury of lumbar and sacral spinal cord and nerves at abdomen, lower back and pelvis level

Injuries classified here include those involving the spinal cord, nerve roots, peripheral nerves, and sympathetic nerves, including nerve plexuses and ganglions located in the region of the lumbar spine, sacrum, abdomen, and pelvis. A plexus or ganglion is a bundle of nerves that serves a particular region of the body. A plexus lies relatively deep in the body as opposed to superficial nerves, which are close to the surface of the skin. Sympathetic nerves along with parasympathetic nerves are part of the autonomic nervous system. The autonomic system is considered to be involuntary, regulating body processes such as breathing, heartbeat, digestion, and orientation in space. The parasympathetic nervous system regulates everyday body processes that restore the body and conserve energy. In contrast, the sympathetic nervous system responds to emergency situations by activating the flight or fight response when there is a perception of danger or harm.

S34.0- Concussion and edema of lumbar and sacral spinal cord

A concussion of the spinal cord is a mild traumatic injury to the spinal cord that results in temporary neurological deficits at the level of the spinal cord injury with full recovery within 72 hours of the occurrence. Spinal cord concussions typically result from a severe blow or jarring injury. Edema is swelling of the spinal cord that can also compromise neurological function.

S34.11- Complete lesion of lumbar spinal cord

A complete lesion of the spinal cord causes immediate total paralysis and sensory loss below the level of the injury. It is sometimes referred to as a complete injury or transverse cord injury. Depending on the site of injury, outcomes vary. Paralysis to both legs and the lower portion of the body is termed paraplegia.

S34.3- Injury of cauda equina

The cauda equina is a bundle of nerve roots that extend below the lumbar level that resembled a horse's tail to early anatomists, hence its name. An injury to these nerves can affect the lower extremities and bladder and bowel function and cause sexual dysfunction.

S35.- Injury of blood vessels at abdomen, lower back and pelvis level

Vascular trauma may result from penetrating or blunt injury. Arterial blood loss manifests as profuse and bright red, while venous loss is steady and dark. Injuries to the larger arteries of the abdomen, lower back, and pelvis are life-threatening.

Focus Point

Traumatic aneurysms are reported with codes for injury to blood vessels. An aneurysm is a weakening in the arterial wall that bulges with the pumping of the blood, posing the threat of rupture. When aneurysms are part of a disease process and not due to trauma, they are reported with codes from Chapter 9 Diseases of the Circulatory System.

S36.- Injury of intra-abdominal organs

Injuries to the following organs are classified here: spleen, liver, gallbladder, pancreas, stomach, small and large intestines, rectum, peritoneum, and retroperitoneum.

Some of the injuries included in this category are contusions, lacerations, and blast injuries.

A blast injury causes damage to organs or tissues caused solely by the direct effect of a blast wave pressure, called overpressurization shockwave, from high order explosives. These injuries are due to anatomical and physiological changes incurred upon the body from the direct or reflected impact of the overpressurization force. The force can emanate from a bomb, gas leak, or any other explosion. Blast injuries are graded as primary, secondary, tertiary, and miscellaneous. A primary blast injury affects air-filled organs, such as the lungs, ears, and bowel. If the tympanic membrane is ruptured, the physician automatically assumes serious organ damage. Secondary injury results from injuries associated with flying objects. Tertiary injuries may result from striking objects while airborne. Morbidity and mortality are greatest if the explosion occurs within a confined space or underwater.

Focus Point

Only primary blast injuries are reported in this category. Secondary and tertiary blast injuries are reported with codes describing the specific injuries sustained.

S36.0- Injury of spleen

The spleen is covered by a thick fibrous membrane, the capsule, which plays a part in grading the severity of splenic injuries. Injury to the spleen may occur as a result of blunt trauma or a penetrating wound.

S36.02- Contusion of spleen

Contusion or bruising of the spleen results from blunt trauma. Contusions are classified based on size with minor contusions being less than 2 cm and major contusions being 2 cm or more in size. Most spleen contusions heal without medical intervention although rest and close monitoring are required to ensure that no complications arise from the spleen injury.

S36.03- Laceration of spleen

The spleen may rupture or tear as a result of blunt trauma or be punctured by the ribs if a rib fracture occurs. The spleen may also be injured as a result of penetrating trauma to the upper left abdomen. Spleen lacerations are classified based on severity. A laceration or tear of the capsule only is classified as a superficial injury as is a laceration that extends less than 1 cm beyond the capsule into the spleen. Moderate lacerations are those that extend 1 to 3 cm in depth beyond the capsule. Major lacerations are those that extend more than 3 cm in depth, involve multiple smaller lacerations, or involve rupture or avulsion of the spleen.

S36.11- Injury of liver

The liver is protected by the fibrous membrane Glisson's capsule. Not all liver injuries need surgical repair. If the patient is stable hemodynamically and has no other intraabdominal injury that requires surgery, nonoperative medical management of the injury may suffice. Liver injuries are classified based on severity, which includes contusion and minor, moderate, or major laceration.

S38.- Crushing injury and traumatic amputation of abdomen, lower back, pelvis and external genitals

Crushing injuries may involve the abdomen, pelvis, or external genitalia. Traumatic amputation may involve the male or female external genitalia or tissue from the abdominal wall, lower back, or pelvis.

S38.0- Crushing injury of external genital organs

S38.1- Crushing injury of abdomen, lower back, and pelvis

A crushing injury occurs when a body part is subjected to a high degree of force or pressure, typically after being pressed between two heavy or motionless objects. Damage related to crush injuries can include lacerations, fractures, bleeding, bruising, and compartment syndrome. Severe crush injuries cause extensive damage to skin, muscle, nerves, bone, and internal organs of the abdomen and pelvis. There may be bleeding, internally and/or externally, or blood supply may be cut off. Plasma may leak from the blood vessels into the damaged tissues, causing swelling and shock. When the crushed part is released, toxic chemicals produced by damaged muscles get into general circulation, which can cause kidney failure in severe cases.

S39.- Other and unspecified injuries of abdomen, lower back, pelvis and external genitals

Strain injuries and lacerations of muscle, fascia, or tendon are classified here. Strains occur when the muscle, fascia, or tendon is stretched or subjected to a level of force beyond its stretching or strength capabilities. A tear of a muscle, fascia, or tendon is classified as a strain. A pulled muscle is also classified as a strain. Symptoms of strains include swelling, bruising, pain at rest and with activity, weakness in the strained muscle, and inability to use the affected body part. A laceration is a deep cut through the soft tissue and into the fascia, muscle, and/or tendon.

> **Focus Point**
>
> *A sprain injury should not be confused with a strain injury. A sprain is an injury to the ligaments, which are the tough fibrous tissues that bind bones together at joints. Sprains of the lumbar spine, sacroiliac joints, and other parts of the pelvis are located in category S33.*

Injuries to the Shoulder and Upper Arm (S40-S49)

Injuries classified here range from minor injuries, such as contusions, abrasions, superficial foreign bodies, and insect bites, to deeper injuries involving the soft tissues to fractures and dislocations.

The categories in this code block are as follows:

S40	Superficial injury of shoulder and upper arm
S41	Open wound of shoulder and upper arm
S42	Fracture of shoulder and upper arm
S43	Dislocation and sprain of joints and ligaments of shoulder girdle
S44	Injury of nerves at shoulder and upper arm level
S45	Injury of blood vessels at shoulder and upper arm level
S46	Injury of muscle, fascia and tendon at shoulder and upper arm level
S47	Crushing injury of shoulder and upper arm
S48	Traumatic amputation of shoulder and upper arm
S49	Other and unspecified injuries of shoulder and upper arm

S42.- Fracture of shoulder and upper arm

A fracture is a break in a bone resulting from two possible causes: the direct or indirect application of undue force against the bone and pathological changes resulting in spontaneous fractures. This chapter includes only those fractures that have arisen as a result of an injury. It includes delayed healing and nonunions of fractured bones. Closed fractures are contained beneath the skin, while open or compound fractures connote an associated open wound. Open fractures are always compound, with a wound leading to the fracture or the broken bone ends protruding through the skin. There is a very high risk of infection with open fractures since the tissues are exposed to contaminants.

> **Focus Point**
>
> *Subcategories identify whether the fracture is displaced or nondisplaced. A fracture not indicated as nondisplaced or displaced should be classified to displaced. The seventh character for an initial encounter specifies whether the fracture is open or closed. If unspecified, the default is closed.*

S42.0- Fracture of clavicle

The clavicle, or collarbone, has a shaft and articulating ends—the sternal and acromial ends. The acromial end articulates with the scapula, which is the shoulder bone. Fractures of the clavicle are classified by site (e.g., the sternal end also called proximal clavicle fractures, the shaft, or the lateral [acromial] end) and by whether the fracture is displaced or nondisplaced. Fractures of the sternal end that are displaced are further differentiated by the direction of the displacement: anterior or posterior. Because the sternal end of the clavicle is near vital intrathoracic structures any fracture of this site may compromise neurovascular or other structures.

S42.1- Fracture of scapula

The scapula articulates with the clavicle and the humerus, the long bone in the upper arm. Its socket, the glenoid fossa, receives the humeral head. The coracoid process superior to the glenoid fossa provides a surface for attachments of muscles and tendons. Scapula fractures are classified by site. The most common fracture site is the body of the scapula, accounting for more than half of all fractures of this bone, with the second most common site being the scapular neck. Other less common fracture sites include the acromial process, coracoid process, and glenoid cavity.

S42.2- Fracture of upper end of humerus

The proximal portion or upper end of the humerus is composed of the humeral head, anatomical neck, lesser tuberosity, greater tuberosity, and surgical neck.

S42.22- 2-part fracture of surgical neck of humerus

S42.23- 3-part fracture of surgical neck of humerus

S42.24- 4-part fracture of surgical neck of humerus

The most common site of fracture in the upper (proximal) end of the humerus is the surgical neck. These fractures are classified by how many other sites, in addition to the surgical neck, are fractured. Other sites that can be involved include the greater tuberosity, anatomical neck, and lesser tuberosity. A two-part fracture involves the surgical neck only and is subclassified as two-part displaced or two-part nondisplaced. A three-part fracture involves the surgical neck and a second fracture line with the bone separated into three parts. A four-part fracture involves the surgical neck and two additional fracture lines with the bone separated into four parts.

Focus Point

The Neer classification is one method of classifying fractures of the proximal-end of the humerus. However, these codes do not strictly conform to the Neer classification. In the Neer classification, the number of parts and the number of displaced fractures are used to classify the fracture as follows:

- *In the two-part, there are fracture lines that involve two to four sites and one is displaced*

- *In the three-part, there are fracture lines that involve three to four sites and two are displaced*

- *In the four-part, fracture lines involve all sites and three are displaced in respect to the fourth*

However in ICD-10-CM, only the number of parts is considered. For example, a two-part surgical neck fracture includes separate codes for two-part displaced and two-part nondisplaced; three-part fractures and four-part fractures do not differentiate between displaced and nondisplaced fractures.

A two-part fracture of the proximal humerus involving only the greater tuberosity is reported with a code from subcategory S42.25-. A two-part fracture of the proximal humerus involving only the lesser tuberosity is reported with a code from subcategory S42.26-.

S42.25- Fracture of greater tuberosity of humerus

The greater tuberosity is the large protuberance on the proximal aspect of the humerus to which the supraspinatus, infraspinatus, and teres minor tendons attach.

Focus Point

An isolated fracture of the greater tuberosity is sometimes called a two-part fracture; however, this should not confused with the two-part fracture described by codes in subcategory S42.22-, which are two-part fractures involving the surgical neck only.

S42.26- Fracture of lesser tuberosity of humerus

The lesser tuberosity is the smaller protuberance on the proximal humerus situated anterior to the greater tuberosity.

Focus Point

An isolated fracture of the lesser tuberosity is sometimes called a two-part fracture; however, this should not confused with the two-part fracture described by codes in subcategory S42.22-, which are two-part fractures involving the surgical neck only.

S42.27- Torus fracture of upper end of humerus

Torus fractures (a.k.a., buckle fracture, incomplete fracture) are common injuries among the pediatric population. It is commonly a result of axial loading on a long bone of an extremity, such as falling on an outstretched hand. This type of fracture is characterized by one side of the bone buckling upon itself without disrupting the other side. This characteristic "buckling" is due to the softer nature of the child's developing bone, allowing for the bone to compress, buckle, or "collapse" on one side, instead of break. Diagnostic imaging readily identifies torus fracture. These are generally quick-healing injuries that are treated with casting or splinting.

S42.3- Fracture of shaft of humerus

The shaft of the humerus begins below the surgical neck at the (proximal) end of the humerus and extends to the supracondylar ridges at the lower (distal) end of the humerus. Humeral shaft fractures are classified based on the type of fracture. Laterality is also a component of the code.

S42.31- Greenstick fracture of shaft of humerus

Greenstick fractures are incomplete fractures with bending and cracking of the bone. They are common in children because of the greater flexibility of children's bones.

S42.32- Transverse fracture of shaft of humerus

Transverse fractures occur in a straight line across the bone at a right angle to the long axis of the bone.

S42.33- Oblique fracture of shaft of humerus

Oblique fractures occur at a diagonal angle across the bone shaft.

S42.34- Spiral fracture of shaft of humerus

Spiral fractures, also called torsion fractures, are caused by a twisting force resulting in a diagonal fracture around and through the bone.

S42.35- Comminuted fracture of shaft of humerus

In a comminuted fracture, the bone is fractured, splintered, or shattered into multiple pieces with many small bone fragments.

S42.36- Segmental fracture of shaft of humerus

In a segmental fracture, the bone is broken in two places leaving at least one segment unattached to the body of bone.

S42.4- Fracture of lower end of humerus

The lower (distal) end of the humerus articulates with the radius and ulna of the forearm forming the elbow joint. The distal humerus has a number of distinct features. The supracondylar region, also called the supraepicondylar region, is the region just above the medial and lateral epicondyles, which are two bony projections on the inner and outer aspect of the distal humerus. Below the epicondyles are two condyles, the medial condyle also called the trochlea and the lateral condyle also called the capitellum. The medial condyle articulates with the ulna, while the lateral condyle articulates with the radius. Codes for fractures of the distal humerus, with the exception of torus fracture, are specific to site.

S42.41- Simple supracondylar fracture without intercondylar fracture of humerus

S42.42- Comminuted supracondylar fracture without intercondylar fracture of humerus

Supracondylar fractures are common in children, particularly children aged 7 or younger, and most often result from a fall from a height with a hyperextended elbow or a fall onto a flexed elbow. A supracondylar fracture without intercondylar extension of the fracture is an extraarticular injury meaning that the fracture does not extend into the joint. Simple fractures may have only a single fracture line with or without displacement of the fracture, while comminuted fractures involve multiple bone fragments that may or may not be displaced.

S42.48- Torus fracture of lower end of humerus

Torus fractures (a.k.a., buckle fracture, incomplete fracture) are common injuries among the pediatric population. It is commonly a result of axial loading on a long bone of an extremity, such as falling on an outstretched hand. This type of fracture is characterized by one side of the bone buckling upon itself without disrupting the other side. This characteristic "buckling" is due to the softer nature of the child's developing bone, allowing for the bone to compress, buckle, or "collapse" on one side, instead of break. Diagnostic imaging readily identifies torus fracture. These are generally quick-healing injuries that are treated with casting or splinting.

S43.- Dislocation and sprain of joints and ligaments of shoulder girdle

This category includes subluxations, dislocations, and sprains of the shoulder region. A subluxation refers to a partial dislocation. A sprain is an injury to the ligaments, which are the tough fibrous tissues that bind bones together at joints.

S43.0- Subluxation and dislocation of shoulder joint

S43.1- Subluxation and dislocation of acromioclavicular joint

S43.2- Subluxation and dislocation of sternoclavicular joint

S43.3- Subluxation and dislocation of other and unspecified parts of shoulder girdle

Luxation is another term used to describe a complete dislocation, one that has separated the articulating surfaces of the joint. An incomplete dislocation, or subluxation, is one in which the joint surfaces maintain some articulation. A simple dislocation is a closed injury without a penetrating or communicating wound. An uncomplicated dislocation is not associated with other significant injuries. Open dislocations are those with an open wound at the site of the joint. Open injuries, also called compound dislocations, are subject to infection. Reduction of a dislocation or subluxation is by manipulation, open or closed. The severity of injury to the acromioclavicular joint is determined by the degree of damage to the acromioclavicular and coracoclavicular ligaments.

S43.4-   Sprain of shoulder joint

S43.5-   Sprain of acromioclavicular joint

S43.6-   Sprain of sternoclavicular joint

S43.8-   Sprain of other specified parts of shoulder girdle

S43.9-   Sprain of unspecified parts of shoulder girdle

A sprain is an injury to the ligaments, which are the tough fibrous tissues that bind bones together at joints. Sprains are graded. A Type I sprain denotes minor ligamentous injury, Type II is an incomplete ligamentous injury, and Type III describes a complete disruption of the ligament. The more ligaments involved in the sprain, the more serious the injury. Sprains manifest with swelling, pain, and limited mobility. A mild sprain may heal in two to six weeks, while a severe sprain may require eight weeks to 10 months to heal.

> **Focus Point**
>
> *A sprain is not identical to a strain, and the two terms should not be used synonymously. A strain is an injury to the muscles or tendons. Codes for strains in the shoulder and upper arm are located in category S46.*

S45.-   Injury of blood vessels at shoulder and upper arm level

Vascular trauma may result from penetrating or blunt injury. Arterial blood loss manifests as profuse and bright red, while venous loss is steady and dark.

> **Focus Point**
>
> *Traumatic aneurysms are reported with codes for injury to blood vessels. An aneurysm is a weakening in the arterial wall that bulges with the pumping of the blood, posing the threat of rupture. When aneurysms are part of a disease process and not due to trauma, they are reported with codes from Chapter 9 Diseases of the Circulatory System.*

S46.-   Injury of muscle, fascia and tendon at shoulder and upper arm level

Strain injuries and lacerations of muscle, fascia, or tendon are classified here. Strains occur when the muscle, fascia, or tendon is stretched or subjected to a level of force beyond its stretching or strength capabilities. A tear of a muscle, fascia, or tendon is classified as a strain. A pulled muscle is also classified as a strain. Symptoms of strains include swelling,

bruising, pain at rest and with activity, weakness in the strained muscle, and the inability to use the affected body part. A laceration is a deep cut through the soft tissue and into the fascia, muscle, and/or tendon.

> **Focus Point**
>
> *A sprain injury should not be confused with a strain injury. A sprain is an injury to the ligaments, which are the tough fibrous tissues that bind bones together at joints. Sprains of the shoulder, acromioclavicular joint, sternoclavicular joint, and other parts of the shoulder girdle are located in category S43.*

S47.-   Crushing injury of shoulder and upper arm

A crushing injury occurs when a body part is subjected to a high degree of force or pressure, typically after being pressed between two heavy or motionless objects. Damage related to crush injuries can include lacerations, fractures, bleeding, bruising, and compartment syndrome. Severe crush injuries cause extensive damage to skin, muscle, nerves, and bone. There may be bleeding, internally and/or externally, or blood supply may be cut off. Plasma may leak from the blood vessels into the damaged tissues, causing swelling and shock. When the crushed part is released, toxic chemicals produced by damaged muscles get into general circulation, which can cause kidney failure in severe cases.

S49.-   Other and unspecified injuries of shoulder and upper arm

Classified here are physeal fractures of the humerus bone, the large bone that spans from the shoulder joint to the elbow joint, as well as other and unspecified injuries occurring in the upper arm area.

S49.0-   Physeal fracture of upper end of humerus

S49.1-   Physeal fracture of lower end of humerus

Physeal fractures are pediatric fractures of the growth plate or physis of the bone. The Salter-Harris classification system is a method of describing the involvement of the physis, metaphysis, and epiphysis of the fracture. The classification helps determine treatment and possible long-term complications. Most of these heal without any disturbance of growth but some may lead to shortening or other deformities.

A Salter-Harris Type I fracture has the following characteristics:

- Transverse fracture through the physis only

- Increases width of physis

- Generally the growing zone is not injured and there is no disturbance to growth

A Salter-Harris Type II fracture has the following characteristics:

- Fracture through the physis and metaphysis
- Most common Salter-Harris fracture
- May cause minimal shortening but rarely results in functional disabilities

A Salter-Harris Type III fracture has the following characteristics:

- Fracture through the physis and the epiphysis, splitting the epiphysis
- Damages the reproductive layer of physis and likely causes some chronic disability
- Rarely results in major deformity; often surgical treatment is done with favorable prognosis

A Salter-Harris Type IV fracture has the following characteristics:

- Fracture through epiphysis, physis, and metaphysis
- Can disrupt growth of cartilage cells causing premature fusion of involved bone
- May lead to deformity of joint and chronic disability

Salter-Harris Fractures

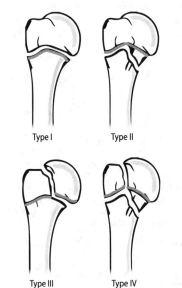

Type I   Type II

Type III   Type IV

Injuries to the Elbow and Forearm (S50-S59)

Injuries classified here range from minor injuries, such as contusions, abrasions, superficial foreign bodies, and insect bites, to deeper injuries involving the soft tissues to fractures and dislocations.

The categories in this code block are as follows:

S50	Superficial injury of elbow and forearm
S51	Open wound of elbow and forearm
S52	Fracture of forearm
S53	Dislocation and sprain of joints and ligaments of elbow
S54	Injury of nerves at forearm level
S55	Injury of blood vessels at forearm level
S56	Injury of muscle, fascia and tendon at forearm level
S57	Crushing injury of elbow and forearm
S58	Traumatic amputation of elbow and forearm
S59	Other and unspecified injuries of elbow and forearm

S52.-   Fracture of forearm

The radius and ulna operate in tandem, with a hinge-like motion for bending and capabilities for pronation and supination for the hand and wrist. In the anatomical position, the hands are supinated. In the pronated position, the palms are down. In some of the codes for open fractures, the required seventh character not only captures the type of encounter and whether the fracture is open or closed, but also identifies the type of open fracture based on the Gustilo classification. Following are the definitions for the open fractures as defined by the Gustilo classification:

Type I:	Low energy injury, clean wound less than 1 cm
Type II:	Wound is more than 1 cm with moderate soft tissue damage
Type III:	High energy wound, greater than 1 cm with extensive soft tissue damage, and subclassified to IIIA, IIIB, and IIIC
Type IIIA:	Adequate soft tissue coverage despite extensive soft tissue damage
Type IIIB:	Inadequate soft tissue coverage usually with severe wound contamination
Type IIIC:	Type III open fracture associated with arterial injury

S52.01- Torus fracture of upper end of ulna

Torus fractures (a.k.a., buckle fracture, incomplete fracture) are common injuries among the pediatric population. It is commonly a result of axial loading on a long bone of an extremity, such as falling on an outstretched hand. This type of fracture is characterized by one side of the bone buckling upon itself without disrupting the other side. This characteristic "buckling" is due to the softer nature of the child's developing bone, allowing for the bone to compress, buckle, or "collapse" on one side, instead of break. These are generally quick-healing injuries that are treated with casting or splinting.

S52.11- Torus fracture of upper end of radius

Torus fractures (a.k.a., buckle fracture, incomplete fracture) are common injuries among the pediatric population. It is commonly a result of axial loading on a long bone of an extremity, such as falling on an outstretched hand. This type of fracture is characterized by one side of the bone buckling upon itself without disrupting the other side. This characteristic "buckling" is due to the softer nature of the child's developing bone, allowing for the bone to compress, buckle, or "collapse" on one side, instead of break. These are generally quick-healing injuries that are treated with casting or splinting.

S52.2- Fracture of shaft of ulna

Ulnar shaft fractures are classified based on the type of fracture. Laterality is also a component of the code.

S52.21- Greenstick fracture of shaft of ulna

Greenstick fractures are incomplete fractures with bending and cracking of the bone. They are common in children because of the greater flexibility of children's bones.

S52.22- Transverse fracture of shaft of ulna

Transverse fractures occur in a straight line across the bone at a right angle to the long axis of the bone.

S52.23- Oblique fracture of shaft of ulna

Oblique fractures occur at a diagonal angle across the bone shaft.

S52.24- Spiral fracture of shaft of ulna

Spiral fractures are also called torsion fractures and are caused by a twisting force resulting in a diagonal fracture around and through the bone.

S52.25- Comminuted fracture of shaft of ulna

In a comminuted fracture, the bone is fractured, splintered, or shattered into multiple pieces with many small bone fragments.

S52.26- Segmental fracture of shaft of ulna

In a segmental fracture, the bone is broken in two places leaving at least one segment unattached to the body of bone.

S52.27- Monteggia's fracture of ulna

A Monteggia's fracture is a common fracture at the proximal end of the ulna that occurs in combination with dislocation of the radial head.

S52.28- Bent bone of ulna

A bent bone, also called a bowing fracture, appears bent without any noticeable fracture line.

S52.3- Fracture of shaft of radius

Radial shaft fractures are classified based on the type of fracture. Laterality is also a component of the code.

S52.31- Greenstick fracture of shaft of radius

Greenstick fractures are incomplete fractures with bending and cracking of the bone. They are common in children because of the greater flexibility of children's bones.

S52.32- Transverse fracture of shaft of radius

Transverse fractures occur in a straight line across the bone at a right angle to the long axis of the bone.

S52.33- Oblique fracture of shaft of radius

Oblique fractures occur at a diagonal angle across the bone shaft.

S52.34- Spiral fracture of shaft of radius

Spiral fractures, also called torsion fractures, are caused by a twisting force resulting in a diagonal fracture around and through the bone.

S52.35- Comminuted fracture of shaft of radius

In a comminuted fracture, the bone is fractured, splintered, or shattered into multiple pieces with many small bone fragments.

S52.36- Segmental fracture of shaft of radius

In a segmental fracture, the bone is broken in two places leaving at least one segment unattached to body of bone.

S52.37- Galeazzi's fracture

A Galeazzi's fracture is a distal radial shaft fracture combined with a dislocation of the distal radioulnar joint.

S52.38- Bent bone of radius

A bent bone, also called a bowing fracture, appears bent without any noticeable fracture line.

S52.5- Fracture of lower end of radius

Fractures of the distal or lower end of the radius typically occur about an inch from the distal end of the bone but depending on the mechanism of injury, the fracture configurations vary. Some common types unique to the radius include Colles' fracture, Smith's fracture, and Barton's fracture. These fractures are also classified based on whether or not they extend into the joint or articular surface of the bone. Fractures that do not extend into the joint are called extraarticular, while those that involve the joint are called intraarticular. Laterality is a component of distal radius fracture codes.

S52.52- Torus fracture of lower end of radius

Torus fractures (a.k.a., buckle fracture, incomplete fracture) are common injuries among the pediatric population. It is commonly a result of axial loading on a long bone of an extremity, such as falling on an outstretched hand. This type of fracture is characterized by one side of the bone buckling upon itself without disrupting the other side. This characteristic "buckling" is due to the softer nature of the child's developing bone, allowing for the bone to compress, buckle, or "collapse" on one side, instead of break. These are generally quick-healing injuries that are treated with casting or splinting.

S52.53- Colles' fracture

A common fracture is Colles' fracture, which is a transverse fracture of the distal radius with backward or dorsal displacement of fracture fragments, displacing the hand. In most cases, it is considered extraarticular but some may extend intra-articularly. This injury typically occurs when an individual puts out a hand to break a fall.

S52.54- Smith's fracture

A Smith's fracture, also called reverse Colles' fracture, is an extraarticular distal radius fracture although intra-articulation extension is common. Smith's fracture involves anterior (volar) displacement of the distal fragments. This type of fracture occurs predominantly in younger people as the result of a high energy injury to the extended wrist.

S52.56- Barton's fracture

Barton's fracture is an intraarticular fracture of the distal radius that also involves the dislocation of the radiocarpal joint. It is generally considered a Colles or Smith's fracture with a dislocation.

S52.6- Fracture of lower end of ulna

Fractures of the lower end of the ulna occur near the wrist joint and are often associated with a concurrent radius fracture.

S52.62- Torus fracture of lower end of ulna

Torus fractures (a.k.a., buckle fracture, incomplete fracture) are common injuries among the pediatric population. It is commonly a result of axial loading on a long bone of an extremity, such as falling on an outstretched hand. This type of fracture is characterized by one side of the bone buckling upon itself without disrupting the other side. This characteristic "buckling" is due to the softer nature of the child's developing bone, allowing for the bone to compress, buckle, or "collapse" on one side, instead of break. These are generally quick-healing injuries that are treated with casting or splinting.

S53.- Dislocation and sprain of joints and ligaments of elbow

This category includes subluxations, dislocations, and sprains of the elbow region. A subluxation refers to a partial dislocation. A sprain is an injury to the ligaments, which are the tough fibrous tissues that bind bones together at joints.

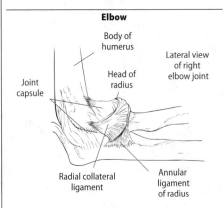

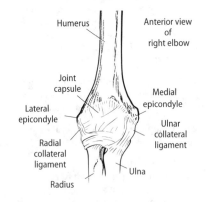

Elbow

S53.0- Subluxation and dislocation of radial head

Luxation is another term used to describe a complete dislocation, one that has separated the articulating surfaces of the joint. An incomplete dislocation, or subluxation, is one in which the joint surfaces maintain some articulation. A simple dislocation is a closed injury without a penetrating or communicating wound. An uncomplicated dislocation is not associated with other significant injuries. Open dislocations are those with an open wound at the site of the joint. Open injuries, also called compound dislocations, are subject to infection. Reduction of a dislocation or subluxation is by manipulation, open or closed.

S53.03- Nursemaid's elbow

Nursemaid's elbow is a common specific type of partial dislocation of the radial head whereby the head of the radius is dislocated from its encirclement by annular ligament, which slips or tears over the radial head. It most commonly occurs in children younger than age 5. The mechanism of injury is often one of a sudden pull on the upper limb. Upon presentation, the injured elbow is often pronated, partially flexed, and held by the side of the body with pain and tenderness over the anterolateral radial head. Manual reduction of the dislocation is often effectively performed in the emergency department, often with an immediate relief of pain. Immobilization may not be necessary if treatment is immediately sought. However, if treatment is delayed, immobilization and splinting may be required.

S53.1- Subluxation and dislocation of ulnohumeral joint

Luxation is another term used to describe a complete dislocation, one that has separated the articulating surfaces of the joint. An incomplete dislocation, or subluxation, is one in which the joint surfaces maintain some articulation. A simple dislocation is a closed injury without a penetrating or communicating wound. An uncomplicated dislocation is not associated with other significant injuries. Open dislocations are those with an open wound at the site of the joint. Open injuries, also called compound dislocations, are subject to infection. Reduction of a dislocation or subluxation is by manipulation, open or closed.

S53.4- Sprain of elbow

A sprain is an injury to the ligaments, which are the tough fibrous tissues that bind bones together at joints. Sprains are graded. A Type I sprain denotes minor ligamentous injury, Type II is an incomplete ligamentous injury, and Type III describes a complete disruption of the ligament. The more ligaments involved in the sprain, the more serious the injury.

Sprains manifest with swelling, pain, and limited mobility. A mild sprain may heal in two to six weeks, while a severe sprain may require eight weeks to 10 months to heal.

> **Focus Point**
>
> *A sprain is not identical to a strain and the two terms should not be used synonymously. A strain is an injury to the muscles or tendons. Codes for strains at the forearm level are located in category S56.*

S55.- Injury of blood vessels at forearm level

Vascular trauma may result from penetrating or blunt injury. Arterial blood loss manifests as profuse and bright red, while venous loss is steady and dark.

> **Focus Point**
>
> *Traumatic aneurysms are reported with codes for injury to blood vessels. An aneurysm is a weakening in the arterial wall that bulges with the pumping of the blood, posing the threat of rupture. When aneurysms are part of a disease process and not due to trauma, they are reported with codes from Chapter 9 Diseases of the Circulatory System.*

S56.- Injury of muscle, fascia and tendon at forearm level

Strain injuries and lacerations of muscle, fascia, or tendon are classified here. Strains occur when the muscle, fascia, or tendon is stretched or subjected to a level of force beyond its stretching or strength capabilities. A tear of a muscle, fascia, or tendon is classified as a strain. A pulled muscle is also classified as a strain. Symptoms of strains include swelling, bruising, pain at rest and with activity, weakness in the strained muscle, and inability to use the affected body part. A laceration is a deep cut through the soft tissue and into the fascia, muscle, and/or tendon.

Posterior View of Right Elbow

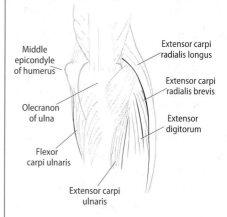

Middle epicondyle of humerus

Olecranon of ulna

Flexor carpi ulnaris

Extensor carpi ulnaris

Extensor carpi radialis longus

Extensor carpi radialis brevis

Extensor digitorum

Focus Point

A sprain injury should not be confused with a strain injury. A sprain is an injury to the ligaments, which are the tough fibrous tissues that bind bones together at joints. Sprains of the elbow are located in category S53.

S57.- Crushing injury of elbow and forearm

A crushing injury occurs when a body part is subjected to a high degree of force or pressure, typically after being pressed between two heavy or motionless objects. Damage related to crush injuries can include lacerations, fractures, bleeding, bruising, and compartment syndrome. Severe crush injuries cause extensive damage to skin, muscle, nerves, and bone. There may be bleeding, internally and/or externally, or blood supply may be cut off. Plasma may leak from the blood vessels into the damaged tissues, causing swelling and shock. When the crushed part is released, toxic chemicals produced by damaged muscles get into general circulation, which can cause kidney failure in severe cases.

S59.- Other and unspecified injuries of elbow and forearm

Physeal fractures involving the lower end of the ulna or the upper or lower end of the radius comprise the bulk of this category. There are also codes for other specified injuries of the elbow and forearm that do not have a more specific code and unspecified injuries of these sites.

S59.0- Physeal fracture of lower end of ulna

S59.1- Physeal fracture of upper end of radius

S59.2- Physeal fracture of lower end of radius

Physeal fractures are pediatric fractures of the growth plate or physis of the bone. The Salter-Harris classification system is a method of describing the involvement of the physis, metaphysis, and epiphysis of the fracture. The classification helps determine treatment and possible long-term complications. Most of these heal without any disturbance of growth but some may lead to shortening or other deformities.

A Salter-Harris Type I fracture has the following characteristics:

- Transverse fracture through the physis only

- Increases width of physis

- Generally the growing zone is not injured and there is no disturbance to growth

A Salter-Harris Type II fracture has the following characteristics:

- Fracture through the physis and metaphysis

- Most common Salter-Harris fracture

- May cause minimal shortening but rarely results in functional disabilities

A Salter-Harris Type III fracture has the following characteristics:

- Fracture through the physis and the epiphysis, splitting the epiphysis

- Damages the reproductive layer of physis and likely causes some chronic disability

- Rarely results in major deformity; often surgical treatment is done with favorable prognosis

A Salter-Harris Type IV fracture has the following characteristics:

- Fracture through epiphysis, physis, and metaphysis

- Can disrupt growth of cartilage cells causing premature fusion of involved bone

- May lead to deformity of joint and chronic disability

Injuries to the Wrist, Hand and Fingers (S60-S69)

Injuries classified here range from minor injuries such as contusions, abrasions, superficial foreign bodies, and insect bites to deeper injuries involving the soft tissues to fractures and dislocations.

The categories in this code block are as follows:

S60	Superficial injury of wrist, hand and fingers
S61	Open wound of wrist, hand and fingers
S62	Fracture at wrist and hand level
S63	Dislocation and sprain of joints and ligaments at wrist and hand level
S64	Injury of nerves at wrist and hand level
S65	Injury of blood vessels at wrist and hand level
S66	Injury of muscle, fascia and tendon at wrist and hand level
S67	Crushing injury of wrist, hand and fingers
S68	Traumatic amputation of wrist, hand and fingers
S69	Other and unspecified injuries of wrist, hand and finger(s)

S62.-   Fracture at wrist and hand level

The distal radius and ulna articulate with the proximal carpals and form part of the wrist joint, although they are classified as the bones of the forearm. The carpals, which form the wrist, are classified with the hand. The eight carpal bones are functionally linked to the placement of each bone and its articulation with adjacent bones. Two rows of bones, with the scaphoid bone common to each row, act as a bridge to provide stability. The first row (proximal) is comprised of the scaphoid, lunate, pisiform, and triquetrum. The second row (distal) is comprised of the scaphoid, trapezium, trapezoid, capitate, and hamate. Carpal fractures usually occur as a result of extreme dorsiflexion or extension of the wrist and require significant force to happen at all.

The metacarpals are the bones of the hand distal to the carpals and proximal to the phalanges (fingers). The numbering convention identifies the first metacarpal as that associated with the thumb and the fifth metacarpal as the one associated with the little finger, sometimes called the pinkie.

The thumb has two bones, the proximal and distal phalanges, while the fingers have three, the proximal, middle, and distal phalanges. The anatomy of each phalanx is described in terms of base, body, and head. The base is the proximal end of the bone, the body is the midsection, and the head is the distal end. The distal phalanx has an additional descriptor, a tuberosity. Two sesamoid bones are located close to the distal joint of the first metacarpal (thumb). Because they project and perform many functions, the metacarpals and phalanges account for 10 percent of all fractures.

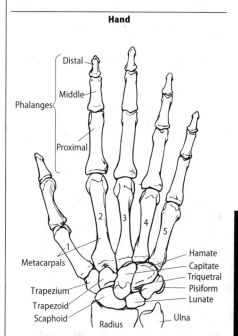

Hand

Focus Point

Many subcategories identify whether the fracture is displaced or nondisplaced. A fracture not indicated as nondisplaced or displaced should be classified to displaced. The seventh character for an initial encounter specifies whether the fracture is open or closed. If unspecified, the default is closed.

S62.21-   Bennett's fracture

Bennett's fracture is caused by a forced abduction of the thumb resulting in a two piece, intraarticular fracture dislocation of the base of the thumb at the carpometacarpal (CMC) joint.

S62.22-   Rolando's fracture

Rolando's fracture consists of a three-part or comminuted intraarticular fracture dislocation of the base of the thumb at the carpometacarpal (CMC) joint. It is often caused by fistfights and is considered an unstable injury requiring surgery.

S63.- Dislocation and sprain of joints and ligaments at wrist and hand level

This category includes subluxations, dislocations, and sprains involving the wrist, hand, and finger joints. A subluxation refers to a partial dislocation. A sprain is an injury to the ligaments, which are the tough fibrous tissues that bind bones together at joints.

S63.0- Subluxation and dislocation of wrist and hand joints

S63.1- Subluxation and dislocation of thumb

S63.2- Subluxation and dislocation of other finger(s)

Luxation is another term used to describe a complete dislocation, one that has separated the articulating surfaces of the joint. An incomplete dislocation, or subluxation, is one in which the joint surfaces maintain some articulation. A simple dislocation is a closed injury without a penetrating or communicating wound. An uncomplicated dislocation is not associated with other significant injuries. Open dislocations are those with an open wound at the site of the joint. Open injuries, also called compound dislocations, are subject to infection. Reduction of a dislocation or subluxation is by manipulation, open or closed.

S63.5- Other and unspecified sprain of wrist

S63.6- Other and unspecified sprain of finger(s)

A sprain is an injury to the ligaments, which are the tough fibrous tissues that bind bones together at joints. Sprains are graded. A Type I sprain denotes minor ligamentous injury, Type II is an incomplete ligamentous injury, and Type III describes a complete disruption of the ligament. The more ligaments involved in the sprain, the more serious the injury. Sprains manifest with swelling, pain, and limited mobility. A mild sprain may heal in two to six weeks, while a severe sprain may require eight weeks to 10 months to heal.

Focus Point

A sprain is not identical to a strain and the two terms should not be used synonymously. A strain is an injury to the muscles or tendons. Codes for strains at the wrist and hand level are located in category S66.

S65.- Injury of blood vessels at wrist and hand level

Vascular trauma may result from penetrating or blunt injury. Arterial blood loss manifests as profuse and bright red, while venous loss is steady and dark.

Focus Point

Traumatic aneurysms are reported with codes for injury to blood vessels. An aneurysm is a weakening in the arterial wall that bulges with the pumping of the blood, posing the threat of rupture. When aneurysms are part of a disease process and not due to trauma, they are reported with codes from Chapter 9 Diseases of the Circulatory System.

S66.- Injury of muscle, fascia and tendon at wrist and hand level

Strain injuries and lacerations of muscle, fascia, or tendon are classified here. Strains occur when the muscle, fascia, or tendon is stretched or subjected to a level of force beyond its stretching or strength capabilities. A tear of a muscle, fascia, or tendon is classified as a strain. A pulled muscle is also classified as a strain. Symptoms of strains include swelling, bruising, pain at rest and with activity, weakness in the strained muscle, and inability to use the affected body part. A laceration is a deep cut through the soft tissue and into the fascia, muscle, and/or tendon.

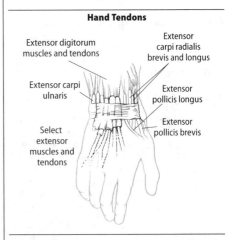

Hand Tendons

Extensor digitorum muscles and tendons

Extensor carpi radialis brevis and longus

Extensor carpi ulnaris

Extensor pollicis longus

Select extensor muscles and tendons

Extensor pollicis brevis

Focus Point

A sprain injury should not be confused with a strain injury. A sprain is an injury to the ligaments, which are the tough fibrous tissues that bind bones together at joints. Sprains of the wrist, hand, thumb, and fingers are located in category S63.

S67.- Crushing injury of wrist, hand and fingers

A crushing injury occurs when a body part is subjected to a high degree of force or pressure, typically after being pressed between two heavy or motionless objects. Damage related to crush injuries can include lacerations, fractures, bleeding, bruising, and compartment syndrome. Severe crush injuries can cause extensive damage to skin, muscle, nerves, and bone. There may be bleeding internally and/or externally, or blood supply may be cut off. Plasma may leak from the blood vessels into the damaged tissues causing swelling and shock. When the crushed part is released, toxic chemicals produced by damaged muscles get into general circulation, which can cause kidney failure in severe cases.

Injuries to the Hip and Thigh (S70-S79)

Injuries classified here range from superficial injuries, such as contusions, abrasions, superficial foreign bodies, and insect bites, to deeper injuries involving the soft tissues to fractures and dislocations.

The categories in this code block are as follows:

S70	Superficial injury of hip and thigh
S71	Open wound of hip and thigh
S72	Fracture of femur
S73	Dislocation and sprain of joint and ligaments of hip
S74	Injury of nerves at hip and thigh level
S75	Injury of blood vessels at hip and thigh level
S76	Injury of muscle, fascia and tendon at hip and thigh level
S77	Crushing injury of hip and thigh
S78	Traumatic amputation of hip and thigh
S79	Other and unspecified injuries of hip and thigh

S72.- Fracture of femur

The proximal femur bears the brunt of accidents leading to fractures, compared to the other bones used for locomotion. Fractures of the femoral shaft are relatively uncommon, while fractures of the neck are among the most frequent. A subcapital or intracapsular fracture of the femoral neck has the highest risk of avascular necrosis, which occurs when a severe injury disrupts the blood supply to the bone. This fracture also is inherently more unstable after surgery than an intertrochanteric fracture since the weakest part of the bone is now supporting the point of greatest stress.

In some of the codes for open fractures, the required seventh character not only captures the type of encounter and whether the fracture is open or closed, but also identifies the type of open fracture based on the Gustilo classification. Following are the definitions for the open fractures as defined by the Gustilo classification:

Type I:	Low energy injury, clean wound less than 1 cm
Type II:	Wound is more than 1 cm with moderate soft tissue damage
Type III:	High energy wound, greater than 1 cm with extensive soft tissue damage, and subclassified to IIIA, IIIB, and IIIC
Type IIIA:	Adequate soft tissue coverage despite extensive soft tissue damage
Type IIIB:	Inadequate soft tissue coverage usually with severe wound contamination
Type IIIC:	Type III open fracture associated with arterial injury

> **Focus Point**
>
> *Radiologists often use the terminology intracapsular and extracapsular when describing fractures of the femoral head and neck. An intracapsular fracture is one that is located within the joint capsule of the hip below the edge of the femoral head but above the insertion of the joint capsule of the hip. An extracapsular fracture is located outside the joint capsule of the hip below the insertion of the joint capsule but no lower than 5 cm below the lesser trochanter.*
>
> *Many subcategories identify whether the fracture is displaced or nondisplaced. A fracture not indicated as nondisplaced or displaced should be classified to displaced. The seventh character for an initial encounter specifies whether the fracture is open or closed. If unspecified, the default is closed.*

S72.0- Fracture of head and neck of femur

Femoral head and neck fractures occur within the joint capsule and may also be referred to as intracapsular fractures. Intracapsular fractures of the femoral neck may occur in the subcapital region, just below the femoral head in the midcervical region, also called the transcervical region, which is the midportion of the femoral neck. They may also occur at the base of the femoral neck, also called the basicervical or cervicotrochanteric region. A femoral head fracture is a rare fracture that typically occurs in conjunction with dislocation of the femur. Femoral neck fractures are more common particularly in the elderly.

> **Focus Point**
>
> *A subcapital fracture of the femur is reported with codes from subcategory S72.Ø1- Unspecified intracapsular fracture of femur.*

S72.1-   Pertrochanteric fracture

A pertrochanteric fracture occurs in the upper (proximal) femur and may involve the greater trochanter, lesser trochanter, apophysis of lesser or greater trochanter, or the intertrochanteric region. These fractures are extracapsular meaning that they occur outside the joint capsule. The greater trochanter is the bony protuberance at the upper outer (lateral) aspect of the hip and is the site of attachment for the hip extensor and abductor tendons. The lesser trochanter is a smaller bony protuberance located in the upper inner (medial) aspect at the hip joint and is the site of attachment of the iliopsoas (flexor muscle). Apophyseal fractures are avulsion fractures at the site of attachment of a tendon. Intertrochanteric fractures occur in the proximal femur between the greater and lesser trochanters.

S72.2-   Subtrochanteric fracture of femur

The subtrochanteric region of the femur is generally defined as the region from the bottom of the lesser trochanter to 5 cm below the lesser trochanter.

S72.3-   Fracture of shaft of femur

Fractures of the femoral shaft may occur anywhere from about 5 cm below the lesser trochanter to the region about 5 cm above the lateral and medial condyles at the distal end of the femur.

S72.32-   Transverse fracture of shaft of femur

Transverse fractures occur in a straight line across the bone at a right angle to the long axis of the bone.

S72.33-   Oblique fracture of shaft of femur

Oblique fractures occur at a diagonal angle across the bone shaft.

S72.34-   Spiral fracture of shaft of femur

Spiral fractures, also called torsion fractures, are caused by a twisting force resulting in a diagonal fracture around and through the bone.

S72.35-   Comminuted fracture of shaft of femur

In a comminuted fracture, the bone is fractured, splintered, or shattered into multiple pieces with many small bone fragments.

S72.36-   Segmental fracture of shaft of femur

In a segmental fracture, the bone is broken in two places leaving at least one segment unattached to the body of bone.

S72.4-   Fracture of lower end of femur

The lower end of the femur is generally defined as the region from about 5 cm above the medial and lateral condyles to the distal end of the bone.

S72.47-   Torus fracture of lower end of femur

Torus fractures (a.k.a., buckle fracture, incomplete fracture) are common injuries among the pediatric population. It is commonly a result of axial loading on a long bone of an extremity, such as falling on an outstretched hand. Less common in the distal femur, it can occur with hyperextension of the knee. This type of fracture is characterized by one side of the bone buckling upon itself without disrupting the other side. This characteristic "buckling" is due to the softer nature of the child's developing bone, allowing for the bone to compress, buckle, or "collapse" on one side, instead of break. These are generally quick-healing injuries that are treated with casting or splinting.

S73.-   Dislocation and sprain of joint and ligaments of hip

This category includes subluxations, dislocation, and sprains involving the hip region. A subluxation refers to a partial dislocation. A sprain is an injury to the ligaments, which are the tough fibrous tissues that bind bones together at joints.

S73.Ø-   Subluxation and dislocation of hip

Luxation is another term used to describe a complete dislocation, one that has separated the articulating surfaces of the joint. An incomplete dislocation, or subluxation, is one in which the joint surfaces maintain some articulation. A simple dislocation is a closed injury without a penetrating or communicating wound. An uncomplicated dislocation is not associated with other significant injuries. Open dislocations are those with an open wound at the site of the joint. Open injuries, also called compound dislocations, are subject to infection. Reduction of a dislocation or subluxation is by manipulation, open or closed.

S73.1-   Sprain of hip

A sprain is an injury to the ligaments, which are the tough fibrous tissues that bind bones together at joints. Sprains are graded. A Type I sprain denotes minor ligamentous injury, Type II is an incomplete ligamentous injury, and Type III describes a complete disruption of the ligament. The more ligaments involved in the sprain, the more serious the injury.

Sprains manifest with swelling, pain, and limited mobility. A mild sprain may heal in two to six weeks, while a severe sprain may require eight weeks to 10 months to heal.

Focus Point

A sprain is not identical to a strain and the two terms should not be used synonymously. A strain is an injury to the muscles or tendons. Codes for strains at the hip and thigh level are located in category S76.

S75.- Injury of blood vessels at hip and thigh level

Vascular trauma may result from penetrating or blunt injury. Arterial blood loss manifests as profuse and bright red, while venous loss is steady and dark.

Focus Point

Traumatic aneurysms are reported with codes for injury to blood vessels. An aneurysm is a weakening in the arterial wall that bulges with the pumping of the blood, posing the threat of rupture. When aneurysms are part of a disease process and not due to trauma, they are reported with codes from Chapter 9 Diseases of the Circulatory System.

S76.- Injury of muscle, fascia and tendon at hip and thigh level

Strain injuries and lacerations of muscle, fascia, or tendon are classified here. Strains occur when the muscle, fascia, or tendon is stretched or subjected to a level of force beyond its stretching or strength capabilities. A tear of a muscle, fascia, or tendon is classified as a strain. A pulled muscle is also classified as a strain. Symptoms of strains include swelling, bruising, pain at rest and with activity, weakness in the strained muscle, and the inability to use the affected body part. A laceration is a deep cut through the soft tissue and into the fascia, muscle, and/or tendon.

Focus Point

A sprain injury should not be confused with a strain injury. A sprain is an injury to the ligaments, which are the tough fibrous tissues that bind bones together at joints. Sprains of the hip are located in category S73.

S77.- Crushing injury of hip and thigh

A crushing injury occurs when a body part is subjected to a high degree of force or pressure, typically after being pressed between two heavy or motionless objects. Damage related to crush injuries can include lacerations, fractures, bleeding, bruising, and compartment syndrome. Severe crush injuries cause extensive damage to skin, muscle, nerves, and bone. There may be bleeding, internally and/or externally, or blood supply may be cut off. Plasma may leak from the blood vessels into the damaged tissues, causing

swelling and shock. When the crushed part is released, toxic chemicals produced by damaged muscles get into general circulation, which can cause kidney failure in severe cases.

S79.- Other and unspecified injuries of hip and thigh

Physeal fractures involving the upper and lower end of the femur comprise the bulk of this category. There are also codes for other specified injuries of the hip and thigh that do not have a more specific code and unspecified injuries of these sites.

S79.0- Physeal fracture of upper end of femur

S79.1- Physeal fracture of lower end of femur

Physeal fractures are pediatric fractures of the growth plate or physis of the bone. The Salter-Harris classification system is a method of describing the involvement of the physis, metaphysis, and epiphysis of the fracture. The classification helps determine treatment and possible long-term complications. Most of these heal without any disturbance of growth but some may lead to shortening or other deformities.

A Salter-Harris Type I fracture has the following characteristics:

- Transverse fracture through the physis only
- Increases width of physis
- Generally the growing zone is not injured and there is no disturbance to growth

A Salter-Harris Type II fracture has the following characteristics:

- Fracture through the physis and metaphysis
- Most common Salter-Harris fracture
- May cause minimal shortening but rarely results in functional disabilities

A Salter-Harris Type III fracture has the following characteristics:

- Fracture through the physis and the epiphysis, splitting the epiphysis
- Damages the reproductive layer of physis and likely causes some chronic disability
- Rarely results in major deformity; often surgical treatment is done with favorable prognosis

A Salter-Harris Type IV fracture has the following characteristics:

- Fracture through epiphysis, physis, and metaphysis
- Can disrupt growth of cartilage cells causing premature fusion of involved bone
- May lead to deformity of joint and chronic disability

Injuries to the Knee and Lower Leg (S80-S89)

Injuries classified here range from minor injuries, such as contusions, abrasions, superficial foreign bodies, and insect bites, to deeper injuries involving the soft tissues to fractures and dislocations.

The categories in this code block are as follows:

S80	Superficial injury of knee and lower leg
S81	Open wound of knee and lower leg
S82	Fracture of lower leg, including ankle
S83	Dislocation and sprain of joints and ligaments of knee
S84	Injury of nerves at lower leg level
S85	Injury of blood vessels at lower leg level
S86	Injury of muscle, fascia and tendon at lower leg level
S87	Crushing injury of lower leg
S88	Traumatic amputation of lower leg
S89	Other and unspecified injuries of lower leg

S82.-   Fracture of lower leg, including ankle

Fractures classified here include those involving the patella, the upper end of the tibia and fibula including intraarticular fractures at the knee joint, tibial and fibular shafts, and the lower end of the tibia and fibula including intraarticular fractures of the ankle joint. Codes for open fractures of the extremities require a seventh character that not only captures the type of encounter and whether the fracture is open or closed, but also identifies the type of open fracture based on the Gustilo classification. Following are the definitions for the open fractures as defined by the Gustilo classification:

Type I:	Low energy injury, clean wound less than 1 cm
Type II:	Wound is more than 1 cm with moderate soft tissue damage
Type III:	High energy wound, greater than 1 cm with extensive soft tissue damage, and subclassified to IIIA, IIIB, and IIIC
Type IIIA:	Adequate soft tissue coverage despite extensive soft tissue damage
Type IIIB:	Inadequate soft tissue coverage usually with severe wound contamination
Type IIIC:	Type III open fracture associated with arterial injury

S82.0-   Fracture of patella

The anatomy of the knee joint and associated muscles, tendons, and ligaments predispose the occurrence of patellar fractures in conjunction with sprains or ruptures of the ligaments. Typically, injuries are due to direct application of force or twisting. A severely injured knee remains prone to reinjury, instability, or arthritis.

S82.01-   Osteochondral fracture of patella

An osteochondral fracture of the patella involves tearing of the overlying cartilage and fracture of the bone on the underside of the patella. This type of injury is most common in adolescents usually from twisting type injuries or direct trauma to the joint as seen in many types of sports injuries. In displaced osteochondral fractures, there is bone and cartilage fragments in the knee joint.

S82.02-   Longitudinal fracture of patella

Longitudinal fractures are also called vertical fractures. These fractures occur in a superior to inferior direction and cause a vertical split in the patella.

S82.03-   Transverse fracture of patella

Fractures that occur in a medial to lateral direction across the patella are called transverse fractures. They are more common in the central portion or distal aspect of the patella.

S82.04-   Comminuted fracture of patella

In a comminuted fracture, the bone is fractured, splintered, or shattered into multiple pieces with many small bone fragments.

S82.1-   Fracture of upper end of tibia

Fractures of the upper or proximal aspect of the tibia are classified by site with the exception of torus fractures. Fractures of the proximal tibia may extend into the joint and involve the articular surface. Fractures that do not extend into the joint are called extraarticular while those that involve the joint are called intraarticular.

S82.16-   Torus fracture of upper end of tibia

Torus fractures (a.k.a., buckle fracture, incomplete fracture) are common injuries among the pediatric population. It is commonly a result of axial loading on a long bone of an extremity, such as falling on an outstretched hand. Less common in the upper tibia, it can occur with hyperextension of the knee, also referred to as toddler's fracture. This type of fracture is characterized by one side of the bone buckling upon itself without disrupting the other side. This characteristic "buckling" is due to the softer nature of the child's developing bone, allowing for the bone to compress, buckle, or "collapse" on one side, instead of break. These are generally quick-healing injuries that are treated with casting or splinting.

S82.2-   Fracture of shaft of tibia

Fractures of the tibial shaft are classified by type and whether or not the fracture is displaced or nondisplaced. Laterality is also a component of the code.

S82.22-   Transverse fracture of shaft of tibia

Transverse fractures occur in a straight line across the bone at a right angle to the long axis of the bone.

S82.23-   Oblique fracture of shaft of tibia

Oblique fractures occur at a diagonal angle across the bone shaft.

S82.24-   Spiral fracture of shaft of tibia

Spiral fractures, also called torsion fractures, are caused by a twisting force resulting in a diagonal fracture around and through the bone.

S82.25-   Comminuted fracture of shaft of tibia

In a comminuted fracture, the bone is fractured, splintered, or shattered into multiple pieces with many small bone fragments.

S82.26-   Segmental fracture of shaft of tibia

In a segmental fracture, the bone is broken in two places leaving at least one segment unattached to the body of bone.

S82.31-   Torus fracture of lower end of tibia

Torus fractures (a.k.a., buckle fracture, incomplete fracture) are common injuries among the pediatric population. It is commonly a result of axial loading on a long bone of an extremity, such as falling on an outstretched hand. Less common in the tibia, it can occur with hyperextension of the knee, also referred to as toddler's fracture. This type of fracture is characterized by one side of the bone buckling upon itself without disrupting the other side. This characteristic "buckling" is due to the softer nature of the child's developing bone, allowing for the bone to compress, buckle, or "collapse" on one side, instead of break. These are generally quick-healing injuries that are treated with casting or splinting.

S82.4-   Fracture of shaft of fibula

Fractures of the shaft of the fibula are classified by type and whether or not the fracture is displaced or nondisplaced. Laterality is also a component of the code.

S82.42-   Transverse fracture of shaft of fibula

Transverse fractures occur in a straight line across the bone at a right angle to the long axis of the bone.

S82.43-   Oblique fracture of shaft of fibula

Oblique fractures occur at a diagonal angle across the bone shaft.

S82.44-   Spiral fracture of shaft of fibula

Spiral fractures, also called torsion fractures, are caused by a twisting force resulting in a diagonal fracture around and through the bone.

S82.45-   Comminuted fracture of shaft of fibula

In a comminuted fracture, the bone is fractured, splintered, or shattered into multiple pieces with many small bone fragments.

S82.46-   Segmental fracture of shaft of fibula

In a segmental fracture, the bone is broken in two places leaving at least one segment unattached to the body of bone.

S82.5-   Fracture of medial malleolus

The medial malleolus is located at the distal end of the tibia on the inner aspect of the ankle. Fractures of the medial malleolus typically require a forceful impact such as landing from a height but can occur with a rolling ankle type of injury as well. Because of the force required for the medial malleolus to break, the type of fracture is usually found in combination with other injuries such as a sprained ankle or other fractures.

S82.6-   Fracture of lateral malleolus

The lateral malleolus is located at the distal end of the fibula on the outer aspect of the ankle. Dupuytren's fracture, which is classified here, is a fracture of the lateral malleolus and dislocation of the ankle with the talus downwardly displaced. The talus is one of the major ankle (tarsal) bones.

S82.81-   Torus fracture of upper end of fibula

S82.82-   Torus fracture of lower end of fibula

Torus fractures (a.k.a., buckle fracture, incomplete fracture) are common injuries among the pediatric population, although it does occur less in the fibula. It is commonly a result of axial loading on a long bone of an extremity, such as falling on an outstretched hand. This type of fracture is characterized by one side of the bone buckling upon itself without disrupting the other side. This characteristic "buckling" is due to the softer nature of the child's developing bone, allowing for the bone to compress, buckle, or "collapse" on one side, instead of break. These are generally quick-healing injuries that are treated with casting or splinting.

S82.84- Bimalleolar fracture of lower leg

A bimalleolar fracture involves two of the three malleoli of the tibia and fibula. The tibia has two malleoli, the medial and posterior, and the fibula has one, the lateral. Typically, the fracture involves the lateral malleolus of the fibula and medial malleolus of the tibia. However, it may instead involve the posterior malleolus and one of the other two malleoli: medial or lateral.

S82.85- Trimalleolar fracture of lower leg

A trimalleolar fracture involves a fracture of all three malleoli of the ankle, the medial and lateral malleoli, and the posterior aspect of the tibia referred to as the posterior malleolus. A trimalleolar fracture is considered an unstable injury and typically requires surgery.

S82.86- Maisonneuve's fracture

This is an unstable spiral fracture of the fibula involving the upper (proximal) aspect of the shaft of the fibula along with an injury to the ankle including disruption of the tibiofibular syndesmosis that may be accompanied by fracture of the medial malleolus, fracture of the posterior malleolus, tear of the anterior inferior tibiofibular ligament, tear in the interosseous ligament, and/or rupture of the deltoid ligament.

S82.87- Pilon fracture of tibia

This is a fracture of the lower end of the tibia or shin bone. The pilon is the weight bearing portion of the tibia that articulates with the talus at the ankle joint. Pilon fractures are considered high energy fractures because it typically takes a stronger force to cause it, such as a car accident or fall from a height. The name comes from the French word *pilon*, which is an instrument that is used for crushing. In many pilon fractures, the bones of the ankle are crushed. Pilon fractures are often accompanied by fibula fracture or other injuries.

Focus Point

When there is a concurrent fracture of the fibula, a separate code is required to report the fibula fracture.

S83.- Dislocation and sprain of joints and ligaments of knee

This category includes subluxations, dislocations, and sprains involving the knee joint. A subluxation refers to a partial dislocation. A sprain is an injury to the ligaments, which are the tough fibrous tissues that bind bones together at joints.

S83.0- Subluxation and dislocation of patella

Luxation is another term used to describe a complete dislocation, one that has separated the articulating surfaces of the joint. An incomplete dislocation, or subluxation, is one in which the joint surfaces maintain some articulation. A simple dislocation is a closed injury without a penetrating or communicating wound. An uncomplicated dislocation is not associated with other significant injuries. Open dislocations are those with an open wound at the site of the joint. Open injuries, also called compound dislocations, are subject to infection. Reduction of a dislocation or subluxation is by manipulation, open or closed. Dislocation of the patella is typically lateral. The choice of open or closed reduction depends on the degree of disruption of the nearby ligaments and tendons. Intraarticular dislocations of the patella usually require open reduction.

S83.1- Subluxation and dislocation of knee

Luxation is another term used to describe a complete dislocation, one that has separated the articulating surfaces of the joint. An incomplete dislocation, or subluxation, is one in which the joint surfaces maintain some articulation. A simple dislocation is a closed injury without a penetrating or communicating wound. An uncomplicated dislocation is not associated with other significant injuries. Open dislocations are those with an open wound at the site of the joint. Open injuries, also called compound dislocations, are subject to infection. Reduction of a dislocation or subluxation is by manipulation, open or closed. Dislocations of the knee are serious injuries, often requiring immediate surgery to offset the risk of vascular complications.

S83.2- Tear of meniscus, current injury

The menisci consist of two tough, rubbery, C-shaped pieces of cartilage below the patella that act as shock absorbers between the femur and the tibia and aid in cushioning and stabilizing the knee joint. One meniscus is located on the outer aspect of the joint and is called the lateral meniscus and the other one is located on the inner aspect and is called the medial meniscus. Injuries to the medial meniscus are more common than injuries to the lateral meniscus because the medial meniscus is firmly attached to medial collateral ligament and the joint capsule while the lateral meniscus is more mobile. Meniscal tears are classified by type of tear, which includes bucket-handle, peripheral, complex, or other type; by which meniscus is injured, lateral or medial; and by laterality. Traumatic tears of the menisci predominately occur from sports injuries.

S83.21- Bucket-handle tear of medial meniscus, current injury

The bucket-handle tear is caused when the meniscus gets trapped between the femur and tibia, which creates a tear in the central part of the interior curve of the C. This creates a bucket-handle configuration with the bucket-handle being displaced into the joint space. Bucket-handle tears tend to be large tears that can limit range of motion of the knee. Surgical repair of the tear or removal of the meniscus is required. Bucket-handle tears occur more frequently on the medial meniscus than on the lateral meniscus.

S83.22- Peripheral tear of medial meniscus, current injury

Peripheral tears of the meniscus occur on the periphery or outer edge of the meniscus. Peripheral tears are the easiest to repair and usually heal well without complications.

S83.23- Complex tear of medial meniscus, current injury

Meniscus tears occur in a variety of different patterns, including longitudinal, bucket-handle, parrot beak, radial, and horizontal. A complex tear is one that involves more than one pattern. Complex tears may also involve complete separation of one or more pieces of the meniscus from the body of the meniscus.

S83.25- Bucket-handle tear of lateral meniscus, current injury

The bucket-handle tear is caused when the meniscus gets trapped between the femur and tibia, which creates a tear in the central part of the interior curve of the C. This creates a bucket-handle configuration with the bucket-handle being displaced into the joint space. Bucket-handle tears tend to be large tears that can limit range of motion of the knee. Surgical repair of the tear or removal of the meniscus is required. Bucket-handle tears occur more frequently on the medial meniscus than on the lateral meniscus.

S83.26- Peripheral tear of lateral meniscus, current injury

Peripheral tears of the meniscus occur on the periphery or outer edge of the meniscus. Peripheral tears are the easiest to repair and usually heal well without complications.

S83.27- Complex tear of lateral meniscus, current injury

Meniscus tears occur in a variety of different patterns, including longitudinal, bucket-handle, parrot beak, radial, and horizontal. A complex tear is one that involves more than one pattern. Complex tears may also involve complete separation of one or more pieces of the meniscus from the body of the meniscus.

S83.4- Sprain of collateral ligament of knee

The collateral ligaments are located on the sides of the knee and control the sideways motion of the knee. The medial collateral ligament is interior and the lateral collateral ligament is on the outside. This type of sprain is generally caused by direct contact sports. A sprain is an injury to the ligaments, which are the tough fibrous tissues that bind bones together at joints. Sprains are graded. A Type I sprain denotes minor ligamentous injury, Type II is an incomplete ligamentous injury, and Type III describes a complete disruption of the ligament. The more ligaments involved in the sprain, the more serious the injury. Sprains manifest with swelling, pain, and limited mobility. A mild sprain may heal in two to six weeks, while a severe sprain may require eight weeks to 10 months to heal.

S83.5- Sprain of cruciate ligament of knee

The cruciate ligaments are located inside the knee joint. The anterior and posterior cross each other and control the back and forth motion of the knee. One of the most common knee injuries is the anterior cruciate ligament (ACL) sprain. It typically occurs in athletes who are involved in high demand sports and usually involves damage to other knee structures. A sprain is an injury to the ligaments, which are the tough fibrous tissues that bind bones together at joints. Sprains are graded. A Type I sprain denotes minor ligamentous injury, Type II is an incomplete ligamentous injury, and Type III describes a complete disruption of the ligament. The more ligaments involved in the sprain, the more serious the injury. Sprains manifest with swelling, pain, and limited mobility. A mild sprain may heal in two to six weeks, while a severe sprain may require eight weeks to 10 months to heal.

S83.6- Sprain of the superior tibiofibular joint and ligament

S83.8- Sprain of other specified parts of knee

S83.9- Sprain of unspecified site of knee

A sprain is an injury to the ligaments, which are the tough fibrous tissues that bind bones together at joints. Sprains are graded. A Type I sprain denotes minor ligamentous injury, Type II is an incomplete ligamentous injury, and Type III describes a complete disruption of the ligament. The more ligaments involved in the sprain, the more serious the injury. Sprains manifest with swelling, pain, and limited mobility. A mild sprain may heal in two to six weeks, while a severe sprain may require eight weeks to 10 months to heal.

> **Focus Point**
>
> *A sprain is not identical to a strain and the two terms should not be used synonymously. A strain is an injury to the muscles or tendons. Codes for strains at the lower leg level are located in category S86.*

S85.-   Injury of blood vessels at lower leg level

Vascular trauma may result from penetrating or blunt injury. Arterial blood loss manifests as profuse and bright red, while venous loss is steady and dark.

Focus Point

Traumatic aneurysms are reported with codes for injury to blood vessels. An aneurysm is a weakening in the arterial wall that bulges with the pumping of the blood, posing the threat of rupture. When aneurysms are part of a disease process and not due to trauma, they are reported with codes from Chapter 9 Diseases of the Circulatory System.

S86.-   Injury of muscle, fascia and tendon at lower leg level

Strain injuries and lacerations of muscle, fascia, or tendon are classified here. Strains occur when the muscle, fascia, or tendon is stretched or subjected to a level of force beyond its stretching or strength capabilities. A tear of a muscle, fascia, or tendon is classified as a strain. A pulled muscle is also classified as a strain. Symptoms of strains include swelling, bruising, pain at rest and with activity, weakness in the strained muscle, and the inability to use the affected body part. A laceration is a deep cut through the soft tissue and into the fascia, muscle, and/or tendon.

Focus Point

A sprain injury should not be confused with a strain injury. A sprain is an injury to the ligaments, which are the tough fibrous tissues that bind bones together at joints. Sprains of the knee are located in category S83.

S87.-   Crushing injury of lower leg

A crushing injury occurs when a body part is subjected to a high degree of force or pressure, typically after being pressed between two heavy or motionless objects. Damage related to crush injuries can include lacerations, fractures, bleeding, bruising, and compartment syndrome. Severe crush injuries cause extensive damage to skin, muscle, nerves, and bone. There may be bleeding, internally and/or externally, or blood supply may be cut off. Plasma may leak from the blood vessels into the damaged tissues, causing swelling and shock. When the crushed part is released, toxic chemicals produced by damaged muscles get into general circulation, which can cause kidney failure in severe cases.

S89.-   Other and unspecified injuries of lower leg

This category includes physeal fractures of the upper and lower tibia and fibula, as well as other specified and unspecified injuries to the lower leg.

S89.0-   Physeal fracture of upper end of tibia

S89.1-   Physeal fracture of lower end of tibia

S89.2-   Physeal fracture of upper end of fibula

S89.3-   Physeal fracture of lower end of fibula

Physeal fractures are pediatric fractures of the growth plate or physis of the bone. The Salter-Harris classification system is a method of describing the involvement of the physis, metaphysis, and epiphysis of the fracture. The classification helps determine treatment and possible long-term complications. Most of these heal without any disturbance of growth but some may lead to shortening or other deformities.

A Salter-Harris Type I fracture has the following characteristics:

- Transverse fracture through the physis only

- Increases width of physis

- Generally the growing zone is not injured and there is no disturbance to growth

A Salter-Harris Type II fracture has the following characteristics:

- Fracture through the physis and metaphysis

- Most common Salter-Harris fracture

- May cause minimal shortening but rarely results in functional disabilities

A Salter-Harris Type III fracture has the following characteristics:

- Fracture through the physis and the epiphysis, splitting the epiphysis

- Damages the reproductive layer of physis and likely causes some chronic disability

- Rarely results in major deformity; often surgical treatment is done with favorable prognosis

A Salter-Harris Type IV fracture has the following characteristics:

- Fracture through epiphysis, physis, and metaphysis

- Can disrupt growth of cartilage cells causing premature fusion of involved bone

- May lead to deformity of joint and chronic disability

Injuries to the Ankle and Foot (S90-S99)

Injuries classified here range from superficial injuries, such as contusions, abrasions, superficial foreign bodies, and insect bites, to deeper injuries involving the soft tissues to fractures and dislocations.

The categories in this code block are as follows:

S90	Superficial injury of ankle, foot and toes
S91	Open wound of ankle, foot and toes
S92	Fracture of foot and toe, except ankle
S93	Dislocation and sprain of joints and ligaments at ankle, foot and toe level
S94	Injury of nerves at ankle and foot level
S95	Injury of blood vessels at ankle and foot level
S96	Injury of muscle and tendon at ankle and foot level
S97	Crushing injury of ankle and foot
S98	Traumatic amputation of ankle and foot
S99	Other and unspecified injuries of ankle and foot

S92.-   Fracture of foot and toe, except ankle

Bones of the foot and toes are divided into the tarsal bones, the metatarsals, and the phalanges. The tarsal bones are the heel bone (calcaneus, os calcis), talus (astragalus), navicular (scaphoid), cuboid, and the lateral, medial, and intermediate cuneiform bones. The metatarsals are the five long bones of the foot extending from the tarsal bones to the phalanges or toes. A fracture is a break in a bone resulting from two possible causes: the direct or indirect application of undue force against the bone and pathological changes resulting in spontaneous fractures. This chapter includes only those fractures that have arisen as a result of an injury. It includes delayed healing and nonunions of fractured bones. Closed fractures are contained beneath the skin, while open or compound fractures connote an associated open wound. Open fractures are always compound, with a wound leading to the fracture or the broken bone ends protruding through the skin. There is a very high risk of infection with open fractures since the tissues are exposed to contaminants.

Focus Point

Subcategories identify whether the fracture is displaced or nondisplaced. A fracture not indicated as nondisplaced or displaced should be classified to displaced. The seventh character for an initial encounter specifies whether the fracture is open or closed. If unspecified, the default is closed.

S93.-   Dislocation and sprain of joints and ligaments at ankle, foot and toe level

This category includes subluxations, dislocation and sprains involving the ankles, feet, and toes. A subluxation refers to a partial dislocation. A sprain is an injury to the ligaments, which are the tough fibrous tissues that bind bones together at joints.

S93.0-   Subluxation and dislocation of ankle joint

S93.1-   Subluxation and dislocation of toe

S93.3-   Subluxation and dislocation of foot

Luxation is another term used to describe a complete dislocation, one that has separated the articulating surfaces of the joint. An incomplete dislocation, or subluxation, is one in which the joint surfaces maintain some articulation. A simple dislocation is a closed injury without a penetrating or communicating wound. An uncomplicated dislocation is not associated with other significant injuries. Open dislocations are those with an open wound at the site of the joint. Open injuries, also called compound dislocations, are subject to infection. Reduction of a dislocation or subluxation is by manipulation, open or closed.

Focus Point

The ankle is seldom dislocated without an accompanying fracture and is easily reduced. Fracture dislocations are reported with fracture codes.

S93.4-   Sprain of ankle

Ankle sprains are common injuries. A sprain is an injury to the ligaments, which are the tough fibrous tissues that bind bones together at joints. Sprains are graded. A Type I sprain denotes minor ligamentous injury, Type II is an incomplete ligamentous injury, and Type III describes a complete disruption of the ligament. The more ligaments involved in the sprain, the more serious the injury. Sprains manifest with swelling, pain, and limited mobility. A mild sprain may heal in two to six weeks, while a severe sprain may require eight weeks to 10 months to heal. Ankle sprains are classified based on which ligament is injured: calcaneofibular, deltoid, tibiofibular, or other ligament.

Focus Point

A sprain is not identical to a strain and the two terms should not be used synonymously. A strain is an injury to the muscles or tendons. A strain at the ankle level is reported with a code from category S96 Injury of muscle and tendon at ankle. Codes for strains at the ankle level are specific to the muscle or tendon injured.

S93.5-   Sprain of toe

A sprain is an injury to the ligaments, which are the tough fibrous tissues that bind bones together at joints. Sprains are graded. A Type I sprain denotes minor ligamentous injury, Type II is an incomplete ligamentous injury, and Type III describes a complete disruption of the ligament. The more ligaments involved in the sprain, the more serious the injury. Sprains manifest with swelling, pain, and limited mobility. A mild sprain may heal in two to six weeks, while a severe sprain may require eight weeks to 10 months to heal. Sprains of the toes are classified based on the joint affected (interphalangeal or metatarsophalangeal), the toe (great or lesser), and laterality.

> **Focus Point**
>
> *A sprain is not identical to a strain and the two terms should not be used synonymously. A strain is an injury to the muscles or tendons. Codes for strains of the toes are located in category S96.*

S93.6-   Sprain of foot

A sprain is an injury to the ligaments, which are the tough fibrous tissues that bind bones together at joints. Sprains are graded. A Type I sprain denotes minor ligamentous injury, Type II is an incomplete ligamentous injury, and Type III describes a complete disruption of the ligament. The more ligaments involved in the sprain, the more serious the injury. Sprains manifest with swelling, pain, and limited mobility. A mild sprain may heal in two to six weeks, while a severe sprain may require eight weeks to 10 months to heal. A sprain of the foot may involve the tarsal ligament, the tarsometatarsal ligament, or another specified site.

> **Focus Point**
>
> *A sprain is not identical to a strain and the two terms should not be used synonymously. A strain is an injury to the muscles or tendons. Codes for strains at the foot level are located in category S96.*

S95.-   Injury of blood vessels at ankle and foot level

Vascular trauma may result from penetrating or blunt injury. Arterial blood loss manifests as profuse and bright red, while venous loss is steady and dark.

> **Focus Point**
>
> *Traumatic aneurysms are reported with codes for injury to blood vessels. An aneurysm is a weakening in the arterial wall that bulges with the pumping of the blood, posing the threat of rupture. When aneurysms are part of a disease process and not due to trauma, they are reported with codes from Chapter 9 Diseases of the Circulatory System.*

S96.-   Injury of muscle and tendon at ankle and foot level

Strain injuries and lacerations of muscle, fascia, or tendon are classified here. Strains occur when the muscle, fascia, or tendon is stretched or subjected to a level of force beyond its stretching or strength capabilities. A tear of a muscle, fascia, or tendon is classified as a strain. A pulled muscle is also classified as a strain. Symptoms of strains include swelling, bruising, pain at rest and with activity, weakness in the strained muscle, and the inability to use the affected body part. A laceration is a deep cut through the soft tissue and into the fascia, muscle, and/or tendon.

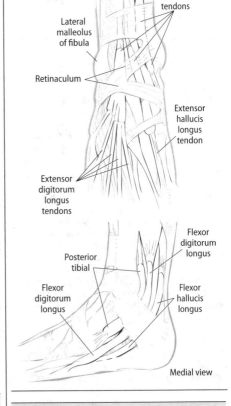

Tendons of Ankle and Foot

Select tendons

Lateral malleolus of fibula

Retinaculum

Extensor hallucis longus tendon

Extensor digitorum longus tendons

Flexor digitorum longus

Posterior tibial

Flexor digitorum longus

Flexor hallucis longus

Medial view

> **Focus Point**
>
> *A sprain injury should not be confused with a strain injury. A sprain is an injury to the ligaments, which are the tough fibrous tissues that bind bones together at joints. Sprains of the ankle, foot, and toes are located in category S93.*

S97.- Crushing injury of ankle and foot

A crushing injury occurs when a body part is subjected to a high degree of force or pressure, typically after being pressed between two heavy or motionless objects. Damage related to crush injuries can include lacerations, fractures, bleeding, bruising, and compartment syndrome. Severe crush injuries cause extensive damage to skin, muscle, nerves, and bone. There may be bleeding, internally and/or externally, or blood supply may be cut off. Plasma may leak from the blood vessels into the damaged tissues, causing swelling and shock. When the crushed part is released, toxic chemicals produced by damaged muscles get into general circulation, which can cause kidney failure in severe cases.

S99.- Other and unspecified injuries of ankle and foot

Classified here are physeal fractures, also known as growth plate fractures, occurring in pediatric patients as they are growing. The physis is the developing tissue at the ends of the long bones. These types of fractures can occur due to injury, overuse, cancer therapy, certain neurologic or metabolic conditions, or genetic predisposition. The Salter-Harris classification system is a method of describing the involvement of the physis, metaphysis, and epiphysis of the fracture. The classification helps determine treatment and possible long-term complications.

This category of codes differentiates between these bones and further classifies the fracture based on the Salter-Harris type to describe the extent of the damage. The following definitions have been standard since the 1960s:

A Salter-Harris Type I fracture has the following characteristics:

- Transverse fracture through the physis only

- Increased width of physis

- Generally no injury to the growing zone with no disturbance to growth

A Salter-Harris Type II fracture has the following characteristics:

- Fracture through the physis and metaphysis

- Most common Salter-Harris fracture

- Sometimes causing minimal shortening but rarely resulting in functional disabilities

A Salter-Harris Type III fracture has the following characteristics:

- Fracture through the physis and the epiphysis, splitting the epiphysis

- Damage to the reproductive layer of physis, likely causing some chronic disability

- Rarely cause of major deformity; often surgical treatment has favorable prognosis

A Salter-Harris Type IV fracture has the following characteristics:

- Fracture through epiphysis, physis, and metaphysis

- Possible disruption of growth of cartilage cells, causing premature fusion of involved bone

- Possible cause of deformity of joint and chronic disability

Most of these fractures heal without any disturbance of growth, but some may lead to shortening or other deformities and may require more than one method of treatment depending on the injury and location. Casts and alignment are typical treatments and, in more severe cases, surgery and physical therapy are also necessary. Complications arise due to decreased bone development at the injured site with more serious complications resulting from damage to nerves or blood vessels in the area.

S99.0- Physeal fracture of calcaneus

The calcaneus is the largest tarsal bone in the foot and is also referred to as the heel bone.

S99.1- Physeal fracture of metatarsal

The metatarsals are the five long bones in the foot between the tarsal bones and the phalanges (toes).

S99.2- Physeal fracture of phalanx of toe

The phalanx is a bone of the digits, in this case, the toes.

Effects of Foreign Body Entering Through Natural Orifice (T15-T19)

Instances of foreign bodies (FB) in orifices are one of the most common reasons for emergency department visits. Complications from the foreign body depend on several factors, including its location within the body, how long it has been in the body, and what the foreign body is composed of. Batteries, for instance, may not cause much pain on ingestion but can be very damaging to the gastrointestinal tract when the corrosive material in the battery leaks out.

The categories in this code block are as follows:

T15	Foreign body on external eye
T16	Foreign body in ear
T17	Foreign body in respiratory tract
T18	Foreign body in alimentary tract
T19	Foreign body in genitourinary tract

T15.- Foreign body on external eye

Foreign bodies in the eye are particularly common. Only a physician should remove a foreign body in the eye because of the danger of damaging the eye. If the foreign body is not removed, or is improperly removed, infection and permanent vision loss can result.

T17.- Foreign body in respiratory tract

A foreign body in the respiratory tract is particularly dangerous because it can cause asphyxiation. Asphyxiation is the insufficient intake of oxygen, resulting in pathological changes brought on by a lack of oxygen perfusion to the tissues or excessive carbon dioxide in the blood, and is a serious complication. Other injuries may include ulcer or abscess formation, perforation, and vascular injury. Foreign bodies are classified based on the type of foreign body, which includes gastric contents, food, or other foreign body. All codes in this category except for the nasal sinus and nostril sites require a sixth character identifying whether the foreign body in the respiratory tract caused asphyxiation or other injury.

T17.5- Foreign body in bronchus

Children frequently aspirate foreign bodies into the right main bronchus. Often the act is not observed, and the child may present with pneumonia or a lung abscess if the foreign body has been present for a long time. Hypoxia may result from objects obstructing breathing. Typically, the foreign body is located by use of the flexible bronchoscope and removed in the operating room with a rigid bronchoscope.

T18.- Foreign body in alimentary tract

The alimentary tract, or what is more commonly referred to as the gastrointestinal (GI) tract, begins at the esophagus and ends at the anus and is divided into an upper and lower segment. The upper GI tract is composed of the esophagus, stomach, and duodenum, which is the first section of the small intestine. The lower GI tract is composed of the other sections of the small intestine (e.g., jejunum and ileum), the entire colon (ascending, transverse, descending, and sigmoid colon), as well as the cecum, rectum, and anal canal. Foreign bodies may enter via the mouth or via the anus.

T18.1- Foreign body in esophagus

A complication of foreign body of the esophagus is compression of the trachea, which results from an extrinsic force (outside the trachea) that narrows the trachea and reduces airflow. This may be due to the FB pushing directly into the trachea or from dilation of the esophagus in response to the FB. Symptoms that are common to trachea compression include stridor or wheezing. Perforation, fistula formation, and strictures are just a few other injuries that may result from an esophageal foreign body. Codes associated with esophageal foreign bodies must identify the type of

foreign body as gastric contents, food, or other foreign body and also whether there is a compression of the trachea or another specified injury associated with the FB.

Burns and Corrosions (T20-T32)

Burn codes are used for reporting thermal burns that come from a heat source and burns associated with electricity and radiation. Corrosion codes are used to report burns related to chemicals. This code block is broken down into three parts based on whether the burn or corrosion injury was to the external body surface (T20-T25), the eye and internal organs (T26-T28), or multiple and unspecified body sites (T30-T32).

> **Focus Point**
>
> When there are burns of the same local site of varying degrees, use the code indicating the highest degree documented in the medical record. Sequence first the code with the highest degree of burn in cases of multiple burns.
>
> The treatment of current, unhealed burns is classified here along with late effects of burns. Late effects are reported with the same code for a current burn, except that the 7th character "S" is used to identify the encounter as a sequela. When coding the late effect of a burn, the appropriate code for describing the sequela (late effect) is coded first, followed by the burn code.
>
> Because of the nature of burns, it is possible for a patient to have healed and non-healed burns during a single encounter. For this reason, it is appropriate to use a code for currently unhealed burns and a code for the sequela.
>
> Sunburns and burns from tanning beds are classified to Chapter 12 Diseases of the Skin and Subcutaneous Tissue.

Burns and Corrosions of External Body Surface, Specified by Site (T20-T25)

Burns and corrosions of the external body surface are classified by the specific sites and the depth (degree) of the burn injury (first degree through third degree). These are defined further as:

First degree: Epidermis (outer layer of skin) only, erythema

Second degree: Epidermis and part of the dermis (inner layer of skin), blisters are common

Third degree: Loss of the epidermis and dermis (full thickness); damage to underlying muscle, tendons, and even bone may occur; pain is often minimal due to damage to nerve endings

Unspecified: Depth is not documented in the medical record

An extensive burn injury has a profound effect on the body. The muscles, nerves, bones, blood vessels, respiratory system function, temperature regulation, joint function, fluid/electrolyte balance, physical appearance, and psychological function are all affected.

Burns and corrosions of the external body surface are arranged into broad categories based on site.

The categories in this code block are as follows:

T20	Burn and corrosion of head, face, and neck
T21	Burn and corrosion of trunk
T22	Burn and corrosion of shoulder and upper limb, except wrist and hand
T23	Burn and corrosion of wrist and hand
T24	Burn and corrosion of lower limb, except ankle and foot
T25	Burn and corrosion of ankle and foot

Burns and Corrosions Confined to Eye and Internal Organs (T26-T28)

This code block captures burns and corrosions of the eye, the internal structures of the ear, as well as internal organs that comprise the respiratory, digestive, and genitourinary tracts.

The categories in this code block are as follows:

T26	Burn and corrosion confined to eye and adnexa
T27	Burn and corrosion of respiratory tract
T28	Burn and corrosion of other internal organs

Burns and Corrosions of Multiple and Unspecified Body Regions (T30-T32)

Categories T31-T32 classify the extent of body surface affected by the burn or corrosion and are useful as an adjunctive set of codes in assessing morbidity and mortality in burn centers. These categories may also be used when no further information is available, as in a patient who is briefly brought to an emergency department, stabilized, and transported to a specialty unit.

The categories in this code block are as follows:

T30	Burn and corrosion, body region unspecified
T31	Burns classified according to extent of body surface involved
T32	Corrosions classified according to extent of body surface involved

Focus Point

Categories T31-T32 are used to classify burns according to the body surface area involved. These codes are used as an additional code for reporting purposes when there are third-degree burns involving 10 percent or more of the body surface or when further information is needed for evaluating burn mortality.

T31.- Burns classified according to extent of body surface involved

T32.- Corrosions classified according to extent of body surface involved

The impact of burn injuries is magnified according to the amount of body surface burned. Children have much smaller thresholds for what is considered severe.

The rule of nines is a method for rapidly estimating the percent of total body surface area affected, which in adult burn victims is a strong predictor of the patient's prognosis. This metric helps emergency clinicians decide whether a patient needs to be transferred to a regional burn center for specialized care and helps in estimating the amount of fluid replacement the patient needs to replace losses from the burned area. Radiation burns are the most dangerous thermal burn injury, though they may have a more benign appearance than a third-degree injury from other types of thermal burns.

The concept of the rule of nines is basically to break the adult body down into smaller anatomical regions. Each anatomical region is roughly 9 percent of the body as a whole. If more than one anatomical area is burned, calculation of total body surface area is as easy as taking the number of anatomical areas affected and multiplying by nine. The anatomical regions include:

- Head
- Left arm
- Right arm
- Upper torso
- Upper back
- Lower torso
- Lower back
- Front of left leg
- Front of right leg
- Back of left leg
- Back of right leg
- Genitals (1%)

The rule of nines cannot be applied to children as they have larger heads and torsos in relation to their extremities.

Frostbite (T33-T34)

Frostbite is the effect of a low environmental temperature reducing blood circulation. When exposed to extreme cold, the body restricts the amount of blood sent to the extremities in order to keep the core body temperature normal, thus protecting vital internal organs. The extremities, particularly the fingers and toes, as well as the nose and ears, are at greatest risk of frostbite. Although direct exposure to extreme cold increases the likelihood of frostbite, skin that is covered may also be affected. Patients who already have poor circulation due to another disease process, such as diabetes, or take certain medications may be more prone to frostbite due to an already compromised circulation.

The categories in this code block are as follows:

T33   Superficial frostbite

T34   Frostbite with tissue necrosis

T33.-   Superficial frostbite

Superficial frostbite may also be referred to as first- or second-degree frostbite. Depth of the injury may involve a portion of the dermis but in most cases it is the surface of the skin only or the epidermis. Blisters may occur in second-degree frostbite and heat or cold intolerance may be experienced.

T34.-   Frostbite with tissue necrosis

Tissue necrosis is the buildup of dead cells and tissue. Frostbite can cause cell death in two ways: the lack of blood circulation to certain areas causes cell death due to lack of oxygen and crystal formation from extremely cold temperatures causes the cells to burst. During normal cellular death, phagocytes are signaled to engulf and recycle the dead cells. Cellular death in necrosis occurs prematurely and the typical signals are not activated, resulting in no phagocytic cell response and a buildup of dead and decomposing cells. Decomposing cells can leak cellular material that is harmful to the healthy cells nearby creating an area of perpetual cell death and healing cannot take place.

Poisoning by, Adverse Effect of and Underdosing of Drugs, Medicaments and Biological Substances (T36-T50)

A poison, in general, is anything that has the potential to kill or injure through some form of chemical action and includes any type of substance, whether meant for human consumption or not. ICD-10-CM classifies poisonings to only those substances intended for human ingestion or contact. Any substance not meant for human consumption results in what is referred to as a toxic effect and toxic effects are reported with codes in categories T51-T65.

> **Focus Point**
>
> *Ethanol is one of a couple of exceptions to the poisoning versus toxic effect classification in ICD-10-CM. Ethanol is a substance that can be and is commonly consumed by humans; however, when complications arise as a result of ethanol ingestion it is recognized only as a toxic effect and not as a poisoning.*

The circumstances in which a poisoning may occur are defined by ICD-10-CM as:

- Error in the drug prescription or in its administration

- Wrong substance given or taken in error

- Intentional overdose

- Nonprescribed drug with correctly prescribed and properly administered drug

- Interaction between drug(s) and alcohol

Poisoning may be accidental (unintentional), intentional self-harm, due to an assault, or undetermined. There are coding guidelines related to assignment of accidental (unintentional) versus undetermined. When no intent is documented, the default is always accidental (unintentional). Undetermined is only used when the documentation specifically states that the physician could not determine the intent.

An adverse effect is a condition, disease process, symptom, or other unusual reaction a patient has to a drug that has been correctly prescribed and properly administered. As with poisonings, only substances intended for human use have the potential to cause an adverse effect.

Underdosing is defined as taking less than the appropriate amount of a medication. This may occur when a patient intentionally or unknowingly takes less than what was prescribed by a doctor; takes less than what is instructed by the manufacturer of the medication; or the patient was under prescribed a medication, meaning the provider prescribed a medication at a lower dose than what was clinically suitable. The consequences of underdosing can often be just as severe as an overdose; withdrawal signs and symptoms can occur with certain drugs that are weaned too soon or too fast and the disease process for which the drug was prescribed can continue to progress leading to extreme exacerbation of the condition itself and/or to secondary adverse conditions.

The categories in this code block are as follows:

T36	Poisoning by, adverse effect of and underdosing of systemic antibiotics	
T37	Poisoning by, adverse effect of and underdosing of other systemic anti-infectives and antiparasitics	
T38	Poisoning by, adverse effect of and underdosing of hormones and their synthetic substitutes and antagonists, not elsewhere classified	
T39	Poisoning by, adverse effect of and underdosing of nonopioid analgesics, antipyretics and antirheumatics	
T40	Poisoning by, adverse effect of and underdosing of narcotics and psychodysleptics [hallucinogens]	
T41	Poisoning by, adverse effect of and underdosing of anesthetics and therapeutic gases	
T42	Poisoning by, adverse effect of and underdosing of antiepileptic, sedative-hypnotic and antiparkinsonism drugs	
T43	Poisoning by, adverse effect of and underdosing of psychotropic drugs, not elsewhere classified	
T44	Poisoning by, adverse effect of and underdosing of drugs primarily affecting the autonomic nervous system	
T45	Poisoning by, adverse effect of and underdosing of primarily systemic and hematological agents, not elsewhere classified	
T46	Poisoning by, adverse effect of and underdosing of agents primarily affecting the cardiovascular system	
T47	Poisoning by, adverse effect of and underdosing of agents primarily affecting the gastrointestinal system	
T48	Poisoning by, adverse effect of and underdosing of agents primarily acting on smooth and skeletal muscles and the respiratory system	
T49	Poisoning by, adverse effect of and underdosing of topical agents primarily affecting skin and mucous membrane and by ophthalmological, otorhinolaryngological and dental drugs	
T50	Poisoning by, adverse effect of and underdosing of diuretics and other and unspecified drugs, medicaments and biological substances	

T36.- Poisoning by, adverse effect of and underdosing of systemic antibiotics

Antibiotics are a group of drugs designed to treat bacterial infections, either by killing the bacteria directly or limiting the growth and/or proliferation of the bacteria. Systemic antibiotics simply indicate that the drug works throughout the body rather than one localized site. Antibiotics are classified based on the mechanism used to destroy or inhibit the bacteria and the type of bacteria they target. Broad-spectrum antibiotics are effective against many different types of bacteria, both gram-positive and gram-negative. Narrow-spectrum antibiotics are more specialized, effective only on select bacterial organisms or groups.

T36.0- Poisoning by, adverse effect of and underdosing of penicillins

Most common drugs: ampicillin, nafcillin, penicillin amoxicillin, amoxicillin + clavulanate (Augmentin), Piperacillin + tazobactam (Zosyn), imipenem.

T36.1- Poisoning by, adverse effect of and underdosing of cephalosporins and other beta-lactam antibiotics

Most common drugs: ceftriaxone (Rocephin), cephalexin (Keflex), cefazolin (Ancef), monobactam (Aztreonam).

T36.3- Poisoning by, adverse effect of and underdosing of macrolides

Patients who are allergic to the penicillin class of drugs may be given this class instead as it works against most of the same types of bacteria but is better tolerated by the patient.

Most common drugs: erythromycin (excludes ophthalmic and topical), azithromycin (Zithromax), clarithromycin.

T36.4- Poisoning by, adverse effect of and underdosing of tetracyclines

Most common drugs: tetracycline, doxycycline (Vibramycin).

T36.5- Poisoning by, adverse effect of and underdosing of aminoglycosides

Most common drugs: gentamicin (excludes ophthalmic and topical), tobramycin, amikacin, streptomycin.

T36.6- Poisoning by, adverse effect of and underdosing of rifampicins

Most common drugs: rifampin, rifabutin.

T36.8- Poisoning by, adverse effect of and underdosing of other systemic antibiotics

Most common drugs: clindamycin (Cleocin), linezolid (Zyvox), metronidazole (Flagyl), vancomycin, ciprofloxacin, levofloxacin, Bactrim.

T37.- Poisoning by, adverse effect of and underdosing of other systemic anti-infectives and antiparasitics

Anti-infective drugs inhibit the growth of or kill microorganisms. Some of the microorganisms targeted by drugs in this category include viruses, protozoa, malaria, mycobacteria, and parasites.

T38.- Poisoning by, adverse effect of and underdosing of hormones and their synthetic substitutes and antagonists, not elsewhere classified

Hormones are molecules used by the body to signal certain cell or organ activity. There are very few processes within the body that can function without involvement of one or more hormones. Digestion, sleep, mood, and reproduction are just a few of the physiological and behavioral activities that may be regulated by hormone production.

The job of a hormone antagonistic drug is to block specific hormones naturally produced by the body. It is a decoy hormone; it looks like a specific hormone so that the receptors on receiving cells will bind with it but does not carry out the actions of the hormone once bound.

T39.- Poisoning by, adverse effect of and underdosing of nonopioid analgesics, antipyretics and antirheumatics

Analgesics are used to treat mild to moderate pain. Nonopioid analgesics are less habit forming so the patient will not become dependent with their use. Fever reducing medications are called antipyretics. Antirheumatics are drugs that slow the progression of or treat the symptoms (pain, swelling) of rheumatoid arthritis.

T39.1- Poisoning by, adverse effect of and underdosing of 4-Aminophenol derivatives

Most common drug: acetaminophen.

T40.- Poisoning by, adverse effect of and underdosing of narcotics and psychodysleptics [hallucinogens]

The primary use for narcotic or opioid medications is to relieve severe pain. Tolerance to the drug does not take long and as such its use is primarily restricted to acute, short-term pain management. Narcotics are also highly addictive.

Psychodysleptic drugs, more formally known as hallucinogens, alter the perceptions, thoughts, and/or feelings of the user. Although there are a few limited uses of psychodysleptic drugs in medicinal or therapeutic settings, most are considered illegal.

T40.5- Poisoning by, adverse effect of and underdosing of cocaine

In the United States, cocaine toxicity is one of the leading causes of drug-related emergency department visits. Cocaine toxicity in combination with other substances, including alcohol, is common. Although nearly all body systems are affected, cocaine users have an exponentially increased risk of stroke, heart attack, seizure, and fatal trauma. Three clinical stages have been reported with acute cocaine toxicity. The progression of symptoms includes:

- Phase 1 (early stimulation): Severe anxiety, headache, nausea and vomiting, vertigo, tremor, high blood pressure, increased respiration, euphoria, and emotional lability

- Phase 2 (advanced stimulation): Seizures, status epilepticus, decreased CNS response to stimuli, hypertension dysrhythmia, hypotension, coagulopathy, hyperthermia, and cyanosis

- Phase 3 (premorbid state): Coma, cardiac arrest, renal failure, respiratory failure

A few medical applications of cocaine do exist mostly as a local numbing agent for some nasal and lacrimal duct surgeries.

T41.- Poisoning by, adverse effect of and underdosing of anesthetics and therapeutic gases

Anesthetics, in general, are drugs used to temporarily invoke a loss of feeling, sensation, or consciousness. There are several types of anesthetics (local versus general) and several routes of administration (inhaled versus intravenous versus topical).

T42.- Poisoning by, adverse effect of and underdosing of antiepileptic, sedative- hypnotic and antiparkinsonism drugs

Antiepileptic drugs (AED) are used to reduce the number, severity, or duration of seizures or prevent seizures altogether. The name can be misleading as these drugs do not in any way alter the epileptic disease itself but only treat a symptom of epilepsy, the seizures. These drugs may also be used for nonepileptic seizures and as such may be better referred to as anticonvulsant or antiseizure medications.

Sedative-hypnotic drugs are central nervous system depressants, meaning they slow body functions down. Do to their calming and sleep inducing affects, they are often used in the treatment of anxiety related disorders and insomnia.

The primary role for most antiparkinsonism drugs is to regulate dopamine levels in the brain. Dopamine is a neurotransmitter that helps control movements and emotions and is produced by dopamine-generating cells in the brain. Symptoms of Parkinson's disease, such as tremor, muscle rigidity, slow movement, behavior, or emotional problems all occur as a result of the death of these cells and lowered dopamine production. It is these symptoms that antiparkinsonism drugs aim to control.

T43.- Poisoning by, adverse effect of and underdosing of psychotropic drugs, not elsewhere classified

Psychotropic drugs and substances may be defined as those that affect or alter mental activity, behavior, perception, or mood. Antidepressants, neuroleptics, and psychostimulants are several psychotropic drugs that are classified here.

As their name implies, antidepressants were primarily developed to treat symptoms related to depression; however, there are a wide range of conditions for which antidepressants may be prescribed. Chemical imbalances in the brain are thought to cause many mood and behavioral conditions and antidepressants work to correct these imbalances.

Neuroleptic drugs, also known as antipsychotics, are primarily used to reduce psychotic manifestations such as hallucinations, delusions, and mania.

Psychostimulants are used to improve mood and overall mental function by enhancing central and peripheral nervous system activity. In general, these drugs work to increase certain chemical levels in the brain including dopamine and norepinephrine.

T43.61- Poisoning by, adverse effect of and underdosing of caffeine

Caffeine is a central nervous system (CNS) stimulant, a mild diuretic, and acts as a mild antidepressant. In excess, it may disrupt behavior in certain substance sensitive individuals. Caffeinated beverages have become popular and are widely available in various forms, including coffee, soft drinks, and energy drinks. Symptoms of overdose and poisoning may vary according to individual tolerances, but may include dizziness, breathlessness, chest discomfort, nervousness, and irritability. Excessive doses may cause more severe multisystemic and potentially fatal symptoms such as arrhythmia, hypertension, seizure, respiratory failure, and cerebral edema.

T50.- Poisoning by, adverse effect of and underdosing of diuretics and other and unspecified drugs, medicaments and biological substances

Along with diuretics, other drugs in this category include appetite depressants, antidotes, chelating agents, diagnostic agents, and vaccines.

Toxic Effects of Substances Chiefly Nonmedicinal as to Source (T51-T65)

A toxic effect can occur from ingestion of or direct contact with a harmful substance. Sources may include gases, metals, plants, food, and even alcohol and tobacco.

The toxicity of a substance is due to its ability to damage or disrupt metabolism. An acutely toxic substance can cause damage as the result of a single or short-duration exposure. A chronically toxic substance causes damage after repeated or long-duration exposure or becomes evident only after a long latency period. Toxicity varies with the route of exposure and the effectiveness with which the material is absorbed. A chemical that enters the body in large quantities but is not easily absorbed is a much lower risk than one that is easily absorbed into the bloodstream.

Skin contact is the most common route of exposure but often the best barrier since the skin guards against the entry of most chemicals. Once a chemical passes through the skin it enters the bloodstream and is carried to all parts of the body.

Inhalation is the most dangerous route of entry because the lungs are ineffective barriers. Chemicals that pass the lung membrane are absorbed into the bloodstream and carried to all parts of the body. Absorption can be extremely rapid. The rate of absorption depends on the concentration of the toxic substance, its solubility in water, the depth of respiration, and the rate of blood circulation.

Ingested materials are absorbed into the bloodstream anywhere along the gastrointestinal tract. If the material cannot be absorbed, it will be eliminated from the body.

A toxic effect can be similar to an allergic reaction but more severe. If the liver is functioning normally, it may allow a small amount of the toxic material to enter the body, but eliminate the rest. If the liver is not functioning normally, the substance may enter the body and cause a toxic chemical overload that may result in blood poisoning and death. Toxemia is a poisoned condition of the blood caused by the presence of toxic materials.

Toxic effect codes, like poisoning codes, specify the intent as accidental (unintentional), intentional self-harm, assault, or undetermined. There are coding guidelines related to assignment of accidental (unintentional) versus undetermined. When no intent is documented, the default is always accidental (unintentional). Undetermined is only used when the documentation specifically states that the physician could not determine the intent.

The categories in this code block are as follows:

T51	Toxic effect of alcohol
T52	Toxic effect of organic solvents
T53	Toxic effect of halogen derivatives of aliphatic and aromatic hydrocarbons
T54	Toxic effect of corrosive substances
T55	Toxic effect of soaps and detergents
T56	Toxic effect of metals
T57	Toxic effect of other inorganic substances
T58	Toxic effect of carbon monoxide
T59	Toxic effect of other gases, fumes and vapors
T60	Toxic effect of pesticides
T61	Toxic effect of noxious substances eaten as seafood
T62	Toxic effect of other noxious substances eaten as food
T63	Toxic effect of contact with venomous animals and plants
T64	Toxic effect of aflatoxin and other mycotoxin food contaminants
T65	Toxic effect of other and unspecified substances

T51.- Toxic effect of alcohol

The major subcategories included here are ethanol, methanol, 2-Propanol (isopropyl alcohol), and fusel oil.

T51.0- Toxic effect of ethanol

Ethanol is a colorless liquid most commonly used as fuel or a fuel additive but it is also used in solvents, antiseptics, cough syrup, mouthwashes, and some rubbing alcohols. Most people relate ethanol however to that used in alcoholic beverages. The effects of alcohol poisoning depend on several factors the most important of which is the amount of alcohol and the timeframe in which the consumption occurred. Minor symptoms include confusion, vomiting, and slow or dulled reflexes and more serious symptoms include slowed breathing and heart rate, seizures, and unconsciousness. Ethanol toxicity more commonly occurs with co-ingestion of other illicit or prescription drugs.

T51.1- Toxic effect of methanol

Methanol, like ethanol, is a colorless flammable liquid primarily used in solvents. Metabolic acidosis is the primary concern with methanol ingestion. Vision loss and movement disorders are also common due to optic nerve and basal ganglia damage respectively.

T51.2- Toxic effect of 2-Propanol

More commonly known as isopropanol or isopropyl alcohol, 2-propanol is used in rubbing alcohol, hand sanitizers, and other cleaning solvents. Isopropanol is another alcohol that works as a central nervous system depressant and can also have damaging effects to the gastrointestinal system. Some symptoms may include dizziness, vomiting, hemorrhagic gastritis, and coma.

T51.8- Toxic effect of other alcohols

Included in this subcategory is ethylene glycol, a common ingredient in antifreeze. Toxic effects of ethylene glycol include altered mental status, acidosis, renal insufficiency, and hypocalcemia.

> **Focus Point**
>
> Not all formulations of ethylene glycol are reported with code T51.8-. See also subcategories T52.3- Toxic effects of glycol, and T52.8- Toxic effect of other organic solvents.

T54.- Toxic effect of corrosive substances

A corrosive substance is one that damages tissue on contact. Chemical burns are often the most common outcome; however, other systemic effects may also occur depending on route of transmission and the specific substance involved.

> **Focus Point**
>
> When chemical burns from corrosive substances are documented, a code from the burn and corrosion categories (T20-T32) in chapter 19 should also be applied. These codes further identify the specific site of the corrosion and, in some cases, the extent of the tissue damage (e.g., first, second, or third degree).

T54.0- Toxic effects of phenol and phenol homologues

Phenol is a sweet smelling acid that can be found in sunscreens, hair coloring, and paint strippers. Introduction into the human body predominantly takes place through direct skin contact or the inhalation of phenol vapors. Inhalation injuries are less common but prolonged exposure may result in lung edema. Phenol is readily absorbed through the skin resulting in severe systemic effects including seizures, breathing difficulties, and changes in heart rhythm.

T54.3- Toxic effects of corrosive alkalis and alkali-like substances

Alkalis are found in various products such as oven cleaners, laundry detergent, ammonia, and alkaline batteries. Toxic effects may include swelling of the throat and trouble breathing, nausea and vomiting, vision loss, low blood pressure, and metabolic acidosis.

T58.- Toxic effect of carbon monoxide

Carbon monoxide is a colorless and odorless but very toxic gas. It is produced as a byproduct of any type of heater, cooking equipment, vehicle, or tool that is powered by carbon-based fuels such as gasoline, propane, methane, or diesel. The effects of carbon monoxide arise as a result of the carbon monoxide combining with the hemoglobin in the blood, essentially paralyzing the hemoglobin so that it is unable to release oxygen. Organs that require a high supply of oxygen to function properly, most importantly the heart and brain, are the most severely affected. Symptomology depends on the length of exposure: acute but limited exposure may result in confusion, flu-like symptoms, and the most common symptom, headache; acute but prolonged exposure can result in hypoxic injury, convulsions, loss of consciousness, and death. Patients may also experience delayed sequelae after acute carbon monoxide poisoning, primarily neurologically related. Manifestations may include amnesia, short-term memory loss, depressed mood, speech disturbances, and dementia. Chronic exposure may result in the loss of teeth, cognitive impairment, and depression. Diagnosing carbon monoxide poisoning can be difficult as most of the symptoms are vague and/or may be similar to what is observed in other conditions, such as a viral infection, and the patient may not even realize that they were exposed to carbon monoxide due to its colorless and odorless state.

T63.- Toxic effect of contact with venomous animals and plants

There are a wide variety of venomous plants and animals across the United States and the world. Some are more toxic than others, some must bite the victim for the venom to be effective, and some venom is deadly on contact.

T63.0- Toxic effect of snake venom

Each of the 48 contiguous states in the United States harbors at least one species of venomous snake. The pit vipers (copperhead, cottonmouth, and rattlesnakes) and coral snakes are two venomous families widely spread in the United States. Snake venoms are rated on a lethality index, with the Mojave rattlesnake having the highest index of any North American snake. Survival often depends on the time it takes to obtain medical help. Envenomation must be assessed whenever a patient presents at the medical center with a snake bite since not all bites from venomous snakes actually involve venom injection. Protocol calls for treating snakebites without envenomation as puncture wounds. If envenomation does occur, the patient presents a complex poisoning picture.

T63.01- Toxic effect of rattlesnake venom

Rattlesnakes inhabit both North and South America. Rattlesnake venom is hemotoxic, meaning it attacks the blood, in this case disrupting how the blood clots. It also can be very damaging to tissues. In addition to hemotoxic venom, several species of rattlesnake also produce neurotoxic venom. Neurotoxic venom acts faster than hemotoxic venom and attacks the nervous system causing paralysis, which can sometimes be severe. Typical symptoms related to rattlesnake venom include pain and swelling at the bite area, numbness, nausea, lightheadedness, and difficulty breathing. Rarely are rattlesnake bites fatal especially if treated quickly.

T63.02- Toxic effect of coral snake venom

Coral snakes have neurotoxic venom generally causing nerve conduction damage and CNS damage. Typically no associated pain or swelling is observed at the site of the bite and with symptoms in humans sometimes taking several hours to appear, the victim may think the bite is not serious. But coral snake venom is deadly and without antivenom can progress rapidly with muscle paralysis, slurred speech, and respiratory and cardiac failure.

T63.1- Toxic effect of venom of other reptiles

The only two lizard species in North America known to produce venom are the Gila monster and the beaded lizard.

T63.11- Toxic effect of venom of gila monster

The Gila monster is native to the southwestern United States and parts of Mexico. The administration of the toxin to the victim is by way of the lower jaw with the Gila monster biting and chewing on its victims in order to get the venom into the wound. The Gila monster venom is a very potent neurotoxin, very similar to the coral snake venom; however, it can only produce the toxin in small amounts. The effects of a Gila monster bite include severe pain, weakness, and low blood pressure, but rarely is the bite fatal to a healthy human.

T63.12- Toxic effect of venom of other venomous lizard

The beaded lizard is a venomous lizard primarily found in Mexico. Similar to its close relative the Gila monster, the beaded lizard bites its victim and makes a chewing motion with its jaws so that the venom in the lower jaw is released. Unlike the Gila monster, the beaded lizard's venom is a weak hemotoxin and not a neurotoxin. The most profound effect the venom has on its victim is the severe pain at and beyond the site of the bite that can last up to 24 hours. Edema, weakness, and low blood pressure may also be experienced.

T63.3- Toxic effect of venom of spider

There are numerous venomous spider species in the United States. Most bites require only local care, although in cases of severe envenomation, the victim must be hospitalized for supportive measures. Fatalities are few, with the greatest risk for children and the elderly. The major players in this subcategory include the black widow, tarantula, and brown recluse spiders and there are specific codes for each of these venomous spiders.

Other and Unspecified Effects of External Causes (T66-T78)

An external cause is a particular circumstance from which a medical condition may come to exist. This code block in particular captures circumstances related to the natural environment, such as weather or air pressure, that may adversely affect a patient. More intimate circumstances are also captured here, including abuse and neglect.

The categories in this code block are as follows:

T66	Radiation sickness, unspecified
T67	Effects of heat and light
T68	Hypothermia
T69	Other effects of reduced temperature
T70	Effects of air pressure and water pressure
T71	Asphyxiation
T73	Effects of other deprivation

T74	Adult and child abuse, neglect and other maltreatment, confirmed
T75	Other and unspecified effects of other external causes
T76	Adult and child abuse, neglect and other maltreatment, suspected
T78	Adverse effects, not elsewhere classified

T66.- Radiation sickness, unspecified

A substance emitting ionizing radiation is capable of creating radiation sickness. Acute radiation sickness is classified as cerebral, gastrointestinal, or hematopoietic. The cerebral syndrome is fatal within a few hours of exposure to a dose in an amount greater than 30 Gy. The gastrointestinal syndrome involves a dose of at least 4 Gy, with death occurring within two or three weeks. The hematopoietic syndrome is also fatal, with neutropenia the contributing cause of death due to lowered immune resistance. The dose is 2 to 10 Gy. Recovery from a radiation accident depends on the size of the dose, the rate at which the dose is received, and the distribution of the dose over the body. While a large dose all at once over the entire body is fatal, the same dose administered therapeutically to a small area for a brief period of time may be repeated over time without fear of fatality. Therapeutic doses may cause radiation sickness, involving nausea, vomiting, and diarrhea with malaise and tachycardia. These symptoms decline spontaneously, over time.

T67.- Effects of heat and light

Heat-related illnesses are classified here from the most deadly to the mildest. Heat stroke has many names and is a major medical emergency, causing death in 10 percent of its victims.

T67.0- Heatstroke and sunstroke

Heatstroke may be described as exertional or classic. Classic heatstroke victims typically are older, debilitated from chronic health problems, sedentary, and do not present with major systemic disorders. Exertional heatstroke, which may cause multiple systemic derangements, more often strikes younger, healthier individuals engaged in strenuous activity.

T67.1- Heat syncope

Heat syncope occurs from dehydration, lack of acclimatization to heat when undertaking exercise, and failure to undergo a cool-down period after exercise. Once the patient is prostrate, recovery is immediate.

T67.3- Heat exhaustion, anhydrotic

T67.4- Heat exhaustion due to salt depletion

T67.5- Heat exhaustion, unspecified

Heat exhaustion is excessive body core temperature in the range of 100.4° to 104.9° Fahrenheit and is primarily seen as a corollary to water depletion or salt depletion, although typically it is a combination of both. Thermoregulation in a human is primarily accomplished through sweating. When a person sweats, liquid is excreted from the sweat glands onto the skin, which then evaporates from the skin, cooling the body. When a person is unable to sweat (anhydrotic), the cooling process does not take place and body temperature rises. Some people develop or are born with anhydrosis while in others it may be secondary to inadequate hydration in extreme heat and/or during vigorous exercise. Salt is a regulatory substance in the body, controlling water levels in the cells. If the ratio of water to salt is too high, too much water enters the cells causing them to swell. Salt depletion often coincides with water depletion, as salt is also excreted in sweat, but it can also be seen in individuals who are adequately hydrated. When only the water is replenished in the body and not the salt, body functions can be compromised.

T67.7- Heat edema

Heat edema is the swelling of the extremities, typically the legs, in hot weather. Exercise and elevation of the affected parts lessens the swelling.

T68.- Hypothermia

Hypothermia is a very low body temperature that occurs when body heat is lost faster than it is produced. Accidental hypothermia can result from conduction, convection, or radiation. Examples of conduction hypothermia are wet clothing and skin freezing upon metal contact. Convection injuries are from wind chill. Radiated heat is the result of body heat lost from body areas unprotected to the elements. Shivering is a very common and important sign in hypothermia because a patient with hypothermia that does not exhibit shivering can be in the severe stages of the condition. Besides shivering, mild hypothermia symptoms can include dizziness, accelerated breathing, lack of coordination, and confusion. Patients in more severe stages of hypothermia may exhibit slurred speech, poor decision making, shallow breathing, and loss of consciousness.

T69.- Other effects of reduced temperature

Maintaining a constant body temperature is an important factor in homeostasis. The extremities, in particular, are the most susceptible to reduced temperatures due to their direct contact with cold surfaces and their higher surface area.

T69.1- Chilblains

This condition is an abnormal reaction to cold temperatures. The extremities, nose, and ears are the most likely places for it to occur and some people are more susceptible to it than others. The hallmark symptoms are very itchy and often painful red bumps on the skin. If severe, blisters and even ulcers can occur but permanent damage is rare. Certain conditions may predispose patients to acquiring this condition, such as diabetes, though in many cases an underlying cause cannot be found.

T70.- Effects of air pressure and water pressure

Pressure is an exertion of weight on an object. Air and water exert different amounts of pressure on the body depending on the particular place in the environment the body is located.

T70.0- Otitic barotrauma

Otitic barotrauma is damage to the ear as a result of rapid pressure changes. Symptoms include pain, hearing loss, rupture of the tympanic membrane, vertigo, and, perhaps the most dangerous manifestation, disorientation, since it can interfere with the ability to move to safety. This condition is mostly seen in aviators, divers, or tunnel workers.

T70.1- Sinus barotrauma

Sinus barotrauma, also called aerosinusitis, occurs when the air pressure in the sinuses is not equal to the pressure outside the body (ambient pressure). The air in the sinuses compresses or expands to try and compensate for the pressure difference, resulting in inflammation and swelling of the lining of the sinuses. Pain and nose bleeds (epistaxis) are the most common symptoms. Sinus barotrauma often coincides with congestion or obstruction in the sinuses, such as sinus infections, allergies, or upper respiratory infections as these obstructions can make it harder to equalize the air pressure in the sinuses.

Focus Point

Patients may develop sinus barotrauma when receiving hyperbaric oxygen therapy. Hyperbaric oxygen therapy is a treatment that involves sitting in a sealed chamber that delivers pure oxygen. The air pressure within the chamber is much higher and if the air-filled cavities in the body do not equalize with the increased air pressure, barotrauma can occur.

T70.2- Other and unspecified effects of high altitude

The effect high altitude has on the body comes down to how much oxygen is in the air; the higher the altitude, the thinner the atmosphere and the greater reduction in oxygen content. To compensate for the lower oxygen levels, the body has to produce a greater number of red blood cells to carry oxygen; however, the body needs time to make this adjustment or acclimatize. When given adequate time at various levels of ascent, most individuals can successfully adapt to the thinner atmosphere. The best and only way to reverse the effects of high altitude is to descend to where the atmospheric pressure is higher. Mild effects of altitude may include headache, dizziness, trouble sleeping, and loss of appetite. The moderate to severe stages can alter mental status or the degree of consciousness and cause ataxia and shortness of breath with cyanosis, all of which can be fatal if the patient is not removed to a lower altitude.

T70.3- Caisson disease [decompression sickness]

Caisson disease occurs as a result of improper decompression, most often related to underwater activities. When a diver ascends too fast nitrogen gas is released into tissues forming potentially lethal bubbles in the body and blood. The bubbles may affect the area where they were initially formed or they may travel throughout the body, resulting in widespread manifestations. In most cases, symptoms occur in the joints and are manifested by pain. Changes in vision, headaches, skin changes, confusion, and paralysis are less common but may also occur.

T71.- Asphyxiation

Asphyxiation occurs when the act of breathing cannot bring enough oxygen into the body. This category specifically classifies causes unrelated to a disease process, noxious gas, or foreign body. Mechanical or traumatic forces, such as being smothered or hanged, as well as environmental factors, such as confined spaces with limited oxygen supply, are just a few causes that are included here.

T75.- Other and unspecified effects of other external causes

Lightning, vibration, electric currents, and gravitation are just a few of the external forces captured in this category that can be harmful to the human body.

T75.0- Effects of lightning

Electrical energy from a lightning strike to a person may be direct, travel along the earth's surface, or travel along a conductive surface such as a metal fence or tree. The nerves, muscles, and blood vessels are excellent electrical conductors, so often when an individual is struck it typically results in cardiac arrest, respiratory arrest, vascular spasm, neurological damage, and autonomic instability.

T75.1- Unspecified effects of drowning and nonfatal submersion

This code is used only when immersion or drowning is documented but the specific effects of the drowning are not.

T75.4- Electrocution

The extent of an injury by electric shock is a function of the amount of voltage delivered, current type, resistance to the current, and the length of contact to the current. If the skin is thick and dry, it presents greater resistance to the current, resulting in extensive burns, though only slight damage to internal organs. Of the two types of current, direct current is the least deadly since it throws the victim, cutting short the exposure to the current. Alternating current is three times more dangerous than direct current since the chances of tetanic contractions multiply threefold. Tetany is likely to occur when the "let-go reflex" is depressed, increasing the victim's length of contact with the current.

T78.- Adverse effects, not elsewhere classified

This category reports various allergic reactions and effects on the body that are not related to medication or prescribed substances. An allergy is a faulty immune system reaction to what is normally a harmless substance. The immune system identifies the harmless substance as a foreign invader and responds by producing antibodies. Upon reexposure to the substance, the antibodies attack the substance releasing chemicals in the body that produce the various allergy-related symptoms. This is why first time exposure to an allergen often does not result in an allergic reaction, as the antibodies need time to buildup and respond to the substance before a reaction is triggered. Anaphylaxis is a very severe and widespread form of an allergic reaction often affecting more than one body system.

> **Focus Point**
>
> *Although clinically indistinguishable, the mechanisms behind anaphylactic and anaphylactoid reactions are different. An anaphylactic reaction is a true allergic reaction caused by the production of antibodies, usually immunoglobulin E (IgE), which are allergen binding antibodies. An anaphylactoid reaction is caused by the substance itself with no immunoglobulin involvement.*

T78.2- Anaphylactic shock, unspecified

Shock is a consequence of decreased blood flow and associated oxygen supply to critical tissues and organs. Hallmark signs include low blood pressure, dizziness, and confusion or loss of consciousness. Anaphylactic shock is a severe anaphylactic reaction that can occur instantly after exposure to the causative allergen and needs prompt medical attention.

T78.3- Angioneurotic edema

Angioneurotic edema is an allergic reaction that manifests itself by one or both of the following: angioedema or urticaria. Angioedema is swelling of the deep layers of skin, often localized to the hands, feet, and face. The swelling in these areas is often painful and can last several days. Mucous membranes of the mouth, throat, and lungs may also become swollen resulting in more serious complications including compromised breathing. Urticaria, or what is commonly referred to as hives, are itchy raised welts or bumps that appear on the surface of the skin. Hives are often less localized appearing across many sites of the body and usually resolve faster than the deeper swelling associated with angioedema.

T78.41- Arthus phenomenon

Arthus phenomenon, also known as Arthus reaction, refers to changes in the skin at the location of intradermal injections of an antigen. Repeated injections of the same antigen result in a proliferation of immune complexes in the walls of blood vessels. These immune complexes trigger an inflammatory response that over time can cause irritation and tissue damage. It is not an acute, immediately overwhelming condition but most often develops over hours or days depending on antibody levels. Localized Arthus reactions are distinguished by pain, swelling, hardening of the soft tissues, and excessive fluid accumulation.

Certain Early Complications of Trauma (T79)

Complications are consequential conditions that in this case occur after the initial trauma and are a direct result of the traumatic injury. Although the site of the complication may be close to the site of injury, it typically affects a completely different body system or body function.

The categories in this code block are as follows:

T79   Certain early complications of trauma

T79.- Certain early complications of trauma, not elsewhere classified

The complications identified in this category are those that occur almost immediately after the trauma occurs, confounding the overall management as well as the prognosis of the patient.

T79.Ø- Air embolism (traumatic)

An air embolism is a bubble of air that forms in or enters the vascular system and can occur in the veins or the arteries. The primary risk associated with an air embolism is the bubble getting lodged in a vessel and stopping the flow of blood to a particular body part. Signs and symptoms related to an air embolism largely depend on what part of the body is compromised, and can range from respiratory failure to stroke to mental changes. If lodged in the brain, heart, or lungs, the results can be deadly.

T79.1- Fat embolism (traumatic)

A fat embolism is the result of fat entering and getting lodged somewhere in the bloodstream. It is typically associated with fracture of one of the long bones, especially the femur.

T79.4- Traumatic shock

Traumatic shock sets in when the heart fails to deliver oxygenated blood and other nutrients to the body, usually because of a high rate of blood loss. The shock triggers other organ failure, with the kidney among the first affected. Blood volume must be restored as soon as possible to prevent traumatic shock and its sequelae.

T79.5- Traumatic anuria

Anuria is the inability to produce urine. Traumatic anuria occurs when there is damage to the kidneys and may occur as a result of direct trauma to the kidneys or as a secondary effect of trauma not related to kidney injury. Traumatic anuria is often seen with crush injuries, where the extremities and/or trunk are compressed under a heavy object. Swelling and neurological compromise to the muscles being compressed results in muscle degradation and the release of harmful byproducts into the bloodstream, which then travel to the kidney causing renal failure. If the renal failure is severe, the production of urine will cease.

T79.6- Traumatic ischemia of muscle

When the blood supply to a specific muscle is blocked or restricted, necessary oxygen cannot reach the muscle resulting in damage or loss of muscle tissue. Many injuries can compromise the blood flow to a muscle, including compression injuries and lacerations. Volkmann's ischemic contracture is a type of traumatic ischemia that can appear in the hand or the foot. In the hand, constriction of the radial artery produces the characteristic pronation and flexion. In the foot, a tibial fracture leading to an embolus or thrombus is more likely to be the causative agent.

T79.7- Traumatic subcutaneous emphysema

Traumatic subcutaneous emphysema is tissue rupture that allows gas bubbles to form beneath the skin, a result of a high-pressure injury.

T79.A- Traumatic compartment syndrome

A compartment is a collection of muscle, nerves, tendons, and blood vessels surrounded by a layer of fascia. There are several compartments in each of the legs and arms as well as other sites throughout the body. Compartment syndrome occurs when there is a buildup of pressure inside one of these compartments. The fascia layer was not made to stretch or expand, so any swelling or blood extravasation into the compartment has nowhere to go and instead puts undue pressure on the structures within the compartment. Pain is a common presenting symptom and is often more severe than what would typically be expected with the related injury.

Complications of Surgical and Medical Care, Not Elsewhere Classified (T80-T88)

Patients may experience idiosyncratic reactions to materials (biological or synthetic) used to support, replace, monitor, assist, or prevent certain functions in the body. Many categories in this code block not only capture the material or device causing the complication but also the specific reaction that resulted.

The categories in this code block are as follows:

T80	Complications following infusion, transfusion and therapeutic injection
T81	Complications of procedures, not elsewhere classified
T82	Complications of cardiac and vascular prosthetic devices, implants and grafts
T83	Complications of genitourinary prosthetic devices, implants and grafts
T84	Complications of internal orthopedic prosthetic devices, implants and grafts
T85	Complications of other internal prosthetic devices, implants and grafts
T86	Complications of transplanted organs and tissue
T87	Complications peculiar to reattachment and amputation
T88	Other complications of surgical and medical care, not elsewhere classified

T80.- Complications following infusion, transfusion and therapeutic injection

Infusions, transfusions, and injections are methods used to introduce a particular substance into the body. Infusions and transfusions typically involve direct placement of the substance into the bloodstream via a vein or artery while injections are typically used for placement of a substance into other various sites from subcutaneous tissue to the epidural space.

T80.21- Infection due to central venous catheter

Central line-associated infections affect an estimated 250,000 hospital patients per annum in the United States. These infections can prolong hospitalizations and increase resource use. The two major categories of

infections due to central venous catheters include local, site-confined infections and systemic infections, each with disparate clinical and epidemiological implications.

T80.211- Bloodstream infection due to central venous catheter

In central line associated bloodstream infections (CLABSI), the infectious organism is seeded into the patient's bloodstream. These infections are defined as laboratory-confirmed bloodstream infections (LCBI) that are not secondary to an infection meeting CDC/NHSN criteria at another body site.

T80.212- Local infection due to central venous catheter

Local catheter infections include exit or insertion site infections, port or reservoir infections, and subcutaneous tunnel infections. Signs of infection may include localized pain, purulence, erythema, or tenderness. Exit site infections occur at the catheter exit or insertion site. Port or reservoir infections are associated with implantable venous access devices and confined to the skin over the reservoir, within the reservoir, or in the subcutaneous pocket. A tunnel infection involves the artificially created path through which the catheter is tunneled underneath the skin. Signs of exit site inflammation or infection may or may not be present in tunnel infections.

T80.81- Extravasation of vesicant agent

When a substance is given intravenously, it is possible for the substance to pass from a blood vessel or organ into the surrounding tissue. Drugs are classified as non-vesicant or irritant, based on their potential to cause local tissue injury. Those drugs classified as vesicant drugs have the capability to induce blister formation and/or cause tissue destruction if extravasation should occur. Due to the nature of antineoplastic agents, many chemotherapy drugs are classified as vesicants; however, there are some other drugs given intravenously that also have vesicant potential. While health care providers have procedures in place to avoid extravasation complications of vesicant chemotherapeutic procedures, it does occasionally occur. Causal factors may include intravenous (IV) catheter or device displacement or IV device separation or breakage. Extravasation of vesicant chemotherapy can cause significant tissue damage. It can be one of the most injurious events occurring in a physician office or hospital outpatient setting. Symptoms can range in severity from localized pain and tissue inflammation to full-thickness necrosis and ulceration of skin and underlying structures. This is often dependent upon the infusion site, condition of the tissue, volume and concentration of vesicant, and efficacy of treatment.

T80.91- Hemolytic transfusion reaction, unspecified incompatibility

Hemolytic transfusion reactions (HTR) are potentially serious transfusion-related complications often attributed to preventable medical error, such as mislabeling or other mismatch. The severity of transfusion reaction depends on the type of transfusion and nature of incompatibility. Presentation may be acute, within the immediate posttransfusion period, or delayed, manifesting from 24 hours to 28 days (one month) following the transfusion.

T80.910- Acute hemolytic transfusion reaction, unspecified incompatibility

Acute hemolytic reactions are life-threatening medical emergencies that can rapidly result in acute renal failure, disseminated intravascular coagulation, multiorgan failure, and shock. Hemolysis is a process of accelerated abnormal red blood cell (RBC) destruction, clinically characterized by fever, chills, dyspnea, urticaria, and rigors. As a complication of transfusion, it is precipitated by an incompatibility between a blood donor and recipient; in this case, the specific incompatibility is not known.

Focus Point

Only acute hemolytic transfusion reaction due to an unspecified incompatibility is included in subcategory T80.910-. If the incompatibility is documented as ABO, or another specific non-ABO incompatibility, or Rh incompatibility, a more specific code from subcategories T80.3-, T80.4-, or T80.A- should be reported.

T81.- Complications of procedures, not elsewhere classified

Conditions classified here are complications that occurred during or as a result of a procedure. This category captures adverse postprocedural conditions from infections to fistula formation.

T81.1- Postprocedural shock

Postoperative shock is a physiological state that can occur as a result of certain complications following major surgery. The state of shock is characterized by a potentially fatal decreased perfusion and oxygenation of the bodily tissues, requiring immediate intervention to prevent cell death, irreversible organ damage, and multi-system organ failure. Initial signs and symptoms of shock include decreased urine output, mental status changes, hypotension, tachycardia, and cool, clammy skin. Certain postoperative complications, such as hypovolemia, heart failure, myocardial infarction, sepsis, and anaphylaxis, can provide the underlying mechanisms that precipitate a state of shock.

T81.10- Postprocedural shock unspecified

The unspecified code is reported when a more specific type of shock is not documented.

T81.11- Postprocedural cardiogenic shock

Cardiogenic shock is a consequence of heart damage that alters its ability to move the appropriate amount of blood to other organs and tissues in the body.

T81.12- Postprocedural septic shock

Septic shock is very low blood pressure that occurs in response to a severe, full body infection. Underlying postoperative infections that originate in the wound, lungs, or blood/vascular catheter can result in septic shock.

T81.19- Other postprocedural shock

Hypovolemic shock occurs as a result of a loss of blood and/or fluid volume. This results in a decreased circulating blood supply and the potential for multiorgan failure. The most common etiology of postprocedural hypovolemic shock is hemorrhaging.

T81.3- Disruption of wound, not elsewhere classified

Disruption (i.e., "dehiscence") of a wound describes the physical separation of a surgical or previously repaired traumatic wound. Wound separation can be a potentially fatal complication, increasing the patient's risk for wound or body cavity infection that could progress to systemic sepsis. Wound dehiscence can occur anywhere on the body where there is an operative or traumatic wound. Associated risks and treatment indications depend on the anatomic site and thickness (penetration) of the wound disruption. For example, a minor (partial thickness) disruption of a wound confined to the skin poses less risk than a major abdominopelvic wound separation. A minor skin wound may require little treatment, whereas a wound disruption that extends into deeper tissues of the body may require meticulous wound care or surgical repair. A full-thickness abdominal cavity wound dehiscence places the patient at considerable risk for intraabdominal contamination or evisceration, an emergent, life-threatening complication whereby the internal organs are exposed and vulnerable to displacement and infection.

T82.- Complications of cardiac and vascular prosthetic devices, implants and grafts

Complications identified in this category involve devices, implants, and grafts used to reinforce a function of the cardiovascular system.

T82.897- Other specified complication of cardiac prosthetic devices, implants and grafts

A complication of stent insertion procedures is the formation of scar tissue at the site of the stent. This is not considered to be a mechanical complication of the stent, as the stent is in working order. The scar tissue formation is the body's natural reaction to the introduction of the stent. There is not a specific code for scar tissue formation so it is reported here.

T83.- Complications of genitourinary prosthetic devices, implants and grafts

This category classifies complications of genitourinary devices. As the genitourinary system comprises the urinary and reproductive organs, some devices and their related complications may be specific to only female (such as an intrauterine contraceptive device) or male (such as a penile prosthesis) patients.

T83.0- Mechanical complication of urinary catheter

Urinary catheters can be placed in the bladder and kidney, as well as other sites along the urinary system, including artificially created openings such as an ileostomy or urostomy. For catheters that reside directly in the bladder, the urinary tube can be placed percutaneously through the abdominal wall, what is referred to as a cystostomy, or via the urethra, referred to as an indwelling urinary catheter. A nephrostomy drains the kidney via catheter that is inserted percutaneously into the back. Artificial openings (stoma) sometimes require the use of a catheter to drain the diverted substances out of the body. These include continent ileostomy, also called a Koch pouch or ileostomy reservoir, and continent urostomy, also called an ileal reservoir or urinary diversion. A urinary catheter, like any other device, can have mechanical problems that may necessitate clinical intervention. Complications included in this subcategory are mechanical breakdown, displacement (migration) of the device, leakage, obstruction protrusion, and perforation of urinary tissues.

T84.- Complications of internal orthopedic prosthetic devices, implants and grafts

This category captures complications related to partial or total replacement of joints, internal fixation devices, and other bone devices. Subcategories capture complications directly related to the device, implant, or graft and secondary effects such as infection.

T84.0- Mechanical complication of internal joint prosthesis

The codes in this subcategory help capture the different causes of mechanical complications related to total or partial joint replacement failure, most often the hip or knee.

T84.02- Dislocation of internal joint prosthesis

Dislocation of a joint replacement is most common with hip replacement procedures among the elderly, older than age 70, who have certain types of arthritic disease, although displacement can occur at any age and with any type of prosthetic joint. Factors such as surgical technique, mechanical device, and health and mobility of the patient play a part in potential subluxation of a prosthetic joint.

T84.03- Mechanical loosening of internal prosthetic joint

Mechanical loosening of a prosthetic joint is the most common cause of long-term failure in hip and knee replacements. Loosening may occur regardless of the fixation material employed.

T84.06- Wear of articular bearing surface of internal prosthetic joint

Wear of the articular bearing surface occurs over time, and is largely dependent on the age and activity level of the patient. One threat associated with wear on the prosthetic surface is the creation of "dust" or debris. This dust can cause a biological response in the natural bone ensuing in the breakdown of the host bone and consequential bone resorption. This may occur in more active patients with total hip replacement, especially those with polyethylene plastics in the implant.

T85.- Complications of other internal prosthetic devices, implants and grafts

This category captures complications related to devices placed in the nervous system, gastrointestinal system, breast, and eye, as well as complications related to other devices such as insulin pumps, sutures, and dialysis catheters.

T85.1- Mechanical complication of implanted electronic stimulator of nervous system

Electrical stimulation can relieve the symptoms of many nervous system conditions—from Parkinson's to gastroparesis. The system consists of two major components: one or more electrodes (leads) and a generator. One end of each electrode is inserted into the brain, a nerve, or a muscle and the other end is connected to a generator that relays an electrical impulse. The generator, a battery-powered device, is placed just under the skin of the chest or lower abdomen. The patient or provider uses a handheld remote to adjust, turn off, or turn on the stimulation.

Brain neurostimulators focus on stimulating areas of the brain that affect movement. Stiffness, tremor, difficulty walking, and slowness of movement describe some of the symptoms treated. Spinal cord and peripheral nerve neurostimulators are used primarily to treat chronic pain. Gastric neurostimulators relieve symptoms related to gastroparesis, specifically nausea and vomiting. Vagal nerve neurostimulators are used principally to reduce seizure frequency in epileptic patients. Complication codes in this subcategory differentiate between those related to the electrode and the generator and include mechanical breakdown, displacement (migration), obstruction, perforation, and protrusion.

T85.613- Breakdown (mechanical) of artificial skin graft and decellularized allodermis

Advances in the treatment of burns and other severe conditions affecting the skin have provided new technologies that are able to permanently regenerate or replace skin layers. These include artificial skin, decellularized allodermis, and cultured epithelial cells. As with any type of graft, complications can occur. Breakdown or mechanical complications occur when the skin substitute does not assimilate with the natural skin around it. This may be due to poor wound bed preparation, fluid buildup between the wound and the graft, infection, and immune system rejection.

T85.623- Displacement of artificial skin graft and decellularized allodermis

Advances in the treatment of burns and other severe conditions affecting the skin have provided new technologies that are able to permanently regenerate or replace skin layers, including artificial skin, decellularized allodermis, and cultured epithelial cells. Displacement of skin substitutes commonly occurs in areas of flexion or extension where repeated movement can disrupt any adherence between the artificial skin and the wound bed.

T85.730- Infection and inflammatory reaction due to ventricular intracranial (communicating) shunt

Ventricular intracranial shunts are typically used to treat hydrocephalus. Shunt infection is one of the most common complications, generally occurring during the first month after implantation. The most common bacterial agents involved are *Staphylococcus epidermidis* and *Staphylococcus aureus*, commonly found on the skin and in hair follicles and sweat glands. Early signs of infection include prolonged postoperative fever, which may progress to sepsis, meningitis, or peritonitis (in cases with ventriculoperitoneal shunts).

T85.731- Infection and inflammatory reaction due to implanted electronic neurostimulator of brain, electrode (lead)

T85.732- Infection and inflammatory reaction due to implanted electronic neurostimulator of peripheral nerve, electrode (lead)

T85.733- Infection and inflammatory reaction due to implanted electronic neurostimulator of spinal cord, electrode (lead)

Neurostimulation is used to treat conditions such as spinal cord injuries, epilepsy, pain, incontinence, tremor disorders, and anxiety. It functions by sending electrical impulses to specific parts of the nervous system to adjust the signals between the brain and affected body area. The electrodes (or leads) are electric terminals specialized for a particular electrochemical reaction that acts as a medium between a body surface and another instrument. An electrode may carry a current of electrical activity from the body to a recording instrument or it may conduct current into the body from a generator source. Because these devices are implanted within the body, complications such as infection and inflammation may occur. This subcategory addresses such complications when the electrode is placed within the brain, a peripheral nerve, or spinal cord.

T85.734- Infection and inflammatory reaction due to implanted electronic neurostimulator, generator

The implantable neurostimulator generator is the device that holds the battery and delivers the electrical current through the electrodes to the desired body location. The generator is placed within various locations as close to the targeted area as practical such as scapula area, abdomen, chest, or back, where a pocket under the skin and subcutaneous tissue is formed to house the generator. As with implantable electrodes, sometimes the pocket or incision becomes infected or inflamed and requires removal and/or reinsertion of the generator.

T85.735- Infection and inflammatory reaction due to cranial or spinal infusion catheter

Cranial or spinal infusion catheters may be inserted to deliver medications and/or to reroute cerebral spinal fluid (CSF). Given that these catheters are placed inside the body, it stands to reason that complications such as infection or inflammation may occur; however, typically the complications result in catheter displacement. Treatment of the complication is determined based on the condition or cause and may include removal and reinsertion of the catheter as well as antibiotic delivery.

Chapter 19. Injury and Poisoning (SØØ-T88)

T86.- Complications of transplanted organs and tissue

Organs commonly transplanted include the kidneys, heart, lungs, and liver. Tissue that is commonly transplanted or grafted may include bone, skin, stem cells, and bone marrow.

Focus Point

Graft-versus-host disease (GVHD) is a complication related to allogeneic organ or tissue, meaning transplanted from another human. The immune cells in the donor tissue identify the cells in the host as foreign and attack the host cells. This is most commonly seen in stem cell or bone marrow transplants. When a complication of a transplanted organ is identified as GVHD, a code from this category should be applied first followed by the appropriate code from subcategory D89.81- in Chapter 3 Diseases of the Blood and Blood-forming Organs.

T86.5 Complications of stem cell transplant

Stem cell transplants pose the potential for complications, including anemia, stem cell (graft) failure, and organ damage. The most common complications resulting from autologous (self) stem cell transplant include bleeding, anemia, infection, interstitial pneumonitis, liver damage, damage to mucosal tissues particularly the mouth and esophagus, cataracts, infertility, and secondary neoplasms. The most common complications resulting from allogeneic (donor) stem cell transplant include graft-versus-host disease (GVHD) and graft rejection where the host rejects the donor cells.

T88.- Other complications of surgical and medical care, not elsewhere classified

This category provides codes that can help characterize complications related to procedures or other medical care that does not fit into previous categories. Codes included here may capture specific complications, such as those related to anesthesia, or provide a means of capturing complications that are not clearly defined in the documentation.

T88.3- Malignant hyperthermia due to anesthesia

Malignant hyperthermia is actually a rare inherited disorder in which a patient is genetically predisposed to having an adverse reaction when a specific environmental trigger, in this case an anesthetic medication, is introduced. As the name implies, a very high body temperature is a hallmark symptom along with muscle rigidity, acidosis, and rapid heart rate. If not treated promptly it can result in multiorgan failure and even death.

T88.52- Failed moderate sedation during procedure

Many minor procedures do not require full general anesthesia and can be satisfactorily managed with moderate (conscious) sedation. However, in some situations, inadequate sedation can occur, resulting in unsafe conditions for the patient. A patient may exhibit an adverse or idiosyncratic response to the sedation, become under- or oversedated, be unable to maintain a patent airway, or experience hemodynamic compromise. These situations may extend beyond the capabilities of the provider administering the sedation. This often requires urgent intervention, such as enlisting the services of an anesthesiologist or other expert to ensure a safe outcome for the patient by administering deep sedation or anesthesia. Patients may have a history of such situations during previous procedures that necessitate planned intervention during subsequent procedures to prevent a similar adverse sedation event.

T88.53- Unintended awareness under general anesthesia during procedure

The purpose of general anesthesia is to induce a loss of consciousness. When placed under general anesthesia, the patient should not respond to or perceive any external stimuli. Unintended awareness during general anesthesia involves sensory perceptions, including auditory, visual, and tactile awareness, during a procedure for which the patient should perceive nothing. The frequency of patients with this awareness is low, one or two adult patients out of 1,000, and not all recollections are negative. However negative recall, such as feeling pain, awareness of surroundings, and feeling paralyzed but unable to communicate, can lead to late psychological symptoms of post-traumatic stress disorder (PTSD). Underlying causes include inadequate primary anesthetic, drug error, or unknown cause. There appears to be a higher incidence of anesthesia awareness during cardiac surgery, major trauma surgery, or obstetrical surgery. Patients with a prior history of anesthesia awareness are also at high risk of developing the condition again. Many surgical facilities have developed policies that address the prevention and management of anesthesia awareness. The latest research in the area is focused on monitoring activities that measure brain activity, not merely physiological responses.

T88.6- Anaphylactic reaction due to adverse effect of correct drug or medicament properly administered

The key to understanding an allergy is to recognize that a previously sensitized individual has been reexposed to a substance. The initial exposure instigated an immune response in the body that later causes the body to react to the substance when reintroduced. Antibiotics, in particular those in the penicillin group, are the most common drugs associated with anaphylactic reaction.

Chapter 20: External Causes of Morbidity (VØØ-Y99)

This chapter classifies external causes of injury and other adverse effects. Common external causes include automobile accidents, falls, bites, fire (flames), smoke, and drowning.

Most often external cause codes are used in conjunction with codes from Chapter 19 Injury, Poisoning, and Certain other Consequences of External Causes; however, these codes can be used with codes from any chapter to provide additional information on conditions that may be a consequence of an external cause.

External cause codes are the means by which data is reported and collected on how an injury occurred (mechanism), what the injured person was doing when the injury occurred (activity), where the injury occurred (place of occurrence), and the status of the person at the time the injury occurred, such as work (e.g., civilian, military, volunteer, or other), leisure, or other non-work. In some cases, intent is also captured by the external cause code. For example, a handgun injury may be accidental, due to an assault, or self-inflicted with the intent of causing self-harm.

About one-third of all emergency department visits are due to injuries. Collecting data related to the external cause of these injuries is important to understanding the circumstances surrounding an injury and in developing policies and procedures to help prevent future injuries. This data may be used by the health care facility, public health departments, employers, and third-party payers to address health care delivery needs, develop public health policy and education resources, address workplace injury risks, and develop strategies to reduce the risk of injury.

External cause codes are organized into several large sections that contain multiple code blocks for related types of external causes, such as transport accidents (VØØ-V99) and other external causes of accidental injury (WØØ-X58). Most of these large sections contain multiple related code blocks.

Because most codes for external causes are self-explanatory, only key points related to the most common external causes of injury are discussed in this chapter.

Transport Accidents (VØØ-V99)

Motor vehicle accidents classified in this section represent the third most common cause of emergency department visits due to injury.

The categories in this code block are as follows:

VØØ-VØ9	Pedestrian injured in transport accident
V1Ø-V19	Pedal cycle rider injured in transport accident
V2Ø-V29	Motorcycle rider injured in transport accident
V3Ø-V39	Occupant of three-wheeled motor vehicle injured in transport accident
V4Ø-V49	Car occupant injured in transport accident
V5Ø-V59	Occupant of pick-up truck or van injured in transport accident
V6Ø-V69	Occupant of heavy transport vehicle injured in transport accident
V7Ø-V79	Bus occupant injured in transport accident
V8Ø-V89	Other land transport accidents
V9Ø-V94	Water transport accidents
V95-V97	Air and space transport accidents
V98-V99	Other and unspecified transport accidents

Other External Causes of Accidental Injury (WØØ-X58)

Falls represent the most common external cause of injury resulting in emergency department visits. Falls (WØØ-W19) may occur on the same level or from one level to another. Falls on the same level may result from slipping, tripping, stumbling, or just losing one's balance. Falls from one level to another include a fall from a bed, playground equipment, sidewalk curb, tree, or cliff. Jumping or diving into water with a resulting injury is also included in this code block.

The second most common external cause of injury resulting in emergency department visits is accidental striking against or being struck by an inanimate object (W20-W22) or animate object (W50-W64). External cause of injury codes in these categories include being accidentally struck by a ball, bat, racquet, hockey stick or puck, or being accidentally run into or struck by a person or animal.

The categories in this code block are as follows:

WØØ-W19	Slipping, tripping, stumbling and falls
W2Ø-W49	Exposure to inanimate mechanical forces

W50-W64 Exposure to animate mechanical forces

W65-W74 Accidental non-transport drowning and submersion

W85-W99 Exposure to electric current, radiation and extreme ambient air temperature and pressure

X00-X08 Exposure to smoke, fire and flames

X10-X19 Contact with heat and hot substances

X30-X39 Exposure to forces of nature

X52-X58 Accidental exposure to other specified factors

Other External Causes (X71-Y38)

External causes of injuries by various means that are intentionally self-inflicted (self-harm) or intentionally caused by another person (assault) are included in code blocks in this section. External causes of injuries by various means for which the intent is specifically documented as undetermined are also classified here.

External causes of injuries that result from an encounter with a law enforcement officer, those incurred during war or military operations, and those that result from an act of terrorism are also included as separate code blocks.

The categories in this code block are as follows:

X71-X83 Intentional self-harm

X92-Y09 Assault

Y21-Y33 Event of undetermined intent

Y35-Y38 Legal intervention, operations of war, military operations, and terrorism

Complications of Medical and Surgical Care (Y62-Y84)

External causes of injuries or other conditions such as adverse reactions resulting from medical or surgical care are included here.

The categories in this code block are as follows:

Y62-Y69 Misadventures to patients during surgical and medical care

Y70-Y82 Medical devices associated with adverse incidents in diagnostic and therapeutic use

Y83-Y84 Surgical and other medical procedures as the cause of abnormal reaction of the patient, or of later complication, without mention of misadventure at the time of the procedure

Supplementary Factors Related to Causes of Morbidity Classified Elsewhere (Y90-Y99)

External cause codes that identify place of occurrence, activity, and external cause status are included in the last code block. The only other codes for supplementary factors related to external cause of injury or other conditions that are included in this code block are those that identify blood alcohol level.

Chapter 21: Factors Influencing Health Status and Contact With Health Services (Z00-Z99)

The purpose of the "Z" codes is not to identify a specific disease process or injury; instead, these codes are more informational. They identify the reason for an encounter and circumstances related to the patient that may impact current disease processes and help depict a more complete picture of the patient's overall health.

As a first listed code, Z codes can capture and justify the reason for a visit to a health care entity. Well child visits, cancer screening, aftercare, and admissions solely for chemotherapy are just a few examples where the Z code can be used to identify the reason for the encounter.

As secondary codes, Z codes identify circumstances related to the patient that could influence health care needs during the current admission or in the future. Family history codes, personal history codes, economic circumstances, blood type, and do not resuscitate status are just a few Z codes that help validate certain treatment options and narrate why a patient was or will be managed a certain way.

The chapter is broken down into the following code blocks:

Z00-Z13	Persons encountering health services for examinations
Z14-Z15	Genetic carrier and genetic susceptibility to disease
Z16	Resistance to antimicrobial drugs
Z17	Estrogen receptor status
Z18	Retained foreign body fragments
Z19	Hormone sensitivity malignancy status
Z20-Z29	Persons with potential health hazards related to communicable diseases
Z30-Z39	Persons encountering health services in circumstances related to reproduction
Z40-Z53	Encounters for other specific health care
Z55-Z65	Persons with potential health hazards related to socioeconomic and psychosocial circumstances
Z66	Do not resuscitate status
Z67	Blood type
Z68	Body mass index (BMI)
Z69-Z76	Persons encountering health services in other circumstances
Z77-Z99	Persons with potential health hazards related to family and personal history and certain conditions influencing health status

Persons Encountering Health Services for Examinations (Z00-Z13)

Codes found in this code block are used to capture general health examinations, follow-up studies, and screenings.

Examinations are used by medical professionals to monitor patients that are currently asymptomatic for precursors to disease, to evaluate the growth and development of children and adolescents, and for administrative purposes for things like sports or military participation.

Follow-up examinations are used to monitor previous disease processes that no longer require treatment. This ensures that the treatment was successful and that the disease itself or a sequela of the disease has not returned.

Screenings are performed as a preemptive strike in the detection of diseases. When caught early, the disease can be managed with typically less intensive treatments and result in better outcomes for the patient. Breast cancer and colon cancer are two conditions that are routinely screened.

The categories in this code block are as follows:

Z00	Encounter for general examination without complaint, suspected or reported diagnosis
Z01	Encounter for other special examination without complaint, suspected or reported diagnosis
Z02	Encounter for administrative examination
Z03	Encounter for medical observation for suspected diseases and conditions ruled out

Z04   Encounter for examination and observation for other reasons

Z05   Encounter for observation and evaluation of newborn for suspected diseases and conditions ruled out

Z08   Encounter for follow-up examination after completed treatment for malignant neoplasm

Z09   Encounter for follow-up examination after completed treatment for conditions other than malignant neoplasm

Z11   Encounter for screening for infectious and parasitic diseases

Z12   Encounter for screening for malignant neoplasms

Z13   Encounter for screening for other diseases and disorders

Z00.- Encounter for general examination without complaint, suspected or reported diagnosis

This category captures routine physicals, well-child visits, and other general health examinations in patients who are currently not symptomatic, even if the exam identifies abnormal findings. A typical general examination covers the history of the patient's health status and lifestyle including family history; vital signs, such as temperature, heart rate, and blood pressure; heart and lung exam to identify abnormal lung sounds or heartbeats; and then a review of the body systems such as ears, eyes, skin, abdomen, extremities, and nervous system. Laboratory tests, such as a complete blood count or chemistry panel, may also be performed.

Z00.1- Encounter for newborn, infant and child health examinations

From the time a child is born to when they become an adolescent their bodies and minds go through tremendous growth and development. In order to ensure that milestones are being met, the recommendation is that the child is seen roughly two to three days or one to two weeks after birth, at two-month intervals until 6 months old, three-month intervals until 2 years old, and at least yearly after the 2-year mark.

Z00.2 Encounter for examination for period of rapid growth in childhood

A period of rapid growth may be a normal variation in childhood growth patterns and not cause for concern or it may be indicative of a disease process that requires additional workup. Rapid growth or growth

acceleration in childhood can be an indicator of a pituitary gland tumor, a genetic condition such as Marfan's syndrome, or other conditions such as precocious puberty.

Z01.- Encounter for other special examination without complaint, suspected or reported diagnosis

During a general examination, most or all of the body systems may be checked to look at the overall health of the patient. In some cases, only a specific body system needs to be investigated, per the request of the patient or the practitioner. Codes in this category are used to capture these encounters. Exams identified here range from routine gynecological exams to dental, vision, or hearing exams to blood typing and allergy testing. Similar to general examinations, these routine exams may turn up abnormal findings, which can be coded in addition to the encounter code.

Z01.8- Encounter for other specified special examinations

Special examinations may include preoperative exams, allergy testing, blood typing, and intelligence testing that is not elsewhere classified.

Z01.81- Encounter for preprocedural examinations

Preprocedural clearance exams are performed prior to surgery or other procedures to ensure the patient is healthy enough to undergo the procedure and is able to tolerate anesthesia. The patient may require a focused examination of the cardiovascular, respiratory, or immune system or laboratory evaluation of blood and/or urine.

Z01.84 Encounter for antibody response examination

Antibody response examinations ensure that persons in need of vaccines receive them and that adequately vaccinated patients are not over immunized. In lieu of adequate vaccination documentation, prevaccination serologic testing assists in determining immunity and eliminating unnecessary vaccinations. Similarly, serologic susceptibility testing may assist in reducing the cost of vaccinating adult populations that have an expected high prevalence of disease. Postvaccination testing for antibody response assists in determining the appropriate postexposure prophylaxis, since medical management of exposures often depends on the patient's immune status.

Z02.- Encounter for administrative examination

Certain administrative entities, such as schools, employers, prisons, insurance programs, and the armed forces, require a health examination prior to the participation or acceptance of an individual. Exams performed for these purposes are captured in this category. Also included here are exams that determine the disability level of a patient, testing to determine paternity, and testing for blood-alcohol or drug levels, as well as exams needed for adoption services.

Z03.- Encounter for medical observation for suspected diseases and conditions ruled out

The codes in this category are used when a patient presents with a suspected medical condition that upon further investigation is determined to not be present, or is ruled out, and that requires no further treatment or follow-up. This category may be used for administrative or legal observations as well.

Z03.7- Encounter for suspected maternal and fetal conditions ruled out

Pregnant patients may be referred to maternal-fetal specialists for further detailed diagnostic tests when an initial prenatal screening test indicates a possible abnormality. However, in many cases the detailed exam does not show an abnormality and the suspected condition is ruled out. Codes in this subcategory assist in supporting the medical necessity of tests and encounters for the purpose of ruling out suspected conditions that, if present, would require a higher level of care.

Z05.- Encounter for observation and evaluation of newborn for suspected diseases and conditions ruled out

The codes in this category are assigned when a newborn is assessed for a suspected condition that is subsequently ruled out. The codes are differentiated by the body system affected or type of condition being evaluated and include the following:

- Cardiac condition

- Infectious condition

- Neurological condition

- Respiratory condition

- Genetic condition

- Metabolic condition

- Immunologic condition

- Gastrointestinal condition

- Genitourinary condition

- Skin and subcutaneous tissue condition

- Musculoskeletal condition

- Connective tissue condition

- Other specified suspected condition

- Unspecified suspected condition

Z08 Encounter for follow-up examination after completed treatment for malignant neoplasm

Z09 Encounter for follow-up examination after completed treatment for conditions other than malignant neoplasm

Follow-up examinations are used to check on a patient following the completion of treatment to verify that the treatment was successful and the disease has not returned. This is especially important for malignancies as their invasive nature can sometimes make it hard to ensure total and complete eradication of the disease.

Z11.- Encounter for screening for infectious and parasitic diseases

An infectious disease is caused by a microorganism that can be transmitted with or without contact. A parasite is an organism that attacks a host but does not contribute to the survival of that host. In some instances, the infectious or parasitic agent may lay dormant within the host, without provoking adverse symptomology. Screening allows the detection of such pathogens while the patient is asymptomatic so that treatment can be started if tests are positive and to limit the spread of the pathogen.

Z11.1 Encounter for screening for respiratory tuberculosis

Tuberculosis (TB) is a bacterial infection, caused by *Mycobacterium tuberculosis*, that usually attacks the lungs, but which may also affect other organs. TB is transmitted by inhaling air droplets exhaled by an infected person or, sometimes, the infection is absorbed by the skin. Asymptomatic individuals who have been exposed to respiratory tuberculosis require screening to ensure that they have not contracted the disease and to allow prompt treatment and prevent further spread if they are infected.

Z12.- Encounter for screening for malignant neoplasms

Age, genetic predisposition, sex, and other factors can predispose a patient to certain types of cancers. As such, certain procedures such as mammograms and colonoscopies are recommended at regular intervals depending on the age and history of the patient. When cancer is detected early, treatment can be started sooner, reducing the chances of the cancer spreading and typically with less adverse effects on the patient.

Z13.- Encounter for screening for other diseases and disorders

Special investigations and screening codes should be reported for examination of a specific body system or screening for a specific disease so that potentially early and adequate treatment can be provided for those who test positive.

Z13.0   Encounter for screening for diseases of the blood and blood-forming organs and certain disorders involving the immune mechanism

Screening for anemia, as well as other diseases of the blood and blood-forming organs and immune mechanism, is included here. An anemia screening may be for a nutritional anemia such as iron deficiency anemia or a hereditary type of anemia such as sickle cell anemia. The term anemia refers to a lower than normal erythrocyte count or level of hemoglobin in the circulating blood. Iron deficiency anemia is almost always caused by blood loss in adults. Sickle-cell anemia is a severe, chronic, and incurable form of anemia occurring in patients who inherit hemoglobin S genes from both parents. Less severe variations of the disease occur when the patient inherits one hemoglobin S gene from one parent and one hemoglobin C, D, or E gene from the other.

Z13.2-   Encounter for screening for nutritional, metabolic and other endocrine disorders

Screening may be performed for malnutrition, such as protein-calorie malnutrition, or for more specific nutritional deficiencies such as a specific vitamin or minerals deficiency. Metabolic disorders occur when the body is not able to break down or utilize certain nutrients. This includes problems with amino-acid transport, carbohydrate transport, and lipoid metabolism. Endocrine disorders involve over- or under-secretion of hormones.

Z13.220   Encounter for screening for lipoid disorders

Lipoid disorders involve abnormal levels of lipoproteins and triglycerides in the blood that put a person at risk for vascular disease, including heart attack and stroke. There are three types of lipoproteins that carry cholesterol through the bloodstream, including high-density lipoproteins (HDL), also known as good cholesterol; low-density lipoproteins (LDL), also known as bad cholesterol; and very low-density lipoproteins (VLDL), also known as very bad cholesterol. Triglycerides are a type of fat present in the blood.

Z13.228   Encounter for screening for other metabolic disorders

Screening for metabolic disorders, including inborn (inherited) metabolic disorders such as cystic fibrosis, galactosemia, and phenylketonuria, is included here. Cystic fibrosis is caused by a defect in the manufacture of cystic fibrosis transmembrane conductance regulator (CFTR). Normally, CFTR forms a channel through which chloride ions transverse the cells lining in the lungs, pancreas, sweat glands, and small intestine. Cystic fibrosis causes thick, sticky mucus that blocks the airway and can interfere with enzyme production in the pancreas. Galactosemia is a congenital condition marked by the body's inability to break down galactose. This is due to an absence of enzymes needed to convert galactose to glucose. Phenylketonuria (PKU) is an inherited error of metabolism affecting phenylalanine. This condition is a failure to break down amino acids found in many foods. This can cause intellectual disabilities and hyperphenylalaninemia.

Z13.29   Encounter for screening for other suspected endocrine disorder

Screening for endocrine disorders may be performed to test for thyroid disease or any other disorder of the endocrine glands with the exception of screening for diabetes mellitus, which has a more specific code.

Z13.4   Encounter for screening for certain developmental disorders in childhood

Developmental disorders may involve intellectual or developmental delays or disabilities. Intellectual disabilities are defined as general intellectual functioning at least two standard deviations below the norm as measured in a standardized intelligence test. It must be accompanied by significant limitation in communication, self-care, home living, interpersonal skills, self-direction, work, leisure, health, or safety. This onset must occur before adulthood. A developmental delay is the failure to obtain developmental milestones that are related to a specific age. This may include sitting, crawling, and walking.

Z13.5   Encounter for screening for eye and ear disorders

Screening of the eye may be performed for cataracts, glaucoma, or other congenital or acquired eye disease. Glaucoma is an increase in intraocular pressure due to an abnormal aqueous humor outflow from the anterior chamber or, rarely, from an above normal rate of aqueous humor production by the ciliary body. If untreated, glaucoma ultimately leads to optic nerve damage and loss of vision. Also included in the code are screening procedures for diseases of the ear.

Z13.6   Encounter for screening for cardiovascular disorders

Screening for cardiovascular disorders includes testing for hypertension, myocardial infarction, other forms of ischemic heart disease, and other vascular conditions. Hypertension is a condition in which the diastolic pressure exceeds 100 mm Hg in persons 60 years of age and older or 90 mm Hg in persons younger than 60 years of age. Hypertension is generally asymptomatic until complications develop, which is why routine screening is needed. Ischemic heart disease is an inadequate flow of blood through the coronary arteries to the tissue of the heart. The predominant etiology of the ischemia is arteriosclerosis. Partially obstructed coronary artery blood flow can manifest in angina pectoris; complete obstruction results in an infarction of the myocardium.

Z13.820 Encounter for screening for osteoporosis

Screening for osteoporosis is performed to determine bone density and to assess the risk for nontraumatic fracture resulting from osteoporosis, which is the loss of bone density. Osteoporosis is generalized bone disease characterized by decreased osteoblastic formation of matrix combined with increased osteoclastic resorption of bone, resulting in a marked decrease in bone mass.

Z13.828 Encounter for screening for other musculoskeletal disorder

Screening for rheumatoid arthritis is included here. Rheumatoid arthritis is a chronic, systemic inflammatory disease of unknown etiology, characterized by a variable but prolonged course with swelling. In early stages, the disease attacks the joints of the hands and feet. As the disease progresses, more joints become involved leading to progressive deformities, which may develop rapidly and cause permanent disability.

Z13.850 Encounter for screening for traumatic brain injury

Screening examinations are often indicated to assess and diagnose mental status changes or other symptoms that might be present following trauma to the head. Depending on the nature and scope of the testing, Traumatic brain injury (TBI) screening exams assist in triaging patients into evaluation, establishing diagnoses and treatment plans, and obtaining appropriate education and clinical resources.

Genetic Carrier and Genetic Susceptibility to Disease (Z14-Z15)

Genes are information carriers passed from a parent to a child. The information or trait a particular gene displays is dependent on the interaction between and the health of the genes passed from the mother and the father, as all genes are paired. If the specific gene from the mother or father has mutated, is missing, or incomplete, it can result in what is called an inherited disease.

The categories in this code block are as follows:

Z14	Genetic carrier
Z15	Genetic susceptibility to disease

Z14.- Genetic carrier

Genetic carriers are individuals who have a gene mutation associated with a certain disease. Although a carrier of a mutated gene has the ability to pass on that gene, carriers typically do not have the disease nor are they at risk for developing the disease. In order for the offspring of the carrier to harbor symptoms of the mutated gene, both parents must be carriers of and pass on the same type of genetic abnormality. If only one parent passes on the abnormal gene, the child will also be a carrier.

Z14.0- Hemophilia A carrier

Hemophilia A is abnormal coagulation characterized by subcutaneous and intramuscular hemorrhage and caused by a gene mutation on chromosome X. Unlike most conditions for which a person is a carrier, some female carriers of hemophilia A are symptomatic for impaired blood coagulation (clotting) while others may exhibit no symptoms. This is a particular risk during pregnancy and childbirth when hemorrhaging can occur due to gene mutation.

Z14.1 Cystic fibrosis carrier

A cystic fibrosis carrier has an abnormal copy of the gene that regulates the secretion of mucus. Cystic fibrosis is caused by a defect in the manufacture of cystic fibrosis transmembrane conductance regulator (CFTR). Normally, CFTR forms a channel through which chloride ions transverse the cell's lining in the lungs, pancreas, sweat glands, and small intestine. Cystic fibrosis causes thick, sticky mucus that blocks the airway and can interfere with enzyme production in the pancreas.

Z15.- Genetic susceptibility to disease

Genetic susceptibility is a red flag to providers, identifying a person who is at a higher risk and/or has a greater chance of getting a disease or malignant growth because of their inborn predisposition. Genetic susceptibility to a specific disease or malignancy may alter screening protocol or it may prompt the person to take prophylactic measures in an effort to reduce the risk of acquiring the disease or malignancy. For example, women with a genetic predisposition to breast or ovarian cancer may elect to have their breasts or ovaries removed prophylactically in the hope that taking such a step will prevent the disease from occurring.

Resistance to Antimicrobial Drugs (Z16)

Antimicrobial drugs are used to kill or prevent the spread of pathogens, such as bacteria, parasites, viruses, and fungi. In order for their survival, all pathogens, but bacteria in particular, have learned to adapt, resisting the effects of commonly used drugs that once were effective in destroying them.

The categories in this code block are as follows:

Z16	Resistance to antimicrobial drugs

Z16.- Resistance to antimicrobial drugs

The increasing prevalence of drug-resistant organisms is the result of overuse or underuse of antimicrobial drugs, from patients not completing treatment as prescribed, and from person-to-person spread of the resistant organisms. Because of this, many common infections that were once effectively treated with antimicrobials have now become untreatable. New drugs have been developed to treat drug-resistant diseases but, in general, these drugs are much more expensive than their predecessors, which may limit their use.

Estrogen Receptor Status (Z17)

In breast cancer, the receptor status of the cancer cells for the hormone estrogen is a feature that is used to help determine treatment and evaluate prognosis.

The categories in this code block are as follows:

Z17   Estrogen receptor status

Z17.- Estrogen receptor status

Estrogen receptor (ER) status is classified as positive (ER+) or negative (ER-). ER+ breast cancer responds to hormone therapies, with the two most common being tamoxifen and aromatase, while ER- breast cancer does not. In addition, ER+ breast cancer cells, which are those that express estrogen receptor in their nuclei, generally have a better prognosis since these cells are better differentiated and can respond to hormonal manipulation.

Retained Foreign Body Fragments (Z18)

This code block contains a single category to report embedded or retained foreign body fragments.

The categories in this code block are as follows:

Z18   Retained foreign body fragments

Z18.- Retained foreign body fragments

This category includes embedded fragment, splinter, or foreign body status. Certain injuries involving retained or embedded fragments or splinters preclude removal due to technical difficulty, number of retained objects, or anatomically-sensitive location in the body. Any embedded object (natural or synthetic) has the potential to cause infection. Some objects may migrate to other areas of the body and interfere with physiologic function. The body's immune response may form fibrotic tissue to encapsulate a foreign body, which can similarly cause health problems or impair function, depending on the affected anatomic site. Certain metals and plastics contain potentially toxic chemical compounds. Chemicals from these fragments

may travel through the bloodstream and affect other parts of the body, posing possible long-term health threats. For these reasons, identifying the chemical composition of fragments and long-term surveillance are often necessary. Retained foreign body fragments are classified by the substance or material, which include radioactive, metal, plastic, organic, and other types, such as glass, stone, or crystalline fragments.

Z18.0- Retained radioactive fragments

The presence of radioactive fragments may be a result of exposure to munitions and armor containing depleted uranium or due to depleted isotope fragments from previous use in the treatment of certain cancers.

Z18.01 Retained depleted uranium fragments

Certain past and ongoing military conflicts have included exposure to munitions and armor containing depleted uranium (DU). When a DU munition passes through body armor or when body armor containing DU is penetrated, small fragments of DU may be inhaled, swallowed, or penetrate the skin and soft tissues. Because even depleted uranium is radioactive, it is a potential health hazard and individuals with retained radioactive fragments may require additional tests and monitoring for adverse effects.

Z18.1- Retained metal fragments

Retained metal fragments are a contraindication to MRI scanning. In military operations, bullets and/or shrapnel fragments composed of a lead core and a copper or brass jacket can cause a systemic toxicity that can have deleterious multisystemic effects. Some munitions contain tungsten alloys and other metals that may also have long-term toxic effects in the body.

Hormone Sensitivity Malignancy Status (Z19)

Hormones are a byproduct of the endocrine system. Endocrine glands produce hormones that the bloodstream carries to various sites within the body. Some hormones influence the growth and activity of certain cells and/or organs. Because cancer is an abnormality that starts at the cellular level, certain types of cancer may need or use the hormones in the cell to grow and divide. For some types of cancer, stopping the production of the hormone within the body or blocking the effect of the hormones on the cancer cells slows or stops cancer growth. When cancer cells respond to these types of therapies, the patient has a hormone-sensitive cancer. Other cancers, even those found in sites or organs that are affected by hormones do not respond to these therapies, and these patients have hormone-resistant cancers.

Z19.1   Hormone sensitive malignancy status

The list of hormone-sensitive cancers is relatively small. Some cancers of the following sites are hormone sensitive:

- Breast
- Ovary
- Uterus (endometrium)
- Prostate
- Kidney

Z19.2   Hormone resistant malignancy status

Hormone-resistant cancers may be classified as resistant, meaning the cancer did not respond to any type of hormone elimination or blocking therapy, or refractory, meaning a cancer that was first responding to hormone therapy subsequently developed a resistance to that therapy. This is seen in prostate cancer. Prostate cancer that does not respond to any type of hormone therapy is called castrate-resistant prostate cancer (CRPC). Prostate cancer that was successfully treated with hormone therapy but that now fails to respond to any of the available hormone therapies is referred to as hormone-refractory prostate cancer (HRPC).

Persons with Potential Health Hazards Related to Communicable Diseases (Z20-Z29)

This category supplies codes that can be used for patients who have been in contact with or had exposure to communicable diseases (e.g., diseases that are transferable from one person to another), are a carrier of an infectious disease, and codes that identify encounters for immunizations or reasons why an immunization was not performed.

The categories in this code block are as follows:

Z20	Contact with and (suspected) exposure to communicable diseases
Z21	Asymptomatic human immunodeficiency virus [HIV] infection status
Z22	Carrier of infectious disease
Z23	Encounter for immunization
Z28	Immunization not carried out and underimmunization status
Z29	Encounter for other prophylactic measures

Z20.-   Contact with and (suspected) exposure to communicable diseases

A communicable disease is one that can be transferred from one person to another or from an animal to a person. In most cases, the patient's immune system can successfully defeat the agent of disease. In this instance, while the patient may test positive for exposure to the disease, they do not show symptoms of an active disease process. Factors that can influence a person's ability to resist a contagious agent are age, underlying diseases, or, in some cases, current medical treatment. Although a majority of the communicable diseases are the result of an infectious organism, such as bacteria and viruses, they also can occur as an infestation. Infestations are the presence of parasitic organisms on the external surfaces of the host, such as lice and mites. The codes in this category are used for patients who have been exposed to or have been in close contact with a contagious agent but are not currently exhibiting symptoms, indicating that they have the disease and require monitoring for a period of time to ensure that they remain disease free.

Focus Point

There are two types of parasites: ectoparasitic and endoparasitic. Ectoparasites primarily live on the external surfaces of their hosts while endoparasites live within the host (internal). The term infestation can be used for both types of parasites but is typically reserved for ectoparasites (external), while endoparasitic invasion (internal) is referred to as an infection.

Z21   Asymptomatic human immunodeficiency virus [HIV] infection status

Human immunodeficiency virus (HIV) is a serious health concern. Two types of HIV are known to exist: HIV-1 and HIV-2. HIV-1 is widespread throughout the world and causes acquired immune deficiency syndrome (AIDS). HIV-2 is found primarily in West Africa and is seldom seen in the United States. There are three stages of HIV. The first is the acute stage, which may present with flu-like symptoms. Most individuals do not test positive for HIV during the acute stage. The second stage is the asymptomatic stage, which may last for 10 years or more. Infected individuals do not exhibit clinical symptoms; however, the virus is replicating and these individuals are infectious and can pass the virus on to others. During the asymptomatic stage, individuals normally test positive for HIV. The third phase is the symptomatic phase. This code (Z21) should be used during the second stage of the disease process when the patient is asymptomatic. This usually occurs four weeks to six months after the acute infection with HIV-1.

Z22.- Carrier of infectious disease

Carriers of an infectious disease have the infectious microorganism in or on their bodies, but do not have a current infectious process from the microorganism. While carriers do not exhibit any signs or symptoms of infection, they are capable of spreading the infectious microorganism to others who may then develop an infectious disease.

Z22.3- Carrier of other specified bacterial diseases

Other bacteria that commonly colonize the skin and other body sites and have the potential to cause infectious disease include meningococci, staphylococci, and streptococci.

Z22.31 Carrier of bacterial disease due to meningococci

Meningococcal infections caused by *Neisseria meningitidis* have the potential to cause serious infections of the spinal cord and brain (meningitis), heart, joints, optic nerve, or bloodstream. Although the bacterium is found in the nasopharynx of 5 percent of the population, only a fraction of carriers ever develop the disease, but they do have the potential to spread the disease, which occurs most often in infants or in epidemics among persons who live in close quarters (barracks, schools).

Z22.32- Carrier of bacterial disease due to staphylococci

Carriers of *Staphylococcus aureus* may be colonized with methicillin susceptible or methicillin resistant strains of *S. aureus*.

Z22.321 Carrier or suspected carrier of Methicillin susceptible Staphylococcus aureus

Carriers of methicillin susceptible *Staphylococcus aureus* have MSSA on their skin or in their body but do not exhibit signs of infection. These individuals are able to pass MSSA on to others who may then develop an infection.

Z22.322 Carrier or suspected carrier of Methicillin resistant Staphylococcus aureus

Carriers of methicillin resistant *Staphylococcus aureus* have MRSA on their skin or in their body but do not exhibit signs of infection. These individuals are able to pass MRSA on to others who may then develop an infection. Carriers of MRSA pose a particular threat of spreading a severe and difficult to treat infection because MRSA strains are resistant to many antibiotics.

Z23 Encounter for immunization

Immunizations are a purposeful stimulation of an immune response through the use of a vaccine, instead of having to acquire and survive the actual disease. Vaccines help prevent specific diseases by introducing weakened or dead bacteria, viruses, or toxins into the body, and allowing the body to create antibodies against the pathogen that is introduced (e.g., immunity). There are two types of vaccines: active and passive. An active vaccine stimulates the immune system to give protection against disease while a passive vaccine takes lymphoid cells or serum from immune individuals and administers them to nonimmune individuals to provide specific immune reactivity. Most vaccines are given during the early childhood years. However, some vaccinations such as for influenza and pneumonia are recommended for adults. Often more than one vaccine is included in one injection.

Z29.- Encounter for other prophylactic measures

This group of codes is assigned when the patient is seen for some form of medication as a preventive encounter, specifically immunotherapy or fluoride treatment.

Z29.1- Encounter for prophylactic immunotherapy

Prophylactic immunotherapy is performed to prevent disease involving the immune system. This subcategory is specific to the prophylactic treatment against conditions such as respiratory syncytial virus, certain poisonous venom, rabies, and others.

Z29.11 Encounter for prophylactic immunotherapy for respiratory syncytial virus (RSV)

This code is used to report the encounter for the administration of prophylactic medication, generally given monthly for certain populations during RSV season. This virus leads to infections within the respiratory tract and is most common in children under the age of 2 years old. While the symptoms may be minor, the condition can be detrimental in premature babies or babies with associated health conditions. The virus can lead to serious complications in patients with heart and lung disorders and weak immunity.

Z29.12 Encounter for prophylactic antivenin

This medication is given to patients exposed to specific toxins from snakes, spiders, or scorpions in order to fight the poison. Although the treatments were once thought to be helpful, there has been little evidence that prophylactic treatments are of benefit and they are not widely used.

Z29.13 Encounter for prophylactic Rho(D) immune globulin

This formula is provided to patients with immune thrombocytopenic purpura (ITP) when the patient has Rh-positive blood. This disorder decreases the amount of platelets, leading to the inability of the blood to clot. The substance may also be given to an Rh-negative patient who was transfused with Rh-positive blood and during pregnancy when the mother is Rh-negative and the baby is Rh-positive. This prophylactic administration allows the body to boost immunity and prevent bleeding.

Z29.14 Encounter for prophylactic rabies immune globin

This administration consists of one dose of human rabies immune globulin (HRIG), which is provided once at the onset of antirabies treatment of an unvaccinated person after initial exposure, allowing the body to produce antibodies. Four doses of rabies vaccinations are also administered, one with the HRIG dose followed by three more given on days 3, 7, and 14. If the HRIG is unavailable and not initially administered, it is still effective if given within seven days of initial vaccination.

Z29.3 Encounter for prophylactic fluoride administration

Fluoride administration is typically provided to children during tooth development to help prevent dental caries. Forms include tablets and varnish, which is typically applied directly to the teeth by a dental provider.

Persons Encountering Health Services in Circumstances Related to Reproduction (Z30-Z39)

Reproduction (procreation) is the biological process necessary to create an offspring. Several categories in this code block feature codes related to the management of procreation, either to help assist an individual and/or couple in procreation or to prevent the creation of an offspring. The other categories are for use in the management of a pregnant patient, from initial pregnancy testing to routine supervision of the pregnancy and the postpartum.

The categories in this code block are as follows:

Z30	Encounter for contraceptive management
Z31	Encounter for procreative management
Z32	Encounter for pregnancy test and childbirth and childcare instruction
Z33	Pregnant state
Z34	Encounter for supervision of normal pregnancy
Z36	Encounter for antenatal screening of mother
Z3A	Weeks of gestation

Z37	Outcome of delivery
Z38	Liveborn infants according to place of birth and type of delivery
Z39	Encounter for maternal postpartum care and examination

Z30.- Encounter for contraceptive management

Contraceptive management is used for patients who are trying to prevent pregnancy. There are many avenues for which contraception may be obtained, including oral medications, intrauterine devices, and surgical procedures for males and females (sterilization).

Codes in this category are assigned not only for the initial introduction or implantation of contraceptives, but also for surveillance and ongoing evaluation of the devices, including counseling by medical personnel and the encounters for removal. A code for an encounter for the sole purpose of surgical sterilization for either male or female is also included here.

Z31.- Encounter for procreative management

Procreative management is the use of health care services to assist or counsel individuals and/or couples in producing offspring. This may involve something as simple as an encounter for advice on natural family planning to an encounter that is more involved, such as reversal of a previous sterilization procedure. The codes reflect the procreative issue that is being investigated or managed.

Z31.7 Encounter for procreative management and counseling for gestational carrier

This code describes management and care of a surrogate mother. The surrogate carries and gives birth to a child for another woman by artificial insemination or embryo implantation.

Z31.8- Encounter for other procreative management

This subcategory captures other procreative assistance or infertility investigations that could not be classified in previous codes from this category.

Z31.84 Encounter for fertility preservation procedure

The incidence of cancer and other diseases in younger populations, coupled with the increase in individuals who wish to start or expand their families later in life, have resulted in many patients seeking measures to preserve the ability to procreate. The effect of disease and its associated treatment on a patient's fertility may be temporary or permanent depending on the nature of the disease or type of cancer, the type and dosage of therapeutic regimens, the route of administration or anatomic site of treatment, and the patient's health and fertility status prior to diagnosis and treatment. Fertility preservation procedures allow the patient to save, for future use, certain reproductive material. For females this may include cryopreservation, which involves the harvesting and freezing of oocytes (eggs), embryos, or ovarian tissue. Eggs may also be harvested via in vitro fertilization prior to the treatment of a medical condition, and then reimplanted after the disease has been eradicated or has gone into remission. Male patients may also use cryopreservation services by donating sperm or testicular tissue to be frozen. This may be the only option available to achieve future fertility for certain male children undergoing treatment for cancer or other disease.

Focus Point

When the purpose or intent of the encounter is only to provide counseling on fertility preservation, only Z31.62 Encounter for fertility preservation counseling, should be coded.

Z36.- Encounter for antenatal screening of mother

Antenatal screening is testing performed during pregnancy to detect disease or disease precursors in the growing fetus or to diagnose any maternal conditions that may affect fetal development, so that early detection and treatment can be provided should the baby test positive for a disease.

Z36.0 Encounter for antenatal screening for chromosomal anomalies

This code classifies a screening encounter for various tests to assess probability of potential chromosomal anomalies such as Down syndrome Trisomy-21 and Trisomy-18.

Z36.1 Encounter for antenatal screening for raised alphafetoprotein level

Encounter for a screening blood test for high levels of alpha-fetoprotein (AFP), which can be done after the sixteenth week of pregnancy, to evaluate the possibility of spina bifida and other neural tube defects, anencephaly, or omphalocele in the fetus.

Z36.2 Encounter for other antenatal screening follow-up

This code is assigned for encounters for follow-up results of other antenatal screens, including prior screens such as ultrasound that failed to visualize certain anatomy.

Z36.3 Encounter for antenatal screening for malformations

As part of a second trimester ultrasound, a fetal anatomic survey can provide valuable information about the fetus. It is performed similarly to a physical exam, with a "head to toe" examination using standard protocol transabdominal or transvaginal approach. A routine fetal anatomic survey includes examination and assessment of the growth and development of the following structures:

Skull:	Head shape, circumference, and biparietal diameter
Brain:	Cerebral ventricles, choroid plexuses, midbrain, and posterior fossa (cerebellum and cisterna magma)
Face:	Orbits, lip, and profile
Neck:	Nuchal fold thickness
Spine:	Longitudinal and transverse views
Heart:	Rate and rhythm, four-chamber view, and outflow tracts
Thorax:	Shape of the thorax, lungs, and diaphragm
Abdomen:	Circumference, stomach, liver, kidneys, bladder, abdominal wall, and umbilicus
Limbs:	Shape and measurement of femur, tibia and fibula, humerus, radius and ulna, hands and feet

Although fetal size, position, movement, and other factors may affect the exam, major body systems are often readily visualized and assessed by 18 weeks gestation. A wide range of congenital anomalies can be diagnosed by fetal anatomic survey, including defects of the central nervous system, heart, anterior abdominal wall, urinary tract, and skeleton. If an anomaly is suspected, a more detailed examination may be indicated.

Z36.4 Encounter for antenatal screening for fetal growth retardation

Prenatal screening for fetal growth retardation (FGR) or intrauterine growth restriction (IUGR) involves identifying any risk factors for slow fetal growth including multiple pregnancies, placenta previa, maternal drug use, or a genetic disorder, and assessing fetal size using detailed sonographic assessment of the fetus, placenta, and amniotic fluid. Fetal growth is a relationship between the size (small or large) and weight (light or heavy) of the fetus at a particular gestational age. Typically, a fetus grows proportionally in relation to the gestational age until about the 37th week, when growth commonly plateaus. When a fetus is not the typical size at a particular gestational week it may be an indicator of an underlying condition.

Z36.5 Encounter for antenatal screening for isoimmunization

Screening for blood type and maternal antibodies is routine prenatal care. Isoimmunization is the incompatibility of Rh and ABO between a mother and a fetus. Rh factor is a protein found on the surface of red blood cells in some individuals. Individuals with Rh factor on the surface of their red blood cells are Rh-positive, while those without Rh factor are Rh-negative. Rh isoimmunization occurs when an Rh-negative mother carries an Rh-positive fetus and the fetal blood crosses the placenta entering the mother's bloodstream. The mother then makes antibodies to the Rh factor, which is identified as a foreign protein in the mother's blood. If these antibodies cross the placenta and enter the fetal blood, they damage and destroy the fetal red blood cells causing Rh isoimmunization.

There are four blood types: A, B, AB, and O. ABO isoimmunization may occur when a mother with one blood type carries a fetus with an incompatible blood type. If blood from a fetus with an incompatible blood type crosses the placenta and enters the mother's bloodstream, the mother's body makes antibodies to the foreign blood type. If these antibodies cross the placenta and enter the fetal blood, they can damage and destroy the fetal red blood cells resulting in ABO isoimmunization.

Z36.8- Encounter for other antenatal screening

Subcategory Z36.8- includes antenatal screening for certain other specified potential conditions such as hydrops fetalis, nuchal translucency, congenital cardiac abnormalities, fetal lung maturity, Streptococcus B, risk of pre-term labor, uncertain dates, large-for-dates, and other specified screening not classified elsewhere.

Z36.81 Encounter for antenatal screening for hydrops fetalis

This code classifies antenatal screening for hydrops fetalis, which includes diagnostic studies such as fetal ultrasounds and maternal blood examination. Hydrops fetalis has several etiologies and presents as an abnormal accumulation of fluid in two or more parts of the fetus such as ascites, effusion of the pleural or pericardial tissues, or edema. The infant mortality rate is high, particularly with premature infants. Hydrops fetalis due to isoimmunization is caused by mother-fetus blood incompatibility. Therapies include exchange blood transfusions, resuscitation and mechanical ventilation at birth, and thoracentesis. Associated conditions include erythroblastosis fetalis, respiratory failure, alloimmune hemolytic anemia, high output cardiac failure, and hypoproteinemia. Nonimmune fetal hydrops can be caused by a wide variety of diseases and disorders involving many different body systems. Therapies include vigorous resuscitation such as mechanical ventilation at birth, thoracentesis for pleural effusion, and diuresis.

Z36.82 Encounter for antenatal screening for nuchal translucency

This screening examination measures translucency of the nuchal fold—a small, clear space beneath the skin of a growing fetus' neck—using ultrasound. It is normally performed between week 11 and week 13 of pregnancy. In babies who are at an increased risk for chromosomal abnormalities such as Down syndrome, trisomy 18, or congenital heart problems, this area tends to accumulate increased fluid and expands in size.

Z36.83 Encounter for fetal screening for congenital cardiac abnormalities

Antenatal screening for fetal congenital cardiac abnormalities/congenital heart defects can be performed during pregnancy using fetal echocardiography. A prenatal congenital heart disease diagnosis can reduce serious complications after the baby is born, give the parents information about the prognosis and treatments that might be required, and sometimes allow for fetal cardiac intervention before birth.

Z36.84 Encounter for antenatal screening for fetal lung maturity

Screening for fetal lung maturity involves testing to determine if the baby's lungs have developed adequately in cases where a medically indicated preterm delivery between 32 to 39 weeks may be indicated.

Z36.85 Encounter for antenatal screening for Streptococcus B

This code classifies screening encounter for testing, usually late in pregnancy at 35 to 37 weeks, for the presence of Streptococcus B (group B streptococcus [GBS]), a type of bacteria normally found in the vagina and rectum in healthy women. Newborns exposed to GBS, however, can develop sepsis, meningitis, pneumonia, blindness, deafness, and even death. If positive, prophylactic antibiotics are administered to the mother to prevent the baby being born with infection.

Z36.86 Encounter for antenatal screening for cervical length

Antenatal screening to measure cervical length using transvaginal ultrasound, typically between 18 and 20 weeks, can be performed to identify pregnant women at high risk of premature delivery due to a shortened cervix (less than 2 cm) in the second trimester of pregnancy. Cervical shortening may pose a risk factor for premature birth, and may alter the course of treatment and management of the pregnancy, yet the patient may carry the fetus to term.

Z36.87 Encounter for antenatal screening for uncertain dates

This type of antenatal screening is performed to evaluate fetal gestational age in cases of uncertain or inconsistent menstrual dates.

Z36.88 Encounter for antenatal screening for fetal macrosomia

Report this code for antenatal screening examination for fetal macrosomia or other large-for-dates fetus. Fetal macrosomia refers to fetal growth significantly larger than average, regardless of gestational age. Some risk factors associated with high neonatal birth weight are multiparity, maternal age 30 to 40 years, and diabetes. Women who are pregnant with large babies are more likely to require cesarean delivery or delivery complicated by birth injuries, shoulder dystocia, chorioamnionitis, fourth-degree perineal lacerations, and postpartum hemorrhage.

Z3A.- Weeks of gestation

Gestation is the fetal age between conception and birth. It is measured in weeks and is typically determined from the first day of the woman's last menstrual cycle to the present date; however, it can also be determined by an early ultrasound. Many OB codes require an additional code to describe the gestational week of the fetus. These secondary only codes are specifically for use on the mother's record, if known.

> **Focus Point**
>
> *When an encounter encompasses overlapping gestational weeks, the week of gestation at the time of the admission should be used.*

Z37.- Outcome of delivery

Codes used to report the outcome of a delivery on the mother's record are used in addition to codes from the obstetric section (Chapter 15) of ICD-10-CM. A code from this category indicates whether the outcome of delivery was a single or multiple birth, as well as identifies whether all of the fetuses were liveborn, some stillborn and some liveborn, or all stillborn. These codes should be used on all maternal delivery records.

Z38.- Liveborn infants according to place of birth and type of delivery

These codes are used as the principal diagnosis on all newborn birth records and only for that first birth encounter. The codes in this category capture whether the newborn was a single birth or part of a multiple birth, whether the delivery was vaginal or cesarean, and whether or not the newborn was born inside or outside of the hospital.

Encounters for Other Specific Health Care (Z40-Z53)

The majority of the categories in this code block provide the justification behind certain postprocedural encounters, with the majority of the codes relating to aftercare and/or fitting and adjustment of a plethora of devices. Encounters related to cosmetic, prophylactic, and reconstructive surgeries are also coded here.

The categories in this code block are as follows:

Z40	Encounter for prophylactic surgery
Z41	Encounter for procedures for purposes other than remedying health state
Z42	Encounter for plastic and reconstructive surgery following medical procedure or healed injury
Z43	Encounter for attention to artificial openings
Z44	Encounter for fitting and adjustment of external prosthetic device
Z45	Encounter for adjustment and management of implanted device
Z46	Encounter for fitting and adjustment of other devices
Z47	Orthopedic aftercare
Z48	Encounter for other postprocedural aftercare
Z49	Encounter for care involving renal dialysis
Z51	Encounter for other aftercare and medical care
Z52	Donors of organs and tissues
Z53	Persons encountering health services for specific procedures and treatment, not carried out

Z40.- Encounter for prophylactic surgery

This category provides codes for prophylactic surgeries performed that are related to malignancy risk factors and other specified and unspecified reasons.

Z40.0- Encounter for prophylactic surgery for risk factors related to malignant neoplasms

Codes in this subcategory are assigned for patients admitted for prophylactic removal of the breasts, ovaries, or other organs who have a family or personal history of cancer or other risk factors related to malignant neoplasms such as genetic susceptibility or for prevention of a new primary malignancy or metastatic disease.

Focus Point

Assign any codes for genetic susceptibility or personal or family history as appropriate in addition to codes from this category. Do not assign codes from this subcategory if the organ removal is for treatment of a malignancy.

Z42.- Encounter for plastic and reconstructive surgery following medical procedure or healed injury

Plastic and/or reconstructive surgery may be performed on patients who have a defect from a previous surgery or healed injury and for which another procedure is required to put the anatomical site back to its natural state.

Z42.1 Encounter for breast reconstruction following mastectomy

When a patient undergoes mastectomy, breast tissue is removed according to the size, location, and nature of the tumor. Patients may request breast reconstruction in order to gain back the symmetry and aesthetic balance they had prior to the mastectomy. Breast reconstruction is commonly performed after treatment (e.g., chemo or other therapy) has been completed and is determined to be successful. Examples of breast reconstructive procedures include insertion of tissue expanders or implants, muscle and/or skin transfers, matching or balancing procedures to mimic the appearance of the native breast, and areolar and nipple grafting or tattooing.

Z43.- Encounter for attention to artificial openings

An artificial opening or ostomy is a surgically created opening connecting an internal organ to the outside of the body (skin). This code can be used for any encounters involving cleaning of the ostomy opening, adjustment or removal of a catheter within the opening, or reforming or closure of the opening.

Z44.- Encounter for fitting and adjustment of external prosthetic device

When a patient is missing a body part due to a congenital condition or secondary to trauma or infection, an artificially manufactured device is sometimes provided to replace the missing body part. External prosthetic devices are created to be as compatible as possible with the patient's specific anatomy and functional requirements. Often the patient needs a team of health care professionals, including physical and occupational therapists, to learn to use and adjust to the prosthetic device. Codes in this category are used only when a prosthetic device is in some way being managed, such as being fitted to the patient, removed, adjusted, or replaced, and only when there are no other complications associated with the device.

Z44.2- Encounter for fitting and adjustment of artificial eye

An artificial eye is placed when the native eye globe has been removed surgically to treat a disease or due to injury/trauma. Fitting and adjustment, which includes removal, of the artificial eye is required for comfort and to ensure optimal cosmetic appearance. Removal by a physician is necessary on at least a yearly basis for polishing due to buildup of concretions that can irritate the eye if they are not removed. Further adjustments may be necessary due to changes in the socket tissues. This code also covers an encounter for instruction provided by the ocularist related to the care and handling of the artificial eye and correct removal and replacement techniques when performed by the patient.

Z45.- Encounter for adjustment and management of implanted device

Most of the implanted devices represented in this category are devices needed to support a biological function that has been damaged or is dysfunctional. These devices are typically going to be a permanent implant, such as a pacemaker or cochlear device that must always be present in order to have optimal functioning of the organ or structure. Also included here are breast prostheses that are implanted under the skin.

Z45.4- Encounter for adjustment and management of implanted nervous system device

Common nervous system devices include implanted neuropacemaker, spinal cord stimulators, and ventriculoperitoneal and lumboperitoneal shunts.

Z45.41 Encounter for adjustment and management of cerebrospinal fluid drainage device

Cerebrospinal fluid drainage devices, more commonly referred to as shunts, are used to divert cerebrospinal (CSF) fluid from the ventricles in the brain or from the subarachnoid space around the brain or spinal cord to another anatomical site. Typically CSF is diverted to the peritoneal cavity but CSF can also be diverted to the atrium of the heart, the lung, or the pleural cavity. The purpose of this diversion is to reduce the amount of CSF in the subarachnoid space or ventricles and alleviate pressure on the brain or spinal cord that can occur when CSF cannot be properly absorbed. Hydrocephalus and idiopathic intracranial hypertension are two conditions for which shunts are commonly used.

Z45.42   Encounter for adjustment and management of neuropacemaker (brain) (peripheral nerve) (spinal cord)

A neuropacemaker is an implanted device that is used to relieve nerve injury pain or to help lessen the symptoms of movement disorders. The entire system is composed of a pacemaker (generator) and one or more electrodes (leads). The pacemaker is inserted in the subcutaneous tissue in the chest or sometimes the abdomen. Depending on the therapeutic purpose of the procedure, electrodes are selectively placed in, near, or around specific sites within the brain, spinal cord, and peripheral or cranial nerves and then tunneled and connected to the pacemaker.

Z46.-   Encounter for fitting and adjustment of other devices

Other types of devices that require regular appointments for evaluation and assessment of the device and/or instruction related to patient use of the device include insulin pumps and nonvascular catheters.

Z46.51   Encounter for fitting and adjustment of gastric lap band

Gastric banding (lap band) is a type of bariatric surgery to treat obesity. A restrictive inflatable silicone ring is placed around the top portion of the stomach, restricting the expansion of the stomach and slowing the passage of food. The silicone ring can be inflated or deflated as necessary to achieve desired weight loss. Tightening of the band is achieved by adding saline to inflate the band. If vomiting or difficulty in swallowing occurs, the band may need to be loosened by reducing the amount of saline. When adjusted optimally, the patient can achieve weight loss by feeling full with less food, slowing digestion, and increasing the feeling of fullness after a meal, yet allowing adequate nutrition. A self-adjusting subcutaneous port is connected to the band, allowing adjustments to be made through the skin with a syringe, adding or releasing saline as necessary. Patients may be allowed to self-adjust the band; however, physician office visits may be necessary for optimal adjustment.

Z46.81   Encounter for fitting and adjustment of insulin pump

Insulin pump training is provided to patients who require insulin for diabetes. The use of an insulin pump is an alternative to daily injections. The insulin pump is an external device with a tube positioned in the subcutaneous tissue. The pump delivers appropriate amounts of insulin continuously, 24-hours a day. Typically a continuous amount of insulin, called a basal rate, is delivered throughout the day along with large boluses given at mealtimes. Patients must be instructed on how to use and program the pump to maintain optimal blood sugar levels.

Z47.-   Orthopedic aftercare

Orthopedic aftercare is a means of monitoring patients who have had an orthopedic surgery performed to ensure any devices placed are working properly and that the surgical sites have healed appropriately. This code is used only for orthopedic aftercare provided for musculoskeletal conditions that are not the result of a current traumatic injury.

Focus Point

If the care provided is for an injury due to a trauma, the correct code for the encounter is an injury code with the appropriate seventh character (e.g., character D for subsequent care), not the aftercare code.

Z47.3-   Aftercare following explantation of joint prosthesis

It is sometimes necessary for a provider to remove a joint prosthesis for reasons related to infection, mechanical malfunction, or other complication related to the prosthetic device. Depending on the nature of the medical condition, it may not be possible to place the new prosthetic device during the same encounter, resulting in what is called a staged procedure. In a staged procedure, the old device is removed during the initial encounter and the new device is inserted in the second (staged) encounter. The codes in this subcategory provide a means of identifying any follow-up care performed to monitor a joint following explantation, as well as codes that validate the admission of a patient for a staged procedure necessary to insert the new prosthetic device.

Z48.-   Encounter for other postprocedural aftercare

Postprocedural aftercare is care following a procedure that may be provided during the healing or recovery phase or for long-term medical care for circumstances related to the procedure.

Z48.2-   Encounter for aftercare following organ transplant

Patients who have had an organ transplant require posttransplant care during the initial healing and recovery phase, as well as long-term medical care to monitor for specific complications that can occur due to the presence of the transplanted organ and the medications needed to prevent rejection of the transplanted organ.

Z51.- Encounter for other aftercare and medical care

This category captures admissions for cancer treatment, including chemotherapy, immunotherapy, and radiation therapy, as well as monitoring certain drug levels for patients on long-term drug therapy.

Z51.0 Encounter for antineoplastic radiation therapy

Antineoplastic radiation therapy is a specific type of high energy radiation that is used to destroy cancer cells. It may be delivered from an external source, implanted in the body within or near the malignant tumor, or delivered intravenously as a radioisotope. Antineoplastic radiation therapy may be performed before, during, or after other treatments for the cancer such as chemotherapy or surgery and may also be delivered over a prolonged period of time in a maintenance dose.

Z51.11 Encounter for antineoplastic chemotherapy

Antineoplastic chemotherapy is used to treat a wide variety of cancers. This treatment modality uses antineoplastic or cytotoxic drugs to destroy cancer cells. Typically the drugs are delivered intravenously, which allows the drugs to reach all parts of the body and destroy any cancer cells that may have seeded to sites remote from the primary malignant neoplasm. In some cases, drugs may be injected directly into a specific body site (e.g., intrathecal) or body cavity (e.g., intrathoracic or intraperitoneal).

Z51.12 Encounter for antineoplastic immunotherapy

Immunotherapy, also called biologic therapy, stimulates the body's own immune defense system to fight infection and disease. Whereas traditional cytotoxic chemotherapies attack the cancer cells themselves, biologic therapy lends support to the body's defenses by mimicking naturally occurring substances that activate the immune system. This stimulates the activity of cells that attack malignant neoplasms.

Z51.5 Encounter for palliative care

Palliative care is a multidisciplinary approach to managing patients with life-threatening conditions. The goal of palliative care is to make the patient comfortable and improve quality of life by managing any adverse symptoms related to the disease, side effects related to the treatment for the disease, and any emotional or psychological problems that may arise. The initiation of palliative care does not mean that treatment for the terminal illness can no longer be pursued, although this code would also be used for such situations. Treatment of the terminal illness may be continued concomitantly with palliative care although typically treatment is aimed more at making the patient comfortable rather than treating the illness itself.

Z51.6 Encounter for desensitization to allergens

An allergy is the body's reaction to a substance (allergen) that the body would not normally treat as an invader. The body reacts to the allergen by stimulating the immune system to attack the allergen. Allergy sufferers can have any number of symptoms, including runny nose, itchy eyes, swelling of airways, nausea, and dizziness. Allergy desensitization is a treatment used to reduce the symptoms of and, in limited cases, cure patients who suffer from certain allergies. The procedure involves introducing the allergic agent to the body in incremental amounts over an extended amount of time. Eventually the allergen is viewed less and less as a hostile invader, effectively switching off the immune system's response to that allergen. Protocols have been developed to treat allergies to many insects, dust mites, animal dander, mold, and pollen.

Z53.- Persons encountering health services for specific procedures and treatment, not carried out

Services and/or procedures may not be carried out when circumstances surrounding the patient's current health status change or increase the risk of the patient experiencing a harmful or adverse event should the service or procedure be performed or continued (e.g., reaction to anesthesia, extremely high blood pressure.) This category is also used when the patient is refusing treatment or leaves the facility without seeing the provider or against the advice of the provider.

Z53.3- Procedure converted to open procedure

In certain instances, procedures performed by scopes are converted to open procedures because the scope cannot perform the procedure (e.g., there are extensive adhesions) or because the procedure is more extensive than originally anticipated. The medical necessity of converting a scope procedure to an open procedure should be well documented in the patient's health record.

Persons with Potential Health Hazards Related to Socioeconomic and Psychosocial Circumstances (Z55-Z65)

Situations such as living in poverty, exposure to adverse or hostile conditions at a work place, or a poor family network can have a substantial influence on the mental and physical wellbeing of a patient. Socioeconomic and psychosocial circumstances codes captured here relate the influence of education, income, occupation, family, and social status on a patient, especially those that could negatively impact a patient's health status.

The categories in this code block are as follows:

Z55	Problems related to education and literacy
Z56	Problems related to employment and unemployment
Z57	Occupational exposure to risk factors
Z59	Problems related to housing and economic circumstances
Z60	Problems related to social environment
Z62	Problems related to upbringing
Z63	Other problems related to primary support group, including family circumstances
Z64	Problems related to certain psychosocial circumstances
Z65	Problems related to other psychosocial circumstances

Z56.- Problems related to employment and unemployment

This category captures encounters for patients who are experiencing problems related to employment, such as the threat of layoff, extreme physical demands, or sexual harassment that could potentially lead to problems with the patient's health or mental stability.

Z56.82 Military deployment status

The health consequences associated with deployment may include physical, psychological, and/or emotional impairments for the deployed individual. These effects may be related to physical injuries, physical stressors, exposure, or psychological trauma, which may manifest as diagnosable medical and mental health conditions. Alternately, other effects of deployment may involve nonspecific symptoms and impairments for which the patient may seek medical care.

> **Focus Point**
>
> *This code is to be used for the deployed individual. For deployment affecting the family or other entities of the deployed individual, use code Z63.31 Absence of family member due to military deployment.*

Z59.- Problems related to housing and economic circumstances

Lack of housing can be a potential health hazard as can inadequate housing, which includes a living situation without access to heat, electricity, or water for bathing. There may also be potential health hazards if the patient is experiencing problems with neighbors, other residents in the same home or facility, or with a landlord. Economic circumstances that can adversely affect overall health and well-being include low income and poverty, which may lead to lack of food and/or the availability of clean drinking water. Stressors such as insufficient social insurance or welfare support, inability to make house payments or other problems with creditors, and isolated location of a home are also included here.

Z62.- Problems related to upbringing

A proper support system is very important during a child's formative years. The codes captured here identify situations during a patient's upbringing, such as abuse or being in foster care, that adversely affect or have the potential to adversely affect the patient's mental and/or physical health. Most of these codes can be used for patients of any age because, in some cases, the life event may not manifest negative effects until later in life.

Z63.- Other problems related to primary support group, including family circumstances

Certain familial disruption circumstances can affect the patient's ability to manage health-related problems and may create stress that can exacerbate a medical or psychological condition. Disruptive or stressful situations (e.g., marital discord, separation, or divorce; death; deployment; substance abuse) can manifest as emotional, behavioral, or health problems and have adverse effects not only for the patient, but for family members as well. In addition, the patient or family members may seek health-related services such as counseling to cope with these circumstances. Sequencing is dependent upon the circumstances of the encounter.

Z63.31　Absence of family member due to military deployment

Absence of a family member, particularly one deployed in the military to a war zone to provide peacekeeping or humanitarian aid, may result in stress for the deployed individual's family and other loved ones.

Z63.71　Stress on family due to return of family member from military deployment

The stress and health consequences associated with a family member returning home from deployment may be simply due to a long absence and the need for both the deployed individual and the family to readjust to having the deployed individual home. Stress may be related to physical injuries, exposures, or psychological traumas suffered by the deployed individual that the family must adapt to.

Do Not Resuscitate Status (Z66)

This code block contains only one valid three-character code that is used to identify patients that do not wish to have life-saving efforts performed should their heart or respirations cease.

The categories in this code block are as follows:

Z66　　Do not resuscitate

Z66　　Do not resuscitate

A do-not-resuscitate (DNR) order consists of a statement by a physician in the medical record informing the medical staff that cardiopulmonary resuscitation (CPR) should not be performed, preventing the unnecessary or unwanted invasive treatment to prolong life, should cardiac arrest occur. Unsuccessful CPR attempts in combination with a patient's medical condition or other frailties may render a patient with permanent brain damage or other debilitating sequelae. For these and other reasons, a DNR order assists in ensuring that the patient experiences a natural death without aggressive resuscitative efforts. The decision to waive CPR may be made by the patient or qualifying surrogates in the event of terminal illness. DNR orders may be written for patients in the hospital, nursing home, or home for those receiving home care.

Body Mass Index [BMI] (Z68)

Body mass index (BMI) is calculated by dividing a person's weight in kilograms by their height in meters squared (kg/M^2). BMI measurements are a guideline for categorizing weight in a more specific manner than relying solely on "overweight" or "obese" terminology.

The BMI is only one factor in determining a patient's risk for acquiring obesity-related diseases or disorders. Practitioners must also take into account the patient's age, sex, and race. Other variances, such as the presence or absence of muscle mass and the distribution of body fat, also need to be taken into consideration. For example, a body builder with an excess of healthy muscle mass will have a higher BMI, often in the range considered to be "overweight." Persons with fat distributed primarily in the upper body or around the waist line are at a higher risk for diseases such as hypertension and cardiovascular disease than those patients with fat mainly distributed in the lower body, below the waist.

The categories in this code block are as follows:

Z68　　Body mass index [BMI]

Z68.-　　Body mass index [BMI]

BMI is used to help determine whether an individual is underweight, a healthy weight, overweight, or obese. The CDC classifies BMI differently depending on whether the individual is an adult (age 21 or older) or a child (age 2 to 20).

Z68.1　　Body mass index (BMI) 19.9 or less, adult

A BMI below 18.5 is considered underweight in CDC weight classifications.

Z68.2-　　Body mass index (BMI) 20-29, adult

A BMI between 18.5 and 24.9 in an adult is designated as normal in CDC weight classifications, while one between 25.0 and 29.9 is designated as overweight.

Z68.3-　　Body mass index (BMI) 30-39, adult

A BMI between 30 and 39 in an adult is designated as obese in CDC weight classifications.

Z68.4-　　Body mass index (BMI) 40 or greater, adult

A BMI more than 40 in an adult suggests morbid obesity and corresponds to a weight that is 80 to 100 pounds above the healthy parameter for weight. Morbid obesity status increases the risk of premature death, diabetes, hypertension, heart disease, cancer, arthritis, and heart failure, among other health problems.

Z68.5-　　Body mass index (BMI) pediatric

The CDC provides four weight classifications for children: underweight, healthy, at risk, and overweight.

Z68.51　　Body mass index (BMI) pediatric, less than 5th percentile for age

A BMI less than the 5th percentile for age is designated as underweight, based on the CDC weight classifications.

Z68.52 Body mass index (BMI) pediatric, 5th percentile to less than 85th percentile for age

A BMI between the 5th percentile to less than the 85th percentile for age is designated as healthy, based on the CDC weight classifications.

Z68.53 Body mass index (BMI) pediatric, 85th percentile to less than 95th percentile for age

A BMI between the 85th percentile to less than the 95th percentile for age is designated as at risk, based on the CDC weight classifications.

Z68.54 Body mass index (BMI) pediatric, greater than or equal to 95th percentile for age

A BMI greater than or equal to the 95th percentile for age is designated as overweight, based on the CDC weight classifications.

Persons Encountering Health Services in Other Circumstances (Z69-Z76)

Codes in this code block may be used as first listed when the patient is primarily seeking counseling or medical advice. Additionally, codes in this code block can provide important supplementary information, as secondary codes, to identify circumstances related to the patient, such as bed confinement status that may alter the patient's care regime or identify risk factors for conditions that are not yet present.

The categories in this code block are as follows:

Z69	Encounter for mental health services for victim and perpetrator of abuse
Z70	Counseling related to sexual attitude, behavior and orientation
Z71	Persons encountering health services for other counseling and medical advice, not elsewhere classified
Z72	Problems related to lifestyle
Z73	Problems related to life management difficulty
Z74	Problems related to care provider dependency
Z75	Problems related to medical facilities and other health care
Z76	Persons encountering health services in other circumstances

Z71.- Persons encountering health services for other counseling and medical advice, not elsewhere classified

Codes in this category are used when a patient or family member receives assistance in the aftermath of an illness or injury, or when support is required in coping with family or social problems. Counseling services may be performed by physicians or other qualified healthcare providers to improve risk factors in the presence or absence of disease, promote healthy living, and/or prevent illness or injury. Counseling may include evaluation of social and family issues, appropriate diet and exercise, high-risk behavior, avoidance of injury, dental issues, and discussion of test results.

Z71.3 Dietary counseling and surveillance

Dietary or nutrition counseling can be done by a certified nutrition consultant or a registered dietitian (RD). These health professionals assess a patient's dietary intake, physical activity, medical therapy such as medications and other treatments, individual preferences, and other factors, and identify areas where change, education, support, and follow-up are needed to promote and maintain dietary changes for healthier eating, a medically therapeutic diet, or to avoid drug interactions. Counseling may be indicated in patients with identified risk factors, malnutrition, or chronic diseases, including cardiovascular disease, diabetes mellitus, hypertension, kidney disease, eating disorders, gastrointestinal disorders, seizures, or chronic obstructive pulmonary disease.

Z71.7 Human immunodeficiency virus [HIV] counseling

Human immunodeficiency virus (HIV) counseling involves a risk assessment and providing advice and accurate medical information to help prevent and reduce HIV acquisition and transmission. Patients are educated on how to reduce the risk of contracting or transmitting HIV, given information regarding the benefits and consequences of testing and how to undergo testing, and receive a detailed explanation of the test results, as well as counseling and referral after positive test results.

Z71.82 Exercise counseling

Exercise counseling helps patients prevent, treat, or manage chronic conditions such as hypertension, high cholesterol or other cardiovascular risk factors, diabetes and prediabetes, kidney disease and other metabolic disorders, muscle weakness due to age or disease, osteoporosis, arthritis, obesity, and stress and anxiety. Providers assess the patient's health status and physical activity levels and make exercise program recommendations, such type of exercise, intensity, and duration, with specific exercise goals based on the patient's physical activity needs and circumstances.

Z71.83   Encounter for nonprocreative genetic counseling

Nonprocreative genetic counseling is generally performed by providers with experience and expertise in genetic medicine and genetic testing methods. It is primarily aimed at patients who may be at risk for inherited disorders. Genetic counselors interpret the results of genetic tests and assist the patient's understanding of the risk factors, benefits and risks of genetic testing, and the potential impact on the patient and/or family members.

Z72.-   Problems related to lifestyle

Most of the lifestyle problems recognized in this category involve negative or self-damaging habits, such as promiscuous sexual behavior, gambling, and irregular or unhealthy sleep habits.

Z72.3   Lack of physical exercise

Z72.4   Inappropriate diet and eating habits

Some experts agree that lack of exercise can be as damaging as smoking a pack of cigarettes every day. Lack of exercise may contribute to heart disease and increase the risk for diabetes and high blood pressure. Inappropriate diet may also contribute to health-related problems.

Z72.5-   High risk sexual behavior

High-risk sexual behaviors are those that put the individual at risk for sexually transmitted diseases or could place an individual in situations where physical and/or mental abuse or assault may occur.

Z72.81-   Antisocial behavior

Antisocial behavior, whether in a child, adolescent, or adult, is behavior that is negative and outside what is perceived as normal. This may include irresponsibility, lack of concern for the feelings of others, inability to maintain relationships, easy frustration and aggression, and the inability to learn from experience.

Z73.-   Problems related to life management difficulty

Many people experience difficulties managing day-to-day personal, school, or work circumstances. This may be attributable to a lack of balance between work and leisure resulting in burn-out or just a generalized feeling of constant stress. Poor interpersonal relationship skills or parenting skills can also result in life management difficulties and conflict.

Z73.81-   Behavioral insomnia of childhood

Behavioral insomnia is common in childhood. Three types are recognized. Sleep onset association type occurs when the child needs a specific object or person present in order to fall asleep initially and get back to sleep if awakened. Limit setting type occurs when the child refuses to go to bed or stalls in an attempt to stay up longer. Attempts to get the child to go to sleep may result in tantrums when the child does not want to go to bed or the child stalling the attempt by requesting water, hugs, or stories. In combined type, the child experiences sleep onset association type and limit setting type.

Z73.82   Dual sensory impairment

Dual sensory impairment is a condition where vision and hearing are significantly impaired. Dual sensory impairment poses significant life management issues for the patient and the family. Dual sensory impairment affects the emotional, mental, and physical needs of the patient and family because it can significantly impact the ability of the patient to communicate and attain developmental milestones when the condition occurs in childhood. When the impairment is acquired later in life, it affects the ability to communicate and to perform activities of daily living.

Z75.-   Problems related to medical facilities and other health care

This category identifies problems related to access to medical facilities, medical services in the home, or certain other health care entities.

Z75.1   Person awaiting admission to adequate facility elsewhere

In some instances, an individual may present to a facility where the appropriate services are not available. In other instances, the acute care given at one facility may be completed but further aftercare may be required at discharge in a setting such as a skilled nursing or rehabilitative facility. The patient may need to be held at the initial facility until arrangements can be made for transfer to a more appropriate facility.

Z75.5   Holiday relief care

Holiday relief care is reported when a patient who normally receives care at home is provided health care in another facility to enable a relative or caretaker to take time away from caretaking duties.

Persons with Potential Health Hazards Related to Family and Personal History and Certain Conditions Influencing Health Status (Z77-Z99)

The categories in this code block help recognize the past medical history of the patient, as well as the medical history related to the patient's family that could have been passed down. Postprocedural history, such as organ transplantation or limb amputation, artificial opening status, and the presence of certain medical devices is also captured with the Z codes in this code block.

The categories in this code block are as follows:

Z77	Other contact with and (suspected) exposures hazardous to health
Z78	Other specified health status
Z79	Long term (current) drug therapy
Z80	Family history of primary malignant neoplasm
Z81	Family history of mental and behavioral disorders
Z82	Family history of certain disabilities and chronic diseases (leading to disablement)
Z83	Family history of other specific disorders
Z84	Family history of other conditions
Z85	Personal history of malignant neoplasm
Z86	Personal history of certain other diseases
Z87	Personal history of other diseases and conditions
Z88	Allergy status to drugs, medicaments and biological substances
Z89	Acquired absence of limb
Z90	Acquired absence of organs, not elsewhere classified
Z91	Personal risk factors, not elsewhere classified
Z92	Personal history of medical treatment
Z93	Artificial opening status
Z94	Transplanted organ and tissue status
Z95	Presence of cardiac and vascular implants and grafts
Z96	Presence of other functional implants
Z97	Presence of other devices
Z98	Other postprocedural states
Z99	Dependence on enabling machines and devices, not elsewhere classified

Z79.-   Long term (current) drug therapy

Codes for long-term (current) drug use can be used for over-the-counter or prescribed medications that a patient is currently taking to treat a medical condition or is receiving as a prophylactic measure, for palliative effect, or for treatment measures. Long-term use of any medication can pose a risk. Risks are related to a person's overall health, the type of medication being used, and how the medications are used. Patients who take drugs on a long-term basis oftentimes need to be monitored to evaluate the continued effectiveness of the drug and to manage any adverse effects.

> **Focus Point**
>
> Code additionally any therapeutic drug level monitoring with code Z51.81.

Z79.01   Long term (current) use of anticoagulants

Anticoagulants disrupt chemical processes in the blood that promote coagulation, which decreases the ability of the blood to clot by reducing fibrin formation and prevents clots already present from getting larger.

Z79.02   Long term (current) use of antithrombotics/antiplatelets

Antithrombotics reduce thrombus formation and antiplatelets prevent the blood from clotting by disrupting platelet aggregation.

Z79.2   Long term (current) use of antibiotics

Antibiotics attack bacteria within the body by eliminating it or reducing the ability of bacteria to multiply. However, antibiotics also alter the makeup of the normal flora in the body, which can have health risks.

Z79.81-   Long term (current) use of agents affecting estrogen receptors and estrogen levels

Many breast tumors are "estrogen sensitive," meaning the hormone estrogen helps them to grow. By reducing estrogen levels, inhibiting the binding of estrogen to cancer cells, or eliminating estrogen production all together these medications reduce the estrogen cancer cell interaction, inhibiting the growth and division of the cancer cells.

Z79.810 Long term (current) use of selective estrogen receptor modulators (SERMs)

Selective estrogen receptor modulators (SERM) inhibit the proliferative effects of estrogen that are mediated through the estrogen receptor (ER). Tamoxifen (also known as Nolvadex®) and raloxifene (also known as Evista®) are examples of this class of drug and have been proven effective in breast cancer prevention and treatment.

Z79.811 Long term (current) use of aromatase inhibitors

Aromatase inhibitors (AI) can help block the growth of breast tumors by lowering the amount of estrogen in the body. Examples of AIs include anastrozole (Arimidex®), exemestane (Aromasin®), and letrozole (Femara®). These drugs do not affect estrogen receptors, but work to reduce estrogen levels.

Z79.818 Long term (current) use of other agents affecting estrogen receptors and estrogen levels

Estrogen-receptor down regulators (ERD) is an option for postmenopausal women with advanced (metastatic) breast cancer that is hormone-receptor-positive and has stopped responding to other antiestrogen therapy.

Z79.891 Long term (current) use of opiate analgesic

This code includes the long term use of methadone, but only if it is being used for pain relief purposes.

Focus Point

Methadone reduces withdrawal symptoms in heroine or other opiate addicts and is used in detoxification and maintenance programs for drug addiction. The appropriate code for the use of methadone for this purpose is located in subcategory F11.2-.

Z80.- Family history of primary malignant neoplasm

People with a family history of certain primary malignant neoplasms have an increased risk of developing the same or a related type of malignancy. This is particularly true of the most common cancers of the breast, colon, ovary, and prostate. Family history codes are frequently used to indicate the need for prophylactic surgery and treatment. Family history codes may also be used with screening codes to justify a test or procedure.

Z82.- Family history of certain disabilities and chronic diseases (leading to disablement)

A family history of certain disabilities and chronic diseases includes visual loss and blindness, hearing loss and deafness, stroke, neurological diseases, ischemic heart disease, other cardiovascular diseases, asthma, other respiratory diseases, arthritis, osteoporosis, other musculoskeletal diseases, polycystic disease, and other congenital conditions. Because many of these diseases are hereditary, knowing the family history can help physicians order the appropriate screening or diagnostic tests, prescribe preventative measures in the absence of current disability or disease, and diagnose and treat any conditions or symptoms that may be indicative of these conditions.

Z82.1 Family history of blindness and visual loss

A family history of blindness or visual loss can alert the physician to inherited disorders or genetic traits that may predispose a patient to certain eye diseases that could put the patient at risk for visual loss or blindness.

Z82.4- Family history of ischemic heart disease and other diseases of the circulatory system

Many types of heart and circulatory system diseases are thought to have a hereditary component. A family history of these conditions may put the patient at risk for developing these diseases and may alter the screening protocol or require prophylactic measures to help prevent the likelihood of developing these conditions.

Z82.41 Family history of sudden cardiac death

Family history is a risk factor for sudden cardiac death. Sudden cardiac death is a death that occurs from any cardiac cause without long-term symptoms and often without a previous diagnosis of a specific cardiac condition. The death typically occurs within a very short time, usually within minutes but not more than an hour, following the onset of symptoms.

Z82.49 Family history of ischemic heart disease and other diseases of the circulatory system

Family history is a risk factor for the development of ischemic heart disease and some other types of circulatory system diseases. Ischemic heart disease is an inadequate flow of blood through the coronary arteries to the tissue of the heart. The predominant etiology of the ischemia is arteriosclerosis.

Z83.- Family history of other specific disorders

A family history of certain other specific conditions includes diabetes mellitus, other endocrine and metabolic diseases, anemia, other blood disorders, colon polyps or other digestive disorders, and infectious and parasitic diseases. Knowing the family history can help physicians order the appropriate screening or diagnostic tests and diagnose and treat the patient's condition or symptoms.

Z83.41 Family history of multiple endocrine neoplasia [MEN] syndrome

This code is used to report that a patient has a family history of multiple endocrine neoplasia syndrome (MEN), which is important to note because many of these syndromes are inherited. MEN syndromes are a group of conditions in which several endocrine glands grow excessively (such as in adenomatous hyperplasia) and/or develop benign or malignant tumors. Tumors and hyperplasia associated with MEN often produce excess hormones, which impede normal physiology. MEN is often due to gene alterations transmitted via family members. There is no cure, but screening can detect the alteration and monitor management of the condition based on the specific gland affected by medication and sometimes surgery. Genetic testing is advised for persons with a family history of the disease or conditions that may be associated with MEN. The specific gene alteration often determines which type of MEN the patient has or will have. All manifest as tumors or overproduction and hyperactivity of the gland affected. Type 1 presents in more than one of the following glands: parathyroid, pancreas, pituitary, thyroid, and adrenal. Type IIA is inherited and presents in more than two of the following glands: thyroid, adrenal, and parathyroid. Type IIB can present as medullary thyroid cancer, pheochromocytomas, and/or neuromas. Abnormalities of the digestive tract, and spine, skull, and limb bones are also common; however, this type is not shown to have a familial connection.

Z83.42 Family history of familial hypercholesterolemia

This code identifies patients with a family history of familial hypercholesterolemia. Familial hypercholesterolemia is a genetic condition due to an anomaly within chromosome 19 that leads to very high levels of low-density lipoprotein (LDL) cholesterol in the bloodstream, leading to narrowing of the arteries. Typically the abnormality is inherited from one parent. However, both parents may carry the mutation and if that is the case, the condition is more serious, leading to a greatly elevated risk of heart disease, including heart attacks in younger patients.

Z83.511 Family history of glaucoma

Glaucoma is characterized by increased intraocular pressure and visual field loss, with potentially associated optic nerve damage. It is the leading cause of blindness in the United States. Certain forms of glaucoma have an asymptomatic presentation. As such, the symptoms can progress without pain, postponing medical intervention. Currently, clinical evaluation for glaucoma entails the assessment of clinical factors in determining risk. A family history of glaucoma places an individual at increased risk for the disease, requiring surveillance. Early diagnosis is imperative to the maintenance of sight. Therefore, regular eye exams with intraocular pressure monitoring are essential.

Z84.- Family history of other conditions

This category captures family history of conditions such as diseases in certain body systems, consanguinity, sudden infant death syndrome, carrier of genetic disease and other specified conditions not otherwise specified in categories Z80.- through Z83.-.

Z84.3 Family history of consanguinity

Consanguinity indicates that the children are a result of closely related bloodlines and is reported when a patient's family history may have bearing on current or future health circumstances. Reproduction within close familial ties can lead to serious genetic disorders in the children. This is especially dangerous when first cousins have children together because it increases risks of autosomal recessive genetic disorders due to having the same grandparents. When a genetic mutation is suspected, screening and counseling services are provided and appropriate even in more distant relations such as third or fourth cousins.

Z84.81 Family history of carrier of genetic disease

This code indicates that a family member may be a carrier of any genetic disease that is not previously classified in another code group.

Z84.82 Family history of sudden infant death syndrome

This code is used when there is a family history of sudden infant death syndrome (SIDS). Also known as crib death, this syndrome typically occurs when an otherwise healthy baby dies in its sleep when under 1 year old. Some believe this may be due to a part of the brain controlling the breathing function and the function of waking up from sleep, while additional factors may include premature birth, respiratory infections, sleeping position, and/or where the infant sleeps. Additional risk factors for SIDS include:

- Male infants
- Ages 2 to 3 months old
- Babies of African American, American Indian, or Alaska Native heritage
- Family history of SIDS in siblings or cousins
- Households exposed to smoking
- Prematurity
- Mothers under the age of 20
- Mothers who are smokers
- Mothers who are drug and/or alcohol users

- Mothers who did not receive regular prenatal care

Evaluation and counseling for this type of family history may cover preventative measures, including instruction on sleeping positions, items to remove from the crib, options for reducing overheating the baby, the benefits of breastfeeding, the appropriate use of baby monitors, and use of a pacifier.

Z85.- Personal history of malignant neoplasm

A personal history of malignant neoplasm identifies a malignancy that has been previously treated or removed but for which there is no current treatment for the condition and no evidence of the disease. Personal history codes may be reported to indicate the need for adjunctive surgery and treatment or to indicate ongoing surveillance or testing for a recurrence. A previous malignant neoplasm may also put the patient at risk for developing a related malignancy, such as breast cancer in the contralateral breast in a patient who has already had breast cancer in one breast.

Z86.- Personal history of certain other diseases

Codes in this category report a personal history of certain other diseases that are no longer present and for which the patient is no longer receiving treatment. However, a past history of these conditions can put the patient at risk for a recurrence of the condition or for other related conditions. Personal history of an in-situ or benign neoplasm; certain infectious or parasitic diseases; diseases of the blood, blood forming organs, or immune system; endocrine, nutritional, and metabolic disorders; mental and behavioral disorders; nervous system and sense organ disorders; and circulatory system disorders are included here.

Z86.14 Personal history of Methicillin resistant Staphylococcus aureus infection

A personal history of MRSA infection can result in an increased susceptibility to future infection thereby affecting treatment. This code should be used when the presence of previous MRSA infection has the potential to impact treatment or outcome of a current illness.

Z86.5- Personal history of mental and behavioral disorders

Mental illness covers a broad range of conditions. The causes of mental illness are not well understood. Some believe it is a functioning of the neurotransmitters in the brain; others believe that stress, drugs, and heredity may play a role in mental illness. An individual with a personal history of mental and behavioral disorders may be at greater risk for a recurrence of these conditions, especially during periods of stress.

Z86.51 Personal history of combat and operational stress reaction

A combat operational stress reaction (COSR) is an acute response to stressful military operations, either inherent in combat or during stability and support operations (SASO), that has physical and emotional manifestations. An individual with a personal history of COSR may be at greater risk for a recurrence of symptoms especially during periods of stress.

Z86.73 Personal history of transient ischemic attack (TIA), and cerebral infarction without residual deficits

A transient ischemic attack (TIA), also known as a mini-stroke, has a rapid onset with a short duration, typically less than five minutes. A TIA occurs when a blood clot temporarily blocks the blood flow within a vessel in the brain. A cerebral infarction occurs due to deficiency in the blood supply to the cerebrum causing lack of oxygen to the brain and resulting in an area of necrosis within the damaged vessels. A cerebral infarction may result in a variety of neurological deficits or resolve without any residual results. This personal history code captures a personal history of TIA or cerebral infarction without lasting effects.

Z87.- Personal history of other diseases and conditions

This category of codes is used to report that the patient had a particular disease that may impact treatment or outcome of current medical care even though the disease is no longer present and the patient is no longer receiving treatment for the disease or condition that was treated in the past.

Z87.31- Personal history of (healed) nontraumatic fracture

Codes in this subcategory identify those patients who have suffered a nontraumatic fracture, such as a fracture due to osteoporosis, a pathologic fracture due to another disease process, or a stress fracture in the past. A patient that has had a previous nontraumatic fracture is at risk for future nontraumatic fractures.

Z87.310 Personal history of (healed) osteoporosis fracture

Patients with osteoporosis or other conditions affecting the integrity of the bone structure are susceptible to pathologic fractures. This increased fracture risk affects clinical treatment and patient care.

Z87.41- Personal history of dysplasia of the female genital tract

Patients with cervical, vaginal, or vulvar dysplasia are tested every four to six months following treatment to verify that there has been no recurrence of dysplastic cells. Patients with dysplasia are at an increased risk for neoplastic changes. This history may be the sole reason for the encounter, which provides surveillance for early detection of potentially premalignant cellular transformations in susceptible patients.

Z87.7- Personal history of (corrected) congenital malformations

Due to advances in surgical technology, many congenital anomalies can be repaired and leave little or no obvious residual deformity or evidence of surgical correction. However, the history of the malformation or surgical intervention may play an important role in influencing the patient's care or relating in some manner to the patient's future health care needs. For example, a history of a corrected congenital malformation of the heart may factor into the management of arteriosclerotic heart disease, conduction abnormalities, or other cardiac interventions in the patient's future.

Z87.891 Personal history of nicotine dependence

This code may be added to an encounter when the patient is known to have had a history of dependence to nicotine, or tobacco. Although quitting reduces risk, previous nicotine dependence can still lead to several related diseases, including heart disease, stroke, and cancer. Capturing this code can also affect meaningful use of data and public health.

Z87.892 Personal history of anaphylaxis

An anaphylactic reaction (anaphylaxis) is a potentially fatal multisystemic allergic hypersensitivity reaction, caused by an immune mediated response to an allergen. A history of anaphylaxis is a risk factor for experiencing anaphylaxis in the future. An anaphylactic reaction can occur in response to a trigger, which is an exposure to a substance by ingestion, injection, or other exposure. The immune system then overreacts to the substance and creates an allergic response. Most cases of allergic responses are not life-threatening, with only minor symptoms that spontaneously resolve or resolve with minimal intervention (e.g., antihistamines, steroid therapy). In anaphylaxis, the allergic response is multisystemic in nature, and more severe in presentation. The immune reaction manifests with integumentary (e.g., hives, pruritus), respiratory (e.g., airway obstruction), gastrointestinal (e.g., vomiting, diarrhea), metabolic (e.g., dehydration), and cardiovascular (e.g., hypotension) symptoms. Severe reactions may be characterized by the presence of rapid onset of shock, which can be fatal without prompt medical intervention. A patient with a history of even a mild allergic reaction in the past may be at increased risk for future anaphylaxis, as subsequent allergic reactions may progress in severity. Depending on the nature of anaphylactic reaction, a patient may undergo immunotherapy to reduce the body's allergic response

and prevent recurrence. Additionally, prevention is enhanced by patient and caregiver education regarding triggers and administration of epinephrine in emergent response to exposure.

Z88.- Allergy status to drugs, medicaments and biological substances

Drug allergies should not be confused with normal side effects of the drug. Drug allergies can be life-threatening. Symptoms of an allergy can be hives, skin rash, itching, wheezing, difficulty breathing, rapid pulse, and swelling of the lips, tongue, or face. Allergic reactions are caused by an increased sensitivity of the immune system to the drug. An allergic reaction may not happen the first time the drug is taken, but as the body's immune system creates antibodies against the drug, the allergic reaction may appear in subsequent use of the drug. Treatment may include oral or topical antihistamines, nebulizer treatments, and epinephrine injections.

Z89.- Acquired absence of limb

Acquired absence of a limb identifies patients who have had a previous amputation due to disease or injury. This category covers acquired absence of part or all of a limb including acquired absence of joint structures only. Patients who have lost a limb may require ongoing care related to the missing limb, such as fitting of prosthetics. Patients may also be receiving ongoing care due to complications of a prosthetic joint, such as infection requiring removal of the prosthesis.

Z89.52- Acquired absence of knee

Knee joint prosthesis complications may require removal of the prosthesis, treatment of the complication, and subsequent reimplantation arthroplasty. This is most often the case in the treatment of joint prosthesis infections. The infected prosthesis is removed, the joint space debrided, antibiotic-impregnated spacers are often implanted within the joint cavity, and the operative wound is closed. The patient is often placed on IV antibiotic therapy until the infection has been eradicated. A new prosthesis may or may not be placed (reimplantation arthroplasty) once the infection has resolved.

Z89.62- Acquired absence of hip

This code reports acquired absence of hip due to disarticulation at the hip joint or due to joint prosthesis complications. Disarticulation is an amputation of the entire leg performed through the hip joint with removal of the entire femur and all soft tissue and bones below the hip level. Alternatively, joint prosthesis complications, most often a joint prosthesis infection, may require removal of the hip prosthesis and any infected or necrotic bone or other tissue. An antibiotic-impregnated spacer is usually implanted within the joint cavity. The patient is then placed on IV antibiotic therapy until the infection has been eradicated. A new prosthesis may or may not be placed (reimplantation arthroplasty) once the infection has resolved.

Z90.-   Acquired absence of organs, not elsewhere classified

Acquired absence of an organ results from surgical removal of a diseased organ or from traumatic injury that requires removal of the damaged organ.

Z90.41-   Acquired absence of pancreas

Several types of pancreatectomy exist, which may include partial or total removal of the pancreas and, in some cases, the adjacent organs (e.g., spleen, portion of bowel, gallbladder). Indications for pancreatectomy include neoplastic disease, chronic inflammation (pancreatitis), and traumatic injury. Total pancreatectomy induces a diabetic state in which the patient requires insulin supplementation to control blood glucose levels and pancreatic enzymes to properly digest food. In certain partial pancreatectomy procedures, the remaining portion of the organ attempts to function normally by continuing to produce and release digestive enzymes and hormones. The long-term effects of partial or total removal of the pancreas depend on the nature of the underlying disease, viability of remaining tissue, comorbid conditions, and the extent of pancreas tissue removed, among other factors. Post-pancreatectomy sequela often includes deficiencies of endocrine and exocrine function whereby replacement therapy, dietary modification, and careful monitoring are required to maintain essential digestive and endocrine function. Furthermore, pain persists in many patients post-pancreatectomy, which poses a significant additional challenge to the patients and caregivers, requiring continued intervention and management to maintain the patient's level of functioning and quality of life. Acquired absence of pancreas is classified as total or partial.

Z90.71-   Acquired absence of cervix and uterus

The cervix and/or uterus may be surgically removed to treat a malignant neoplasm or other disease process or as a result of a complication of pregnancy. Sometimes the cervix and uterus are removed, but in some instances only the uterus or cervix requires removal. These codes assist in supporting medical necessity of Pap smears for this population of patients. Women who have had a full hysterectomy no longer need cervical Pap smears, but they do require vaginal smears to test for vaginal malignancies. Women with a cervical stump following a hysterectomy still require cervical Pap smears.

Z91.-   Personal risk factors, not elsewhere classified

This category classifies the presence of personal risk factors such as a personal history of allergies, noncompliance with medical treatment or therapy, abuse or psychological trauma, self-harm, falling, military deployment, wandering, or dental caries. These risk factors can influence healthcare needs during the current admission or in the future or are clinically important in that they help validate certain treatment options and narrate why a patient was or will be managed a certain way.

Z91.4-   Personal history of psychological trauma, not elsewhere classified

This subcategory classifies personal history of adult physical, sexual, or psychological abuse including domestic abuse and rape, or other adult abuse and neglect, as well as other personal history of psychological trauma not classified elsewhere. Psychological trauma is the psychological damage or injury from emotional response to extremely stressful, life-threatening or traumatic events, or ongoing stressors which may manifest as diagnosable medical and mental health conditions or affect treatment options.

Focus Point

This subcategory is not intended to classify personal history of child abuse and neglect (Z62.81-) or current adult physical or sexual abuse (T74.11, T76.11).

Z91.84-   Oral health risk factors

Dental caries, or tooth decay, is breakdown or demineralization of the tooth enamel caused by acids produced by bacteria, particularly *Streptococcus mutans*. This subcategory was created to classify a patient's personal risk of developing dental caries with three severity levels: low, moderate, and high. These risk levels assist dental providers with identifying etiological factors, determining treatment modalities, clinical data collection, and monitoring and research. Risk management can reduce patient risk of developing advanced disease or arrest the disease process. Primary prevention measures include fluoride therapy, fissure-sealant therapy, dietary counseling, and oral-hygiene measures.

Z92.-   Personal history of medical treatment

This category captures the history of various medical treatments, from previous contraceptive use to immunosuppression or radiation therapy.

Z92.81 Personal history of extracorporeal membrane oxygenation (ECMO)

A personal history of extracorporeal membrane oxygenation (ECMO) describes a history of respiratory support by circulating blood through an artificial lung, consisting of two compartments separated by a gas-permeable membrane, with blood on one side and the ventilating gas on the other. This is typically given to babies, but may be used in adults with acute respiratory distress.

Z92.82 Status post administration of tPA (rtPA) in a different facility within the last 24 hours prior to admission to current facility

Tissue plasminogen activator (tPA) is a drug administered to break up blood clots in specific patients experiencing myocardial infarction or stroke and is the most utilized drug for immediate treatment of these conditions. In order to decrease the damage to the heart or brain, it must be administered within the first few hours of symptom onset. This code is reported by the receiving facility when the patient received tPA at one facility on an emergent basis prior to being transferred to the receiving facility where more specialized intensive acute care services were available.

Focus Point

Code Z92.82 should be used secondary to the code for the condition requiring the tPA administration, such as the stroke or MI.

Z92.83 Personal history of failed moderate sedation

A patient who has exhibited failed moderate sedation during past interventional episodes may require precautionary measures to ensure optimal outcome. Such past situations may have included over or under sedation, adverse reactions to medications, or other respiratory or hemodynamic responses. In these cases, nonroutine services may be necessary to prevent another failed sedation episode (e.g., medication change, specialist services).

Z92.84 Personal history of unintended awareness under general anesthesia

Unintended awareness during general anesthesia involves sensory perceptions, including auditory, visual, and tactile awareness, during a procedure for which the patient should perceive nothing. Because there is a high risk of patients with a history of anesthesia awareness to develop the condition again, it is important for the patient and the providers to know that such a history exists.

Z93.- Artificial opening status

These codes should be used only to indicate the presence, without need for care, of an artificial opening such as a tracheostomy, colostomy, or cystostomy and should only be reported as secondary diagnoses.

Focus Point

When the encounter is for attention or management of an artificial opening or when care is given, the appropriate codes are located in category Z43. If there are complications of an external stoma, the correct codes are located in the appropriate body system chapter (e.g., J95.0-, K94.-, or N99.5-).

Z94.- Transplanted organ and tissue status

Codes in this category should be used when organs or tissue from oneself (autologous), another person (homologous), or from another animal species (heterologous or xenogenic) have been removed and transplanted. Transplant status codes indicate that a person has had an organ replaced but there are no current complications with the transplant. The presence of a transplanted organ or tissue may necessitate additional screening and monitoring services and may alter the care requirements for other medical conditions.

Z94.7 Corneal transplant status

A corneal transplant is performed to preserve or restore vision in a patient with certain eye diseases or injury to the cornea.

Z95.- Presence of cardiac and vascular implants and grafts

Cardiac and vascular implants and grafts are used to treat a wide variety of cardiovascular disease. Implants in this category include mechanical devices (cardiac pacemaker, cardiac defibrillator, heart assist device, artificial heart) and tissue or synthetic implants or grafts (heart valve, arterial and venous grafts, and intracoronary stents).

Z95.1 Presence of aortocoronary bypass graft

This code indicates a patient has had an aortocoronary bypass procedure and currently has a venous, arterial, or synthetic bypass graft in situ that has replaced or bypassed a diseased coronary artery.

Z95.2 Presence of prosthetic heart valve

Z95.3 Presence of xenogenic heart valve

Z95.4 Presence of other heart-valve replacement

Diseased heart valves are commonly replaced with porcine valves, which are a type of xenogenic heart valve obtained from pigs (porcine), cows (bovine), or by synthetic or mechanical heart valves. The presence of a replaced heart valve may have health implications warranting additional screening or monitoring for any complications specific to the presence of the heart valve. In addition, patients with heart valves may require prophylactic measures prior to certain medical interventions.

Z96.- Presence of other functional implants

Functional implants replace or supplement organs or tissues that have been removed due to disease or injury.

Z96.1 Presence of intraocular lens

Pseudophakos is the term used to describe replacement of the native intraocular lens (IOL) with an implant that functions like the native lens. A replacement lens may be inserted when the native lens has been irreparably injured or diseased (e.g., cataract). An artificial IOL may also be inserted to correct serious vision disorders, such as myopia, hyperopia, and astigmatism.

Z97.- Presence of other devices

Devices classified here do not fit well into other more specific categories.

Z97.Ø Presence of artificial eye

Eye globe replacement is indicated when the natural eyeball has been removed (enucleated) to treat a disease, such as a malignant neoplasm, or when a traumatic injury has caused extensive damage to the eye with loss of vision. An implant replaces the eyeball, restores the space within the eye socket, and provides a cosmetic appearance to the eye. Extraocular muscles may be attached to the prosthesis so that it moves in conjunction with the contralateral healthy eye.

Z98.- Other postprocedural states

A history of a procedure can affect the health status of the patient and impact future care and management.

Z98.4- Cataract extraction status

Codes in this subcategory indicate that the patient has had a cataract removed. Extraction is the only definitive treatment for cataract and the inherent clouding of the lens and progressive vision associated with this condition.

Z98.83 Filtering (vitreous) bleb after glaucoma surgery status

One type of surgical procedure performed to treat the excess intraocular fluid and elevated intraocular pressure associated with glaucoma is filtration. Filtration surgery involves opening a passage in the sclera, the white part of the eye, for draining excess fluid. A small bubble, called a bleb, forms over the opening, which is a sign that the fluid is draining out in a controlled manner and collecting under the conjunctiva where it is eventually reabsorbed by the tissue. The presence of the filtering bleb is an indication that the opening is patent and that excess fluid is continuing to drain. The presence of the filtering bleb may need to be monitored to ensure that it is functioning properly.

Z98.87- Personal history of in utero procedure

Fetal surgery enables treatment of certain fetal conditions and anomalies previously considered untreatable. However, these procedures are not without risk for the fetus and the mother, depending on the nature of the diagnosis and type of intervention. Two codes are available. One code reports the mother's postsurgical status and provides a causal link to any associated complications or conditions resulting from the procedure. The other code reports the same information related to procedures performed on a fetus that may have the potential to affect the health status of the individual throughout life.

NOTES

NOTES

NOTES

NOTES

NOTES

NOTES

NOTES

NOTES